Heart Failure

The Expert's Approach

Heart Failure

The Expert's Approach

Editors

Alan S Maisel MD
Professor of Medicine
Director, CCU and HF Program
Department of Medicine and Cardiology
VA Medical Center, University of California
San Diego, California, USA

Gerasimos S Filippatos MD FESC
Heart Failure Unit, Department of Cardiology
Attikon University Hospital, University of Athens
School of Medicine, Athens, Greece

JAYPEE

JAYPEE BROTHERS MEDICAL PUBLISHERS (P) LTD.

New Delhi • London • Philadelphia • Panama

Jaypee Brothers Medical Publishers (P) Ltd

Headquarters

Jaypee Brothers Medical Publishers (P) Ltd
4838/24, Ansari Road, Daryaganj
New Delhi 110 002, India
Phone: +91-11-43574357
Fax: +91-11-43574314
Email: jaypee@jaypeebrothers.com

Overseas Offices

J.P. Medical Ltd
83 Victoria Street, London
SW1H 0HW (UK)
Phone: +44-2031708910
Fax: +02-03-0086180
Email: info@jpmedpub.com

Jaypee Medical Inc
The Bourse
111 South Independence Mall East
Suite 835, Philadelphia, PA 19106, USA
Phone: +1 267-519-9789
Email: joe.rusko@jaypeebrothers.com

Jaypee Brothers Medical Publishers (P) Ltd
Bhotahity, Kathmandu, Nepal
Phone: +977-9741283608
Email: kathmandu@jaypeebrothers.com

Jaypee-Highlights Medical Publishers Inc
City of Knowledge, Bld. 237, Clayton
Panama City, Panama
Phone: +1 507-301-0496
Fax: +1 507-301-0499
Email: cservice@jphmedical.com

Jaypee Brothers Medical Publishers (P) Ltd
17/1-B Babar Road, Block-B, Shaymali
Mohammadpur, Dhaka-1207
Bangladesh
Mobile: +08801912003485
Email: jaypeedhaka@gmail.com

Website: www.jaypeebrothers.com
Website: www.jaypeedigital.com

Heart Failure *The Expert's Approach* / Eds. Alan S Maisel and Gerasimos S Filippatos

First Edition: **2014**

ISBN 978-93-5090-949-2

Printed at Ajanta Offset & Packagings Ltd

Dedicated to

Fran, Amanda, Naomi, Max, Samantha, and Sofie
and
My students and fellows

Alan S Maisel

Maria and Angela
and
My students and fellows

Gerasimos S Filippatos

Contributors

Editors

Alan S Maisel MD
Professor of Medicine
Director, CCU and HF Program
Department of Medicine and Cardiology
VA Medical Center, University of California
San Diego, California, USA

Gerasimos S Filippatos MD FESC
Heart Failure Unit, Department of Cardiology
Attikon University Hospital
University of Athens
School of Medicine, Athens, Greece

Contributing Authors

Eric Adler MD
Associate Professor of Medicine and
Medical Director of Cardiac Transplant
Department of Medicine, Division of Cardiology
University of California
San Diego, California, USA

Ali Ahmed MD MPH
Professor of Medicine and Epidemiology
University of Alabama at Birmingham
Birmingham, Alabama, USA

Nancy M Albert PhD CCNS CHFN CCRN NE-BC FAHA FCCM
Associate Chief Nursing Officer
Research and Innovation, Nursing Institute
Cleveland Clinic Health System and
Clinical Nurse Specialist
Heart and Vascular Institute, Cleveland Clinic
Cleveland, Ohio, USA

Khwaja S Alim MD
Practicing Internal Medicine
St. Martin Dominican Hospital
Las Vegas, Nevada, USA

Lora AlKhawam MD
Department of Emergency Medicine
Northwestern University Feinberg School of Medicine
Chicago, Illinois, USA

Inder S Anand MD FRCP D Phil
Professor of Medicine
University of Minnesota Medical School
Director, Heart Failure Program, VA Medical Center
Minneapolis, Minnesota, USA

Hermineh Aramin MD
Research Assistant
VA Health Care Center
San Diego, California, USA

Eloisa Arbustini MD
Director of the Transplant Research Area
Director of the Centre for
Inherited Cardiovascular Diseases
Director of the Molecular Genetic Laboratory
Fondazione IRCCS Policlinico San Matteo
Pavia, Italy

Ajay Bahl MD DNB MRCP DM
Associate Professor
Department of Cardiology
Postgraduate Institute of Medical Education and Research
Chandigarh, India

Manish Bansal MD DNB FASE FISCU
Senior Consultant Cardiology
Department of Cardiology
Medanta - The Medicity
Gurgaon, Haryana, India

Denise D Barnard MD FACC
Clinical Professor of Medicine
Advanced Heart Failure, Cardiac Transplantation and
Mechanical Assist Device Program
UCSD Health Sciences and UCSD School of Medicine
San Diego, California, USA

Tyler W Barrett MD MSCI FACEP
Associate Professor
Department of Emergency Medicine
Vanderbilt University Medical Center
Nashville, Tennessee, USA

Tina Baykaner MD
Cardiology Fellow
Department of Cardiology
University of California
San Diego, California, USA

Vassiliki Bistola MD PhD
Heart Failure Unit, Attikon University Hospital
University of Athens
Athens, Greece

Daniel G Blanchard MD FACC
Professor of Clinical Medicine
Director, UCSD Cardiology Fellowship Program
UCSD Sulpizio Cardiovascular Center
San Diego, California, USA

Rudolf A de Boer MD PhD FESC
Department of Cardiology
University Medical Center Groningen
University of Groningen
Groningen, The Netherlands

Harleah G Buck PhD RN CHPN FPN
Assistant Professor
College of Nursing
The Pennsylvania State University
State College, Pennsylvania, USA

Javed Butler MD MPH
Professor of Medicine
Emory Cardiovascular Clinical Research Institute
Atlanta, Georgia, USA

Jeffrey Chan MD
Physician
University of California, San Diego Medical Center
San Diego, California, USA

Jia Hoong Chi BPharm
Pharmacist
Lorong Bersatu, Off Jalan Damai
Luyang, Sabah, Malaysia

Anthony Choi MD
Department of Cardiology
Naval Medical Center San Diego
San Diego, California, USA

Rajiv Choudhary MPH MD
Internal Medicine Resident
Department of Internal Medicine
Capital Health Regional Medical Center – Fuld
Trenton, New Jersey, USA

John GF Cleland MD PhD FRCP FESC FACC
Professor of Clinical Cardiology
National Heart and Lung Institute
Royal Brompton and Harefield Hospitals, Imperial College
London, England, UK

Robert T Cole MD
Assistant Professor of Medicine
Emory Cardiovascular Clinical Research Institute
Atlanta, Georgia, USA

Maria R Costanzo MD FACC FAHA
Medical Director
Midwest Heart Specialists-Advocate Medical Group
Heart Failure and Pulmonary Arterial Hypertension Programs
Medical Director
Edward Hospital Center for Advanced Heart Failure
Naperville, Illinois, USA

Justin Cox MD
Cardiology Fellow
Naval Medical Center San Diego
San Diego, California, USA
Assistant Professor of Medicine
Uniformed Services University of the Health Sciences
Bethesda, Maryland, USA

Lori B Daniels MD MAS
Director
Coronary Care Unit
Associate Professor of Medicine
Division of Cardiology
University of California
Sulpizio Cardiovascular Center
San Diego, California, USA

Eugene C DePasquale MD
Ahmanson-UCLA Cardiomyopathy Center
David Geffen School of Medicine
Los Angeles, California, USA

Benjamin Dicken MBBS MRCP
Department of Cardiology
Hull York Medical School
Castle Hill Hospital, University of Hull
Kingston-upon-Hull, England, UK

Riet Dierckx MD
Clinical Lecturer Telehealth
Academic Department of Cardiology
Hull York Medical School
Kingston upon Hull, England, UK

Mary A Dolansky PhD RN
Associate Professor
Case Western Reserve University
Frances Payne Bolton School of Nursing
Cleveland, Ohio, USA

Christos Dresios MD
Centre for Cardiovascular Sciences
City Hospital, University of Birmingham
Birmingham, England, UK

Lothar Faber MD FESC FAHA
Cardiologist, Expert for HCM, Cardiac Imaging
Heart and Diabetes Center NRW
Bad Oeynhausen, North Rhine-Westphalia, Germany

Gregg C Fonarow MD FACC FAHA
Eliot Corday Professor of Cardiovascular Medicine and Science
Director, Ahmanson-UCLA Cardiomyopathy Center; Co-Chief of Clinical Cardiology, UCLA Division of Cardiology
Co-Director, UCLA Preventative Cardiology Program
Los Angeles, California, USA

Nancy J Gardetto PhD FNP-BC
Clinical Nurse Practitioner
Nurse Researcher, Heart Failure and Cardiac Transplantation Program
VA San Diego Healthcare System
San Diego, California, USA

Luna Gargani MD
Cardiologist
Researcher, Institute of Clinical Physiology
National Research Council
Chair of the TTE Sub-Committee
European Association of Cardiovascular Imaging
Pisa, Italy

Maurizia Grasso PhD
Centre for Inherited Cardiovascular Diseases
Fondazione IRCCS Policlinico San Matteo
Pavia, Italy

Barry Greenberg MD
Professor of Medicine
University of California, San Diego
Director, Advanced Heart Failure Treatment Program for the UCSD Health System
San Diego, California, USA

Erik A Green BA
VA Hospital
San Diego, California, USA

Hardeep K Grewal PGDCC FCNIC
Attending Consultant Cardiology
Department of Cardiology
Medanta - The Medicity
Gurgaon, Haryana, India

Meghana G Halkar MD
Clinical Associate Staff
Cleveland Clinic
Cleveland, Ohio, USA

J Thomas Heywood MD
Director, Heart Failure Research and Recovery
Director, Left Ventricular Assist Device Program
Scripps Clinic
San Diego, California, USA

Erin Higginbotham BS
Medical Student
Keck School of Medicine
University of Southern California
Los Angeles, California, USA

Scott Hopkins MD
Cardiology Fellow
Naval Medical Center San Diego
San Diego, California, USA

Connie Huberty MS RN APN-BC CHFN
Heart Failure Nurse Practitioner
Edward Hospital
Naperville, Illinois, USA

Fatima Iqbal MD
Research Associate
VA San Diego Healthcare System
San Diego, California, USA

Navaid Iqbal MD
Research Coordinator
VA San Diego Healthcare System
San Diego, California, USA

Affan Irfan MD
Resident
Internal Medicine Program
University of Illinois – Urbana Champaign
Champaign, Illinois, USA

Shiro Ishihara MD
Inserm U942
Nippon Medical School Musashi-Kosugi Hospital
Paris, France

Tiny Jaarsma PhD RN
Professor
Department of Social and Welfare Studies
Linköping University
Linköping, Sweden

Allan S Jaffe MD
Professor of Medicine
Professor of Laboratory Medicine and Pathology
Mayo Clinic
Rochester, Minnesota, USA

Ewa A Jankowska MD PhD FESC
Department of Heart Diseases
Wroclaw Medical University
Cardiology Department, Military Hospital
Wroclaw, Poland

James L Januzzi Jr MD FACC FESC
Director
Cardiac Intensive Care Unit
Massachusetts General Hospital
Boston, Massachusetts, USA

Brian E Jaski MD
San Diego Cardiac Center
Medical Director
Advanced Heart Failure/Cardiac Transplant
Sharp Memorial Hospital
San Diego, California, USA

Robert L Jesse MD PhD
Principal Deputy Under Secretary for Health
Veterans Health Administration
Richmond, Virginia, USA

Mariell Jessup MD
Advanced Heart Failure and Transplant Cardiologists
Division of Cardiovascular Medicine
Department of Medicine
University of Pennsylvania School of Medicine
Philadelphia, Pennsylvania, USA

Corrine Y Jurgens PhD RN ANP-BC FAHA
Associate Professor, Director of Cardiovascular Research
School of Nursing, Stony Brook University
Stony Brook, New York, USA

Ravi R Kasliwal MD DM FIMSA MNAMS
Chairman
Clinical and Preventive Cardiology Community Outreach and Education Program
Medanta Heart Institute
Medanta - The Medicity
Gurgaon, Haryana, India

Matt M Kawahara BA
Staff Research Associate
VA San Diego Healthcare System
San Diego, California, USA

Basem Khishfe MD
Department of Emergency Medicine
Cook County Hospital
Chicago, Illinois, USA

Fatima Khusro MD
Research Associate
VA San Diego Healtcare System
San Diego, California, USA

Benjamin A Kipper BS
VA Medical Center La Jolla
San Diego, California, USA
Oakland University William Beaumont School of Medicine
Rochester, Michigan, USA

Takahide Kodama MD PhD
Cardiovascular Center
Toranomon Hospital
Toranomon, Tokyo, Japan

David E Krummen MD
Associate Professor of Medicine
University of California, San Diego and
VA San Diego Healthcare System
San Diego, California, USA

Vijaya A Kumar MD FAAFP
Assistant Professor
Department of Emergency Medicine
Wayne State University School of Medicine
Detroit, Michigan, USA

Dick Kuo MD FACEP
Baylor College of Medicine
Houston, Texas, USA

Rashid Kysia MD MPH
Department of Emergency Medicine
Cook County Hospital
Chicago, Illinois, USA

Jennifer LaCorte RN MSN CCRN
Technical Clinical Trainer
Baxter-Gambro Renal, Aquapheresis Systems
Naperville, Illinois, USA

Gautam G Lalani MD
Fellow, Cardiac Electrophysiology
University of California
San Diego, California, USA

Carolyn SP Lam MBBS MRCP MS
Associate Professor, Department of Internal Medicine
National University of Singapore
Consultant, Cardiac Department
National University Hospital, Singapore
Director, Women's Heart Health Clinic, National University Heart Centre, Singapore

Elizabeth Lee BS
Research Coordinator
Maisel Cardiology Research Lab
Saratoga, California, USA

Phillip D Levy MD MPH
Associate Professor of Emergency Medicine
Assistant Director of Clinical Research
Cardiovascular Research Institute
Associate Director of Clinical Research
Department of Emergency Medicine
Wayne State University School of Medicine
Detroit, Michigan, USA

Siow-Yen Liau MPharm PhD
Pharmacist, Pharmacy Department
Queen Elizabeth Hospital II, Ministry of Health
Kota Kinabalu, Sabah, Malaysia

Houng-Bang Liew MB BCh BAO FRCP FNHAM
Head, Department of Cardiology
Queen Elizabeth Hospital II, Ministry of Health
Kota Kinabalu, Sabah, Malaysia

Gregory YH Lip MD FRCP FESC FACC
Centre for Cardiovascular Sciences
City Hospital, University of Birmingham
Birmingham, England, United Kingdom

Alexander R Lyon MA BM BCh MRCP PhD
Senior Lecturer and Consultant Cardiologist
Royal Brompton Hospital
London, England, UK

Josep Masip MD PhD FESC
ICU Director
Hospital Sant Joan Despí Moisès Broggi
Consorci Sanitari Integral
Associate Professor of Cardiology
University of Barcelona
Barcelona, Spain

Patrick McCann MD
Fellow in Cardiac Failure
Department of Medicine, Division of Cardiology
University of California
San Diego, California, USA

Alexandre Mebazaa MD PhD
Department of Anesthesia and Critical Care
U942 Inserm, Lariboisière-Saint-Louis Hospital
University Paris Diderot
Paris, France

Hirsch S Mehta MD
Physician, Stanford University School of Medicine
Stanford, California, USA

Wouter C Meijers MD
Department of Cardiology
University Medical Center Groningen
University of Groningen
Groningen, The Netherlands

Wayne L Miller MD PhD
Mayo Clinic
Rochester, Minnesota, USA

Rajeev C Mohan MD
Division of Cardiology
Scripps Clinic
San Diego, California, USA

Andrew C Morley-Smith MA MB BChir MRCP
Clinical Research Fellow
Imperial College London and
Royal Brompton and Harefield NHS Foundation Trust
London, England, UK

Nupoor Narula MD
Centre for Inherited Cardiovascular Diseases
Fondazione IRCCS Policlinico San Matteo
Pavia, Italy
Department of Medicine, Mayo Clinic
Rochester, Minnesota, USA

Silvia Navarin MD
Emergency Medicine Postgraduate School Resident
Department Medical-Surgery Sciences and Translational Medicine
Post Graduate School of Emergency Medicine
Sapienza University, Sant'Andrea Hospital
Rome, Italy

Keshav R Nayak MD FACC FSCAI
Director, Cardiac Catheterization Laboratory
Naval Medical Center San Diego
San Diego, California, USA

Michel Noutsias MD FESC
Department of Cardiology – Internal Medicine
University Hospital of Jena
Jena, Thuringia, Germany

Peter S Pang MD MSCI FACEP FAAEM FACC FAHA
Associate Chief, Associate Professor
Department of Emergency Medicine and Medicine
Northwestern University Feinberg School of Medicine
Chicago, Illinois, USA

John T Parissis MD
Associate Professor of Cardiology
Heart Failure Clinic
Attikon University Hospital, University of Athens
Athens, Greece

Sunaina Parsons MBChB MRCP
Clinical Research Fellow
Centre for Cardiovascular and Metabolic Research
Hull York Medical School
Kingston-upon-Hull, England, UK

Kanan Patel MBBS MPH
Academic Specialist
University of California
San Francisco, California, USA

Minal V Patel BSc
Research Coordinator
Department of Medicine, Cardiology
University of California, San Diego
VA San Diego Healthcare System
San Diego, California, USA

W Frank Peacock MD FACEP
Professor, Emergency Medicine
Associate Chair and Research Director
Baylor College of Medicine
Houston, Texas, USA

Pierpaolo Pellicori MD FESC
Clinical Research Fellow
Department of Academic Cardiology
Castle Hill Hospital
Kingston upon Hull, England, UK

Bertram Pitt MD
School of Medicine, University of Michigan
Ann Arbor, Michigan, USA

Piotr Ponikowski MD PhD FESC
Department of Heart Diseases
Wroclaw Medical University
Cardiology Department, Military Hospital
Wroclaw, Poland

Christian Prinz MD FESC
Cardiologist, Expert for HCM, Cardiac Imaging, Cardiac Biomarkers
Heart and Diabetes Center NRW
Bad Oeynhausen, North Rhine-Westphalia, Germany

Sonal Sarkariya MD
Internal Medicine Resident Physician
University of California
San Diego, California, USA

Michelle Schlueter Pharm D
Department of Cardiology
University of California, San Diego School of Medicine
San Diego, California, USA

Amir A Schricker MD MS
Cardiac electrophysiology fellow
University of California, San Diego Medical Center
VA San Diego Healthcare System
San Diego, California, USA

Alessandra Serio MD PhD
Cardiologist
Centre for Inherited Cardiovascular Diseases
Fondazione IRCCS Policlinico San Matteo
Pavia, Italy

Abhishek S Shah MD
University of California
San Diego, California, USA

Kevin S Shah MD
Resident Physician
Department of Internal Medicine
University of California
San Diego, California, USA

Ahmad Shoaib MBBS MRCP
Honorary Senior Clinical Tutor, Hull York Medical School
Clinical Research Fellow
Department of Cardiology
Division of Cardiovascular and Respiratory Studies
Post Graduate Medical Institute
Castle Hill Hospital
Kingston-upon-Hull, England, UK

Salvatore D Somma MD PhD
Professor of Medicine
Director Emergency Medicine
Chairman Postgraduate School of Emergency Medicine
Department of Medical-Surgery Sciences and Translational Medicine
Sapienza University, Sant'Andrea Hospital
Rome, Italy

Anna Strömberg PhD RN
Professor, Division of Nursing
Department of Medical and Health Sciences
Linköping University
Linköping, Sweden

José Tallaj MD
University of Alabama at Birmingham
Veterans Affairs Medical Center
Birmingham, Alabama, USA

WH Wilson Tang MD
Professor of Medicine
Cleveland Clinic
Cleveland, Ohio, USA

Allart R van der Velde MD
Department of Cardiology
University Medical Center Groningen
University of Groningen
Groningen, The Netherlands

Joyce W Wald DO
Advanced Heart Failure and Transplant Cardiologists
Division of Cardiovascular Medicine
Department of Medicine
University of Pennsylvania School of Medicine
Philadelphia, Pennsylvania, USA

Brian S Wasserman MD
Department of Emergency Medicine
Vanderbilt University Medical Center
Nashville, Tennessee, USA

Sandra Williams MD DO MPH
Baylor College of Medicine
Houston, Texas, USA

Joel R Wilson MD
Assistant Professor of Medicine
Department of Internal Medicine
Division of Cardiology and
Department of Radiology
University of California
San Diego, California, USA

Raymond CC Wong MBBS MRCP
Senior Consultant
National University Heart Centre
Singapore

Yu Xie MD
Chief Medical Resident of
the Internal Medicine Program
University of California
San Diego, California, USA

Yang Xue MD
Medical Center for Cardiovascular Medicine
University of California
San Diego, California, USA

Jian Zhang MD PhD
Professor
Heart Failure Center
Fuwai Cardiovascular Hospital
National Center for Cardiovascular Diseases
Chinese Academy of Medical Sciences and
Peking Union Medical College
Beijing, China

Yuhui Zhang MD
Associate Professor
Heart Failure Center
Fuwai Cardiovascular Hospital
National Center for Cardiovascular Disease
Chinese Academy of Medical Sciences and
Peking Union Medical College
Beijing, China

Preface

It is clear to every healthcare practitioner that heart failure has become a worldwide epidemic. The scourge of obesity and heart disease and the ageing of the population have certainly contributed to this phenomenon as has the longer survival following therapeutic interventions for acute myocardial infarction and cardiac disease in general. Thus, with the increasing prevalence of heart failure, it is important to examine the newest data as well, as the latest treatment paradigms.

It was our idea to make this a hands-on book; that is, something you could not only sit down for a leisurely read, but could open up to succinct chapters as the occasion arose, and come right to important information on the workup and treatment of all aspects of heart failure. To this end, we had instructed our expert contributors to punctuate their chapters with new and improved algorithms that one could immediately use at the bedside or the office. "How to really do it right" was the mantra used. We also had the idea to write small chapters with brief text, many figures and treatment algorithms, and a small number of selected references. This was easy to do in some chapters like conventional drug therapy. In more controversial areas with lower level of evidence, we thought that the reader would benefit from more extensive information and suggested literature to read.

Professor Peter Pang from Northwestern University handled Section 1 on the Emergency Department. In this section, we have covered the spectrum of what one would see and do in the emergency. From the early evaluation of the dyspneic patient, to the diagnostic techniques, including biomarkers, echocardiography and impedance, to appropriate triage, risk stratification, and treatment of the patient, we offer practical suggestions to simplify diagnosis and management in this urgent care setting.

Section 2 deals with Heart Failure in the Hospital, which includes the use of biomarkers, the latest medical treatments, and the associated comorbidities, such as hyponatremia, coronary artery disease, and cardiorenal syndromes.

Section 3 deals with how to take care of Chronic Heart Failure Patients in the Outpatient Setting. There are chapters on monitoring with echocardiography and biomarkers, as well as strategic chapters on preserved ejection fraction, atrial fibrillation, and issues with anticoagulation.

Section 4 deals with Special Issues in Heart Failure. This includes, age, gender, sex and ethnic issues, along with heart failure in other countries as well as the Veterans Systems. We also deal with heart failure in the Nursing home setting and get a good nursing perspective.

Section 5 deals with the approach to End-stage Heart Failure, and the final section deals with practical recommendations for diagnosis and management of cardiomyopathies.

We hope the readers, whether they be primary care physicians, house officers, practicing cardiologists, or nurses, will both learn and enjoy the contents of this book.

Alan S Maisel
Gerasimos S Filippatos

Acknowledgments

I would like to first acknowledge the now deceased Dr Ralph Shabetai, who as my first chief of cardiology gave me his time and advice and turned my interests towards challenges of the heart failure patient. Never have I met a more selfless and giving man than Ralph. Second, I would like to thank my laboratory personnel without whose help and support I would never have been productive. A special thanks to my lab director, Steve Carter, for 25 years of unwavering loyalty. I would like to thank the Publishers M/s Jaypee Brothers Medical Publishers for being incredibly supportive to this long endeavor, in particular, Dr Neeraj Choudhary for his friendship and advice. Finally, I would be completely remiss if I did not thank my five children, who last summer lost their mother and on a daily basis remind me of why God put me on Earth. And Fran, my lovely wife, thanks for putting up with my long hours, extensive travel, and crazy sense of humor.

Alan S Maisel

Acknowledgments

I would like to acknowledge Professor George Baltopoulos, who trained me in critical care and helped me, from my first steps in research to my doctoral degree, more than 25 years ago. I also owe much to Professor Lambros Anthopoulos, former Chair of the Department of Cardiology at Evangelismos Hospital, who gave me the opportunity to develop and direct the Heart Failure Unit and the Intensive Cardiac Care Unit at Evangelismos Hospital in the mid-1990s; and to Professor Dimitrios Kremastinos, founder of the Attikon University Hospital, who asked me 10 years ago to organize and run the Heart Failure Unit of the Department. However, my biggest supporters are my wife Maria and my daughter Angela. It is difficult to make space for a life away from work. This becomes impossible if you are trying to find time to write a book on the top of the other activities. Thank you for your support.

Gerasimos S Filippatos

Contents

Section 1: The Emergency Department

1. **How to Evaluate Dyspnea in the Emergency Department** 3
   W Frank Peacock, Dick Kuo, Sandra Williams
2. **Heart Failure Disposition: When to Admit, When to Observe, and When to Discharge Home** 8
   Phillip D Levy, Vijaya A Kumar
3. **The Treatment of Acute Heart Failure in the Emergency Department** 15
   Lora AlKhawam, Peter S Pang
4. **Management of Atrial Fibrillation in Patients with Heart Failure and Preserved and Low Ejection Fractions** 21
   Brian S Wasserman, Tyler W Barrett
5. **How to Use Natriuretic Peptides in the Emergency Department** 32
   Yang Xue, Jeffrey Chan, Sonal Sarkariya, Erik A Green, Alan S Maisel
6. **How to Use New Biomarkers in the Emergency Department** 40
   Navaid Iqbal, Rajiv Choudhary, Erin Higginbotham, Fatima Khusro, Alan S Maisel
7. **The Role of Ultrasound in the Management of Acute Heart Failure** 54
   Luna Gargani
8. **Use of Bioelectrical Impedance Vector Analysis in the Dyspneic Patient** 66
   Salvatore D Somma, Silvia Navarin
9. **Mechanical Ventilation in Acute Heart Failure: The Role of Noninvasive Ventilation** 73
   Josep Masip
10. **Emergency Department Observation Unit: Management of Congestive Heart Failure** 80
    Basem Khishfe, Rashid Kysia
11. **When to Employ Cardiac Magnetic Resonance Imaging and Cardiac Computed Tomography in the Evaluation of Heart Failure** 86
    Joel R Wilson
12. **When to Discharge the Heart Failure Patient** 101
    Benjamin A Kipper, Matt M Kawahara

Section 2: Heart Failure in the Hospital

13. **How to Use Natriuretic Peptides in the Inpatient Setting?** 109
Jeffrey Chan, Abhishek S Shah, Alan S Maisel

14. **Approaches to Diuretics in the Hospital** 117
Meghana G Halkar, WH Wilson Tang

15. **Vasodilators in Acute Heart Failure** 127
Shiro Ishihara, Alexandre Mebazaa

16. **When and How to Use Inotropes?** 130
John T Parissis, Vassiliki Bistola

17. **New Cardiovascular Disease Biomarkers in Hospital Medicine: Neutrophil Gelatinase-associated Lipocalin** 139
Jeffrey Chan, Alan S Maisel

18. **Practical Approach to Hyponatremia in Heart Failure** 143
Hirsch S Mehta, Rajeev C Mohan, J Thomas Heywood

19. **Heart Failure and Acute Coronary Syndrome** 151
Jeffrey Chan, Kevin S Shah, Alan S Maisel

20. **The ABCs of Isolated Venovenous Ultrafiltration in Fluid-overloaded Heart Failure Patients** 158
Maria R Costanzo, Connie Huberty, Jennifer LaCorte

21. **Who Should Receive a Pulmonary Artery Catheter** 178
Robert T Cole, Javed Butler

Section 3: Chronic Heart Failure in the Outpatient Setting

22. **Outpatient Follow-up—What Should We Monitor** 187
Tina Baykaner, Yu Xie, Michelle Schlueter, Barry Greenberg

23. **Echocardiography: Getting It Right** 197
Daniel G Blanchard

24. **A Practical Guide for Reducing Readmissions in Heart Failure** 203
Eugene C DePasquale, Gregg C Fonarow

25. **Initiation of Angiotensin-converting Enzyme Inhibitors and Beta Blockers in Heart Failure: Putting Evidence into Practice** 213
Jeffrey Chan, Alan S Maisel

26. **Mineralocorticoid Receptor Antagonists in Patients with Heart Failure and a Reduced Left Ventricular Ejection Fraction: How to Do It Right** 218
Bertram Pitt

27. **Atrial Fibrillation Done Right** 225
Amir A Schricker, David E Krummen

28. **Ventricular Tachycardia Done Right** 232
Gautam G Lalani, David E Krummen

29. **Issues in Anticoagulation** 238
Christos Dresios, Gregory YH Lip

30. **Management of the Patient with Heart Failure with Preserved Ejection Fraction** 255
Alan S Maisel, Gerasimos S Filippatos, Kevin S Shah, Jeffrey Chan

31. **Implantable Cardioverter-defibrillator and Cardiac Resynchronization Therapy in Heart Failure Patients: How to Choose the Right Device for the Right Patients** 261
Khwaja S Alim, Erik A Green

32. **Clinical Decision-making in the Outpatient Setting: The Use of Galectin-3** 267
Allart R van der Velde, Wouter C Meijers, Rudolf A de Boer

33. **Guiding Heart Failure Care with Natriuretic Peptides** 273
James L Januzzi Jr

34. **ST2: How to Really Do It Right** 283
Lori B Daniels

35. **Using Cardiac Troponin to Assist in the Management of Patients with Congestive Heart Failure—A Practical Guide** 289
Affan Irfan, Wayne L Miller, Allan S Jaffe

36. **Biomarkers on the Horizon for Chronic Heart Failure** 298
Christian Prinz

Section 4: Special Issues in Heart Failure

37. **Sex Differences in Heart Failure: Implications for Clinical Practice** 311
Nancy J Gardetto, Denise D Barnard

38. **Chronic Heart Failure in Geriatric Patients** 322
José Tallaj, Kanan Patel, Ali Ahmed

39. **How to Diagnose and Treat Anemia in Patients with Heart Failure** 333
Ewa A Jankowska, Piotr Ponikowski

40. **Diabetes Management in Heart Failure** 340
Rajiv Choudhary, Alan S Maisel

41. **Heart Failure in Europe** 347
John GF Cleland, Pierpaolo Pellicori, Benjamin Dicken, Ahmad Shoaib, Sunaina Parsons, Riet Dierckx

42. **Heart Failure in Southeast Asia** 369
Raymond CC Wong, Carolyn SP Lam

43. **Heart Failure in India** 380
Ajay Bahl, Inder S Anand

44. **Heart Failure in India: Clinical Perspective** 387
Hardeep K Grewal, Manish Bansal, Ravi R Kasliwal

45. **Heart Failure in China** 396
Yuhui Zhang, Jian Zhang

46. **Heart Failure from the US Veterans Health Administration Perspective: A Patient-centered Approach to Care** 402
Robert L Jesse

47. Heart Failure in the Nursing Home Setting 407
Corrine Y Jurgens, Mary A Dolansky, Harleah G Buck

48. Heart Failure from the Nursing Perspective 415
Nancy M Albert

49. Developing Heart Failure Service in a Developing Nation: Borneo Malaysia Perspective 425
Houng-Bang Liew, Siow-Yen Liau, Jia Hoong Chi

Section 5: Advanced Heart Failure

50. Approach to the End-stage Heart Failure Patient 437
Joyce W Wald, Mariell Jessup

51. Left Ventricular Assist Device Versus Transplantation: How to Decide 443
Patrick McCann, Eric Adler

52. Approach to Left Ventricular Assist Devices and Follow-up in Advanced Congestive Heart Failure 451
Anthony Choi, Keshav R Nayak, Brian E Jaski

53. How to Approach Palliative and End-of-life Care 461
Tiny Jaarsma, Anna Strömberg

54. Percutaneous Mechanical Circulatory Support in Cardiogenic Shock 468
Scott Hopkins, Justin Cox, Keshav R Nayak

Section 6: Cardiomyopathies: Practical Recommendations to Diagnosis and Management

55. New Onset Cardiomyopathy: Biopsy or MRI and Other Imaging Modalities 477
Khwaja S Alim, Matt M Kawahara

56. Hypertrophic Cardiomyopathy 485
Christian Prinz, Lothar Faber, Alan S Maisel

57. Takotsubo Cardiomyopathy 494
Andrew C Morley-Smith, Alexander R Lyon

58. Myocarditis 506
Michel Noutsias

59. When is Genetic Testing Necessary? 522
Nupoor Narula, Maurizia Grasso, Alessandra Serio, Takahide Kodama, Eloisa Arbustini

60. AIDS-induced Cardiac Abnormalities and Heart Failure 541
Khwaja S Alim, Hermineh Aramin, Minal V Patel, Elizabeth Lee

61. Prohormone Levels in Heart Failure 546
Navaid Iqbal, Rajiv Choudhary, Fatima Iqbal, Erik A Green, Alan S Maisel

Appendix 551

Index 555

1

SECTION

The Emergency Department

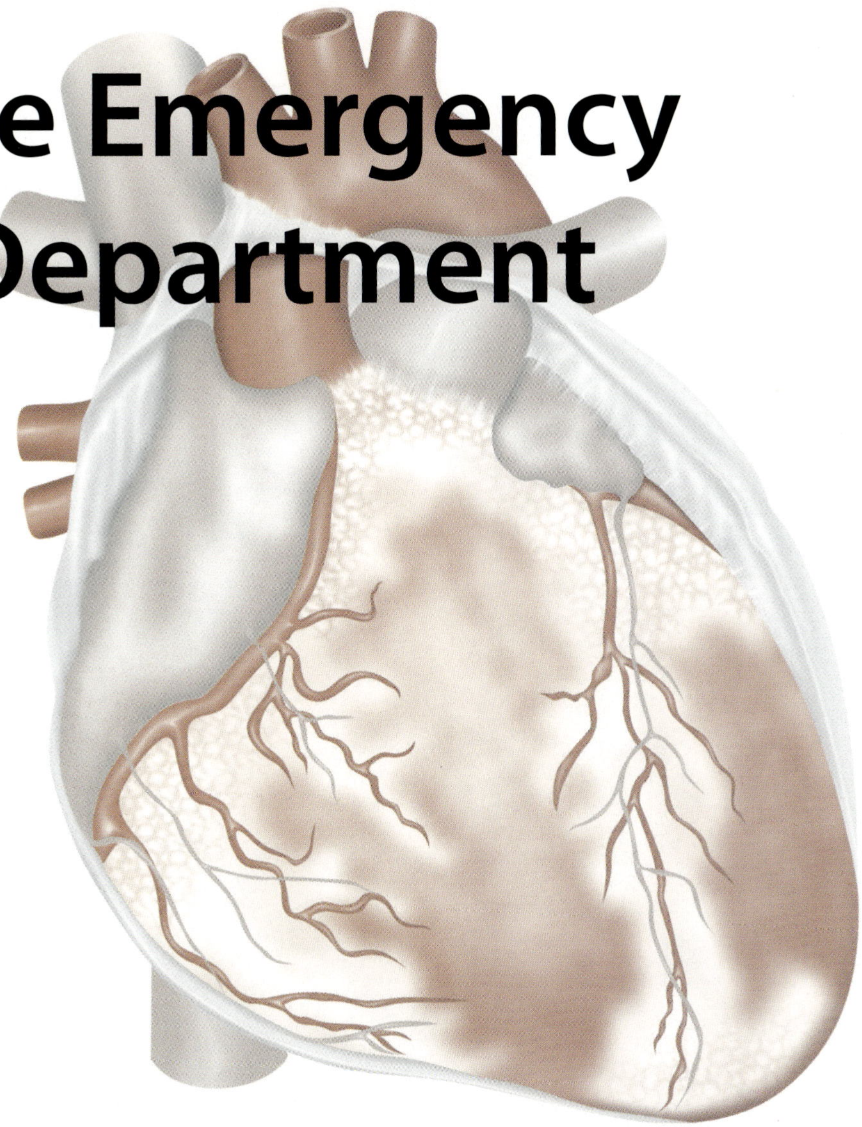

Chapter 1

How to Evaluate Dyspnea in the Emergency Department

W Frank Peacock, Dick Kuo, Sandra Williams

ABSTRACT

Dyspnea, the subjective complaint of breathlessness, is a normal symptom of heavy exertion but becomes pathological if it occurs in unexpected situations (Box 1). A completely subjective symptom, dyspnea can be rated numerically, the results of which can be used to evaluate the effectiveness of therapy. While the sensation of dyspnea may be the result of normal physiologic processes it is also the common final pathway for many fatal and high-risk events of concern in early emergency department (ED) evaluation. In 85% of cases, it is either due to asthma, pneumonia, cardiac ischemia, interstitial lung disease, congestive heart failure, chronic obstructive pulmonary disease, or psychogenic causes. The acuity of the patient's presentation determines if an immediate therapeutic intervention is required, or if a more measured response may be employed as is preferable if the patient is more clinically stable. Treatment typically depends on the underlying cause. Much of the ED determination of the underlying etiology depends upon vital sign measurement, observation of the breathing pattern, physical examination findings, and the evaluation of selected laboratory or radiographic testing. Newer tools now available to evaluate dyspnea include bioimpedance vector analysis and bedside ultrasound.

INTRODUCTION

The discomfort associated with the sensation of breathlessness is nearly primordial in its universal abhorrence. Transcending race, gender, and age, it is the one common experience that can supersede all. No activity may be continued in the face of mounting dyspnea. Nothing is more important than air. In fact, when surveying the general public on "what would make you go to the emergency department (ED) at 3 am?", the surprisingly shortlist is either dyspnea or severe pain. But dyspnea is king. While even moderate dyspnea may prompt an early morning emergency room (ER) visit, moderate pain is insufficient to force a patient from the comfort of the bed. It is for this reason that dyspnea is one of the most common reasons for presentation to the ED.

Like pain, dyspnea is a completely subjective experience. There are no objective measures to determine the severity of the patient's complaint. Thus to define the severity of the patient's initial complaint and to determine the impact of interventions on the relief of dyspnea, recording the patient's numerical report of their symptoms is of utility. A common method to be able to rate and track the patient's dyspnea is the visual analog scale (VAS). To perform this, the patient indicates their degree of discomfort by drawing an indicator on a

Box 1: Definition of dyspnea

Dyspnea (pronunciation: djspniY/*disp-NEE-Y*; also dyspnoea; Latin: *dyspnoea*; Greek: *äýóðíïéá, dýspnoia*), shortness of breath, or air hunger, is the subjective symptom of breathlessness.

It is a normal symptom of heavy exertion but becomes pathological if it occurs in unexpected situations. In 85% of cases it is due to either asthma, pneumonia, cardiac ischemia, interstitial lung disease, congestive heart failure, chronic obstructive pulmonary disease, or psychogenic causes. Treatment typically depends on the underlying cause[1]

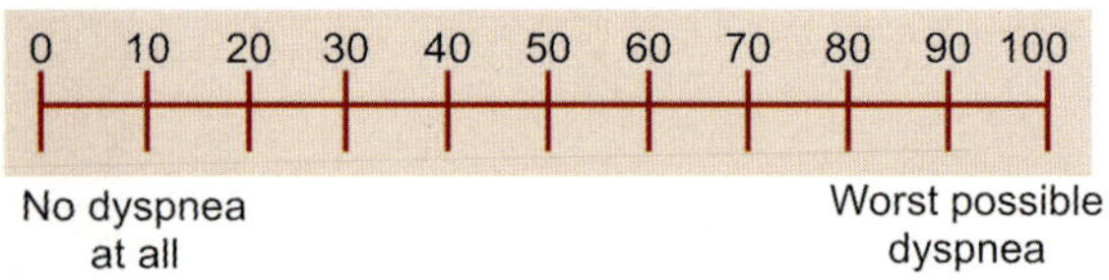

Fig. 1 Visual analog scale showing degree of discomfort, rate, and track the patient's dyspnea

Box 2: Relative dyspnea score

- Markedly better
- Moderately better
- Minimally better
- Unchanged
- Minimally improved
- Moderately improved
- Markedly improved

TABLE 1: Categorical examples of the causes of dyspnea

Mechanical	*Metabolic*	*Hemodynamic*
Foreign body/ anaphylaxis	Acidosis (e.g., DKA)	HF/AMI
Asthma/COPD	Anemia	Septic shock
Trauma (e.g. pneumothorax, rib fractures)	Toxin (e.g., cyanide)	Hemorrhagic shock
Airspace pus (pneumonia) or blood (trauma)		Cardiogenic shock
Pulmonary embolus		Shunts
Neurologic (ALS)		

DKA, diabetic ketoacidosis; HF, heart failure; AMI, acute myocardial infarction; COPD, chronic obstructive pulmonary disease; ALS, amyotrophic lateral sclerosis

100 mm line, where 0 is "no dyspnea" and 100 is "worst possible dyspnea" (Fig. 1). Prior data from the pain literature suggests that clinically relevant change should exceed 13 mm.[2] This method simply records what the patient's experience is at the exact moment the scale is administered. A second method of dyspnea evaluation uses a relative dyspnea report by asking the patient "compared to a prior time (e.g., ED presentation), your symptoms have changed in what fashion". Examples of potential responses are found in box 2. Inherent in this type of measure, because the patient is rating them as such, all changes documented by this scale are clinically relevant. However, relative scales cannot evaluate dyspnea at presentation, and tend to be less sensitive for smaller changes in dyspnea than VAS scoring.

While the sensation of dyspnea may be the result of normal physiologic processes (e.g., aggressive physical activity) it is also the common final pathway for many fatal and high-risk events of concern in the early evaluation (Box 2). Ultimately, regardless of the cause, failure of the body to ventilate and oxygenate in a fashion sufficient to meet its metabolic requirements results in the sensation of dyspnea. Because the list is extensive and lugubrious, the challenge for the emergency physician is to rapidly identify and reverse the underlying causes of dyspnea (Table 1). And to complicate this further, purely psychiatric complaints may manifest with a complaint of dyspnea. This last caveat represents a serious clinical challenge, especially when patients with severe morbidity suffer concurrent psychiatric complications.

VITAL SIGNS

Presentation of vital signs, including pulse oximetry, represents the earliest objective measure of the extent of distress that may be obtained. Although extremely insensitive when near the normal range, increasing deviations of the vital signs are associated with a logarithmically increasing probability of serious underlying pathology (Box 3). When considering respiratory status, excessively low respiratory rates [<6 breaths per minute (bpm)] are generally a premorbid condition, with immediate therapeutic intervention (e.g., endotracheal intubation, naloxone) necessary to obviate a fatality. Figure 2 demonstrates an algorithmic approach to the nonapneic patient. Likewise, excessively high respiratory rates (>30 bpm) may be initially tolerated but cannot be maintained for long periods as they ultimately lead to respiratory failure if prompt intervention does not reverse underlying pathology. If respiratory rates are closer to normal range, pulse oximetry may provide additional objective measures as to the adequacy of oxygen transport. As the ability of hemoglobin to transport oxygen drops precipitously with saturation levels below 90%, levels

Box 3: Normal vital sign ranges for the average healthy adult while resting[3]

- Blood pressure: 90/60 mmHg to 120/80 mmHg
- Breathing: 12–18 breaths/minute (bpm)
- Pulse: 60–100 beats/minute
- Temperature: 97.8–99.1°F/average 98.6°F

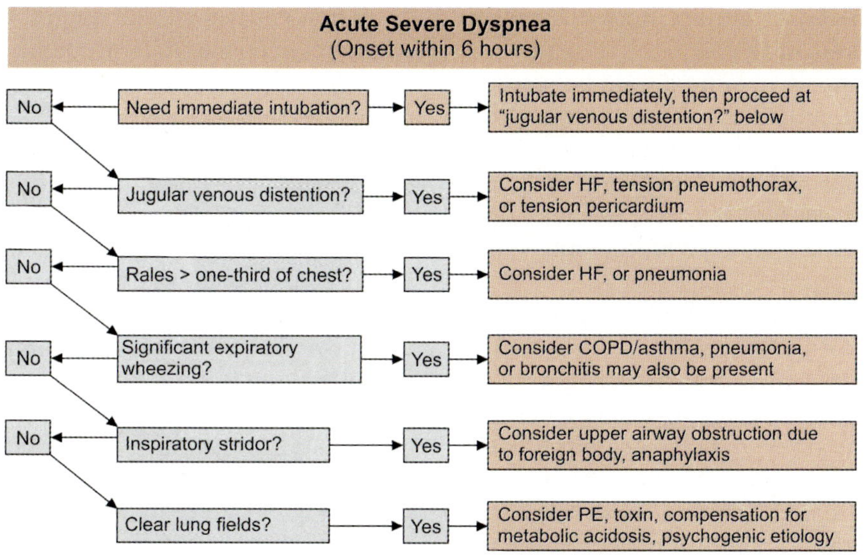

HF, heart failure; COPD, chronic obstructive pulmonary disease; PE, pulmonary embolism; BiPap, bilevel positive airway pressure; CPAP, continuous positive airway pressure

Fig. 2 An approach to the patient presenting with acute severe dyspnea. The patient's process of breathing should be observed for several respiratory cycles. If afterward the physician is assured, at least a modicum of time is available before immediate endotracheal intubation is required, the following algorithm may be considered. While it is presented in a stepwise fashion, the entire process is performed in less than 15 seconds, while listening to the lung sounds

The decision to intubate a patient with severe dyspnea is not determined by the results of any objective testing. Rather it is a clinical decision based solely on the physicians' impression that the patient is either currently, or imminently will, suffer acute respiratory failure. In cooperative but distressed patients, a limited trial of BiPap or CPAP may allow enough time for immediate therapeutic interventions to take effect, thus avoiding the need for more invasive measures. However, noninvasive ventilatory measures are not definitive airway management and should be considered as short term temporary adjuncts. If improvement in clinical status is not seen relatively quickly after their implementation, endotracheal intubation should be considered.

below this should prompt an immediate evaluation and interventions to correct hypoxia. While pulse oximetry is a rapid, noninvasive, inexpensive, objective measure of total function of the body's oxygen delivery system, it suffers from several caveats. First, abnormalities of hemoglobin from some toxins (e.g., cyanide, carbon monoxide) may imply normal oxygen transport capability when in fact tissue oxygen delivery is distinctly impaired. Second, the presence of adequate oxygenation does not reflect on ventilatory status, which must be considered independently.

Blood pressure is a critical value in determining the potential etiology in patients presenting with dyspnea. The presence of dyspnea and hypertension, associated with the appropriate lung findings, is highly suggestive of acute pulmonary edema, and immediate therapy aimed at rapid blood pressure reduction is warranted. This is true for all HF, even with blood pressures as low as 140 mmHg, as due to their poor myocardial performance, their tolerance for hypertension is extremely limited. In patients with lower blood pressures, with less evidence of volume overload and with concurrent pulmonary wheezes, the diagnosis is more likely to be COPD. Finally, patients with very low blood pressure (<90 mmHg), require immediate intervention as the acute mortality rate for HF patients presenting to the ED with blood pressure below 90 mmHg approximates 70%.

OBSERVATION

When patients present with a complaint of dyspnea, observing the mechanics of breathing is a critical intervention and should occur as soon as possible. Watching the patient is a frequently underrated, but extremely valuable, intervention. The parameters to consider include the respiratory pattern, the apparent depth of the patient's inhalation, and an estimate of how much effort the patient is expending to breathe.

The normal pattern of breathing involves an apparently effortless inhalation/exhalation timing relationship of approximately 1:3. Perturbations in this pattern can provide early diagnostic clues. For example, distress on inhalation suggests upper airway pathology (e.g., foreign body, anaphylaxis), while extended expiration suggests lower respiratory tract obstruction as may occur with asthma or COPD.

Secondly, the depth of breathing can be used to approximate minute ventilation (minute ventilation = tidal volume × bpm). Increased minute ventilation occurs with respiratory compensation for underlying metabolic acidosis from various causes, but can be seen with anemia, and may also be the result of presentations from severe anxiety.

Third, an estimate of the work of breathing is critical. Accessory muscle use, an upright position and abdominal muscle use are all consistent with increased effort. The number of words that the patients may speak between breaths can provide an index of their apparent distress. Patients who are diaphoretic as a result of the effort to breathe are likely to tire and suffer an acute respiratory arrest unless the clinical presentation is rapidly addressed. Finally, non-pulmonary observations may provide diagnostic clues as well. For example, the presence of persistent jugular venous distention is consistent with HF, tension pneumothorax, or pericardial tamponade.

PHYSICAL EXAMINATION

After the initial vital signs have been obtained and the patient's respiratory status observed, if immediate treatment is not needed, a physical examination is warranted. This begins by specifically noticing any smells that may emanate from the patient (e.g., spearmint suggests dyspnea is resulting from acidosis compensation as occurs from aspirin poisoning secondary to oil of wintergreen ingestion) and touching the patient to determine if they are febrile (consistent with pneumonia or sepsis), or if they are cold and wet as a result of compensatory peripheral vasoconstriction (as occurs in certain phenotypes of HF and acute hemorrhagic shock).

Lung sounds are a useful determination in the patient presenting with undefined dyspnea. Asymmetry of auscultatory findings is consistent with asymmetric pathologies (e.g., pneumonia, pneumothorax, pleural effusion). While the presence of basilar rales is not particularly useful diagnostically, the extent of their manifestation is suggestive of the severity of the presentation. Finally, thoracic percussion may be helpful in identifying the presence of a pulmonary effusion when breath sounds are difficult to discern.

The last part of significance of the physical examination to evaluate dyspnea involves a general inspection of the naked patient. Clues to look for include the presence or absence of jugular venous distention, abdominal distention consistent with ascites, and the presence and symmetry of any peripheral edema.

EMERGENCY DEPARTMENT INVESTIGATIONS

Laboratory

A number of laboratory tests may be obtained; however, in the severely ill patient the focus should be on the obtainable history and physical examination as laboratories take time and generally only confirm what was already suspected and initially acted based on clinical findings. In patients with less acute severity of presentation, where immediate intervention is not required, consideration of specific laboratories may be of utility. This includes measuring troponin, natriuretic peptides, and obtaining a D-dimer in selected cases. Additionally, chemistry analysis may be helpful for risk stratification and to plan future diagnostic studies (e.g., creatinine). They may identify potential complications resulting from prior outpatient therapy (e.g., hypokalemia), and selected drug levels may be necessary (e.g., digoxin).

It should be specifically noted that, while arterial blood gases (ABGs) may be of use to determine acid-base status, and when managing an intubated patient, their results are rarely of any diagnostic assistance in the acute setting. ABGs should not be used to evaluate the airway or the need for intubation at the acute presentation. While they may be of use later in the management, at the time of presentation the time wasted obtaining ABGs is better spent performing a clinical assessment and initial interventions.

Bioimpedance Vector Analysis

Bioimpedance vector analysis is the technology of determining total body water by the measurement the body's electrical conductive properties. This has been shown to provide rapid noninvasive, inexpensive, reproducible and objective values that correlate with total body water, the need for diuretic therapy, and the probability of hospitalization after an ED visit. While knowledge of perturbations in total body water is not diagnostic in and of itself, it is useful when considered in combination with other bedside findings.

Radiology

Chest radiography is an extremely useful tool. Although the chest X-ray does suffer from a number of limitations

TABLE 2: Well's criteria

Clinical findings	*Points*
Clinical signs and symptoms of DVT?	+3
PE is number one diagnosis, or equally likely	+3
Heart rate >100 beats/minute	+1.5
Immobilization at least 3 days, or surgery in the previous 4 weeks	+1.5
Previous, objectively diagnosed PE or DVT?	+1.5
? Hemoptysis	+1
Malignancy with treatment within 6 months, or palliative	+1

DVT, deep vein thrombosis; PE, pulmonary embolism

(e.g., delayed manifestations, insensitivity when done by portable technique, exposure to radiation, relatively more expensive), it can be performed rapidly and at the bedside. A relatively normal finding should markedly change the differential diagnosis if acute heart failure (AHF) is suspected.

Pulmonary computed tomography (CT) angiography has now become the gold standard for evaluation of suspected pulmonary embolus.[4] However, it should be obtained in only a minority of dyspneic patients as it is unnecessary in most. Its greatest use in the patient presenting with acute dyspnea is when the clinical diagnosis is likely acute pulmonary embolism (PE). Pretest probability scoring, using the Well's criteria (Table 2),[5] is generally of use in assessing a patient's risk for PE. While patients with higher scores are more likely to suffer acute PE, in those with low scores (<3) and a negative qualitative D-dimer test, PE can be safely excluded. Severely ill hemodynamically unstable patients, and those too dyspneic to lie flat, are not be candidates for CT evaluation. This latter population may be best served by empiric treatment.

Ultrasound

Bedside ultrasound, when performed by the emergency physician, provides a rapid, noninvasive, inexpensive measure to assist in determining the etiology of dyspnea. Ultrasound can evaluate for the presence of pneumothorax, provide information on myocardial contractility, and determine the presence of a pericardial effusion (Fig. 3). By looking at the lungs themselves, ultrasound can help differentiate between the HF and the COPD patient by the identification of B-lines. It may also give information on pulmonary volume overload by direct

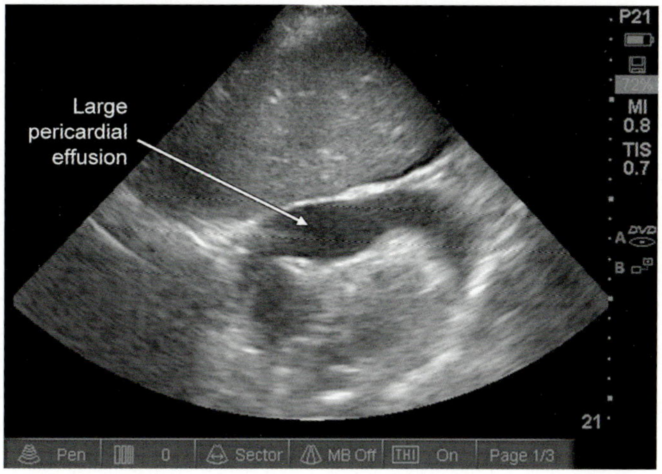

Fig. 3 Subxiphoid view of a pericardial effusion

lung imaging or by the evaluation of vena cava diameter changes that occur as a result of the respiratory cycle.

CONCLUSION

Dyspnea, the most common reason that most AHF patients present to the hospital, is the final common pathway for a myriad of pathologies. Determining what, if any, immediate intervention is required is driven by the acuity of the presentation and the diagnostic certainty of the practitioner. Thus, in severe presentations, initial clinical decisions may be entirely based upon vital signs, observation of the patient's breathing cycle, their level of discomfort and the physical examination. However, if the patient's distress can tolerate investigations preceding therapy, then selected laboratory tests, bioimpedance measures, ultrasound or radiographic testing, may greatly limit the differential diagnosis and add to diagnostic certainty.

REFERENCES

1. Wikipedia, The Free Encyclopedia. (2013). Dyspnea. [online] Available from: en.wikipedia.org/wiki/Dyspnea. [Accessed November, 2013].
2. Todd KH, Funk KG, Funk JP, et al. Clinical significance of reported changes in pain severity. Ann Emerg Med. 1996;27(4):485-9.
3. Medline Plus. (2013). Vital signs. [online] Available from: www.nlm.nih.gov/medlineplus/ency/article/002341.htm. [Accessed November, 2013].
4. Wells PS, Anderson DR, Rodger M, et al. Excluding pulmonary embolism at the bedside without diagnostic imaging: management of patients with suspected pulmonary embolism presenting to the emergency department by using a simple clinical model and d-dimer. Ann Intern Med. 2001;135(2):98-107.
5. Wolf SJ, McCubbin TR, Feldhaus KM, et al. Prospective validation of Wells Criteria in the evaluation of patients with suspected pulmonary embolism. Ann Emerg Med. 2004;44(5):503-10.

Chapter 2

Heart Failure Disposition: When to Admit, When to Observe, and When to Discharge Home

Phillip D Levy, Vijaya A Kumar

ABSTRACT

Disposition of the emergency department (ED) patient with acute heart failure (AHF) can be anxiety provoking. Patients sent home inappropriately can contribute to already excessive postdischarge event rates while unnecessary admission to the hospital adds significantly to health care costs. Finding the right balance requires a solid understanding of existing and evolving evidence with systematic incorporation into a streamlined treatment pathway. In this chapter, we provide real-world insight into the process of ED disposition and propose a simplified approach to decision-making built on a foundation of multilevel, evidence-based risk-stratification.

THE BIG PICTURE

Appropriate disposition of the emergency department (ED) patient with acute heart failure (AHF) is a clinical challenge. While few who present to the ED with AHF are severely ill[1] and many respond well to initial therapeutic intervention;[2] the default pathway remains admission to the hospital. Much of this is driven by uncertainty regarding postdischarge events and fear associated with the implications (medicolegal and others) of perceived negligence; a circumstance compounded by the relative lack of outcome data, and an absence of validated, evidence-based decision support tools derived specifically from ED patients.[3]

While it has been suggested that hospitalization could be safely avoided in up to 50% of AHF patients,[4] concerns about the postdischarge course are not entirely unfounded with data from both Canada[5] and the United States[6] showing higher mortality rates and excessive treatment failure through 90 days in those who are directly discharged from the ED. Largely reflective of poor care coordination postdischarge and underutilization of guideline-based chronic drug therapy,[7] at least some of these events could probably have been prevented by admission to the hospital.

Clearly, a better approach to ED disposition for AHF patients is needed. In their 2010 Comprehensive Practice Guidelines, the Heart Failure Society of America did propose criterion upon which hospitalization is either recommended or should be considered (Box 1), but the selected variables are loosely defined and based entirely on expert consensus (strength of evidence = C).[8] What then should clinicians use to bolster their decision-making?

RISK STRATIFICATION

From the ED perspective, every disposition involves a calculated risk and risk assessment is a multistep process. Foremost is to identify patients who, absent acute intervention, are at most likely to suffer an immediate adverse event. Clinically, accessible hemodynamic, cardiopulmonary, and renal parameters including blood pressure (BP), heart rate/rhythm, perfusion status, respiratory rate, oxygen saturation, work of breathing, and urine output are particularly important and provide important clues as to the necessary type, intensity, and urgency of treatment.[9] Without any further information, certain patient subtypes (i.e., hypotensive, cardiogenic shock, myocardial infarction, respiratory distress or

Box 1: Heart Failure Society of America admission criteria[8]

- Hospitalization recommended:
  - Evidence of severe ADHF, including:
    - Hypotension
    - Worsening renal function
    - Altered mentation
  - Dyspnea at rest, as evidenced by:
    - Resting tachypnea
    - Oxygen saturation <90%
  - Hemodynamically significant arrhythmia including:
    - New onset of rapid atrial fibrillation
  - Acute coronary syndromes
- Hospitalization should be considered:
  - Worsened congestion:
    - With or without dyspnea
  - Signs and symptoms of pulmonary or systemic congestion:
    - With or without weight gain
  - Major electrolyte disturbance
  - Associated comorbid conditions:
    - Pneumonia
    - Pulmonary embolus
    - Diabetic ketoacidosis
    - Cerebrovascular disease
  - Repeated ICD firings
  - New-onset heart failure

ADHF, acute decompensated heart failure; ICD, implantable cardioverter-defibrillator

failure, unstable dysrhythmias, hypertensive emergency) will be designated for an intensive care unit admission.

For those who appear relatively stable at first pass, additional considerations such as HF etiology, underlying cardiac dysfunction (especially ejection fraction), suspected precipitant (i.e., hypertension, arrhythmia, myocardial ischemia, worsening renal function), and degree of volume overload provide the next level of stratification and help to ensure that management is properly aligned with the needs of the patient. Clinical response to initial treatment is an important indicator of likely disposition. Patient profiles can change dramatically within a few hours of ED arrival[10] and frequent (for those who are critically ill) or periodic (for those with less severe symptoms) reassessment involving both physical examination and laboratory investigation should be performed. Patients without high-risk features (described in greater detail below) who rapidly improve and return to (or close to) their baseline status may be eligible for ED discharge, in lieu of or after a brief period of observation.[11]

On the other hand, patients who experience minimal improvement or a worsening of symptoms after initial ED care are poor candidates for discharge and should be promptly triaged to an inpatient unit for more extensive management.[10]

Less certain is the management of those who fall between these extremes, with a partial but incomplete response to early therapy. With continued treatment, these individuals may improve enough to go home, but this often requires more time than is usually acceptable in the ED setting necessitating an in-patient or observation unit stay. However, unlike diseases, such as asthma or chronic obstructive pulmonary disease (COPD) where symptoms and their response to therapy tell most of the story, AHF represents a complex interplay of multiple organ systems and perturbations in one or more can have a profound impact on the subsequent clinical course. Thus, it may be possible to temporize overt manifestations of AHF, especially breathlessness, with acute therapy, such as diuresis or afterload reduction while failing to recognize or address ongoing and potentially lethal pathophysiology. Accordingly, a second tier of risk assessment involving a search for additional factors associated with worse (or better) outcomes is routinely employed. From the ED perspective, this rarely involves invasive monitoring or advanced imaging, instead focusing on variables that are readily attainable and interpretable at the point of care in the ED setting.

High Risk Features

Numerous attempts have been made using clinical trial,[12] registry,[13-19] and regional cohort data[20,21] to define high-risk features for admitted patients with AHF. The majority of these have targeted in-hospital or short-term (up to 90-day) mortality as the outcome measure and, despite varying methodologies, have demonstrated remarkable consistency with lower presenting BP, decreased serum sodium, renal dysfunction, and myocardial injury or stress showing the strongest association. As such, in addition to BP assessment, electrocardiography along with measurement of serum electrolytes, renal function [i.e., blood urea nitrogen (BUN) and serum creatinine], and cardiac biomarkers [i.e., troponin and natriuretic peptides (NP)] is considered essential in the evaluation of AHF patients with relative abnormalities (Table 1) serving as important indicators of risk.[11] In general, patients who are found to have high-risk features should be admitted to the hospital for ongoing treatment and, depending on the circumstance, a more exhaustive search for a

TABLE 1: Evidence-based markers of acute heart failure risk[11]

Marker	*Threshold for risk*
Systolic blood pressure	<100 mmHg
Respiratory rate	<32 breaths/minute
Electrocardiography	New ischemic changes
Renal function:	
Blood urea nitrogen	>40 mg/dL
Creatinine	>3.0 mg/dL
Serum sodium	<135 mmoL/L
Cardiac-specific troponin	Any value > 99th percentile (varies by assay)
Natriuretic peptides:	
Brain natriuretic peptide	>1,000 pg/mL
N-terminal-pro-BNP	>5,000 pg/mL

TABLE 2: Emergency heart failure mortality risk grade model[21]

*Variable**	*Unit or measure*	*Mathematical adjustment†*
Age	Continuous in years	Multiply by 2
Transported by emergency medical service	Categorical	Add 60 if yes
Systolic blood pressure	Continuous in mmHg (maximum = 160 mmHg)	Multiply by −1
Heart rate	Continuous in bpm (minimum = 80, maximum = 120 bpm)	Multiply by 1
Oxygen saturation	Continuous as % (Maximum = 92%)	Multiply by −2
Creatinine	Continuous as mg/dL (divide by 88.4 if reported as µmoL/L)	Multiply by 20
Potassium	Categorical: • 4.0–4.5 mmoL/L • ≥4.6 mmoL/L • ≤3.9 mmoL/L	If yes: • Add 0 • Add 30 • Add 5
Troponin	Categorical	Add 60 if > upper limit of normal
Active cancer	Categorical	Add 45 if yes
Metolazone at home	Categorical	Add 60 if yes
Adjustment factor	—	Add 12

*Based on initial or triage measurement

†Score derived from sum of all variables, including the adjustment factor:

- Very low-risk ≤ −15.9
- Low risk = −15.8–17.9
- Intermediate risk = 18.0–56.5
- High risk = 56.6–89.3
- Very high-risk ≥89.4

reversible underlying cause of or contributor to acute decompensation.

While mortality is, for obvious reasons, the major focal point of risk assessment, it is not the only end-point to consider. Patients with AHF are also at-risk for other serious, but nonfatal events, such as worsening renal function, worsening HF, delayed myocardial infarction, atrial or ventricular arrhythmias, respiratory failure, cardiogenic shock, and cardiac arrest. Unfortunately, such outcomes have been insufficiently explored and defining in whom they are more likely to develop is difficult. Not surprisingly, in the limited studies that have been conducted, factors associated with an increase in the risk of death also correlate with composite measures of nonfatal events.[22] Other variables including heart rate, respiratory rate, blood glucose, white blood cell count, and arterial pH have also been evaluated and, when abnormal, appear to portend a higher-risk profile.[23]

Low-risk Features

Though outcomes are clearly better for AHF patients who lack high-risk features, this does not necessarily mean that they are at low-risk.[24] Further, perspectives on risk differ according to individual tolerance for uncertainty and what one defines as low-risk may be above another's threshold. Understanding this is important to the consideration of ED disposition but increasingly, efforts are being directed toward identification of variables that truly reflect what most would consider a low-risk profile. A 10-item scale [the Emergency Heart Failure Mortality Risk Grade (EHMRG)] has recently been developed and validated in a retrospectively derived cohort of 12,500 non-dialysis dependent ED patients with AHF.[3] By combining these 10 variables into a single model (Table 2), a score can be generated that provides a reasonably reliable (C-statistic = 0.807 and 0.803 in the derivation and validation groups, respectively) estimation of mortality risk within 7 days of discharge. Based on this preliminary work, as many as 25% of such patients may be classifiable as very low-risk (<0.5%) and up to 50% as low-risk (<1.1%) for early, postdischarge death. While such data are encouraging for the future of evidence-based ED disposition, further investigation of EHMRG is needed, particularly a prospective outcomes study.

No-risk Features

Given the known decrease in life-expectancy that accompanies this disorder, few if any AHF patients can truly be considered no-risk. However, there are some individuals who, lacking insurance or other financial means necessary to access outpatient care, come to the ED simply for medication refills or a semblance of care continuity. Often, these patients have been recently discharged from the hospital and report indolent symptoms, such as increasing edema or mild but persistent dyspnea. While some (if not all) of this can be attributed to medication or dietary noncompliance, a search for potential contributors, such as worsening renal function or interval development of myocardial injury should be pursued. Absent evidence of newly developed high risk features (i.e., elevated but unchanged creatinine in a patient with known chronic kidney disease), these patients have a relatively stable risk profile that is unlikely to be modified by hospitalization. Despite this, they may still benefit from a reevaluation of their medications, perhaps with short-term uptitration of diuretic dosing or addition of previously unprescribed, evidence-based therapy such as an aldosterone antagonist or a dual action beta-blocker. Further HF-specific education with emphasis on the importance of disease self-management may also be needed. While it may be possible to accomplish this entirely within the ED encounter, socioeconomics will have critical bearing on the success of outpatient management and related disposition decisions for these seemingly "no-risk" patients should be made with this all-important consideration in mind.

WHEN SHOULD YOU ADMIT?

The primary goal of hospitalization is to provide continued therapy in the acute and subacute phase of AHF in an effort to optimize volume and hemodynamic status, thereby decreasing symptoms and facilitating a return to baseline. Hospitalization also provides an opportunity to more extensively investigate potential worrisome contributors to the AHF episode, such as coronary artery disease. Appropriate timing of hospitalization requires a careful balance to ensure that adequate initial treatment has been started and a sufficient risk-assessment period has transpired. As noted above, for patients who are clearly critical, there is little reason to delay transition from the ED to an intensive care setting and the process of admission should be initiated concurrent with stabilizing measures. That said, some critically ill patients may improve while waiting for an intensive care unit bed to become available enabling a discontinuation of certain therapies, such as intravenous nitroglycerin or noninvasive positive pressure ventilation in the ED and a potential downgrade in the level of necessary in-patient care. In spite of this, there is a general reluctance on the part of ED physicians to withdraw vasoactive therapy over concerns about potential rebound symptoms and in most hospitals, AHF patients initially admitted to the intensive care unit end up in a critical care bed.

For more stable patients, it is common to wait for completion of the initial work-up prior to contacting an admitting service or physician. Once that has occurred, the presence of any high-risk features generally warrants admission and should prompt discussion of the need for continuous cardiac monitoring (i.e., telemetry) or, depending on the circumstance and hospital policy, possible admission to a step-down unit. Cardiac-specific troponin (especially when measured serially using a contemporary or high-sensitivity assays) has particular relevance, providing independent prognostic and diagnostic information for AHF patients.[17,25,26] Hemodynamically stable patients without high-risk features who have marked peripheral edema with or without residual dyspnea will likely require ongoing intravenous diuretic therapy and should be designated for a nonmonitored in-patient stay.

WHEN TO DISCHARGE HOME?

Those patients with improved dyspnea and a low or very low-risk profile may be eligible for extended management in an observation unit or, depending on social circumstances and the ability to arrange outpatient follow-up, discharge home. In the vast majority of patients who present with AHF, dyspnea is a consequence of central congestion related to volume overload and the primary cause of their ED visit.[19] Signs of fluid overload include elevated jugular venous pressure, peripheral edema, and weight-gain. Dyspnea, orthopnea, dizziness, and decreased exercise tolerance are key symptoms and their presence has been associated with an increase rate of adverse events postdischarge.[19] Therefore, comprehensive evaluation for and alleviation of these findings are crucial steps when considering whether a patient is stable for discharge. Improved symptoms related to congestion coupled with hemodynamic evidence of decreased volume overload are reasonable end-points to consider when deciding if a patient is clinically suitable for discharge.

Dyspnea Resolution

While objective improvement in fluid overload can be identified on physical examination by specific findings including a reduction in jugular venous pressure, resolution of pulmonary rales, a decrease in peripheral edema, diminished body weight, and an increase in urine output, there is no validated measure to assess dyspnea.[27] Most clinical trials have used 5-point or 7-point Likert scales and 100 mm visual analogue scales (VAS), both of which appear to adequately capture changes over time for supine patients.[2,27] Typically used in patients with chronic pulmonary disease, peak expiratory flow rate (PEFR) has also been evaluated as a way to standardize dyspnea measurement with data suggesting that it may be complimentary to Likert scales, especially within the first 24 hours of treatment.[28] However, none of these measures provides a sufficient evaluation of orthopnea, an important but often overlooked component of clinical congestion. Provocative dyspnea assessment (PDA), a recently developed approach where patients self-report shortness of breath symptoms in the upright and, after a brief equilibration period, supine positions, may address this gap-enabling identification of "hidden" symptoms of persistent dyspnea.[2,27] Though further validation is needed, PDA may ultimately prove to be an important tool in the appraisal of dyspnea and its resolution in ED patients with AHF.

Despite improvements in dyspnea at rest, symptoms may still be present on exertion and serve as a marker of residual congestion. Orthostatic hypotension manifesting as postural light-headedness may also be seen, especially when overly aggressive diuresis or BP reduction has occurred in a short period of time. As such, the patient's ability to ambulate without dyspnea or dizziness should be assessed by having the walk around the ED. How far and how long they should be able to ambulate prior to discharge has not been established, but in stable angina patients, the 6-minute walk test (6MWT), where the maximal ambulatory distance is measured over 6 minutes and compared to age-adjusted population norms, is considered a valid metric of cardiovascular risk.[29] While the 6MWT has not been formally tested as a metric of "dischargeability", a modified version involving 3 minutes of ambulation with concurrent monitoring of heart rate, respiratory rate, pulse oximetry, and subjective dyspnea may be useful, helping to distinguish ED patients with AHF at-risk for worse outcome in a small, single center feasibility study (n = 40).[30] Bottom line: even without a formal approach to assessment, treated AHF patients who cannot ambulate due to dyspnea or dizziness for even a brief period in the ED are likely to suffer from ongoing or worsening debility at home, making them poor candidates from discharge.

Is There a Role for Natriuretic Peptides?

As noted throughout this textbook, NP play an important role in the management of AHF patients, providing prognostic and diagnostic information both on admission[16,31,32] and at discharge.[33] However, from a disposition perspective, there is uncertainty regarding the incremental value of repeated measurement with studies showing little apparent correlation between a reduction in NP levels and dyspnea relief over the first 72 hours for admitted AHF patients.[34] Further, in an ED-based trial of AHF treatment, no differences in hospital length of stay, 30-day readmissions, or all-cause mortality were found for patients randomized to serial B-type NP testing (baseline followed by repeat measurement at 3, 6, 9, and 12 hours then daily) versus usual care.[35] In addition, the interval decrement in B-type NP levels over the first 24 hours in both experimental and control patients was modest (54 pg/mL and 95 pg/mL, respectively) suggesting limited utility of short-term NP reassessment as measure of discharge suitability.

Other Considerations

In addition to dyspnea resolution, several other milestones should be considered prior to discharge including: Identification of the reason for acute decompensation with at least partial reversal; demonstrated diuresis of at least 1 L for those with volume overload with successful transition from intravenous to oral diuretic; provision of disease-specific education to the patient and their family; achievement of medication reconciliation with reappraisal and alignment of the outpatient pharmacologic regimen based on existing guidelines; and development of transitional care plan that incorporates a follow-up evaluation, ideally with a HF cardiologist, within 5–7 days.[36] Lastly, for patients who have not had an echocardiogram within the preceding 6-months and for those who meet criteria for cardiac resynchronization therapy, appropriate referrals should be provided. Inability to facilitate an outpatient work-up for such patients, even when a dramatic improvement in symptoms has occurred, should prompt consideration of an observation unit or in-patient stay.

PUTTING IT ALL TOGETHER

As shown in the accompanying flowchart 1, disposition decision-making for ED patients with AHF can be greatly enhanced by incorporating an evidence-based, multilevel approach to risk stratification. Unstable patients and those deemed to be at high-risk on initial evaluation or subsequent to therapeutic intervention should be directed toward early hospital admission, most often in a monitored setting. For stable patients who lack high-risk features, disposition can be guided by a comprehensive reassessment of congestion with a specific focus on completeness of dyspnea resolution. Contrary to conventional practice, a number of patients may be suitable for discharge home, provided they meet low or very low-risk criteria and an individually appropriate, achievable transitional care plan has been developed.

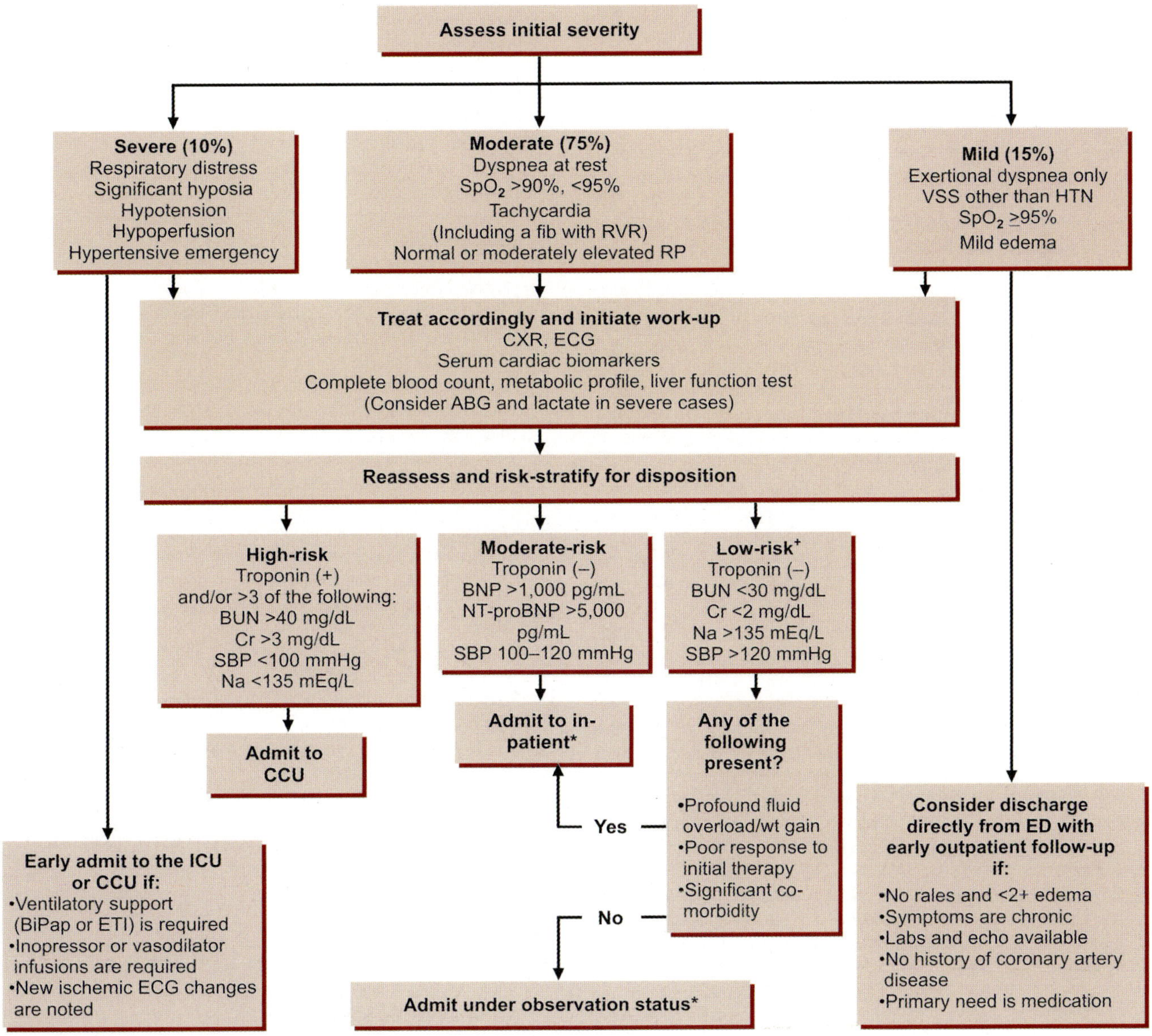

⁺Consider modified approach using EMHRG score

*Telemetry criteria: arrhythmia; ICD firing; syncope; active chest pain; potassium ≤2.5 or ≥6.0; magnesium ≤1 mEq/L

SpO_2, saturated oxygen; RVR, rapid ventricular response; BUN, blood urea nitrogen; BP, blood pressure; CXR, chest X-ray; ECG, electrocardiogram; ABG, arterial blood gas; Cr, creatinine; SBP, systolic blood pressure; Na, sodium; NT, N-terminal; BNP, brain natriuretic peptide; EHMRG, Emergency Heart Failure Mortality Risk Grade; CCU, critical care unit; ICU, intensive care unit; BiPap, bilevel positive airway pressure; ETI, endotracheal intubation; ICD, implantable cardioverter-defibrillator; ED, emergency department

Flowchart 1 Sample evidence-based algorithm for acute heart failure patient disposition from the emergency department

REFERENCES

1. Fonarow GC, Heywood JT, Heidenreich PA, et al. Temporal trends in clinical characteristics, treatments, and outcomes for heart failure hospitalizations, 2002 to 2004: findings from Acute Decompensated Heart Failure National Registry (ADHERE). Am Heart J. 2007;153(6):1021-8.
2. Mebazaa A, Pang PS, Tavares M, et al. The impact of early standard therapy on dyspnoea in patients with acute heart failure: the URGENT-dyspnoea study. Eur Heart J. 2010;31(7):832-41.
3. Lee DS, Stitt A, Austin PC, et al. Prediction of heart failure mortality in emergent care: a cohort study. Ann Intern Med. 2012;156(11):767-75.
4. Collins SP, Pang PS, Fonarow GC, et al. Is hospital admission for heart failure really necessary?: the role of the emergency department and observation unit in preventing hospitalization and rehospitalization. J Am Coll Cardiol. 2013;61(2):121-6.
5. Lee DS, Schull MJ, Alter DA, et al. Early deaths in patients with heart failure discharged from the emergency department: a population-based analysis. Circ Heart Fail. 2010;3(2):228-35.
6. Rame JE, Sheffield MA, Dries DL, et al. Outcomes after emergency department discharge with a primary diagnosis of heart failure. Am Heart J. 2001;142(4):714-9.
7. Lee DS, Stukel TA, Austin PC, et al. Improved outcomes with early collaborative care of ambulatory heart failure patients discharged from the emergency department. Circulation. 2010;122(18):1806-14.
8. Lindenfeld J, Albert NM, Boehmer JP, et al. HFSA 2010 Comprehensive Heart Failure Practice Guideline. J Card Fail. 2010;16(6):e1-194.
9. Gheorghiade M, Braunwald E. A proposed model for initial assessment and management of acute heart failure syndromes. JAMA. 2011;305(16):1702-3.
10. Collins SP, Lindsell CJ, Storrow AB, et al. Early changes in clinical characteristics after emergency department therapy for acute heart failure syndromes: identifying patients who do not respond to standard therapy. Heart Fail Rev. 2012;17(3):387-94.
11. Peacock WF, Fonarow GC, Ander DS, et al. Society of Chest Pain Centers recommendations for the evaluation and management of the observation stay acute heart failure patient-parts 1-6. Acute Card Care. 2009;11(1):3-42.
12. O'Connor CM, Mentz RJ, Cotter G, et al. The PROTECT in-hospital risk model: 7-day outcome in patients hospitalized with acute heart failure and renal dysfunction. Eur J Heart Fail. 2012;14(6):605-12.
13. Abraham WT, Fonarow GC, Albert NM, et al. Predictors of in-hospital mortality in patients hospitalized for heart failure: insights from the Organized Program to Initiate Lifesaving Treatment in Hospitalized Patients with Heart Failure (OPTIMIZE-HF). J Am Coll Cardiol. 2008;52(5):347-56.
14. O'Connor CM, Abraham WT, Albert NM, et al. Predictors of mortality after discharge in patients hospitalized with heart failure: an analysis from the Organized Program to Initiate Lifesaving Treatment in Hospitalized Patients with Heart Failure (OPTIMIZE-HF). Am Heart J. 2008;156(4):662-73.
15. Fonarow GC, Adams KF Jr., Abraham WT, et al. Risk stratification for in-hospital mortality in acutely decompensated heart failure: classification and regression tree analysis. JAMA. 2005;293(5):572-80.
16. Fonarow GC, Peacock WF, Phillips CO, et al. Admission B-type natriuretic peptide levels and in-hospital mortality in acute decompensated heart failure. J Am Coll Cardiol. 2007;49(19):1943-50.
17. Peacock WF 4th, De Marco T, Fonarow GC, et al. Cardiac troponin and outcome in acute heart failure. N Engl J Med. 2008;358(20):2117-26.
18. Gheorghiade M, Abraham WT, Albert NM, et al. Relationship between admission serum sodium concentration and clinical outcomes in patients hospitalized for heart failure: an analysis from the OPTIMIZE-HF registry. Eur Heart J. 2007;28(8):980-8.
19. Gheorghiade M, Abraham WT, Albert NM, et al. Systolic blood pressure at admission, clinical characteristics, and outcomes in patients hospitalized with acute heart failure. JAMA. 2006;296(18):2217-26.
20. Auble TE, Hsieh M, Gardner W, et al. A prediction rule to identify low-risk patients with heart failure. Acad Emerg Med. 2005;12(6):514-21.
21. Lee DS, Austin PC, Rouleau JL, et al. Predicting mortality among patients hospitalized for heart failure: derivation and validation of a clinical model. JAMA. 2003;290(19):2581-7.
22. Auble TE, Hsieh M, McCausland JB, et al. Comparison of four clinical prediction rules for estimating risk in heart failure. Ann Emerg Med. 2007;50(2):127-35.
23. Hsieh M, Auble TE, Yealy DM. Validation of the Acute Heart Failure Index. Ann Emerg Med. 2008;51(1):37-44.
24. Weintraub NL, Collins SP, Pang PS, et al. Acute heart failure syndromes: emergency department presentation, treatment, and disposition: current approaches and future aims: a scientific statement from the American Heart Association. Circulation. 2010;122(19):1975-96.
25. Kociol RD, Pang PS, Gheorghiade M, et al. Troponin elevation in heart failure prevalence, mechanisms, and clinical implications. J Am Coll Cardiol. 2010;56(14):1071-8.
26. O'Connor CM, Fiuzat M, Lombardi C, et al. Impact of serial troponin release on outcomes in patients with acute heart failure: analysis from the PROTECT pilot study. Circ Heart Fail. 2011;4(6):724-32.
27. Hogg KJ, McMurray JJ. Evaluating dyspnoea in acute heart failure: progress at last! Eur Heart J. 2010;31(7):771-2.
28. Ezekowitz JA, Hernandez AF, O'Connor CM, et al. Assessment of dyspnea in acute decompensated heart failure: insights from ASCEND-HF (Acute Study of Clinical Effectiveness of Nesiritide in Decompensated Heart Failure) on the contributions of peak expiratory flow. J Am Coll Cardiol. 2012;59(16):1441-8.
29. Beatty AL, Schiller NB, Whooley MA. Six-minute walk test as a prognostic tool in stable coronary heart disease: data from the heart and soul study. Arch Intern Med. 2012;172(14):1096-102.
30. Pan AM, Stiell IG, Clement CM, et al. Feasibility of a structured 3-minute walk test as a clinical decision tool for patients presenting to the emergency department with acute dyspnoea. Emerg Med J. 2009;26(4):278-82.
31. Januzzi JL, van Kimmenade R, Lainchbury J, et al. NT-proBNP testing for diagnosis and short-term prognosis in acute destabilized heart failure: an international pooled analysis of 1256 patients: the International Collaborative of NT-proBNP Study. Eur Heart J. 2006;27(3):330-7.
32. Maisel A, Hollander JE, Guss D, et al. Primary results of the Rapid Emergency Department Heart Failure Outpatient Trial (REDHOT). A multicenter study of B-type natriuretic peptide levels, emergency department decision making, and outcomes in patients presenting with shortness of breath. J Am Coll Cardiol. 2004;44(6):1328-33.
33. Kociol RD, Horton JR, Fonarow GC, et al. Admission, discharge, or change in B-type natriuretic peptide and long-term outcomes: data from Organized Program to Initiate Lifesaving Treatment in Hospitalized Patients with Heart Failure (OPTIMIZE-HF) linked to Medicare claims. Circ Heart Fail. 2011;4(5):628-36.
34. Kociol RD, McNulty SE, Hernandez AF, et al. Markers of Decongestion, Dyspnea Relief and Clinical Outcomes Among Patients Hospitalized with Acute Heart Failure. Circ Heart Fail. 2013;6(2):240-5.
35. Singer AJ, Birkhahn RH, Guss D, et al. Rapid Emergency Department Heart Failure Outpatients Trial (REDHOT II): a randomized controlled trial of the effect of serial B-type natriuretic peptide testing on patient management. Circ Heart Fail. 2009;2(4):287-93.
36. Bonow RO, Ganiats TG, Beam CT, et al. ACCF/AHA/AMA-PCPI 2011 performance measures for adults with heart failure: a report of the American College of Cardiology Foundation/American Heart Association Task Force on Performance Measures and the American Medical Association-Physician Consortium for Performance Improvement. Circulation. 2012;125(19):2382-401

Chapter 3

The Treatment of Acute Heart Failure in the Emergency Department

Lora AlKhawam, Peter S Pang

ABSTRACT

In the emergency department (ED), rapid diagnosis and treatment of acute heart failure (AHF) is critical to ensure optimal outcomes. Failure to diagnose and treat promptly is associated with worse morbidity and mortality. In this chapter, we review the initial approach to AHF management, utilizing systolic blood pressure (SBP) as a guide to treatment. Intravenous (IV) loop diuretics and vasodilators are the primary pharmacological treatment options for the vast majority of AHF patients, and we discuss how to utilize these agents effectively in the ED.

Current treatment recommendations are based on smaller studies and expert consensus. However, over the last 10 years, our understanding of the diagnosis, prognosis, and pathophysiology of early AHF has evolved, suggesting a new framework upon which to base treatment recommendations. In this chapter, we present a clinical approach to AHF management.

BACKGROUND

Of the 1 million hospitalizations for acute heart failure (AHF) every year, approximately 800,000 will initially be managed in the ED. Although the signs and symptoms of heart failure (HF) are the hallmark of the AHF patient [i.e., dyspnea, fatigue, edema, rales, and jugular venous distension (JVD)], the heterogeneity of the patient population in regards to underlying etiology of HF, cardiac structure and function, acute precipitant, cardiovascular, and non-cardiovascular comorbidities, is tremendous. Contrary to traditional belief, approximately half of the AHF population presents with preserved ejection fraction (EF) and this group experiences a post-discharge event rate similar to patients with impaired systolic function.[1] Although for the purposes of this review we will define AHF broadly, individualizing therapy based on the unique pathophysiologic profile of each patient is an area of intense research focus.

DEFINITION

There is no universally accepted definition of AHF. Herein, the definition established by consensus in 2005 for AHF is used: patients with HF signs and symptoms in need of urgent or emergent therapy.[2]

INITIAL APPROACH (TABLE 1)

Diagnosis and management commonly occur in parallel in the ED setting; patients who present in need of immediate intervention highlight the importance of this approach. Recognition and treatment of the precipitant, if it can be identified, is paramount and cannot be overemphasized. Given the lack of evidence to make strong recommendations, the initial approach to AHF in the ED is based on the current best available evidence and is highlighted in flowchart 1.[3]

TABLE 1: Initial management for acute heart failure syndrome*

Treat immediate life-threatening conditions	Immediate resuscitative or lifesaving measures may precede or parallel diagnostic evaluation (i.e., unstable arrhythmia, flash pulmonary edema, and STEMI)
Establish the diagnosis	Based on medical history, signs (JVD, S3, and edema), symptoms (dyspnea), and biomarkers (BNP)
Determine clinical profile	Key components include HR, BP, JVP, presence of pulmonary congestion, ECG, CXR, renal function, troponin, BNP, pulse oximetry, and history of CAD
Determine and manage the precipitant	Management of precipitants, such as ischemia, hypertension, arrhythmias, acute valvular pathologies, worsening renal function, uncontrolled diabetes and/or infectious etiologies is critical to ensure maximal benefits from HF management
Alleviate symptoms (e.g., dyspnea)	Usually a diuretic with or without other vasoactive agents. Morphine may also be used†
Myocardial and renal protection/preservation	Avoid hypotension or increase in HR. Use of inotropes should be restricted to those with low-output state (low BP or organ hypoperfusion). Risk for myocardial injury is greater in those with underlying CAD
Disposition	Majority of patients are admitted to telemetry, with a small, but significant number discharged home. Robust evidence to support risk stratification and disposition in terms of admission to the hospital or safe discharge with close outpatient follow-up is lacking

*These steps usually occur in parallel, not series

†Retrospective data suggests morphine is associated with worse outcomes

STEMI, ST-segment elevation myocardial infarction; JVD, jugular venous distention; BNP, brain natriuretic peptide; HR, heart rate; BP, blood pressure; JVP, jugular venous pressure; ECG, electrocardiogram; CXR, chest X-ray; CAD, coronary artery disease; HF, heart failure

Source: Adapted from Gheorghiade H, Pang PS. Acute heart failure syndromes. J Am Coll Cardiol. 2009;53(7):557-73, *with permission*

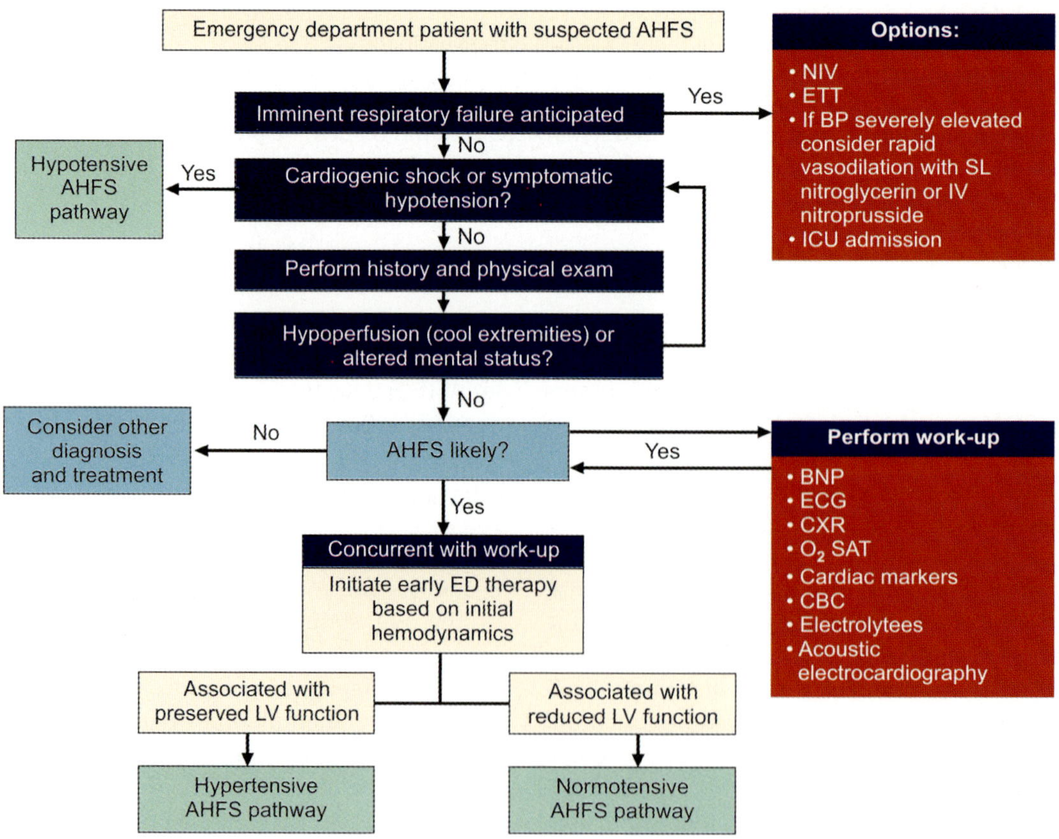

AHFS, acute heart failure syndrome; NIV, noninvasive ventilation; ETT, endotracheal tube; BP, blood pressure; SL, sublingual; IV, intravenous; ICU, intensive care unit; BNP, brain natriuretic peptide; ECG, electrocardiogram; CXR, chest X-ray; CBC, complete blood count; ED, emergency department; LV, left ventricular

Flowchart 1 Emergency department patient with suspected acute heart failure syndrome

Source: Adapted from Collins S, Storrow AB, Kirk JD, et al. Beyond pulmonary edema: diagnostic, risk stratification, and treatment challenges of acute heart failure management in the emergency department. *Ann Emerg Med*. 2008;51(1):45-57, *with permission*

RATIONALE FOR ACUTE HEART FAILURE MANAGEMENT USING SYSTOLIC BLOOD PRESSURE

Systolic blood pressure (SBP) is a key prognostic indicator; the higher the BP, the better the outcome.[4] With the exception of the patient in cardiogenic shock, this may be counterintuitive in the ED setting as patients with extremes of BP (i.e., the hypertensive flash pulmonary edema patient) often appear the most severe. However, rapid, effective management of these patients often leads to near complete resolution of symptoms after the ED phase of management, leading to a downgrade from critical care to usual care. Contrary to traditional belief, a wide range of SBP is seen in AHF, with only a smaller segment of the population having a low SBP, defined as less than 90 mmHg.[5] BP in AHF is also useful in that it allows for a crude estimate of EF.[6] Ultimately, we recommend use of BP to guide clinicians in selecting a vasodilator intensive versus diuretic intensive approach to initial therapy.

The following three flowcharts (Flowcharts 2–4) outline an approach to hypertensive (SBP >140 mmHg), normotensive (SBP >90 mmHg) and hypotensive AHF (SBP <90 mmHg).

PATHOPHYSIOLOGIC RATIONALE

For patients who present with higher SBP, it has been suggested that AHF signs and symptoms stem less from total volume overload and more from volume redistribution.[7,8] The "flash" pulmonary edema patient is representative of this concept. These patients have a dramatic and sudden presentation as opposed to days of slowly progressive weight gain, peripheral edema, or fatigue. While vasodilators are potentially of value in all congested patients, for AHF patients with hypertension, their capacity for both preload and afterload reduction are key in mitigating congestion's effect on a weakened heart.

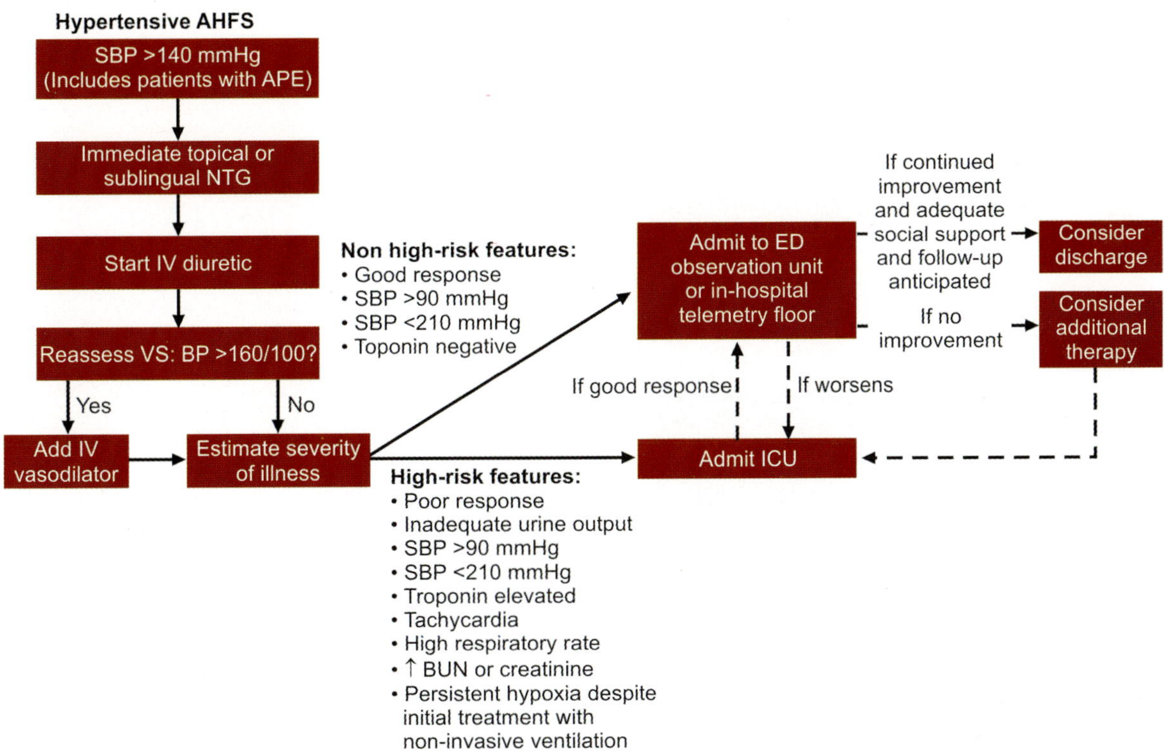

AHFS, acute heart failure syndrome; SBP, systolic blood pressure; APE, acute pulmonary embolism; NTG, nitroglycerin; IV, intravenous; BP, blood pressure; ED, emergency department; ICU, intensive care unit; BUN, blood urea nitrogen

Flowchart 2 Hypertensive acute heart failure syndrome pathway

Source: Adapted from Collins S, Storrow AB, Kirk JD, et al. Beyond pulmonary edema: diagnostic, risk stratification, and treatment challenges of acute heart failure management in the emergency department. *Ann Emerg Med.* 2008;51(1):45-57, *with permission*

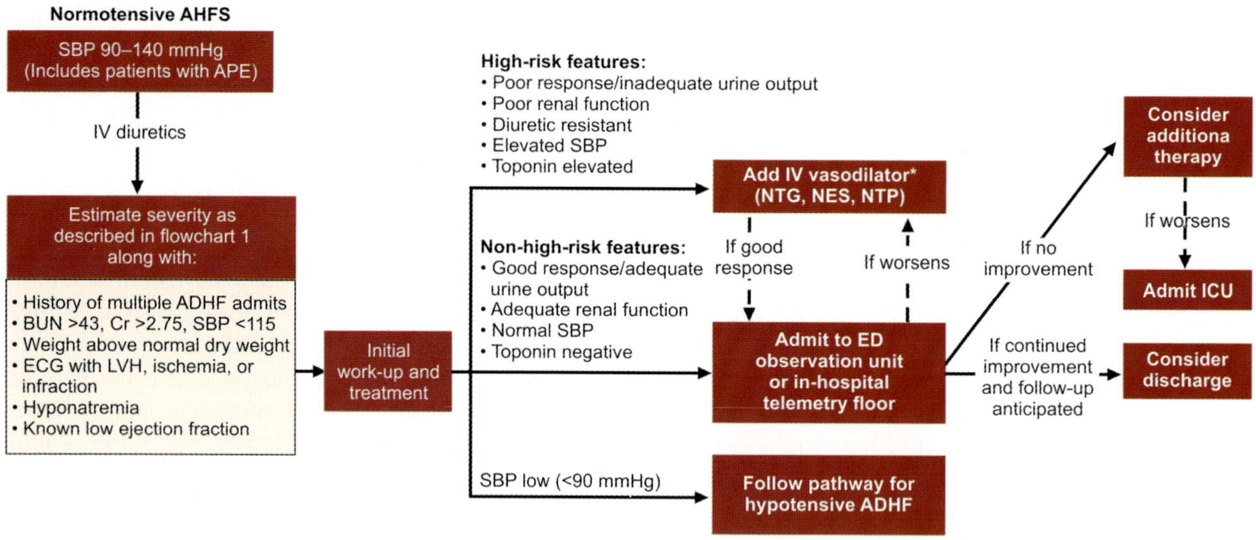

*Recommend caution unless certain of diagnosis and congested state

AHFS, acute heart failure syndrome; SBP, systolic blood pressure; APE, acute pulmonary embolism; IV, intravenous; ADHF, acute decompensated heart failure; BUN, blood urea nitrogen; Cr, creatinine; ECG, electrocardiogram; LVH, left ventricular hypertrophy; NES, nesiritide; NTG, nitroglycerin; NTP, nitroprusside; ED, emergency department; ICU, intensive care unit

Flowchart 3 Normotensive acute heart failure syndrome pathway

Source: Adapted from Collins S, Storrow AB, Kirk JD, et al. Beyond pulmonary edema: diagnostic, risk stratification, and treatment challenges of acute heart failure management in the emergency department. *Ann Emerg Med.* 2008;51(1):45-57, *with permission*

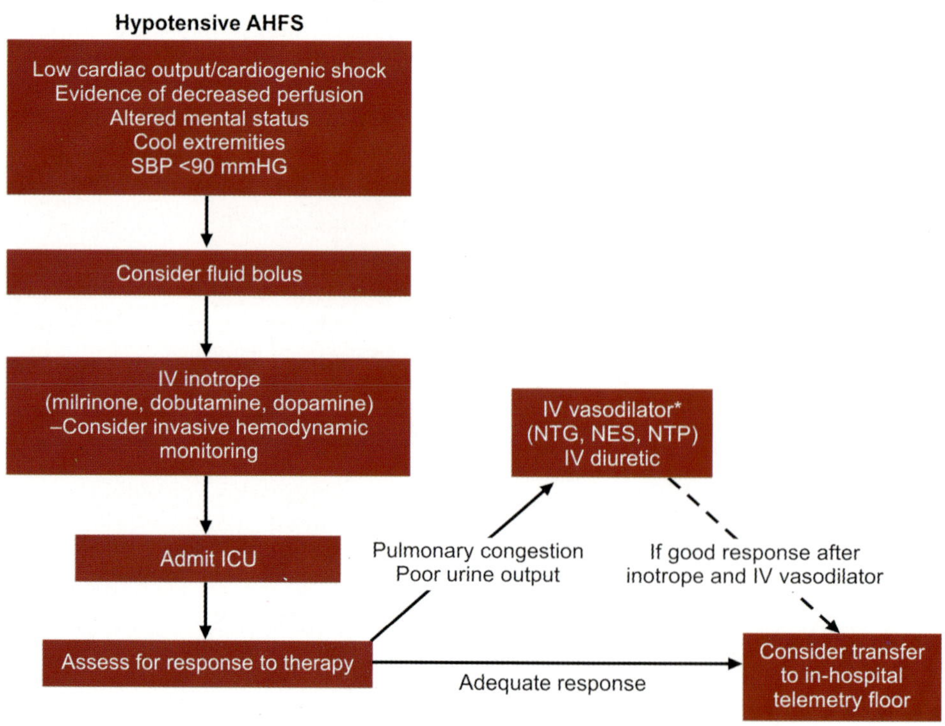

*Recommend caution unless certain of diagnosis and congested state

AHFS, acute heart failure syndrome; SBP, systolic blood pressure; IV, intravenous; NES, nesiritide; NTG, nitroglycerin; NTP, nitroprusside; ICU, intensive care unit

Flowchart 4 Hypotensive acute heart failure syndrome pathway

Source: Adapted from Collins S, Storrow AB, Kirk JD, et al. Beyond pulmonary edema: diagnostic, risk stratification, and treatment challenges of acute heart failure management in the emergency department. *Ann Emerg Med.* 2008;51(1):45-57, *with permission*

THERAPIES FOR HYPERTENSIVE AND NORMOTENSIVE ACUTE HEART FAILURE

Noninvasive Ventilation

Noninvasive ventilation (NIV) is recommended in all patients with cardiogenic pulmonary edema who have any degree of respiratory distress, assuming they have the appropriate mental status to protect their airway, and can comply.[9] Specifically, NIV can be initiated in the ED with 10–15 cm H_2O of positive pressure. Among the benefits of NIV are its noninvasive nature and its ability to be quickly removed if clinical improvement or deterioration occurs.

This recommendation in favor of NIV is made in spite of the findings of the Three Interventions in Cardiogenic Pulmonary Edema (3CPO) trial, which found no difference in intubation rates or mortality at 7 days when compared to standard oxygen therapy.[10] Smaller studies and meta-analyses suggest the benefit of NIV.[9,11] Anecdotally, NIV appears to prevent intubation when applied rapidly. Importantly, NIV is safe when used in patients with intact mental status. We generally start with continuous positive airway pressure (CPAP) only, as there is a potential association between bilevel positive airway pressure (BiPap) and myocardial infarction (MI).[12] However, the 3CPO study also found no differences between CPAP and BiPap on the rate of MI.

INTRAVENOUS NON-POTASSIUM SPARING LOOP DIURETICS

We recommend doubling the dose of chronic oral diuretic as the first IV dose. For example, if a patient is taking 40 mg of oral furosemide twice a day (BID), 80 mg of IV should be given as a bolus.

Intravenous diuretic therapy remains the cornerstone of AHF treatment. Yet despite its longstanding use, the evidence in its support reaches only level B, as there have been no large, definitive clinical trials testing its efficacy and safety. The Diuretic Optimization Strategies in Acute Heart Failure (DOSE-AHF) study demonstrated the short-term safety and efficacy of higher dose IV diuretic therapy; the trial was not powered to definitively answer long-term safety, though no long-term safety concerns were observed.[13] Higher dose was defined as 2.5 times the chronic oral dose, divided by the usual schedule of IV bolus at your institution. For example, if a patient was taking 40 mg BID and your hospital doses IV bolus diuretic thrice a day (TID), then the initial dose would be approximately 65 mg ($2.5 \times 80 = 200 \div 3$). Higher dose treated patients had greater dyspnea relief, urine output, and weight loss.[13] The DOSE-AHF trial also explored the relative benefits of continuous versus bolus infusion and found no difference between the two strategies.

VASODILATORS

For hypertensive AHF patients, we recommend the immediate use of nitroglycerin (NTG) to reduce congestion through vasodilation.

Nitroglycerin is the most widely used vasodilator, and can be administered via the sublingual, topical, or IV route. Similar to all other early AHF therapies, the data supporting its use does not reach the highest level of evidence required to make strong recommendations. However, smaller studies support its safety and efficacy, and potential value to improve outcomes.[14-16] The European Society of Cardiology (ESC) 2012 guidelines provide a table for initial dosing and titration. In general, we recommend starting low and titrating rapidly, every 1–2 minutes, as needed.

Use of nesiritide (NES) has decreased considerably, yet the data surrounding NES is arguably stronger than that for any other vasodilator. Although there was initial enthusiasm for NES following the Vasodilation in the Management of Acute Congestive Heart Failure (VMAC) trial, meta-analyses suggested its potential harm.[17,18] The Acute Study of Clinical Effectiveness of Nesiritide in Decompensated Heart Failure (ASCEND-HF) trial, the largest AHF trial conducted to date, demonstrated that NES was safe.[19] However, NES's clinical efficacy continues to be debated. Depending on the perspective, one could argue that NES has "more evidence" than NTG based on modern day clinical trials and smaller studies that demonstrate its hemodynamic activity. Whether it is "better" than NTG remains debated; however, its safety is arguably more strongly established. At the present time, we recommend NES as second-line therapy.

Early use of angiotensin-converting enzyme inhibitors (ACEI) has been suggested due to its known antihypertensive effects. Although ACEI have proven benefits in chronic heart failure (CHF), there have been no definitive studies in AHF. The ESC currently recommends against the use of early ACEI for initial AHF management;[20] however, the ACEP clinical policy committee supports its use by expert consensus, based on smaller studies. Although ACEI reduce SBP, whether or not they have a deleterious effect on short- or long-term outcomes is not well known. Other therapies such as NTG and NES have better data to support their use.

In general, morphine is no longer recommended for the ED treatment of AHF. However, the data in favor or against its use is largely retrospective, with no definitive trials to suggest it is unsafe. Similar to loop diuretic analyses that suggest higher doses are associated with worse outcomes; secondary analyses of morphine may be confounded by a sicker patient population. Regardless, morphine is not a first-line agent and if used, careful attention to respiratory depression is mandatory.

CONCLUSION

At the present time, robust evidence to guide early therapeutic treatment of AHF is lacking. We stress the importance of identification and treatment of the precipitant of AHF during the ED phase of management. For patients with normal to elevated SBP, an emphasis on either vasodilators (high SBP) or diuretics (normotensive SBP) is recommended. Oftentimes, use of vasodilators is overlooked, despite their benefits in appropriate patients. Ultimately, frequent reassessment of the patient to ensure continued improvement is critical to guide therapy.

REFERENCES

1. Fonarow GC, Stough WG, Abraham WT, et al. Characteristics, treatments, and outcomes of patients with preserved systolic function hospitalized for heart failure: a report from the OPTIMIZE-HF Registry. J Am Coll Cardiol. 2007;50(8):768-77.
2. Gheorghiade M, Zannad F, Sopko G, et al. Acute heart failure syndromes: current state and framework for future research. Circulation. 2005;112(25): 3958-68.
3. Collins S, Storrow AB, Kirk JD, et al. Beyond pulmonary edema: diagnostic, risk stratification, and treatment challenges of acute heart failure management in the emergency department. Ann Emerg Med. 2008;51(1):45-57.
4. Gheorghiade M, Abraham WT, Albert NM, et al. Systolic blood pressure at admission, clinical characteristics, and outcomes in patients hospitalized with acute heart failure. JAMA. 2006;296(18):2217-26.
5. Gheorghiade M, Vaduganathan M, Ambrosy A, et al. Current management and future directions for the treatment of patients hospitalized for heart failure with low blood pressure. Heart Fail Rev. 2013;18(2):107-22.
6. Styron JF, Jois-Bilowich P, Starling R, et al. Initial emergency department systolic blood pressure predicts left ventricular systolic function in acute decompensated heart failure. Congest Heart Fail. 2009;15(1):9-13.
7. Cotter G, Felker GM, Adams KF, et al. The pathophysiology of acute heart failure—is it all about fluid accumulation? Am Heart J. 2008;155(1): 9-18.
8. Cotter G, Metra M, Milo-Cotter O, et al. Fluid overload in acute heart failure—re-distribution and other mechanisms beyond fluid accumulation. Eur J Heart Fail. 2008;10(2):165-9.
9. Vital FM, Saconato H, Ladeira MT, et al. Non-invasive positive pressure ventilation (CPAP or bilevel NPPV) for cardiogenic pulmonary edema. Cochrane Database Syst Rev. 2008;(3):CD005351.
10. Gray A, Goodacre S, Newby DE, et al. Noninvasive ventilation in acute cardiogenic pulmonary edema. N Engl J Med. 2008;359(2):142-51.
11. Masip J, Roque M, Sanchez B, et al. Noninvasive ventilation in acute cardiogenic pulmonary edema: systematic review and meta-analysis. JAMA. 2005;294(24):3124-30.
12. Silvers SM, Howell JM, Kosowsky JM, et al. American College of Emergency Physicians. Clinical policy: Critical issues in the evaluation and management of adult patients presenting to the emergency department with acute heart failure syndromes. Ann Emerg Med. 2007;49(5):627-69.
13. Felker GM, Lee KL, Bull DA, et al. Diuretic strategies in patients with acute decompensated heart failure. N Engl J Med. 2011;364(9):797-805.
14. Publication Committee for the VMAC Investigators (Vasodilatation in the Management of Acute CHF). Intravenous nesiritide vs nitroglycerin for treatment of decompensated congestive heart failure: a randomized controlled trial. JAMA. 2002;287(12):1531-40.
15. Peacock WF, Fonarow GC, Emerman CL, et al. Impact of early initiation of intravenous therapy for acute decompensated heart failure on outcomes in ADHERE. Cardiology. 2007;107(1):44-51.
16. Cotter G, Metzkor E, Kaluski E, et al. Randomised trial of high-dose isosorbide dinitrate plus low-dose furosemide versus high-dose furosemide plus low-dose isosorbide dinitrate in severe pulmonary oedema. Lancet. 1998;351(9100):389-93.
17. Sackner-Bernstein J, Kowalski M, Fox M, et al. Short-term risk of death after treatment with nesiritide for decompensated heart failure. JAMA. 2005;293(15):1900-5.
18. Sackner-Bernstein JD, Skopicki HA, Aaronson KD. Risk of worsening renal function with nesiritide in patients with acutely decompensated heart failure. Circulation. 2005;111(12):1487-91.
19. O'Connor CM, Starling RC, Hernandez AF, et al. Effect of nesiritide in patients with acute decompensated heart failure. N Engl J Med. 2011; 365(1):32-43.
20. McMurray JJ, Adamopoulos S, Anker SD, et al. ESC Guidelines for the diagnosis and treatment of acute and chronic heart failure 2012: The Task Force for the Diagnosis and Treatment of Acute and Chronic Heart Failure 2012 of the European Society of Cardiology. Developed in collaboration with the Heart Failure Association (HFA) of the ESC. Eur Heart J. 2012;33(14):1787-847.

Chapter 4

Management of Atrial Fibrillation in Patients with Heart Failure and Preserved and Low Ejection Fractions

Brian S Wasserman, Tyler W Barrett

ABSTRACT

Atrial fibrillation (AF) is the most common sustained arrhythmia with an estimated prevalence in the developed world of 1.5–2% of the general population. AF and heart failure have a complex relationship, and patients with heart failure provide specific challenges and limitations in management. As many as 40% of patients with AF or heart failure develop the other condition and having both diseases is associated with increased mortality. International cardiology guidelines recommend that the management of patients with AF focus on three objectives: (1) rate control, (2) prevention of thromboembolism, and (3) correction of the rhythm disturbance. This chapter provides recommendations for the acute management of AF in patients with heart failure and preserved and low ejection fractions.

INTRODUCTION

Atrial fibrillation (AF) is the most common sustained arrhythmia with an estimated prevalence in the developed world of 1.5–2 fold of the general population.[1] The estimated prevalence in the United States ranges from 2.7 million to 6.1 million in 2010 and that number is expected to nearly double by 2050.[2] AF is associated with a fivefold increase in the risk of stroke, a threefold increase in the risk of developing heart failure and 1.5–2 fold increased risk of death.[3-7] The prevalence of AF increases as individuals age; 5.9% of those over 65 years of age, and 9% of individuals over 80 years are diagnosed with AF.[2,5] The lifetime risk for development of AF is estimated to be one in four for individuals 40 years of age and older.[2,6] Similar risk factors are associated with developing AF and heart failure. Among patients with new onset AF or heart failure in the Framingham Heart Study, 21% were newly diagnosed with both AF and heart failure on the same day.[8] The study also reported that 40% of patients with AF or heart failure developed the other condition and having both diseases was associated with increased mortality.[8]

Atrial fibrillation is defined as a "supraventricular tachyarrhythmia characterized by uncoordinated atrial activity with consequent deterioration of atrial mechanical function".[9] Atrial flutter is an atrial tachycardia characterized by a pattern of saw-tooth regular atrial activation on an electrocardiogram.[9] Atrial flutter may degenerate into AF and it commonly occurs together in patients with AF. Therefore, the 2008 American College of Cardiology (ACC)/American Heart Association (AHA) guidelines group the two arrhythmias together with regard to performance measures recommendations.[9] Previous landmark trials regarding treatment of AF have included patients with atrial flutter.[10,11] Given the significant association and the similar emergency department (ED) management and disposition, our recommendations for the acute management of patients with AF and heart failure will also apply to those patients with acute atrial flutter and heart failure unless specifically stated to the contrary.

The number of ED visits for complaints related to AF increased by 88% between 1993 and 2003 and now account for nearly 1% of all ED visits in the United States.[12,13] The ACC/AHA/European Society of Cardiology

(ESC) 2006 guideline for the management of patients with AF states that management involves three objectives: (1) rate control, (2) prevention of thromboembolism, and (3) correction of the rhythm disturbance.[14] Patients with heart failure provide specific challenges and limitations when managing acute AF exacerbations.

Atrial fibrillation and heart failure have a complex, bidirectional relationship. Heart failure commonly causes structural remodeling of the atria that increases susceptibility to development of AF and decreases the likelihood of the successful maintenance of sinus rhythm. Heart failure is a risk factor for stroke in patients with AF and an indication for anticoagulation. Conversely, prolonged rapid AF (or any other supraventricular arrhythmia) is known to cause a tachycardia-mediated cardiomyopathy and beget the development of heart failure. In these patients, cardiac function usually improves over time, even normalizing, with rate control.[15]

Box 1: Initial diagnostic workup for patients with atrial fibrillation

The ABC's of treating atrial fibrillation in patients with heart failure:

A: Airway—Ensure a patent and protected airway

B: Breathing—Evaluate for adequate ventilation and listen for signs of pulmonary edema or a precipitating pneumonia

C: Circulation and cardiac monitoring—Determine hemodynamic stability and decide on a rate vs rhythm control treatment strategy

D: Defibrillator/pacing pads—Apply to anterior/posterior chest early in ED evaluation for unstable patient—diuresis (in the patient with volume overload)

E: Electrocardiogram (12-lead) and evaluate risk for thromboembolism and need for anticoagulation (CHA_2DS_2-VASc)

CHA_2DS_2-VASc, congestive heart failure, Hypertension, Age ≥75 years, Diabetes mellitus, Stroke, Vascular disease, Age 65–74 years, Female Sex category

Atrial Fibrillation Classifications

Atrial fibrillation is characterized by the duration of the arrhythmia. This has implications for workup and therapy. In general, the longer the duration of AF, the lower the likelihood of a successful cardioversion from AF to sustained sinus rhythm. On the initial presentation, AF is classified as *first detected.* Paroxysmal AF is defined as two or more lifetime episodes that terminate spontaneously in less than 7 days (and usually <24 hours). *Persistent* AF episodes last longer than 7 days and may require cardioversion to terminate. *Permanent* AF refers to the treating clinician no longer attempting to restore sinus rhythm.[14] Patients with longstanding persistent and permanent AF may be difficult to differentiate without continuous rhythm monitoring. The term *lone AF* refers to patients younger than 60 years of age who have AF without clinical or echocardiographic evidence of cardiopulmonary disease, including hypertension.[14]

INITIAL ASSESSMENT OF THE PATIENT WITH ATRIAL FIBRILLATION AND HEART FAILURE IN THE EMERGENCY DEPARTMENT

The first priority in the ED management of patients with AF and heart failure is determining the stability of the patient with primary attention to airway, breathing and circulation (Box 1). Patients who are hemodynamically unstable directly related to their AF should be emergently cardioverted regardless of their anticoagulation status or duration of symptoms.

Unfortunately, making this determination is not always as clear as presented in Case Study 1 and the treating physician should follow a standard approach when treating all patients with acute AF to provide the most optimal care. While the physician is evaluating the patient's airway, breathing, and circulatory status, the nurse or paramedic should establish a large-bore (e.g., 14–16 gauge) IV access and attach the patient to the cardiac monitor. Consider administering supplemental oxygen, by nasal cannula or nonrebreather facemask, in patients with low oxygen saturations.

Airway

The physician caring for the patient should ensure that the patient's airway is patent and protected. An easy way to assess airway patency is to ask the patient to say their name. A patient who can speak their name fluently without garbled or gasping breaths has a patent airway at that time. Frequent reassessments of airway status are critical in the ED as a patient's airway status can rapidly deteriorate secondary to progression of their disease process or in response to administered medications. When a patient's airway is not protected, whether due to a primary respiratory process (e.g., critical pulmonary edema or hypercapnia) or cerebral hypoperfusion from circulatory collapse, the ED physician must secure the patient's airway preferably by intubating the patient with an appropriately sized endotracheal tube.

Case Study 1

A 77-year-old male arrives in your ED in severe respiratory distress. His blood pressure is 70/40 mmHg and his pulse is rapid and irregular at a rate of 140–170 beats/min. He is breathing nearly 30 times per minute and his pulse oximeter reads 88% on 6 L of oxygen by nasal cannula. He speaks in two to three word sentences but has obvious jugular venous distention, audible rales in both posterior lung bases and 3+ pitting lower extremity edema. His wife reports that he has known severe heart failure (EF <15%), hypertension, diabetes but no prior AF diagnosis. He was in his usual state of health until this morning when he reported palpitations. His 12-lead electrocardiogram shows AF. How should this patient be treated?

Treatment: This patient is clearly unstable and in acute decompensated heart failure with pulmonary edema that may be precipitated or worsened by his new AF with rapid ventricular response. Patients with severely impaired heart failure may decompensate quickly when their heart rhythm decompensates secondary to losing the atrial kick contribution to their already tenuous stroke volume. This patient needs emergent cardioversion and potentially advanced airway management with either noninvasive positive pressure ventilation or endotracheal intubation and mechanical ventilation. Our practice would be to administer a short-acting sedative [e.g., etomidate 0.15 mg/kg by intravenous (IV) route] and perform emergent synchronized cardioversion with a biphasic defibrillator at 200 Joules. Following successful cardioversion, this patient will require hospitalization to treat his decompensated heart failure as well as evaluation for long-term anticoagulation given his CHA_2DS_2-VASc score of 5.

Breathing

Once the patient's airway is stabilized, attention shifts to the patient's breathing and ventilatory effort. AF should not directly impair a patient's respiratory status unless the arrhythmia and associated diminished stroke volume compromises cerebral circulation resulting in diminished respiratory drive or AF causes acute decompensated heart failure and pulmonary edema. Consider initiating ventilatory support with noninvasive positive pressure ventilation early in the ED management of patients with signs of impaired ventilation (e.g., tachypnea, mild hypoxia, and use of accessory muscles) but who are mentating and protecting their airway. The early initiation of noninvasive positive pressure ventilation may provide sufficient ventilatory assistance for the patient, while other treatments for their AF and heart failure are administered and take effect.

Circulation

The initial evaluation of a patient's circulatory stability includes palpation of pulses, capillary refill, and signs of hypoperfusion (Flowchart 1). When a patient is obtunded and distal radial or pedal pulses are not palpable, then immediately palpate femoral and carotid pulses to ensure that the patient is not in pulseless electrical activity. Measure the patient's blood pressure and make an initial determination on whether the patient appears hypovolemic (e.g., dehydration secondary to a gastrointestinal illness or over diuresis), euvolemic, or hypervolemic (i.e., in volume overload). Patients who are hypovolemic should be volume resuscitated with a rapid infusion of 500–1,000 mL of IV normal saline or lactated Ringers' solution followed by reassessment of their circulatory status. Patients with a known low EF might require smaller crystalloid volumes and a slower infusion rate. Likewise, stable patients with signs of volume overload may benefit from diuresis and consideration of early cardioversion if they are dependent on their atrial kick to maintain adequate cardiac output. Once the clinician has stabilized the patient's respiratory and hemodynamic status, then they should perform a complete history including a detailed review of current medications, recent changes and medication compliance, a head-to-toe physical examination and order diagnostic studies that might identify specific risk factors for AF (e.g., thyroid studies, urine drug screen, and electrolytes) and determine the best individualized treatment for that individual's AF.

PRIORITIES IN MANAGING ATRIAL FIBRILLATION IN THE ACUTE SETTING

There are three main goals for the management of patients with AF in the acute setting: (1) ventricular rate control, (2) prevention of thromboembolism, and (3) correction of the arrhythmia.[14] Rate control refers to the use of atrioventricular (AV) nodal blockade to control the ventricular response to the atrial activity. The foremost thromboembolic complication is a cerebral embolism. Stroke prevention includes an assessment of the patient's risk for embolic events and prescription of the most optimal anticoagulation regimen when indicated. Heart failure and left ventricular dysfunction is a major risk factor for stroke and included in both the $CHADS_2$ and CHA_2DS_2-VASc scores.[16,17] Correction of the arrhythmia, or rhythm control, refers to maintenance of sinus rhythm via pharmacological or electrical means.

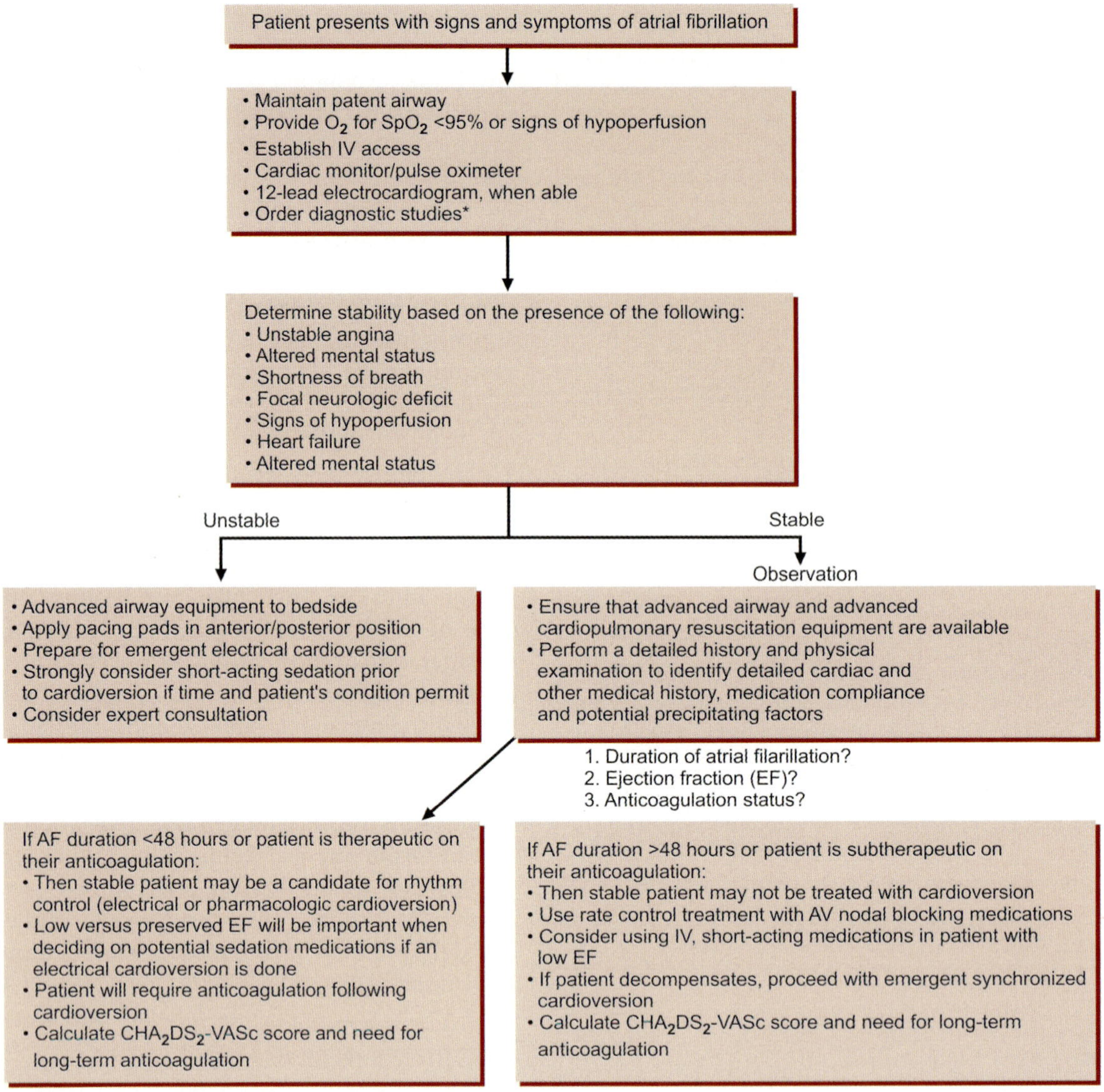

*Diagnostic Studies should include a chest radiograph, possible transthoracic or transesophageal elctrocardiogram based on clinical presentation. Laboratory studies may include the following (only to be ordered when clinically indicated): complete blood count with differential, basic metabolic panel (includes electrolytes), urinalysis, cardiac enzymes, brain natriuretic peptide, thyroid function studies and a urine or serum toxicology screen

O_2, oxygen; SpO_2, saturated oxygen; IV, intravenous; CHA_2DS_2-VASc, Congestive heart failure, Hypertension, Age ≥75 years, Diabetes mellitus, Stroke, Vascular disease, Age 65–74 years, Female Sex category; AV, atrioventricular

Flowchart 1 The acute management of patients with atrial fibrillation and heart failure in the emergency department

RATE VERSUS RHYTHM CONTROL: WHICH TREATMENT IS BETTER?

Deciding between a rate versus rhythm control treatment strategy in the stable patient with AF and heart failure in the ED should be based on a number of important questions: (1) duration of this AF episode; (2) anticoagulation status; (3) current treatment regimen and response to prior rhythm control treatments; and (4) details of this specific AF episode.

- *Determine when this AF episode started*
  First, how long has the patient been in AF? Patients who are clearly aware of when their AF begins may be able to provide an accurate determination of the duration of their symptoms. Individuals whose duration of AF is less than 48 hours may be candidates for cardioversion in the ED with the estimated risk of stroke reported to be less than 1%.[18] Individuals whose symptoms have been ongoing for longer than 48 hours and those who are unaware of the duration

of their AF are at higher risk for stroke if cardioverted with estimates as high as 7%.[18]

- *Is the patient on anticoagulation and, if so, is it therapeutic?*
  Patients with known AF who are adequately anticoagulated [i.e., international normalized ratio (INR) between 2 and 3 if on warfarin or documented compliance with oral thrombin or factor Xa inhibitor agent] may also be safely cardioverted in the ED. Verifying compliance with the newer oral thrombin or factor Xa inhibitors is more challenging without an objective laboratory measure available in most EDs. The physician may need to decide on a case-by-case basis whether they trust the patient's report of medication compliance prior to attempting cardioversion in the stable patient. The physician should have a detailed discussion with the patient informing them of the increased risk of stroke in patients who are not adequately anticoagulated prior to the procedure. A signed written consent documenting these risks prior to the cardioversion is also important, especially in litigious nations such as the United States. Hemodynamically stable individuals who are not adequately anticoagulated should undergo a transesophageal echocardiogram to exclude an apical thrombus prior to cardioversion.
- *Is the patient already being treated with rate or rhythm control? How did the patient respond to prior cardioversion attempts?*
  Patients with AF are most often treated with either a rate control or rhythm control medication regimen with some patients taking both classes of medications. Large international multicenter trials compared outcomes with rate control and rhythm control strategies and found no significant difference in efficacy between the two options.[19,20] A personalized approach may identify patients who could benefit from a rhythm control strategy, such as those starting treatment for AF, who are symptomatic despite adequate rate-control, or who experience side effects of rate control medications. Patients whose cardiologist has chosen a rhythm control treatment and prefers maintenance of sinus rhythm should preferentially be cardioverted (electrically or pharmacologically) if there are not specific contraindications (e.g., subtherapeutic INR or not stable for sedation). Likewise, patients who have failed multiple prior cardioversion attempts may be treated with a rate control approach by their cardiologists and this would be the preferred treatment protocol in an acute AF exacerbation.
- *Are there specific events relative to this episode of AF that might impact your acute treatment?*
  Patients with paroxysmal AF might occasionally experience AF while suffering from infections such as pneumonia or gastroenteritis that causes profound volume depletion and electrolyte disturbances including hypokalemia. In patients with preserved EFs, an initial treatment with volume resuscitation with intravenous crystalloid (1–2 L of normal saline or lactated Ringers solution may be required) and repletion of electrolyte losses may result in improved ventricular rate control and spontaneous conversion back to sinus rhythm. Another patient who presents with crushing chest pain and first detected AF in the setting of an acute ST-segment elevation myocardial infarction (STEMI) is likely best served going immediately to the cardiac catheterization laboratory for coronary angiography and percutaneous coronary intervention rather than their reperfusion being delayed by an attempted cardioversion in the ED. In addition to the standard STEMI medications and discussion with your interventional cardiologist, the best initial treatment may be administering a short-acting beta-blocker intravenously to decrease ventricular rate and myocardial oxygen demand.

Case Study 2

A 66-year-old female with a history of paroxysmal AF and New York Heart Association (NYHA) class I heart failure with preserved EF presents to the ED with 12 hours of AF with ventricular rates in 110–120's. She is on warfarin and her INR is stable at 2.3. She denies any other symptoms and has been successfully cardioverted following her last AF episode 2 years ago. How would you treat this patient?

Recommended treatment: Given that this patient gives a detailed AF duration, is adequately anticoagulated with a therapeutic INR, and is normally in sinus rhythm, she is an excellent candidate for cardioversion in the ED. Physician and patient preference and the patient's prior response to cardioversion methods should determine whether electrical or pharmaceutical cardioversion is chosen. Following successful cardioversion, this patient should continue her warfarin and is a candidate for discharge home with outpatient cardiology follow-up.

WHEN RATE CONTROL TREATMENT IS BEST FOR YOUR PATIENT WITH HEART FAILURE AND ACUTE ATRIAL FIBRILLATION

Patients with acute AF often have signs and symptoms that are due to rapid ventricular rate rates including

TABLE 1: Overview of intravenous rate control agents[14]

Drugs	*Mechanism*	*IV loading dose*	*IV maintenance*	*Side effects*
Metoprolol	β1 antagonism	2.5–5 mg (up to three doses 5 min apart)	Not applicable	Heart failure, hypotension, bradycardia, heart block, asthma
Esmolol	β1 antagonism	500 μg/kg	600 μg/kg/min	Heart failure, hypotension, bradycardia, heart block, asthma
Diltiazem	L-type Ca^{2+} channel blockade	0.25 mg/kg IV	5–15 mg/hour	Heart failure, hypotension, bradycardia, heart block
Verapamil	L-type Ca^{2+} channel blockade	0.075–0.15 mg/kg	Not applicable	Heart failure, hypotension, bradycardia, heart block
Digoxin	Na^+/K^+ exchange inhibitor, vagotonic	0.25 mg Q2h to total dose of 1.5 mg	0.125–0.375 mg/day	Bradycardia, heart block, digitalis toxicity

IV, intravenous; Q2h, every 2 hour

palpitations, dyspnea, angina/demand ischemia, and pulmonary edema. Patients with heart failure and preserved AF may be more symptomatic and cognizant of their AF onset as they are often without significant baseline cardiopulmonary complaints. Patients with severe heart failure and low EFs at baseline may report only a gradual worsening of their symptoms or an acute decompensation based on the contribution of the synchronized atrial contraction to their cardiac output. These often improve or resolve with adequate ventricular rate control through AV nodal blockade. Rapid ventricular rate frequently causes decreased stroke volume due to loss of atrial kick and inadequate diastolic filling times, especially in patients with inadequate reserve.

Rate control therapy may be delivered through multiple routes. The most commonly used forms for acute administration are IV administration, and continuous IV infusion (see Table 1 for detailed discussion on medications). Oral dosing is often given after stabilization. The patient's stability and comorbidities often dictate the choice of agent and route administered. There is some debate about the ideal heart rate target. Previously, a typical long-term goal was a ventricular rate of 60–80 beats/min; however, recent data suggests that lenient rate control with ventricular rates less than 110 beats/min may be adequate.[21] The presence of systolic dysfunction limits the therapeutic options for control of the ventricular rate. Digoxin can be used, however, it is rarely effective as monotherapy in patients with significant tachycardia, and has a slower onset than the other rate control agents. Patients with renal dysfunction also have increased risk of digoxin toxicity. In addition, recent data suggests that patients with AF on chronic digoxin therapy both with and without heart failure may have increased all-cause mortality.[22] Beta-blockers can be used in the absence of acute decompensated heart failure. However, in the acute setting these medications can negative inotropes and might incite or worsen heart failure symptoms. Small (e.g., 2.5 mg) doses of metoprolol or an esmolol infusion are preferred to assess hemodynamic tolerance. The non-dihydropyridine calcium channel blockers (CCB) (diltiazem, verapamil) are negative inotropes, and should be avoided in patients with reduced EF.

Case Study 3

A 75-year-old gentleman with a history of hypertension and mild heart failure (EF 40% on last ECG) presents to the ED with a complaint of palpitations and irregular heart beating for the past month. Today, he experienced near syncope when he arose from bed to use the bathroom. He did not lose consciousness but noticed his pulse was fast and called an ambulance. He denies chest pain, shortness of breath, or worsening lower extremity edema. His blood pressure on arrival was 145/95 mmHg; his pulse was irregular and measured at 137 beats/min. The patient takes only a daily 81 mg aspirin and is not on oral anticoagulants. He reports prior palpitations but has not been formally diagnosed with AF. His 12-lead electrocardiogram shows AF with rapid ventricular rate in 130s, evidence of LV hypertrophy but no signs of acute ischemia. How would you treat this patient? How might your treatment regimen change if the patient's EF was recently found to be only 15%?

Treatment: The initial priority in the acute management of AF is to determine stability. Although this patient's tachycardia is concerning, he appears hemodynamically stable and shows no signs of impaired perfusion to his vital organs based on the initial history and physical examination. The patient reports that his irregular heart beating has been ongoing on for at least a month and he is not on any oral anticoagulation. Therefore, he is at increased risk for a thromboembolic event if he were to be cardioverted and a rate control strategy is the best initial treatment option. Depending on the patient's antihypertensive regimen, acute AV nodal blockade with either an IV beta-blocker (e.g. metoprolol) or CCB (e.g. diltiazem or verapamil) would be the preferred initial treatments to slow the ventricular rate. If a single or repeat dose of the chosen rate control medications does not adequately reduce the ventricular rate, then the physician may proceed to a continuous infusion of the AV nodal blocker medication. Alternatively, adding a second agent such as digoxin or amiodarone may be necessary although amiodarone does have the potential to convert the rhythm to sinus.

If the patient had a low EF, our recommendation would still be to use a rate control treatment regimen but we would instead use short-acting AV nodal blockers agents such as esmolol that may be quickly titrated up or down depending on the patient's hemodynamics. Remember that if the patient decompensates and becomes hemodynamically unstable with impaired perfusion to vital organs, then emergent synchronized cardioversion is the recommended treatment.

Common side effects of AV nodal blocking are related to their mechanism of action. While hypotension often improves with rate control, some patients may experience lowered blood pressure due to beta-receptor or calcium channel blockade. Bradycardia and heart block can also be seen, especially when agents from different classes are combined or multiple doses are given in succession. Patients with existing conduction system disease, including the elderly, are more susceptible to these side effects.

Caution: Special consideration for Wolff-Parkinson-White or other pre-excitation syndrome must be given to patients with AF and signs of pre-excitation, including wide QRS complex, delta waves and very fast ventricular rates. AV nodal blockade can lead to preferential conduction down the accessory pathway, which can cause AF to degenerate into ventricular fibrillation and death. Drugs that should be avoided in patients with AF and pre-excitation include CCBs, adenosine, digoxin, and beta-blockers. IV procainamide and ibutilide have been used in this situation. IV amiodarone has also been given with good results despite lack of formal approval for acute AF. Cardioversion is also commonly used to restore sinus rhythm.

WHEN RHYTHM CONTROL TREATMENT IS BEST FOR YOUR PATIENT WITH HEART FAILURE AND ACUTE ATRIAL FIBRILLATION

In the acute setting, rhythm control refers to treatment intended to convert the patient from AF to sinus rhythm. This can be accomplished via electrical or pharmacologic means. Electrical cardioversion is the treatment of choice for unstable patients with AF, and is also used to restore sinus rhythm electively. The success of maintaining sinus rhythm depends on multiple patient factors. Patients who have longstanding persistent AF, significant structural heart disease, an unaddressed underlying cause and heart failure are less likely to remain in sinus rhythm after cardioversion. In addition, rhythm control is less successful in the elderly.

The major side effect of cardioversion is increased risk of thromboembolism, with stroke being the most devastating complication. This is because after conversion from AF to sinus rhythm, the atria are "stunned" for a time leading to increased thrombus formation. In addition, the change in rhythm from AF to sinus may cause already formed thrombus to dislodge and embolize. This increased stroke risk is present after spontaneous, electrical and pharmacologic cardioversion. The stroke risk is dependent on the duration of the AF episode and the patient's anticoagulation status. Patients with AF for less than 48 hours or for greater than 48 hours on adequate anticoagulation have an incidence of stroke after electrical cardioversion of less than 1%,[23] whereas patients with permanent AF not on anticoagulation have a stroke rate up to 7%.[18] Oral anticoagulation with warfarin or one of the newer thrombin or factor Xa inhibitors is recommended for at least 4 weeks after cardioversion. In unstable patients without contraindication, unfractionated heparin or low-molecular-weight heparin should be started as soon as possible. In stable patients for whom the duration of AF is unknown or greater than 48 hours, left atrial thrombus should be excluded by transesophageal echocardiogram or empiric anticoagulation given for 3–4 weeks prior to cardioversion. In stable patients for whom the duration of AF is known to be less than 48 hours, cardioversion can safely be performed without prior anticoagulation. Due to the fact that patients may be asymptomatic and thus the true duration unknown, some clinicians will still perform a transesophageal electrocardiogram. Another adverse effect of cardioversion is patient discomfort. The use of procedural sedation for the cardioversion procedure minimizes patient discomfort; however, these medications may induce hypotension, oversedation, respiratory suppression and delirium. The physician performing the sedation must carefully select the appropriate analgesic and sedative medications based on the patient's history, hemodynamics and in accordance with their institutional protocols. The risk of intracranial hemorrhage increases significantly (up to tenfold) with a preprocedure INR above 3.5.[24]

Electrical Cardioversion

Synchronized direct-current cardioversion is one option for rhythm control treatment in the ED. Patients should be consented, when time and conditions permit, prior to the procedure and adequately sedated. Common sedation choices at our institution include etomidate and propofol but the choice of appropriate sedation medication should be determined based on a careful review of the patient's medical history, allergies and individual institutional protocols. The initial waveform energy is a subject of debate but the 2006 ACC/AHA/ESC guidelines recommend using an initial energy of 200 Joules or greater with monophasic defibrillators.[14] Our preference is to apply the defibrillator pads in an anteroposterior position and perform a synchronized cardioversion using 200 Joules with biphasic defibrillator. Patients undergoing electrical cardioversion have an increased stroke risk due to atrial stunning, and post-cardioversion oral anticoagulation is indicated. Furthermore, unless prolonged sinus rhythm is documented on a loop recorder, many clinicians will continue anticoagulation in patients on a rhythm control strategy due to the possibility of periods of asymptomatic AF.

Pearl: It is sometimes difficult to determine whether a patient truly is able to differentiate when their rhythm converts from sinus to AF or when they develop rapid ventricular rate related to their AF. Many patients may not be able to tell when they are in AF without rapid ventricular rate, and are still at increased risk for thrombus formation during these instances. If the physician has any concern that the AF duration may exceed 48 hours in a patient who is not adequately anticoagulated, err on the side of caution and perform a transesophageal electrocardiogram prior to cardioversion.

Pharmacologic Cardioversion

There are multiple antiarrhythmic drugs that can be used to restore sinus rhythm in patients with AF (Table 2). If a rhythm control strategy with pharmacologic cardioversion is to be pursued, a critical distinction is the presence of any structural heart disease. For patients without structural heart disease, flecainide, propafenone and sotalol are first-line agents; however, these are contraindicated in patients with left ventricular hypertrophy and coronary artery disease. Procainamide has shown to be about 50% effective in converting patients to sinus rhythm with a low incidence of side effects.[25]

The presence of heart failure and other comorbidities limits the available agents. The class III (potassium channel blocking) antiarrhythmics dofetilide, ibutilide and sotalol increase the QT interval and are associated with *torsades de pointes.* Sotalol is contraindicated in uncontrolled heart failure. Sotalol and dofetilide are contraindicated with changing renal function or severe renal dysfunction. Amiodarone is also a class III agent; however, it rarely causes *torsades de pointes.* Amiodarone can be given to patients with heart failure, and has the advantage of having beta-blocking properties in patients who remain in AF. The chronic toxicities of amiodarone including pulmonary, liver and thyroid dysfunction as well as the multitude of drug interactions with amiodarone make it a suboptimal chronic rate control medication. Consider switching a patient to a beta-blocker medication from amiodarone when AF persists. Class IC (sodium channel blocking) antiarrhythmic medications are contraindicated due to increased risk of death.[26]

Although electrical and pharmacologic cardioversion have not been compared head-to-head, in general it is

TABLE 2: Overview of rhythm control agents

Drugs	*Class*	*Side effects*	*Contraindications*
Procainamide	IA	Hypotension, nausea, QT prolongation, drug-induced systemic lupus erythematosus	Systemic lupus erythematosus
Flecainide	IC	Ventricular tachycardia/ventricular fibrillation	Heart failure, left ventricular hypertrophy
Propafenone	IC	Ventricular tachycardia/ventricular fibrillation	Heart failure, left ventricular hypertrophy
Amiodarone	III	QT prolongation, pulmonary, liver, thyroid toxicity, drug interactions	Baseline pulmonary, liver, thyroid dysfunction
Ibutilide	III	QT prolongation	Long QT, hypokalemia
Dofetilide	III	QT prolongation	Long QT, creatinine clearance <20 mL/min
Sotalol	III	QT prolongation, bradycardia	Long QT, uncontrolled heart failure

thought that electrical cardioversion is more efficacious.[14] There is a role in certain patients for treatment with antiarrhythmic drugs prior to cardioversion; however, this is best done in conjunction with experts in arrhythmia management due to the risk of precipitating a potentially lethal arrhythmia.

STROKE PREVENTION

Thromboembolic phenomena, particularly stroke, are among the most feared complications of permanent AF. Stasis of blood in the left atrium, especially the left atrial appendage, may lead to thrombus formation that can then embolize distally to the cerebrovascular circulation. Stroke risk and treatment recommendations for patients with nonvalvular can be determined by the CHA_2DS_2-VASc clinical prediction score (Tables 3 and 4). Patients with valvular AF are at higher risk of stroke, and should be anticoagulated in the absence of contraindications.

Platelet inhibition is inferior to anticoagulation for stroke prevention in non-low risk patients with AF. Aspirin has uncertain benefit in very low risk (CHA_2DS_2-VASc = 0); however, it has not been shown superior to placebo. Current guidelines do not recommend aspirin for patients with a CHA_2DS_2-VASc score of 0 in the absence of another indication. Aspirin plus clopidogrel was shown to be superior to aspirin alone in high-risk patients who could not (or refused) to be treated with warfarin.[27] Stroke prevention with this combination was inferior to warfarin with similar bleeding risk, however.[28]

Warfarin has been widely studied for stroke prevention in AF. When a large meta-analysis showed that the average stroke rate per year for patients on warfarin was around 2%.[29] The mechanism of action for warfarin is inhibition of the vitamin K epoxide reductase complex 1 (VKORC1), which prevents activation of coagulation factors II, VII, IX, X. Warfarin has a high degree of inter- and intrapatient variation due to multiple drug interactions, dietary interactions and genetic variation in metabolism. Variations in VKORC1 can cause a variable response to warfarin.[30] Hepatic cytochrome P450 enzymes, primarily CYP2C9, metabolize warfarin and inhibition by drugs or genetic variation can have profound effects on elimination.[31] Increases in vitamin K intake can decrease the INR and dietary counseling is given to patients on warfarin. Numerous antibiotics can increase the effect of warfarin, due to alteration in the gut flora that activates vitamin K. For these reasons, patients on warfarin require frequent monitoring of the INR, with corresponding dose adjustment.

TABLE 3: Congestive heart failure, Hypertension, Age ≥75 years, Diabetes mellitus, Stroke, Vascular disease, Age 65–74 years, Female Sex category score[14]

Category	Score
CHF/left ventricular dysfunction	1
Hypertension	1
Age 65–74 years	1
Age >75 years	2
Diabetes	1
Stroke/TIA/thromboembolism	2
Vascular disease (MI, PAD, or aortic plaque)	1
Sex (female)	1

CHF, congestive heart failure; TIA, transient ischemic attack; MI, myocardial infarction; PAD, peripheral arterial disease

TABLE 4: Stroke risk/year by Congestive heart failure, Hypertension, Age ≥75 years, Diabetes mellitus, Stroke, Vascular disease, Age 65–74 years, Female Sex category score[14]

	Score (%)
1	1.3
2	2.2
3	3.2
4	4.0
5	6.7
6	9.8
7	9.6
8	6.7
9	15.2

The major side effect of all oral anticoagulants is bleeding and warfarin is among the top drugs implicated in serious adverse events and death. There are numerous clinical risk factors for bleeding. The 2012 update to the ESC guidelines recommend formal bleeding risk assessment in patients with AF for whom anticoagulation is being considered with a HAS-BLED [Hypertension, Abnormal renal/liver function, Stroke, Bleeding history or predisposition, Labile INR, Elderly (age > 65 years), Drugs/alcohol] score greater than or equal to 3.[1] Compared to the newer oral anticoagulants, warfarin does have the benefit of reversibility in the case of a bleeding event or overanticoagulation by using multifactor prothrombin complex concentrates, fresh frozen plasma and vitamin K.

Recently, new classes of oral anticoagulants have been released. Dabigatran, a direct thrombin inhibitor, as well as rivaroxaban and apixaban, both factor Xa inhibitors, have all been evaluated in clinical trials versus warfarin for prevention of AF, with favorable efficacy and safety profiles.[32-34] The role that these drugs will have in management of stroke prevention in AF is still evolving. They offer a potential benefit to patients who will require a defined period of anticoagulation (such as peri-cardioversion). The lack of rapid reversal agents for these newer anticoagulants is a primary concern when patients taking these medications present to the ED with uncontrolled bleeding.[35]

ADDITIONAL ACUTE MANAGEMENT CONSIDERATIONS

Investigation Additional Etiologies of First Detected Atrial Fibrillation

Although heart failure and its associated risk factors are both associated with the development of AF, the astute physician should also consider alternative underlying etiologies for first detected AF. In up to 50% of cases of acute AF, an underlying cause can be identified.[14] This is important for diagnosis as well as treatment. Often times treatment of the underlying condition will improve symptoms related to AF, whereas therapies that address only the AF are unlikely to succeed. Common underlying causes of acute AF include:

- Hyperthyroidism (including subclinical hyperthyroidism)
- Pericardial disease (pericarditis/effusion)
- Hypertensive urgency/emergency
- Ingestions: Cocaine, methamphetamine, theophylline, caffeine, alcohol
- Infection
- Pulmonary embolism.

While AF is common post-MI, it is rarely the only sign of ischemia or infarction. Evaluation for ischemia should be directed by other clinical factors and stress testing is not routinely recommended for patients with AF without other coronary artery disease risk factors.

SPECIAL CONSIDERATIONS

Patients with AF may present to the ED for complaints related to symptomatic bradycardia including AF with inappropriately slow ventricular response. The symptomatic bradycardia may result in insufficient cardiac output resulting in syncope, near syncope or decreased exercise tolerance. The bradycardia may be a consequence of worsening cardiac conduction disease. AF is associated with the development of sinus node dysfunction.[36-38] Among AF patients, a history of heart failure triples the odds of developing symptomatic bradycardia requiring permanent pacemaker implantation.[39] Symptomatic bradycardia may also be an iatrogenic complication of medications used for rate control. Medication-associated bradycardia may be due to an unexpected exaggerated response to proper adherence to dosing recommendations; however, intentional and unintentional overdose must be considered. A classic finding in digoxin overdose is AF with a slow ventricular response. Physicians should measure a digoxin level in patients taking digoxin who present with AF and slow ventricular rates to exclude digoxin toxicity.

EMERGENCY DEPARTMENT DISPOSITION AND FOLLOW-UP

The 2006 ACC/AHA/ESC guidelines are clear that a patient with a first-documented episode of AF, who achieves rate control, does not need a hospital admission.[14] Patients with underlying heart failure who present to the ED with first detected AF and acute decompensated heart failure most often require hospitalization in part to monitor their response to new rate or rhythm control medications. Discharge home from the ED with outpatient cardiology follow-up is appropriate for individuals without acute decompensated heart failure and who achieve ventricular rate control or convert to normal sinus rhythm. Patients who are discharged home from the ED must have their stroke risk assessed. The 2012 focused update of the ESC guidelines for the management of AF recommends using the CHA_2DS_2-VASc score for determining a patient's risk for stroke and thromboembolism and deciding on appropriate anticoagulation treatment.[1] Patients with AF who have CHA_2DS_2-VASc score greater than or equal to 1 should be started on either warfarin or one of the new, approved oral thrombin or factor Xa inhibitors.[1] Patients with underlying heart failure and AF, whether a new or established diagnosis, benefit from being followed closely as outpatients by both an arrhythmia specialist and a cardiologist expert in heart failure management.

REFERENCES

1. Camm AJ, Lip GY, De Caterina R, et al. 2012 focused update of the ESC Guidelines for the management of atrial fibrillation: an update of the 2010 ESC Guidelines for the management of atrial fibrillation—developed with the special contribution of the European Heart Rhythm Association. Europace. 2012;14(10):1385-413.

2. Go AS, Mozaffarian D, Roger VL, et al. Heart disease and stroke statistics—2013 update: a report from the American Heart Association. Circulation. 2013;127(1):e6-e245.
3. Benjamin EJ, Wolf PA, D'Agostino RB, et al. Impact of atrial fibrillation on the risk of death: the Framingham Heart Study. Circulation. 1998;98(10):946-52.
4. Krahn AD, Manfreda J, Tate RB, et al. The natural history of atrial fibrillation: incidence, risk factors, and prognosis in the Manitoba Follow-Up Study. Am J Med. 1995;98(5):476-84.
5. Stewart S, Hart CL, Hole DJ, et al. A population-based study of the long-term risks associated with atrial fibrillation: 20-year follow-up of the Renfrew/Paisley study. Am J Med. 2002;113(5):359-64.
6. Wolf PA, Abbott RD, Kannel WB. Atrial fibrillation as an independent risk factor for stroke: the Framingham Study. Stroke. 1991;22(8):983-8.
7. Wolf PA, Dawber TR, Thomas HE, et al. Epidemiologic assessment of chronic atrial fibrillation and risk of stroke: the Framingham study. Neurology. 1978;28(10):973-7.
8. Wang TJ, Larson MG, Levy D, et al. Temporal relations of atrial fibrillation and congestive heart failure and their joint influence on mortality: the Framingham Heart Study. Circulation. 2003;107(23):2920-5.
9. Estes NA, Halperin JL, Calkins H, et al. ACC/AHA/Physician Consortium 2008 clinical performance measures for adults with nonvalvular atrial fibrillation or atrial flutter: a report of the American College of Cardiology/American Heart Association Task Force on Performance Measures and the Physician Consortium for Performance Improvement (Writing Committee to Develop Clinical Performance Measures for Atrial Fibrillation): developed in collaboration with the Heart Rhythm Society. Circulation. 2008;117(8):1101-20.
10. Wyse DG, Waldo AL, DiMarco JP, et al. A comparison of rate control and rhythm control in patients with atrial fibrillation. N Engl J Med. 2002;347(23):1825-33.
11. Van Gelder IC, Hagens VE, Bosker HA, et al. A comparison of rate control and rhythm control in patients with recurrent persistent atrial fibrillation. N Engl J Med. 2002;347(23):1834-40.
12. Scott PA, Pancioli AM, Davis LA, et al. Prevalence of atrial fibrillation and antithrombotic prophylaxis in emergency department patients. Stroke. 2002;33(11):2664-9.
13. McDonald AJ, Pelletier AJ, Ellinor PT, et al. Increasing US emergency department visit rates and subsequent hospital admissions for atrial fibrillation from 1993 to 2004. Ann Emerg Med. 2008;51(1):58-65.
14. Fuster V, Ryden LE, Cannom DS, et al. ACC/AHA/ESC 2006 Guidelines for the Management of Patients with Atrial Fibrillation: a report of the American College of Cardiology/American Heart Association Task Force on Practice Guidelines and the European Society of Cardiology Committee for Practice Guidelines (Writing Committee to Revise the 2001 Guidelines for the Management of Patients With Atrial Fibrillation): developed in collaboration with the European Heart Rhythm Association and the Heart Rhythm Society. Circulation. 2006;114(7):e257-354.
15. Shinbane JS, Wood MA, Jensen DN, et al. Tachycardia-induced cardiomyopathy: a review of animal models and clinical studies. J Am Coll Cardiol. 1997;29(4):709-15.
16. Gage BF, Waterman AD, Shannon W, et al. Validation of clinical classification schemes for predicting stroke: results from the National Registry of Atrial Fibrillation. JAMA. 2001;285(22):2864-70.
17. Lip GY, Nieuwlaat R, Pisters R, et al. Refining clinical risk stratification for predicting stroke and thromboembolism in atrial fibrillation using a novel risk factor-based approach: the euro heart survey on atrial fibrillation. Chest. 2010;137(2):263-72.
18. Kinch JW, Davidoff R. Prevention of embolic events after cardioversion of atrial fibrillation. Current and evolving strategies. Arch Intern Med. 1995;155(13):1353-60.
19. Wyse DG, Waldo AL, DiMarco JP, et al. A comparison of rate control and rhythm control in patients with atrial fibrillation. N Engl J Med. 2002;347(23):1825-33.
20. Van Gelder IC, Hagens VE, Bosker HA, et al. A comparison of rate control and rhythm control in patients with recurrent persistent atrial fibrillation. N Engl J Med. 2002;347(23):1834-40.
21. Van Gelder IC, Groenveld HF, Crijns HJGM, et al. Lenient versus strict rate control in patients with atrial fibrillation. N Engl J Med. 2010;362(15):1363-73.
22. Whitbeck MG, Charnigo RJ, Khairy P, et al. Increased mortality among patients taking digoxin--analysis from the AFFIRM study. Eur Heart J. 2013;34(20):1481-8.
23. Gentile F, Elhendy A, Khandheria BK, et al. Safety of electrical cardioversion in patients with atrial fibrillation. Mayo Clin Proc. 2002;77(9):897-904.
24. Singer DE, Chang Y, Fang MC, et al. Should patient characteristics influence target anticoagulation intensity for stroke prevention in nonvalvular atrial fibrillation?: the ATRIA study. Circ Cardiovasc Qual Outcomes. 2009;2(4):297-304.
25. Stiell IG, Clement CM, Symington C, et al. Emergency Department Use of Intravenous Procainamide for Patients with Acute Atrial Fibrillation or Flutter. Acad Emerg Med. 2007;14(12):1158-64.
26. Echt DS, Liebson PR, Mitchell LB, et al. Mortality and morbidity in patients receiving encainide, flecainide, or placebo. The Cardiac Arrhythmia Suppression Trial. N Engl J Med. 1991;324(12):781-8.
27. ACTIVE Investigators, Connolly SJ, Pogue J, et al. Effect of clopidogrel added to aspirin in patients with atrial fibrillation. N Engl J Med. 2009;360(20):2066-78.
28. ACTIVE Writing Group of the ACTIVE Investigators, Connolly S, Pogue J, et al. Clopidogrel plus aspirin versus oral anticoagulation for atrial fibrillation in the Atrial fibrillation Clopidogrel Trial with Irbesartan for prevention of Vascular Events (ACTIVE W): a randomised controlled trial. Lancet. 2006;367(9526):1903-12.
29. Agarwal S, Hachamovitch R, Menon V. Current trial-associated outcomes with warfarin in prevention of stroke in patients with nonvalvular atrial fibrillation: a meta-analysis. Arch Intern Med. 2012;172(8):623-31.
30. D'Andrea G, D'Ambrosio RL, Di Perna P, et al. A polymorphism in the VKORC1 gene is associated with an interindividual variability in the dose-anticoagulant effect of warfarin. Blood. 2005;105(2):645-9.
31. Bodin L, Verstuyft C, Tregouet DA, et al. Cytochrome P450 2C9 (CYP2C9) and vitamin K epoxide reductase (VKORC1) genotypes as determinants of acenocoumarol sensitivity. Blood. 2005;106(1):135-40.
32. Connolly SJ, Ezekowitz MD, Yusuf S, et al. Dabigatran versus warfarin in patients with atrial fibrillation. N Engl J Med. 2009;361(12):1139-51.
33. Patel MR, Mahaffey KW, Garg J, et al. Rivaroxaban versus warfarin in nonvalvular atrial fibrillation. N Engl J Med. 2011;365(10):883-91.
34. Granger CB, Alexander JH, McMurray JJ, et al. Apixaban versus warfarin in patients with atrial fibrillation. N Engl J Med. 2011;365(11):981-92.
35. Kaatz S, Kouides PA, Garcia DA, et al. Guidance on the emergent reversal of oral thrombin and factor Xa inhibitors. Am J Hematol. 2012;87 (Suppl 1):S141-S5.
36. Steinbach M, Douchet MP, Bakouboula B, et al. Outcome of patients aged over 75 years who received a pacemaker to treat sinus node dysfunction. Arch Cardiovas Dis. 2011;104(2):89-96.
37. Li H, Lakkireddy D, Korlakunta H, et al. Pacemaker utilization during permanent atrial fibrillation in patients who received pacemaker implantation for sinus node dysfunction. Am J Cardiol. 2005;96(7):942-5.
38. Sweeney MO, Bank AJ, Nsah E, et al. Minimizing ventricular pacing to reduce atrial fibrillation in sinus-node disease. N Engl J Med. 2007;357(10):1000-8.
39. Barrett TW, Abraham RL, Jenkins CA, et al. Risk factors for bradycardia requiring pacemaker implantation in patients with atrial fibrillation. Am J Cardiol. 2012;110(9):1315-21.

Chapter 5

How to Use Natriuretic Peptides in the Emergency Department

Yang Xue, Jeffrey Chan, Sonal Sarkariya, Erik A Green, Alan S Maisel

ABSTRACT

Acute heart failure is a common diagnosis among patients hospitalized in the United States. Although acute dyspnea is a common presenting symptom among patients with acute heart failure, differentiating between patients with pulmonary diagnosis and acute heart failure remains a challenge. Natriuretic peptides (NPs) are highly effective in assisting the diagnostic evaluation of patients with acute heart failure in the emergency department (ED). NP can not only increase the diagnostic accuracy of acute heart failure and decrease diagnostic uncertainty in the ED, but they can also decrease ED and hospital length of stay without increasing risk for adverse outcomes. Furthermore, level of NPs can be used to guide therapy for acute heart failure patients in the ED.

INTRODUCTION

Acute heart failure is the leading diagnosis among hospitalized patients in the United States.[1,2] Clinically, heart failure is a complex syndrome that results from a variety of conditions that prevent the left ventricle from properly filling and ejecting blood. Despite major advances in the therapy of heart failure, challenges still remain in the timely diagnosis of acute heart failure. The use of biomarkers in acute heart failure diagnosis stemmed from the need for a fast and reliable test with high sensitivity and specificity to aide the diagnostic workup of patients with acute dyspnea. Differentiating between pulmonary and cardiac causes of acute dyspnea has traditionally been a challenge as the history, physical examination, laboratory, and radiographic findings of the two conditions often overlap. Delayed or erroneous diagnosis for acute heart failure not only causes increased length of hospital stay and healthcare cost, but also leads to increased morbidity and mortality, making the accurate diagnosis imperative. Biomarkers, with their objectivity, reproducibility, and widespread availability have an indispensible role in assisting the diagnostic workup of patients with acute dyspnea.

Among the biomarkers available today, natriuretic peptides (NPs) are the most validated and accepted in the diagnostic evaluation for acute heart failure. The relevant biomarkers in the NP family are B-type natriuretic peptide (BNP), amino-terminal pro-B-type natriuretic peptide (NT-proBNP), atrial natriuretic peptide (ANP), and mid-region pro-atrial natriuretic peptide (MR-proANP). BNP was first isolated from the porcine brain, leading to its original name "brain natriuretic peptide". It is a 32 amino acid peptide hormone derived from the prohormone B-type natriuretic peptide (proBNP). NT-proBNP is a 76 amino acid cleavage product of proBNP. ANP is a 28 amino acid peptide hormone first isolated from the atrial tissue of rats. ANP is a product of the 126 amino acid precursor prohormone ANP (proANP).[3] MR-proANP is a cleavage fragment of proANP. ANP is made in the atria as well as the cardiac ventricles in humans while BNP is made predominantly in the cardiac ventricles.[4] Among the four, BNP and NT-proBNP are more validated by clinical trials and more widely used in today's clinical practice (Table 1). In general, BNP has a much slower clearance than ANP. The circulating half-life of ANP is 3–5 minutes while the circulating half-life of BNP is about 20–30 minutes. NT-proBNP has a much longer circulating half-life, about

TABLE 1: Characteristics of B-type natriuretic peptide and amino N-terminal prohormone B-type natriuretic peptide

	BNP	*NT-proBNP*
Components	BNP molecule	NT fragments (1–76) NT-proBNP (1–108)
Molecular weight	4 kilodaltons	8.5 kilodaltons
Genesis	Cleavage from NT-proBNP	Release from ventricular myocytes
Half-life	20 minutes	120 minutes
Clearance mechanism	Neutral endopeptidase clearance receptors	Renal clearance
Increase with normal aging	+	++++
Correlation with estimated glomerular filtration rate	- 0.20	- 0.60
Approved cutoff(s) for CHF diagnosis	100 pg/mL	Age <75: 125 pg/mL Age >75: 450 pg/mL
Studies completed	1,370	39
Entry on US market	November, 2000	December, 2002

BNP, B-type natriuretic peptide; NT-proBNP, amino N-terminal prohormone B-type natriuretic peptide; CHF, chronic heart failure

60–90 minutes. Comparing to ANP, MR-proANP is much more stable and has a considerably longer half-life (up to 50 minutes). Physiologically, ANP and BNP are protective hormones that counteract the physiologic abnormalities of acute heart failure. Their functions include increasing glomerular filtration rate (GFR), increasing sodium and water excretion, relaxing arterioles and venules, increasing diastolic relaxation, decreasing myocardial fibrosis, inhibiting cardiac hypertrophy, as well as inhibiting renin and aldosterone secretion. As for clearance, ANP and BNP are removed via multiple mechanisms, including receptor mediated degradation, proteolytic degradation by neutral endopeptidases, and excretion by the kidneys. Both NT-proBNP and MR-proANP are fragments of prohormones which play no significant physiologic roles. Thus, their clearance is mostly via the kidneys. Elevations of NP concentrations correlate well with elevated pulmonary capillary wedge pressure (PCWP) and increased left ventricular wall stress.[5-8] For example, in patients with severe aortic stenosis, BNP concentrations correlated very well with left ventricular wall stress both pre- and post-aortic valve replacement. This correlation between NPs and PCWP is also seen in patients with heart failure (Fig. 1).[9,10] The reason NP levels correlate so well with increased left ventricular wall stress and PCWP lies in its origin. ANP and BNP are produced

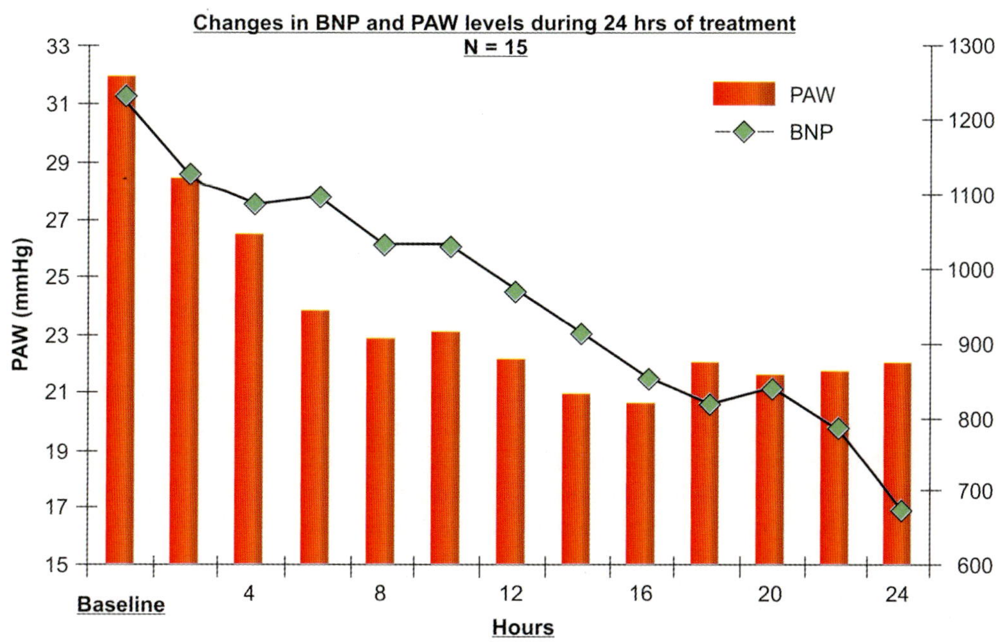

Fig. 1 Correlation between B-type natriuretic peptide (BNP) and pulmonary artery wedge (PAW) pressure

Source: Adapted from Kazanegra R, Cheng V, Garcia A, et al. A rapid test for B-type natriuretic peptide correlates with falling wedge pressures in patients treated for decompensated heart failure: a pilot study. *J Card Fail.* 2001;7(1):21-9, *with permission*

mostly by the cardiac ventricles, with the left ventricle being the predominant source. Increased ventricular wall stress leads to upregulation and increased production of ANP and BNP by ventricular myocytes. This upregulation can be seen histologically in patients with hypertrophic cardiomyopathy. The strong correlation between elevated NP and PCWP and left ventricular wall stress provides the physiological basis for using NPs in the diagnostic evaluation of patients with acute heart failure.

B-TYPE NATRIURETIC PEPTIDE: THE EVIDENCE

Although BNP was first isolated in 1988, its role as a biomarker in acute heart failure was not established until 2002. The multicenter Breathing Not Properly trial demonstrated the effectiveness of BNP in the diagnostic workup of patients presenting to the ED with acute dyspnea.[11] In this study, 1,586 patients with acute dyspnea as their chief complaint to the ED were enrolled from seven international sites. The gold standard diagnosis of acute heart failure was made by two cardiologists who were blinded to BNP measurements. There were 883 male and 773 female patients in this study. Acute heart failure was diagnosed in 744 patients. In patients with acute heart failure, BNP levels were 675 ± 450 pg/mL while patients without acute heart failure had BNP levels of 110 ± 225 pg/mL. BNP was the single best predictor of acute heart failure with an area under the receiver-operating-characteristic curve (AUC) of 0.91 (95% confidence interval: 0.90–0.93, $p < 0.001$). A BNP cutoff of 100 pg/mL had a sensitivity of 90%, specificity of 75% and diagnostic accuracy of 83%. BNP levels less than 50 pg/mL were associated with a negative predictive value of 96%. In multiple logistic-regression analysis, BNP above a cutoff of 100 pg/mL was the strongest independent predictor of acute heart failure with an odds ratio of 29.6.

N-TERMINAL PRO-B-TYPE NATRIURETIC PEPTIDE: THE EVIDENCE

N-terminal-proBNP is also commonly used in the diagnostic evaluation of patients with acute heart failure. Its effectiveness in the diagnosing patients with acute heart failure was demonstrated by the ProBNP Investigation of Dyspnea in the Emergency Department (PRIDE) study.[12] This study included 599 patients who presented to the ED with acute dyspnea. The study design was very similar to the Breathing Not Properly trial. Among the 599 patients enrolled, 209 had a final diagnosis of acute heart failure. Among patients with acute heart failure, the average NT-proBNP level was 4,054 pg/mL while the average NT-proBNP level in patients without acute heart failure was 131 pg/mL. The AUC for NT-proBNP for the diagnosis of acute heart failure was 0.94 ($p < 0.0001$). As NT-proBNP levels varied significantly based on age, different cut points were selected for patients less than 50 years old and over 50 years old. For patients less than 50 years of age, NT-proBNP cutoff of 450 pg/mL had a sensitivity of 93%, specificity of 95%, and diagnostic accuracy of 95% for acute heart failure. For patients over 50 years of age, a NT-proBNP cutoff of 900 pg/mL had a sensitivity of 91%, specificity of 80%, and diagnostic accuracy of 85% for acute heart failure. When the cutoff of 900 pg/mL was applied to the whole patient population, the sensitivity was 90%, specificity was 85% and diagnostic accuracy was 87%. NT-proBNP concentration less than 300 pg/mL had a sensitivity of 99% and negative predictive value of 99%. By multivariate analysis, NT-proBNP was the strongest predictor of acute heart failure with an odds ratio of 44.0 ($p < 0.0001$). NT-proBNP was better than clinician estimated likelihood for the diagnosis of acute heart failure (AUC = 0.94 vs. AUC = 0.90). Adding NT-proBNP to clinician estimated likelihood of acute heart failure improved the AUC from 0.90 to 0.96. Among patients with the physician estimated acute heart failure likelihood of 0–25%, NT-proBNP by optimal cut point had a sensitivity of 96% and specificity of 88% for acute heart failure. Among patients with physician estimated acute heart failure likelihood of 25–75%, NT-proBNP by optimal cut point had a sensitivity of 93% and specificity of 85% for acute heart failure. In patients with physician estimated acute heart failure likelihood range of greater than 75%, the sensitivity of NT-proBNP by optimal cut point was 93% and specificity was 84% for acute heart failure.

ATRIAL NATRIURETIC PEPTIDE AND MID-REGION PRO-ATRIAL NATRIURETIC PEPTIDE: THE EVIDENCE

Although elevations of both BNP and ANP have been associated with acute heart failure, ANP was inferior to BNP in head to head studies. For example, in one study by Cowie et al. the AUC of acute heart failure was 0.96 for BNP and 0.93 for ANP. The sensitivity for ANP was 97%, specificity was 72% and positive predictive value was 55% for acute heart failure. In comparison, the sensitivity of BNP was 97%, specificity was 84%, and positive predictive value was 70% for acute heart failure.[13] The suboptimal result for ANP was due in part to its rapid clearance, which made reliable measurements difficult

TABLE 2: Mid-region prohormone atrial natriuretic peptide versus B-type natriuretic peptide for diagnosis of acute heart failure in the biomarkers in acute heart failure trial[14]

Measure	*Sensitivity*	*Specificity*	*Accuracy*
MR-proANP 120 pmol/L	95.56	59.85	72.64
BNP 100 pg/mL	96.98	61.90	73.50
Difference	1.42	2.05	0.86
Upper 95% limit	2.82	3.84	2.10
Non-inferiority p	<0.0001	<0.0001	<0.0001

Abbreviations: MR-proANP, mid-region prohormone atrial natriuretic peptide; BNP, B-type natriuretic peptide.

in typical clinical settings, thus limiting ANP's clinical application. Recently, biochemical assays targeting a stable mid-region fragment of proANP, MR-proANP became available. MR-proANP is a much more stable and degradation resistant molecule than the active ANP with substantially longer serum half-life. The diagnostic utility of MR-proANP in acute heart failure was demonstrated in the Biomarker in Acute Heart Failure (BACH) trial, which demonstrated that MR-proANP at cut point of 120 pmol/L was non-inferior to BNP at 100 pg/mL for the diagnosis for the acute heart failure. The correlation between MR-proANP and both BNP and NT-proBNP was 0.92. BNP at the 100 pg/mL cut point had a sensitivity of 95.6%, specificity of 61.9%, diagnostic accuracy of 73.6%, positive predictive value of 57%, and a negative predictive value of 96.4%. In comparison, MR-proANP with a cut point of 120 pmol/L had a sensitivity of 97%, specificity of 59.9%, diagnostic accuracy of 72.7%, positive predictive value of 56%, and a negative predictive value of 97.4 (Table 2). Furthermore, elevated MR-proANP added significantly to elevated BNP, increasing the C-statistic from 0.787 to 0.816 ($p < 0.001$). Requiring both MR-proANP and BNP to be elevated increased the overall diagnostic accuracy from 73.6% for BNP alone to 76.6% for the combined diagnosis. In patients with intermediate BNP levels and obesity, MR-proANP added incremental predictive value to BNP for the prediction of acute heart failure. In patients with intermediate NT-proBNP levels, renal insufficiency (Creatinine > 1.6 mg/dL), obesity, age more than 70 years, and edema, MR-proANP also added incremental predictive value to NT-proBNP for the prediction of acute heart failure (Flowchart 1). In the subgroup of patients where the ED physicians were uncertain of the diagnosis, defined as 20–80% probability of acute heart failure on a visual analog scale, the addition of MR-proANP reduced indecision by 29%.[14]

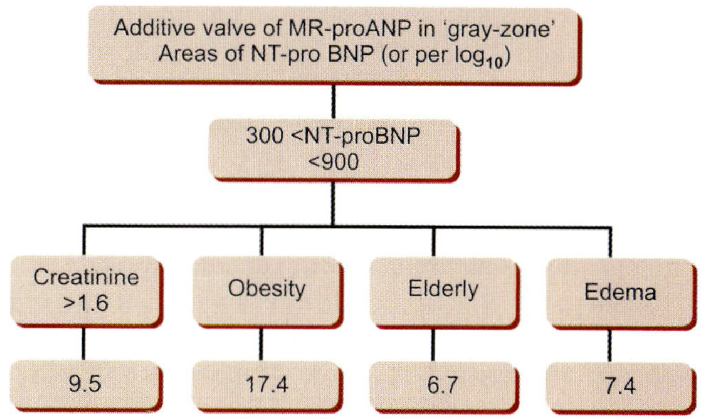

MR-proANP, mid-region prohormone atrial natriuretic peptide; NT-proBNP, N-terminal prohormone B-type natriuretic peptide

Flowchart 1 Incremental predictive value of adding mid-region prohormone atrial natriuretic peptide to gray zone amino N-terminal prohormone B-type natriuretic peptide for the diagnosis of acute heart failure

USING NATRIURETIC PEPTIDES IN THE EMERGENCY DEPARTMENT

For patients presenting to the ED with acute dyspnea, the goal of the initial evaluation is timely diagnosis of the etiology of the acute dyspnea, as delays in the initiation of effective therapy are associated with significantly worse outcomes. While acute dyspnea is the most common presenting symptom of acute heart failure, it is certainly not unique to acute heart failure. Other common etiologies of acute dyspnea include pneumonia, viral syndromes, chronic obstructive pulmonary disease, asthma, and pulmonary emboli. While history, physical examination, laboratory, and imaging studies can often provide the clinician with clues, the diagnosis is not always clear during the initial evaluation, which leads to significant delays. This is where NPs come in.

As shown by the evidence outlined above, NPs are excellent independent diagnostic biomarkers for acute heart failure. NPs carry the advantage of wide spread availability, high reproducibility, and relative low cost. NPs can be used to diagnose both acute systolic heart failure and acute diastolic heart failure. If they are added to the initial panel of laboratory tests when the patient arrives at the ED with acute dyspnea, by the time the clinician completes the history and physical examination, the results would become available. As shown by prior studies, NPs not only have high sensitivity and specificity for acute heart failure, but they also have high discriminatory power in cases where the physician diagnosis of acute heart failure is indeterminant. As the NP assays are fast and reliable, they can lead to significantly reduced ED evaluation time, hospital admission rates, hospital length of stay, and overall healthcare cost without increasing mortality or morbidity. Therefore, we advocate for the incorporation of NPs to the routine evaluation of all patients presenting to the ED with acute dyspnea.

When using NPs in the ED to evaluate patients with acute dyspnea who do not have known heart failure, we propose the following algorithm. In patients with acute dyspnea and inconclusive diagnosis by history and physical examination, NP levels should be used to assist the diagnostic evaluation. In patients with BNP levels less than 100 pg/mL or NT-proBNP less than 300 pg/mL, the diagnosis of acute heart failure is very unlikely (<2% likelihood). These patients should be further evaluated for an alternative etiology for their acute dyspnea, such as chronic obstructive pulmonary disease exacerbation, asthma exacerbation, pneumonia, sepsis, pulmonary embolism, cardiac tamponade, constrictive pericarditis, or acute coronary syndrome. In patients with acute dyspnea and BNP levels above 500 pg/mL or NT-proBNP levels above an age dependent cutoff (>450 pg/mL in patients <50 years old or >900 pg/mL in patients between 50 years and 75 years of age or >1,800 pg/mL in patients >75 years of age), acute heart failure is very highly (>95% likelihood). In these patients, therapy should be initiated for acute heart failure without delay. All patients with acute heart failure should receive diuretics to reduce the intravascular volume and left ventricular preload. In patients without evidence of cardiogenic shock, vasodilators can be added if they are hypertensive. Inotropes can also be considered in these patients if they experience poor tissue perfusion and to aide diuresis. In patients with evidence of cardiogenic shock, inotrope and vasodilators may both be necessary in order to improve cardiac output by increasing contractility and decreasing afterload. In patients with NP levels in the gray zone (all ages: BNP between 100 pg/mL and 500 pg/mL; age <50 years: NT-proBNP between 300 pg/mL and 450 pg/mL, age between 50 years and 75 years: NT-proBNP between 300 pg/mL and 900 pg/mL; age >75 years: NT-proBNP between 300 pg/mL and 1,800 pg/mL), if they had a history of heart failure or left ventricular dysfunction or strong evidence of acute heart failure, then acute heart failure is highly probable (90% likelihood). These patients should receive empiric treatment for acute heart failure with diuretics and vasodilators as needed and observed closely. If there is no history of heart failure or strong evidence for acute heart failure or left ventricular dysfunction, then an evaluation for acute coronary syndrome, cor pulmonale, or acute pulmonary embolism should be considered. Patients with electrocardiogram (ECG) and biomarker evidence of acute coronary syndrome should be treated accordingly. Similarly, patients with imaging evidence of acute pulmonary embolism should be initiated on anticoagulation immediately. If there is evidence of existing left ventricular dysfunction or cor pulmonale, then the gray zone NP levels are unlikely to represent acute heart failure (<25% likelihood), as these patients tend to have higher NP levels during acute heart failure. These patients should be closely observed and evaluated for an alternative diagnosis. In patients without baseline left ventricular dysfunction, cor pulmonale, acute coronary syndrome, or acute pulmonary embolism, gray zone NP levels may still represent acute heart failure (>75% likelihood). Empiric therapy for acute heart failure should be initiated in these patients and they should be observed closely (Flowchart 2). Although not widely available, MR-proANP can also be used for the diagnostic evaluation of patients with acute dyspnea. Patients with MR-proANP levels below 120 pg/mL are unlikely to have acute heart failure. Patients with MR-proANP levels above 600 pg/mL are very highly to have acute heart failure. The gray zone for MR-proANP is between 120 pg/mL and 600 pg/mL. When available, MR-proANP levels should be checked in patients with BNP or NT-proBNP levels in the diagnostic gray zone to increase the diagnostic accuracy of NPs in patients with obesity (intermediate BNP levels), renal insufficiency (intermediate NT-proBNP levels), and advanced age (intermediate NT-proBNP levels) (Flowchart 1).

In patients with known chronic heart failure, the diagnosis of acute heart failure with NPs can pose a particular challenge. Patients with existing heart failure can have significantly elevated NP levels at baseline owing to chronically elevated PCWP due to the severe underlying heart failure and renal dysfunction that is commonly associated with heart failure. It is not uncommon to see BNP levels greater than 500 pg/mL and NT-proBNP levels greater than 1,800 pg/mL in patients with existing heart failure who do not have acute heart failure. In these patients, it would be very helpful to know their optivolemic or "dry" NP levels when they are clinically euvolemic. If their presenting NP levels are elevated more than 50% from baseline, then acute heart failure is likely. Empiric therapy for acute heart failure should be implemented as soon as possible. However, if their presenting NP levels are not elevated more than 50%

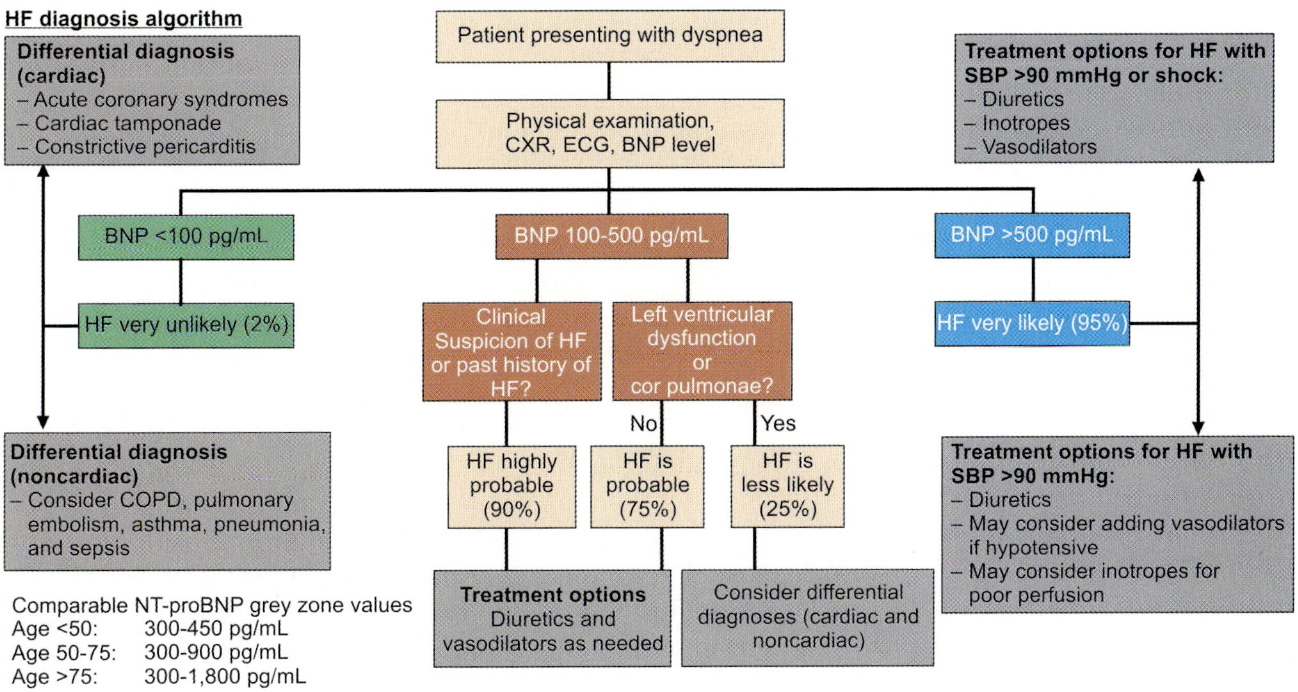

CXR, chest X-ray; HF, heart failure; ECG, electrocardiography; BNP, B-type natriuretic peptide; COPD, chronic obstructive pulmonary disease; NT-proBNP, N-terminal prohormone B-type natriuretic peptide; SBP, systolic blood pressure

Flowchart 2 Algorithm on using B-type natriuretic peptide and amino N-terminal prohormone B-type natriuretic peptide levels to rule in and rule out acute heart failure

Source: Adapted from Maisel A. B-type natriuretic peptide measurements in diagnosing congestive heart failure in the dyspneic emergency department patient. *Rev Cardiovas Med.* 2002;3(Suppl 4):S10-7, *with permission*

from baseline, then acute heart failure is unlikely. These patients should be observed (Flowchart 3).

As NPs are biomarkers of left ventricular preload and wall stress, a change in NP levels during serial measurement is a reflection of left ventricular preload and wall stress. Thus serial measurements of NP can be used to guide therapy for acute heart failure. While the evidence for NP guided therapy is not as robust as the evidence for using them in the diagnostic evaluation of acute heart failure, serial NPs measurements should be considered while managing patients with acute heart failure in the ED. We propose the following algorithm for NP guided therapy in acute heart failure patients in the ED. In patients with BNP levels greater than 1,000 pg/mL or NT-proBNP levels greater than 900 pg/mL for age less than 50 years or greater than 1,800 pg/mL for age between 50 years and 75 years or greater than 3,600 pg/mL for age greater than 75 years, the acute heart failure is likely severe and these patients would benefit from inpatient therapy. However, if the patient's BNP level is between 500 pg/mL and 1,000 pg/mL or NT-proBNP level between 300 pg/mL and an age dependent upper limit (>900 for age <50 years, >1,800 pg/mL for age between 50 years and 75 years, and >3,600 pg/mL for age > 75 years), an intensive treatment approach with diuretics and vasodilators in the ED can be considered. NP levels should be checked every 3 hours during this trial of intensive therapy. If the patient experiences improvement in symptoms and a reduction in NP levels, then they can be discharged with close outpatient follow-up. Conversely, if the patient does not experience any improvement in symptoms or if there is no change to NP levels, then the patient should be admitted for further therapy. For patients with known heart failure who presents with acute dyspnea and natriuretic levels that are 50% higher than baseline, inpatient therapy is often necessary, especially if their presenting BNP level is greater than 1,000 pg/mL or NT-proBNP level is greater than an age dependent cutoff (>900 pg/mL for age <50 years, >1,800 pg/mL for age between 50 years and 75 years, and >3,600 pg/mL for age >75 years). Finally, for patients with gray zone NP levels (BNP between 100 pg/mL and 500 pg/mL, age <50 years: NT-proBNP between 300 pg/mL and 450 pg/mL, age between 50 years and 75 years: NT-proBNP between 300 pg/mL and 900 pg/mL,

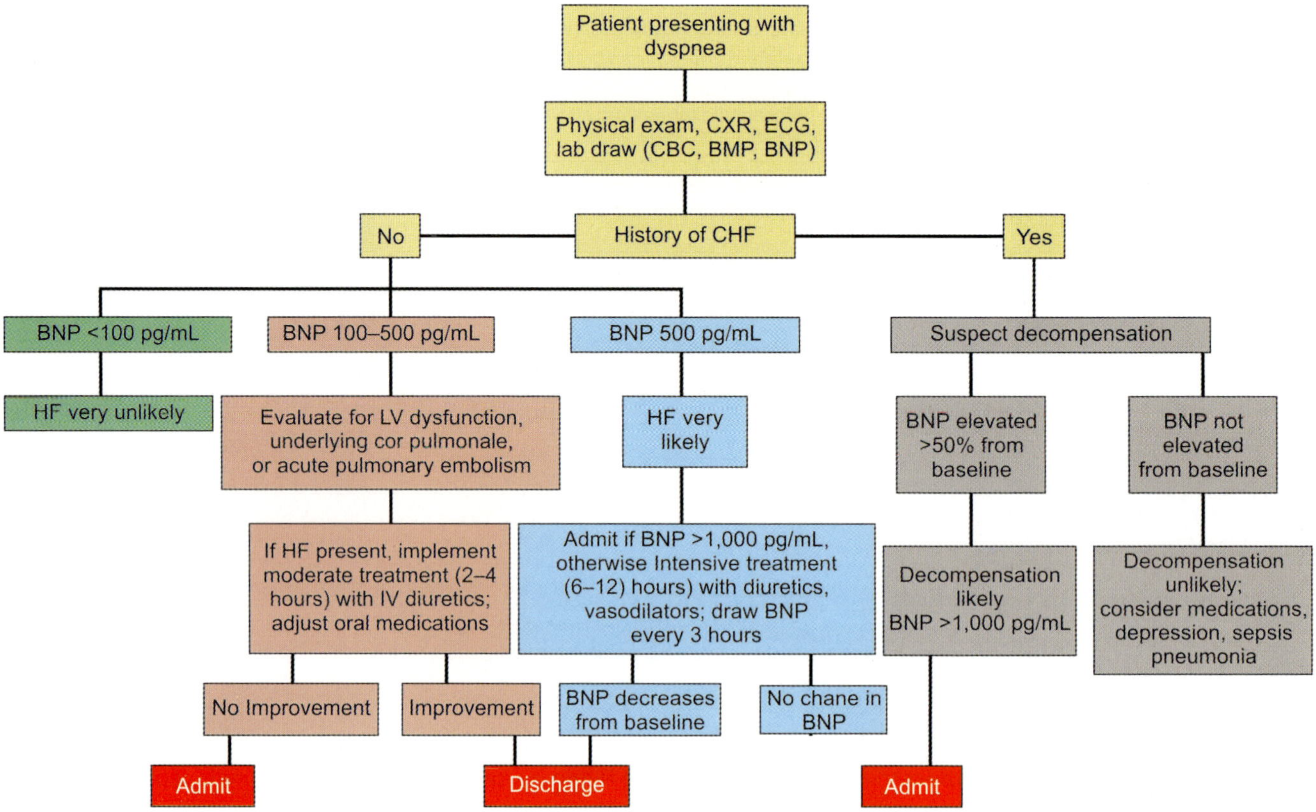

CXR, chest X-ray; ECG, electrocardiogram; CBC, complete blood count; BMP, basic metabolic panel; BNP, B-type natriuretic peptide; CHF, chronic heart failure; HF, heart failure; LV, left ventricular

Flowchart 3 Algorithm for the management of heart failure in an emergency department setting

Source: Adapted from Bhalla V, Maisel AS. B-type natriuretic peptide in the neurohormonal hierarchy in heart failure. *Cardiovasc Rev Rep*. 2004;25(3):100-4, *with permission*

and age >75 years: NT-proBNP between 300 pg/mL and 1,800 pg/mL) who do not have an alterative explanation for their acute dyspnea, such as acute pulmonary embolism, pneumonia, or chronic obstructive pulmonary disease exacerbation, empiric therapy for acute heart failure should be attempted in the ED. If they experience improvement in their symptoms with empiric acute heart failure therapy, then they can be discharged with close outpatient follow-up and further evaluation for heart failure. If they do not experience improvement in their symptoms, then they should be admitted for continued observation and evaluation (Flowchart 3).

When using NPs, there are some important caveats that clinicians must keep in mind. First and foremost, NP elevations are not pathognomonic for AHF. Thus, NPs levels should never be used in isolation during the diagnostic evaluation of patients with acute dyspnea. As shown by prior studies, NP levels can increase due to variety of other reasons. As mentioned above, patients with chronic heart failure can have significantly elevated NP levels even though they are clinically euvolemic. NP levels can also increase during acute coronary syndrome as left ventricular dysfunction develops during acute myocardial ischemia. NP levels can also be elevated due to acute and chronic right heart failure secondary to pulmonary diseases, such as chronic pulmonary hypertension and acute pulmonary embolism. Patients in high cardiac output states, such as sepsis, cirrhosis, and hyperthyroidism can also have elevated NP levels without acute heart failure. Other caveats for using NP include advanced age, female gender, obesity, and renal dysfunction. Baseline levels of both BNP and NT-proBNP increase with age. The effect of age on NT-proBNP levels is more profound, thus leading to the age dependent cutoffs for the diagnostic evaluation of acute dyspnea patients. For unclear reasons, NP levels are higher in women than men. NP levels can also be elevated in patients with renal dysfunction. As a significant amount of NPs clearance occurs in the kidneys, impaired renal function (GFR <60 mL/min/1.7 m^2) is associated with inappropriately elevated NP levels. In addition, patients with renal disease are also more likely to have coronary artery disease, left ventricular hypertrophy, and hypertension, which can all cause increases to left ventricular filling pressure and further chronic elevation in NP levels. As NT-proBNP is primarily cleared in the kidneys, the effect of renal impairment is stronger on NT-proBNP than on BNP. Interestingly, obese patients tend to have inappropriately low BNP levels. The exact mechanism of this inverse relationship between obesity and BNP levels is unknown and may be related to increased tissue clearance by membrane-bound NP receptors and decreased production of BNPs in obese patients. As a rule of thumb, BNP levels should be multiplied by a factor of 2 to 3 in obese patients to account for this inappropriate depression of BNP levels. As NT-proBNP is not cleared by membrane bound NP receptors, its levels are less affected by obesity. Another aspect of NP levels that the clinician must keep in mind is that although there is a correlation between PCWP and NP levels, NP levels do not change "instantaneously". Only a very small amount of NP is stored in myocytes. In situations of acute increases in left ventricular filling pressure, there is a delay in the rise of NPs as the intracellular production of NPs is ramped up. Thus in patients with clear evidence of flash pulmonary edema, a low NP level cannot be used to rule out acute heart failure. Lastly, not all heart failure is caused by increases in left ventricular filling pressures. Conditions, such as mitral stenosis and constrictive pericarditis can cause significant heart failure symptoms without causing elevations of left ventricular filling pressures. Thus the NP levels may be low in these cases.

CONCLUSION

Natriuretic peptides with their low cost, objectivity, reproducibility, and accessibility are excellent adjuncts to physical examination, standard laboratory, and imaging studies in diagnosing acute heart failure in the ED. By providing us with insight into one of the most important pathophysiologic processes in acute heart failure, NPs have revolutionized the evaluation of the patients with acute dyspnea, improving diagnostic accuracy, and efficiency of acute heart failure in a variety of clinical settings. They have been widely accepted by clinicians and will continue to play a significant role in the management of patients with acute dyspnea in the ED.

REFERENCES

1. American Heart Association. Heart Disease and Stroke Statistics: 2010 Update. Dallas, TX: American Heart Association; 2010.
2. Haldeman GA, Croft JB, Giles WH, et al. Hospitalization of patients with heart failure: National Hospital Discharge Survey, 1985 to 1995. Am Heart J. 1999;137(2):352-60.
3. Xu-Cai YO, Wu Q. Molecular forms of natriuretic peptides in heart failure and their implications. Heart. 2010;96(6):419-24.
4. Yasue H, Yoshimura M, Sumida H, et al. Localization and mechanism of secretion of B-type natriuretic peptide in comparison with those of A-type natriuretic peptide in normal subjects and patients with heart failure. Circulation. 1994;90(1):195-203.
5. Ikeda T, Matsuda K, Itoh H, et al. Plasma levels of brain and atrial natriuretic peptides elevate in proportion to left ventricular end-systolic wall stress in patients with aortic stenosis. Am. Heart J. 1997;133(3):307-14.
6. Yoshimura M, Yasue H, Okumura K, et al. Different secretion patterns of atrial natriuretic peptide and brain natriuretic peptide in patients with congestive heart failure. Circulation. 1993;87(2):464-9.
7. Lang CC, Choy AM, Turner K, et al. The effect of intravenous saline loading on plasma levels of brain natriuretic peptide in man. J Hypertens. 1993;11(7):737-41.
8. Haug C, Metzele A, Kochs M, et al. Plasma brain natriuretic peptide concentrations correlate with left ventricular end-diastolic pressure. Clin Cardiol. 1993;16(7):553-7.
9. Massie B, Ports T, Chatterjee K, et al. Long-term vasodilator therapy for heart failure: clinical response and its relationship to hemodynamic measurements. Circulation. 1981;63(2):269-78.
10. Kazanegra R, Cheng V, Garcia A, et al. A rapid test for B-type natriuretic peptide correlates with falling wedge pressures in patients treated for decompensated heart failure: a pilot study. J Card Fail. 2001;7(1):21-9.
11. Maisel AS, Krishnaswamy P, Nowak RM, et al. Rapid measurement of B-type natriuretic peptide in the emergency diagnosis of heart failure. N Engl J Med. 2002;347(3):161-7.
12. Januzzi JL, Camargo CA, Anwaruddin S, et al. The N-terminal Pro-BNP investigation of dyspnea in the emergency department (PRIDE) study. Am J Cardiol. 2005;95(8):948-54.
13. Cowie MR, Struthers AD, Wood DA, et al. Value of natriuretic peptides in assessment of patients with possible new heart failure in primary care. Lancet. 1997;350(9088):1349-53.
14. Maisel A, Mueller C, Nowak R, et al. Mid-region pro-hormone markers for diagnosis and prognosis in acute dyspnea: results from the BACH (Biomarkers in Acute Heart Failure) trial. J Am Coll Cardiol. 2010;55(19):2062-76.

Chapter 6

How to Use New Biomarkers in the Emergency Department

Navaid Iqbal, Rajiv Choudhary, Erin Higginbotham, Fatima Khusro, Alan S Maisel

ABSTRACT

In patients with heart failure (HF), biomarkers like B-type natriuretic peptide (BNP) and N-terminal fragment of the BNP precursor peptide are still the gold standard for prognostic and diagnostic information. However, biomarker testing is rapidly expanding. Biomarkers are reflecting pathophysiological events at a cellular level. New biomarkers like galectin-3, procalcitonin, and others can be used on its own or in combination in order to improve diagnostic accuracy, particularly when other clinical and diagnostic parameters seem unclear. Furthermore, it was demonstrated that monitoring biomarker levels can provide incremental information on disease progression. Therefore, future research seems required for improving diagnosis and treatment of HF patients.

INTRODUCTION

Cardiovascular (CV) disease in the United States continues to be a growing epidemic affecting millions of people.[1] Heart failure (HF) is a significant part of the CV disease spectrum. Biomarker research in the past decade has shown exciting advances in managing HF in the emergent setting. Several clinical trials have demonstrated the efficacy of cardiac and noncardiac biomarkers in the diagnosis and risk stratification of patients with HF presenting to the emergency department (ED).[2-4] According to national HF registry databases, almost 75% of patients with HF present through the ED. Given the nature of the condition, rapid diagnosis is crucial in this setting.

The advances in the field of biomarker research have led to a more in-depth understanding of the ongoing pathophysiology in HF. Moreover, their utility in the emergent setting has broadened in the last few years. Natriuretic peptides (NPs) remain the most established and widely tested biomarkers in the ED for use in the diagnosis of HF. Translational research and clinical trials have shown that NPs significantly improve diagnostic accuracy and provide strong prognostic information on impending adverse outcomes of death or rehospitalization.[5,6] The growing utility of biomarkers in HF is partly due to the changes in its levels in response to treatment, allowing clinicians to chart severity of disease and institute treatment accordingly.

Biomarkers provide timely diagnosis and allow appropriate triaging in the ED. Moreover, their use in the ED can decrease morbidity and mortality, reduce in-hospital stay, decrease readmission rates, and as a result lower the burden of health care. The growing breadth of biomarker research has identified several such robust markers reflecting pathophysiological changes, which can be used to improve management of HF in the ED. This chapter briefly discusses the most important biomarkers relevant to managing HF patients presenting to the ED. Figure 1 provides a schematic overview of the concerned biomarkers.

NATRIURETIC PEPTIDES

Natriuretic peptides refer to a class of circulating peptides released from the heart in response to increased, volume

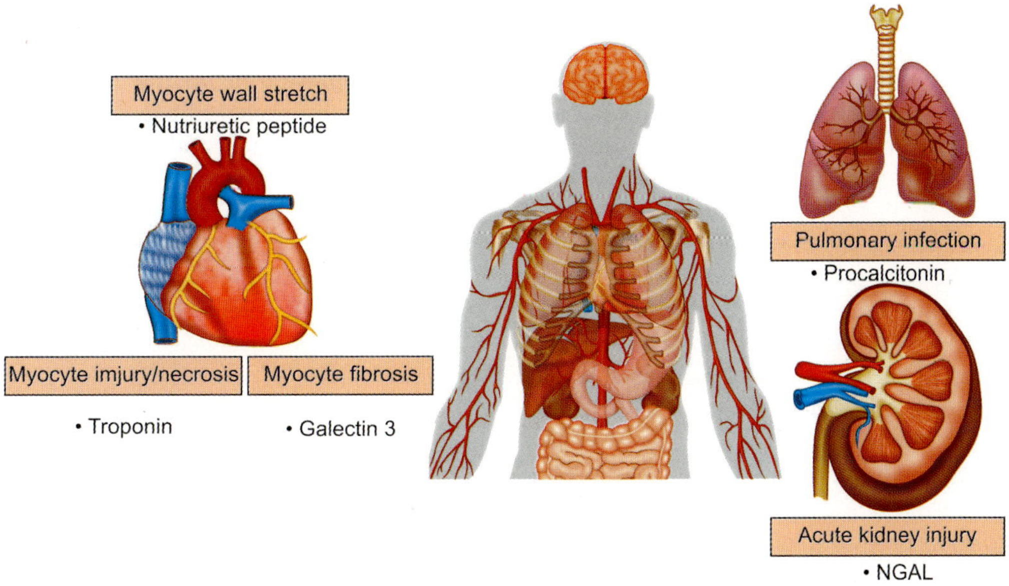

Fig. 1 Overview of cardiac and noncardiac markers which can be utilized in the emergency department to improve diagnostic accuracy and detect concomitant conditions in heart failure patients

and pressure.[7-9] In HF patients presenting to the ED, NP testing in conjunction with clinical judgment and ancillary testing has significantly improved diagnostic accuracy and management.[10,11] Some of the factors that make NPs a valuable commodity in the diagnosis and prognosis of HF in the ED are it's relatively low cost and a rapid turnaround time. Most physicians rely on conventional tools, such as radiographic imaging (chest X-ray) and physical signs to diagnose and also estimate the severity of HF.[12] However, these tools lack sensitivity and specificity.[12,13] Using NP levels in conjunction with these tests has been shown to greatly improve diagnostic uncertainty and prevent misdiagnosis of HF in the ED. Studies have demonstrated a positive correlation between reductions in NP levels in response to HF treatment. Appropriate and effective NP use in the ED can directly impact healthcare costs by reducing in-hospital stay and by lowering readmission rates.

In the acute setting, HF patients presenting to the ED can be classified as acute decompensated heart failure (ADHF), which is acute worsening of preexisting chronic HF, or as new-onset or de novo HF also termed acute heart failure (AHF), which is the first episode of HF in the absence of preexisting disease.[14,15] Unfortunately, based solely on the clinical symptoms and signs at presentation to the ED, it is difficult to distinguish between the types of HF. The majority of these patients present with a common chief complaint of acute dyspnea or shortness of breath.[16] Distinguishing between the types of HF is crucial in order to effectively tailor therapy to achieve positive outcomes, improve response to treatment, and lower costs.

Natriuretic Peptide Pathophysiology

Natriuretic peptides are a family of structurally related polypeptides consisting of atrial-natriuretic peptide (ANP), brain or B-type natriuretic peptide (BNP), C-type NP, and most recently identified D-type NP. Of these, the most widely studied and now part of mainstream use in clinical diagnosis and management of HF are BNP and the N-terminal fragment of the BNP precursor peptide (NT-proBNP).[17,18] First isolated from the porcine brain, BNP has been referred to as the cardiac hormone since its primary site of secretion is the cardiac ventricle of a HF patient. Physiological studies have convincingly demonstrated that the atrial secretory granules located in the atrial myocytes are the primary site of BNP secretion in healthy individuals wherein once secreted they remain under normal levels.[19,20]

Left ventricular (LV) dysfunction either due to impaired contraction (systolic failure) or impaired relaxation (diastolic failure) leads to poor cardiac output. Furthermore, the presence of poorly controlled hypertension (HTN) (wherein the myocardium undergoes structural changes), ischemic events, such as myocardial infarctions (MIs) and/or presence of valvular disorders can further exacerbate this problem by affecting cardiac contractility. The end result is elevated end-diastolic filling pressures. BNP gene activation occurs in ventricular myocytes in response to this increase in pressure and volume.[14,15]

The myocyte stretch signals the activation of the BNP gene that leads to the transcription of the BNP precursor peptide, which contains a C (carboxy) terminal and an N (amino) terminal.[17,20] Translational modification and cleavage of this precursor peptide by a protein-cleaving enzyme, yields the cleavage product, bioactive BNP (the C-terminal portion). The intact N-terminal fragment of the precursor peptide, the NT-proBNP molecule, also circulates in the plasma along with bioactive BNP. The BNP molecule consists of 32 amino acid residues and has a half-life of 20 minutes in the plasma whereas the NT-proBNP molecule contains 76 amino acid residues and circulates in the plasma for almost 90–120 minutes. BNP and NT-proBNP are renally cleared after binding-specific clearance receptors.[17,20]

Natriuretic Peptides Function

The elevated filling pressures and increased ventricular volume activates various compensatory mechanisms which act to restore sodium and water balance, and work to maintain perfusion to the tissues by increasing cardiac output.[21,22] These mechanisms include the activation of the renin-angiotensin-aldosterone system (RAAS), the sympathetic system, the inflammatory pathway, and the neurohormonal system. The NPs are part of the neurohormonal system, and are secreted into the circulation to counteract the decreased cardiac output by causing natriuresis (sodium and water excretion), kaliuresis (potassium excretion), vasodilation, and inhibition of the RAAS. These changes collectively result in ventricular remodeling in the long run.[22,23] Unabated insult results in a positive feedback loop leading to an increase in these compensatory mechanisms and finally results in a vicious cycle further worsening existing disease.

Utility in the Emergency Department

The utility of NPs in the ED is manifold. One of the main concerns for patients with AHF presenting through the ED is the misdiagnosis and improper triage of such patients, leading to inappropriate treatment and high readmission rates.

The Breathing Not Properly study[24] demonstrated that adding BNP to clinical judgment in diagnosing HF in patients presenting to the ED with acute dyspnea, significantly improved diagnostic accuracy from 74% to 81%. Moreover, using BNP cutoff of 100 pg/mL, the negative predictive value was 90%. BNP had a better predictive value than National Health and Nutrition Examination Survey (NHANES) and the Framingham criteria for diagnosing HF. Several studies thus far have shown how BNP levels are able to improve diagnostic capabilities by positively correlating with New York Heart Association (NYHA) functional class, LV dysfunction and also mirroring changes in pulmonary capillary wedge pressures.

The Rapid Emergency Department Heart Failure Outpatient (REDHOT) trial[25] was a crucial study demonstrating a "disconnect" that existed between the perceived severity of HF and of that determined by BNP levels. Statistical analyses revealed that BNP levels were stronger in predicting 90-day adverse outcomes than the ED physician's intention to admit or discharge the patient. Similarly, the utility of NT-proBNP has garnered much attention in aiding diagnosis and prognosis in the AHF patient. The N-Terminal Pro-BNP Investigation of Dyspnea in the Emergency Department (PRIDE) study[26] was one of the earliest studies to stratify NT-proBNP values according to age providing appropriate cutoff values in ruling out HF. NT-proBNP levels of less than 300 pg/mL achieved a negative predictive value of 99%. Table 1 provides an outline of the calculated sensitivities and specificities of NT-proBNP stratified by age. The Canadian Multicenter Improved Management of Patients with Congestive Heart Failure (IMPROVE-CHF) trial[27] demonstrated that utilizing NT-proBNP levels were able to reduce duration of the ED visit, lower rehospitalization rates, and improve direct medical costs. Moreover, NT-proBNP levels used to aid clinical decision making improved diagnostic accuracy to 0.904 on receiver operating curve (ROC) analysis. Flowchart 1 is a proposed NP algorithm which can be used in the ED to reliably "rule in" or "rule out" HF.

Discharging the Acute Heart Failure Patient

Earlier studies conducted by investigators assessing the utility of NPs in the HF patient revealed that they were not only able to aid physicians in discharge planning, but also predicted adverse outcomes based on discharge levels.

The Italian Research Emergency Department (RED) study[28] demonstrated that a reduction in BNP levels

TABLE 1: Optimal cutpoints for N-terminal pro-B type natriuretic peptide use in the emergency department[31]

Rule in						
Age strata	***Optimal cut-point***	***Sensitivity***	***Specificity***	***PPV***	***NPV***	***Accuracy***
All <50 years (n = 183)	450 pg/mL	97%	93%	76%	99%	95%
All 50–75 years (n = 554)	900 pg/mL	90%	82%	82%	88%	85%
All 75 years (n = 519)	1800 pg/mL	85%	73%	92%	55%	93%
Overall average		92%	84%	88%	66%	93%
Rule out						
Rule out	***Optimal cut-point***	***Sensitivity***	***Specificity***	***PPV***	***NPV***	***Accuracy***
Rule out	300 pg/mL	99%	62%	55%	99%	83%

PPV, positive predictive value; NPV, negative predictive value

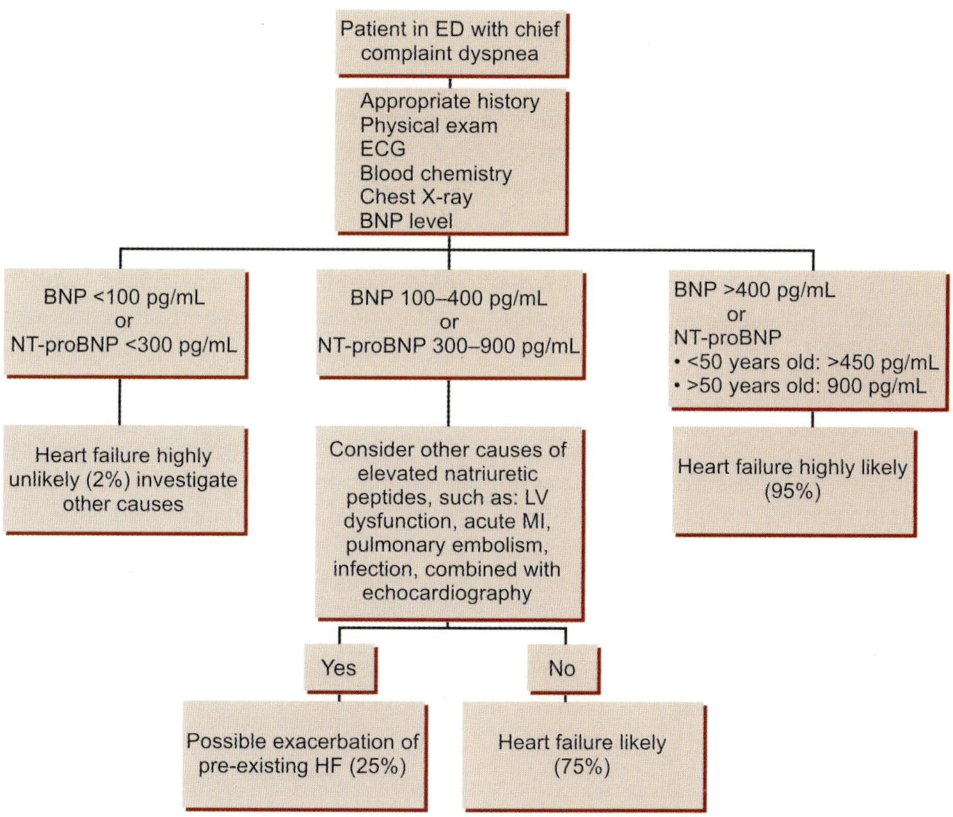

ED, emergency department; ECG, electrocardiography; BNP, B-type natriuretic peptide; NT-proBNP, N-terminal pro-B type natriuretic peptide; LV, left ventricular; MI, myocardial infarction; HF, heart failure

Flowchart 1 Proposed natriuretic peptide algorithm for use in the emergency department

by greater than 46% achieved from the admission BNP level in conjunction with an absolute BNP value of less than 300 pg/mL was able to significantly lower future cardiovascular events [odds ratio 4.77 vs. 9.61 ($p < 0.002$) in those with <46% BNP reduction and >300 pg/mL BNP level at discharge]. In the REDHOT trial those with discharge BNP levels greater than 200 pg/mL had a higher adverse event rate compared to those with BNP levels less than 200 pg/mL. Assessing a smaller cohort of patients with ADHF, variations in NT-proBNP levels significantly predicted readmission rates and 6-month mortality after discharge. In patients with 30% increase or more in NT-proBNP levels during admission had the worst prognosis. The more recently published post-hoc analysis of the Irbesartan in Heart Failure with Preserved Ejection Fraction (I-PRESERVE) trial[29] demonstrated that in HF patients with preserved EF and treated with angiotensin-receptor blocker (ARB), those with NT-proBNP levels greater than 339 pg/mL had increased rate of adverse events.

Cost-effective Utility in the Emergency Department

A randomized controlled trial assessing the role of BNP measurement in patients with AHF presenting to the ED revealed that the use of rapid bedside assay to measure BNP levels proved to be cost-effective by reducing length of stay and lowering treatment cost by 26%.[30] Patients who were randomly assigned to be evaluated based on BNP levels, had significantly shorter time to discharge compared to those who were evaluated using standard care (8 days vs. 11 days) achieved a lowering of total cost of treatment $5,410 in the BNP arm versus $7,264 in the standard care arm. Almost similar results were obtained in the IMPROVE-CHF trial,[27] which evaluated the diagnostic capability of NT-proBNP in HF patients presenting to the ED. The results revealed a cost savings of 25% over 180 days.

Natriuretic peptides function as a surrogate marker for HF. Using NP levels in the acute setting allows a clinician to diagnose underlying HF, especially when clinical signs are inconclusive. Moreover, monitoring NP levels to chart progression of HF may aid pharmacological titration of treatment and achieve better control of HF symptoms.

Elevations in Concomitant Conditions

As the quality of clinical studies have evolved significantly over the last decade, they provide a more in-depth understanding of the underlying pathophysiological mechanisms leading to elevated NP levels in the plasma. We now know that NP levels can be elevated in non-AHF conditions. It has become increasingly crucial to identify these conditions in order to accurately interpret NP levels in the appropriate setting.

Several concomitant conditions seen in AHF patients can result in elevated or lowered NP levels. These NP values are referred to as "gray-zone" values and such patients must be critically observed to rule out other causes of the elevated or lowered NP levels.[31] NP levels must be interpreted as continuous variables and should not be considered as standalone tests but should be used along with blood chemistry values, X-ray and imaging, physical presentation and clinical judgment to achieve the highest diagnostic accuracy in treating AHF. Conditions associated with "gray-zone" NP values include, renal dysfunction, pulmonary disease [acute exacerbation of chronic obstructive pulmonary disease (AECOPD), pulmonary embolism, pulmonary HTN], diastolic dysfunction, acute coronary syndrome (ACS), and neurohormonal stimulation due to other pathophysiological conditions (sepsis, valvular disorders, myocardial remodeling and fibrosis). The following guide may be used to interpret NP levels in concomitant conditions (Table 2).

TABLE 2: Concomitant conditions that can affect B-type natriuretic peptide levels

Condition	*Condition defined*	*Change in NP levels*	*Underlying cause of NP change*	*Adjusted treatment strategy*
Renal dysfunction	GFR <60 mL/min per 1.73 m^2	Increases	Acute renal-tubular injury leading to decreased NP clearance	BNP <200 pg/mL can rule out HF
Obesity	BMI >35 kg/m^2	Decreases	Higher clearance rate of NP via adipocytes	BNP <50 pg/mL can rule out HF. BNP x 2 is reflective of "true" value
Pulmonary disease	Pneumonia, COPD, pulmonary HTN, etc.	Increases	Increased ventricular strain	N/A. Reassess patient with repeat laboratory values
Valvular disorders	Mitral and aortic stenosis/regurgitation	Potential baseline decreases	Absence of high ventricular wall stress	N/A. Reassess with repeat laboratory values, ancillary testing and imaging
Diastolic dysfunction	Diastolic heart failure (HF)	Decreases	Absence of high ventricular wall stress	N/A. Use BNP value to determine severity rather than HF classification

NP, natriuretic peptide; GFR, glomerular filtration rate; BNP, B-type natriuretic peptide; BMI, body mass index; COPD, chronic obstructive pulmonary disease; HTN, hypertension; N/A, not applicable

Renal Dysfunction

More often than not patients with acute decompensation of HF presenting to the ED have renal dysfunction, which could be acute or chronic. In patients with renal dysfunction, defined as glomerular filtration rate (GFR) less than 60 mL/minutes per 1.73 m^2, raising the BNP cutoff value to 200 pg/mL may improve diagnostic accuracy in ruling out AHF in the ED. Worsening of existing renal dysfunction can occur in the acute setting mostly due to the administration of angiotensin-converting enzyme inhibitors (ACEI), intravenous (IV) contrast, and uncontrolled diuresis. Although the underlying pathophysiology leading to elevated NP levels is multifactorial, acute renal-tubular injury leading to decreased NP clearance seems plausible. Moreover, in states of worsening renal dysfunction increased cardiac stress may cause elevated secretion of NPs and thus elevated NP levels in such patients must be seen as mark of worsening HF and should be investigated further.

Obesity

In patients with body mass index (BMI) greater than 35 kg/m^2, BNP levels are lower irrespective of HF severity due to a higher clearance rate of NP via adipocytes. Thus, higher the BMI, lower is the NP level. In such patients with BMI greater than 35 kg/m^2, a BNP level of 50 pg/mL may be used to rule out HF. Conversely to improve diagnostic accuracy in obese patients with BMI greater than 35 kg/m^2 with AHF, multiplying their BNP level by two to correct for the increased BMI must be done.

Pulmonary Disease

In the AHF patient with concomitant pulmonary disease, such as pneumonia, chronic obstructive pulmonary disease (COPD), pulmonary HTN, and NP levels are elevated due to increased right ventricular strain. Moreover, left HF precipitates right HF and thus in such cases elevated NP levels may indicate worsening right HF, and in some cases, the presence of life-threatening conditions, such as pulmonary embolism. Furthermore, the use of multiple biomarkers, such as D-dimers, procalcitonin (PCT) levels may help identify those at risk of emboli versus underlying infection. Generally, in patients with pulmonary disease, NP levels lie in the "gray-zone" and as mentioned before must be investigated further.

Valvular Disorders

Clinical studies have demonstrated that NP levels significantly correlate with atrial and ventricular dysfunction in the presence of valvular disorders, such as mitral and aortic stenosis/regurgitation. In the AHF patient, the initial NP levels might not be elevated due to the absence of significantly high ventricular wall stress. Thus, although the NP levels remain lower in such conditions, the presence of clinical symptoms and signs together with ancillary testing and imaging must be done to evaluate the progression of valvular dysfunction.

Diastolic Dysfunction

Natriuretic peptide levels are unable to distinguish between systolic and diastolic type of HF. Although NPs form an effective surrogate for volume overload, interpreting NP levels in the presence of HF might provide information on the severity of the disease rather than the classification or type of acute HF.

The Optivolemic B-type Natriuretic Peptide

A thorough physical examination in AHF is crucial in identifying presence of HF signs and extent of severity. Furthermore, accurate estimation of the hemodynamic profile in the AHF patient may guide HF therapy. Based on this, the hemodynamic profile of the AHF patient can be categorized as "warm" or "cold" indicating vascular perfusion or hypoperfusion, and "dry" or "wet" indicating the level of congestion.[32,33]

Perfusion refers to maintenance of adequate cardiac output in order to effectively perfuse organs and tissues, thus on examination cool pale extremities, altered pulse pressures may identify a hypoperfused patient as "cold" and treatment should be directed in improving cardiac output and achieving a "warm" hemodynamic profile. Congestion refers to signs of fluid overload due to right-sided HF, such as elevated jugulovenous pulse, hepatojugular reflux, pulmonary rales, peripheral edema, and hepatic congestion indicating a "wet" hemodynamic profile. In such patients, treatment should be directed to adequately diurese in order to relieve fluid overload and achieve a "dry" state. This being said, BNP levels in fluid overloaded patients represent their "wet" BNP component.[32-34]

Acute HF treatment in the ED should be titrated to bring the "wet" component closer to the "dry" component, which refers to the patient's "optivolemic" BNP. In the acute HF patient, BNP levels can be referred to as "dry BNP", which signifies the patient's true BNP level in the absence of fluid overload or in other words his euvolemic BNP. Similarly, in the presence of fluid overload, the elevated BNP is referred to as the "wet BNP" signifying the presence of true volume overload leading to elevations in NP levels. Thus HF therapy should be aimed at reducing the "wet BNP" closer to the "dry BNP" so as to achieve true euvolemia at discharge.[35,36]

HIGH SENSITIVITY TROPONINS

Coronary artery disease (CAD) is one of the main triggers for AHF onset and decompensation of preexisting HF.[37] Life-threatening CADs requiring prompt treatment and high level of care include MI—ST-segment elevation myocardial infarction (STEMI) or non-ST-segment elevation myocardial infarction (NSTEMI) and unstable angina. Collectively, these manifestations of CAD leading to STEMI, NSTEMI, and unstable angina, forming the ACS.

Cardiac troponins (cTn) are one of the established biomarkers utilized in the ED for the diagnosis and risk stratification of patients presenting with ACS. The cardiac troponin complex consists of three-structural proteins of which cardiac troponin I (cTnI) and cardiac troponin T (cTnT) are specific to the cardiac muscle.[38,39] They function as regulatory proteins controlling calcium-mediated interaction of the actin and myosin filaments, part of the contractile apparatus of the heart. Conditions other than ACS causing elevated troponins include pulmonary embolism, stroke, infections, inflammatory cardiac conditions, such as myocarditis, takotsubo cardiomyopathy, sympathomimetic drugs, cardiac contusion, and renal dysfunction.

Conventionally used assays to measure troponin levels in the blood performed suboptimally in the acute period, unable to detect low rising troponin leaks. The redefinition of acute MI by American College of Cardiology (ACC)/European Society of Cardiology (ESC) joint commission incorporated positive diagnosis if troponin values were greater than the 99th percentile of a healthy population and an assay imprecision of less than 10%.[40,41] High sensitivity troponin assays provide a high level of precision while maintain a low coefficient of variation and a diagnostic cutoff at the 99th percentile of the general population.[42] This allows detection of even minute amounts of troponin leaks into the plasma in an event of myocyte injury. As the saying goes "Time is Myocardium", high sensitivity troponin assays allow a faster estimation of slowly rising troponin levels.

Interpretation of High Sensitivity Troponins

In ACS patients presenting to the ED, rapid diagnosis is the key to prevent further worsening of myocardial function. Similarly, it is important to rule out cases of ACS in order to prevent mistreatment.

Importantly, AHF can also result in elevated troponins due to increased myocyte stretch leading to an increase in wall permeability and leaking of the cytosolic proteins. Ascertaining the cause of troponin elevations is important in order to effectively tailor treatment. Several tools exist in the ED to appropriately triage and risk-stratify patients presenting with acute chest pain and dyspnea to the ED. Currently, clinicians base decisions on clinical symptoms and signs, specific electrocardiography (ECG) changes, elevation in non-troponin cardiac markers, such as creatine kinase-myoglobin (CK-MB) and myoglobin, and evaluation of the percentage change in cardiac troponin elevations above the 99th percentile of the general population.[43,44]

While interpreting cardiac troponins using high sensitivity assays, analytical variability must be considered. The most commonly used high sensitivity assay is by Roche Elecsys [awaiting Food and Drug Administration (FDA) approval in the US] with a value of 14 ng/mL and 8% CV (<10%) at the 99th percentile. Other assays have demonstrated different values at the 99th percentile level. Clinical studies have shown that myocyte death in the presence of ischemia is not immediate and can take up to 20 minutes. Moreover, complete myocyte necrosis depends on several factors, such as size of the infarct, the presence of collateral circulations and can vary from 2 hours to 4 hours.[45] A recent study on cardiac troponin measured using a high sensitivity assay with a cutoff of 14 ng/mL measured within 2 hours of presentation carried a 92.2% sensitivity and 79.7% specificity for diagnosing NSTEMI.[46]

Biological variability is significant in patients with low troponin values measured by high sensitive assays. In such patients serial monitoring of troponin changes might allow ascertaining the etiology. As mentioned before, several conditions can cause elevated troponin values. It must be remembered that any high (>10%) rise in the baseline or subsequent troponin elevations are highly indicative of ongoing MI, and these patients should transferred immediately to cardiac catheterization. In patients with troponin values around the 99th percentile,

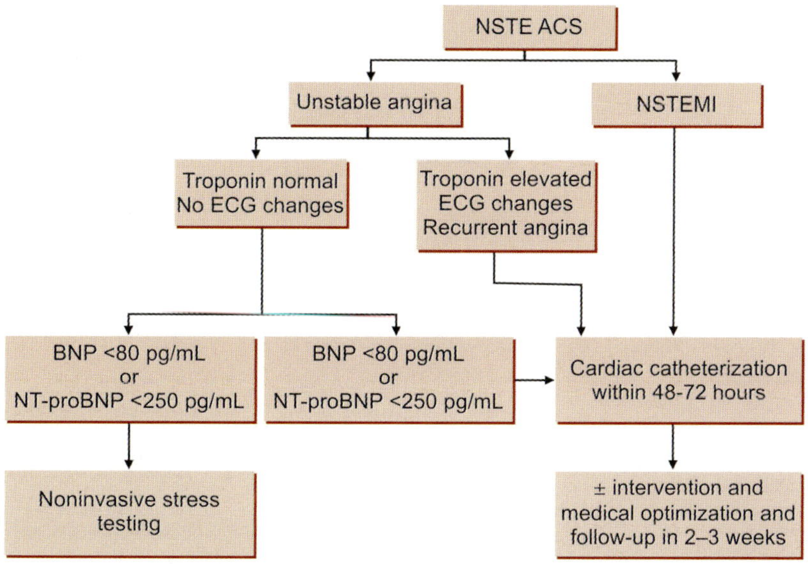

NSTE-ACS, non-ST elevation acute coronary syndrome, NSTEMI, non-ST-segment elevation myocardial infarction; ECG, electrocardiography; BNP, B-type natriuretic peptide; NT-proBNP, N-terminal pro-B type natriuretic peptide

Flowchart 2 Proposed algorithm of natriuretic peptides in acute coronary syndrome[13]

further investigation is required to identify the cause, by looking at other conditions, such as use of cardiotoxic drugs, infection, renal dysfunction, etc. NPs may also be used in conjunction with elevated troponins in non-ST elevated ACSs, to improve diagnostic uncertainty.[45] Flowchart 2 provides a hypothesized algorithm for NP use in conjunction with troponins in patients with ACS.

NEUTROPHIL GELATINASE-ASSOCIATED LIPOCALIN

There is an indisputable connection between HF and kidney injury in patients presenting to the ED with dyspnea. Often when patients present with underlying kidney disease or decreased renal function, HF treatment can exacerbate these issues and lead to worse outcomes. Using renal biomarkers to guide AHF treatment in the ED is a quick and useful way to avoid acute kidney injury (AKI).

Neutrophil gelatinase-associated lipocalin (NGAL) stands as a basic, but useful marker for elucidating, which patients are at high risk for AKI. NGAL is 25 kDa glycoprotein involved in inflammatory response of various tissues and has been implicated in producing cellular changes in the renal epithelium and nephrons.[47,48] Clinical studies have already demonstrated NGAL functions as a biomarker of both AKI and furthermore, Dent et al. illustrated that plasma NGAL spikes significantly preceded creatinine rises suggesting NGAL is an early biomarker of AKI.[49-51] The case has been made for the use of NGAL as a biomarker in patients with AHF. The GALLANT [NGAL EvaLuation Along with B-type NaTriuretic Peptide in acutely Decompensated Heart Failure] trial measured NGAL levels in AHF patients and effectively demonstrated that patients with an increased number of events during a 30-day follow-up period had higher levels of NGAL than those without the same measured outcomes ($P < 0.001$) and that NGAL was a significant independent predictor of events ($P = 0.001$).[52] These results were supported with Alvelos et al. study of 121 AHF patients.[53] Currently, NGAL is approved for prognostic ED use in Europe but is awaiting approval for routine use in the United States.

We have developed a simple algorithm to facilitate the assessment of HF patients' AKI risk based on plasma NGAL levels (Flowchart 3). This biomarker has the potential as a prognostic tool for clinicians to guide HF therapy such that risk of AKI and other renal events is minimized. Patients with an NGAL greater than 200 ng/mL are at a high risk of AKI. We strongly suggest avoiding contrast dye, nonsteroidal anti-inflammatory drugs (NSAIDs) and nephrotoxic antibiotics. Additionally, clinicians should be cautious to not over diurese these patients, but titrate medications with repeated NGAL and other renal biomarker levels. Unless necessary, we suggest holding

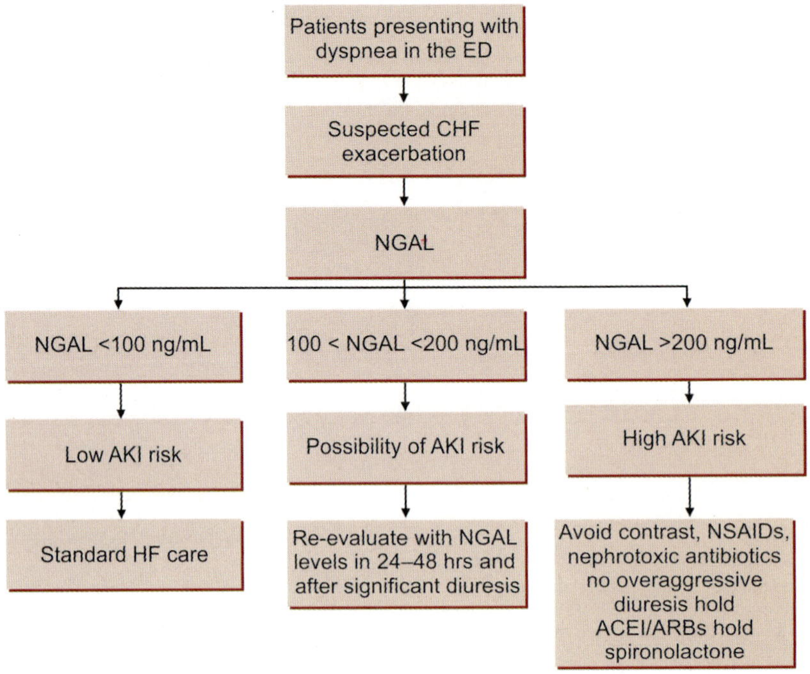

ED, emergency department; CHF, congestive heart failure; NGAL, neutrophil gelatinase-associated lipocalin; AKI, acute kidney injury; HF, heart failure; NSAIDs, nonsteroidal anti-inflammatory drugs; ACEI, angiotensin-converting enzyme inhibitor; ARBs, angiotensin-receptor blockers

Flowchart 3 Patients presenting with dyspnea in the emergency department

ACEI and ARBs, and avoid spironolactone to prevent further kidney damage. Patients with NGAL levels less than 200 ng/mL but greater than 100 ng/mL should be reevaluated in 24–48 hours, or after significant diuresis, to redetermine AKI risk. Finally, patients with NGAL less than 100 ng/mL are at low risk for AKI and standard HF treatment can be carried out.

The solidification of this biomarker as an early indicator of AKI in both human and animal studies, as well as results from European EDs suggests great potential for routine use of NGAL.[48-51,54,55] Further studies of NGAL using varied patient populations could provide more insight into its utility. We suggest this simple NGAL algorithm as a supplement when determining a diagnosis and course of care such that ultimately, clinicians can avoid worse renal outcomes for their HF patients.

PROCALCITONIN

It is a well-known fact that patients presenting to the ED suffer from both cardiac and noncardiac etiologies that are difficult to diagnose and treat. Dyspnea is one of the most common symptoms that a patient presents with to the ED.[56] It can be caused by both cardiac (e.g., HF, ACS, arrhythmias, etc.) and noncardiac (e.g., pneumonia, COPD, sepsis, etc.) etiologies making the diagnosis of dyspnea challenging and cumbersome in emergency settings. The conventional diagnostic tools used nowadays to rule in/rule out the exact cause of dyspnea are time consuming, expensive, and not routinely available.

Procalcitonin is a peptide encoded by the CALC1 gene located on the short-arm of chromosome 11. Expression of this gene is upregulated in the presence of bacterial endotoxin.[57,58] Experimental models have shown that the marked rise in PCT in infective states is due to infection-specific response elements within the promoter region of the CALC1 gene. PCT contains a 116 amino acid structure and a low molecular weight of 12.8 kDa. Besides bacterial endotoxin, inflammatory cytokines, such as tumor necrosis factor-alpha (TNF-α), interleukin-1 beta (IL-1β), and IL-6 can stimulate PCT release. In healthy individuals, PCT secretion is restricted to C cells of the thyroid gland wherein posttranslational modification leads to production of biologically active calcitonin.[57,58]

Procalcitonin can be used to diagnose and guide therapy in lower respiratory tract infections, pneumonia, and sepsis.[59,60] However, PCT has not been used on a large scale to diagnose these conditions in patients presenting

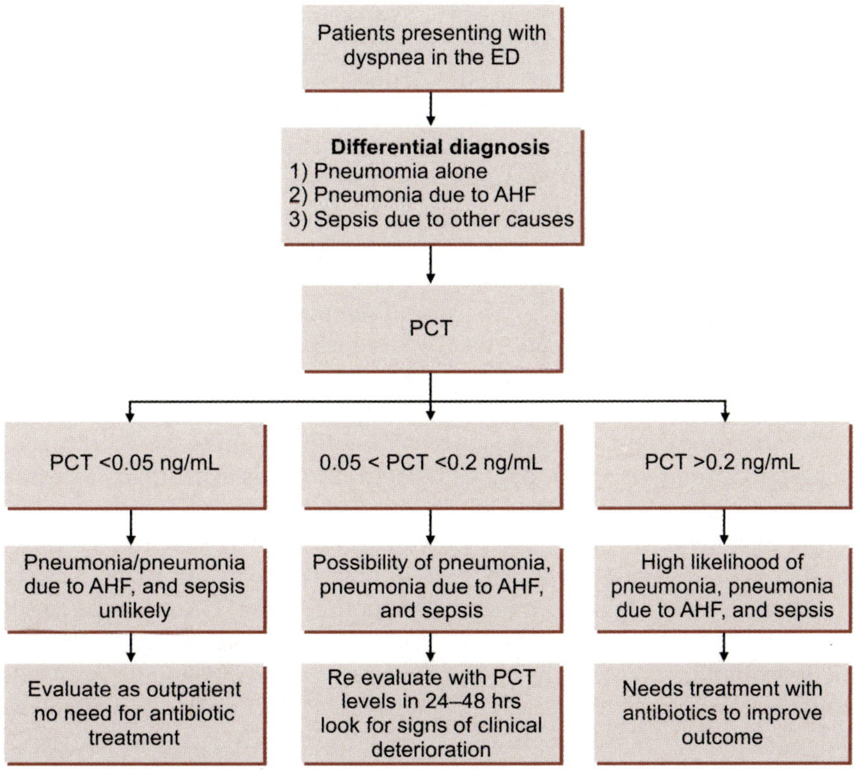

ED, emergency department; AHF, acute heart failure; PCT, procalcitonin

Flowchart 4 Patients presenting with dyspnea in the emergency department

with dyspnea due to AHF. The reason being that detecting superimposed infections like pneumonia in patients with AHF is difficult due to lack of sensitivity and specificity of the clinical tests used today. A rational clinical approach along with the use of an ideal biomarker that is cost-effective like PCT is required in order to correctly diagnose and treat patients with dyspnea. We have hypothesized (Flowchart 4) an algorithm for using PCT in the ED which can help interns, ED physicians and cardiologists involved with the care of patients presenting with HF and superimposed respiratory infection. We think that PCT can play a pivotal role in enhancing a clinician's ability to diagnose pneumonia or sepsis whether occurring in isolation or in conjunction with AHF. We suggest that patients with PCT concentration greater than 0.2 ng/mL are at increased risk of developing pneumonia or sepsis due to cardiac (AHF) or noncardiac causes and are at significantly worse survival if not adequately treated with antibiotics.

Similarly those patients with a PCT value of less than 0.05 ng/mL or falling between 0.05–0.2 ng/mL are not at substantial risk of developing pneumonia or sepsis and should be followed as outpatients or reevaluated with repeat PCT measurements to look for signs of clinical deterioration.

The above data extends the knowledge from previous work[61-63] evaluating the clinical implications of PCT in the diagnosis and management of patients with dyspnea, who are at increased risk of developing pneumonia or sepsis due to cardiac and noncardiac reasons. We think there is a strong likelihood that in acute conditions, PCT will be able to guide physicians in delineating the most frequent cause of dyspnea (infectious or noninfectious) and guide antibiotic therapy. Our clinical approach and conclusions are exploratory and need validation through randomized clinical trials. If this is proven, a logical next phase might then be a study treating according to biomarker stratification.

GALECTIN-3

Heart failure continues to be one of the most complicated and challenging medical and epidemiological problem that is associated with high morbidity and mortality, and is of major concern for the physicians around the globe. Managing this life-threatening condition is difficult, and requires significant utilization of health care resources due to frequent hospital admissions of HF patients. There are several pathologic mechanisms that participate in HF development and progression and there is compelling evidence to support the prominent role of fibrosis and changes in the intracellular matrix in the pathogenesis of HF.[64,65] The use of a biomarker that is directly linked to inflammation and fibrosis could potentially help in improving diagnostic and prognostic yield in patients with HF.

Galectin-3 (GAL-3) is an FDA approved blood test available for clinical use in AHF and chronic HF. It appears to be a promising biomarker that is associated with fibrotic processes.[64,66-69] Increased GAL-3 expression induces cardiac fibroblasts to proliferate and deposit type 1 collagen, contributing to myocardial fibrosis and adverse remodeling.[70] Clinical studies have demonstrated that patients with elevated GAL-3 levels have worse prognosis and are at increased risk of mortality and rehospitalization as compared to patients with low GAL-3 levels providing critical information that will help the clinicians to refine treatment.

The availability of GAL-3 testing can be used to provide best treatment options for patients presenting with symptoms of AHF or chronic HF. We think that GAL-3 levels greater than 17.8 ng/mL predicts two pathways: either there is presence of GAL-3 mediated fibrosis or adverse remodeling; and increase risk of adverse outcomes (i.e., increase mortality and rehospitalization). Knowledge of adverse outcomes may contribute in helping a clinician in decision-making, such as selecting patients with high GAL-3 levels for appropriate disease management through self-management skills, medication compliance and adherence programs as well as evaluating them for advance therapeutic options (e.g., cardiac resynchronization therapy, implantable cardiodefibrillators, ventricular assist devices, cardiac transplantation, etc.).

Similarly, increase in fibrosis and remodeling will help clinicians to arrange more frequent outpatient visits for these patients in order to follow them closely and to treat them appropriately with aldosterone blockers if necessary, as there is recent data supporting the hypothesis that GAL-3 leads to salt and water retention through angiotensin-aldosterone pathway and these patients might benefit from aldosterone antagonist therapy. For patients with GAL-3 levels less than 17.8 ng/mL, we suggest that they should be followed as usual care group (Flowchart 5).

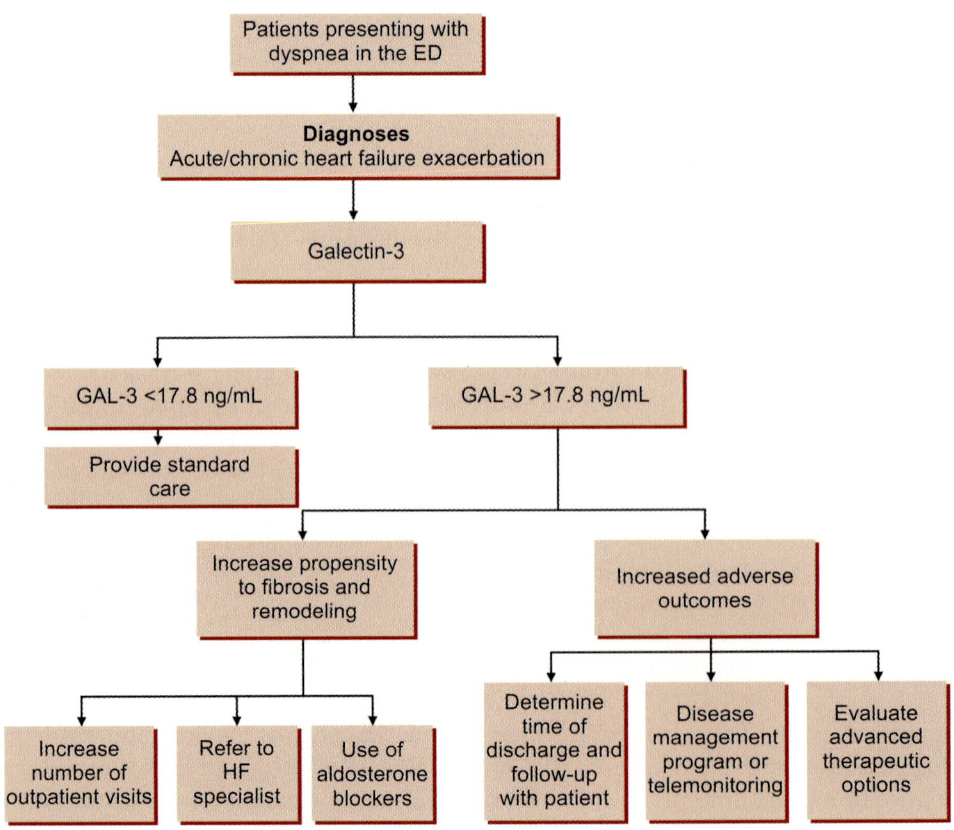

ED, emergency department; GAL-3, galectin-3; HF, heart failure

Flowchart 5 Patients presenting with dyspnea in the emergency department

With increasing hospitalizations due to HF complications each year around the world, the postdischarge morbidity and mortality rates highlight an unmet need. Circulating GAL-3 levels can predict future events in patients with AHF and chronic HF and help to identify those at high risk even before symptoms appear. Thus, measuring GAL-3 levels is a simple way to identify patients who have a significantly higher risk of unplanned readmission[71,72] and may be a cost-effective way to improve outcomes.

CONCLUSION

Biomarkers certainly have carved their niche in HF management. Reflecting ongoing pathophysiological changes, biomarkers are a reliable surrogate of HF progression. They not only provide valuable information improving diagnostic accuracy, but also monitoring their levels, provides strong prognostic information and may lower rehospitalizations and improve CV mortality.

REFERENCES

1. McMurray JJ, Adamopoulos S, Anker SD, et al. ESC Guidelines for the diagnosis and treatment of acute and chronic heart failure 2012: The Task Force for the Diagnosis and Treatment of Acute and Chronic Heart Failure 2012 of the European Society of Cardiology. Developed in collaboration with the Heart Failure Association (HFA) of the ESC. Eur Heart J. 2012;33(14):1787-847.
2. Januzzi JL, Sakhuja R, O'donoghue M, et al. Utility of amino-terminal pro-brain natriuretic testing for prediction of 1-year mortlity in patients with dyspnea treated in the emergency department. Arch Intern Med. 2006;166(3):315-20.
3. Fonarrow GC, Peacock WF, Phillips CO, et al. Admission b-type natriuretic peptide levels and in-hospital mortality in acute decompensated heart failure. J Am Coll Cardiol. 2007;49(19):1943-50.
4. deFilippi CR, Christenson RH, Kop WJ, et al. Left ventricular ejection fraction assessment in older adults: An adjunct to natriuretic peptide testing to identify risk of new onset heart failure and cardiovascular death? J Am Coll Cardiol. 2011;58(14):1497-506.
5. Nouveanu M, Breidthardt T, Potocki M, et al. Direct comparison of serial B-type natriuretic peptide and NT-proBNP levels for the prediction of short- and long-term outcome in acute decompensated heart failure. Crit Care. 2011;15(1):R1.
6. Bettencourt P, Azevedo A, Pimenta J, et al. N-terminal-pro-brain natriuretic peptide predicts outcome after hospital discharge in heart failure patients. Circulation. 2004;110(15):2168-74.
7. Levin ER, Gardner DG, Samson WK. Natriuretic peptides. N Engl J Med. 1998;339(5):321-8.
8. Misono KS, Philo JS, Arakawa T, et al. Structure, signaling mechanism and regulation of the natriuretic peptide receptor guanylate cyclase. FEBS J. 2011;278(11):1818-29.
9. Kemp CD, Conte JV. The pathophysiology of heart failure. Cardiovasc Pathol. 2012;21(5):365-71.
10. Nieminem MS, Böhm M, Cowie MR, et al. Executive summary of the guidelines on the diagnosis and treatment of acute heart failure: the Task Force on Acute Heart Failure of the European Society of Cardiology. Eur Heart J. 2005;26(4):384-416.
11. Weintraub NL, Collins SP, Pang PS, et al. Acute heart failure syndromes: emergency department presentation, treatment, and disposition: current approaches and future aims: a scientific statement from the American Heart Association. Circulation. 2010;(19)122:1975-96.
12. Stevenson LW, Perloff JK. The limited reliability of physical signs for estimating hemodynamics in chronic heart failure. JAMA. 1989; 261(6):884-8.
13. Maisel AS, Nakao K, Ponikowski P, et al. Japanese-Western consensus meeting on biomarkers. Int Heart J. 2011;52(5):253-65.
14. De Luca L, Fonarow GC, Adams KF, et al. Acute heart failure syndromes: clinical scenarios and pathophysiologic targets for therapy. Heart Fail Rev. 2007;12(2):97-104.
15. Cotter G, Felker GM, Adams KF, et al. The pathophysiology of acute heart failure-is it all about fluid accumulation? Am Heart J. 2008;155(1):9-18.
16. Fonarow GC, Heywood JT, Heidenreich PA, et al. Temporal trends in clinical characteristics, treatments, and outcomes for heart failure hospitalizations, 2002 to 2004: findings from Acute Decompensated Heart Failure National Registry (ADHERE). Am Heart J. 2007;153(6):1021-28.
17. Yasue H, Yoshimura M, Sumida H, et al. Localization and mechanism of secretion of B-type natriuretic peptide in comparison with those of A-type natriuretic peptide in normal subjects and patients with heart failure. Circulation. 1994;90(1):195-203.
18. Vanderheyden M, Bartunek J, Goethals M. Brain and other natriuretic peptides: molecular aspects. Eur J Heart Fail. 2004;6(3):261-8.
19. de Bold AJ, Borenstein HB, Veress AT, et al. A rapid and potent natriuretic response to intravenous injection of atrial myocardial extract in rats. Life Sci. 1981;28(1):89-94.
20. Potter LR, Abbey-Hosch S, Dickey DM. Natriuretic peptides, their receptors, and cyclic guanosine monophosphate-dependent signaling functions. Endocr Rev. 2006;27(1):47-72.
21. Richards AM, Troughton RW. Use of Natriuretic Peptides to Guide and Monitor Heart Failure Therapy. Clin Chem. 2012;58(1):67-71.
22. Kim HN, Januzzi JL. Natriuretic peptide testing in heart failure. Circulation. 2011;123(18):2015-9.
23. Green SM, Green JA, Januzzi JL. Natriuretic peptide testing for heart failure therapy guidance in the inpatient and outpatient setting. Am J Ther. 2009;16(2):171-7.
24. Maisel AS, Krishnaswamy P, Nowak RM, et al. Rapid measurement of B-type natriuretic peptide in the emergency diagnosis of heart failure. N Engl J Med. 2002;347(3):161-7.
25. Maisel A, Hollander JE, Guss D, et al. Primary results of the rapid emergency department heart failure outpatient trial (REDHOT). A multicenter study of B-type natriuretic peptide levels, emergency department decision making, and outcomes in patients presenting with shortness of breath. J Am Coll Cardiol. 2004;44(6):1328-33.
26. Januzzi JL, Camargo CA, Anwaruddin S, et al. The N-terminal Pro-BNP investigation of dyspnea in the emergency department (PRIDE) study. Am J Cardiol. 2005;95(8):948-54.
27. Moe GW, Howlett J, Januzzi JL, et al. N-terminal pro-B-type natriuretic peptide testing improves the management of patients with suspected acute heart failure: primary results of the Canadian prospective randomized multicenter IMPROVE-CHF study. Circulation. 2007;115(24):3103-10.
28. Di Somma S, Magrini L, Pittoni V, et al. In-hospital percentage BNP reduction is highly predictive for adverse events in patients admitted for acute heart failure: the Italian RED study. Crit Care. 2010;14(3):R116.
29. Anand IS, Rector TS, Cleland JG, et al. Prognostic value of baseline plasma amino-terminal pro-brain natriuretic peptide and its interactions with

irbesartan treatment effects in patients with heart failure and preserved ejection fraction: findings from the I-PRESERVE trial. Circ Heart Fail. 2011;4(5):569-77.
30. Mueller C, Scholer A, Laule-Kilian K, et al. Use of B-type natriuretic peptide in the evaluation and management of acute dyspnea. N Engl J Med. 2004;350(7):647-54.
31. Maisel A, Mueller C, Adams K, et al. State of the art: using natriuretic peptide levels in clinical practice. Eur J Heart Fail. 2008;10(9):824-39.
32. Drexler B, Heinsch C, Balmelli C, et al. Quantifying cardiac hemodynamic stress and cardiomyocyte damage in ischemic and nonischemic acute heart failure. Circ Heart Fail. 2012;5(1):17-24.
33. Pimenta J, Paulo C, Mascarenhas J, et al. BNP at discharge in acute heart failure patients: is it all about volemia? A study using impedance cardiography to assess fluid and hemodynamic status. Int J Cardiol. 2010;145(2):209-14.
34. Binanay C, Califf RM, Hasselbad V, et al. Evaluation study of congestive heart failure and pulmonary artery catheterization effectiveness: The ESCAPE trial. JAMA. 2005;294(13):1625-33.
35. Valle R, Aspromonte N, Milani L, et al. Optimizing fluid management in patients with acute decompensated heart failure (ADHF): the emerging role of combined measurement of body hydration status and brain natriuretic peptide (BNP) levels. Heart Fail Rev. 2011;16(6):519-29.
36. Thomas SS, Nohria A. Hemodynamic classifications of acute heart failure and their clinical application: an update. Circ J. 2012;76(2):278-86.
37. Adams KF, Fonarow GC, Emerman CL, et al. Characteristics and outcomes of patients hospitalized for heart failures in the United States: rationale, design, and preliminary observations from the first 100,000 cases in the Acute Decompensated Heart Failure National Registry (ADHERE). Am Heart J. 2005;149(2):209-16.
38. Missov E, Mair J. A novel biochemical approach to congestive heart failure: cardiac troponin T. Am Heart J. 1999;139 (1 Pt 1):95-9.
39. Lee TH, Rouan GW, Weisberg MC, et al. Clinical characteristics and natural history of patients with acute myocardial infarction sent home from the emergency room. Am J Cardiol. 1987;60(4):219-24.
40. Wu AH, Lu QA, Todd J, et al. Short-and long-term biological variation in cardiac troponin I measured with a high-sensitivity assay: implications for clinical practice. Clin Chem. 2009;55(1):52-58.
41. Apple FS, Jesse RL, Newby LK, et al. National Academy of Clinical Biochemistry and IFCC Committee for Standardization of Markers of Cardiac Damage Laboratory Medicine Practice Guidelines: Analytical issues for biochemical markers of acute coronary syndromes. Circulation. 2007;115(13):e352-5.
42. Twerenbold R, Reischlin T, Reiter M, et al. High-sensitive cardiac troponin: friend or foe? Swiss Med Wkly. 2011;141:w13202.
43. Thygesen K, Alpert JS, Jaffe AS, et al. Third universal definition of myocardial infarction. J Am Coll Cardiol. 2012;60(16):1581-98.
44. Agewell S, Giannitis E, Jernberg T, et al. Troponin elevation in coronary vs. non-coronary disease. Eur Heart J. 2011;32(4):404-11.
45. Thygesen K, Alpert JS, White HD, et al. Universal definition of myocardial infarction. Eur Heart J. 2007;28(20):2525-38.
46. Aldous SJ, Richards M, Cullen L, et al. Diagnostic and prognostic utility of early measurement with high-sensitivity troponin T assay in patients presenting with chest pain. CMAJ. 2012;184(5):E260-8.
47. Yang J, Goetz D, Li JY, et al. An iron delivery pathway mediated by a lipocalin. Mol Cell. 2002;10(5):1045-56.
48. Mori K, Leet HT, Rapoport D, et al. Endocytic delivery of lipocalin-siderophore-iron complex rescues the kidney from ischemia-reperfusion injury. J Clin Invest. 2005;115(3):610-21.
49. Zappitelli M, Washburn KK, Arikan AA, et al. Urine neutrophil gelatinase-associated lipocalin is an early marker of acute kidney injury in critically ill children: a prospective cohort study. Crit Care. 2007;11(4):R84.
50. Mishra J, Dent C, Tarabishi R, et al. Neutrophil gelatinase-associated lipocalin (NGAL) as a biomarker for acute renal injury after cardiac surgery. Lancet. 2005;356(9466):1231-38.
51. Dent CL, Ma Q, Dastrala S, et al. Plasma neutrophil gelatinase-associated lipocalin predicts acute kidney injury, morbidity and mortality after pediatric cardiac surgery: a prospective uncontrolled cohort study. Crit Care. 2007;11(6):R127.
52. Maisel AS, Mueller C, Fitzgerald R, Brikhan R, Hiestand BC, Iqbal N, et al. Prognostic utility of plasma neutrophil gelatinase-associated liopcalin in patients with acute heart failure: the NGAL EvaLuation Along with B-type NaTriuretic Peptide in acutely decompensated heart failure (GALLANT) trial. Eur J Heart Fail. 2011;13(8):846-51.
53. Alvelos M, Lourenco P, Dias C, et al. Prognostic value of neutrophil gelatinase-associated lipocalin in acute heart failure. Int J Cardiol. 2013;165(1):51-5.
54. Mishra J, Ma Q, Prada A, et al. Identification of NGAL as a novel early urinary marker for ischemic renal injury. J Am Soc Nephrol. 2003;14(10):2534-43.
55. Mishra J, Mori K, Ma Q, et al. Amelioration of ischemic acute renal injury by neutrophil gelatinase-associated lipocalin. J Am Soc Nephrol. 2004;15(12):3073-82.
56. Nawar EW, Niska RW, Xue J. National Hospital Ambulatory Medical Care Survey: 2005 emergency department summary. Adv Data. 2007;386:1-32.
57. Nijsten MW, Olinga P, The TH, et al. Procalcitonin behaves as a fast responding acute phase protein in vivo and in vitro. Criti Care Med. 2000;28(2):458-61.
58. Fillon S, Soulis K, Rajasekaran S, et al. Platelet-activating factor receptor and innate immunity: uptake of gram-positive bacterial cell wall into host cells and cell-specific pathophysiology. J Immunol. 2006;177(9):6182-91.
59. Christ-Crain M, Jaccard-Stolz D, Bingisser R, et al. Effect of procalcitonin-guided treatment on antibiotic use and outcome in lower respiratory tract infections: cluster-randomized, single-blinded intervention trial. Lancet. 2004;363(9409):600-7.
60. Schuetz P, Christ-Crain M, Thomann R, et al. Effect of procalcitonin-based guidelines vs standard guidelines on antibiotic use in lower respiratory tract infections: the ProHOSP randomized-controlled trial. JAMA. 2009;302(10):1059-66.
61. Schuetz P, Christ-Crain M, Wolbers M, et al. Procalcitonin guided antibiotic therapy and hospitalization in patients with lower respiratory tract infections: a prospective, multicenter, randomized controlled trial. BMC Health Serv Res. 2007;7:102.
62. Gogos CA, Drosou E, Bassaris HP, et al. Pro versus anti-inflammatory cytokine profile in patients with severe sepsis: a marker for prognosis and future therapeutic options. J Infect Dis. 2000;181(1):176-80.
63. Maisel A, Neath SX, Landsberg J, et al. Use of procalcitonin for the diagnosis if pneumonia in patients presenting with a chief complaint of dyspnea: results from the BACH (Biomarkers in Acute Heart Failure) trial. Eur J Heart Failure. 2012;14(3):278-86.
64. Sharma UC, Pokharel S, van Brakel TJ, et al. Galectin-3 marks activated macrophages in failure-prone hypertrophied hearts and contributes to cardiac dysfunction. Circulation. 2004;110(19):3121-8.
65. Weber Kt, Gerling IC, Kiani MF, et al. Aldosteronism in heart failure: a proinflammatory/fibrogenic cardiac phenotype. Search for biomarkers and potential drug targets. Curr Drug Targets. 2003;4:505-16.

66. Henderson NC, Mackinnon AC, Farnworth SL, et al. Galectin-3 regulates myofibroblast activation and hepatic fibrosis. Proc Natl Acad Sci USA. 2006;103(13):5060-5.
67. Milting H, Ellinghaus P, Seewald M, et al. Plasma biomarkers of myocardial fibrosis and remodeling in terminal heart failure patients supported by mechanical circulatory support devices. J Heart Lung Transplant. 2008;27(6):589-96.
68. Reifenberg K, Lehr HA, Torzewski M, et al. Interferon-gamma induces chronic active myocarditis and cardiomyopathy in transgenic mice. Am J Pathol. 2007;171(2):463-72.
69. Sano H, Hsu DK, Apgar JR, et al. Critical role of galectin-3 in phagocytosis by macrophages. J Clin Invest. 2003;112(3):389-97.
70. de Boer RA, Yu L, van Veldhuisen DJ. Galectin-3 in cardiac remodeling and heart failure. Curr Heart Fail Rep. 2010;7(1):1-8.
71. de Boer RA, van Veldhuisen DJ, deFilippi C, et al. Plasma galectin-3 is associated with near-term rehospitalization in heart failure: a meta-analysis. J Card Fail. 2011;17(8):S93.
72. McCullough PA, Olobatoke A, Vanhecke TE. Galectin-3: a novel blood test for the evaluation and management of patients with heart failure. Rev Cardiovasc Med. 2011;12(4):200-10.

Chapter 7

The Role of Ultrasound in the Management of Acute Heart Failure

Luna Gargani

ABSTRACT

Echocardiography has a crucial role in the management of acute heart failure. The technique has the advantage of being readily and widely available at the bedside, noninvasively providing critical information for the management of patients, from diagnosis to follow-up, to prognostic stratification. Echocardiography offers an immediate and comprehensive assessment of cardiovascular morphology, function and hemodynamics, with minimal discomfort or risk for the patient, without using contrast material or ionizing radiation. The portability and immediacy of this technique, whose information can be readily used at the bedside, may significantly shorten the decision making process. The possibility to estimate in a few minutes systolic and diastolic left ventricular function, wall motion abnormalities, pericardium, valvular function, right heart morphology and function, and more recently also pulmonary congestion by evaluation of sonographic B-lines, makes this examination the single most versatile and cost-effective imaging technique to assess unstable patients with cardiovascular diseases.

INTRODUCTION

Ultrasound is the imaging technique of choice in emergencies, since it is readily and widely available at the bedside, noninvasively providing crucial information for the management of patients. Although ultrasound can be easily employed for the assessment of many different organs, transthoracic echocardiography (TTE) is the most commonly used sonographic examination in patients with acute heart failure (AHF), since it offers immediate and comprehensive assessment of cardiovascular morphology, function and hemodynamics, with minimal discomfort or risk for the patient, without using contrast material or ionizing radiation.[1] For these reasons, echocardiography has been defined by the 2009 American College of Cardiology/American Heart Association Guidelines for the diagnosis and management of heart failure—the single most useful diagnostic test in the evaluation of patients with heart failure (HF).[2]

Echocardiography in emergencies poses many clinical challenges. Physicians must interpret suboptimal studies and have limited time for consultations with colleagues. In these circumstances, professional medical errors are more likely to occur and can lead to serious consequences. Thus, recognition of echocardiography's advantages and limitations in particular clinical situations is essential for correct interpretation and to avoid potentially catastrophic diagnostic errors.[3]

Echocardiography in AHF can be useful at all stages of a patient's in-hospital management: immediately at admission, for in-hospital follow-up and at discharge.

AT ADMISSION

In patients admitted for AHF, the main aim of echocardiography is to identify the cause of decompensation. Two-dimensional and Doppler echocardiography have markedly improved our understanding of the pathophysiology of AHF, providing a noninvasive technique for accurate diagnosis of underlying causes, hemodynamic evaluation at baseline and during medical intervention, and prognostic information to guide further

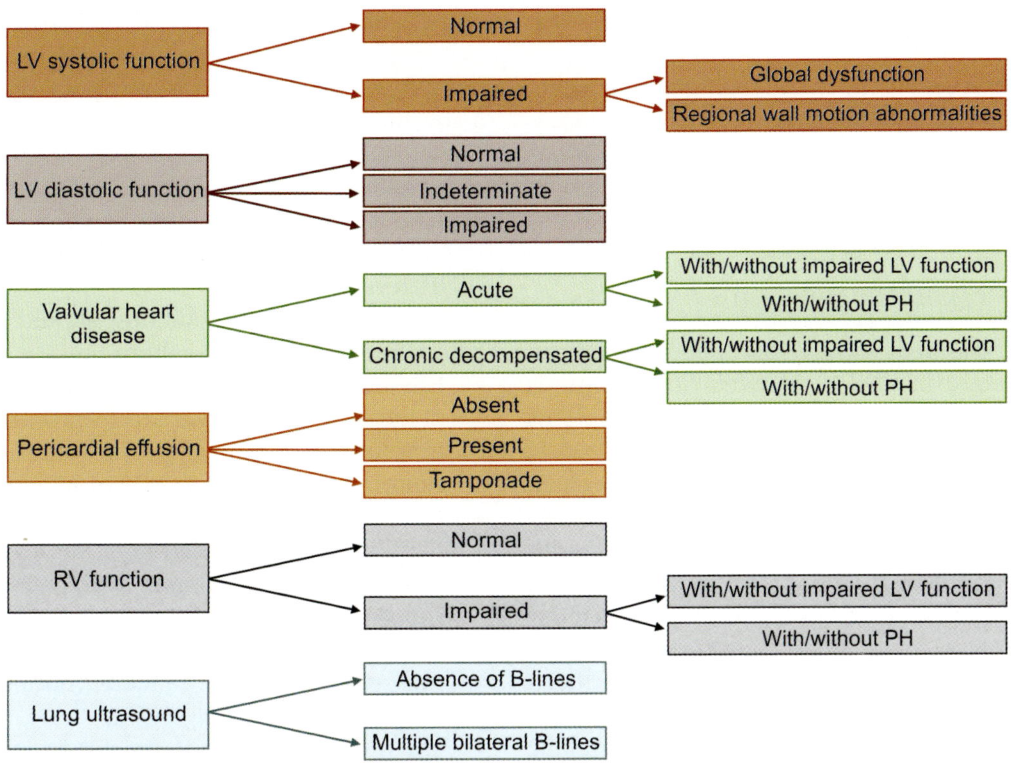

LV, left ventricle; RV, right ventricle; PH, potential hydrogen

Flowchart 1 Schematic overview of the main echocardiographic parameters to evaluate in AHF patients at admission

management. Early understanding of the etiology of the acute condition is mandatory in order to initiate appropriate therapy. The extremely heterogeneous nature of patients with AHF precludes a "one-size-fits-all" approach.

There are many parameters that should be evaluated by TTE in AHF patients in order to establish the cause and characterize of severity of decompensation (Flowchart 1).

Left Ventricular Systolic Function

The quantitation of left ventricular (LV) systolic function, size and geometry is critical for the proper evaluation and management of patients with AHF.[4] When assessing systolic function in AHF, we should be able to answer these fundamental questions:

- Is LV systolic function normal or reduced?
- What is the severity of LV systolic dysfunction (mild, moderate or severe)?
- Has the LV systolic function changed from a previous assessment (if present)?
- Is it a global LV systolic reduction or a localized wall motion abnormality?

This last issue is crucial in identifying subjects with an acute coronary syndrome underlying AHF. For the assessment of LV wall motion abnormalities, the 17-segment model including the apical cap should be used.[5]

Echocardiographic features of systolic HF include a reduced LV ejection fraction (EF) (EF <45–50%), dilatation of the LV (end-diastolic diameter >60 mm, end-systolic diameter >45 mm), diffuse or regional wall motion abnormalities, functional mitral and/or tricuspid regurgitation (TR), low cardiac output (CO) (aortic outflow tract velocity integral <15 cm). Although the need for quick evaluation in an acute patient would suggest eyeballing assessment of the EF, in some circumstances it is advisable to measure LV volumes in 4- and 2-chamber views to perform a proper EF estimation according to the modified Simpson's rule. This is especially crucial in situations when understanding whether systolic function is normal or not is not always straightforward, for example:

- Bradycardic patients, whose systolic function may appear lower than expected
- Patients with frequent supraventricular or ventricular premature beats: it is important to remember not to

perform any measurement during the premature beat or during the beat immediately following
- Patients with severe acute mitral regurgitation, where an EF less than 60% should suggest LV dysfunction.

An echocardiographic LV EF less than 40–45% has been reported to be a powerful predictor of cardiac origin in patients presenting with acute dyspnea.[6,7]

Left Ventricular Diastolic Function

Noninvasive assessment of LV diastolic function at presentation before institution of adequate therapy is particularly relevant for patients with severe symptoms and inconclusive clinical, radiographic and biochemical data with preserved LV EF and without a clear, evident cause of decompensation at first glance by echocardiography. In these patients, heart failure with preserved systolic function (HFPSF) may be the diagnosis.

The ratio of flow Doppler mitral E wave peak velocity and early diastolic velocity of the mitral annulus (E/e') obtained by Tissue Doppler Imaging (TDI) has been proposed as a noninvasive surrogate to establish LV filling pressures.[8] Nowadays, almost all echocardiographic platforms are equipped with TDI analysis, which allows quick estimation of E/e' ratio. Numerous clinical studies have shown a positive relation of E/e' with invasively determined mean LV diastolic pressure, regardless of LV EF, rhythm and heart rate.[9-14] Some studies have also established that variations in E/e' accurately track changes in LV diastolic pressures under unloading therapy.[14-17] For this reason, E/e' recordings after institution of appropriate unloading therapy may lead to inconclusive results.

In patients with depressed LV systolic function, the mitral inflow pattern by itself can be used to estimate filling pressures with reasonable accuracy.[18] In case of impaired relaxation patterns and peak E velocities less than 50 cm/s, LV filling pressures are usually normal. In patients with E/A ratios ≥1 to less than 2, the use of additional Doppler parameters is recommended, such as a systolic peak velocity/diastolic peak velocity ratio in pulmonary venous flow less than 1, Ar - A duration ≥30 ms, E/e' ≥15, and pulmonary artery systolic pressure ≥35 mmHg (in the absence of pulmonary disease) can be used to infer the presence of increased filling pressures.[19]

In patients with normal EF, as in HFPSF, E/e' ratio should be calculated for the estimation of LV filling pressures. An average ratio ≤8 identifies patients with normal LV filling pressures, whereas a ratio ≥13 indicates increased LV filling pressures. When the ratio is between 9 and 13, other measurements are necessary.[18] An E/e' ratio ≥15 can predict a pulmonary capillary wedge pressure (PCWP) ≥15 mmHg with a sensitivity of about 86% and a specificity of 88%.[16] Based on these premises, bedside tissue Doppler echocardiography has been confirmed to be useful for the emergency diagnosis of acute HFPSF in patients with longstanding hypertension,[20] as well as in patients with inconclusive B-type natriuretic peptide (BNP) levels.[21]

However, some limitations should be considered before interpreting these values:
- E/e' and e' are influenced by the mitral annular side of measurement (septal e' is usually lower than lateral e' velocity), so a mean of the values obtained at the septum and the lateral wall is advisable
- E/e' allows only a semi-quantitative assessment of LV filling pressures. Therefore, values of ≥12, ≥15, and ≥13 for lateral, septal, and average E/e', respectively, can be proposed for predicting pulmonary capillary pressure greater than 15 mmHg in the presence of preserved LV systolic function, but the correlation is not necessarily linear
- The E/e' ratio is not accurate as an index of LV filling pressures in normal subjects,[22] in patients with heavy annular calcification, surgical rings, mitral valve disease,[23] basal LV wall motion abnormalities related to left bundle branch block, paced-rhythm, myocardial infarction, cardiopulmonary bypass,[24] and constrictive pericarditis.[25]

Hemodynamics

In addition to LV filling pressure estimation, echocardiographic Doppler techniques are the modality of choice for the noninvasive evaluation of hemodynamics.[26] A noninvasive hemodynamic assessment may be especially valuable in those AHF patients in whom the physical examination is limited or discordant with symptoms, and can be used to monitor the patients after initiating appropriate therapy.

Noninvasive hemodynamic variables that can be useful in AHF are mainly:
- Stroke volume (SV) and CO by pulsed-wave (PW) Doppler of the left ventricular outflow tract (LVOT). The rate of flow through an orifice is equal to the product of flow velocity and cross-sectional area (CSA) of that orifice. Two-dimensional and Doppler imaging can measure both CSA and flow velocity, providing a noninvasive measure of the rate of flow. It is essential to remember that a CSA must be measured

at the same point in space where the Doppler signal is sampled.

Accordingly, SV is calculated as:

$SV = CSA_{(LVOT)} \times TVI_{(LVOT)}$

where TVI is the time-velocity integral of flow measured by PW Doppler in 5-chamber apical view at LVOT.

Cross-sectional area of the respective site is obtained by the formula:

$CSA_{(LVOT)} = \pi \times radius^2$ (Since radius = Diameter/2)

$$CSA_{(LVOT)} = 3.14 \times \left(\frac{Diameter_{(LVOT)}^2}{2}\right)$$

$$CSA_{(LVOT)} = 3.14 \times \left(\frac{Diameter_{(LVOT)}^2}{4}\right)$$

$$CSA_{(LVOT)} = 0.785 \times Diameter_{(LVOT)}^2$$

A zoomed image should be used to visualize the LVOT, allowing a more precise measurement during early systole. The largest of 3–5 measurements should be taken because the inherent error of the tomographic plane is to underestimate the annulus diameter. When serial measurements of SV and CO are being performed to monitor patients' hemodynamics, the baseline annulus measurement can also be used for the repeated studies, since little change in annulus size occurs in adults over time.[27]

- Pulmonary capillary wedge pressure by the following regression equation:[28]
  $PCWP = [1.24 \times (E/e')] + 1.9$
  where E/e' should be calculated by using the average e'
- Right ventricular systolic pressure (RVSP), right atrial pressure (RAP) and pulmonary artery systolic pressures (PASP) from tricuspid valve velocity and inferior vena cava (IVC) dimension and collapsibility.

Right ventricular systolic pressure can be easily assessed in most subjects who present some degree of TR. The velocity recorded across the regurgitant jet corresponds to the right ventricular-right atrial gradient.

Right atrial pressure can be estimated from the end-expiratory diameter and respiratory changes of the IVC as follows:[29]

- Normal diameter (≤2.1 cm) and inspiratory collapse (>50%), RAP = 3 mmHg (range: 0–5 mmHg)
- Dilated IVC (≥2.1 cm) with reduced respiratory variation (<50%), RAP = 15 mmHg (range: 10–20 mm Hg)
- Inferior vena cava diameter and respiratory variation unfitting the previous paradigm, without resolving hepatic flow pattern (absence of prevalent systolic or diastolic flow component) or tricuspid E/e' wave ratio, RAP = 8 mmHg (range: 5–10 mmHg)
- Pulmonary artery systolic pressures can be obtained by adding RVSP to mean RAP

PERICARDIAL EFFUSION

The pericardium surrounds all four chambers of the heart and extends 1–2 cm up the great vessels, and around the pulmonary veins. Normally, there is a very small amount of fluid (5–10 mL) between the two pericardial layers—visceral and parietal. Pericardial effusion (PE) is an increased amount of fluid between the two layers, and can be visible as an echo-free space localized in the dependent zones (in case of free effusion). When the effusion is bigger, the echo-free space extends circumferentially around the heart, and its size depends on the amount of fluid in the pericardial sac.[30]

Echocardiography is the technique of choice for the diagnosis of PE. By echocardiography it is possible to discover from a very small amount of PE to a large PE, and also to guide pericardiocentesis in case of cardiac tamponade.

It is crucial, especially in acute conditions, to:

- Differentiate between pericardial effusion and pericardial fat. Isolated anterior (under the right ventricle) echo-free space may be due to mediastinal fat. This condition does not have acute pathological consequences, and can be differentiated from PE because of its higher density and "sparkling" appearance
- Differentiate between pericardial and pleural effusion (PE). Echo-free space located anteriorly from the descending thoracic aorta in parasternal long axis (PLAX) view is PE, whereas if there is echo-free space posteriorly from descending aorta it is usually PE (Fig. 1).

Pericardial effusion in AHF can be an additional sign of decompensation. In these circumstances, it rarely causes tamponade, but contributes to the poor systo-diastolic function.

VALVULAR DYSFUNCTION

Valvular dysfunction can be a cause and a consequence of AHF.

- Acute valvular heart disease can be the cause of AHF in a previously healthy patient (e.g., chordal rupture)
- Chronic valvular heart disease can be the cause of AHF in case of decompensation

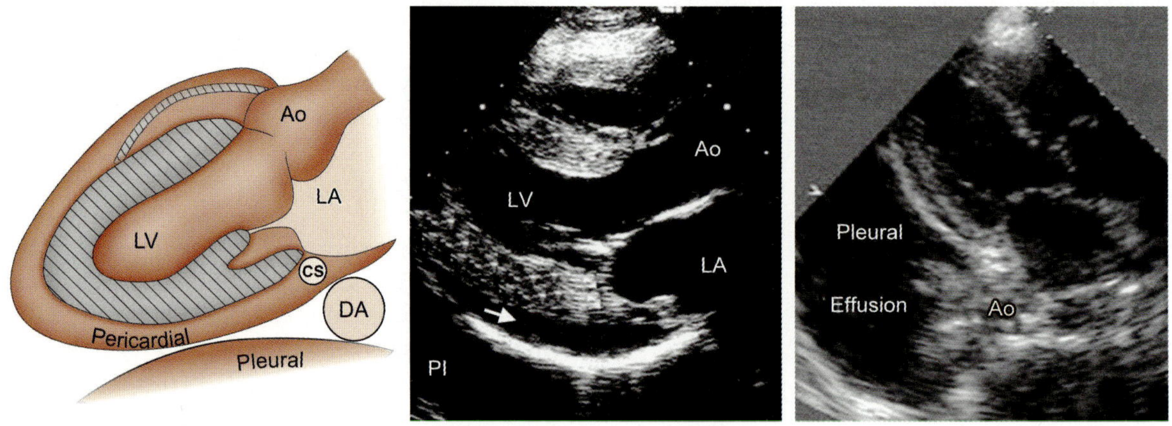

LV, left ventricle; LA, left atrium; DA, dopamine; Ao, aorta.

Fig. 1 Pleural and pericardial effusions can be differentiated by their position relative to the descending thoracic aorta (pleural is posteriorly and pericardial effusion is anteriorly located from the aorta). Moreover, pleural effusion is always visible beyond the atrioventricular junction

- Valvular heart disease can be the consequence of AHF, when functional mitral or TR occurs in the setting of dilated cardiomyopathy or ischemic cardiac disease.

ACUTE MITRAL REGURGITATION

When assessing mitral regurgitation (MR) in a patient with AHF, it is crucial to provide answers to the following key questions:

- Is MR severe?
- Is MR organic or functional?
- Is it acute MR or chronic decompensated MR?
- What is the cause of MR?
- Is MR amenable to surgical intervention?
- How urgent is surgical repair or replacement?

In acute severe MR, the left atrium (LA) and LV must face a sudden volume overload, which increases LV preload, allowing for a modest increase in total SV, but with reduced forward SV.[31] At the same time, the LA and LV cannot accommodate the regurgitant volume (RV), which results in pulmonary congestion. Therefore, the patient has both reduced forward output and pulmonary edema. In these cases, the hemodynamic overload often cannot be tolerated, and mitral valve (MV) repair or replacement must often be performed urgently. TTE allows evaluating the anatomy of the MV and helps providing semiquantitative information on lesion severity. However, inadequate imaging of the color flow jet may sometimes lead to underestimation of the severity. Thus, in the case of hyperdynamic LV systolic function in a patient with AHF, the suspicion of severe MR should always be raised.

Most frequent causes of acute MR are:

- Ischemic MR due to rupture of a papillary muscle. The rupture of the posterior papillary muscle (supplied by a single coronary artery) is the most common. A partial or complete flail of the mitral valve is observed at TTE, with a triangular mobile structure representing the head of the papillary muscle attached to the tip of the flail leaflet prolapsing into the LA during systole. Color Doppler usually shows an eccentric jet directed away from the defective leaflet (anteroseptally directed jet in case of posterior flail leaflet)
- Ischemic MR due to regional LV dysfunction with abnormal contraction of papillary muscle or underlying ventricular wall, with restricted valve leaflet motion and tenting of the mitral valve during systole
- Spontaneous chordal rupture (in degenerative or rheumatic mitral valve disease)
- Infective endocarditis, generally associated with visible vegetations, which can also involve other valves (especially the mitral valve)
- Blunt chest trauma, which can occasionally cause breakage of the chordae tendineae or papillary muscles
- Prosthetic valve dysfunction.

Color flow imaging, although not highly accurate, is the most common technique for assessing MR severity. The general assumption is that as MR severity increases, the size of the jet into the LA also increases. However, this relation presents a large range of variability, because in addition to regurgitation severity, the color flow display depends on many technical and hemodynamic factors. The detection of a large eccentric jet adhering, swirling and reaching the posterior wall of the LA is in favor of significant MR.

When feasible, the measurement of the vena contracta—the narrowest region of the regurgitant jet—is recommended to quantify MR. It can be used in both central and eccentric jets. When MR is severe, the vena contracta should be ≥7 mm (preferably in the PLAX view). In case of intermediate vena contracta values (3–7 mm), confirmation by a more quantitative method is advised.

The flow convergence method by evaluation of the proximal isovelocity surface area (PISA) is now by far the most recommended quantitative approach to evaluating the severity of MR. Although it will not always be feasible in emergencies, it is recommended especially in those patients where MR is not clearly severe. It can be used in both central and eccentric jets. An effective regurgitant orifice area (EROA) ≥40 mm^2 or an RV ≥60 mL indicates severe organic MR. In functional ischemic MR, an EROA ≥20 mm^2 or an RV ≥30 mL identifies a subset of patients at increased risk of cardiovascular events.[32]

Because transesophageal echocardiography can more accurately assess the color flow jet,[33] it should be performed if mitral valve morphology and regurgitant severity are still in question after TTE. Transesophageal echocardiography can also be helpful in demonstrating the anatomic cause of acute severe MR and directing successful surgical repair.[34]

ACUTE AORTIC REGURGITATION

Similarly to MR, when assessing aortic regurgitation (AR) in a patient with AHF, it is crucial to provide answers to the following key questions:

- Is AR severe?
- Is AR organic or consequent to aortic root dilation?
- Is it acute AR or chronic decompensated AR?
- What is the cause of AR?
- Is AR amenable to surgical intervention?
- How urgent is surgical replacement?

In acute severe AR a sudden large RV is imposed on an LV of normal size that has not had time to accommodate the volume overload. With an abrupt increase in end-diastolic volume, LV end-diastolic, and LA pressures may increase rapidly and dramatically, resulting in pulmonary congestion and concomitant decrease in forward SV. Echocardiography is indispensable in confirming the presence and severity of the regurgitation, determining its cause and estimating the degree of pulmonary hypertension.

Most frequent causes of acute AR are:

- Infective endocarditis, generally associated with visible vegetations, that can involve also other valves (especially the mitral valve)
- Blunt chest trauma
- Aortic root dissection, which is a surgical emergency that requires prompt identification and management. Transesophageal echocardiography is indicated when aortic dissection is suspected.[35-37] In those settings when transesophageal echocardiography is not readily available, computed tomographic imaging or magnetic resonance imaging should be performed.[35,36,38] A thorough evaluation of the entire aorta is advisable
- Prosthetic valve dysfunction.

Color flow Doppler provides a qualitative approach to evaluating AR severity. The parasternal views are preferred for visualizing the regurgitant jet into the LV in diastole, due to better axial resolution. The color jet area is weakly correlated with the degree of AR, since it is affected by the aortic to LV diastolic pressure gradient and LV compliance, so it should only be used for a visual assessment of AR.[39]

The vena contracta—the smallest flow diameter at the level of the aortic valve in the LVOT, immediately below the flow convergence region—provides a semiquantitative estimation of the size of the EROA. A vena contracta greater than 6 mm indicates severe AR. Similarly to MR, the vena contracta can often be obtained in eccentric jet. In case of multiple jets, the respective values of vena contracta width are not additive; in case of intermediate values (3–6 mm), confirmation by a more quantitative method, when feasible, is needed.[39]

Diastolic flow reversal in the descending aorta is a qualitative approach to diagnosing severe AR. The flow reversal is best imaged by suprasternal view and PW Doppler, by placing the sample volume distal to the origin of the left subclavian artery. The Doppler filter should be decreased to allow detection of low velocities (<10 cm/s). With milder degrees of regurgitation, there is a brief reversal of flow limited to early diastole. As the degree of the regurgitation increases, the duration and velocity of the reversal flow increases and becomes sustained throughout diastole at velocities exceeding 20 cm/s in severe AR. Significant holodiastolic reversal in the abdominal aorta is also a sensitive sign of severe AR.[39]

The flow convergence method has been less extensively performed in AR than in MR,[40,41] due to low feasibility. An EROA ≥30 mm^2 or an RV ≥60 mL indicates severe AR. In eccentric AR jets, it is recommended to use the parasternal long-axis view.

The rate of deceleration of the diastolic AR jet and the derived pressure-half time (PHT) is related to the pressure difference between the aorta and the LV during diastole, reflecting both the degree of regurgitation and the ventricular end-diastolic pressures. As the degree of AR increases, the aortic diastolic pressure decreases and the LV end-diastolic pressure increases.[42] A PHT less than 200 ms is consistent with severe AR. It is best obtained from the apical 5-chamber view.

DECOMPENSATED CHRONIC VALVULAR HEART DISEASE

Patients with chronic valvular heart disease may survive in a compensated phase for a long time, until a concomitant alteration of the cardiopulmonary homeostasis leads to rapid decompensation, such as in hypertensive crisis, sodium or volume overload, decreased compliance with medical therapy, anemia, exacerbation of chronic obstructive pulmonary disease, inflammation, or infection.

In presence of a heavily calcified mitral valve, mitral stenosis (MS) should always be suspected. Severe MS is characterized at TTE by a valve area less than 1.0 cm^2, mean gradient greater than 10 mmHg, or PASP greater than 50 mmHg.[34-43]

In decompensated chronic MR, the forward SV decreases and the LA pressure increases significantly. However, the LV EF may still be in the low normal range despite significant muscle dysfunction. In these patients, TTE generally show LA dilation in response to chronic volume and pressure overload, with atrial fibrillation being relatively common when indexed LA volume is greater than 40 mL/m^2. A normal-sized LA is not generally associated with significant MR unless it is acute. The presence of TR permits the estimation of PASP, which is generally high. In case of functional MR due to non-ischemic conditions, the LV is generally dilated and with significantly impaired systolic dysfunction, the regurgitant jet is typically central, following global LV dilation and remodeling, with displacement of both anterolateral and posteromedial papillary muscles. In case of functional MR due to ischemic conditions, the LV can be dilated but may also show normal dimensions with regional wall motion abnormalities. Asymmetric tethering with eccentric jet may occur.

Decompensated chronic aortic stenosis (AS) is a relatively frequent cause of AHF in the elderly population, especially with concomitant systolic dysfunction. Severe hypertension is a common precipitating factor. The valve appears severely calcified with extensive thickening, increased echogenicity and a prominent acoustic shadow.

The primary hemodynamic parameters recommended to evaluate AS severity are:

- Aortic stenosis jet maximum velocity and mean transaortic gradient measured by continuous wave (CW) Doppler.

  A smooth velocity curve with a dense outer edge should be recorded. Usually, three beats are averaged in sinus rhythm, or more with irregular rhythms. Special care must be taken to avoid postextrasystolic beats
- Valve area by continuity equation.

  When LV systolic dysfunction coexists with severe AS, the AS velocity and gradient may be low, despite a small valve area, a condition termed "low-flow low-gradient AS". In these patients, calculation of the stenotic orifice area or aortic valve area (AVA) is helpful because it is flow-independent. AVA is calculated based on the continuity-equation, according to the following formula:

$$AVA = \frac{Area_{LVOT} \times VTI_{LVOT}}{VTI_{AV}}$$

which results in:

$$AVA = \frac{0.785 \times (diameter_{LVOT})^2 \times VTI_{LVOT}}{VTI_{AV}}$$

Calculation of continuity-equation valve area requires three measurements:

1. Aortic valve TVI by CW Doppler in 5-chamber apical view.
2. Left ventricular outflow tract time-velocity integral of flow by PW Doppler in 5-chamber apical view.
3. Left ventricular outflow tract diameter from parasternal long axis view (zoomed image).

Another approach to reducing error related to LVOT diameter measurements is removing CSA from the simplified continuity equation. This dimensionless ratio expresses the size of the valvular effective area as a proportion of the CSA of the LVOT and can be performed by using either velocity time integral (VTI) or jet maximum velocities.

$$VTI\ ratio = \frac{VTI_{LVOT}}{VTI_{AV}}$$

or

$$\text{Velocity ratio} = \frac{\text{Vel max}_{LVOT}}{\text{Velmax}_{AV}}$$

In the absence of valve stenosis, the ratio approaches 1, with smaller numbers indicating more severe stenosis. Severe stenosis is present when the ratio is 0.25 or less, corresponding to a valve area 25% of normal.[44]

- Aortic valve area planimetry.

Multiple studies have evaluated the method of measuring anatomic AVA by direct visualization of the valvular orifice.[45] AVA planimetry may be an acceptable alternative when Doppler estimation of flow velocities is unreliable. However, planimetry may be inaccurate when valve calcification causes shadows or reverberations limiting identification of the orifice.

THE RIGHT VENTRICLE

The presence of right ventricular (RV) failure in patients with AHF is often under-recognized,[46] and the actual prevalence of RV failure resulting from LV failure is unknown. When performing an echocardiogram to an AHF patient at admission, the right heart should always be addressed.

The questions to be answered are:

- Is the RV dilated and is RV systolic function normal?
- Is there a specific right heart abnormality?
- Is there pulmonary hypertension?

In patients with LV dysfunction, pulmonary venous hypertension leads to an increase in RV afterload, which may precipitate RV failure. In these patients, RV dysfunction is strongly associated with the severity of LV diastolic dysfunction and increased PASP, and can predict decreased survival.[47] Functional TR is very frequent, and PASP values can be useful for hemodynamic monitoring after institution of adequate therapy. In the case of abnormal RV function without evidence of LV dysfunction or valvular heart disease in a patient admitted with shortness of breath, the suspicion of pulmonary embolism should be raised. In a patient with chest pain and suspected acute coronary syndrome, a dysfunctional RV can be concomitant to inferior ischemia/infarction. Recognition of this is crucial, since in presence of RV dysfunction, medical therapy should not include vasodilators, and diuretics should be administered with caution.

Arrhythmogenic right ventricular dysplasia (ARVD) is a rare cause of isolated RV dysfunction. This condition is characterized by thinning and hypokinesis of the RV free wall with regional or, in cases of extensive dysplasia, global systolic dysfunction.

Techniques that can be employed at bedside to evaluate right ventricular dysfunction include calculation of tricuspid annular plane systolic excursion (TAPSE) and tricuspid systolic annular TDI velocity.[48,49] Serial assessment of RV function can be obtained from the calculation of right ventricular fractional area change (FAC), obtained by the end-diastolic and end-systolic RV areas (FAC = end-diastolic area - end-systolic area/end-diastolic area). Echocardiographic assessment of RV function may help to risk-stratify patients with AHF: a TDI velocity less than 10.8 cm/sec provides additional prognostic information, even in patients with extremely dilated left ventricles.[49]

PULMONARY CONGESTION

In the last few years, lung ultrasound (LUS) has been proposed for the evaluation of pulmonary congestion in patients with HF, through the assessment of B-lines. B-lines are sonographic reverberation artifacts, which originate from water-thickened pulmonary interlobular septa. Bilateral multiple B-lines are present in pulmonary congestion, and may help in the management of AHF by detection, semiquantification and monitoring of extravascular lung water.[50]

B-lines are useful for the differential diagnosis of cardiogenic versus non-cardiogenic dyspnea,[51] with accuracy not significantly inferior to natriuretic peptides.[52-54] They could be a plausible alternative in acute settings where natriuretic peptide analysis is not readily available, or when natriuretic peptide levels are in the "gray zone". Their negative predictive value to exclude the presence of pulmonary edema is particularly high.[52-54] In less than 10 years, the proposal to use B-lines to evaluate pulmonary congestion has moved from a research setting to the clinical arena, and it is now entering recommendation papers.[55,56]

B-line assessment has the advantages of being rapid, quick to learn, easy to perform, inexpensive, and repeatable at the bedside. The examination can be performed with any type of echographic platform, from fully equipped machines to pocket-size devices.[57] Convex or micro-convex probes are the most appropriate, but cardiac and linear probes can also be successfully employed. Although some specific methods have been proposed to scan the lung,[58,59] in emergency situations a quick evaluation of the dependent zones (posterior chest bases or axillary lines for bedridden patients), just by

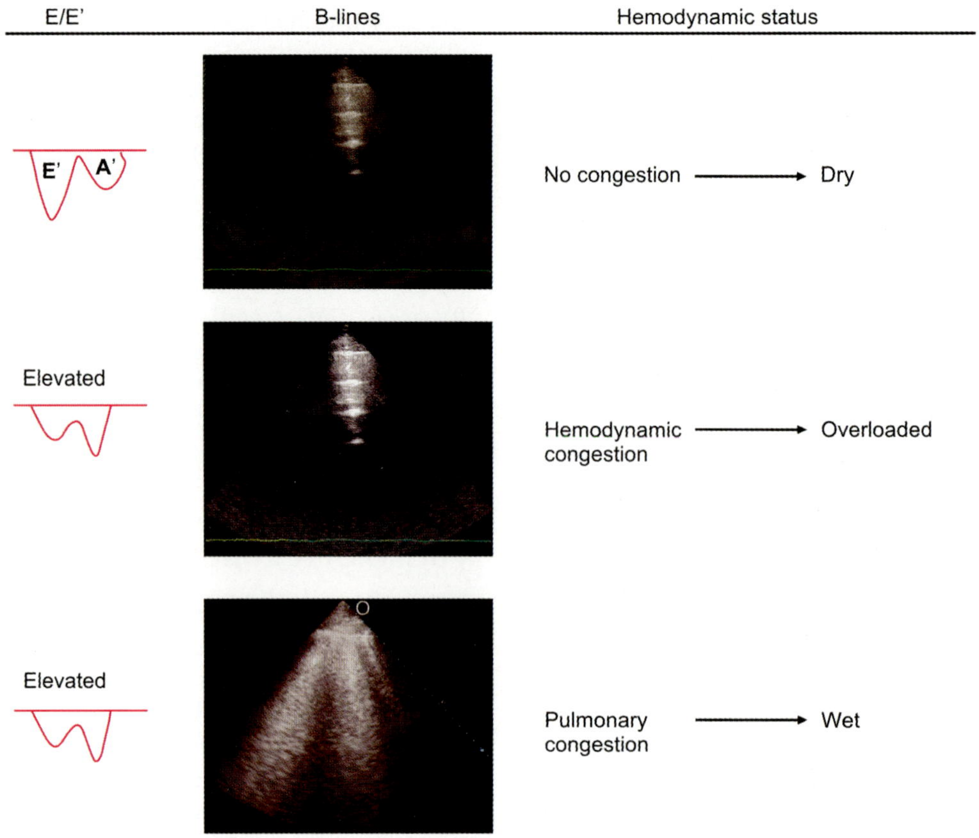

Fig. 2 B-lines may differentiate "hemodynamic congestion" (increased left ventricular filing pressures) from "pulmonary congestion" (pulmonary interstitial edema)[50]

laying the probe along the intercostal spaces, is advisable. An important limitation of B-lines is the lack of specificity. B-lines are a sign of pulmonary interstitial syndrome, so they are a very sensitive but not specific sign of cardiogenic pulmonary edema. As with most biomarkers, B-lines should be evaluated within the clinical context and integrated with the patient's history.[50]

In HF patients, LUS may also enable the detection of PE, the most established application of LUS.[60] The effusion should first be sought in dependent zones. In presence of a radiopacity on chest X-ray, LUS is able to better differentiate PE from atelectasis, consolidations, masses or an elevated hemidiaphragm, and can be repeated serially at the bedside. LUS has better sensitivity and reliability than bedside chest X-ray for the diagnosis of PE,[61] and may detect the effusion, evaluate its extension, and indicate the appropriate area for an eventual thoracentesis.

The addition of LUS to echocardiography, in an integrated cardiopulmonary ultrasound evaluation, provides additional insight into patients with AHF, allowing the distinction between hemodynamic and pulmonary congestion.[62] Hemodynamic congestion, i.e. increased left ventricular filling pressure, can be represented by noninvasive PCWP estimation. The next step in the congestion cascade, characterized by redistribution of excess fluid within the lungs—"pulmonary congestion"—can be visualized by sonographic B-lines. This approach builds on Forrester's classification of "wet" and "dry" patients,[63] to further distinguish between "dry" (no significantly increased PCWP, no significant B-lines), "congested" (increased PCWP, no significant B-lines) and "wet" (increased PCWP and multiple bilateral B-lines) patients (Fig. 2). Differentiation into "cold" (low CO) and "warm" (normal CO) patients can be further added to these three categories.

FOLLOW-UP AND DISCHARGE

It can be useful to noninvasively monitor the patient by ultrasound during the hospital stay. This allows evaluation of the response to therapies, potentially guiding further interventions. A focused TTE can be repeated in-hospital to assess whether CO has increased, whether E/e' and PASP have decreased, and if functional mitral and tricuspidal regurgitation are less severe. Pericardial and PE can also show significant changes, and the number of B-lines as a sign of pulmonary congestion is known to decrease very rapidly after diuretic therapy,[58,59] or when the patient has undergone hemodialysis.[64,65]

Some of these parameters have also shown prognostic value when assessed at discharge. Left ventricular ejection fraction (LVEF) is the main index for predicting the prognosis in patients with HF.[66] Several studies have shown that E/e' is also an independent prognostic predictor of major adverse cardiac events in patients hospitalized with AHF,[67] both alone and in combination with EF.[68] On the right side, PASP and TAPSE have recently proved to improve risk stratification in patients with HF,[69] and bedside evaluation of IVC dimensions and collapsibility as a sign of RAP identifies patients admitted with AHF who are more likely to be readmitted to the hospital.[70]

CONCLUSION

Being readily available at the bedside, echocardiography is the imaging technique of choice in patients with AHF. The critical information about left and right ventricular morphology and function, valvular function, pericardium and noninvasive hemodynamics can be crucial to establish, the correct etiology of the acute decompensation, and to start appropriate treatment. More recently, LUS has also emerged as a simple sonographic method to quickly assess extravascular lung water, thus helping with the differential diagnosis of acute dyspnea, and supporting the physician to titrate medical therapy in acute patients.

Physicians and sonographers performing echocardiography in acute settings must be aware of the many challenges they may encounter: images are often suboptimal due to lack of time and patient's compliance, with limited time for consultations with colleagues: in these circumstances medical errors are more likely to occur and can lead to serious consequences. An accurate knowledge and recognition of echocardiography's advantages and limitations in specific clinical situations is thus essential to avoid potentially catastrophic diagnostic errors.

REFERENCES

1. Popescu BA, Andrade MJ, Badano LP, et al. European Association of Echocardiography recommendations for training, competence, and quality improvement in echocardiography. Eur J Echocardiogr. 2009;10(8): 893-905.
2. Jessup M, Abraham WT, Casey DE, et al. 2009 focused update: ACCF/AHA Guidelines for the Diagnosis and Management of Heart Failure in Adults: a report of the American College of Cardiology Foundation/American Heart Association Task Force on Practice Guidelines: developed in collaboration with the International Society for Heart and Lung Transplantation. Circulation. 2009;119(14):1977-2016.
3. Neskovic AN, Hagendorff A, Lancellotti P, et al. Emergency echocardiography: the European Association of Cardiovascular Imaging recommendations. Eur Heart J Cardiovasc Imaging. 2013;14(1):1-11.
4. Otto C. Textbook of Clinical Echocardiography, 4th edition. Elsevier; 2009.
5. Lang RM, Bierig M, Devereux RB, et al. Recommendations for chamber quantification: a report from the American Society of Echocardiography's Guidelines and Standards Committee and the Chamber Quantification Writing Group, developed in conjunction with the European Association of Echocardiography. J Am Soc Echocardiogr. 2005;18(12):1440-63.
6. Steg PG, Joubin L, McCord J, et al. B-type natriuretic peptide and echocardiographic determination of ejection fraction in the diagnosis of congestive heart failure in patients with acute dyspnea. Chest. 2005;128(1):21-9.
7. Logeart D, Saudubray C, Beyne P, et al. Comparative value of Doppler echocardiography and B-type natriuretic peptide assay in the etiologic diagnosis of acute dyspnea. J Am Coll Cardiol. 2002;40(10):1794-800.
8. Nagueh SF, Appleton CP, Gillebert TC, et al. Recommendations for the evaluation of left ventricular diastolic function by echocardiography. Eur J Echocardiogr. 2009;10(2):165-93.
9. Ommen SR, Nishimura RA, Appleton CP, et al. Clinical utility of Doppler echocardiography and tissue Doppler imaging in the estimation of left ventricular filling pressures: a comparative simultaneous Doppler-catheterization study. Circulation. 2000;102(15):1788-94.
10. Nagueh SF, Sun H, Kopelen HA, et al. Hemodynamic determinants of the mitral annulus diastolic velocities by tissue Doppler. J Am Coll Cardiol. 2001;37(1):278-85.
11. Arques S. Usefulness of combined Doppler indexes in predicting left ventricular filling pressures in patients with acute heart failure. Am J Cardiol. 2003;92(5):649-50.
12. Nagueh SF, Mikati I, Kopelen HA, et al. Doppler estimation of left ventricular filling pressure in sinus tachycardia. A new application of tissue Doppler imaging. Circulation. 1998;98(16):1644-50.
13. Nagueh SF, Lakkis NM, Midleton KJ, et al. Doppler estimation of left ventricular filling pressures in patients with hypertrophic cardiomyopathy. Circulation. 1999;99(2):254-61.
14. Sundereswaran L, Nagueh SF, Vardan S, et al. Estimation of left and right ventricular filling pressures after heart transplantation by tissue Doppler imaging. Am J Cardiol. 1998;82(3):352-7.
15. Bouhemad B, Nicolas-Robin A, Benois A, et al. Echocardiographic Doppler assessment of pulmonary capillary pressure in surgical patients with postoperative circulatory shock and acute lung injury. Anesthesiology. 2003;98(5):1091-100.
16. Dokainish H, Zoghbi WA, Lakkis NM, et al. Optimal noninvasive assessment of left ventricular filling pressures. A comparison of tissue Doppler echocardiography and B-type natriuretic peptide in patients with pulmonary artery catheters. Circulation. 2004;109(20):2432-9.
17. Arques S, Roux E, Luccioni R. Current clinical applications of spectral tissue Doppler echocardiography (E/E' ratio) as a noninvasive surrogate

for left ventricular diastolic pressures in the diagnosis of heart failure with preserved left ventricular systolic function. Cardiovasc Ultrasound. 2007;5:16.
18. Nagueh SF, Appleton CP, Gillebert TC, et al. Recommendations for the evaluation of left ventricular diastolic function by echocardiography. Eur J Echocardiogr. 2009;10(2):165-93.
19. Rivas-Gotz C, Manolios M, Thohan V, et al. Impact of left ventricular ejection fraction on estimation of left ventricular filling pressures using tissue Doppler and flow propagation velocity. Am J Cardiol. 2003;91(6):780-4.
20. Arques S, Roux E, Sbragia P, et al. Comparative accuracy of color M-mode and tissue Doppler echocardiography in the emergency diagnosis of congestive heart failure in chronic hypertensive patients with normal left ventricular ejection fraction. Am J Cardiol. 2005;96(10):1456-9.
21. Huang CH, Tsai MS, Hsieh CC, et al. Diagnostic accuracy of tissue Doppler echocardiography for patients with acute heart failure. Heart. 2006;92(12):1790-4.
22. Firstenberg MS, Levine BD, Garcia MJ, et al. Relationship of echocardiographic indices to pulmonary capillary wedge pressures in healthy volunteers. J Am Coll Cardiol. 2000;36(5):1664-9.
23. Diwan A, McCulloch M, Lawrie GM, et al. Doppler estimation of left ventricular filling pressures in patients with mitral valve disease. Circulation. 2005;111(24):3281-9.
24. D'Souza KA, Mooney DJ, Russell AE, et al. Abnormal septal motion affects early diastolic velocities at the septal and lateral mitral annulus, and impacts on estimation of the pulmonary capillary wedge pressure. J Am Soc Echocardiogr. 2005;18(5):445-53.
25. Ha JW, Oh JK, Ling LH, et al. Annulus paradoxus: transmitral flow velocity to mitral annular velocity ratio is inversely proportional to pulmonary capillary wedge pressure in patients with constrictive pericarditis. Circulation. 2001;104(9):976-8.
26. Nohria A, Mielniczuk LM, Stevenson LW. Evaluation and monitoring of patients with acute heart failure syndromes. Am J Cardiol. 2005; 96(6A):32G-40G.
27. Quiñones MA, Otto CM, Stoddard M, et al. Recommendations for quantification of Doppler echocardiography: a report from the Doppler Quantification Task Force of the Nomenclature and Standards Committee of the American Society of Echocardiography. J Am Soc Echocardiogr. 2002;15(2):167-84.
28. Nagueh SF, Middleton KJ, Kopelen HA, et al. Doppler tissue imaging: a noninvasive technique for evaluation of left ventricular relaxation and estimation of filling pressures. J Am Coll Cardiol.1997;30(6):1527-33.
29. Rudski LG, Lai WW, Afilalo J, et al. Guidelines for the echocardiographic assessment of the right heart in adults: a report from the American Society of Echocardiography endorsed by the European Association of Echocardiography, a registered branch of the European Society of Cardiology, and the Canadian Society of Echocardiography. J Am Soc Echocardiogr. 2010;23(7):685-713.
30. Galiuto L, Badano L, Fox K, Sicari R, Zamorano JL (Eds). The EAE Textbook of Echocardiography, 1st edition. New York, USA: Oxford University Press; 2011.
31. Carabello BA. Mitral regurgitation: basic pathophysiologic principles, part 1. Mod Concepts Cardiovasc Dis. 1988;57:53-8.
32. Lancellotti P, Moura L, Pierard LA, et al. European Association of Echocardiography recommendations for the assessment of valvular regurgitation. Part 2: mitral and tricuspid regurgitation (native valve disease). Eur J Echocardiogr. 2010;11(4):307-32.
33. Castello R, Fagan L, Lenzen P, et al. Comparison of transthoracic and transesophageal echocardiography for assessment of left-sided valvular regurgitation. Am J Cardiol. 1991;68(17):1677-80.
34. Bonow RO, Carabello BA, Chatterjee K, et al. 2008 focused update incorporated into the ACC/AHA 2006 guidelines for the management of patients with valvular heart disease: a report of the American College of Cardiology/American Heart Association Task Force on Practice Guidelines (Writing Committee to revise the 1998 guidelines for the management of patients with valvular heart disease). Endorsed by the Society of Cardiovascular Anesthesiologists, Society for Cardiovascular Angiography and Interventions, and Society of Thoracic Surgeons. J Am Coll Cardiol. 2008;52(13):e1-142.
35. Cigarroa JE, Isselbacher EM, DeSanctis RW, et al. Diagnostic imaging in the evaluation of suspected aortic dissection. Old standards and new directions. N Engl J Med. 1993;328(1):35-43.
36. Nienaber CA, von Kodolitsch Y, Nicolas V, et al. The diagnosis of thoracic aortic dissection by noninvasive imaging procedures. N Engl J Med. 1993;328(1):1-9.
37. Smith MD, Cassidy JM, Souther S, et al. Transesophageal echocardiography in the diagnosis of traumatic rupture of the aorta. N Engl J Med. 1995;332(6):356-62.
38. Rahimtoola SH. Recognition and management of acute aortic regurgitation. Heart Dis Stroke. 1993;2(3):217-21.
39. Lancellotti P, Tribouilloy C, Hagendorff A, et al. European Association of Echocardiography recommendations for the assessment of valvular regurgitation. Part 1: aortic and pulmonary regurgitation (native valve disease). Eur J Echocardiogr. 2010;11(3):223-44.
40. Pouleur AC, le Polain de Waroux JB, Goffinet C, et al. Accuracy of the flow convergence method for quantification of aortic regurgitation in patients with central versus eccentric jets. Am J Cardiol. 2008;102(4):475-80.
41. Detaint D, Messika-Zeitoun D, Maalouf J, et al. Quantitative echocardiographic determinants of clinical outcome in asymptomatic patients with aortic regurgitation: a prospective study. JACC Cardiovasc Imaging. 2008;1(1):1-11.
42. Samstad SO, Hegrenaes L, Skjaerpe T, et al. Half time of the diastolic aortoventricular pressure difference by continuous wave Doppler ultrasound: a measure of the severity of aortic regurgitation? Br Heart J. 1989;61(4):336-43.
43. Baumgartner H, Hung J, Bermejo J, et al. Echocardiographic assessment of valve stenosis: EAE/ASE recommendations for clinical practice. Eur J Echocardiogr. 2009;10(1):1-25.
44. Oh JK, Taliercio CP, Holmes DR, et al. (Prediction of the severity of aortic stenosis by Doppler aortic valve area determination: prospective Doppler-catheterization correlation in 100 patients. J Am Coll Cardiol. 1988;11(6):1227-34.
45. Okura H, Yoshida K, Hozumi T, et al. Planimetry and transthoracic two-dimensional echocardiography in noninvasive assessment of aortic valve area in patients with valvular aortic stenosis. J Am Coll Cardiol. 1997;30(3):753-9.
46. Zakir RM, Al-Dehneh A, Maher J, et al. Right ventricular failure in patients with preserved ejection fraction and diastolic dysfunction: an underrecognized clinical entity. Congest Heart Fail. 2007;13(3):164-9.
47. Berkowitz R, Alhaj E, Manchikalapudi RB, et al. Determinants of right ventricular failure in patients admitted with acute left heart failure. Congest Heart Fail. 2010;16(6):243-8.
48. Ghio S, Recusani F, Klersy C, et al. Prognostic usefulness of the tricuspid annular plane systolic excursion in patients with congestive heart failure secondary to idiopathic or ischemic dilated cardiomyopathy. Am J Cardiol. 2000;85(7):837-42.
49. Meluzin J, Spinarova L, Dusek L, et al. Prognostic importance of the right ventricular function assessed by Doppler tissue imaging. Eur J Echocardiogr. 2003;4(4):262-71.

50. Gargani L. Lung ultrasound: a new tool for the cardiologist. Cardiovasc Ultrasound. 2011;9:6.
51. Lichtenstein D, Meziere G. A lung ultrasound sign allowing bedside distinction between pulmonary edema and COPD: the comet-tail artifact. Intensive Care Med. 1998;24(12):1331-4.
52. Gargani L, Frassi F, Soldati G, et al.(Ultrasound lung comets for the differential diagnosis of acute cardiogenic dyspnoea: a comparison with natriuretic peptides. Eur J Heart Fail. 2008;10(1):70-7.
53. Liteplo AS, Marill KA, Villen T, et al. Emergency thoracic ultrasound in the differentiation of the etiology of shortness of breath (ETUDES): sonographic B-lines and N-terminal pro-brain-type natriuretic peptide in diagnosing congestive heart failure. Acad Emerg Med. 2009;16(3): 201-10.
54. Prosen G, Klemen P, Štrnad M, et al. Combination of lung ultrasound (a comet-tail sign) and N-terminal pro-brain natriuretic peptide in differentiating acute heart failure from chronic obstructive pulmonary disease and asthma as cause of acute dyspnea in prehospital emergency setting. Crit Care. 2011;15(2):R114.
55. Gheorghiade M, Follath F, Ponikowski P, et al. Assessing and grading congestion in acute heart failure: a scientific statement from the acute heart failure committee of the heart failure association of the European Society of Cardiology and endorsed by the European Society of Intensive Care Medicine. Eur J Heart Fail. 2010;12(5):423-33.
56. Volpicelli G, Elbarbary M, Blaivas M, et al. International evidence-based recommendations for point-of-care lung ultrasound. Intensive Care Med. 2012;38(4):577-91.
57. Bedetti G, Gargani L, Corbisiero A, et al. Evaluation of ultrasound lung comets by hand-held echocardiography. Cardiovasc Ultrasound. 2006; 4:34.
58. Picano E, Frassi F, Agricola E, et al. Ultrasound lung comets: a clinically useful sign of extravascular lung water. J Am Soc Echocardiogr. 2006; 19(3):356-63.
59. Volpicelli G, Mussa A, Garofalo G, et al. Bedside lung ultrasound in the assessment of alveolar-interstitial syndrome. Am J Emerg Med. 2006;24(6):689-96.
60. Longo DL, Fauci AS, Kasper DL, et al. Harrison's Principles of Internal Medicine, 18th edition. New York, USA: McGraw-Hill; 2011.
61. Eibenberger KL, Dock WI, Ammann ME, et al: Quantification of pleural effusions: sonography versus radiography. Radiology. 1994;191(3):681-4.
62. Gheorghiade M, Filippatos G, De Luca L, et al. Congestion in acute heart failure syndromes: an essential target of evaluation and treatment. Am J Med. 2006;119(12 Suppl 1):S3-10.
63. Forrester JS, Diamond GA, Swan HJ. Correlative classification of clinical and hemodynamic function after acute myocardial infarction. Am J Cardiol. 1977;39(2):137-45.
64. Noble VE, Murray AF, Capp R, et al. Ultrasound assessment for extravascular lung water in patients undergoing hemodialysis. Time course for resolution. Chest. 2009;135(6):1433-9.
65. Mallamaci F, Benedetto FA, Tripepi R, et al. Detection of pulmonary congestion by chest ultrasound in dialysis patients. JACC Cardiovasc Imaging. 2010;3(6):586-94.
66. Pfeffer MA, Braunwald E. Ventricular remodeling after myocardial infarction. Experimental observations and clinical implications. Circulation. 1990;81(4):1161-72.
67. Ho SJ, Feng AN, Lee LN, et al. Predictive value of predischarge spectral tissue Doppler echocardiography and n-terminal pro-B-type natriuretic peptide in patients hospitalized with acute heart failure. Echocardiography. 2011;28(3):303-10.
68. Hirata K, Hyodo E, Hozumi T, et al. Usefulness of a combination of systolic function by left ventricular ejection fraction and diastolic function by E/E' to predict prognosis in patients with heart failure. Am J Cardiol. 2009;103(9):1275-9.
69. Ghio S, Temporelli PL, Klersy C, et al. Prognostic relevance of a non-invasive evaluation of right ventricular function and pulmonary artery pressure in patients with chronic heart failure. Eur J Heart Fail. 2013;15(4):408-14.
70. Goonewardena SN, Gemignani A, Ronan A, et al. Comparison of hand-carried ultrasound assessment of the inferior vena cava and N-terminal pro-brain natriuretic peptide for predicting readmission after hospitalization for acute decompensated heart failure. JACC Cardiovasc Imaging. 2008;1(5):595-601.

Chapter 8

Use of Bioelectrical Impedance Vector Analysis in the Dyspneic Patient

Salvatore D Somma, Silvia Navarin

ABSTRACT

Dyspnea is one of the most frequent symptoms of admission in the emergency department (ED) but it still represents a challenge for physicians in several conditions.

By now, dyspnea was classified in cardiogenic or non-cardiogenic on the base of history, physical examination, electrocardiogram, chest X-ray and on the basis of innovative methods such as natriuretic peptides and lung ultrasound, whose diagnostic accuracy was proved to be improved by the combination with bioelectrical impedance vector analysis (BIVA) measurements.

The BIVA method assesses the opposition of body tissues to the flow of an alternating current, called bioelectrical impedance, administered by four surface electrodes, two on the wrist and two on the ipsilateral ankle. The results are obtained in 30 seconds and they can be displayed in two ways, as a vector or as a single number expressed in percentage.

Due to its characteristics of manageability, the use of BIVA for assessing hydration status is spreading outside from its original application in the nephrology to all departments, and especially to the emergency rooms, where BIVA has found its role in the dyspnea differential diagnosis. Moreover, in several trials it was showed BIVA predictive value, independently from other variables.

Despite further trials about BIVA measurements in patients with shortness of breath are required to standardize its diagnostic and prognostic role, BIVA technique, as a rapid, noninvasive and accurate method, has already proved its additive value for the management of dyspneic patients.

INTRODUCTION

The bioelectrical impedance vector analysis (BIVA) method measures the opposition of body tissues to the flow of an alternating current of 300 μA, called bioelectrical impedance, administered by four surface electrodes at an operating frequency of 50 kHz. This bioelectrical impedance (Z) consists of two components: (1) resistance (Rz) and (2) reactance (Xc).[1,2] In order to simplify the measurement, the human body is approximated as a sum of five interconnected cylinders that act as conductors in parallel and, while the resistance (Rz) is inversely related with the amount of total body water, the reactance is considered proportional to body mass.[3,4] BIVA device is handy and portable and it can be applied in every critical setting, such as the emergency department (ED), because it does not require to be plugged and it can be easily carried at the patient's bedside (Fig. 1A). Four cutaneous electrodes, two on the wrist and two on the ipsilateral ankle, are applied with an inter-electrodes distance of at least 5 cm to prevent electrodes interaction (Fig. 1B). The subject must be supine and avoid skin contacts with the trunk or with the stretcher[3] (Fig. 1C). Free fluid in thorax and abdomen, as pleural effusion, ascites, and urine does not influence BIVA assessment.[5]

The bioelectrical impedance is measured in 30 seconds and the results can be displayed in two ways, as a vector or as a single number expressed in percentage in a scale, called hydrograph (or hydrogram). The first method represents the bivariate vector with its two

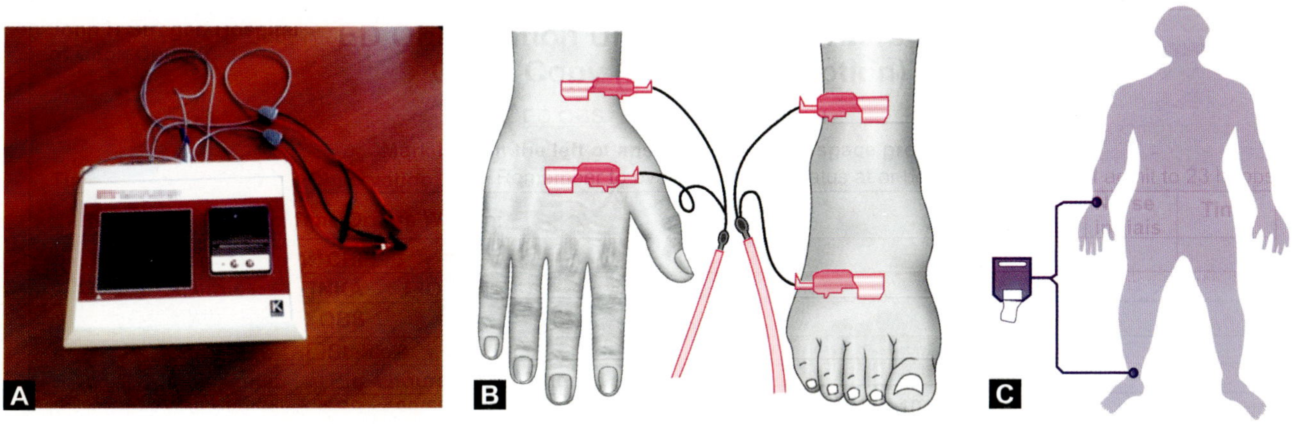

Fig. 1 **A,** Bioelectrical impedance vector analysis device; **B,** Electrodes' application; and **C,** Subject's position

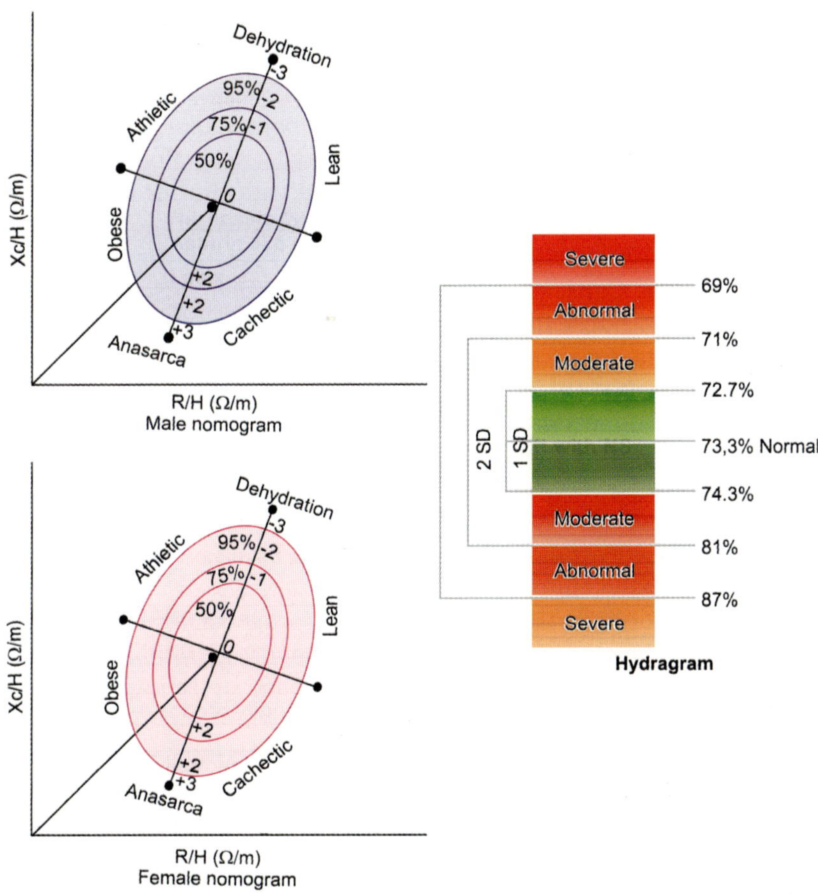

Fig. 2 Bioelectrical impedance vector analysis results design

components (Rz and Xc), adjusted by the patient's height, in a nomogram that is different for men and women.[6] In the same coordinate system, three tolerance ellipses are plotted and they correspond to the 50th, 75th, and 95th vector percentile of the healthy reference population.[1] The major axis of this tolerance ellipses represents hydration status while the minor axis reflects tissue mass. In the second method the 50th percentile corresponds to the values included in the range between 72.7% and 74.3% (Fig. 2).

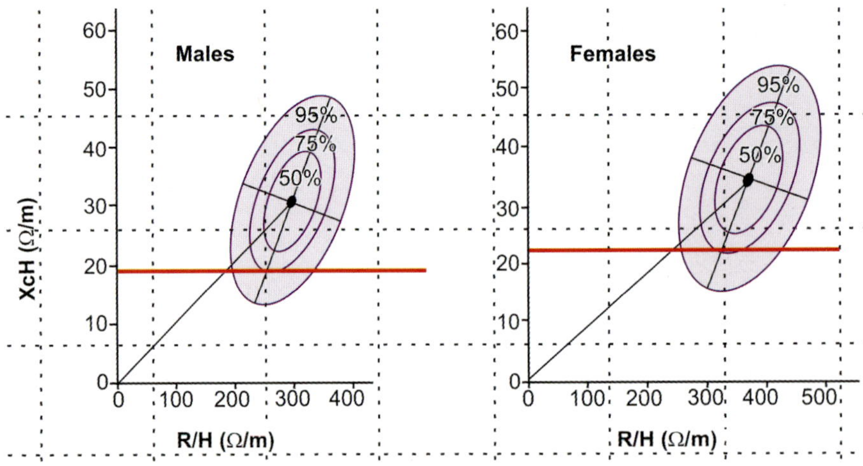

Fig. 3 Nomogram: boundary of normal hydration at 75% of tolerance ellipse

Bioelectrical impedance vector analysis results are very easy and rapid to be interpreted. As previously discussed, fluids are good conductors so the length of Z vector, which represents body's impedance, is inversely related to fluid volume. Moreover, several studies have agreed on the delineation of the 75% tolerance ellipse as the boundary of normal tissue hydration.[1] Consequently, vectors outside the upper pole of the 75% ellipse indicate dehydration, whereas vectors outside the lower pole of 75% confidence ellipse represent overhydration (Fig. 3), and shorter is the vector, more severe is the condition of fluid overload.[7,8] However, it has been suggested that the window of tolerance for hyperhydration or dehydration may vary in patients with different diseases.[9] BIVA also allows to stratify the severity of both overhydration and dehydration subdividing these two classes into mild, moderate, or severe volume abnormalities.[10]

Furthermore, BIVA technique has shown to be able to detect the change of the amount of body fluid. For example, it has been demonstrated the lengthening of the vector not only in chronic renal failure patients after hemodyalysis[7] and after peritoneal dialysis[1] ($P < 0.001$ in men, $P = 0.03$ in women) but also in acute heart failure (AHF) patients after diuretic therapy[5,9] (Fig. 4).

Due to its characteristics of manageability, cheapness, accuracy and velocity, the use of BIVA for assessing hydration status is spreading outside from its original application in the nephrology to all departments, and especially to the emergency rooms.[11]

In intensive care unit patients, BIVA measurements were related to the central venous pressure (CVP). CVP values are significantly and inversely correlated with individual impedance vector components ($r^2 = 0.28$ and 0.27 with resistance and reactance, respectively), and with both vector components together ($r^2 = 0.31$). Particularly, CVP values higher than 12 mmHg were associated with shorter BIVA vectors in 93% of patients, reflecting overhydration. On the other hand, CVP values lower than 3 mmHg were associated with longer vectors in 10% of patients, indicating dehydration. Moreover, the progressive increase of CVP values was associated with shorter and down-sloping impedance vectors on the nomogram.[12]

Moreover, an Italian trial[5] showed the significant difference of BIVA data between decompensated AHF patients and controls at admission to the ED ($P < 0.0007$). AHF patients had a significantly higher value of hydration status (77% ± 4%) as compared with controls (73% ± 2%). The results of this study also proved the potential prognostic role of BIVA, showing a significant correlation of hydration values higher than 80% with events (death or rehospitalization) at 3 months after admission.[5] Moreover, in other trials it was showed BIVA predictive value, independently from other variables.[9,13,14]

The evaluation of total body fluid by BIVA showed its utility in patients with cardiorenal syndrome too.[15]

Moreover, the use of BIVA and several biomarkers has been shown to be useful in evaluating clinical diagnosis of body fluid overload.[16]

USE OF BIVA IN THE DYSPNEIC PATIENTS

All over the world dyspnea is one of the most frequent symptoms of admission in the ED.[17] Despite the growing, innovative and advantageous introduction in the last years in the clinical practice of lung ultrasound and of

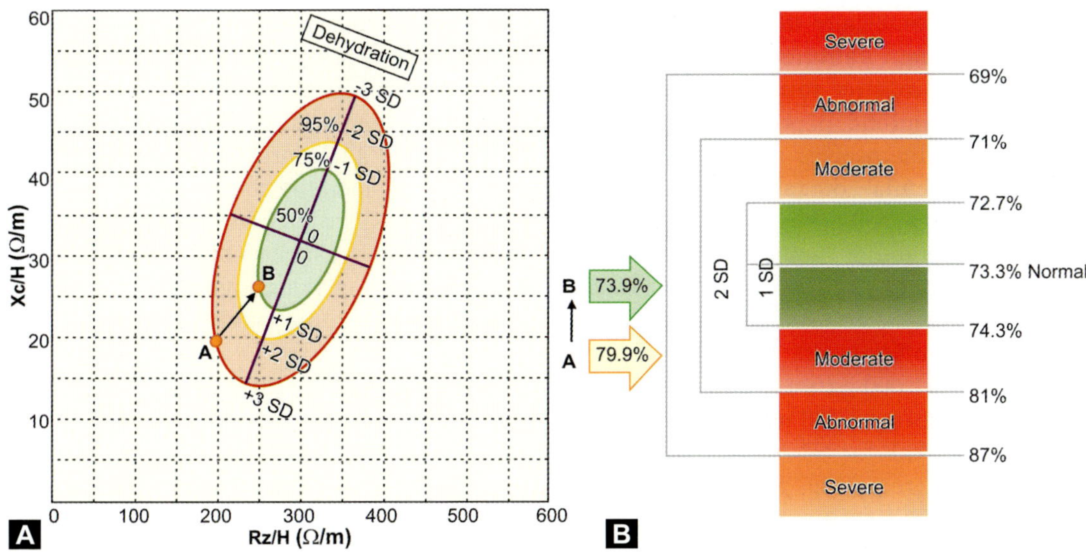

SD, standard deviation

Fig. 4 Graphic representation of the nomogram (left panel) and the numerical scale (right panel) for bioelectrical impedance vector analysis. A typical example of vector migration (A to B) in response to aggressive fluid depletion therapy[9]

natriuretic peptides (NPs),[18,19] dyspnea still represents a challenge for physicians in several conditions. First of all, it is important to classify the type of dyspnea on the base of the onset time (acute or chronic), of the main respiratory phase involved (inspiratory or expiratory) and, particularly, of the etiology (cardiac, respiratory, mixed, etc.).[20] It is well known that dyspnea can hide severe, life-threatening or fatal diseases and that the treatment must be started as soon as possible. Moreover, the population aging has led to an increase of comorbidities. By now, physicians classified dyspnea in cardiogenic or noncardiogenic on the base of the classical methods, such as physical examination, electrocardiogram, chest X-ray, NPs and lung ultrasound, because standardized guidelines to assess properly dyspnea still lack. The typical clinical signs of volume overload due to heart failure, such as elevated jugular venous pressure, third heart sound, rales, and peripheral edema[21-23] have only poor diagnostic reliability, because several studies demonstrated that these signs are present in just few patients with cardiogenic dyspnea.[24,25] Therefore, despite the unquestionable importance of clinical judgment, it seems to be essential to resort to other tools. Although chest X-rays are usually performed in every patient referring to the ED for shortness of breathe, it has been showed that radiography can be seldom diagnostic.[26]

In this complex scenario, BIVA has found its fundamental role in the dyspnea differential diagnosis as a rapid, noninvasive, and accurate method. In several trials BIVA has already showed its efficacy in distinguishing between cardiogenic and noncardiogenic dyspnea[27] (Fig. 5), especially if associated with other variables.

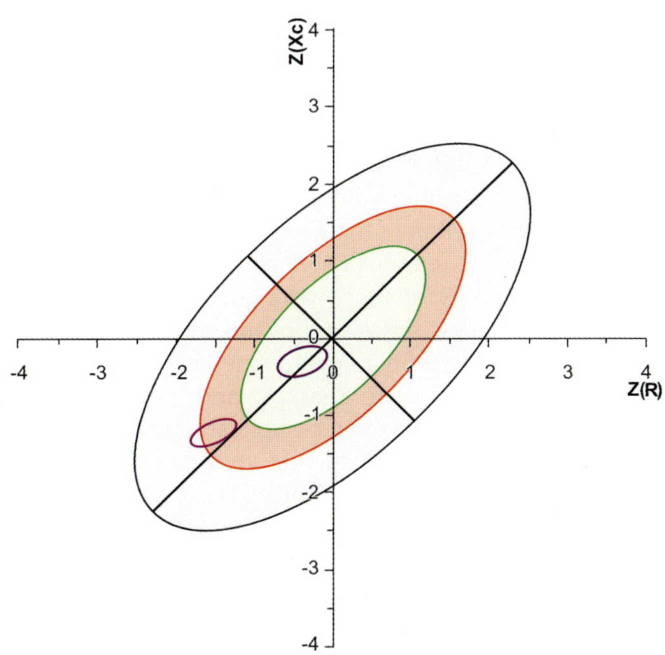

Fig. 5 Distribution of vectors by dyspnea. The blue ring represent patients with noncardiogenic dyspnea, while the black one reflect the average of patients with cardiogenic dyspnea

Natriuretic peptides, especially the 32 amino acids active hormone, called brain natriuretic peptide (BNP), and the 76 amino acids inactive form, named amino-terminal pro-B-type natriuretic peptide (NT-proBNP), have already confirmed themselves as useful aids not only for dyspnea differential diagnosis but also for stratifying the risk in the ED, predicting death and rehospitalization, and guiding therapy.[28,29] A cut-off value for BNP less than 100 pg/mL (and <400 pg/mL for NT-proBNP) is traditionally used to rule out cardiogenic dyspnea, whereas a cut-off value of BNP greater than 400 pg/mL (NT-proBNP >2,000 pg/mL) to rule in. Values of BNP between 100 pg/mL and 400 pg/mL (or between 400 pg/mL and 2,000 pg/mL for NT-proBNP) represent the "gray zone", thus requiring further analysis.[18] However, NPs show their measurement limitations in certain conditions, including renal dysfunction, obesity, and atrial fibrillation. Moreover, it has been recently proposed an interesting differentiation of BNP levels in AHF patients into two components: a baseline value, called BNP dry, which reflects heart failure, and a BNP wet value that increases in acute decompensation and is related to volume or pressure overload.[29] BIVA played a fundamental role in detecting this BNP dichotomy.[5] In fact, it was recently proved the additive diagnostic and prognostic role of HI obtained by BIVA measurements for AHF patients with BNP values in the "grey-zone".[30]

Thus, it was internationally recognized that the combined application of BIVA and BNP evaluations may improve the management of AHF patients in the ED when compared to BNP alone,[31] distinguishing cardiogenic and noncardiogenic dyspnea. Both measures, BIVA and BNP, proved their utility to guide emergency physician's decisions about diuretic therapy and preventing its overuse,[5] thus reducing renal complications.[9]

Another promising tool for dyspnea differential diagnosis is thoracis ultrasound (TUS), despite it is still considered a relatively new imaging technique.[32] It identifies interstitial and/or alveolar edema by sonographic artifact, called B-lines or comet tails. These artifacts reflect a condition of congestion, typically caused by AHF and they thus allow to distinguish cardiogenic from noncardiogenic dyspnea.[33] One more time BIVA assessments, coupled with TUS, proved to improve the effectiveness in discriminating dyspnea (69% sensitivity, 79% specificity).[27]

Further trials and additional publications about BIVA measurements in patients with shortness of breath are required to standardize its diagnostic and prognostic role in the management of dyspneic patients. BIVA proved to be more accurate and more reliable than other impedance methods, such as segmental or whole body bio-impedance analysis (BIA), because BIVA is a faster and easier method that gives clear results. The combined use of BIVA plus NPs showed to improve the management of patients with AHF. In fact, the standardized combination of BIVA results plus NPs values could allow to assess different but complementary aspects of heart failure decompensation, BIVA measuring the congestion and NPs reflecting the pressure and volume overload.[16]

CONCLUSION

Nowadays, BIVA technique has proved to be a promising method for the management of dyspneic patients, obviously in addition to the classical methods, such as clinical judgment and chest X-ray, and to the emerging tools, as NPs and TUS (Flowchart 1).

Bioelectrical impedance vector analysis widespread availability is due to its favorable characteristics of accuracy, noninvasiveness, cheapness, velocity, and manageability. It only requires few seconds to give the results of body tissue impedance that is inversely proportional to fluid overload. As every physician knows, cardiogenic dyspnea is caused by pulmonary congestion, that is first interstitial and then alveolar fluid retention. Thus, total body water assessment by BIVA produces a measure of body congestion, disclosing the cause of dyspnea. This pathophysiological mechanism explains the emerging role of BIVA in the management of dyspneic patients. In fact, this device allows to distinguish between cardiogenic and noncardiogenic dyspnea, because in the first condition BIVA vector is placed outside the lower pole of the 75% tolerance ellipse and it is a shorter vector.[27] Other trials showed the diagnostic power of hydration index too, independently from the vector and without differences between men and women.[5] A hydration index value higher than 74.3% suggests a condition of cardiogenic dyspnea caused by congestion.[5] However, BIVA device can show its results in the both ways to permit to better understand the degree of congestion.

The application of NPs in every day clinical practice has already carried fundamental and undisputed advantages not only for the dyspnea differential diagnosis but also for the risk stratification of AHF patients. However, the main reason of rehospitalization in these kinds of patients is the worsening of congestion, easily and clearly detected by BIVA assessment. Thus, the combined use of BIVA plus NPs could help

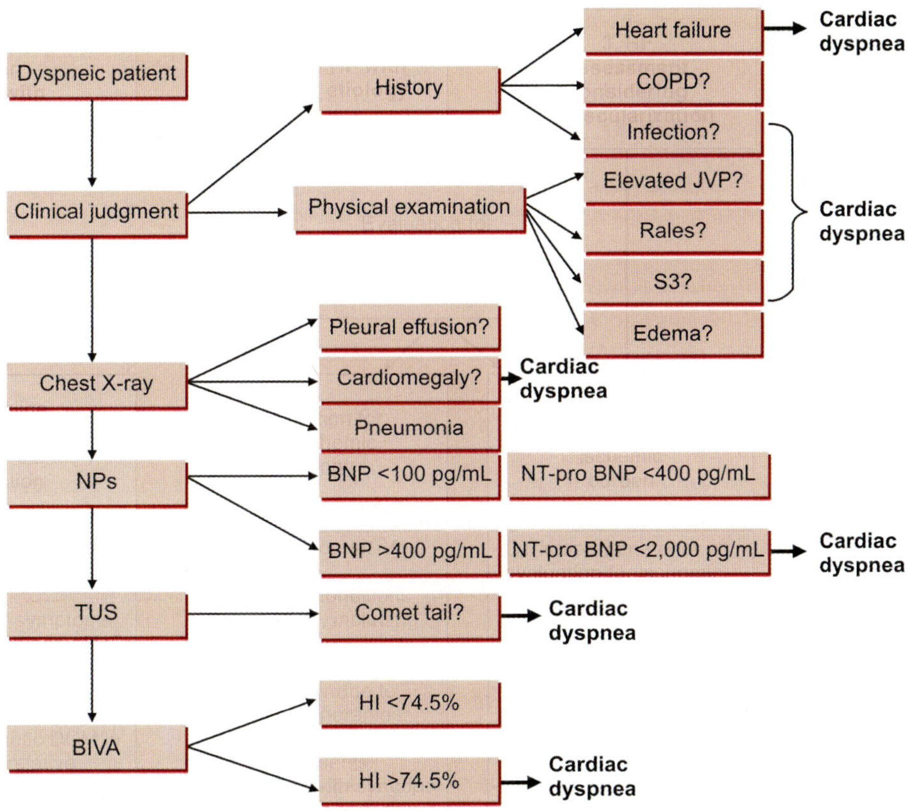

NPs, natriuretic peptides; TUS, thoracis ultrasound; BIVA, bioelectrical impedance vector analysis; BNP, brain natriuretic peptide; NT-proBNP, amino-terminal pro-B-type natriuretic peptide; COPD, chronic obstructive pulmonary disease; JVP, jugular venous pressure

Flowchart 1 Proposal of diagnostic algorithm for dyspneic patients

to prematurely recognize the mechanism of heart decompensation as the cause of dyspnea.[16] Last but not least, BIVA demonstrated its predictive value in order to stratify the risk of dyspneic patients, to guide a proper therapy, and to avoid death or rehospitalization[34] but an international recognized cut-off value of bad prognosis still lacks.

REFERENCES

1. Piccoli A, Italian CAPD-BIA Study Group. Bioelectric impedance vector distribution in peritoneal dialysis patients with different hydration status. Kidney Int. 2004;65(3):1050-63.
2. Lukaski HC, Johnson PE, Bolonchuk WW, et al. Assessment of fat-free mass using bioelectrical impedance measurements of the human body. Am J Clin Nutr. 1985;41(4):810-7.
3. Kushner RF. Bioelectrical impedance analysis: a review of principles and applications. J Am Coll Nutr. 1992;11(2):199-209.
4. Talluri T, Lietdke RJ, Evangelisti A, et al. Fat-free mass qualitative assessment with bioelectric impedance analysis (BIA). Ann N Y Acad Sci. 1999;873:94-8.
5. Di Somma S, De Berardinis B, Bongiovanni C, et al. Use of BNP and bioimpedance to drive therapy in heart failure patients. Congest Heart Fail. 2010;16(Suppl 1):S56-61.
6. Bosy-Westphal A, Danielzik S, Dörhöfer RP, et al. Patterns of bioelectrical impedance vector distribution by body mass index and age: implications for body-composition analysis. Am J Clin Nutr. 2005;82(1):60-8.
7. Piccoli A. Identification of operational clues to dry weight prescription in hemodialysis using bioimpedance vector analysis. The Italian Hemodialysis-Bioelectrical Impedance Analysis (HD-BIA) Study Group. Kidney Int. 1998;53(4):1036-43.
8. Bozzetto S, Piccoli A, Montini G, et al. Bioelectrical impedance vector analysis to evaluate relative hydration status. Pediatr Nephrol. 2010;25(2):329-34.
9. Valle R, Aspromonte N, Milani L, et al. Optimizing fluid management in patients with acute decompensated heart failure (ADHF): the emerging role of combined measurement of body hydration status and brain natriuretic peptide (BNP) levels. Heart Fail Rev. 2011;16(6):519-29.
10. Piccoli A, Rossi B, Pillon L, et al. A new method for monitoring body fluid variation by bioimpedance analysis: the RXc graph. Kidney Int. 1994;46(2):534-9.
11. Tuy T, Peacock F. Noninvasive volume assessment in the emergency department: a look at B-type natriuretic peptide and bioimpedance vector analysis. Contrib Nephrol. 2011;171:187-93.

12. Piccoli A, Pittoni G, Facco E, et al. Relationship between central venous pressure and bioimpedance vector analysis in critically ill patients. Crit Care Med. 2000;28(1):132-7.
13. Drazner MH, Rame JE, Stevenson LW, et al. Prognostic importance of elevated jugular venous pressure and a third heart sound in patients with heart failure. N Engl J Med. 2001;345(8):574-81.
14. Bagshaw SM, Brophy PD, Cruz D, et al. Fluid balance as a biomarker: impact of fluid overload on outcome in critically ill patients with acute kidney injury. Crit Care. 2008;12(4):169.
15. Di Somma S, Gori CS, Salvatori E. How to manage cardiorenal syndromes in the emergency room. Contrib Nephrol. 2010;165:93-100.
16. Di Somma S, Navarin S, Giordano S, et al. The emerging role of biomarkers and bio-impedance in evaluating hydration status in patients with acute heart failure. Clin Chem Lab Med. 2012;50(12):2093-105.
17. Fauci AS, Braunwald E, Kasper DL, Hauser SL, Longo DL, Jameson JL, Loscalzo J (Eds). Harrison Principi Di Medicina Interna, 17th edition. McGraw Hill.
18. Maisel AS, Nakao K, Ponikowski P, et al. Japanese-Western consensus meeting on biomarkers. Int Heart J. 2011;52(5):253-65.
19. Brunetti M, Pregno S, Schünemann H, et al. Economic evidence in decision-making process in laboratory medicine. Clin Chem Lab Med. 2011;49(4):617-21.
20. Ray P, Birolleau S, Lefort Y, et al. Acute respiratory failure in the elderly: etiology, emergency diagnosis and prognosis. Crit Care. 2006;10(3):R82.
21. Butman SM, Ewy GA, Standen JR, et al. Bedside cardiovascular examination in patients with severe chronic heart failure: importance of rest or inducible jugular venous distension. J Am Coll Cardiol. 1993;22(4):968-74.
22. Wang CS, FitzGerald JM, Schulzer M, et al. Does this dyspneic patient in the emergency department have congestive heart failure? JAMA. 2005;294(15):1944-56.
23. Drazner MH, Rame JE, Stevenson LW, et al. Prognostic importance of elevated jugular venous pressure and a third heart sound in patients with heart failure. N Engl J Med. 2001;345(8):574-81.
24. Tsuyuki RT, McKelvie RS, Arnold JM, et al. Acute precipitants of congestive heart failure exacerbations. Arch Intern Med. 2001;161(19):2337-42.
25. Stevenson LW, Perloff JK. The limited reliability of physical signs for estimating hemodynamics in chronic heart failure. JAMA. 1989;261(6): 884-8.
26. Collins SP, Lindsell CJ, Storrow AB, et al. Prevalence of negative chest radiography results in the emergency department patient with decompensated heart failure. Ann Emerg Med. 2006;47(1):13-8.
27. Piccoli A, Codognotto M, Cianci V, et al. Differentiation of cardiac and noncardiac dyspnea using bioelectrical impedance vector analysis (BIVA). J Card Fail. 2012;18(3):226-32.
28. Daniels LB, Maisel AS. Natriuretic peptides. J Am Coll Cardiol. 2007; 50(25):2357-68.
29. Maisel A, Mueller C, Adams K, et al. State of the art: using natriuretic peptide levels in clinical practice. Eur J Heart Fail. 2008;10(9):824-39.
30. Di Somma S, Lalle I, Magrini L, Russo V, Navarin S, Castello L, et al. Additive diagnostic and prognostic value of Bioelectrical Impedance Vector Analysis (BIVA) to brain natriuretic peptide 'grey-zone' in patients with acute heart failure in the emergency department. Eur Heart J Acute Cardiovasc Care. 2014 Feb 12. [Epub ahead of print].
31. Parrinello G, Paterna S, Di Pasquale P, et al. The usefulness of bioelectrical impedance analysis in differentiating dyspnea due to decompensated heart failure. J Card Fail. 2008;14(8):676-86.
32. Lichtenstein D, Mézière G, Biderman P, et al. The comet-tail artifact. An ultrasound sign of alveolar-interstitial syndrome. Am J Respir Crit Care Med. 1997;156(5):1640-6.
33. Liteplo AS, Marill KA, Villen T, et al. Emergency thoracic ultrasound in the differentiation of the etiology of shortness of breath (ETUDES): sonographic B-lines and N-terminal pro-brain-type natriuretic peptide in diagnosing congestive heart failure. Acad Emerg Med. 2009;16(3):201-10.
34. Di Somma S, Lukaski HC, Codognotto M, et al. Consensus paper on the use of BIVA (bioelectrical impedance vector analysis) in medicine for the management of body hydration. ECJ. 2011;4:6-14.

Chapter 9

Mechanical Ventilation in Acute Heart Failure: The Role of Noninvasive Ventilation

Josep Masip

ABSTRACT

A substantial proportion of patients with acute hear failure (AHF) develop severe acute respiratory failure (ARF) requiring ventilatory support. Traditionally, it was provided by ventilators via endotracheal intubation (EI) and sedation. However, in the last decades noninvasive ventilation (NIV) via an interface (mask, pillow, cannula, helmet, etc.) has been progressively used in these patients. There are two main modalities: continuous positive airway pressure (CPAP) and pressure support ventilation, which is usually applied with a positive end expiratory pressure (bilevel). Both techniques and some others recently introduced in the market integrating some technological innovations, have extensively demonstrated a faster improvement of ARF, facilitating the release of conventional mechanical ventilation, frequently avoiding EI and in some cases, reducing mortality. AHF is currently the second indication of this technique. NIV is used in a wide range of acute settings, such as critical care units, emergency departments and in pre-hospital care. The appropriate selection of patients and the adaptation to the technique are the keys to success.

INTRODUCTION

Mechanical ventilation (MV) with positive pressure was the technological innovation that led to the development of intensive care units (ICUs) in the second half of the 20th century. Initially applied under sedation after endotracheal intubation (EI), it began being used in conscious patients using masks in the last several decades, in what was called noninvasive ventilation (NIV).

Nowadays, in general ICUs, MV with EI, or "invasive" (IMV) is used in the majority of patients to treat acute respiratory failure (ARF), whereas in the remaining cases, it is used in patients with coma or exacerbations of chronic diseases (Box 1).[1] Conversely, in cardiac intensive care units (CICUs) the diseases that require IMV are essentially cardiogenic shock, acute pulmonary edema (APE), cardiopulmonary arrest and postoperative cardiac surgery.[2]

While IMV has largely remained limited to critical care units or the operating room, NIV spread as a regular practice to other areas (emergency department, intermediate units, hospital wards, the prehospital setting and, in chronic patients, even in homes). Although used to treat multiple respiratory disorders, exacerbation of chronic obstructive pulmonary disease (COPD) and APE are the main indications. By contrast, in the CICU, NIV is used almost exclusively in patients with APE and in selected cases as a support for ventilator weaning.

Overall, the aim of MV is to decrease the work of breathing and to reverse acute hypoxemia and progressive acidosis. The reduction in the work of breathing, which in severe acute situations may involve 20–50% of the total body oxygen consumption, allows the recovery of respiratory muscles.[3]

INVASIVE MECHANICAL VENTILATION IN PATIENTS WITH HEART FAILURE

Patients with heart failure (HF) and reduced systolic function may have significant hemodynamic instability resulting in abnormal responses to MV. First, EI is poorly tolerated since the loss of adrenergic stimuli and

Box 1: Main diseases treated with mechanical ventilation according to the type of critical care unit

Intensive care units

- Acute respiratory failure (65%)
  - Pneumonia
  - Sepsis
  - Trauma
  - Surgical complications
  - Heart failure
  - Acute respiratory distress syndrome
- Coma
- Chronic obstructive pulmonary disease
- Neuromuscular disorders
- Postoperative high risk interventions

Cardiovascular intensive care unit

- Cardiogenic shock (acute coronary syndromes or myocarditis)
- Acute pulmonary edema
- Cardiorespiratory arrest
- Postoperative cardiac surgery

the vasodilation produced by sedative agents lead to a more pronounced hypotension, which often requires the administration of vasoactive drugs. Second, during IMV, patients with HF have frequent oscillations in blood pressure (BP) and higher incidence of rhythm disturbances, especially atrial fibrillation, complicating ventilation. Hemodynamic instability induced by IMV is greater if it is associated with myocardial ischemia. Third, some patients, especially those with preserved systolic function, may experience an increase in cardiac output when applying MV due to the decrease in left ventricle preload and afterload, which are usually elevated in patients with HF. Positive intrathoracic pressure acts in most cases as a protection for HF and when removed, acute decompensation may occur.[4] This is common in weaning. It has been reported that 30–40% of weaning failures are due to HF. In these cases, baseline B-type natriuretic peptide (BNP) is elevated and shows further increase during the procedure.[5] Adequate compensation with previous fluid negative balance, the administration of vasodilators and diuretics, avoiding hypertension and/or using NIV in some cases, are measures that may prevent this complication. Finally, it should be emphasized that the prognosis of patients with APE treated with IMV does not depend on the severity of ARF but on myocardial injury and the consequent degree of myocardial dysfunction.[6]

NONINVASIVE VENTILATION

The first device with widespread use of NIV was the iron lung. It consisted of a bulky ventilator, which enveloped the patient's body, producing an external negative pressure that expanded the thorax. These devices were providential in the polio epidemics of the early 20th century. However, with the proliferation of IMV with EI and positive pressure, these techniques were abandoned, only to reappear in recent decades in the form of positive pressure through masks.

Currently, NIV can be defined as the application of positive intrathoracic pressure without EI. There are three components: (1) a source of oxygen or air (generally a ventilator), (2) transmission tubes, and (3) the interface, which is the key element of the technique. There are multiple interfaces: masks, helmets, oral clamps, or nasal pillows (Figs. 1A to G). The most commonly used are masks, which can be nasal, oronasal, partial face or total face.

When using a ventilator, synchronization between the ventilator and the patient's inspiratory effort is fundamental. The majority of current ventilators have mechanisms that facilitate ventilation, including leakage compensation, modulation of pressure ramp, trigger, inspiration time, and cycling-off time.

With few exceptions, when using NIV, respiratory rate (RR) is not programmed, because it is the patient who activates the system with his inspiratory effort. This requires a sufficient level of awareness and collaboration, one of the primary advantages of NIV. Avoiding sedation and EI, NIV permits interruptions, communication, and oral feeding.

Noninvasive ventilation is more effective than conventional oxygen therapy in the improvement of ARF with reduced need for EI, which may decrease the length of stay in critical care units, and mortality in some cases. Furthermore, another potential advantage is the reduction of infections and especially the incidence of ventilator associated pneumonia (VAP) that has been found in retrospective analyses of large cohort series.[7] However, NIV may produce several complications (Box 2); it is uncomfortable to a greater or lesser degree, does not protect the airway and does not achieve the same level of ventilation than IMV. Therefore, NIV and IMV are not equivalent and the use of NIV is restricted to cases with less severity and for relatively short periods of time. There is a therapeutic window[8] in which NIV is indicated that is located in the boundaries between good response to conventional oxygen therapy and extremely

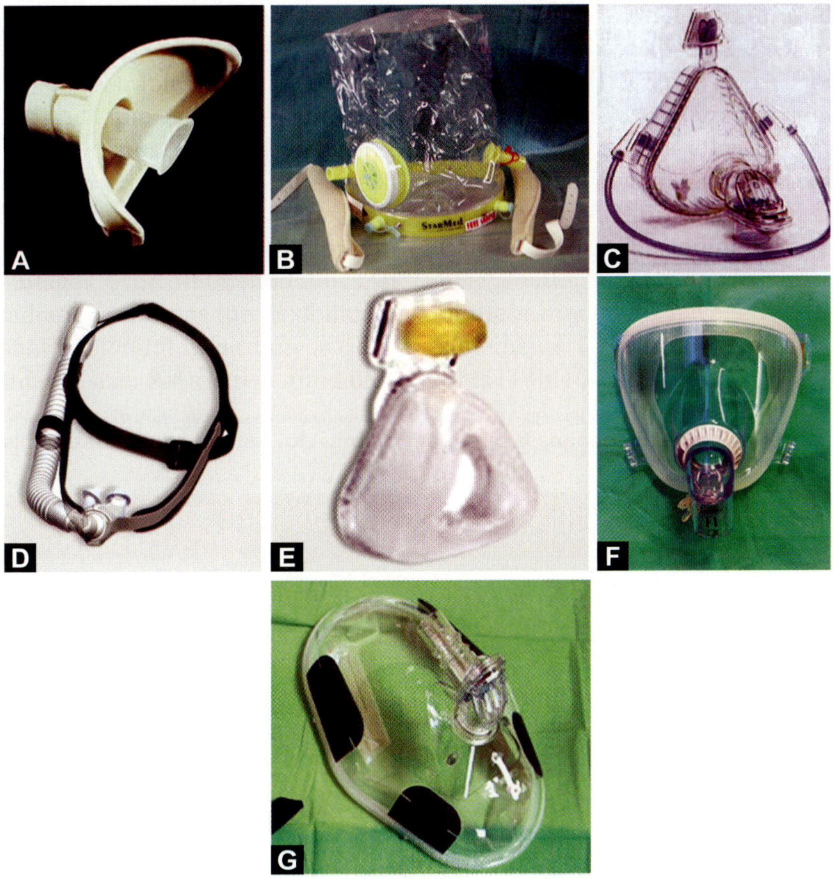

Fig. 1 Interfaces. **A,** Mouthpiece; **B,** Helmet; **C,** Oro-nasal; **D,** Nasal pillows; **E,** Nasal mask; **F** and **G,** Total face masks

Box 2: Inconvenients and complications of noninvasive ventilation

Related to the mask

- Discomfort
- Facial erythema
- Claustrophobia
- Skin ulcers

Related to flow or pressure

- Nasal congestion
- Sinus or ear pain
- Dryness (nasal/oral)
- Ocular irritation
- Gastric distension

Severe Complications

- Aspiration pneumonia
- Hypotension
- Pneumothorax

severe situations requiring immediate EI (Fig. 2). It is important to identify early patients unresponsive to NIV. Continuous monitoring of physiological variables and evaluation of patient status minutes is crucial, at minimum every 1–2 hours, to avoid undue delay in EI for poor responders as such a delay may worsen the prognosis in some cases.[9]

MODALITIES OF NONINVASIVE VENTILATION

There are two main modalities: one is continuous positive airway pressure (CPAP) and the other is pressure support ventilation (PS). PS is usually applied with positive end expiratory pressure (PEEP), also called bilevel, two levels of pressure, or BIPAP.

Continuous positive airway pressure: Although all portable or ICU ventilators have both modalities, CPAP can be applied without the aid of a ventilator, only requiring a source of air or oxygen to renew the air and a hermetical mask equipped with a PEEP valve or with

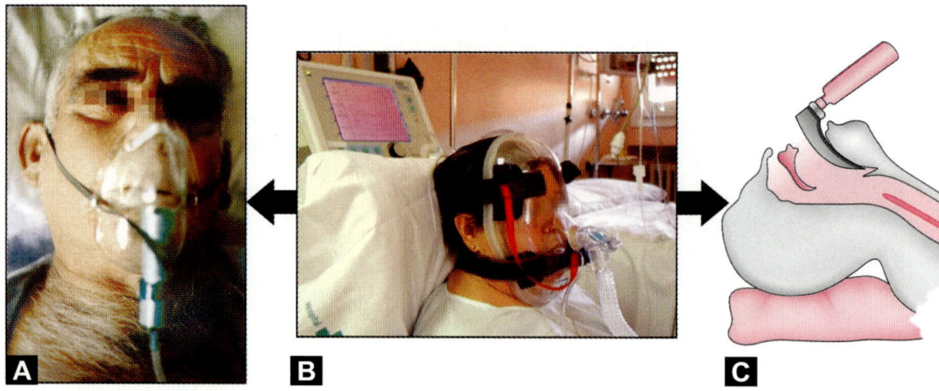

Fig. 2 Therapeutic window for noninvasive ventilation. **A,** Revolution acute respiratory failure; **B,** Moderate-to-severe respiratory distress, absence of contraindication; and **C,** Endotracheal intubation

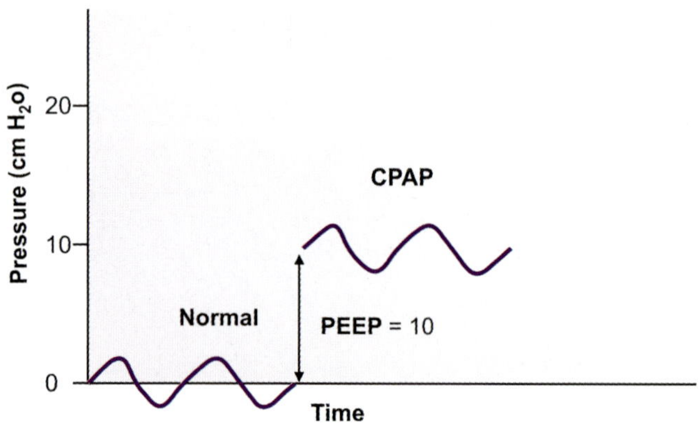

CPAP, continuous positive airway pressure; PEEP, positive end expiratory pressure

Fig. 3 Pressure/time curve of a patient with CPAP

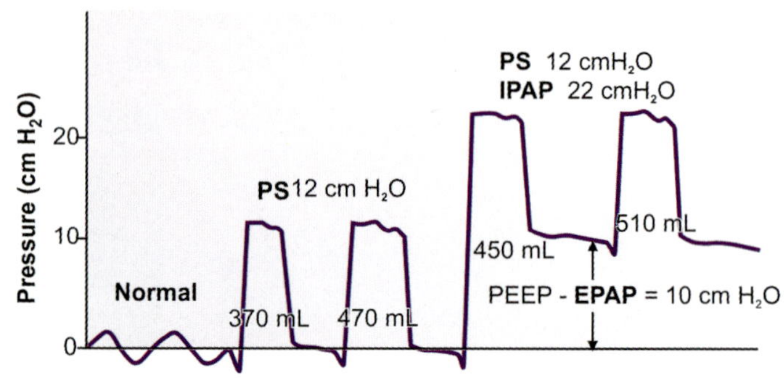

PEEP, positive end expiratory pressure; PS, pressure support; IPAP, inspiratory positive airway pressure; EPAP, expiratory positive airway pressure

Fig. 4 Pressure support ventilation. Pressure-time curves of a patient breathing normally, with pressure support and after the application of PEEP (bilevel)

a Boussignac system, which generates PEEP through a transversal high flow that creates a barrier effect. CPAP is therefore the simplest technique (Fig. 3).

Pressure support ventilation-positive end expiratory pressure or BIPAP: This modality, the foundation of NIV, requires a ventilator. It is usually programmed with two levels of pressure: (1) expiratory pressure (EPAP) (similar to CPAP) and (2) inspiratory pressure (IPAP) (Fig. 4). When the patient starts the inspiratory effort, the ventilator delivers pressure support using a decelerated flow, which keeps the prefixed inspiratory pressure constant (IPAP). When the patient finishes the inspiratory effort or the flow has decreased below a preset percentage of its maximum value (usually 25%), the ventilator assistance ceases and the pressure drops down to the predetermined EPAP. Tidal volumes (Vt) change with each breath according to the patient's effort. The end result is CPAP with inspiratory assistance. This method requires some experience for setting the ventilator to the changing needs of the patient. Adequate synchrony is essential.

OTHER MODALITIES

Proportional assist ventilation (PAV) has been introduced in recent years. In this case, the inspiratory support is regulated by integrating the elastance and resistance of the patient's lung, delivering assisted ventilation proportional to the patient's effort. Although this modality has shown to be more comfortable for patients in some studies, it is quite complex and subject to a wide variability of mismatching. It is not commonly used in clinical practice.

Pressure assisted-controlled ventilation: Two levels of pressure (EPAP or PEEP and IPAP) are delivered as in NIPSV but at a pre-set respiratory rate.

High-flow nasal cannula: The system delivers an oxygen-gas mixture via nasal cannula, which usually exceeds patients' spontaneous inspiratory demand, generating a low level of CPAP, a washout effect in nasopharyngeal and a reduction of upper airway resistance. It has been used in neonates and in mild to moderate ARF in adults.
Neurally adjusted ventilatory assist (NAVA): The electrical diaphragm activity is captured by an esophageal catheter that triggers the inspiratory cycle of the ventilator.
Adaptative-pressure-control (APC) or average volume-assured pressure support (AVAPS). The ventilator provides progressively higher or lower PSV, according to patient's inspiratory effort to ensure a target tidal volume. It has been used in adults with COPD and severe hypercapnic encephalopathy.
Adaptive servoventilation (ASV): Used in complex sleep disturbances. The ventilator compensates central apneas by regulation of the inspiratory and expiratory pressure, treating upper airway obstruction by auto adjustments of the end expiratory pressure.

CURRENT INDICATIONS FOR NONINVASIVE VENTILATION

Although home NIV is used extensively in chronic patients with obstructive sleep-apnea and pulmonary or neuromuscular diseases, the technique is used primarily in patients with ARF (Box 3).

Noninvasive ventilation has been shown to be superior to conventional oxygen therapy in terms of reduced mortality in COPD exacerbations, in APE, hypercapnic COPD patients with pneumonia, immunocompromised patients (hematologic or post-solid organ transplantation), and in weaning. It has also proved useful in terms of faster ARF improvement or decrease in hospitalization, in patients with asthma or pneumonia, in the postoperative period (especially after lung resection or abdominal surgery) and as a palliative measure in "do not intubate" patients. In regard to weaning, the results have been favorable as a preventive measure of post-extubation ARF in individuals at risk and as a direct method of weaning in patients who have failed several spontaneous breathing trials. It has not proven to be useful in treating post-extubation ARF once established.[9]

Box. 3: Acute diseases with some evidence of benefit with the use of noninvasive ventilation

- COPD exacerbation
- Acute pulmonary edema
- Severe asthma
- Pneumonia*
- Acute respiratory distress syndrome at initial phases
- Weaning:
  - Direct method in difficult weaning
  - To prevent post-extubation ARF
- ARF in immunocompromised patients
- Postoperative patients
- Do not intubate patients

*Especially in COPD and hypercapnic patients

COPD, chronic obstructive pulmonary disease; ARF, acute respiratory failure

NONINVASIVE VENTILATION IN ACUTE HEART FAILURE

Although NIV has been successfully used to treat chronic breathing disorders in patients with HF (Obstructive sleep apnea and Cheyne-Stokes), the technique in acute HF is restricted to APE or in initial low cardiac output states.

Most patients with APE present with a mixed acidosis. It has been reported that hypercapnia and improvement after the first hour of NIV are predictors of a good response to the technique in these patients.[10]

As previously mentioned, the salutary effects of positive intrathoracic pressure in APE on preload and afterload may lead to an increase of cardiac output in patients with HF. Currently, APE is the second most frequent indication for NIV, primarily in the emergency room. For APE patients, use of nasal masks is not recommended due to severity of dyspnea driving patients to breathe orally, making airway pressurization impossible. However, there is experience with both modalities of NIV.

Continuous positive airway pressure: The CPAP level used in APE patients varies between 5 cmH_2O and 15 cmH_2O, although the most common pressure used in clinical practice is 10 cmH_2O. FiO_2 is usually recommended to be high (50–100%) and should be titrated according to clinical status and evaluation.

There have been numerous published randomized studies comparing CPAP with conventional oxygen therapy. Although the population of these studies was small individually, several showed a significant decrease in the rate of EI, while none showed an impact on hospital mortality. Conversely, there were several published meta-analyses showing that CPAP reduced mortality and EI.[11] The low cost of the technique and the fact that it does not need special training, makes this mode in limited-resources environments preferable. As a result, the early use of CPAP in the prehospital setting improves oxygenation and reduces the rate of EI with respect to conventional oxygen therapy.[12]

Pressure support ventilation-positive end expiratory pressure: Commonly used inspiratory pressure support is 10–20 cmH_2O and expiratory pressure (PEEP) of 4–7 cmH_2O with high FiO_2 (50–100%). It is convenient to start with lower pressures and increase PS progressively as patient's adaptation improves, to ensure Vt ≥350–500 mL. In ventilators with a single tube, EPAP or PEEP ≥4 cmH_2O should be used to prevent rebreathing. Different types of masks should be available to check optimal adjustment to patients' faces. Modern ventilators are equipped with leakage compensation and display screens, with a wide set of alarms and curves. It is essential to achieve and maintain good synchronicity between patient and ventilator. Every effort must be followed by an inspiratory cycle. In tachypneic patients, it may be useful to reduce the IPAP, with the shortest ramp and inspiratory time possible. In many cases, while giving instructions to the patient, manual support of the mask to the face is recommended at the onset, to reduce excessive leakage (>30 L/m). In those who are very anxious or show excessive tachypnea, supplemental doses of morphine or remifentanil may be useful to decrease RR and achieve better synchrony. In any case, the application of NIV should not delay the concomitant administration of vasodilators and diuretics.

The use of PS-PEEP expanded in the 1990s and the first randomized study of APE was published in the year 2000.[13] Despite being the "genuine" technique of NIV, the collective experience with PS-PEEP is somewhat lower than CPAP. Several smaller studies have demonstrated a reduction in the EI rate and a better response in hypercapnic patients.

In the new European Society of Cardiology (ESC) Guidelines from 2012, NIV is considered Class IIa, level of evidence B for APE.[14]

CONTROVERSIES

In 2008, the 3CPO (cardiogenic pulmonary edema) trial, the largest study ever done on NIV was published.[15] This study was carried out in emergency departments in Britain and included more than 1,000 patients with APE and pH <7.35, divided into three groups according to the type of oxygen therapy: (1) CPAP, (2) PS-PEEP and (3) conventional. Patients in both groups of NIV showed faster improvement in ARF but no difference in mortality at 30 days, which was the primary endpoint. The very low rate of EI in this study (2.9%), the absence of hypoxemia

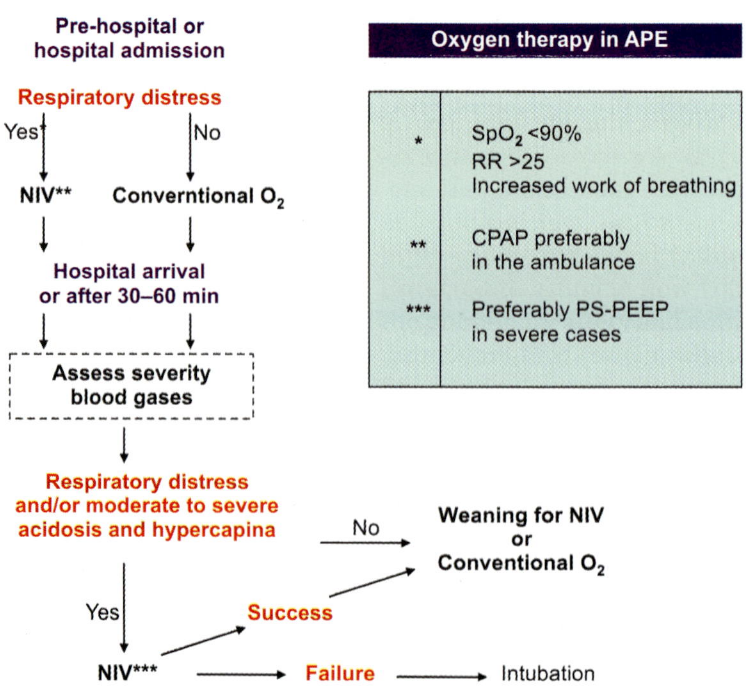

NIV, noninvasive ventilation; RR, relative risk; CPAP, continuous positive airway pressure; PS, pressure support; PEEP, positive end expiratory pressure; APE, acute pulmonary edema.

Flowchart 1 Algorithm for oxygen therapy and NIV in patients with acute pulmonary edema at study entry (average PaO_2 was 100 mmHg in the three groups), the high rate of crossovers (the conventional group was significantly higher due to respiratory distress), the high rate of intolerance to NIV (up to 25%) equating low experience with technique, determined these results. Despite the discrepancy with previous meta-analyses, some new meta-analyses including the 3CPO have shown that both methods reduce the rate of EI and that CPAP also reduces mortality by about 30%.[16] No differences have been demonstrated in the outcomes in trials comparing CPAP and PS-PEEP. However, since a more significant improvement of some respiratory parameters has been described with the use of PS-PEEP compared to CPAP in some randomized studies, and PS-PEEP has been usefully applied as rescue therapy when CPAP has failed in others, PS-PEEP may be preferable in patients with fatigue or significant hypercapnia. No study has shown that NIV can precipitate a higher rate of myocardial infarction, rather, NIV has been successfully used in these patients.

Early NIV treatment (CPAP preferably in the ambulance) is recommended in appropriate patients with APE who show respiratory distress (increased work of breathing, SpO_2 <90% and RR >25), particularly those already treated with conventional oxygen therapy (Flowchart 1). In patients with persistent respiratory distress after 30–60 minutes and particularly in those with acidosis and hypercapnia, NIV (either CPAP or PS-PEEP) must be continued or initiated, if it had not been started yet. PS-PEEP may be preferably in severe cases with significant hypercapnia or in patients with signs of fatigue or CPAP failure. Unlike CPAP, PS-PEEP requires experience and expertise with the equipment and the technique.

CONCLUSION

In conclusion, for the treatment of APE, currently available evidence supports the benefit of NIV compared to conventional treatment in terms of improvement from ARF, reduction in the rate of EI and even death in some cases.

REFERENCES

1. Esteban A, Anzueto A, Frutos F, et al. Characteristics and outcomes in adult patients receiving mechanical ventilation: a 28-day international study. JAMA. 2002;287(3):345-55.
2. Masip J. The Patient Who Needs Mechanical Ventilation. In the Session: The Difficult Patient in the CICU. Paris: European Congress of Cardiology; 2011.
3. Tobin MJ. Mechanical ventilation. New Engl J Med. 1994;330(15):1056-61.
4. Pinsky MR, Summer WR, Wise RA, et al. Augmentation of cardiac function by elevation of intrathoracic pressure. J Appl Physiol Respir Environ Exerc Physiol. 1983;54(4):950-5.
5. Zapata L, Vera P, Roglan A, et al. B-type natriuretic peptides for prediction and diagnosis of weaning failure from cardiac origin. Intensive Care Med. 2011;37(3):477-85.
6. Fedullo AJ, Swinburne AJ, Wahl GW, et al. Acute cardiogenic pulmonary edema treated with mechanical ventilation. Factors determining in-hospital mortality. Chest. 1991;99(5):1220-6.
7. Girou E, Schortgen F, Delcalux C, et al. Association of non-invasive ventilation with nosocomial infection and survival in critical ill patients. JAMA. 2000;284(18):2361-7.
8. Liesching T, Kwok H, Hill NS. Acute applications of noninvasive positive pressure ventilation. Chest. 2003;124(2):699-713.
9. Esteban A, Frutos-Vivar F, Ferguson ND, et al. Noninvasive positive-pressure ventilation for respiratory failure after extubation. N Engl J Med. 2004;350(24):2452-60.
10. Rodríguez Mulero L, Carrillo Alcaraz A, Melgarejo Moreno A, et al. Predictive factors related to success of noninvasive ventilation and mortality in the treatment of acute cardiogenic pulmonary edema. Med Clin (Barc). 2005;124(4):126-31.
11. Masip J, Roque M, Sánchez B, et al. Noninvasive ventilation in acute cardiogenic pulmonary edema: systematic review and meta-analysis. JAMA. 2005;294(24):3124-30.
12. Ducros L, Logeart D, Vicaut E, et al. CPAP for acute cardiogenic pulmonary oedema from out-of-hospital to cardiac intensive care unit: a randomised multicentre study. Intensive Care Med. 2011;37(9):1501-9.
13. Masip J, Betbesé AJ, Páez J, et al. Non-invasive pressure support ventilation versus conventional oxygen therapy in acute cardiogenic pulmonary edema: a randomized study. Lancet. 2000;356(9248):2126-32.
14. McMurray JJ, Adamopoulos S, Anker SD, et al. ESC guidelines for the diagnosis and treatment of acute and chronic heart failure 2012: the Task Force for the Diagnosis and Treatment of Acute and Chronic Heart Failure 2012 of the European Society of Cardiology. Developed in collaboration with the Heart Failure Association (HFA) of the ESC. Eur J Heart Fail. 2012;14(8):803-69.
15. Gray A, Goodacre S, Newby DE, et al. Noninvasive ventilation in acute cardiogenic pulmonary edema. N Engl J Med. 2008;359(2):142-51.
16. Weng CL, Zhao YT, Liu QH, et al. Meta-analysis: noninvasive ventilation in acute cardiogenic pulmonary edema. Ann Intern Med. 2010;152(9):590-600.

Chapter 10

Emergency Department Observation Unit: Management of Congestive Heart Failure

Basem Khishfe, Rashid Kysia

ABSTRACT

Acute heart failure (HF) is a very common presentation to the emergency deparment (ED). Hospital admission is warranted for a high percentage of patients with decompensated HF. The emergency department observation unit could provide a safe alternative in reducing the length of hospital stay and the cost burden of acutely decompensated HF.

INTRODUCTION AND EPIDEMIOLOGY

Heart failure (HF) is a pathophysiologic state of the heart being unable to pump sufficient blood to meet the body's metabolic requirements. A complex neurohormonal regulatory relationship exists between the heart and multiple organ systems. Feedback loops mediated through a variety of vasoactive substances secreted by the kidneys, autonomic nervous system, adrenals, lungs and vascular endothelium are most important.

Alterations of function in any of these organs affect the rest of the organs. HF is a progressive disease. It usually starts long before overt signs and symptoms manifest.

In many circumstances, HF occurs as a consequence of renal, vascular or pulmonary pathologies.

The degree of HF depends on both the functional status of the other organ systems and the amount of primary myocardial disease.

Heart failure is increasing in our society, and it is a very common cause of poor life quality and premature death.

Acute HF is a very common presentation in the emergency department (ED). It is responsible for more than 1 million admissions in the United States per year, with annual cost estimates of \$20–30 billion.[1] It is considered the greatest expense for the medical system in the United States. Given the improvement in outcomes for myocardial infarction and the increasing aged population, HF prevalence is tremendously increasing. Progressive hemodynamic deterioration accounts for approximately 50% of deaths, but sudden death resulting from malignant ventricular dysrhythmias occurs in up to half of the patients. Medical therapy has not significantly decreased sudden dysrhythmia deaths but has improved overall outcomes from pump failure. Multiple pharmacologic therapies, including beta blockers decrease the death rate by improving functional status and slowing progression of pump dysfunction.

Hospital admission is warranted for a high percentage of patients presenting with acutely decompensated heart failure (ADHF). The emergency department observation unit (EDOU) has been used successfully to treat ADHF in certain patients. The EDOU could provide a safe alternative in reducing the length of hospital stay and the cost burden of ADHF exacerbation.

PATIENT SELECTION

Most HF patients are stabilized within the first couple of hours from presentation with adequate diuresis. However, once patients are admitted, the mean hospital stay is 6 days; therefore, EDOU monitoring and management is advantageous for selected patients. Deciding which patients are candidates for EDOU admission versus inpatient admission is crucial. Better outcomes are dependent on appropriate selection of the candidate patients. A protocol should be implemented to ensure that those patients will benefit from a 24-hour expedited management.

Recent reports suggest that EDOU admissions had reduced 90-day ED revisit rate in addition to reduction in HF hospital readmission. Some studies also reported that the 90-day mortality rate was decreased. This could be attributed to a detailed treatment protocol that delivers timely effective management.

DIAGNOSIS

Diagnosing ADHF can be challenging, especially in the ED where rapid decision making is based on limited history and frequently without access to the patient's medical records. The emergency physician must be able to determine the etiology of symptoms in patients with suspected ADHF based on the history, examination, and adjunct diagnostic studies (laboratory data, electrocardiogram, and radiography).

History and Physical Examination

Most patients present with dyspnea; however, dyspnea is nonspecific to ADHF and is very common in the presentation of many other etiologies. History taking should address the presence of orthopnea, paroxysmal nocturnal dyspnea (PND) and decreased exercise tolerance, which increases the likelihood of ADHF. A very important part of the history is previous diagnosis of HF.

Auscultation of crackles or rales on lung examination or S3 gallop on heart examination, and assessment for jugular venous distention (JVD) and lower extremity edema should be included in the examination of a suspected ADHF patient. The absence of these signs decreases the likelihood of ADHF.

Adjunct Diagnostic Studies

Chest radiographs should be performed to assess for pulmonary venous congestion, cardiomegaly, alveolar edema and/or interstitial edema; however, absence of these findings should not exclude the ADHF diagnosis.

Electrocardiography (ECG) is routinely performed on patients with dyspnea and suspicion of HF to identify etiologies of HF exacerbation, such as arrhythmias and/or acute coronary syndrome.

Assembling all the information from adjunct testing in addition to the findings from history and physical examination should help lead the diagnosis of ADHF. In certain cases, even with all those information, it is still challenging to diagnose or exclude ADHF. B-type natriuretic peptide (BNP) measurement is a helpful blood test in diagnosing ADHF. A BNP measurement cutoff of 100 pg/mL has a sensitivity of 90% and specificity of 76%. The addition of BNP level to the physicians' clinical judgment increases the diagnostic accuracy to 81.5%.

CLASSIFICATION OF HEART FAILURE

There are many different methods for the classification of HF, including high versus low output, right-sided versus left-sided, and systolic versus diastolic. Early in the disease progression, these may be useful clinical descriptors suggesting particular causes and treatments; however, these distinctions blur late in the disease.

High-output versus Low-output Failure

High-output failure is a hyperdynamic state with increased cardiac output and decreased oxygen extraction ratio (low arteriovenous oxygen difference). Over time, persistent hyperdynamic state results in myocardial damage.

The hyperdynamic state may result from preload increase as in increased salt and water retention and/or decreased systemic vascular resistance as in arteriovenous (AV) fistulas, cirrhosis, thyrotoxicosis, Paget's disease, and beriberi. Early recognition may allow effective therapy of the underlying condition and thus preventing HF development.

Low-output failure is characterized by low cardiac output and an increased systemic oxygen extraction. It is more common and usually is a result of ischemic heart disease, valvular disease, and/or cardiomyopathies.

Right-sided versus Left-sided Heart Failure

The concept that one cardiac chamber can fail independently of the other is false. The left and right circulations are connected and dysfunction in one chamber has an impact on the other. In addition to the direct effect of one chamber on the other, abnormal catecholamine response will affect all the chambers. Despite this, the terms are commonly used. Patients with "right-sided HF" often present with symptoms of systemic venous congestion, such as hepatomegaly, jugular venous distension and lower extremities edema; while patients with "left-sided HF" present with pulmonary congestion.

Systolic versus Diastolic Dysfunction

Systolic dysfunction is the impairment of contractility leading to reduced stroke output. It is usually secondary to myocyte destruction. Diastolic dysfunction is the inability of the ventricles to fully relax and fill normally. Many patients with diastolic dysfunction have preserved or supranormal ejection fractions, while most cases of systolic dysfunction involve some degree of diastolic dysfunction. Diastolic dysfunction is usually seen in patients with hypertrophic and restrictive cardiomyopathies, aortic stenosis, and hypertension. Diastolic dysfunction is usually a result of increased wall thickness or impaired relaxation.

RISK STRATIFICATION

Many clinical variables are useful for ED risk stratification. ED data can be used to identify low, moderate and high risk HF patient groups. Patients in the ED with systolic blood pressure (SBP) below 100 mmHg have higher mortality rate and warrant inpatient admission possibly to a critical care unit. Hyponatremia upon admission (serum sodium below <135 mmoL/L) has been associated with increased in-hospital and postdischarge mortality, which may warrant inpatient admission. Furthermore, renal dysfunction has been associated with increased mortality rates. Those clinical variables in addition to ischemic changes on ECG or elevated troponins serve as a good foundation for identifying higher-risk patients. In summary, patients with hyponatremia, elevated blood urea nitrogen (BUN) or creatinine, ischemic changes on ECG, low SBP and/or elevated troponin may not be appropriate candidates for EDOU admission. Moreover, other exclusion criteria for EDOU admission are patients with new onset ADHF with poor social support or follow-up, patients on actively titrated intravenous drips, significant hyperventilation or requirement of noninvasive ventilation (NIV) at the time of admission, signs of poor perfusion and/or acutely active comorbidities (Fig. 1).

PROTOCOL FOR TREATMENT

A protocolized approach to the treatment of ADHF is key to successful ADHF-EDOU programs. Treatment algorithms can be divided into subgroups: monitoring care, medical therapy (Box 1), diagnostic procedures, and educational services.

The focus of EDOU management should involve an assessment of the HF exacerbating factors, which may include ischemia, hypotension or hypertension, arrhythmias, valvular heart disease, worsening renal function, uncontrolled diabetes, or infectious etiologies, as well as medication and dietary nonadherence.

Diagnostic procedures may be necessary to assess the progression of disease or determine the precipitant cause of the ADHF. However, the more numerous and complex the diagnostics become, the more likely the patient will require an inpatient evaluation. For this reason, the patient who has a clear, reversible cause of their acute symptoms, such as diet or medication nonadherence, often is the best EDOU candidate.

DIAGNOSTICS

Diagnostic studies should be directed toward searching for etiologies of decompensation, evaluating disease progression, and measuring therapy response. Echocardiogram should be performed on all patients newly diagnosed with HF and in those with no echocardiogram within the previous 6 months.

Serial cardiac biomarkers monitoring is recommended for diagnostic and prognostic purposes; ADHF patients with elevated troponin have higher mortality when compared with patients with undetected troponin. Patients with ECG changes suggestive of ischemia should not be admitted to EDOU units. Serum chemistries should be serially followed to monitor for electrolyte shifts that is commonly found with diuresis and ADHF treatment.

THERAPY

Therapy should be tailored toward diuresis, blood pressure management, and optimization of the outpatient therapy.

Oxygen Therapy

Oxygen supplementation is indicated for most patients presenting with ADHF. Patients with mild distress will need supplementation via nasal cannula, while patients with moderate distress will need a non-rebreather face mask.

As for patients with severe distress and patients with pulmonary edema, ventilator support is often required. NIV using continuous positive airway pressure (CPAP) or bilevel positive airway pressure (BiPAP) has proved effective in reducing the need for intubation. NIV should always be considered in alert and intact mental status patients in distress.

John H Streger, Hospital
of Cook County

ED Observation Unit Provider Orders - CHF
Chart Copy (not a prescription)

Unit: ED OBS Room/Bed ________

Mark box on the left of answers or print in space proived

Time Admitted for 23 HR Observation Remember to evaluate patient status at or before 20 hours post admit to 23 hr obs.

R X	Date/Time Orders Written:	Nurse initiais	Time
	Diagnosis(es): CHF		
	Allergies: ☐NKA ☐Other: ________		
	Admit: ☐ED OBS		
	Condition: ☐Stable ☐Other ________		
	Vital signs: ☐q 4 hours ☐Other ________		
	Call physician if BP <100/50, >170/100; P <50, >140; RR<10, >30; Temp> 101; Chest pain		
	Diet: ☐ Low Salt, Low Cholesterol ☐Other: ________		
	Activity: ☐ Bedrest ☐Other ________		
	Treatments: ☐ Continuous cardiac monitoring		
	☐ Record input and output		
	☐Daily weight		
	☐Oxygen ______ liters via nasal cannula		
	Medications: Patient weight: ________ Lbs/kg		
	☐Nitropaste ½inch to chest wall q 6 hours		
	☐Aspirin 325 mg PO q day		
	☐Lasix ______ mgs IVP Q ______ hr		
	IV fluids: ☐ Maintain saline lock and irrigate q shift with NS		
	☐ Other: ________		
	Labs orders: ☐ MI Screen #2 at ________		
	☐ MI Screen #3 at ________		
	EKG: ☐EKG # 2 at ________		
	☐EKG # 3 at ________		
	Patient to go for 2-d echocardiogram ________ at 8 AM		
	Special Patient Interventions/Observations:		
	☐One to One Observation		
	☐Restrict Visit or Privileges to: ________		
	Provider Print/Sign Name ________ Pager #: ________		

Initials	Print / Sign Name	Title
________	________	
________	________	
________	________	

Patient Name

Fig. 1 Emergency department observation chart for patient

Box 1: Protocol for management of acutely decompensated heart failure with volume overload (normal/elevated systolic blood pressure)

1. Aspirin

   Contraindication: Aspirin allergy   Other__________

   Aspirin 4 (four) 81 mg tablets po × 1 chew and swallow

   If allergic to aspirin, give clopidogrel 75 mg orally × 1
2. Diuretics: IV furosemide

   Take patient's total home daily PO dose and give as slow IVP (maximum initial dose 100 mg)

   If total home daily dose is unknown or patient naive, start furosemide 40 mg slow IVP.
   - Expected UOP response in first 2 hours: 250–500 mL

   If response is inadequate in first 2 hours UOP less than 250–500 mL: double previous IV furosemide dose
   - Maximum total dose in first 6 hours: 240 mg
   - Consider continuous furosemide infusion in discussion with a cardiologist
3. Vasodilators

   Nitroglycerin (NTG)
   - If no respiratory distress, apply 1 inch nitropaste to anterior chest wall
   - If patient is in respiratory distress, consider sublingual or NTG drip instead:

   Sublingual NTG 0.4 mg prn

   NTG drip: Start at 20 mcg/minute
   - Increase by 10–20 mcg/min every 5 minute
   - Maximum dose 300 mcg/minute (or SBP <90 mmHg)
   - Titrate to symptom improvement
4. Morphine: Consider if severe respiratory distress requiring BiPAP/CPAP 2–4 mg IVP
5. Ventilation

   Mild respiratory distress
   - O_2 via nasal cannula

   Moderate-severe respiratory distress: CPAP and BiPAP equally effective

   "May cause decreased blood pressure due to decreased preload"
   - CPAP: 10 mmHg
   - BiPAP: 10/5 mmHg

   Indications for intubation/contraindications to NIV
   - Hemodynamic instability
   - Aspiration risk
   - Decreased level of consciousness
   - Not cooperative with CPAP/BiPAP

ADHF, acutely decompensated heart failure; SBP, systolic blood pressure; IV, intravenous; PO, per os; IVP, intravenous pyelogram; UOP, urinary output; BiPAP, bilevel positive airway pressure; CPAP, continuous positive airway pressure; NIV, noninvasive ventilation; po, per oral

Source: Cook County Hospital ED Obs CHF Guidlines, Nava Geula, Nihja Gordon, Jordan Moskoff, Lauren Smith, Michael Sunu, Joanne C. Witsil RN, for the Department of Emergency Medicine

Patients with signs of impending respiratory failure such as severe dyspnea, diaphoresis, fatigue and acute maxillary sinusitis (AMS) will require invasive ventilation. Some objective parameters may indicate potential need for mechanical ventilation include persistent hypoxia (SaO_2 <90) despite supplemental oxygen, hypercarbia ($PaCO_2$ >55 mmHg), and acidosis (pH <7.25).

Diuretics

Loop diuretics are usually the first-line approach to relieve symptoms of dyspnea and to reduce fluid overload. Despite their importance to the management and symptoms relief, diuretics have serious potential side effects; including hypotension, renal impairment and electrolyte derangements.

Even though diuretics have been used for decades in the ADHF management, and they are included in all guidelines of HF management, there are no large-scale randomized controlled trials to delineate the optimal dose and duration of use. Dosing is usually empiric and depends on the patient response.

Vasodilators

Vasodilator therapy includes a diverse group of agents, such as nitrates, nesiritide and nitroprusside. They are usually part of the ADHF management in patients with normal or elevated blood pressure.

Nitroglycerin works by relaxing the vascular smooth muscles leading to venodilation at low dosages and to arteriolar dilation at higher dosages. Nitroglycerin is available in intravenous (IV), sublingual, and topical preparations.

Headache and abdominal pain are common adverse events with nitroglycerin use.

Nesiritide is a recombinant form of human BNP. It works by preventing excess water and salt retention and by inducing vascular relaxation.

Angiotensin-converting enzyme inhibitors (ACEIs) have also been used in the setting of ADHF. ACEIs are effective antihypertensives and provide antagonism of the renin-angiotensin-aldosterone system, making them ideal for the management of HF. Abundant data demonstrate their benefit in chronic HF management; however, there are limited data on their use in acute settings. Recent studies are demonstrating promising results in rapid symptom improvement in acute settings. Since there are still no large, placebo-controlled trials, and the potential for adverse events, such as hypotension and renal dysfunction, ACE inhibitors are not currently considered standard of care in the management of ADHF.

Morphine sulfate is another common medication that has been traditionally used as a vasodilator. It is thought that morphine produces mild venodilatation with preload reduction. Moreover, morphine would decrease the patient's agitation and induce respiratory relaxation.

DISCHARGE CRITERIA

The decision of discharge should be based upon overall assessment of the patient's improvement. Criteria should be validated for ADHF patients discharge from the EDOU. The criteria should include the need of adequate symptom relief and alleviation of ADHF signs. However, it is crucial to realize that there can be improvement in signs and symptoms in patients while still they have an ongoing elevation in cardiac filling pressures.

Improvement in congestive symptoms coupled with hemodynamic evidence of decreased volume overload is a realistic goal for the management of ADHF patients in the EDOU.

Reduction or resolution of jugular venous pressure, orthopnea, edema, and reduction in the patients' weight are objective measurements of improvement. It is also important that the patient is able to function and ambulate without significant symptoms at the time of discharge.

The underlying reason for acute decompensation should be identified and reversed. Patient education should address and the patient's outpatient oral medication regimen adjusted or implemented. Moreover, a follow-up visit should be arranged prior to discharge.

PATIENT EDUCATION

In the United States, the most commonly reported causes of acute HF decompensation are medication noncompliance, dietary indiscretion or failure to seek medical care for worsening symptoms.

Educational strategies to improve adherence and compliance to medications and lifestyle modifications to increase awareness of worsening signs and symptoms will decrease morbidity and mortality rates of HF, in addition to reducing readmission rates.

REFERENCES

1 Fermann GJ, Collins SP. Observation units in the management of acute heart failure syndromes. Curr Heart Fail Rep. 2010;7(3):125-33.
2 Burkhardt J, Peacock WF, Emerman CL. Predictors of emergency department observation unit outcomes. Acad Emerg Med. 2005;12(9): 869-74.
3 Heart Failure Executive Committee, Peacock WF, Fonarow GC, et al. Society of Chest Pain Centers Recommendations for the evaluation and management of the observation stay acute heart failure patient: a report from the Society of Chest Pain Centers Acute Heart Failure Committee. Crit Pathw Cardiol. 2008;7(2):83-6.
4 Christenson J, Innes G, McKnight D, et al. A clinical prediction rule for early discharge of patients with chest pain. Ann Emerg Med. 2006;47(1): 1-10.

Chapter 11

When to Employ Cardiac Magnetic Resonance Imaging and Cardiac Computed Tomography in the Evaluation of Heart Failure

Joel R Wilson

ABSTRACT

Cardiac magnetic resonance imaging (CMRI) and computed tomography (CT) provide both diagnostic and prognostic information in ischemic and nonischemic cardiomyopathies (CMs). CT and magnetic resonance imaging (MRI) techniques can quantify left ventricular (LV) myocardial mass, biventricular (BiV) volumes and blood flow, to determine the significance of coronary artery disease (CAD) and likelihood of functional recovery after revascularization, and characterize diseases of myocardium. This chapter reviews the indications and contraindications for advanced cardiovascular imaging studies and provides an algorithm for when to order an advanced imaging study. Focusing primarily on the role of CMRI in the initial diagnosis of patients with heart failure (HF), the utility of each modality is framed in terms of the most common questions faced in clinical practice. These scenarios include how advanced cardiovascular imaging can help in determining etiology for systolic dysfunction, evaluating causes and significance of LV and right ventricular (RV) chamber enlargement and structural heart disease, elucidating etiology of increased LV wall thickness/hypertrophy, evaluating patients with biomarker abnormalities but nonobstructive CAD, differentiating constrictive pericarditis from restrictive CM, and evaluating LV masses and thrombus.

INTRODUCTION

Advanced cardiovascular imaging using computed tomography (CT) and magnetic resonance imaging (MRI) are valuable tools in the initial diagnosis, risk stratification and management of patients with heart failure (HF). Cardiac magnetic resonance imaging (CMRI) is considered to be a gold standard for quantification of biventricular (BiV) volumes and systolic function, with standard errors of around 5%.[1-3] CMRI is unencumbered by sonographic windows, allowing for complete visualization of the blood pool and myocardium. Myocardial fibrosis, myocardial edema/inflammation and iron deposition can be readily identified with MRI.[1-5] The presence and pattern of findings helps differentiate between ischemic and nonischemic etiologies, and further distinguishes between subtypes of nonischemic cardiomyopathy (CM).[1,6-17] Additionally, the presence of myocardial fibrosis has prognostic implications in nearly every form of HF.[6-16] If ischemic CM is known or suspected, stress testing with CMRI can be performed either with myocardial perfusion imaging using gadolinium-contrast agent during vasodilator administration, or with functional imaging by assessing contractile response to graded rates of dobutamine infusion. CMRI can quantify blood flow velocities, allowing for evaluation of cardiac output and shunt severity in patients with anatomic defects.[3] Although cardiac CT has less of a role than CMRI in the management of patients with HF, it is well suited for the evaluation of coronary arteries and for delineating morphologic abnormalities. It can also accurately quantify BiV volumes and function in patients with contraindications to CMRI.[18]

The specific test to order, CMRI versus cardiac CT, will not only depend upon the diagnostic question but also on what technologies and expertise are available. The 2013 Appropriate Utilization of Cardiovascular Imaging in Heart Failure document outlines time points

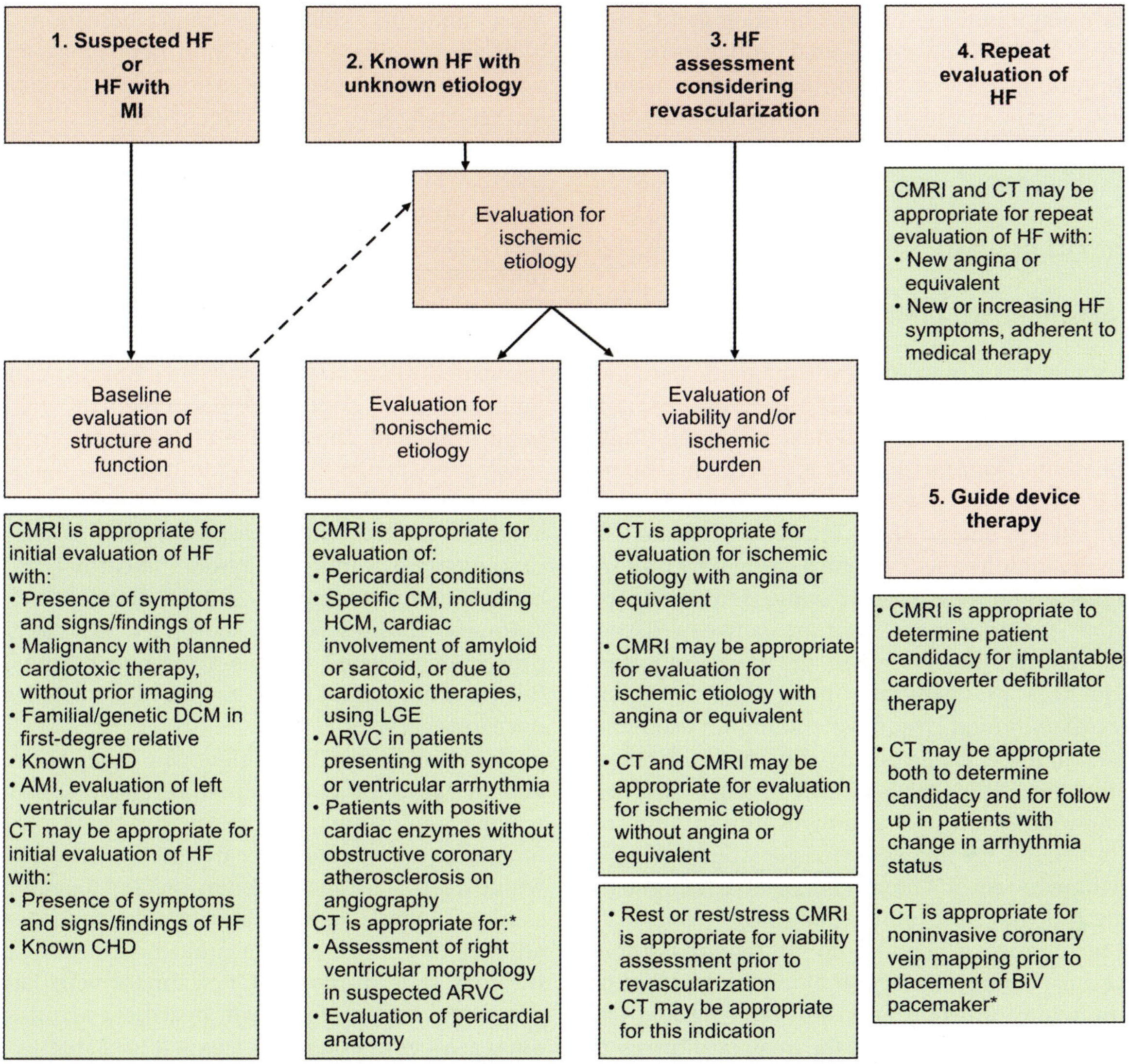

*Indications included in the Flowchart that were not covered by the American College of Cardiology Foundation (ACCF)/American College of Radiology (ACR) document were taken from ACCF/ACR/Society of Cardiovascular Computed Tomography (SCCT)/Society for Cardiovascular Magnetic Resonance (SCMR)/American Society of Nuclear Cardiology (ASNC)/North American Society for Cardiac Imaging (NASCI)/Society for Cardiovascular Angiography and Interventions (SCAI)/Society of Interventional Radiology (SIR) 2010 appropriateness criteria for cardiac computed tomography (CT) and cardiac magnetic resonance imaging (CMRI)[18]

HF, heart failure; MI, myocardial infarction; CMRI, cardiac magnetic resonance imaging; CT, computed tomography; DCM, dilated cardiomyopathy; CHD, congenital heart disease; AMI, acute myocardial infarction; CM, cardiomyopathy; HCM, hypertrophic cardiomyopathy; LGE, late gadolinium enhancement; ARVC, arrhythmogenic right-ventricular cardiomyopathy; BiV, biventricular

Flowchart 1 Five time points at which imaging studies may be indicated for evaluation of heart failure and the relevant appropriateness criteria for use of cardiac magnetic resonance imaging and cardiac computed tomography. Nonischemic cardiomyopathies were not specifically summarized in this document, and are to be addressed in a forthcoming separate work[19]

during the care of HF patients when imaging techniques are typically employed (Flowchart 1). This document covers appropriate utilization of echocardiography, radionucleotide ventriculography, single photon emission computed tomography (SPECT), positron-emission tomography (PET) and invasive angiography in addition to CMRI and cardiac CT.[19] Advanced cardiovascular imaging techniques are rarely the first tests employed in the evaluation of patients with HF. Approximately two-thirds of patients referred for CMRI have undergone transthoracic echocardiography and quarters have had prior invasive angiography.[20] Advanced cardiovascular imaging is usually indicated when the etiology of HF it is not well established on the basis of initial tests; e.g., when echocardiography is suboptimal or did not fully address the specific question, or when results will affect management such as when considering implantation of cardiodefibrillators.

IMAGE ACQUISITION

Cardiac Magnetic Resonance Imaging

An MRI scanner has a powerful static magnetic field that is measured in units of Tesla (T). Most MRI scanners used in CMRI are 1.5 T or 3 T field strengths. Pulse sequences are the combination of radiofrequency bursts and perturbations in magnetic field that stimulate protons to change energy state. Images are created by measuring the radiofrequency signals emitted by protons during pulse sequences. Specific pulse sequences are employed to provide image contrast between tissues of differing compositions. Among the most important pulse sequences to CMRI are those used to obtain cines of cardiac motion. The most commonly used cine imaging technique is called steady-state free precession (SSFP) imaging. This method offers high intrinsic contrast between blood pool and myocardium; thus, no contrast is needed for analysis of myocardial function. Similarly, there are several methods available to highlight myocardial edema and other pathology, called T_2-weighted techniques, which also do not require contrast agent. The most common images that require gadolinium contrast to acquire include perfusion imaging and late gadolinium enhancement (LGE) for imaging fibrosis or damaged myocardium.

Many pulse sequences used in cardiac studies are designed to be played out over a number of heartbeats. Patients are attached to a cardiac monitor in order to acquire images timed to the cardiac cycle (cardiac gating). Additionally, patients are asked to hold their breath during image acquisition to keep the diaphragm immobile. In patients who are unable to hold their breath adequately or who have arrhythmias or frequent ectopy, a limited number of alternative pulse sequences are available that are acquired in real time generally at the cost of decreased spatial resolution.

Cardiac Computed Tomography

Like CMRI, cardiac CT images are also cardiac-gated and breath-held. For evaluation of coronary arteries, most patients without a contraindication to beta-blockade receive a dose of oral beta blocker about an hour prior to the procedure. If needed, the heart rate is further lowered with the patient on the CT table using intravenous (IV) beta-blockade to achieve goal heart rate less than 60 beats per minute (bpm). Once in the scanner, a noncontrast volume of the heart is usually acquired first to assess for coronary calcification and for planning purposes. Patients who are undergoing evaluation of coronary arteries are then premedicated with 0.4 mg nitroglycerin sublingually. Then, contrast and saline are injected through a peripheral IV. Image acquisition is timed for peak contrast enhancement of the structure being evaluated. The number of images acquired during a single study depends upon the indication. A gated cardiac CT used to evaluate cardiac morphology and function acquires multiple full volume images of the heart at multiple time points throughout the cardiac cycle during a single contrast injection. If the indication is to evaluate coronary arteries using coronary CT angiography, prospectively gated images are typically only acquired during a portion of diastasis in order to limit radiation dose exposure.

Most modern CT scanners can cover between 4 cm and 16 cm in the craniocaudal direction (Z-axis) during a single acquisition. This means the heart is completely imaged using between 1 heartbeat and 4 heartbeats. The whole heart is reconstructed by piecing together separate slabs of image data. Image quality can therefore be affected by arrhythmias for multi-heartbeat acquisitions, whereas state-of-the-art CT scanners with large Z-axis coverage allowing for single heartbeat acquisitions can often achieve adequate image quality (Table 1).

PATIENT SCREENING

Metallic Implants

Prior to an MRI examination, all patients are screened for devices that have potential to interact with the magnetic fields or radiofrequency pulses during an MRI examination. These interactions can produce movement of the device, current induction or heating. Compatibility depends in part on the field strength of the MRI, so some implants may be MRI compatible at 1.5 T but not at 3 T. Most but not all non-electronic implanted metallic devices are compatible with the MRI environment at 1.5 T field strengths. Compatible devices at 1.5 T include prosthetic heart valves, coronary and peripheral stents, aortic stent grafts, sternal wires, epicardial pacing

TABLE 1: Questions to be asked before cardiac magnetic resonance imaging and cardiac computed tomography

Questions to ask before CMRI	*If yes*
Does the patient have an implanted pacemaker, cardiac defibrillator or retained transvenous leads?	CMRI is contraindicated
Does patient require a thermodilution Swan-Ganz catheter?	Study must be deferred until catheter can be removed or exchanged for an MRI compatible device
Is the patient's ability to hold their breath and/or lay supine compromised, for example by volume overload?	Consider deferring CMRI until HF is compensated
Does the patient have severe claustrophobia?	Consider premedication with a benzodiazepine
Is atrial fibrillation present?	Consider deferring until after cardioversion, if planned. If not, proceed with study
Does the patient have acute renal failure, or stable chronic renal failure with eGFR <30 mL/min?	Either defer CMRI until renal function stabilizes, or proceed with noncontract study
Does the patient have a history of an allergic-type reaction to gadolinium-based contrast agents?	Consider premedication, e.g., prednisone 50 mg PO Q6H three times (preferred) or hydrocortisone 200 mg IV Q6H three times (second line) ending 1 hour prior to procedure; plus diphenhydramine 50 mg PO or IV one time with final dose of steroid
Questions to ask before cardiac CT	*If yes*
Is atrial fibrillation present?	Consider deferring until after cardioversion, if planned. If not, consult the advanced imaging practitioner regarding feasibility
Is resting heart rate >55 bpm?	Most patients should be premedicated with beta-blockade, e.g., 50–100 mg of metoprolol, for optimal image quality unless contraindicated
Are beta-blockers contraindicated?	Consider premedication with diltiazem to suppress heart rate to <60 bpm unless contractile function is tenuous
Does the patient have a history of a moderate-to-severe allergic-type reaction to iodinated contrast?	Consider premedication, e.g., prednisone 50 mg PO Q6H three times (preferred) or hydrocortisone 200 mg IV Q6H three times (second line) ending 1 hour prior to procedure; plus diphenhydramine 50 mg PO or IV one time with final dose of steroid
Does patient take metformin?	Metformin should be held for 48 hours or more starting at the time of CT scan in most patients with HF to prevent lactic acidosis.
Is acute renal insufficiency or moderate-to-severe CRI present?	Risks of contrast-induced nephropathy must be weighed against information to be gained. Some experts recommend a threshold for creatinine of 2 mg/dL in patients with stable CRI. Anuric patients on hemodialysis can undergo contrast study[21]

CMRI, cardiac magnetic resonance imaging; eGFR, estimated glomerular filtration rate; HF, heart failure; CT, computed tomography; bpm, beats per minute; CRI, chronic renal insufficiency; PO, per orally; Q6H, every 6 hour; IV, intravenous

wires, septal occluder devices and coils, artificial joint replacements and Harrington rods. Some devices require further investigation regarding the specific type of device. For example, some inferior vena cava filters are weakly ferromagnetic and MRI should be deferred for 6 weeks after implantation of such devices. Cerebral aneurysm clips may be a contraindication to MRI depending upon the specific type of clip used. Devices that are contraindications for MRI include implanted cardiodefibrillators (ICD), retained endovascular pacing wires, intra-aortic balloon pumps, the most neurostimulators and thermodilution Swan Ganz catheters. Although some research suggests that MRIs can be safely performed in patients with pacemakers at 1.5 T,[22] pacemakers currently remain a strong relative contraindication for MRI in clinical practice.[23] Additionally, while MRI conditional pacemakers have been developed, they are not approved for cardiothoracic studies. The American Heart Association (AMA) has issued a scientific statement on safety of cardiovascular devices during MRI,[23] and an extensive list of implanted medical devices and their MRI compatibility is maintained at website (www.MRISafety.com).

Contrast Agents

Gadolinium Chelate Agents for Magnetic Resonance Imaging

Gadolinium chelate contrast agents are used for perfusion imaging, tissue characterization (e.g., when assessing for ventricular thrombus) and for assessing for myocardial fibrosis, but as mentioned previously are not necessary for functional or structural assessment. Patients with chronic renal failure and a glomerular filtration rate (GFR) of less than 30 mL/min or acute renal failure cannot undergo gadolinium-enhanced CMRI due to the rare and life-threatening complication of nephrogenic systemic sclerosis[21] (Fig. 1). Immediate hypersensitivity reactions to gadolinium-contrast agents are rare and tend to be mild, with acute reactions occurring in about 0.17% of injections, although reaction rates may vary slightly according to the specific gadolinium chelate agent used.[24] Severe reactions occur at a rate of less than 0.01%. There is not an increased risk of hypersensitivity cross-reaction between iodinated contrast agents and gadolinium chelate agents. However, as with low osmolar iodinated contrast agents, a history of allergic-type reactions to medications in general increases the risk of an allergic-type reaction. Patients with a history of allergic-type reaction to gadolinium contrast agents should be premedicated prior to subsequent exposures in a manner similar to that described above for iodinated agents.[21]

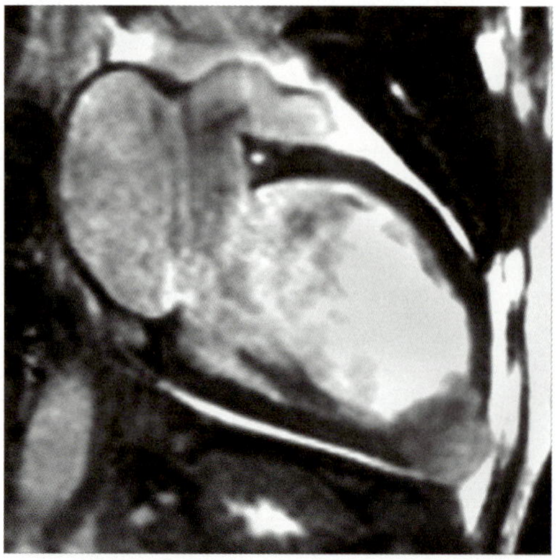

Fig. 1 Metastatic renal cell carcinoma in patient referred for evaluation of apical thrombus. Gadolinium was contraindicated due to severe renal dysfunction. This noncontrast image clearly demonstrates that the mass extends through the apical left ventricular wall. The patient was subsequently found to have metastatic renal cell carcinoma

Iodinated Contrast for Computed Tomography

Iodinated contrast is required for virtually all cardiac assessments. The severity of renal insufficiency should be considered prior to performing cardiac CT. Baseline renal insufficiency is the most consistently identified risk factor for developing contrast-induced nephropathy (CIN). Interestingly, the risk of CIN may not be related to the dose of contrast when given intravenously, although this differs from data from invasive angiography.[21] There is no established threshold for creatinine above which IV contrast becomes a strict contraindication. The risk of worsening renal dysfunction with contrast exposure must be balanced against the value of the information to be gained. A threshold of 2.0 mg/dL has been recommended by some authorities as safe in most patients with chronic stable renal dysfunction.[21] Immediate hypersensitivity reactions to low osmolar iodinated contrast agents occur between 0.18% and 0.7% of administrations, with serious reactions at a rate of 0.04%.[21] For patients requiring contrast-enhanced CT scans, patients with a history of allergic-type reaction should be premedicated prior to CT angiography. Typical premedication regimens include prednisone 50 mg by mouth (PO) every 6 hours (Q6H) for three doses ending 1 hour prior to procedure (start 13 hours in advance), plus diphenhydramine 50 mg PO or intravenously once with the final dose of steroid. Oral prednisone is preferable to IV steroid, but 200 mg hydrocortisone IV may be substituted for prednisone if required. Premedication is not completely effective at preventing breakthrough reactions, however. When breakthrough reactions occur, they are usually similar to the index event.[21]

Claustrophobia

Mild claustrophobia is relatively common, but may be less common in newer generation scanners.[25] It is severe enough to prevent completion of the MRI study in less than 1% of cases, but approximately 2% of patients will require sedation with benzodiazepines to complete the study.[25]

GENERAL UTILITY OF ADVANCED IMAGING

Cardiac MRI has a demonstrable impact on the management majority of the time it is used and only about 15% of patients require subsequent imaging.[20] A large German registry indicates results of CMRI suggest an entirely new diagnosis about 16% of the time, and result in a change in medications over 23% of the time.[20] CMRI has several advantages over other modalities. It does not use ionizing radiation, and has the flexibility to characterize tissues, quantify blood flow and myocardial perfusion, strain and infarct size. As a stress modality, it has higher special resolution than SPECT and is not limited by attenuation artifact. Both CMRI and cardiac CT have the advantage over echocardiography of having no limitations to tomographic planes. Both also have the ability to quantify cardiovascular performance measures like ventricular volumes and mass to accurately represent anatomy, including coronary artery course and origins.[1,18] Cardiac CT has the additional advantage of being helpful in evaluating for coronary atherosclerosis.[18] The strengths of these modalities have led to the creation of guideline statements for a number of indications related to HF/CMs (Table 2).

TABLE 2: Selected guideline statements for use of cardiac magnetic resonance imaging in patients with heart failure or cardiomyopathy[2,5,26]

Condition	*Year*	*Strength of recommendation*	*LOE*	*Society*	*Statement*
General	2012	Class I	C	ESC	CMRI is recommended to evaluate cardiac structure and function, to measure LVEF, and to characterize cardiac tissue in selected patients, especially in subjects with inadequate echocardiographic images or where the echocardiographic findings are inconclusive or incomplete (but taking account of cautions/contraindications to CMRI)
	2013	Class IIa	C	ACC/AHA	CMRI can be useful to assess LVEF and volume when echocardiography is inadequate
		Class I	C	ACC/AHA	Repeat measurement of EF and measurement of the severity of structural remodeling are useful to provide information in patients with HF who have had a significant change in clinical status; who have experienced or recovered from a clinical event; or who have received treatment, including GDMT, that might have had a significant effect on cardiac function; or who may be candidates for device therapy
HCM	2011	Class I	B	ACC/AHA	CMRI is indicated in patients with suspected HCM when echocardiography is inconclusive for diagnosis
		Class I	B	ACC/AHA	CMRI is indicated in patients with known HCM when additional information that may have an impact on management or decision making regarding invasive management, such as magnitude and distribution of hypertrophy or anatomy of the mitral valve apparatus or papillary muscles, is not adequately defined with echocardiography
		Class IIa	B	ACC/AHA	CMRI is reasonable in patients with HCM to define apical hypertrophy and/or aneurysm if echocardiography is inconclusive
		Class IIb	C	ACC/AHA	In selected patients with known HCM, when SCD risk stratification is inconclusive after documentation of the conventional risk factors, CMRI with assessment of LGE may be considered in resolving clinical decision making
		Class IIb	C	ACC/AHA	CMRI may be considered in patients with LV hypertrophy and the suspicion of alternative diagnoses to HCM, including cardiac amyloidosis, Fabry disease and genetic phenocopies such as *LAMP2* CM
		Class IIb		ACC/AHA	The usefulness of CMRI with LGE as a potential SCD risk modifier is unclear but might be considered in selected patients with HCM for whom risk remains borderline after documentation of conventional risk factors

Contd...

Contd...

Condition	Year	Strength of recommendation	LOE	Society	Statement
Infiltrative CMs	2013	Class IIa	B	ACC/AHA	CMR is reasonable when assessing myocardial infiltrative processes or scar burden
Ischemic CM	2012	Class IIa	C	ESC	Myocardial perfusion/ischemia imaging (echocardiography, CMRI, SPECT, or PET) should be considered in patients thought to have CAD, and who are considered suitable for coronary revascularization, to determine whether there is reversible myocardial ischemia and viable myocardium
	2013	Class IIa	C	ACC/AHA	Noninvasive imaging to detect myocardial ischemia and viability is reasonable in patients presenting with de novo HF who have known CAD and no angina unless the patient is not eligible for revascularization of any kind
	2013	Class IIa	B	ACC/AHA	Viability assessment is reasonable in select situations when planning revascularization in HF patients with CAD
Valvular	2008	Class I	B	ACC/AHA	Radionuclide angiography or MRI is indicated for the initial and serial assessment of LV volume and function at rest in patients with AR and suboptimal echocardiograms
		Class IIa	B	ACC/AHA	MRI is reasonable for the estimation of AR severity in patients with unsatisfactory echocardiograms

LOE, Level of Evidence; HCM, hypertrophic cardiomyopathy; CM, cardiomyopathy; ESC, European Society of Cardiology; CMRI, cardiac magnetic resonance imaging; LVEF, left ventricular ejection fraction; ACC, American College of Cardiology; AHA, American Heart Association; EF, ejection fraction; HF, heart failure; GDMT, Guideline-directed Medical Therapy; SCD, sudden cardiac death; LGE, late gadolinium enhancement; LV, left ventricular; *LAMP2, Lysosomal-Associated Membrane Protein 2*; SPECT, single photon emission computed tomography; PET, positron-emission tomography; CAD, coronary artery disease; AR, autosomal recessive

UTILITY OF ADVANCED IMAGING IN SPECIFIC INDICATIONS

Determining the Etiology of Systolic Heart Failure

Cardiac MRI and cardiac CT are helpful in determining etiology of HF in several respects. Initially, these modalities can help distinguish between ischemic and nonischemic causes of systolic dysfunction. Once this determination has been made, CMRI offers information to further refine diagnosis.[1,2,5,6] Analysis of regional function and morphology can identify wall motion abnormalities or LV aneurysms within a coronary distribution that would suggest an ischemic etiology. Secondly, CMRI can accurately image chronic myocardial fibrosis using the technique called LGE. The pattern of fibrosis on LGE images further helps to distinguish ischemic from nonischemic etiologies; a subendocardial-based scar within a coronary distribution is highly suggestive of myocardial infarction (MI), whereas enhancement in the mid-myocardium or epicardium suggests a nonischemic etiology (Fig. 2).[1,17,27] Finally, there are several options for further evaluating the significance of coronary atherosclerosis. An anatomic assessment can be performed using coronary CT angiography in low-to-intermediate risk patients to rule out obstructive coronary artery disease (CAD).[18] Alternatively, two methods of stress testing are available using CMRI: gadolinium first pass myocardial perfusion stress imaging with a coronary vasodilator such as adenosine, or dobutamine stress CMRI. The former identifies stress-induced myocardial perfusion defects, the latter assesses dobutamine-induced wall motion abnormalities indicative of ischemia.[28,29] Indications and cautions for these tests are analogous to vasodilator SPECT myocardial perfusion imaging and dobutamine stress echocardiography, respectively, with additional considerations regarding patient selection for CMRI mentioned above. Patients at high risk for CAD should be referred for invasive angiography. Noninvasive angiography by MRI generally not robust enough to adequately exclude obstructive CAD.[1]

Ischemic Cardiomyopathy and Viability Assessment

Myocardial infarction can be identified in nearly all patients whose systolic dysfunction is primarily due to

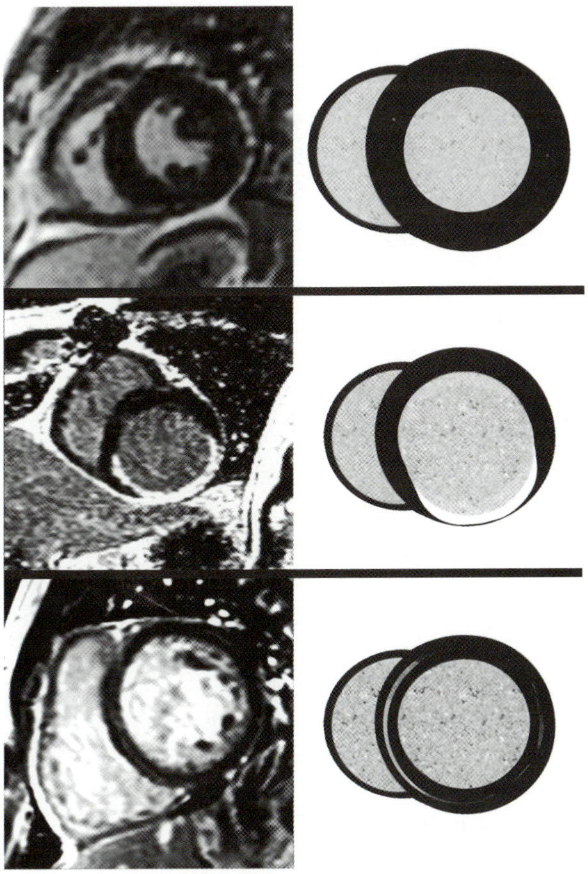

Fig. 2 Patterns of late gadolinium enhancement (LGE) that help distinguish ischemic from nonischemic etiologies. After intravenous infusion, gadolinium distributes in the extracellular space and thus is present in the highest concentrations in fibrotic tissue and other regions of high extracellular volume fraction. Higher concentrations of gadolinium are whiter on LGE images. Normal myocardium is set to appear black (top). A subendocardial-based scar within a coronary distribution is highly suggestive of myocardial infarction (middle), whereas enhancement in the mid-myocardium or epicardium suggests a nonischemic etiology (bottom)

CAD.[27,30] Mortality is directly related to both the end systolic volume index and the extent of left ventricular (LV) fibrosis in patients with ischemic CM [ejection fraction (EF) <40%].[15] After establishing the presence of ischemic CM, viability testing may be indicated in patients being considered for revascularization. Randomized imaging trials are currently underway to elucidate the role of viability testing in patients with ischemic CM after the nonrandomized Surgical Treatment for Ischemic Heart Failure (STICH) viability substudy failed to indicate a mortality benefit for patients with viable myocardium following revascularization with coronary artery bypass surgery (CABG) compared to medical therapy alone.[31,32] However, presently viability assessment remains an appropriate and common indication for CMRI.[19,20]

There are two primary methods of viability assessment in clinical practice using CMRI. The first uses a determination of the transmural extent of fibrosis by LGE, which is the ratio between infarcted to noninfarcted myocardium expressed as a percentage of wall thickness. This parameter is inversely related to the likelihood of functional recovery following revascularization; infarcts with greater than 50% transmural extent are unlikely to improve.[15,29,33-35] The second method uses low dose dobutamine CMRI stress testing, analogous to dobutamine echocardiography viability assessment. Myocardium that improves function with dobutamine stimulation is viable "hibernating" myocardium that is likely to recover following revascularization (Fig. 3).[36]

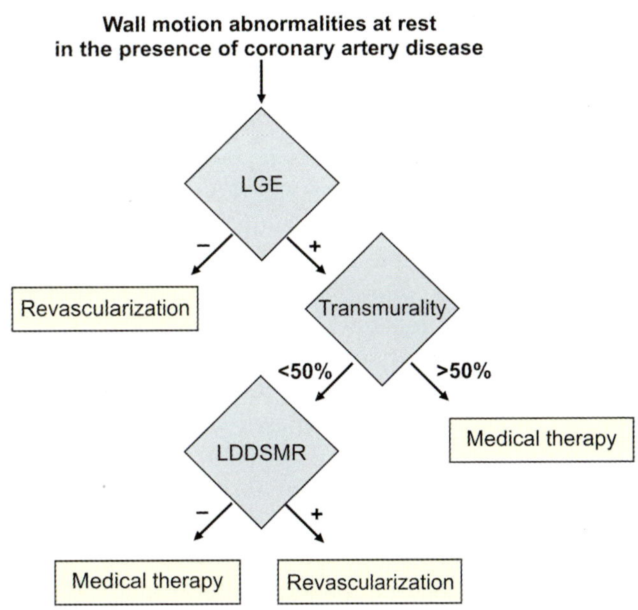

LGE, late gadolinium enhancement; LDDSMR, low-dose dobutamine stress magnetic resonance

Fig. 3 Proposed algorithm for viability testing using cardiac magnetic resonance imaging in patients with coronary artery disease and systolic dysfunction. If myocardial infarction/fibrosis is absent on late gadolinium enhancement, there is a high likelihood of recovery of function following revascularization (~78%). Conversely, if scar transmurality is greater than 50%, there is a low likelihood of functional recovery (~8%). For intermediate scar transmurality of 1–50%, there is an intermediate chance of functional recovery (~53%). Further testing with low-dose dobutamine stress magnetic resonance testing may be indicated to assess contractile reserve as a separate metric of viability in these instances[36]

This technique has the advantage of not requiring a gadolinium contrast agent.[29] Conversely, worsening wall motion with dobutamine may indicate an adverse prognosis (increased cardiac death and MI) in subset of patients referred for dobutamine stress CMRI with mild-to-moderate reductions in EFs (40–55%).[37]

Nonischemic Cardiomyopathies

After exclusion of ischemic CM, further clinical or imaging clues usually suggest a differential diagnosis to be considered. These indicators include the presence of ventricular chamber enlargement, structural or valvular disorder, abnormal wall thickness, biomarker abnormalities in absence of obstructive coronary atherosclerosis, HF with preserved systolic function, or predisposing factor such as hemochromatosis or family history of CM. Subsequent sections will detail how imaging assists in the evaluation of each of these scenarios.

Determining the Etiology of Cardiac Chamber Enlargement

Cardiac MRI is the gold standard for evaluating BiV size and function.[2] This quantitative information is obtained using multiple spatially contiguous cine slices covering the entire LV or right ventricle (RV) (volumetric coverage). The endocardial borders are then manually traced offline at end systole and end diastole to give end-systolic volume, end-diastolic volume, stroke volume and EF (Table 3). In approximately a quarter to a third of patients with nonischemic systolic dysfunction and LV enlargement, a thin stripe of fibrosis within the mid-myocardium can be demonstrated (Fig. 2, bottom). This finding, which is thought to be a marker of prior myocarditis or idiopathic dilated cardiomyopathy (DCM), is associated with adverse clinical outcomes, including a composite of cardiac death, appropriate ICD firings and hospitalizations for HF.[9,16]

Left ventricular or right ventricular (RV) enlargement may otherwise commonly be due to structural or valvular heart disease. Although echocardiography remains the modality of choice for most valvular disorders, CMRI may be considered when echocardiography images are suboptimal or equivocal, especially for aortic valve disorders.[38] A technique called phase contrast imaging provides data complementary to volumetric information for the calculation of regurgitant volumes/fractions or shunt fractions. Each voxel (three-dimensional pixel) of a phase contrast image is encoded with velocity estimates for the blood within that voxel which can be extracted to estimate flow volumes. Images transecting the pulmonary artery and aorta estimate the net forward pulmonary flow (or Qp, where Q stands for volumetric flow and p stands for pulmonary) and net forward flow (Qs), respectively, for use in either shunt fraction calculations or regurgitant volume calculations. When an anatomic shunt is identified, such as an atrial septal defect, phase contrast imaging can also be used directly interrogate the volume and direction of flow through the shunt. Cardiac CT has superior spatial resolution compared to CMRI, making it well suited for the evaluation of many anatomic lesions such as pulmonary venous drainage anomalies. While volumetric data can also be acquired from cardiac CT, CMRI is the preferred method for this in the absence of contraindications as it avoids ionizing radiation exposure.

TABLE 3: Parameters derived from cardiac magnetic resonance imaging with utility in patients with suspected heart failure

Systolic function (LV and RV)	• End-diastolic volume/index • End-systolic volume/index • Stroke volume/index • Ejection fraction • Cardiac output/index • Regional and global systolic wall thickening
Morphology	• LV mass/index • Mean and maximal myocardial wall thickness • Pericardial assessment (thickness, adherence and functional significance)
Wall stress and myocardial strain*	• End-systolic wall stress • Regional/global myocardial strain • Circumferential strain and strain rate
Diastolic function*	• E/A ratio • End-diastolic forward flow in pulmonary veins • Peak untwisting rate
Reversible acute injury	• Edema assessment
Irreversible injury, prognosis	• LGE for myocardial fibrosis

*Primarily in research settings

LV, left ventricular; RV, right ventricular; E/A, early to late ratio; LGE, late gadolinium enhancement

Right ventricular enlargement may also be due to pulmonary hypertension, severe prolonged tricuspid regurgitation or rarely arrhythmogenic right-ventricular cardiomyopathy (ARVC). In the case of ARVC, CMRI findings can fulfill a major criterion for diagnosis if regions of RV akinesia or dyskinesia or dyssynchronous contraction are present and either RV EF is less than 40% or RV volume index is elevated (>110 mL/m^2 for men, >100 mL/m^2 for women).[39] Fibrous or fatty infiltration of RV or LV myocardium can also sometimes be seen by CMRI, but this is not currently a diagnostic criteria for ARVC.[1] Because the diagnosis of ARVC requires at least two major criteria or one major plus two minor criteria, CMRI is best utilized in the evaluation of ARVC in patients with at least one preexisting risk factor.

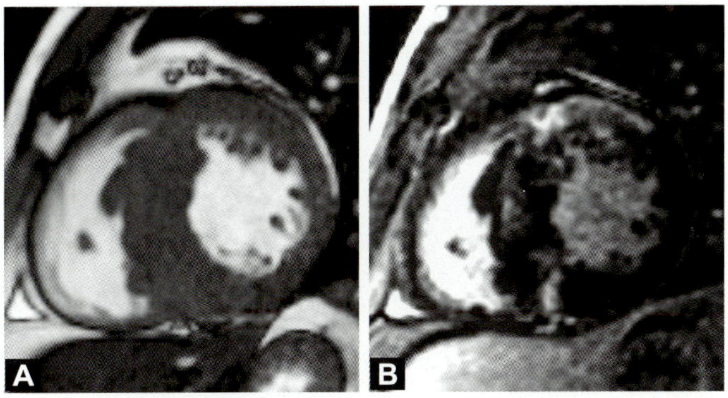

Fig 4 A, Steady-state free precession (SSFP) image and **B,** late gadolinium enhancement (LGE) in patient with hypertrophic cardiomyopathy. SSFP cine images delineate anatomic structure and function. LGE image shows typical distribution of fibrosis within the mid-wall concentrated at the right ventricular insertion sites in regions of hypertrophy

Determining the Etiology of Increased Left Ventricular Wall Thickness

Cardiac MRI is well suited for differentiating LV hypertrophy from infiltrative CMs. It can accurately describe distribution of hypertrophy and quantify maximal wall thickness and myocardial mass. With the exception of hypertensive heart disease, abnormalities in LGE are common amongst infiltrative disorders like cardiac amyloidosis and cardiac sarcoidosis and genetic disorders such as hypertrophic cardiomyopathy (HCM) and the lysosomal storage disorder Fabry disease. Perfusion abnormalities and myocardial edema can also be demonstrated in some cases, providing supportive evidence for a given diagnosis.[1]

Cardiac MRI is playing an increasing role in the diagnosis and management of HCM.[26] Approximately 60% of patients with HCM will have evidence of fibrosis on CMRI.[11] Fibrosis tends to localize to the mid-wall within the regions of hypertrophy and often especially prominent at the RV insertion sites (Fig. 4).[17] The presence of myocardial fibrosis in patients with HCM has been associated with adverse outcomes including cardiac death in several studies.[10-13,40] It may prove to be useful as an additional risk stratification tool for risk stratification for patients whose clinical risk profile does not clearly indicate whether ICD is advisable, but research is not yet conclusive in this regard.[12,26] In addition to presence of LGE, CMRI can also accurate localize regions of hypertrophy, identify systolic anterior motion of the mitral valve, and demonstrate apical aneurysms. Perfusion abnormalities and myocardial edema may also be present.[41] While the cardiac variant of Fabry disease can have hypertrophy in a pattern than can mimic variants of HCM, the pattern of LGE along the basal inferolateral wall can help distinguish these entities.[17]

Cardiac amyloidosis can sometimes be difficult to distinguish from hypertensive heart disease and HCM on the basis of morphology alone. The hallmark of cardiac amyloidosis by CMRI is a diffuse abnormality in LGE such that normal myocardium is often difficult to identify in patients with concentric hypertrophy and impaired ventricular function. Between 67% and 97% of patients with cardiac amyloidosis will demonstrate abnormal LGE.[14,42] In some cases, abnormalities in LGE can precede LV hypertrophy. Contrast kinetics between myocardium and blood pool are frequently altered[1] (Fig. 5). In patients with systemic amyloidosis, these findings allow a high degree of accuracy in diagnosing cardiac infiltration.[1]

Cardiac MRI is an emerging gold standard for the evaluation of cardiac sarcoidosis. Of patients with extracardiac sarcoidosis, approximately 5% of patients have signs or symptoms suggestive of cardiac involvement. However by autopsy and by CMRI studies, evidence of cardiac involvement is present in approximately one quarter of patients with extracardiac sarcoidosis.[17] The pattern of LGE in cardiac sarcoidosis can be variable. Fibrosis often has a focal or nodular type of appearance, but may mimic transmural MI.[43] The presence of myocardial fibrosis in patients with systemic sarcoidosis is associated with death, aborted sudden cardiac death (SCD) and appropriate ICD discharge.[7] Abnormalities in myocardial edema indicating active inflammation can be seen, and may resolve with clinical improvement indicating a potential role for longitudinal follow-up of these patients.[44]

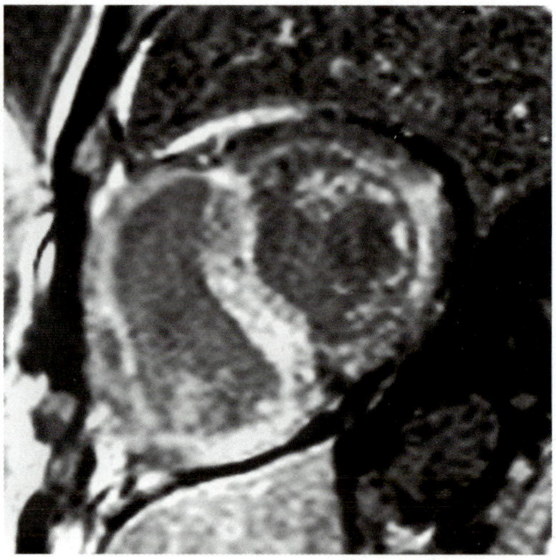

Fig. 5 Typical diffuse pattern of myocardial late gadolinium enhancement (LGE) in cardiac amyloidosis. Blood pool to myocardium contrast is decreased, indicating abnormal gadolinium kinetics. A small pericardial effusion is black on this phase-sensitive LGE image. This patient had normal QRS voltage on electrocardiogram

Evaluating Patients with Biomarker Abnormalities and Nonobstructive Coronary Artery Disease

The differential for systolic dysfunction in patients with abnormalities in cardiac biomarkers including troponin in patients with nonobstructive CAD most commonly includes myocarditis and stress-induced (takotsubo) CM, although other conditions such as pulmonary embolism should also be considered. Often the pretest probability for one entity versus the other is greatly influenced by clinical factors such as gender, age of presentation, predisposing factors such as preceding viral illness or extreme emotional stressor and ECG abnormalities. Most commonly coronary arteries will have been evaluated with invasive angiography, but in select patients with presentation highly suggestive of myocarditis cardiac CT angiography may be an appropriate alternative.[19]

Cardiac MRI can provide additional diagnostic and prognostic informations to the clinical data. The hallmark of most stress-induced CM is regional systolic dysfunction which does not reflect a single coronary distribution. Most commonly there is preservation of systolic function at the base, but hypokinesis of mid and apical segments, although variations have been described with preserved apical function alone. Myocardial edema can be demonstrated by T_2-weighted imaging.[45] The determination as to whether the wall motion abnormality could be attributable to ischemia can often be complicated in patients with primarily apical hypokinesis and a large apical recurrent branch from the left anterior descending. The absence of LGE on CMRI does not completely rule out an ischemic etiology, but would indicate a high likelihood of recovery of systolic function nonetheless, whereas the presence of subendocardial or transmural LGE is not consistent with stress-induced CM but rather MI.[45]

Cardiac MRI has high diagnostic accuracy in patients with suspected myocarditis. Abnormal LGE is present in approximately 53% of patients with biopsy proven myocarditis. It characteristically involves the epicardium and mid-myocardium, sparing the endocardium. Pericardial enhancement may also be demonstrated. The presence of myocardial edema may be suggested by abnormalities in T_2-weighted imaging with or without abnormal LGE. Taking into account morphology, function and T_2 abnormalities combined with LGE, the overall diagnostic accuracy of CMRI to detect myocarditis with biopsy as the reference standard is approximately 84% (Fig. 6).[8]

Differentiating Restrictive Cardiomyopathy from Constrictive Pericarditis

In patients with HF signs and symptoms out of proportion to the degree of systolic dysfunction, CMRI can be very helpful in distinguishing restrictive CM from constrictive pericarditis. Restrictive CM, when due to cardiac amyloidosis, can usually be identified by the presence and pattern of LGE described previously.

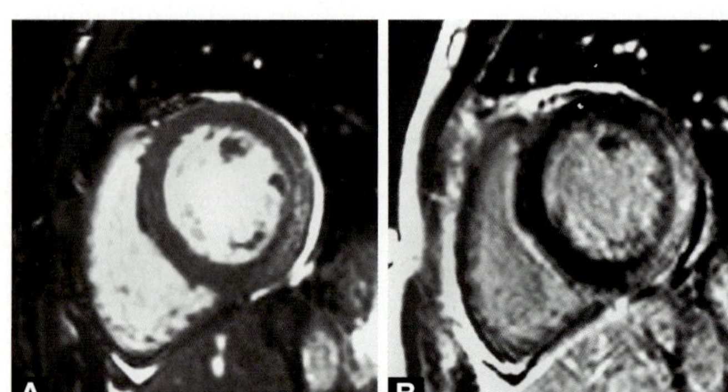

Fig. 6 Myocarditis. **A,** Edema is seen as brighter signal intensity on T_2-weighted images (bright blood technique) in the lateral wall in the image on the left; **B,** The image on the right demonstrates epicardial and mid-myocardial enhancement on late gadolinium enhancement (LGE) images. LGE in the acute setting may represent damaged myocytes rather than fibrosis

In cases where LGE is either absent or when restrictive and constrictive physiology may be overlapping, CMRI can delineate anatomic and physiologic effects of pericardial disease. CMRI can evaluate pericardial thickness (>4 mm is abnormal), presence of pericardial effusion and pericardial enhancement. The shape of the ventricle may be visibly distorted due to circumferential pericardial constriction. Using a specialized technique called myocardial tagging to augment typical cine techniques, regions where pericardium is adherent to myocardium can be identified.[1] Exaggerated ventricular interdependence can be demonstrated using real-time free breathing cine images. An extended cine loop, typically acquired in a short axis orientation in the mid-ventricle, is obtained while the patient takes exaggerated deep breaths. Inversion of the curvature of the interventricular septum early during inspiration is highly suggestive of pericardial disease over restrictive disease (Figs 7A and B).[46] Cardiac CT is superior to other modalities for evaluating the presence of pericardial calcification, and is also probably more accurate than CMRI in gauging pericardial thickness due to its superior spatial resolution. Physiologic assessment of pericardial disease by cardiac CT is not routine, however.

Evaluation of Left Ventricular Masses and Thrombus

Tissue characterization techniques take advantage of the differences in MRI signal between tissues of varying composition. These techniques include T_1- and T_2-weighted imaging, fat suppression or fat/water separation imaging, perfusion imaging and LGE imaging. In the setting of HF, mass assessment commonly involves evaluating for intracardiac thrombus (Fig. 1). Chronic thrombus typically does not enhance with gadolinium. Other contextual clues such as presence of severe global systolic dysfunction or a regional wall motion abnormality or MI in association with a mass help confirm presence of thrombus. There are limited studies to suggest that CMRI is superior to echocardiography in the detection of intramyocardial thrombus.[47,48]

Other Conditions

Cardiac Magnetic Resonance Imaging Prior to Device Implantation

One of the primary considerations when a patient is being evaluated for ICD placement is the EF, but other informative information can be acquired from CMRI and cardiac CT, including the presence of ventricular thrombus and description of venous anatomy for implantation of BiV devices. CMRI can also visualize potential arrhythmogenic substrate. Scar present near LV lead placement sites predict lack of response to cardiac resynchronization therapy (CRT).[19]

Iron Overload Cardiomyopathy

Cardiac MRI placed a unique role in the initial diagnosis of iron overload CM, and in evaluating the efficacy of chelation therapy in chronic myocardial siderosis. Using a specialized technique called T_2^*-weighting

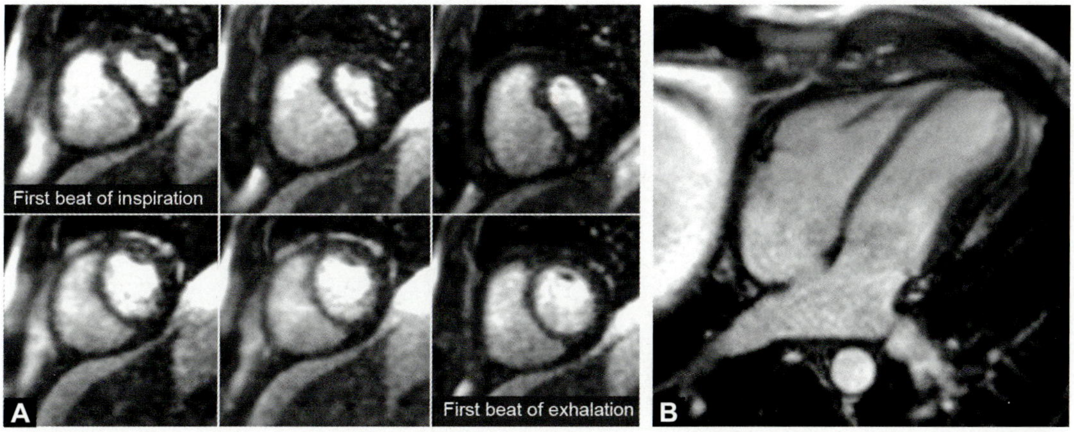

Fig. 7 Constrictive pericarditis. **A,** The still frames on the left represent diastolic frames during a respiratory cycle starting at upper left and progressing clockwise. Exaggerated leftward movement of the interventricular septum during early inspiration indicates exaggerated ventricular interdependence, a hallmark of constrictive pericarditis **B,** The image at the right is a still shot of a cine loop demonstrating a tubular-shaped left ventricle with pericardial thickening along the mid-lateral wall

(pronounced "T_2 star"), myocardial iron concentrations can be accurately and reproducibly quantified. The rate of decrease in MRI signal from myocardium imaged with T_2^*-weighting is dictated by the decay constant T_2^*, which is the time in milliseconds (ms) for signal to decay to 63% of maximum. T_2^* decay constant values below 20 ms are abnormal and predict increased likelihood of arrhythmia. A T_2^* time below 10 ms is the single most important predictor of developing HF in patients with transfusion-dependent thalassemia major.[4] Change in T_2^* time during chelation therapy is a better predictor of therapeutic efficacy than are iron concentration estimates derived from serial liver biopsies.[49] Lengthening of T_2^* rate constant over time correlates with improvements in EF.[49] The adoption of the T_2^* technique in diagnosing iron overload and in guiding therapy is one major reason for the improvement in cardiovascular mortality in transfusion-dependent patients with thalassemia major.[4,49]

Noncompaction Cardiomyopathy

Noncompaction CM has been increasingly recognized in recent years. It is characterized by an increase in the trabecular layer of myocardium relative to normal myocardium, thought due to arresting of normal myocardial compaction during embryologic development. One of the more commonly applied diagnostic criteria for noncompaction CM by CMRI is the ratio of trabeculated to compacted myocardium of greater than 2.4 in end diastole. However, it has been suggested that this criteria lacks specificity, leading to overdiagnosis.[50] In addition to a relative increase in trabecular myocardium relative to compacted myocardium, papillary muscles may be indiscrete. Global systolic dysfunction should be present to increase confidence in the diagnosis. Wall motion abnormalities may be associated with noncompacted regions. In addition to aiding in diagnosis, CMRI can identify ventricular thrombus which is relatively common in this entity. While the optimal diagnostic strategy for this entity has not been established and there is phenotypic overlap with entities such as DCM, in severe cases the diagnosis is obvious.

Congenital Heart Disease

Evaluation and management of adults with CHD is recommended to be performed at specialized centers of expertise where advanced imaging modalities should be available.[3] Advanced imaging is extremely helpful in accurately delineating the anatomy of newly-diagnosed patients with congenital defects. As outlined above, CMRI can identify anatomic shunts and characterize the hemodynamic impact through both phase contrast and volumetric approaches. Because of the lack of ionizing

TABLE 4: Selected 2008 American College of Cardiology/American Heart Association Guideline Statements for use of cardiac magnetic resonance imaging in adults with congenital heart disease[3]

Condition		*Strength of recommendation*	*LOE*	*Statement*
Tetralogy of Fallot		Class I	C	Patients with tetralogy of Fallot should have echocardiographic examinations and/or MRIs performed by staff with expertise in ACHD
Dextro-transposition of the great arteries (d-TGA)	After atrial baffle operation	Class I	B	Additional imaging with TEE, CT, or MRI, as appropriate, should be performed in a regional ACHD center to evaluate the great arteries and veins, as well as ventricular function, in patients with prior atrial baffle repair of d-TGA
	After arterial switch operation	Class IIa	C	Periodic MRI or CT can be considered appropriate to evaluate the anatomy and hemodynamics in more detail
Congenitally corrected transposition of the great arteries (ccTGA)		Class I	C	CMRI is recommended as part of the diagnostic evaluation for patients with ccTGA
		Class I	C	Echocardiography-Doppler study and/or MRI should be performed yearly or at least every other year by staff trained in imaging complex CHD
CHD-related PAH		Class I	C	Diagnostic cardiovascular imaging via TTE, TEE, MRI, or CT as appropriate

LOE, Level of Evidence; CHD, congenital heart disease; PAH, pulmonary arterial hypertension; MRI, magnetic resonance imaging; ACHD, adults with congenital heart disease; TEE, transesophageal echocardiogram; CT, computed tomography; TTE, transthoracic echocardiogram radiation, CMRI in particular is also often employed in serial evaluations when accurate assessments of volumes or function are often necessary. For example, in patients with congenitally corrected transposition of the great arteries (ccTGA), CMRI can characterize severity of regurgitation of the systemic atrioventricular valve and quantify degree of dysfunction of the systemic RV. Following repair of tetralogy of Fallot, CMRI can identify pulmonic or sub-pulmonic stenosis or regurgitation. CMRI has been employed in evaluation of baffle leak or stenosis in patients with prior Mustard or Senning procedures for complete transposition of the great arteries (TGA).[3] A listing of guideline statements relevant to advanced cardiovascular imaging in adults with CHD is listed in Table 4.[3] A complete appraisal of the utility of CMRI in complex CHD is outside the scope of this chapter.

CONCLUSION

Cardiac MRI and to a lesser extent cardiac CT play an important role in the diagnosis and management of HF. When to order an advanced cardiovascular imaging study and what type of examination to order are directed by pretest probability, prior imaging findings and local availability of technologies and expertise. A number of expert consensus documents, guideline and consensus statements exist to help define when further imaging testing is indicated. Both techniques offer significant advantages over other imaging modalities like echocardiography by providing a comprehensive assessment of anatomy in any tomographic imaging plane, and providing accurate volumetric assessments of BiV function that are not based on geometric assumptions. Using CMRI, LGE provides powerful diagnostic and prognostic insights in HF.

REFERENCES

1. Hundley WG, Bluemke DA, Finn JP, et al. ACCF/ACR/AHA/NASCI/SCMR 2010 expert consensus document on cardiovascular magnetic resonance: a report of the American College of Cardiology Foundation Task Force on Expert Consensus Documents. J Am Coll Cardiol. 2010; 55(23):2614-62.
2. McMurray JJ, Adamopoulos S, Anker SD, et al. ESC guidelines for the diagnosis and treatment of acute and chronic heart failure 2012: The Task Force for the Diagnosis and Treatment of Acute and Chronic Heart Failure 2012 of the European Society of Cardiology. Developed in collaboration with the Heart Failure Association (HFA) of the ESC. Eur J Heart Fail. 2012;14(8):803-69.
3. Warnes CA, Williams RG, Bashore TM, et al. ACC/AHA 2008 guidelines for the management of adults with congenital heart disease: a report of the American College of Cardiology/American Heart Association Task Force on Practice Guidelines (Writing Committee to Develop Guidelines on the Management of Adults With Congenital Heart Disease). Developed in Collaboration With the American Society of Echocardiography, Heart Rhythm Society, International Society for Adult Congenital Heart Disease, Society for Cardiovascular Angiography and Interventions, and Society of Thoracic Surgeons. J Am Coll Cardiol. 2008;52(23):e143-263.
4. Pennell DJ, Udelson JE, Arai AE, et al. Cardiovascular function and treatment in beta-thalassemia major: A Consensus Statement from the American Heart Association. Circulation. 2013;128(3):281-308.
5. Yancy CW, Jessup M, Bozkurt B, et al. 2013 ACCF/AHA guideline for the management of heart failure: a report of the American College of Cardiology Foundation/American Heart Association Task Force on Practice Guidelines. J Am Coll Cardiol. 2013;62(16):e147-239.
6. Flett AS, Westwood MA, Davies LC, et al. The prognostic implications of cardiovascular magnetic resonance. Circ Cardiovasc Imaging. 2009;2(3):243-50.
7. Greulich S, Deluigi CC, Gloekler S, et al. CMR imaging predicts death and other adverse events in suspected cardiac sarcoidosis. JACC Cardiovasc Imaging. 2013;6(4):501-11.
8. Grun S, Schumm J, Greulich S, et al. Long-term follow-up of biopsy-proven viral myocarditis: predictors of mortality and incomplete recovery. J Am Coll Cardiol. 2012;59(18):1604-15.
9. Wu KC, Weiss RG, Thiemann DR, et al. Late gadolinium enhancement by cardiovascular magnetic resonance heralds an adverse prognosis in nonischemic cardiomyopathy. J Am Coll Cardiol. 2008;51(25):2414-21.
10. Greulich S, Schumm J, Grun S, et al. Incremental value of late gadolinium enhancement for management of patients with hypertrophic cardiomyopathy. Am J Cardiol. 2012;110(8):1207-12.
11. Green JJ, Berger JS, Kramer CM, et al. Prognostic value of late gadolinium enhancement in clinical outcomes for hypertrophic cardiomyopathy. JACC Cardiovasc Imaging. 2012;5(4):370-7.
12. Bruder O, Wagner A, Jensen CJ, et al. Myocardial scar visualized by cardiovascular magnetic resonance imaging predicts major adverse events in patients with hypertrophic cardiomyopathy. J Am Coll Cardiol. 2010;56(11):875-87.
13. O'Hanlon R, Grasso A, Roughton M, et al. Prognostic significance of myocardial fibrosis in hypertrophic cardiomyopathy. J Am Coll Cardiol. 2010;56(11):867-74.
14. Syed IS, Glockner JF, Feng D, et al. Role of cardiac magnetic resonance imaging in the detection of cardiac amyloidosis. JACC Cardiovasc Imaging. 2010;3(2):155-64.
15. Kwon DH, Hachamovitch R, Popovic ZB, et al. Survival in patients with severe ischemic cardiomyopathy undergoing revascularization versus medical therapy: association with end-systolic volume and viability. Circulation. 2012;126(11 Suppl 1):S3-8.
16. Assomull RG, Prasad SK, Lyne J, et al. Cardiovascular magnetic resonance, fibrosis, and prognosis in dilated cardiomyopathy. J Am Coll Cardiol. 2006;48(10):1977-85.
17. Mahrholdt H, Wagner A, Judd RM, et al. Delayed enhancement cardiovascular magnetic resonance assessment of non-ischaemic cardiomyopathies. Eur Heart J. 2005;26(15):1461-74.
18. Taylor AJ, Cerqueira M, Hodgson JM, et al. ACCF/SCCT/ACR/AHA/ASE/ASNC/NASCI/SCAI/SCMR 2010 appropriate use criteria for cardiac computed tomography. A report of the American College of Cardiology Foundation Appropriate Use Criteria Task Force, the Society of Cardiovascular Computed Tomography, the American College of Radiology, the American Heart Association, the American Society of Echocardiography, the American Society of Nuclear Cardiology, the North American Society for Cardiovascular Imaging, the Society for Cardiovascular Angiography and Interventions, and the Society for Cardiovascular Magnetic Resonance. J Am Coll Cardiol. 2010;56(22):1864-94.

19. Patel MR, White RD, Abbara S, et al. 2013 ACCF/ACR/ASE/ASNC/SCCT/SCMR appropriate utilization of cardiovascular imaging in heart failure: a joint report of the American College of Radiology Appropriateness Criteria Committee and the American College of Cardiology Foundation Appropriate Use Criteria Task Force. J Am Coll Cardiol. 2013;61(21):2207-31.
20. Bruder O, Schneider S, Nothnagel D, et al. EuroCMR (European Cardiovascular Magnetic Resonance) registry: results of the German pilot phase. J Am Coll Cardiol. 2009;54(15):1457-66.
21. American College of Radiology. (2013). ACR Manual on Contrast Media: ACR Committee on Drugs and Contrast Media, Version 9. [online] Available from www.acr.org/~/media/ACR/Documents/PDF/QualitySafety/Resources/Contrast%20Manual/2013_Contrast_Media.pdf. [Accessed January, 2014].
22. Zikria JF, Machnicki S, Rhim E, et al. MRI of patients with cardiac pacemakers: a review of the medical literature. AJR Am J Roentgenol. 2011;196(2):390-401.
23. Levine GN, Gomes AS, Arai AE, et al. Safety of magnetic resonance imaging in patients with cardiovascular devices: an American Heart Association scientific statement from the Committee on Diagnostic and Interventional Cardiac Catheterization, Council on Clinical Cardiology, and the Council on Cardiovascular Radiology and Intervention: endorsed by the American College of Cardiology Foundation, the North American Society for Cardiac Imaging, and the Society for Cardiovascular Magnetic Resonance. Circulation. 2007;116(24):2878-91.
24. Bruder O, Schneider S, Nothnagel D, et al. Acute adverse reactions to gadolinium-based contrast agents in CMR: multicenter experience with 17,767 patients from the EuroCMR Registry. JACC Cardiovasc Imaging. 2011;4(11):1171-6.
25. Dewey M, Schink T, Dewey CF. Claustrophobia during magnetic resonance imaging: cohort study in over 55,000 patients. J Magn Reson Imaging. 2007;26(5):1322-7.
26. Gersh BJ, Maron BJ, Bonow RO, et al. 2011 ACCF/AHA Guideline for the Diagnosis and Treatment of Hypertrophic Cardiomyopathy: a report of the American College of Cardiology Foundation/American Heart Association Task Force on Practice Guidelines. Developed in collaboration with the American Association for Thoracic Surgery, American Society of Echocardiography, American Society of Nuclear Cardiology, Heart Failure Society of America, Heart Rhythm Society, Society for Cardiovascular Angiography and Interventions, and Society of Thoracic Surgeons. J Am Coll Cardiol. 2011;58(25):e212-60.
27. McCrohon JA, Moon JC, Prasad SK, et al. Differentiation of heart failure related to dilated cardiomyopathy and coronary artery disease using gadolinium-enhanced cardiovascular magnetic resonance. Circulation. 2003;108(1):54-9.
28. Greenwood JP, Maredia N, Younger JF, et al. Cardiovascular magnetic resonance and single-photon emission computed tomography for diagnosis of coronary heart disease (CE-MARC): a prospective trial. Lancet. 2012;379(9814):453-60.
29. Arai AE. The cardiac magnetic resonance (CMR) approach to assessing myocardial viability. J Nucl Cardiol. 2011;18(6):1095-102.
30. Soriano CJ, Ridocci F, Estornell J, et al. Noninvasive diagnosis of coronary artery disease in patients with heart failure and systolic dysfunction of uncertain etiology, using late gadolinium-enhanced cardiovascular magnetic resonance. J Am Coll Cardiol. 2005;45(5):743-8.
31. Bonow RO, Maurer G, Lee KL, et al. Myocardial viability and survival in ischemic left ventricular dysfunction. N Engl J Med. 2011;364(17):1617-25.
32. E OM, Mielniczuk LM, Wells GA, et al. Alternative Imaging Modalities in Ischemic Heart Failure (AIMI-HF) IMAGE HF Project I-A: study protocol for a randomized controlled trial. Trials. 2013;14(1):218.
33. Selvanayagam JB, Kardos A, Francis JM, et al. Value of delayed-enhancement cardiovascular magnetic resonance imaging in predicting myocardial viability after surgical revascularization. Circulation. 2004;110(12):1535-41.
34. Schwitter J, Arai AE. Assessment of cardiac ischaemia and viability: role of cardiovascular magnetic resonance. Eur Heart J. 2011;32(7):799-809.
35. Kim RJ, Wu E, Rafael A, et al. The use of contrast-enhanced magnetic resonance imaging to identify reversible myocardial dysfunction. N Engl J Med. 2000;343(20):1445-53.
36. Nagel E, Schuster A. Myocardial viability: dead or alive is not the question! JACC Cardiovasc Imaging. 2012;5(5):509-12.
37. Dall'Armellina E, Morgan TM, Mandapaka S, et al. Prediction of cardiac events in patients with reduced left ventricular ejection fraction with dobutamine cardiovascular magnetic resonance assessment of wall motion score index. J Am Coll Cardiol. 2008;52(4):279-86.
38. Bonow RO, Carabello BA, Chatterjee K, et al. 2008 focused update incorporated into the ACC/AHA 2006 guidelines for the management of patients with valvular heart disease: a report of the American College of Cardiology/American Heart Association Task Force on Practice Guidelines (Writing Committee to revise the 1998 guidelines for the management of patients with valvular heart disease). Endorsed by the Society of Cardiovascular Anesthesiologists, Society for Cardiovascular Angiography and Interventions, and Society of Thoracic Surgeons. J Am Coll Cardiol. 2008;52(13):e1-142.
39. Marcus FI, McKenna WJ, Sherrill D, et al. Diagnosis of arrhythmogenic right ventricular cardiomyopathy/dysplasia: proposed modification of the task force criteria. Circulation. 2010;121(13):1533-41.
40. Nojiri A, Hongo K, Kawai M, et al. Scoring of late gadolinium enhancement in cardiac magnetic resonance imaging can predict cardiac events in patients with hypertrophic cardiomyopathy. J Cardiol. 2011;58(3):253-60.
41. Noureldin RA, Liu S, Nacif MS, et al. The diagnosis of hypertrophic cardiomyopathy by cardiovascular magnetic resonance. J Cardiovasc Magn Reson. 2012;14:17.
42. Maceira AM, Joshi J, Prasad SK, et al. Cardiovascular magnetic resonance in cardiac amyloidosis. Circulation. 2005;111(2):186-93.
43. Patel MR, Cawley PJ, Heitner JF, et al. Detection of myocardial damage in patients with sarcoidosis. Circulation. 2009;120(20):1969-77.
44. Vignaux O, Dhote R, Duboc D, et al. Clinical significance of myocardial magnetic resonance abnormalities in patients with sarcoidosis: a 1-year follow-up study. Chest. 2002;122(6):1895-901.
45. Eitel I, von Knobelsdorff-Brenkenhoff F, Bernhardt P, et al. Clinical characteristics and cardiovascular magnetic resonance findings in stress (takotsubo) cardiomyopathy. JAMA. 2011;306(3):277-86.
46. Francone M, Dymarkowski S, Kalantzi M, et al. Assessment of ventricular coupling with real-time cine MRI and its value to differentiate constrictive pericarditis from restrictive cardiomyopathy. Eur Radiol. 2006;16(4):944-51.
47. Weinsaft JW, Kim RJ, Ross M, et al. Contrast-enhanced anatomic imaging as compared to contrast-enhanced tissue characterization for detection of left ventricular thrombus. JACC Cardiovasc Imaging. 2009;2(8):969-79.
48. Joshi SB, Connelly KA, Jimenez-Juan L, et al. Potential clinical impact of cardiovascular magnetic resonance assessment of ejection fraction on eligibility for cardioverter defibrillator implantation. J Cardiovasc Magn Reson. 2012;14:69.
49. Modell B, Khan M, Darlison M, et al. Improved survival of thalassaemia major in the UK and relation to T2* cardiovascular magnetic resonance. J Cardiovasc Magn Reson. 2008;10:42.
50. Stacey RB, Andersen MM, St Clair M, et al. Comparison of systolic and diastolic criteria for isolated LV noncompaction in CMR. JACC Cardiovasc Imaging. 2013;6(9):931-40.

Chapter 12

When to Discharge the Heart Failure Patient

Benjamin A Kipper, Matt M Kawahara

ABSTRACT

As sedentary lifestyle and poor diet become more common in the United States and other parts of the world, the prevalence of cardiac disease has increased. Heart failure (HF) is one of the leading causes of hospitalization, morbidity, and mortality, and as such hospital readmission rates are high, with one in four HF patients being readmitted within the first 30 days of discharge. Hospital readmission rates have been shown to correlate with increased risk of death, and as such, it is increasingly important that HF patients are medically optimized prior to discharge.[1] This chapter aims to discuss specific aspect of determining when to discharge patients with HF, including: determination of the causative event, management of symptoms, trending biomarkers, appropriate pharmacology and functional assessment. These criteria will benefit the health care community financially by decreasing the costs associated with HF readmission and urgent care. Medically, these criteria will translate into improved medical care and decreased rates of morbidity and mortality.

INTRODUCTION

Heart failure is one of the leading causes of hospital admission, morbidity, and mortality in the United States. Many of the challenges associated with managing a HF patient are associated with acute exacerbations and adverse events secondary to cardiac dysfunction, which often lead to hospital admission. Once admitted and stabilized the next question in managing these patients is determining when they can be discharged. One in four patients hospitalized with HF is readmitted within the first 30 days and many of these hospitalizations can be prevented if care is optimized prior to the patient leaving the hospital. This problem is further complicated by the fact that the frequency of hospitalizations is directly correlated with risk of death.[1] By preventing future hospital readmissions we can decrease the risk of death for many of these patients as well as improve the management and progression of HF. Reducing readmission rates also decrease the financial burden faced by many of these patients and can save the health care system (both private and governmental) millions, if not billions, of dollars. This chapter aims at identifying specific parameters that indicate ideal discharge conditions.

INITIAL PATIENT EVALUATION

Precipitating Event

This is what brought the patient into the hospital in the first place and can be a range of symptoms including, but not limited to, shortness of breath, lower extremity edema, palpitations, and weight gain. Regardless of the symptoms, it is vital to determine the underlying cause of the exacerbation. Whether it is poorly managed medication, an acute cardiovascular event, secondary comorbidity, or another medical condition, treating the underlying cause of the patient's symptoms is necessary. If left untreated, patients may return to the hospital again and again for exacerbations that may have been prevented had the causative factor been previously addressed. By treating the underlying condition we can prevent future adverse events caused by HF and thus prevent future hospital readmissions.

Biomarker Abnormalities

Upon admission to the hospital patients presenting with acute exacerbations of HF and cardiovascular disease have laboratories drawn. These laboratories include specific biomarkers that are highly prognostic and diagnostic of HF, one such marker is known as brain natriuretic peptide (BNP). This and other markers can be used to determine disease severity and deviation from patient baseline values (if previously assessed), providing an important tool in the assessment and management of patients with HF.

Weight Gain/Fluid Retention

Many patients with chronic and acute HF are hemodynamically compromised and suffer from renal dysfunction. As such, many patients arriving to the hospital may show signs of fluid retention; this can be seen in the form of elevated jugular venous pressure (JVP), fluid in the lungs, lower extremity edema, or rapid weight gain. Normalizing patient fluid status is vital in determining when patients should be discharged.

Secondary Comorbidities

Many patients with HF are suffering from ailments that are contributory to their cardiac dysfunction. Commonly these are diabetes, respiratory infections, and renal disease. Because many of these comorbidities can be detrimental to patient health it is vital to determine if they are present, and careful and attentive treatment of these comorbidities is vital to successful patient outcomes.

Cognitive Assessment

Many times patients presenting with a HF exacerbation can demonstrate cognitive impairment due to lack of blood flow to the brain. This can be confused with other conditions, such as dementia or drug use. Thus, when patients with HF are admitted to the hospital, a cognitive assessment should be performed to ensure that the brain is being adequately perfused and mental impairment is not being caused by a condition secondary to cardiac dysfunction.

When to Discharge

Trending Biomarkers Brain Natriuretic Peptide

The classic biomarker for HF and hypervolemia is BNP and is now commonly used clinically as a means of assessing HF exacerbations. In a normal patient, BNP levels are usually below 100 pg/mL; however, during a HF exacerbation levels often rise to greater than 400 pg/mL. These cutoff points are considered ideal; however, many patients presenting with HF exacerbations have a baseline level of BNP that is well above the 100 pg/mL mark. This makes it increasingly important to determine a baseline or "dry" value of BNP that allows physicians to determine significant deviations that may indicate excess fluid retention. A BNP level that is significantly deviated from baseline and thus indicates fluid retention and HF exacerbation is known as a "wet" BNP. Because BNP is a strong predictor of adverse events, it is vital that high values can be driven down prior to discharge.[2] This helps prevent future adverse events and recurrent hospital admissions. If BNP values remain elevated at discharge (>400 pg/mL) this may indicate a high "dry" BNP value or a need for further diuresis. Additionally, aldosterone blockers can be considered along with home monitoring and a return visit within 1 week to reduce readmission rates. Thus, BNP should be used not only as a guide for treatment, but also as a guide for appropriate discharge timing. Once a patient's BNP level returns to near baseline, discharge may be considered (Fig. 1).

Other Biomarkers to be Considered

Recent evidence has identified additional biomarkers useful in the management of patients with HF. These include markers such as: ST-2, neutrophil gelatinase-associated lipocalin (NGAL), galectin-3, and midregional-proadrenomedullin (MR-proADM). High levels of these markers have all been shown to correlate with high mortality rates, some even outperforming the HF standard BNP.[3-5] These markers are not currently used regularly in the clinical setting; however, they are available and can be ordered if standard diagnostic and prognostic markers for HF are noninformative.

Symptom Management

One of the keys to determine if a patient with HF is ready for discharge is symptom management and control. Symptoms that should be adequately managed are listed below:

- *Orthopnea*: Patients should be able to lie flat (or at least near their baseline), comfortably, before being discharged from the hospital
- *Chest pain*: Chest pain is not a common symptom of chronic HF, although it is indicative of possible coronary artery disease. Prior to discharge patients should be experiencing no chest pain

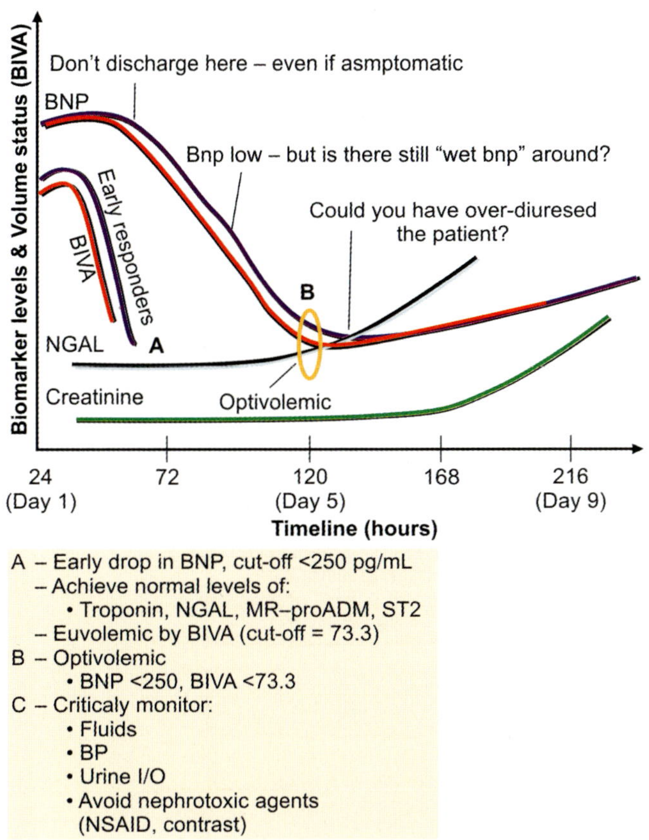

BNP, brain natriuretic peptide; NGAL, neutrophil gelatinase-associated lipocalin; MR-proADM, midregional-proadrenomedullin; BIVA, biomarker levels and volume status; BP, blood pressure; NSAID, non-steroidal anti-inflammatory drug

Fig. 1 Finding the optivolemic level before discharge

- *Hypertension*: Many patients with HF also have associated hypertension. Patients with orthostatic or malignant hypertension should have these issues addressed prior to discharge to prevent future adverse events caused by these conditions
- *Arrhythmia*: Arrhythmia is a common finding in patients with HF and while not all arrhythmias require treatment prior to discharge, many require appropriate precautions and medical management. Patients should receive medications to control problematic dysrhythmias and to prevent emboli formation, if indicated
- *Oxygen saturation*: Prior to discharge patients should have oxygen saturation levels above 90%, with or without additional oxygen, depending on if they were previously using supplemental oxygen (again, knowledge of baseline value is helpful)
- *Ambulatory capacity*: Patients being prepared for discharge should have their ambulatory capacity determined prior to leaving the hospital. Unfortunately, many patients with HF are confined to a wheelchair or have difficulty in walking, but if possible, patients should be able to move from bed to toilet with minimal assistance, particularly if they will be taking a diuretic
- *Weight gain*: One of the key symptoms that is associated with HF is weight gain primarily due to hypervolemia and fluid retention. Prior to discharge patients should be returned to their baseline weight and optimal volume status; this is usually achieved through aggressive diuresis
- *Treatment of secondary medical issues*: Exacerbations of HF are one of the main reasons for hospitalization in these patients; however, other medical conditions can lead to hospital admission. This can include conditions, such as pneumonia, urinary tract infection, gout, chronic obstructive pulmonary disease (COPD), etc. Prior to discharge these conditions should be adequately managed and treated
- *Renal function assessment*: One of the main comorbidities associated with HF is renal dysfunction. The heart's lack of ability to perfuse the kidneys often leaves them vulnerable, particularly when potent diuretics are being administered. This makes it vital to determine renal function prior to discharge. This is usually done via renal biomarkers, such as creatinine and blood urea nitrogen (BUN), although recent evidence has identified other biomarkers, such as NGAL that may identify kidney injury and dysfunction much sooner than the traditional markers (Flowchart 1).[6-8]

Pharmacologic Management and Education

Medical management of HF patients is paramount to them leaving the hospital. Management of these patients involves a variety of cardioactive and vasoactive drugs along with diuretics. Standard guidelines state that patients with HF should be started on an angiotensin-converting enzyme (ACE) inhibitor and beta-blocker, particularly if there is reduced left ventricular (LV) ejection fraction. Additionally, before being discharged, patients should demonstrate tolerance to their medications and should be successfully transitioned from intravenous to oral diuretics. In combination with optimal management, patients should receive education regarding their prescribed medications.

Complicated drug regimens that are used to treat HF and other comorbidities are very specific and sensitive to dosage timing. These complex schedules

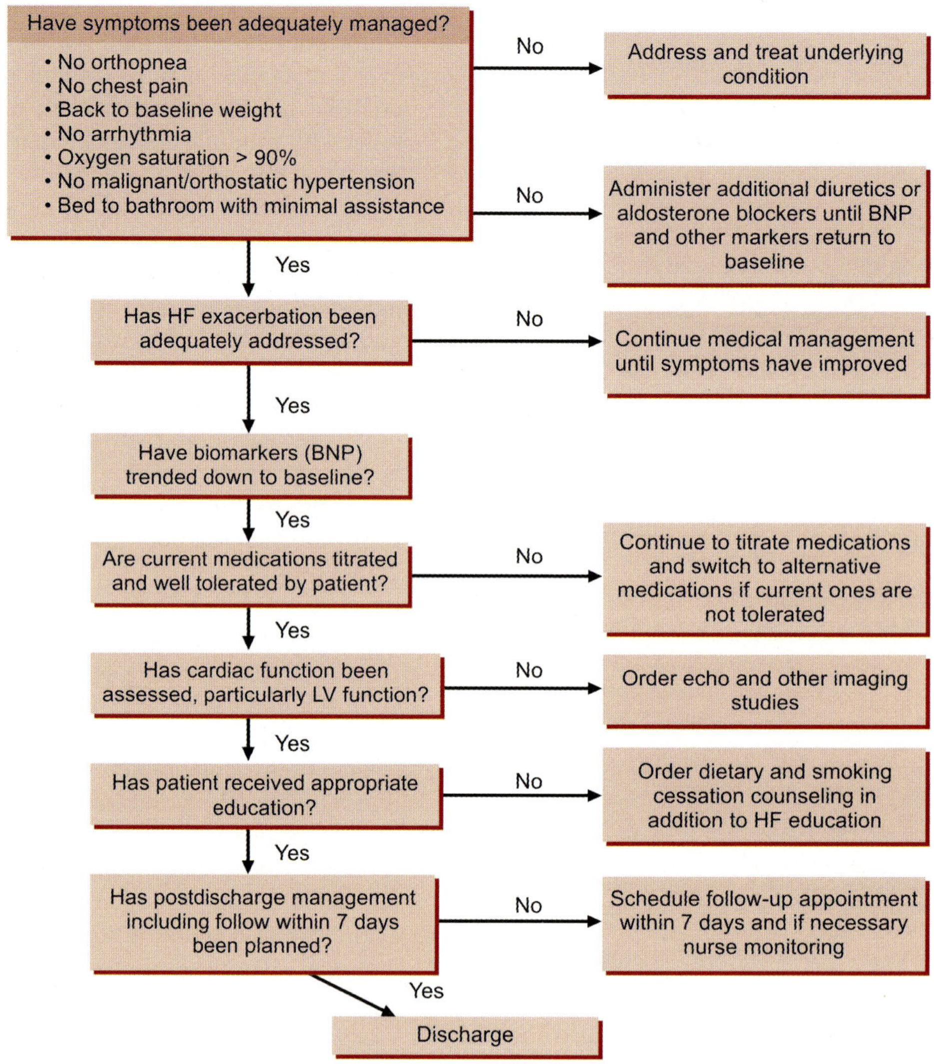

BNP, brain natriuretic peptide; HF, heart failure; LV, left ventricular

Flowchart 1 When to discharge heart failure patient algorithm

can be conducive to mistakes as well as nonadherence. Medication nonadherence is a growing concern and is a leading cause of negative patient outcomes, higher readmission rates, and higher health care costs.[9] Frequently, it may be important for the patient to be educated by the treating staff about the medications they will be taking and about the health consequences of nonadherence. Postdischarge follow-up appointments should be scheduled before discharge which should include reminders of drug schedules and adherence reports. Additionally, much research is being conducted to develop effective pre- and postdischarge systems to help patients take their medications correctly.[10] Reducing medication nonadherence is a challenging task, but it does significantly improve patient outcomes and reduce hospital readmissions.

Assessment of Cardiac Function

Patients coming into the hospital for exacerbations of HF often have previously documented assessments of cardiac function. However, if undocumented, it is vitally important to determine baseline cardiac parameters, particularly LV ejection fraction. This type of useful information can often be achieved through echocardiography, electrocardiogram, biomarker levels, and magnetic resonance imaging. This allows physicians to determine if patients are presenting with new abnormalities and pathologies during future clinical visits and hospital readmissions.

Assessing Functional Status

Physical and cognitive functional status is an important consideration when planning to discharge a patient with HF. Common among patients with HF are frailty, cognitive impairment, and limited social and financial support. Depression is also a common condition among patients with HF. Because of these factors, patients can find it difficult to comply with plans for new lifestyle changes they may need to make or with their new and often complicated medication regimens. In this situation, a multidisciplinary team is especially useful in addressing each difficulty in hopes of increasing motivation and overall compliance.

Management of Other Comorbidities

Especially in elderly patients, comorbidities can further complicate HF treatment. Improper management of these complications can ultimately contribute to readmission rates. Common comorbidities, such as respiratory disease, renal dysfunction, and diabetes mellitus need to be monitored closely by the treating staff.[11] Polypharmacy is often unavoidable when treating patients with HF and multiple comorbidities. Because of this, systems need to be in place which allow the treating staff to review a patient's medication list, ensure efficacy of the medications, and to identify and avoid adverse drug interactions. Properly recognizing and treating any and all comorbidities does significantly improve outcome for patients with HF.

Patient Education

An important factor in preventing readmission rates in patients with HF is the implementation of a system of structured patient and family education. Detailed education regarding essential considerations, such as diet, smoking cessation, and exercise is vital to improving patient outcomes. Often, patients with HF are discharged with an inadequate understanding about their health, medications, and plan of action; this is where the difference between simply communicating information and actual patient education becomes critical.[12] Compliance with low salt diets, exercise regimens, smoking cessation, and medication schedules requires lifestyle changes which can be very difficult. By engaging with the patient and their support group in two-way communication, trained staff can more effectively tailor education sessions to best fit the needs of the patient. Many studies have also shown that using a multidisciplinary approach to therapy can boost compliance.[12,13] A multidisciplinary team can help a patient understand the complexities of HF and it is therapy at a more in depth level. Ensuring that a patient and their family are thoroughly educated before discharge, will help to reduce readmission rates significantly.

An additional benefit to provide disease education to patients with HF is that it allows them to take responsibility and personal control over their condition. This provides a sense of self-care along with physician care can greatly improve patient compliance to their medications and required changes in habits (i.e., not smoking) and greatly improving overall patient outcome. Patient education has been shown to greatly improve rates of survival after hospital discharge and thus should always be an integral component of discharging any patient.

Postdischarge Management

Postdischarge management of patients with HF is crucial, not only to decrease the number of hospital readmissions, but also to prevent future mortality and morbidities in a non-hospital setting. Discharge management includes patient monitoring via telephone within 3 days of discharge, clinical follow-up within 1 week, scale administration to monitor in-home weight values, and on occasion blood pressure monitoring. Studies have shown that only 37.5% of patients discharged from the hospital with HF receive a follow-up appointment within 7 days.[14] This number is not ideal, as recent evidence has shown that hospitals that have low rates of early physician follow-up have higher rates of rehospitalization compared to those with higher rates of early physician follow-up.[14] Adequate postdischarge management is necessary for patients with HF as it can help prevent many of the adverse events associated with readmission.

CONCLUSION

Determining when to discharge patients with HF should include a variety of considerations, many of which are predicated on the patient's baseline status. Treatment and management of exacerbating factors is necessary and paramount prior to discharge. Additionally, patient functional and physiological status along with medication regimen understanding and tolerance should be assessed. Lastly, patients should receive adequate disease and lifestyle education in combination with planned postdischarge care prior to leaving the hospital. If these guidelines are followed, medical care of these patients will be improved and future hospital admissions can be prevented. Financially, this will translate into a decreased economic burden for both patient and the health care system, which can potentially, decreases the costs of health care in general. Medically, this will translate into higher rates of survival and decreased numbers of adverse events in patients with HF and an improvement in quality of life.

REFERENCES

1. Setoguchi S, Stevenson LW, Schneeweiss S. Repeated hospitalizations predict mortality in the community population with heart failure. Am Heart J. 2007;154(2):260-6.
2. Logeart D, Thabut G, Jourdain P, et al. Predischarge B-type natriuretic peptide assay for identifying patients at high risk of re-admission after decompensated heart failure. J Am Coll Cardiol. 2004;43(4):635-41.
3. van Kimmenade RR, Januzzi JL Jr, Ellinor PT, et al. Utility of amino-terminal pro-brain natriuretic peptide, galectin-3, and apelin for the evaluation of patients with acute heart failure. J Am Coll Cardiol. 2006;48(6):1217-24.
4. Maisel AS, Mueller C, Fitzgerald R, et al. Prognostic utility of plasma neutrophil gelatinase-associated lipocalin in patients with acute heart failure: The NGAL EvaLuation along with B-type NaTriuretic peptide in acutely decompensated heart failure (GALLANT) trial. Eur J Heart Fail. 2011;13(8):846-51.
5. Maisel A, Mueller C, Nowak R, et al. Mid-region pro-hormone markers for diagnosis and prognosis in acute dyspnea: Results from the BACH (biomarkers in acute heart failure) trial. J Am Coll Cardiol. 2010;55(19):2062-76.
6. Macdonald S, Arendts G, Nagree Y, et al. Neutrophil gelatinase-associated lipocalin (NGAL) predicts renal injury in acute decompensated cardiac failure: A prospective observational study. BMC Cardiovasc Disord. 2012;12:8.
7. Damman K, Masson S, Hillege HL, et al. Clinical outcome of renal tubular damage in chronic heart failure. Eur Heart J. 2011;32(21):2705-12.
8. Aghel A, Shrestha K, Mullens W, et al. Serum neutrophil gelatinase-associated lipocalin (NGAL) in predicting worsening renal function in acute decompensated heart failure. J Card Fail. 2010;16(1):49-54.
9. Ho PM, Bryson CL, Rumsfeld JS. Medication adherence: Its importance in cardiovascular outcomes. Circulation. 2009;119(23):3028-35.
10. Jaarsma T. Inter-professional team approach to patients with heart failure. Heart. 2005;91(6):832-8.
11. Lang CC, Mancini DM. Non-cardiac comorbidities in chronic heart failure. Heart. 2007;93(6):665-71.
12. Paul S. Hospital discharge education for patients with heart failure: What really works and what is the evidence? Crit Care Nurse. 2008;28(2):66-82.
13. Phillips CO, Wright SM, Kern DE, et al. Comprehensive discharge planning with postdischarge support for older patients with congestive heart failure: A meta-analysis. JAMA. 2004;291(11):1358-67.
14. Hernandez AF, Greiner MA, Fonarow GC, et al. Relationship between early physician follow-up and 30-day readmission among medicare beneficiaries hospitalized for heart failure. JAMA. 2010;303(17):1716-22.

2 SECTION

Heart Failure in the Hospital

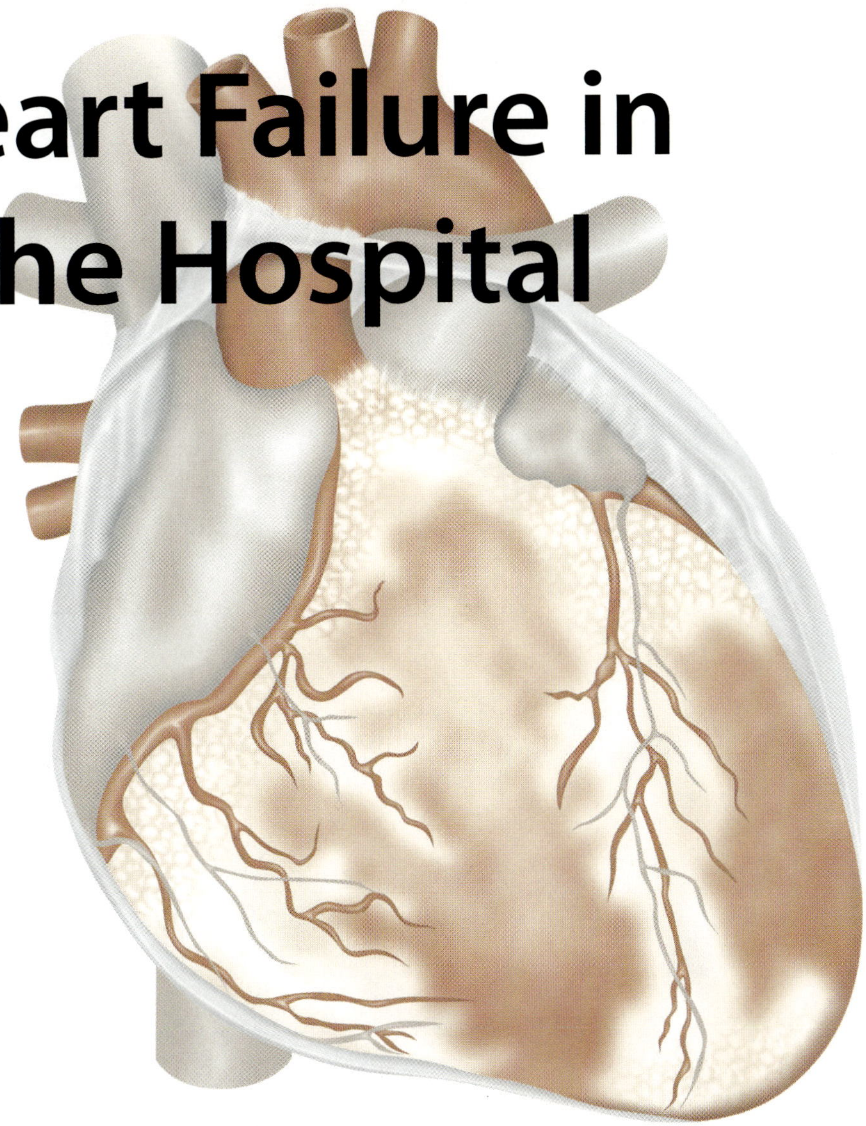

Chapter 13

How to Use Natriuretic Peptides in the Inpatient Setting?

Jeffrey Chan, Abhishek S Shah, Alan S Maisel

ABSTRACT

Given the burden of heart failure (HF) in today's healthcare system, accurate and timely diagnosis of this condition will improve both the delivery of health care while decreasing its costs. Brain natriuretic peptide (BNP) is an established marker for diagnosing HF and left ventricular (LV) dysfunction. However, while the application of natriuretic peptides (NPs) in the emergency room (ER) has been extensively covered and studied, the use of these markers in the general inpatient setting is less well defined and established. Similarly, the use of NPs for daily medical management decisions in the intensive care unit (ICU) for critically ill patients is also quite nebulous and less studied. This chapter provides a basic introduction to the common NPs that have shown promises through evidence-based studies as markers of cardiac dysfunction. However, the bulk of this chapter focuses on providing a simple algorithmic framework for clinicians on how to utilize these biomarkers in the general inpatient setting once a patient is already admitted for general or intensive medical care. As this chapter describes, the value of NPs encompasses not simply diagnosis, but also the guidance of medical management and a variety of noncoronary avenues for application in the ICU.

INTRODUCTION

As demographics shift over the next few decades with aging of the baby boomer generation, heart failure (HF) will become a more prevalent disease. According to the National Health and Nutrition Examination Survey (NHANES) study from 2007 to 2010, an estimated 5.1 million Americans older than 20 years of age have HF.[1] By 2030, HF prevalence will increase by 25% over 2013 levels with incidence increasing with age.[2] Given the burden of HF, accurate and timely diagnosis of this condition will improve both delivery of health care and decrease costs. This chapter briefly reviews the evidence and background for four types of natriuretic peptides (NPs) [i.e., B-type natriuretic peptide (BNP), N-terminal pro-B-type natriuretic peptide (NT-proBNP), atrial natriuretic peptide (ANP) and mid-region proatrial natriuretic peptide (MR-proANP)] and subsequently describes a practical approach for using NPs in the general inpatient hospital setting. Our goal is to provide the reader with a practical, evidence-based, clinical framework for using BNP to deliver cost-effective quality care to patients.

B-TYPE NATRIURETIC PEPTIDE

The clinical utility of BNP measurement was first demonstrated by the Breathing Not Properly Multinational Study in 2002.[3-8] In that study, when less than 50 pg/mL, BNP demonstrated a negative predictive value (NPV) of 96%. In practice, values less than 100 pg/mL are routinely used as the rule out threshold and values greater than 400 pg/mL are used as indicating that HF is very probable.[9,10] However, there are important exceptions to the cutoffs used for diagnosis. BNP values in obese patients have been known to show an inverse relationship with increasing body mass index (BMI) and have reduced sensitivity for diagnosis.[11] Patients with renal failure also have a decreased rate of BNP clearance and thus higher baseline values.

Besides its utility for diagnosis of HF, BNP measurements can provide important prognostic information as well. A systematic review done in 2005 of studies assessing BNP values and prognosis showed a relative risk of all-cause mortality of 1.37 per 100 pg/mL that BNP was elevated.[12] Combined event rate [congestive heart failure (CHF) visits or admissions and mortality] at 90 days in patients admitted with BNP less than 200 pg/mL was 9% and 29% in those with BNP greater than 200 pg/mL. Similarly, the higher the BNP value, the higher the in-hospital mortality rate.

With rising costs in our current healthcare environment, cost-effective approaches are increasingly espoused. Methods that increase diagnostic efficiency enable the delivery of efficient, directed, and evidence-based care as evidenced in a major study of 452 patients randomly assigned to a rapid BNP measurement arm or a standard arm (where BNP was not measured) that noted decreased hospitalization rates, faster median discharge times, and not surprisingly, reduced costs that occurred with the use of BNP.[13]

N-TERMINAL PRO-B-TYPE NATRIURETIC PEPTIDE

Proteolytic cleavage of the precursor proBNP molecule yields BNP with the n-terminal fragment termed NT-proBNP. While it is produced in an equimolar fraction to BNP, its plasma concentration is higher than that of BNP due to comparatively decreased clearance.[14] The biologic utility of NT-proBNP however is still unknown.

Cutoff values for NT-proBNP studied in 2004 in a pooled analysis found that a cutoff value of greater than 300pg/mL has a NPV of 99% and a sensitivity/specificity of 99%/62%, respectively.[15,16] A NT-proBNP levels greater than 450 pg/mL in those less than 50 years had a positive predictive value (PPV) of 76% for HF.[16] Similarly, levels greater than 900 pg/mL in 50–75 year-olds had a PPV of 82% and levels greater than 1,800 pg/mL in more than 75 year-olds had a PPV of 92% for HF. Similarly, a prospective study done with 600 patients evaluated for dyspnea in the emergency room (ER) showed that an NT-proBNP level of greater than 900 pg/mL had a PPV of 77% in the cohort of greater than 50 years of age, reinforcing the age dependent relationship of NT-proBNP.[17,18]

As with BNP, NT-proBNP also provides prognostic information. In an analysis of 1,256 patients admitted with acute decompensated HF showed that an NT-proBNP value of greater than 5,180 pg/mL was 68% sensitive and 72% specific for predicting 76-day mortality, with a PPV of 19% and an NPV of 96%.[19]

ATRIAL NATRIURETIC PEPTIDE

Atrial natriuretic peptide is primarily released in atrial tissue, though at times of increased myocardial stretch, is also released from ventricular tissue like BNP.[20] As with BNP, ANP antagonizes the renin–angiotensin–aldosterone system (RAAS) system to promote vasodilation, diuresis, and natriuresis.[21] Not surprisingly, ANP also helps prevent the remodeling process that is so deleterious to long-term survival in HF patients and evidence suggests this is mediated in part through direct inhibitory effects on myocyte and fibroblast proliferation.[22]

To date, ANP has been overshadowed by BNP in terms of research effort and thus clinical utility. Part of this was due to reduced stability of ANP compared to its counterparts.[23] Additionally, early pilot studies showed decreased statistical performance of ANP to BNP. A study done in 1996 showed an area under the receiver-operating characteristic (ROC) curve for BNP of 0.880 which was significantly greater than the value for ANP which was 0.761.[24] The same study showed a sensitivity of 100% for BNP and 90% for ANP at the study cut-off values. Most of these studies showed that ANP was less reliable a marker than its twin n-terminal proANP (n-ANP) which is derived from precursor proANP (which is cleaved into ANP and n-ANP).[25] As such, much of the utility of the family of ANPs comes from a proteolytic product of n-ANP.

MID-REGION PROATRIAL NATRIURETIC PEPTIDE

Mid-region proatrial natriuretic peptide detection assays are directed against a specific mid-portion of the proANP molecule (residues 58–90 in the BRAMHS AG assay) which is a total of 98 amino acids long.[26] In the Biomarkers in Acute Heart failure (BACH) trial, investigators reported noninferiority of MR-proANP compared to BNP at cutoff values of 120 pmol/L and 100 pg/mL, respectively.[27] Specifically, MR-proANP had a sensitivity of 97%, specificity of 59.9%, and a NPV of 97.4%. MR-proANP also had a similar area under curve (AUC) for the ROC curve as BNP. It also conferred a positive odds ratio (OR), though not as dramatically, for patients more than 70 years old, patients with renal insufficiency, and patients with obesity. MR-proANP was also found to confer a positive OR for indeterminate

NT-proBNP values (300–900 pg/mL). Thus, when the diagnosis of HF is uncertain and the BNPs are indeterminate, MR-proANP has been shown to of use as an adjunctive test.[28]

With regards to prognostication, increasing levels of MR-proANP have been shown to confer increased risk of mortality.[29] Levels greater than 460 pmol/L conferred a risk ratio of 3.73. BNP conferred a risk ratio of 3.22 for values greater than 1,250 ng/L. Interestingly, MR-proANP has been shown to be a stronger predictor of death than even BNP and NT-proBNP.

USE OF BNP IN THE GENERAL INPATIENT SETTING

Application of Natriuretic Peptide in the Diagnostic Algorithm for Heart Failure

The application of NPs begins with the diagnostic workup of a patient presenting to the hospital with symptoms of acute onset dyspnea. Depending on the general approach to patient evaluation unique to a particular hospital, the application of BNP begins either in the ER or immediately in the admitted inpatient setting, wherever the initial process of medical diagnostics begins. While the application of NPs in the ER is covered in greater depth in other chapters of this manuscript, we propose the same diagnostic algorithm for the inpatient setting as the initial step of NP utilization to evaluate new patients with an inconclusive diagnosis by history and physical examination if not already performed in the ER.

In patients with BNP levels less than 100 pg/mL or NT-proBNP less than 300 pg/mL, the diagnosis of acute HF is very unlikely (less than 2% likelihood). These patients should be further evaluated for an alternative etiology for their acute dyspnea, such as chronic obstructive pulmonary disease exacerbation, asthma exacerbation, pneumonia, sepsis, pulmonary embolism (PE), cardiac tamponade, constrictive pericarditis, or acute coronary syndrome. In patients with acute dyspnea and BNP levels above 500 pg/mL or NT-proBNP levels above an age-dependent cutoff (greater than 450 pg/mL in patients less than 50 years old or greater than 900 pg/mL in patients between 50 years and 75 years of age or greater than 1,800 pg/mL in patients greater than 75 years of age), acute HF is very likely (greater than 95% likelihood) and therapy should be initiated for acute HF without delay. All patients with acute HF should receive diuretics to reduce the intravascular volume and left ventricular preload. In patients without evidence of cardiogenic shock, vasodilators can be added if they are hypertensive. Inotropes can also be considered in these patients if they experience poor tissue perfusion and to aide diuresis. In patients with evidence of cardiogenic shock, inotropes and vasodilators are both necessary in order to improve cardiac output by increasing contractility and decreasing afterload. In patients with NP levels in the gray zone (all ages: BNP between 100 pg/mL and 500 pg/mL; age less than 50 years: NT-proBNP between 300 pg/mL and 450 pg/mL; age between 50 years and 75 years: NT-proBNP between 300 pg/mL and 900 pg/mL; age greater than 75 years: NT-proBNP between 300 pg/mL and 1,800 pg/mL), a history of HF or left ventricular dysfunction or strong evidence of acute HF make acute HF highly probable (90% likelihood). These patients should receive empiric treatment for acute HF with diuretics and vasodilators as needed and observed closely. If there is no history of HF or strong evidence for acute HF or left ventricular dysfunction, then an evaluation for acute coronary syndrome, cor pulmonale, or acute PE should be considered. Patients with electrocardiography (ECG) and biomarker evidence of acute coronary syndrome should be treated accordingly. Similarly, patients with imaging evidence of acute PE should be initiated on anticoagulation immediately. If there is evidence of existing left ventricular dysfunction or cor pulmonale, then the gray zone NP levels are unlikely to represent acute HF (less than 25% likelihood), as these patients tend to have higher NP levels during acute HF. These patients should be closely observed and evaluated for an alternative diagnosis. In patients without baseline left ventricular dysfunction, cor pulmonale, acute coronary syndrome or acute PE, gray zone NP levels may still represent acute HF (greater than 75% likelihood). Empiric therapy for acute HF should be initiated in these patients and they should be observed closely. Although not widely available, MR-proANP can also be used for the diagnostic evaluation of patients with acute dyspnea. Patients with MR-proANP levels below 120 pg/mL are unlikely to have acute HF. Patients with MR-proANP levels above 600 pg/mL are very likely to have acute HF. The gray zone for MR-proANP is between 120 pg/mL and 600 pg/mL. When available, MR-proANP levels should be checked in patients with BNP or NT-proBNP levels in the diagnostic gray zone to increase the diagnostic accuracy of NPs in patients with obesity (intermediate BNP levels), renal insufficiency (intermediate NT-proBNP levels), and advanced age (intermediate NT-proBNP levels). Flowchart 1 depicts the algorithmic application of BNP we proposed in initial diagnostics. Flowchart 2 takes a

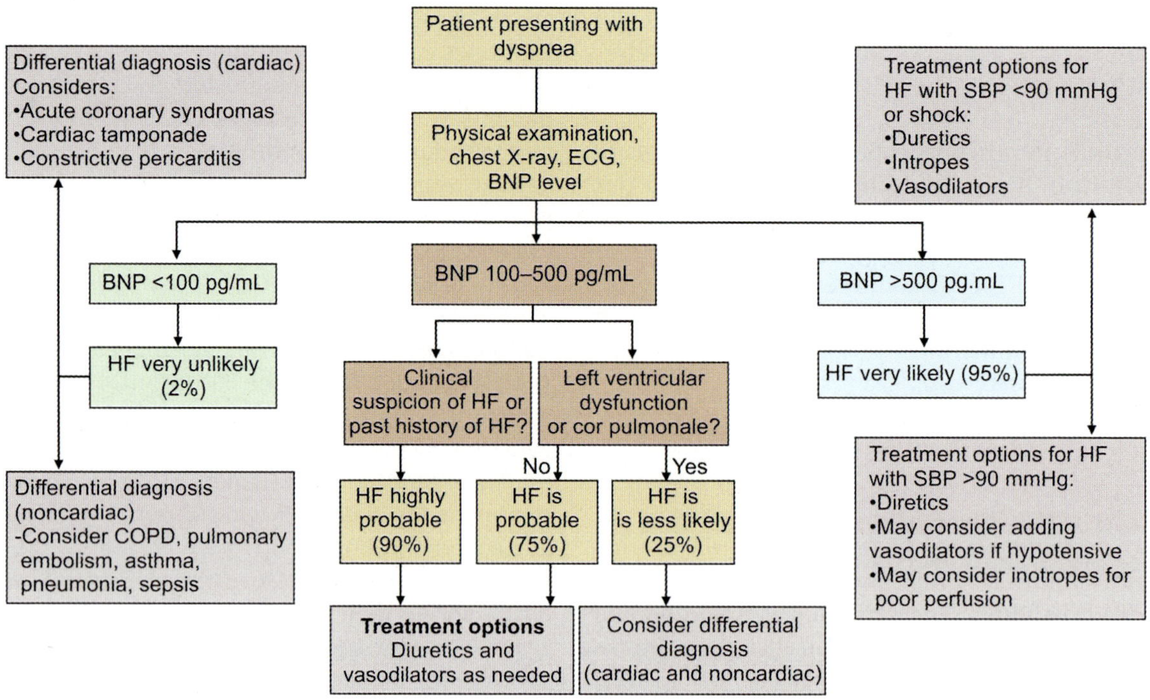

ECG, electrocardiography; COPD, chronic obstructive pulmonary disease; HF, heart failure; BNP, B-type natriuretic peptide; SBP, systolic blood pressure

Flowchart 1 Algorithm using B-type natriuretic peptide to rule in and rule out congestive heart failure

Source: Adapted from Maisel A. B-type natriuretic peptide measurements in diagnosing congestive heart failure in the dyspneic emergency department patient. *Rev Cardiovas Med.* 2002;3:S10-7

different focus and illustrates the application of BNP to the initial treatment of HF that we proposed as well.

Conceptual Framework of Natriuretic Peptide Level Once a Patient Admitted

Overall, the use of NP once a patient has been admitted has been studied less extensively as compared to the use in the emergency department (ED). However, once the initial diagnostic steps and necessary stabilizing interventions in the early evaluation of patients has taken place, we propose that emphasis should be directed towards understanding the full interpretation of the patient's current NP level. Conceptually, the NP of a patient admitted with decompensated HF is comprised of two components, that of a baseline (dry) NP level and that occurring from acute pressure or volume overload (wet) NP level. At a point of decompensation, a patient's NP level is the sum of the baseline NP level plus what volume overload adds. As Table 1 illustrates, we define a wet NP level as any level 25–50% over what the patient's dry BNP level is. On the contrary, we define dry NP level as the level once optimum fluid status is reached.

Approach to Nondeclining BNP Levels Despite Treatment

Despite following algorithmic guidelines in the treatment of HF, often times NP levels do not decline in various patients. In such situations, various clinical scenarios should be considered. First, and generally most importantly, consistently high NP levels may actually represent the patient's dry NP level due to persistent increased ventricular wall stress, even after resolution of acute episodes of volume overload. Additionally, it may be possible that with excessive diuretic treatment, intravascular dehydration may induce subsequent prerenal states; decreased glomerular filtration rates have known to result in increased levels of BNP and NT-proBNP. Additionally, another possibility explaining non-declining NP levels despite diuretic treatment that should always be considered is the situation where patients with concomitant right-sided HF and significant ascites and/or edema who require diuresis of many liters of fluid before subsequent changes in NP levels are actually demonstrated. In these cases, the initial lag period during which no change in NP levels are noted are due to the

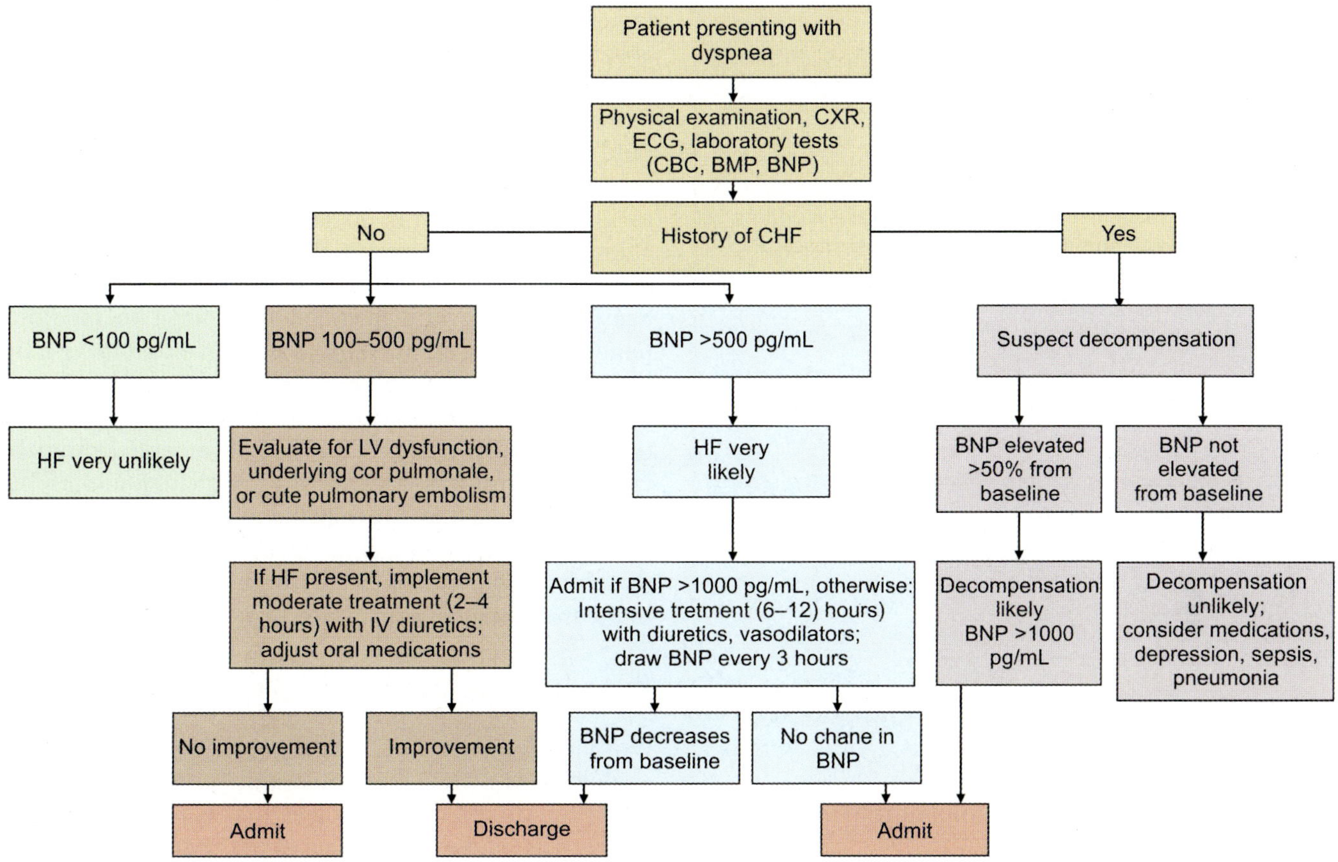

ECG, electrocardiogram; CBC, complete blood count; BMP, basic metabolic panel; BNP, B-type natriuretic peptide; HF, heart failure; LV, left ventricular

Flowchart 2 Algorithm for the use of natriuretic peptides in the inpatient management of heart failure

Source: Adapted from Bhalla V, Maisel AS. B-type natriuretic peptide in the neurohormonal hierarchy in heart failure. *Cardiovasc Rev Rep.* 2004;25:100-4

mobilization of third-space fluid rather than lowering of cardiac filling pressures. Lastly, clinicians should also consider scenarios in which treatment simply does not effectively reduce central cardiac hemodynamics and therefore does not improve cardiomyocyte stress nor does it induce any decline in NP levels.

TABLE 1: Wet versus dry natriuretic peptide levels

Wet NP level	*Dry NP level*
• Any NP level 25–50% over the patient's euvolemic BNP level • In the ER, often >600 pg/mL for BNP and >900 pg/mL for NT-proBNP • Declines rapidly with treatment	• NP level once optimal fluid status is attained • Correlated with functional class and prognosis • May be 20–20,000 pg/mL depending on the severity of disease • Declines slowly with treatment

NP, natriuretic peptide; BNP, B-type natriuretic peptide; NT-proBNP, N-terminal pro-B-type natriuretic peptide

We additionally recommend that NP levels be routinely measured not simply at the time of admission, but also prior to discharge. Measuring discharge NP levels have been shown to increase prognostic information.[30,31] In fact, the lower the discharge NP level, the lower the risk of death and rehospitalization. However, the precise relationship between discharge BNP levels and long-term outcomes is still unclear. Ultimately, while some studies have shown that a relative drop (approximately 30%) in BNP levels is associated with good short-term prognosis,[32] the absolute BNP level at discharge appears to be a better reflection of the state of the ventricle and whether a dry baseline status has been reached. Predischarge BNP levels appear to be more cost-effective as well. Repeated NP measurements while still as an inpatient should only be considered in the event of clinical deterioration or to evaluate adequacy of therapy.

Box 1: Practical recommendations for the use of natriuretic peptides in the general inpatient setting

- NP levels substantially above prior levels (>50%) usually reflect volume overload
- A patient admitted with acute dyspnea due to HF and a high BNP level (generally >600 pg/mL for BNP and 6000 pg/mL for proBNP) usually has high filling pressures secondary to volume overload, and a treatment-induced decrease in PCWP will usually lead to a rapid drop in NP levels
- NP levels should be interpreted together with renal function
- NP levels should be measured on admission and prior to discharge
- Reduction in NP levels in response to treatment is important, but the final NP level appears to the most accurate predictor of death/readmission
- BNP <350–400 pg/mL or NT-proBNP <4000 pg/mL at discharge in setting of euvolemia predicts a stable post-hospital course
- If NP levels fail to decrease, consider more aggressive in-hospital treatment or outpatient monitoring

PCWP, pulmonary capillary wedge pressure; NP, natriuretic peptide; NT-proBNP, N-terminal pro-B-type natriuretic peptide

Practical Recommendations and Summary for Inpatient NP Use

Practical recommendation and summary for inpatient NP use described in Box 1.

USE OF NATRIURETIC PEPTIDES IN THE INTENSIVE CARE UNIT

The role of NPs in medical management in intensive care units (ICUs) is only recently receiving greater attention as we are beginning to appreciate the syndrome of HF in the ICU. The major differences in patient characteristics, disease severity, comorbidity, and therapies between the ICU and the general inpatient levels of care require that the potential clinical use of NP levels in the ICU be defined by specific ICU studies. While NP levels seem to also have high accuracy in the identification of cardiac dysfunction in the ICU, the rule-out levels may be higher, around greater than 150 pg/mL in the case of BNP.[33] In fact, a BNP of less than 150 pg/mL in ICU patients had been shown to have a NPV of 97% for the presence of cardiac dysfunction. However, despite appearing as relatively straightforward, the challenge of translating both the diagnostic and prognostic value of NPs from the general inpatient setting to a consistent role in the critically ill patient is more complex and still relatively unclear. In the critically ill ICU patient, multiple comorbidities, particularly renal failure or sepsis can confound laboratory interpretation by causing elevation of serum levels of NPs in the absence of HF. Figure 1 illustrates the variety of factors in the typical ICU patient that may influence serum NP levels in a single patient. Proper consideration of current fluid management, mechanical ventilation settings, and pharmacologic medications must be thoroughly reviewed to properly interpret measured serum BNP levels. Numerous studies have sought to clarify a role for NPs as prognostic marker in the ICU setting, yet the results have been conflicting and insufficiently robust to modify a patient's management.[34-38] Although an elevated NP most likely represents cardiac dysfunction even in the critically ill patient, it lacks discriminating power to identify what type of cardiac dysfunction is present and cannot be compared with echocardiography, which should always be routinely used in critically ill patients with underlying heart dysfunction. In fact, an in-depth review concluded that the utilization of NPs did not have a substantive role in the management of critically ill patients in the ICU.[39]

Potential Noncardiac Uses of NPs in the ICU

Cardiac biomarkers have also begun to show potential usefulness in the diagnosis and prognostication of noncoronary artery pathologies that commonly present in the ICU as well, including acute pulmonary emboli, sepsis, and acute lung injury. Elevation of cardiac troponin (cTn) are seen in acute PE as it is elevated secondary to increased metabolic demand and reduced myocardial perfusion, which causes right ventricular ischemia. More specifically, the increased wall stress often results in an elevation of NPs as well. In fact, a cTn below the cutoff required to diagnose an acute myocardial infarction or a BNP less than 50 ng/mL have a greater than 98% NPV for in-hospital death by PE.[40] NPs have also been known to be elevated, however, controversy still remains as to whether the information they yield alters outcomes.[41] Interestingly, despite being a cardiac biomarker, BNP has also demonstrated effectiveness in the diagnosis of hypoxic respiratory failure and determining optimal timing for extubation. It has been shown that a BNP level less than 250 pg/mL supports the diagnosis of acute lung injury (AUC = 0.71) with improved accuracy when renal failure is excluded.[42] Similarly, in a study of over 100 patients undergoing spontaneous breathing trials before extubation, a baseline cutoff BNP level of 263 ng/L and NT-proBNP level of 1,343 ng/L prior to commencing spontaneous breathing trial (SBT) or an increase of 48 ng/L and 21 ng/L, respectively predicted patients who failed extubation as a result of underlying cardiac failure.

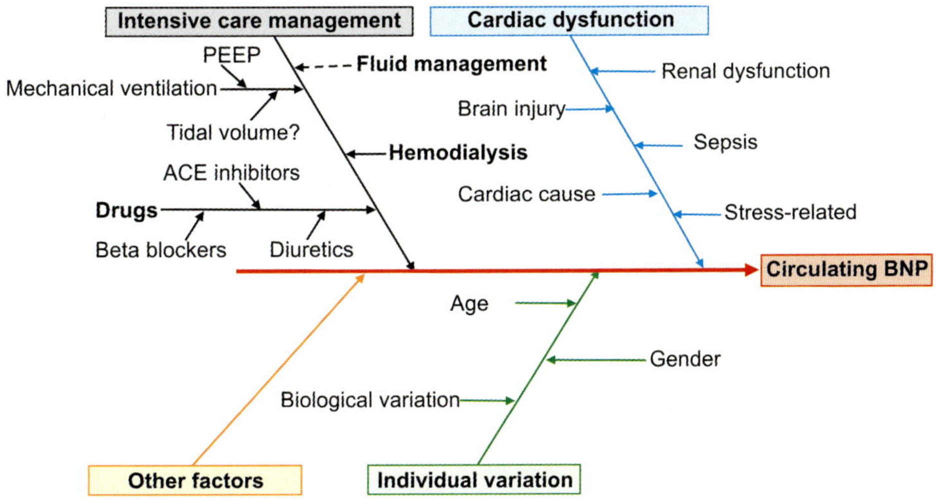

Fig. 1 Variables in the critically ill patient that influence natriuretic peptide levels
Source: Adapted from Mclean AS, Huang SJ. Cardiac biomarkers in the intensive care unit. *Ann Intensive Care*. 2012;2:8

Ultimately, the advantages to applying NPs in the general inpatient setting or cardiology wards are not always as clear or shared in the ICU where confounders frequently make for a more cautious interpretation before careful consideration of subsequent management decisions are made. However, when confounders are taken into consideration, as are other common variables of critically ill patients including fluid status and active medications, value assessments on patient hemodynamics can still be made from measured NP levels.

Practical Recommendations and Summary

Practical recommendation and summary for NP use in the ICU are described in Box 2.

Box 2: Practical recommendations for the use of natriuretic peptides (NPs) in the intensive care unit

Practical recommendations and summary

- NP levels identify cardiac dysfunction in the intensive care unit but at higher rule-out values
- NP levels may be useful in distinguishing between cardiogenic and noncardiogenic pulmonary edema
- NP levels are elevated in severe sepsis, septic shock, and cardiogenic shock and are therefore not useful in the differential diagnosis of shock
- NP levels may be helpful in the timing of extubation
- NP levels predict perioperative cardiac complications

REFERENCES

1. Go AS, Mozaffarian D, Roger VL, et al. Heart disease and stroke statistics—2013 update: a report from the American Heart Association. Circulation. 2013;127:e6-e245.
2. Hall MJ. Hospitalization for congestive heart failure: United States, 2000-2010. Centers for Disease Control and Prevention; 2012.
3. Sudoh T, Kangawa K, Minamino N, et al. A new natriuretic peptide in porcine brain. Nature. 1988;332:78-81.
4. Harris PJ, Thomas D, Morgan TO. Atrial natriuretic peptide inhibits angiotensin-stimulated proximal tubular sodium and water reabsorption. Nature. 1987;326:697-8.
5. Gunning M, Ballermann BJ, Silva P, et al. Brain natriuretic peptide: interaction with renal ANP system. Am J Physiol. 1990;258:F467-72.
6. Hobbs RE, Mills RM. Endogenous B-type natriuretic peptide: a limb of the regulatory response to acutely decompensated heart failure. Clin Cardiol. 2008;31:407-12.
7. Semenov AG, Seferian KR. Biochemistry of the human B-type natriuretic peptide precursor and molecular aspects of its processing. Clin Chim Acta. 2011;412:850-60.
8. Maisel AS, Krishnaswamy P, Nowak RM, et al. Rapid measurement of B-type natriuretic peptide in the emergency diagnosis of heart failure. NEJM. 2002;347:161-7.
9. Maisel A, Mueller C, Adams K, et al. State of the art: using natriuretic peptide levels in clinical practice. Eur J Heart Fail. 2008;10:824-39.
10. Maisel AS, Daniels LB. Breathing not properly 10 years later: what we have learned and what we still need to learn. J Am Coll Cardiol. 2012;60:277-82.
11. Krauser DG, Lloyd-Jones DM, Chae CU, et al. Effect of body mass index on natriuretic peptide levels in patients with acute congestive heart failure: a ProBNP Investigation of Dyspnea in the Emergency Department (PRIDE) substudy. Am Heart J. 2005;149:744-50.
12. Doust JA, Pietrzak E, Dobson A, et al. How well does B-type natriuretic peptide predict death and cardiac events in patients with heart failure: systematic review. BMJ. 2005;330:625.
13. Mueller C, Scholer A, Laule-Kilian K, et al. Use of B-type natriuretic peptide in the evaluation and management of acute dyspnea. N Engl J Med. 2004;350:647-54.

14. Pemberton CJ, Johnson ML, Yandle TG, et al. Deconvolution analysis of cardiac natriuretic peptides during acute volume overload. Hypertension. 2000;36:355-9.
15. McDonagh TA, Holmer S, Raymond I, et al. NT-proBNP and the diagnosis of heart failure: a pooled analysis of three European epidemiological studies. Eur J Heart Fail. 2004;6:269-73.
16. Maisel A, Hollander JE, Guss D, et al. Primary results of the Rapid Emergency Department Heart Failure Outpatient Trial (REDHOT). A multicenter study of B-type natriuretic peptide levels, emergency department decision making, and outcomes in patients presenting with shortness of breath. J Am Coll Cardiol. 2004;44:1328-33.
17. Fonarow GC, Peacock WF, Phillips CO, et al. Admission B-type natriuretic peptide levels and in-hospital mortality in acute decompensated heart failure. J Am Coll Card. 2007;49:1943-50.
18. Januzzi JL, Kimmenade R, Lainchbury J, et al. NT-proBNP testing for diagnosis and short-term prognosis in acute destabilized heart failure: an international pooled analysis of 1256 patients: the International Collaborative of NT-proBNP Study. Eur Heart J. 2006;27:330-7.
19. Yoshimura M, Yasue H, Ogawa H. Pathophysiological significance and clinical application of ANP and BNP in patients with heart failure. Can J Physiol Pharmacol. 2001;79:730-5.
20. Baxter JD, Lewicki JA, Gardner DG. Atrial natriuretic peptide. Nature Biotechnology. 1988;6:529-46.
21. Gardner DG. Natriuretic peptides: markers or modulators of cardiac hypertrophy? Trends Endocrinol Metab. 2003;14:411-6.
22. Cowie MR, Struthers AD, Wood DA, et al. Value of natriuretic peptides in assessment of patients with possible new heart failure in primary care. Lancet. 1997;350:1349-53.
23. NC Davidson, AA Naas, JK Hanson, et al. Comparison of atrial natriuretic peptide, and N-terminal proatrial natriuretic peptide as indicators of left ventricular systolic dysfunction. Am J Cardiol. 1996;77:828-31.
24. Omland T, Aakvaag A, Vik-Mo H. Plasma cardiac natriuretic peptide determination as a screening test for the detection of patients with mild left ventricular impairment. Heart. 1996;76:232-7.
25. Morgenthaler NG, Struck J, Thomas B, et al. Immunoluminometric assay for the midregion of pro-atrial natriuretic peptide in human plasma. Clin Chem. 2004;50:234-6.
26. Maisel A, Mueller C, Nowak R, et al. Mid-region pro-hormone markers for diagnosis and prognosis in acute dyspnea: results from the BACH (Biomarkers in Acute Heart Failure) trial. J Am Coll Card. 2010;55: 2062-76.
27. Dieplinger B, Gegenhuber A, Haltmayer M, et al. Biomarkers and heart disease: evaluation of novel biomarkers for the diagnosis of acute destabilized heart failure in patients with shortness of breath. Heart. 2009;95:1508-13.
28. Gegenhuber A, Struck J, Dieplinger B, et al. Comparative evaluation of b-type natriuretic peptide, mid-regional pro-a-type natriuretic peptide, mid-regional pro-adrenomedullin, and copeptin to predict 1-year mortality in patients with acute destabilized heart failure. J Card Fail. 2007;13:42-9.
29. Moertl D, Berger R, Struck J, et al. Comparison of mid-regional pro-atrial and B-type natriuretic peptides in chronic heart failure: influencing factors, detection of left ventricular systolic dysfunction, and prediction of death. J Am Coll Cardiol. 2009:53:1783-90.
30. Dokainish H, Zoghbi WA, Lakkis NM, et al. Incremental predictive power of B-type natriuretic peptide and tissue Doppler echocardiography in the prognosis of patients with congestive heart failure. J Am Coll Cardiol. 2005;45:1223-6.
31. Logeart D, Saudubray C, Beyne P, et al. Comparative value of Doppler echocardiography and B-type natriuretic peptide assay in the etiologic diagnosis of acute dyspnea. J Am Coll Cardiol. 2002;40:1794-800.
32. Cowie MR, Jourdain P, Maisel A, et al. Clinical applications of B-type natriuretic peptide (BNP) testing. Eur Heart J. 2003;24:1710-8.
33. McLean AS, Tang B, Nalos M, et al. Increased B-type natriuretic peptide (BNP) level is a strong predictor for cardiac dysfunction in intensive care unit patients. Anaesth Intensive Care. 2003;31:21-7.
34. McLean A, Huang S, Hyams S, et al. Prognostic values of B-type natriuretic peptide in severe sepsis and septic shock. Crit Care Med. 2007;35: 1019-26.
35. Varpula M, Pulkki K, Karlsson S, et al. Predictive value of N-terminal pro-brain natriuretic peptide in severe sepsis and septic shock. Crit Care Med. 2007;35:1277-83.
36. Phua J, Koay E, Lee K. Lactate, procalcitonin, and amino-terminal pro-B type natriuretic peptide versus cytokine measurements and clinical severity scores for prognostication in septic shock. Shock. 2008;29:328-33.
37. Kandil E, Burack J, Sawas A, et al. B-type natriuretic peptide: a biomarker for the diagnosis and risk stratification of patients with septic shock. Arch Surg. 2008;143:242-6.
38. Cuthbertson B, Patel R, Croal B, et al. B-type natriuretic peptide and the prediction of outcome in patients admitted to intensive care. Anesthesia. 2005;60:16-21.
39. Christenson RH. What is the value of B-type natriuretic peptide peptide testing for diagnosis, prognosis, or monitoring of the critically ill adult patients in intensive care? Clin Chem Lad Med. 2008;46:1524-32.
40. Kucher N, Goldhaber S. Cardiac biomarkers for risk stratification of patients with acute pulmonary embolus. Circulation. 2003;108:2191-4.
41. Post F, Weilemann L, Messow C, et al. B-type natriuretic peptide as a marker for sepsis-induced myocardial depression in intensive care patients. Crit Care Med. 2008;36:3030-7.
42. Rana R, Vlahakis NE, Daniels CE, et al. B-type natriuretic peptide in the assessment of acute lung injury and cardiogenic pulmonary edema. Crit Care Med. 2006;34:1941-6.

Chapter 14

Approaches to Diuretics in the Hospital

Meghana G Halkar, WH Wilson Tang

ABSTRACT

Relief of congestion ultimately resulting in improvement of subjective symptoms; while trying to optimize objective, measurable markers has been the central theme in acute decompensated heart failure (ADHF). While diuretics have held their place as core drugs for the acutely decompensated patient, given the unrelenting pattern of heart failure readmissions often related to worsening renal function (WRF), it becomes very important to understand how to use them favorably to tide over the acute hospitalization.

With the expanding practice of evidence-based medicine, multiple clinical trials continue to be shed light on the effectiveness of various strategies for decongestion as well as minimization of side effects. We seek to provide a simplified logical approach to optimal diuretic therapy in the hospital, with the goal of serving as an aid to implementing best practice methods among our fellow physicians.

While guidelines have provided us with a right direction to pursue, there are no specific recommendations on diuretic dosing methods, and it continues to be tailored to the individual scenario. A thorough understanding of the underlying pathophysiology and varied clinical presentations will thus help steer adequate therapy, as briefly outlined herein.

INTRODUCTION

Patients with heart failure often get admitted to the hospital when they have symptoms of worsening congestion, fluid retention, dyspnea, or failure to thrive. Others get admitted due to complications of treatment or an adverse event (such as myocardial infarction or a defibrillator discharge). As such, treatment to relieve congestion is still the mainstay. For the goal to remove salt and volume, diuretic drugs (particularly loop diuretics) are very effective. However, how best to achieve adequate and sustained relief of congestion without adverse consequences; in other words, how much to remove, what methods to use and at what pace to facilitate their removal, continues to be a challenge.

Although not commonly considered, diuretics are essentially "poisons" of channels that shuttle electrolytes across tubular cells at different levels (Fig. 1). Thus, diuretics should be judiciously utilized as their overuse and abuse may lead to many unwanted consequences. Table 1 illustrates the different classes of diuretics, their pharmacokinetic characteristics and recommended dosages. Currently, there are a wide range of diuretic drugs that can be used to effectively achieve salt and volume removal, but they are often administered in a subjective "sliding scale" format per the discretion of the treating clinician:

- Loop diuretics (such as furosemide, torsemide, bumetanide): They act at the level of the medullary portion of the thick ascending loop of Henle on the sodium potassium chloride cotransporter and inhibit the reabsorption of sodium, which is normally reabsorbed at the rate of about 25%. This enhances the level of sodium delivered to the distal tubule and collecting duct with consequent decrease in reabsorption of water due to the relative hypotonicity of the interstitium, thereby, causing both natriuresis and diuresis. Loop diuretics are also known to

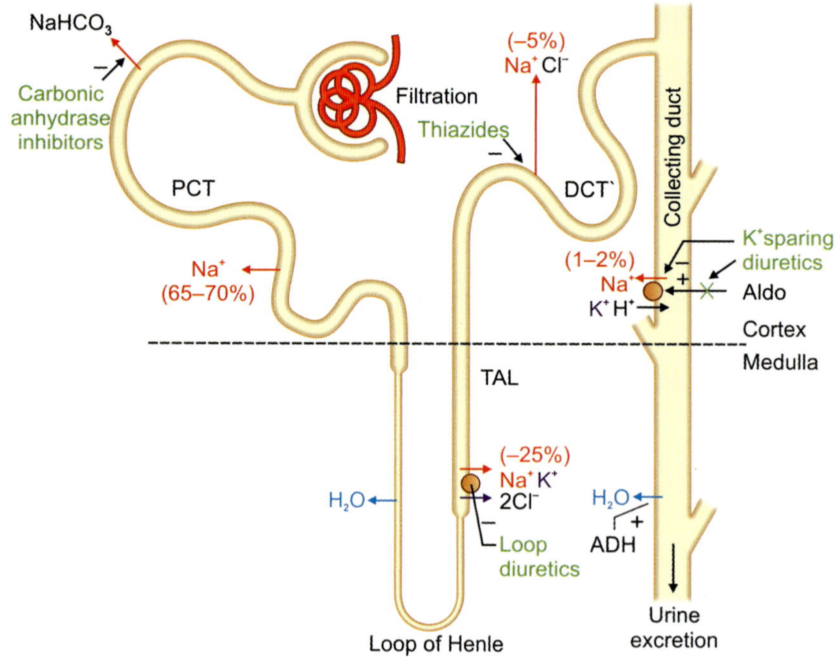

PCT, proximal convoluted tubule; DCT, distal convoluted tubule; TAL, thick ascending limb; ADH, antidiuretic hormone

Fig. 1 Different types of diuretics and their sites of action in the nephron

upregulate prostaglandin production, which in turn causes increased renal blood flow by dilation of the afferent arteriole and redistribution of the circulation to the glomerular cortex. Prostaglandins also cause a dilation of the peripheral vasculature and venodilation. This makes loop diuretics, the most powerful diuretics and is widely used to overcome fluid overload in heart failure

- Thiazide diuretics (such as hydrochlorothiazide, metolazone): They act at the level of the distal tubule inhibiting the sodium chloride cotransporter inhibiting the absorption of sodium, normally absorbed at the rate of roughly 5%. They cause hypokalemia by two distinct mechanisms: the first being activation of the aldosterone-sensitive sodium pump which leads to increased sodium absorption in exchange for potassium and hydrogen ion losses. The second is activation of the renin–angiotensin–aldosterone system (RAAS) from the decrease in intravascular volume and pressure, which leads to increased secretion of aldosterone causing greater conservation of sodium in exchange for potassium and hydrogen ions. Thiazides being less effective than loop diuretics are not used primarily by themselves in the treatment of heart failure except in combination with loop diuretics to achieve effective diuresis by overcoming diuretic resistance in patients with refractory fluid overload despite loop diuretic therapy[1]
- Potassium-sparing diuretics (such as spironolactone, triamterene): This class of diuretics includes drugs, which act either in an aldosterone-dependent or aldosterone-independent manner to enhance the excretion of sodium and water by the collecting duct. Triamterene and amiloride act independent of the level of aldosterone on the aldosterone-dependent sodium channel in the distal tubule to inhibit the reabsorption of sodium, thereby, enhancing the delivery to the collecting duct causing decreased water reabsorption leading to diuresis. Spironolactone and eplerenone act by nonselectively and selectively antagonizing the aldosterone receptors on the sodium–potassium–hydrogen pump in the distal tubule, thereby, reducing the reabsorption of sodium and sparing the excretion of potassium. They are weak diuretics and are used in conjunction with loop and thiazide diuretics for their potassium-sparing effects to prevent hypokalemia induced by others

TABLE 1: Pharmacokinetics and dosing of diuretics

Diuretics	*Bioavailability*	*Onset of action*		*Time to peak*		*Elimination of half-life ($t_{1/2}$)*			*Duration of action*		*Oral dose*	
						Normal subjects	*Patients with renal insufficiency*	*Patients with congestive heart failure*				
	Oral	*Oral*	*IV*	*Oral*	*IV*	*Oral*	*Oral*	*Oral*	*Oral*	*IV*	*Initial dose*	*Maximal dose*
Loop diuretics												
Bumetanide	80–100%	30–60 minutes	2–3 minutes	1–2 hours	15–30 minutes	1 hour	1.6 hours	1.3 hours	4–6 hours	2–3 hours	1 mg QD or BID	10 mg/day
Furosemide	60–64%	30–60 minutes	5 minutes	1–2 hours	30 minutes	1.5–2 hours	2.8 hours	2.7 hours	6–8 hours	2 hours	40 mg QD or BID	400 mg/day
Torsemide	80%	<60 minutes	<10 minutes	1–2 hours	<1 hour	3–4 hours	4–5 hours	6 hours	18–24 hours	18–24 hours	10 mg QD or BID	200 mg/day
Thiazide diuretics												
Chlorthiazide	30–50%	2 hours	15 minutes	4 hours	30 minutes	45–120 minutes	Prolonged	No change	6–12 hours	6–12 hours	500 mg	1,000 mg
Chlorthalidone	64%	2 hours	NA	2–6 hours	NA	40 hours	Prolonged	ND	48–72 hours	NA	50–100 mg/day	200 mg/day
Hydrochlor-thiazide	65–75%	2 hours	NA	4–6 hours	NA	5–14 hours	Prolonged	No change	6–12 hours	NA	25 mg QD	200 mg/day
Indapamide	93%	1–3 hours	NA	2 hours	NA	Biphasic 14 and 25 hours	ND	ND	36 hours	NA	2.5 mg QD	5 mg/day
Metolazone	40–65%	1 hour	NA	2 hours	NA	14 hours	Prolonged	No change	12–24 hours	NA	2.5–5 mg QD or BID	20 mg/day
Potassium-sparing diuretics												
Amiloride	15–25%	2–3 hours	NA	6–10 hours	NA	17–26 hours	100 hours	ND	24 hours	NA	5 mg QD	15–20 mg/day
Eplerenone	69%	Unknown	NA	1.5 hours	NA	4–6 hours	No change	Oral	Unknown	NA	25 mg QD	50 mg/day
Spironolactone	65%	Unknown	NA	3–4 hours	NA	1.4 hours	No change	No change	2–3 days	NA	12.5–25 mg QD	25–50 mg/day
Triamterene	50%	2–4 hours	NA	3 hours	NA	2–5 hours	Prolonged	ND	7–9 hours	NA	100 mg BID	300 mg/day
Carbonic anhydrase inhibitors												
Acetazolamide		2 hours	2 minutes	2–4 hours	15 minutes	3–6 hours	Prolonged	Unknown	8–12 hours	4–5 hours	250–375 mg QD	375 mg/day
Vasopressin antagonists												
Conivaptan	100%	NA	Unknown	NA	2–4 hours	5–8 hours	No change	Unknown	NA	12 hours	NA	NA
Tolvaptan	ND	2–4 hours	NA	4–8 hours	NA	5–12 hours	No change	No change	24 hours	NA	15 mg QD	60 mg/day

IV, intravenous; NA, not applicable; ND, not determined; QD, once daily; BID, twice daily

- Vasopressin receptor antagonists (VRAs) (such as tolvaptan, conivaptan): In heart failure, there is an increase in arginine vasopressin release through nonosmotic mechanisms leading to increased water reabsorption with hyponatremia and also vasoconstriction causing increased afterload and myocyte hypertrophy. The role of VRA drugs is mainly to overcome hyponatremia in heart failure. Among those studied, which included conivaptan, tolvaptan, lixivaptan, satavaptan and reclovaptan, only conivaptan as intravenous (IV) formulation and tolvaptan as oral formulation have been US Food and Drug Administration (FDA) approved for use in euvolemic and hypervolemic hyponatremia[2]
- Carbonic anhydrase inhibitors (such as acetazolamide): They act mainly at the proximal tubule inhibiting the absorption of bicarbonate, leading to a greater delivery of bicarbonate, sodium and water to the distal nephron for excretion. Being weak diuretics, they are not routinely used in heart failure therapy except rarely as an option in patients with central sleep apnea in congestive heart failure who do not tolerate continuous positive airway pressure if closely monitored. The second rare occasion for its use was demonstrated in a study showing effective treatment of hypochloremic normokalemic alkalosis in patients treated with loop diuretics and aldosterone in severe refractory CHF.

Evidence-based Medicine for Using Diuretics in the Hospital

The approach to the use of diuretics has been largely guided by expert opinion, but over the past few years, several landmark studies in this subject have shed light on how to utilize loop diuretics in the hospital and two particular studies will be reviewed here in greater detail. Both studies are reassuring regarding the relative safety of aggressive loop diuretic use in the decompensated setting. Interestingly, in both cases left ventricular ejection fraction was not a criterion for enrollment.

The first one, Diuretic Optimization Strategies Evaluation in Acute Heart Failure (DOSE-AHF) study was the only prospective, double-blind and randomized control trial that compared the effectiveness of low dose (daily oral loop diuretic dose) versus high dose (2.5 times daily oral loop diuretic dose) of intravenous loop diuretics. The study also compared the effectiveness of continuous versus intermittent bolus (every 12 hours) infusion of IV loop diuretics in a 2 × 2 factorial design. The outcomes measured were global assessment of symptoms and mean change in creatinine at 72 hours. There was no significant difference in outcome among the bolus versus infusion strategy. However, the high-dose strategy provided a trend towards more effective than the low-dose in improving global assessment of symptoms and was also associated with a greater efficacy of secondary endpoints of dyspnea, net diuresis and weight loss. Interestingly, there was a transient worsening of creatinine in the high-dose group which resolved at the time of discharge and did not pose additional adverse consequences.[3]

Although not strictly testing the appropriate use of loop diuretics, the Cardiorenal Rescue Study in Acute Decompensated Heart Failure (CARRESS-HF) study tested a volume-targeted approach using either a stepped pharmacologic care strategy versus ultrafiltration (mechanical removal of salt and volume) in decompensated patients with worsening renal function (WRF, often defined by a rise in creatinine ≥0.3 mg/dL) despite persistent congestion. Interestingly, adequate urine output became the guidance of therapy (~3–5 L of urine/day) for the stepped pharmacologic care arm via the use of continuous infusion strategies, add-on thiazide and/or vasoactive drugs. Overall, an impressive average of 12 pounds of weight loss was achieved with congestion as the therapeutic target, which was comparable with the ultrafiltration arm. Meanwhile, there were no detrimental consequences to renal function with this aggressive approach, and both groups had comparable 60-day event rates.[4]

GENERAL CONCEPTS

In order to better appreciate how diuretics can be effectively utilized, one has to first determine when is the most appropriate time to use it rather than a reflexive response to tackle congestion. Like pain management and glycemic control, a delicate balance act ensures maximizing benefits and minimizing risks. The overarching treatment goal should always be long term maintainence of euvolemia, rather than simply seeking short term gratification without considering adverse consequences.

In general, several important concepts need to be appreciated:

- It is important to distinguish between intravascular versus total-body volume overload at the bedside. Diuretics can only be effective if there is excess of salt and fluid in the body and if such excess is accessible and "refills" through the vasculature. Estimating the "degree" of congestion is therefore very important and should be performed consistently to ensure careful monitoring of progress. On the other hand, some conditions like restrictive or constrictive cardiomyopathies may have far less reserve for aggressive diuresis since their "mobilizable" volume is often reduced. Very often, the pace at which salt and volume is being removed, is a major determinant of effective diuresis and thus needs to be individualized. In other words, how a patient responds to a specific diuretic dose needs to be carefully studied. This often becomes a delicate balance between maintaining adequate perfusion and the desire to remove volume

- It is important to have a thorough understanding of the pharmacokinetics and pharmacodynamics of diuretics as it pertains to the individual patient. Often overlooked in everyday clinical practice is the ability of the drugs to exert their actions, their half-lives and their interactions (Table 1). It is important for drugs to reach their sites of action and for such sites (in the kidneys) to be responsive to the drugs and this problem can often be overcome by increasing dosages
- It is important to recognize that not all congestive signs and symptoms require immediate and unrelenting diuretic therapy, and the goal is to maintain long-term euvolemia rather than how quickly one can reach euvolemic state. Obviously, prompt relief of congestion is important, yet the balancing act to maintain end-organ perfusion can be very challenging. Sometimes, congestion (with associated diuretic response) is even unrelated to underlying cardiac issues and therefore careful assessments of diuretic responses are important. Peripheral or dependent edema develops over weeks to months and both are often less hazardous than central or pulmonary edema. Furthermore, peripheral edema can sometimes be effectively treated even with nonpharmacologic measures. On the other hand, hypotension caused by aggressive diuretic therapy in response to fluid retention may hinder the uptitration of antagonists of the renal angiotensin aldosterone system, thereby limiting the ability to counter the root cause and driver of congestive signs and symptoms. Therefore, confounding causes leading to fluid retention (such as adverse consequences of drugs, e.g., dihydropyridine calcium channel blockers or thiazolidinediones) should be identified and eliminated.

APPROACH TO USING DIURETIC THERAPY IN THE HOSPITAL

The general approach to using diuretic therapy in the hospital is outlined in Flowchart 1.

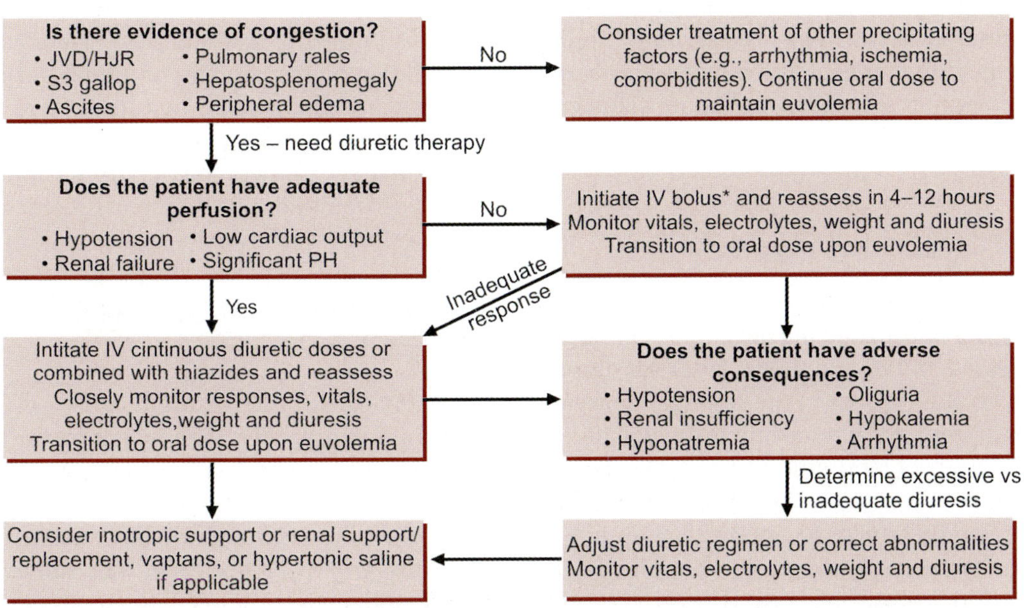

*Treatment dose: 1–2.5 x home oral daily in IV (DOSE-AHF); Goal: target 2–3 L/day urine output (CARRESS-HF)

JVD, jugular venous distention; HJR, hepatojugular reflux; IV, intravenous; PH, pulmonary hypertension; DOSE-AHF, Diuretic Optimization Strategies Evaluation in Acute Heart Failure study; CARRESS-HF, Cardiorenal Rescue Study in Acute Decompensated Heart Failure

Flowchart 1 General approach to using diuretic therapy in the hospital

Does the Patient Actually Need Intravenous Diuretics?

This might seem oddly phrased and a self-fulfilling question when approaching a patient with heart failure, but not all patients admitted to the hospital with a history of worsening heart failure have congestion as the underlying cause. Also, there are situations where congestion is either minimal or easily amenable to oral regimens, which can be administered without causing adverse consequences, and there may also be some patients [particularly in those with heart failure and preserved ejection fraction (HFpEF)] who are so "volume-sensitive" that even a single administration of IV diuretics may lead to adverse consequences.

Does the Patient Have Evidence of Congestion?

This is a fundamental question and needs objective validation prior to initiation of diuretics. There is always a constant temptation to remove any visible edema. However, a fact to be kept in mind is that patients admitted with acute heart failure may not have overt volume overload (e.g., acute-onset rapid atrial fibrillation or defibrillator shock with worsening symptoms). For example, acute "flash" pulmonary edema (as a result of volume redistribution rather than excess) may require more vasodilators than diuretics. If the patient is already using oral diuretic drugs at home and without significant fluid retention, continuing their drugs during the hospital course is the norm.

Is the Degree of Congestion Amenable to Removal?

This is perhaps the most difficult question, sometimes not easily addressed without an actual "trial" of diuretic therapy. The issue often comes in the setting of marginal hemodynamics or underlying renal impairment, whereby a continuous infusion of loop diuretics is often initiated rather than bolus injections. The DOSE-AHF study, however, illustrates that such an approach may not be necessary for routine administration, yet it may be helpful in initiating the initial "push" of diuresis especially when patients are already receiving high doses of oral diuretics at home and still admitted with obvious congestion. Also remember that adequate renal perfusion is necessary for effective diuresis and thus evidence of jugular venous distention (JVD), a third heart sound (S3) and hepatosplenomegaly are far more indicative of the need for diuretic therapies.

How Should Diuretics Be Started?

The overall goals of diuresis should first be established in order to construct an effective treatment plan. That would include a careful assessment of volume status and the parameters that can be followed over the course of the treatment.

How Can the Kidney Handle the Diuretics?

Once the need for diuretics is established, the next step includes picking the drug or drugs to use, their dosages and their routes of administration. An important task is to appreciate the functionality of the organ which diuretics are dependent on—the kidneys. There is a wide range of opinions and hence limited consensus. Unlike heparin or insulin, there is no "standard" dosing or regimen, and the amount of drugs given is often determined by adequate needs based on previous exposures and standing home dosages, which are essentially surrogates of renal responsiveness. For most instances, IV loop diuretics (such as furosemide or bumetanide) are the most common choices of initial therapy. In the case of furosemide with a bioavailability of 50% for oral drugs, a 1:1 conversion to bolus IV dosing is a safe start whereby many elect for 2–2.5 times higher amount as initial dosing. The DOSE-AHF study demonstrated that there were no detrimental consequences and a trend towards more prompt symptomatic relief with higher dosing approach. In many instances, bolus administration of diuretics several times a day may further achieve decongestive purposes.

How Much Volume Does One Aim to Remove and over How Long?

Like any drug intervention, there is a therapeutic window for diuretics that needs to be individualized. In congestive states, patients can easily achieve a 1–2 L net negative fluid balance that corresponds to 1–3 kg drop in body weight. Both tracking methods however may be grossly inaccurate and therefore inquiring about subjective improvement in congestive signs and symptoms are often helpful. The pace and duration of decongestive therapy will depend largely on determining how to remove the maximal amount of fluid safely without jeopardizing end-organ perfusion or electrolyte imbalance.

How Does the Patient Respond?

Initiation of therapy is only the first step and patients often get into trouble either because they do not mount any responses or they responded too much. The first 4–12 hours of diuresis are perhaps the most important, because interim decisions have to be made in order to tailor the therapeutic regimen to an individual patient's condition and response. In many instances due to the care transition from the emergency department to the hospital floor, meticulous monitoring of drug responses may be interrupted, thereby potentially jeopardizing the care and should be avoided. Inadequate responses may be evident with a few hours after administering IV loop diuretics and may require dose increase or transition to continuous infusion strategies as mentioned before.

What to Monitor during Diuresis?

Since the objective of administering diuretics is to relieve congestion, monitoring of diuretic efficacy is perhaps of the utmost importance. Urine output, weight loss and symptomatic relief should be evaluated hours after administration and dose adjustments may be necessary. Hypotension should be avoided by slowing down diuresis or temporarily adjusting concomitant drugs. Electrolytes (particularly sodium and potassium) should be watched carefully, the latter requires supplementation if excess potassium loss occurs (often with magnesium as well). Contraction metabolic alkalosis often ensues, sometimes even with a touch of azotemia. Occasionally, indirect evidence of hemoconcentration (such as increase in hemoglobin, total protein or serum albumin) can be indicative of effective diuresis. These measures; however, are neither sensitive nor specific, and are only reserved for confirmatory purposes.

How to Handle Excessive Diuresis?

Patients, who have overzealous volume loss, may experience asymptomatic (or even symptomatic) hypotension as well as precipitation of azotemia and even proceed toward acute kidney injury (often in the form of acute tubular necrosis). Besides holding existing diuretic therapy, occasionally immediate fluid replenishment (in the form of bolus saline infusions), or even temporarily withholding neurohormonal antagonists may be necessary. In extreme cases, temporary infusions of pressors are required, although some may favor the use of IV dopamine with its presumed favorable renovascular effects even though supportive evidence is still somewhat lacking. The recent "ROSE-AHF" study established that routine administration of dopamine in renally insufficient patients with acute heart failure has no benefit in preventing renal compromise or improving clinical outcomes.

How to Handle Inadequate Diuresis?

The concept of "diuretic resistance" is actually quite elusive, as there is no formal definition other than a phenomenon recognized by clinicians, an inability to achieve euvolemia despite high or increasing diuretic dosing. Most cases of inadequate diuresis are due to simply inadequate loop diuretics and can be overcome by higher doses, greater frequencies or more consistent administration (e.g., continuous infusion). In more serious instances, the so-called "acute (or type 1) cardiorenal syndrome" may develop, whereby progressive renal insufficiency in the setting of decongestive therapy may preclude effective diuresis.

- The first task to tackle "diuretic resistance" is to determine if inadequate renal perfusion is the cause, which may result in diminished drug delivered to the kidney and impaired pharmacodynamics. In such scenarios increasing the dose often produces a better output, but inadequacies in frequency of dosing could result in a rebound reabsorption of sodium during the interval that the diuretic is not administered thus nullifying the effect. Adequate timing and interval of dosing the drug as well as adequate systemic pressures are thus important to minimize this
- Another phenomenon called "braking phenomenon" occurs in chronic diuretic therapy where the distal tubular cells undergo hypertrophy resulting in increased sodium and water reabsorption at that level. This is the scenario whereby pretreatment with thiazides in combination with loop diuretics may be effective
- The act of intravascular volume depletion driven by diuretic therapy may lead to activation of the RAAS and sympathetic nervous system, causing a vasoconstrictor response and further decreased renal perfusion thereby worsening resistance.

A common method used to overcome resistance is concurrent use of two diuretics like thiazides or acetazolamide added to loop diuretics which lead to sequential blockade of different sites on the nephron, thus achieving more effective diuresis. Adverse effects to be monitored closely include hypokalemia, hyponatremia and even metabolic acidosis with acetazolamide. Often mineralocorticoid receptor antagonist is added to minimize the potassium loss; yet intravascular volume depletion often exacerbates hyperkalemia and should be carefully monitored.

What Should Be Done When the Creatinine Rises?

With chronic exposure to loop diuretics, some patients with heart failure may develop WRF by way of progressive rising serial creatinine levels. This decreased response to the drug could be due to many reasons. The most important step is to make the decision as to whether there is still persistent congestion. Sometimes even flattening of the JVD does not necessarily mean that an individual is euvolemic, particularly when there is still overt evidence that may suggest volume overload. Examples include body weight still above regular "dry" weight, markedly elevated natriuretic peptide levels above and beyond that in stable conditions or still persistently symptomatic upon exertion associated with congestive symptoms. In these scenarios, the main determinant is not to stop diuretics, but to try one of two strategies to reduce the pace to which diuretics are being administered. This has been validated by findings from the CARRESS-HF study, whereby a volume-directed, stepwise administration of either diuretics or ultrafiltration in the setting of persistent congestion and WRF can achieve substantial removal of salt and fluid.

- Sometimes, a long-acting and more bioavailable oral loop diuretic (such as torsemide) may be initiated; at other times, temporarily holding a dose of diuretic for better "refill" and restarting at lower doses might also help. Both will depend on whether the kidneys are still effectively responding to the loop diuretics. There is also a temptation to replenish fluids when azotemia is the prime suspect. While that may be reasonable, in most cases in the absence of hypovolemia simply stopping a dose of diuretics may suffice
- One of the biggest mistakes is to withhold neurohormonal antagonists (especially upon discharge) in the setting of rising creatinine with the "fear" of detrimental effects despite adequate ongoing diuresis while maintaining perfusion (i.e., adequate blood pressure). In fact, one of the most common reasons for deterioration and discontinuation of lifesaving neurohormonal antagonists is the abrupt withholding of drugs during acute changes related to aggressive diuresis
- When the evidence of intravascular depletion is clear, temporarily holding diuresis to reestablish plasma refill may be necessary. At present, options include:
  - Holding diuretics
  - Holding nephrotoxic drugs
  - Holding renin–angiotensin–aldosterone antagonists
  - Giving bolus infusions of saline.

The appropriate strategy is not entirely clear, and it likely will depend on individual circumstances. The key, however, is to carefully monitor and determine how to reestablish guideline-based therapies and achieve euvolemia prior to discharge.

What Side Effects Need to Watch for?

Aggressive diuretic therapy in heart failure is accompanied frequently by both reversible and irreversible side effects. Due to the decreased reabsorption of sodium along the various sites of the nephron as described before, diuretics have the propensity to cause hyponatremia, hypokalemia, hypochloremia with or without metabolic alkalosis due to decreased excretion of bicarbonate. Goals of therapy during the hospitalized period must include optimization of electrolytes to prevent life threatening cardiac arrhythmias in the already decompensated patients.[5-8]

- Hypokalemia in particular can lead to lethal arrhythmias. A common goal in practice is to aim for a potassium level greater than 4 mEq/L and an adequate whole-body magnesium level (not easily measurable as it does not correlate with serum magnesium levels)
- Although patients with volume overload can often present with hypervolemic hyponatremia in the acute setting, diuretics often result in the resolution of hyponatremia. An increase in water excretion compared to sodium can cause hypernatremia which needs to be carefully watched for. Hypotension and hypovolemia are also common leading to a decreased renal perfusion causing acute kidney injury. Although, studies had shown higher doses of loop diuretics to be associated with a greater tendency to cause renal injury, the DOSE-AHF trial demonstrated that high doses of loop diuretics was associated with a transient worsening of renal function that resolved by the time of discharge. There is activation of the RAAS and sympathetic nervous system, which can cause an increase in the left ventricular filling pressures by retention of water due to release of aldosterone and also a systemic vasoconstriction. Inhibition of sodium

chloride uptake at the macula densa also leads to a secretion of renin causing activation of RAAS
- Hyperuricemia is a well-known side effect of thiazides in particular and is caused by both decreased excretion of solutes, including uric acid due to reduced glomerular filtration rates, and also decreased secretion of uric acid into the tubular lumen during diuretic administration. Hyperuricemia can also lead to attacks of acute gout during therapy for heart failure. During the episode, diuresis is typically continued while treating the underlying gout flare-up
- Ototoxicity is seen with loop diuretics particularly ethacrynic acid, which has been associated with irreversible damage, thus, minimizing its use except in rare occasions with allergy to other loop diuretics. Furosemide and bumetanide also result in hearing loss, which is mostly reversible. Dose-dependent increase in ototoxic potential have been identified in studies with rapid infusion of IV bolus doses being associated with more risk of inner ear damage than slow infusions. The mechanisms of damage are mediated by a decrease in electrochemical potassium gradient across the lymphatic membranes.

How and When Should Home Dosing Be Transitioned?

Like any good treatment plan, there should be some initial expectations of the "best-case scenario" with diuretics, with an important forward-looking plan to maintain euvolemia.

When to Transition from Intravenous to Oral Drug Regimens?

Most often oral drug regimens will be restarted after patients approach euvolemia in order to provide adequate maintenance of intravascular volume. There are currently no clear conversion guidelines on how to best achieve a successful transition, and most have followed a reverse IV to oral equivalent dosing conversion.

What Else May Contribute to Recurrent Congestion?

Noncompliance with salt restriction leads to ineffective diuresis due to a positive sodium balance. Drugs like nonsteroidal anti-inflammatory drugs can further worsen heart failure by decreasing prostaglandin production, which normally causes vasodilation of the afferent arteriole. These factors need to be thoroughly discussed and counseled at the time of discharge and promptly recognized once patients leave the hospital. However, recurrent congestion may also be indicative of more advanced cardiorenal compromise that may warrant more invasive strategies (e.g., replacement therapies) or palliative care.

What We Still Do Not Know?

Despite the best technologies and drug choices, there are still major gaps in our knowledge regarding diuretic dosing. First, we have very limited appreciation of how diuretic response can be assessed. This is in part due to the fact that there is no reliable *in vivo* measure of natriuresis and fluid intake and output are often inaccurate. For now, changes in weight have been the best surrogate, yet it is also highly variable. Second, we have limited understanding as to whether different modalities of removing salt and water make any differences in long-term consequences. In other words, one may effectively remove congestion at the expense of aggravating sodium avidity and neurohormonal activation. Third, what is effective in a few days of aggressive therapy may not directly translate into long-term maintenance of euvolemia and thus the initial diuretic choices may not have major impact on prognosis in the absence of reliable identification and correction of modifiable factors leading to acute heart failure syndrome.

CONCLUSION

Diuretics have been the core of acute heart failure therapy and their use has largely been guided by expert opinion. The DOSE-AHF trial has helped us in understanding the permissible use of high-dose loop diuretics with a finite yet tolerable detrimental effect on renal function. This has so far served as an important tool in managing patients with acute decompensated heart failure (ADHF), but optimal management strategies still remain a challenge due to lack of long randomized control trials evaluating specific diuretic protocols, especially with respect to cardiorenal syndrome. Cardiorenal syndrome continues to remain a challenge in diuretic therapy; the precise role of ultrafiltration besides salvage therapy still remains to be determined. Further studies are required to answer the question of minimizing WRF and mortality while treating the volume overload effectively in this progressive syndrome. Until then, the best practice would be based on expert opinion and individualized to the clinical scenario.[9]

REFERENCES

1. Volz EM, Felker GM. How to use diuretics in heart failure. Curr Treat Options Cardiovasc Med. 2009;11(6):426-32.
2. Cavalcante JL, Khan S, Gheorghiade M. EVEREST study: Efficacy of Vasopressin Antagonism in Heart Failure Outcome Study with Tolvaptan. Expert Rev Cardiovasc Ther. 2008;6(10):1331-8.
3. Felker GM, Lee KL, Bull DA, et al. Diuretic strategies in patients with acute decompensated heart failure. N Engl J Med. 2011;364(9):797-805.
4. Bart BA, Goldsmith SR, Lee KL, et al. Ultrafiltration in decompensated heart failure with cardiorenal syndrome. N Engl J Med. 2012;367(24): 2296-304.
5. Jessup M, Abraham WT, Casey DE, et al. 2009 focused update: ACCF/AHA Guidelines for the Diagnosis and Management of Heart Failure in Adults: a report of the American College of Cardiology Foundation/American Heart Association Task Force on Practice Guidelines: developed in collaboration with the International Society for Heart and Lung Transplantation. Circulation. 2009;119(14):1977-2016.
6. Heart Failure Society of America, Lindenfeld J, Albert NM, et al. HFSA 2010 Comprehensive Heart Failure Practice Guideline. J Card Fail. 2010; 16(6):e1-194.
7. Abraham WT, Hasan A. Diagnosis and management of heart failure. In: Fuster V, Walsh RA, Harrington RA (Eds). Hurst's the Heart, 13th edition. McGraw Hill Companies, Inc.; 2011.
8. McMurray JJ, Adamopoulos S, Anker SD, et al. ESC Guidelines for the diagnosis and treatment of acute and chronic heart failure 2012: The Task Force for the Diagnosis and Treatment of Acute and Chronic Heart Failure 2012 of the European Society of Cardiology. Developed in collaboration with the Heart Failure Association (HFA) of the ESC. Eur Heart J. 2012; 33(14):1787-847.
9. Brater DC. Update in diuretic therapy: clinical pharmacology. Semin Nephrol. 2011;31(6):483-94.

Chapter 15

Vasodilators in Acute Heart Failure

Shiro Ishihara, Alexandre Mebazaa

ABSTRACT

Vasodilators (VDs) mainly reduce filling pressure in patients with acutely decompensated heart failure (ADHF). The European Society of Cardiology guidelines recommend VD use in ADHF patients with normal to high blood pressure at the time of admission. VDs have favorable effects on hemodynamic profile in patients with ADHF, including reduction in preload and afterload and increase in stroke volume. It should be used with cautions or avoided in ADHF patients with hypotension. Furthermore, excessive drop in systolic blood pressure should be avoided, as it is associated with poor prognosis.

WHAT IS ACUTELY DECOMPENSATED HEART FAILURE?

Acutely decompensated heart failure (ADHF) is a disease related to the accumulation of blood, upstream the left and the right ventricles. This induces lung, kidney, or liver congestion with maintained cardiac output (CO). In addition to organ's congestion, ADHF may be associated with catecholamine release, sympathetic tone stimulation and arterial vasoconstriction (rise in systemic vascular resistance) that can worsen increase in left ventricular end-diastolic pressure (LVEDP) and pulmonary congestion. In parallel, venous vasoconstriction may lead to increase in venous pressure and worsen congestion and organ dysfunction.[1-4]

Beneficial immediate hemodynamic effects of VDs are mostly related to the relief of vasoconstriction. Venodilation leads to increase in venous capacitance, decrease in venous pressure and increase in organ's (kidney or liver) flow. Furthermore, a decrease in left ventricular (LV) afterload can lead to decrease in LVEDP and increase in CO. Reduction in right ventricular (RV) and LV afterload and improvement in heart load conditions often leads to an additional improvement in stroke volume. Accordingly, VDs can relief symptoms of dyspneic patients with ADHF faster than diuretics do.

Because of these favorable effects, the European Society of Cardiology guidelines[5] and practical recommendations[6] for the management of ADHF recommend vasodilator use with normal to high blood pressure (BP) at the time of admission.

CURRENTLY AVAILABLE VASODILATORS IN ACUTELY DECOMPENSATED HEART FAILURE AND HOW TO USE IT?

Spray, Sublingual, and Intravenous Nitroglycerin

Nitroglycerin (NTG) is very easy to use. It mainly acts on venous side and also acts on arterial side. NTG can unload the heart through lowering preload and afterload and increase CO, when given appropriate dose. When BP is adequate, two sprays of NTG may be given once under the tongue, while introducing the intravenous (IV) treatment. Effects of NTG occur immediately after initiation and

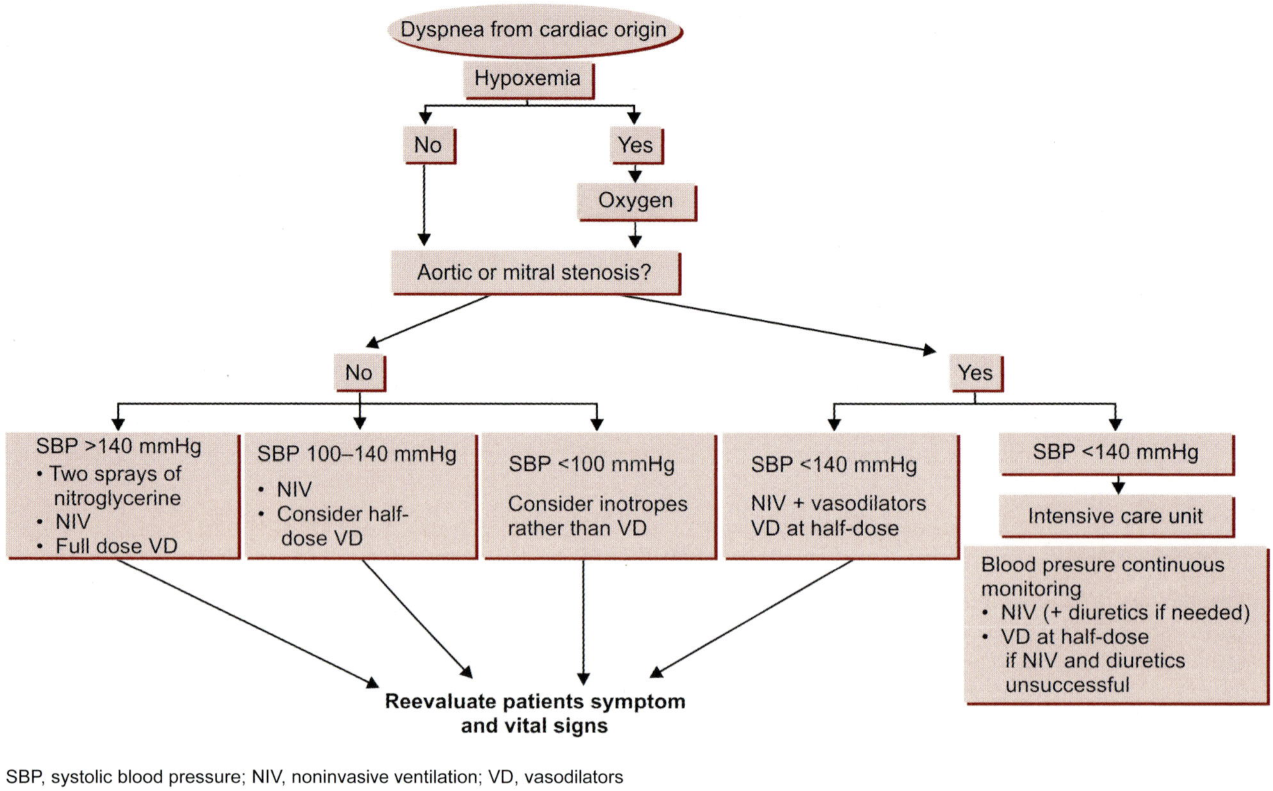

Flowchart 1 Algorithm for early management of patients with acutely decompensated heart failure

TABLE 1: Recommended dose of vasodilators[5]

Drugs	*Full starting dose*	*Half-dose*
Nitroglycerine	Start with 10 μg/min, increase if needed	Start with 5 μg/min, increase if needed
Nesiritide	Bolus 2 μg/kg + infusion 0.01 μg/kg/min*	Bolus 1 μg/kg + infusion 0.005 μg/kg/min*
Nitroprusside	Start with 0.3 μg/kg/min	Start with 0.15 μg/kg/min

*Nesiritide can be initiated without bolus

eliminate immediately after cessation. IV NTG starts 10 μg/min and titrates until improvement of symptoms, getting favorable hemodynamic responses, side effects, or maximum dose (200 μg/min). Tachyphylaxis can be developed within 24 hours, and tolerance can be occurred on continuous use, which leads us to titrate to get sufficient efficacy (Flowchart 1 and Table 1).

Nesiritide

Nesiritide, human B-type natriuretic peptide (BNP), has variable effects including urinary output and sodium excretion. However, its main action is vasodilatory effect. Nesiritide can also reduce preload and afterload, and increase CO. Nesiritide does not have tachyphylaxis.[7]

Sodium Nitroprusside

Sodium nitroprusside is very difficult to use. It acts on arterial side and venous side with balanced fashion. Nitroprusside can also reduce preload and afterload, and increase CO. Invasive hemodynamic monitoring is recommended to avoid hypotension. In general, nitroprusside starts 0.3 μg/kg/min and titrates gradually until improvement of symptoms. Nitroprusside must be covered because of its light sensitivity. Long-term use, in high doses, or renal dysfunction have been associated with the risk of isocyanate toxicity. To avoid rebound vasoconstriction, nitroprusside must be tapered gradually.

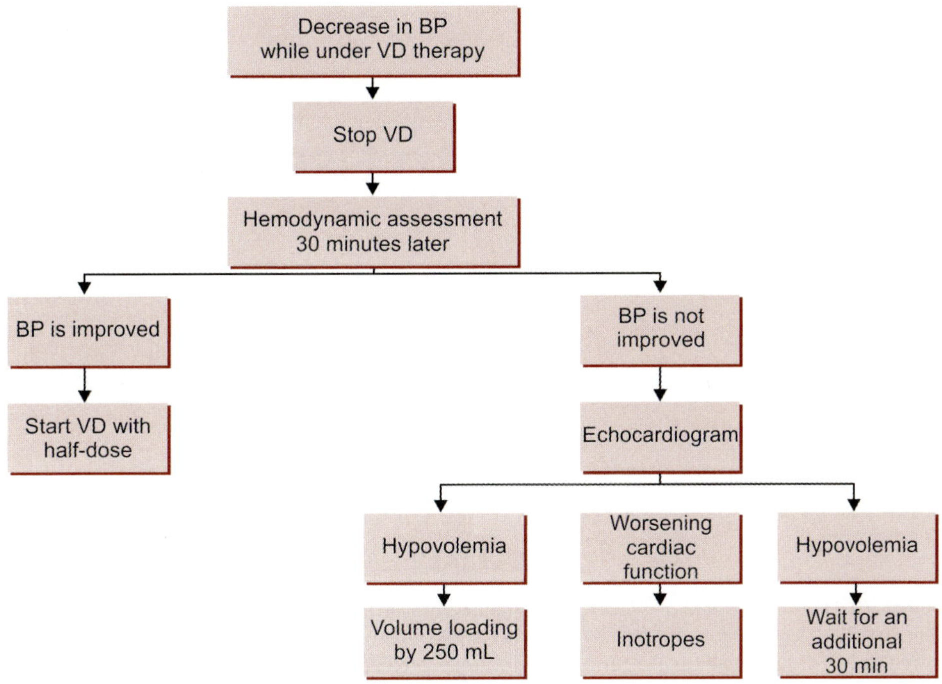

BP, blood pressure; VD, vasodilators

Flowchart 2 Algorithm for the management of vasodilators-induced decrease in blood pressure

IN CASE OF VASODILATORS-INDUCED HYPOTENSION

All VDs listed here have a possibility to cause hypotension. Patients with ADHF are treated with diuretics to alleviate volume overload. BP can drop abruptly after few hours. Excessive early drop of BP is known as one of the determinant of developing worsening renal function.[8] Management of decreased BP is seen in Flowchart 2.

HOW LONG SHOULD WE USE VASODILATORS?

Dyspnea should be measured every 2–6 hours on a visual analogue scale (VAS): 0 (no dyspnea) to 100 mm (maximum dyspnea). VDs can be stopped when VAS is below 20 mm.

CONCLUSION

Vasodilators are powerful tools to relief symptom of dyspneic patients with ADHF, because it can decrease in preload and afterload, and to increase in CO. However, VDs should be used with enough caution with BP.

REFERENCES

1. Dilley JR, Corradi A, Arendshorst WJ. Glomerular ultrafiltration dynamics during increased renal venous pressure. Am J Physiol. 1983;244(6):F650-8.
2. Nohria A, Hasselblad V, Stebbins A, et al. Cardiorenal interactions: insights from the ESCAPE trial. J Am Coll Cardiol. 2008;51(13):1268-74.
3. Mullens W, Abrahams Z, Francis GS, et al. Importance of venous congestion for worsening of renal function in advanced decompensated heart failure. J Am Coll Cardiol. 2009;53(7):589-96.
4. Nikolaou M, Parissis J, Yilmaz MB, et al. Liver function abnormalities, clinical profile, and outcome in acute decompensated heart failure. Eur Heart J. 2013;34(10):742-9.
5. McMurray JJ, Adamopoulos S, Anker SD, et al. ESC Guidelines for the diagnosis and treatment of acute and chronic heart failure 2012: The Task Force for the Diagnosis and Treatment of Acute and Chronic Heart Failure 2012 of the European Society of Cardiology. Developed in collaboration with the Heart Failure Association (HFA) of the ESC. Eur Heart J. 2012;33(14):1787-847.
6. Mebazaa A, Gheorghiade M, Piña IL, et al. Practical recommendations for prehospital and early in-hospital management of patients presenting with acute heart failure syndromes. Crit Care Med. 2008;36(1 Suppl):S129-39.
7. Publication Committee for the VMAC Investigators (Vasodilatation in the Management of Acute CHF). Intravenous nesiritide vs nitroglycerin for treatment of decompensated congestive heart failure: a randomized controlled trial. JAMA. 2002;287(12):1531-40.
8. Voors AA, Davison BA, Felker GM, et al. Early drop in systolic blood pressure and worsening renal function in acute heart failure: renal results of Pre-RELAX-AHF. Eur J Heart Fail. 2011;13(9):961-7.

Chapter 16

When and How to Use Inotropes?

John T Parissis, Vassiliki Bistola

ABSTRACT

Acute heart failure (AHF) encompasses a broad spectrum of clinical presentations, ranging from decompensation of chronic heart failure (HF) to low cardiac output–hypoperfusion syndromes with cardiogenic shock (CS) at the extreme end of this side. Inotropes are pharmacological agents that enhance cardiac contractility, thereby, increasing cardiac output. Currently, there are three major classes of inotropes in clinical use with distinct mechanisms of action: beta-adrenergic agonists, phosphodiesterase III inhibitors (PDEIs) and the calcium sensitizer levosimendan. Inotropes are indicated in AHF patients with either CS (usually with coadministration of a vasoconstrictor) or low output syndromes with vital organ hypoperfusion as a short-term treatment to stabilize patient's hemodynamic condition and maintain/restore peripheral perfusion. Inotropes can cause serious cardiovascular adverse effects, most commonly tachyarrhythmias, hypotension/hypertension and myocardial ischemia and are associated with increases in medium- and long-term mortality in HF. Therefore, intense patient monitoring is necessary during their administration, while long-term administration is contraindicated with the exception of end-stage HF patients in whom they are used as a bridge to a definitive treatment (transplantation, or ventricular assist device implantation) or as palliative therapy. New inotropic agents (e.g., cardiac myosin activators and istaroxime) are currently being tested in phase II clinical trials for their efficacy and safety in AHF.

INTRODUCTION

Acute heart failure (AHF) is characterized by the recent onset or change in the severity of symptoms and signs of HF. In most cases, AHF is a result of the deterioration of the clinical status of patients previously diagnosed with HF, while it can also be the first presentation of HF. The clinical presentations of patients with AHF encompass a broad spectrum of conditions that range from gradually (over days or even weeks) worsening dyspnea or peripheral edema to the critical states of pulmonary edema or CS. Accordingly, in-hospital mortality varies widely between 2% in low-risk patients and 22% in high-risk patients, stratified according to their vital signs [low versus high systolic blood pressure (SBP)] and laboratory data (normal versus abnormally elevated blood urea nitrogen and creatinine levels) measured upon hospital admission.[1,2] Currently, no available pharmacologic strategies have a proven efficacy to reduce medium- and long-term morbidity and mortality in AHF. Therefore, the treatment goals remain symptomatic relief by reducing elevated ventricular filling pressures, stabilization of the patient's hemodynamic condition to preserve vital end-organ function, and probably, reduction of the length of hospital stay, rehospitalizations and short-term mortality.[3] Loop diuretics are first-line agents for the relief of dyspnea and edema; in hypertensive and normotensive AHF, vasodilators are used to reduce ventricular afterload and indirectly increase cardiac output. Inotropes and inodilators directly enhance cardiac contractility; therefore, they increase cardiac output, which is reduced acutely in a subset of AHF patients. However, these agents have been shown to induce adverse cardiovascular effects including myocardial ischemia, tachyarrhythmias and have been associated with increases in medium- and long-term mortality. Therefore, their routine use in unselected AHF patients is not recommended, while they remain as a necessary short-term treatment option in patients who display evidence of low cardiac output and peripheral hypoperfusion.

CLASSES OF INOTROPES AND MECHANISM OF ACTION

Currently, there are three major classes of inotropes in clinical use for the management of patients with AHF: beta-adrenergic agonists (dopamine, dobutamine, epinephrine, norepinephrine), PDEIs (milrinone) and the calcium sensitizer levosimendan (Table 1).

Beta-adrenergic Agonists

Beta-adrenergic agonists mediate their cardiac inotropic effect through stimulation of sarcolemmal beta 1 adrenergic receptors of cardiac myocytes, which, in turn, activates the intracellular adenyl cyclase system resulting in increased cAMP formation. cAMP then activates Ca^{2+} channels located in the sarcolemmal membrane and the sarcoplasmic reticulum membrane, causing a massive release of Ca^{2+} from the sarcoplasmic reticulum through the Ca^{2+}-induced Ca^{2+} release effect. The increase in the levels of sarcoplasmic Ca^{2+} increases the strength of actin-myosin-troponin interaction, enhancing myocardial contraction.

Dopamine

Dopamine is an endogenous molecule that acts through the dopaminergic types 1 and 2 and beta 1 and alpha 1 adrenergic receptors. At low doses (0.5–2.5 μg/kg/minute), it causes renal and splanchnic vasodilation through the postsynaptic type 1 and presynaptic type 2 dopaminergic receptors, respectively. By this mechanism it increases the renal blood flow independently of the increase in cardiac output. The clinical significance of the renal effects of low dose dopamine remains controversial, since it does not increase glomerular filtration rate and a renal protective effect has not been demonstrated.[4] At moderate doses (3–5 μg/kg/minute), it exerts primarily its inotropic and chronotropic effects through the cardiac beta 1 receptors. At higher doses (>5 μg/kg/minute), it acts mainly on alpha 1 receptors causing vasoconstriction. Important side effects include tachyarrhythmias, which become more frequent at doses of 10 μg/kg/minute and above and hypertension.

Dobutamine

Dobutamine is a synthetic analogue of dopamine that in order of decreasing strength stimulates beta 1, beta 2 and alpha 1 adrenergic receptors. By binding to cardiac beta 1 receptors, dobutamine primarily increases cardiac contractility with weaker chronotropic effects, while in the vasculature it causes a net mild vasodilation due to a combined alpha 1 receptor agonism and antagonism and beta 2 stimulation. Overall, dobutamine increases cardiac output with concomitant mild vasodilation that is evident particularly at low infusion doses (<5 μg/kg/minute). At high doses peripheral vasoconstriction predominates through stimulation of alpha 1 receptors. Dobutamine is administered at doses starting from 1–2 μg/kg/minute up to 20 μg/kg/minute, but higher doses are administered occasionally (up to 40 μg/kg/minute). The potential disadvantages of dobutamine are that it may not be as effective as anticipated in patients already receiving beta blockers and that tolerance develops after just a few days of therapy. Dobutamine is associated with increased risk of tachyarrhythmias at any infusion dose.

Norepinephrine

Norepinephrine has a prominent agonist effect on vascular alpha 1 adrenergic receptors, with a modest cardiac beta 1 agonist activity. Therefore, it is considered primarily a potent vasoconstrictor and less a cardiac inotropic agent. In clinical practice, it increases systolic, diastolic and pulse pressure without significantly affecting cardiac output. In HF patients, it is used in conjunction with inotropic agents in CS or in patients treated with an inodilator to avoid hypotension. Norepinephrine is usually administered at doses of 0.01–0.03 μg/kg/minute, but doses as high as 1 μg/kg/minute may be required. Prolonged infusions can be directly toxic to the myocardium through the induction of cardiomyocyte apoptotic cell death. Adverse effects include arrhythmias, myocardial ischemia, and hypertension.

Epinephrine

Epinephrine stimulates cardiac beta 1 and vascular beta 2 and alpha 1 adrenoreceptors. At low doses (<0.01 μg/kg/minute) beta 2-induced vasodilation predominates decreasing arterial blood pressure (BP), while doses greater than 0.2 μg/kg/minute produce a mixed inotropic and vasoconstrictor effect that overall increases

TABLE 1: Pharmacological properties of inotropic agents and useful "tips" for their administration[26-28]

Properties	*Dobutamine*	*Dopamine*	*Norepinephrine*	*Epinephrine*	*Levosimendan*	*Milrinone*
Mechanism of action	β1 > β2 > α	Dopaminergic > β; high-dose α	β1 > α > β2	β1 = β2 > α	Calcium sensitizer; high dose PDE inhibitor	PDE inhibitor
Elimination $t_{1/2}$ (minute)	2.4	2.0	3.0	2.0	Active metabolite: 4,800	150
Infusion dose	2–20 µg/kg/minute	• <3 µg/kg/minute: renal effect • 3–5 µg/kg/minute: inotropic • >5 µg/kg/minute vasoconstrictor	0.2–10 µg/kg/minute	0.05–0.5 µg/kg/minute	0.05–0.2 µg/kg/minute	0.375–0.75 µg/kg/minute
Bolus dose	No	No	No	1 mg can be given IV during resuscitation every 3–5 minutes	12 µg/kg/minute over 10 minutes (optional)	25–75 µg/kg/minute over 10–20 minutes
Inotropic effect	↑↑	↑↑	↑	↑↑	↑	↑
Arterial vasodilatation	↑	↑↑ (LD)	0	↑	↑↑	↑↑
Vasoconstriction	↑ (HD)	↑↑ (HD)	↑↑	↑ (HD)	0	0
Pulmonary vasodilatation	↑ or 0		↓ or 0 (at high PVR)	↓ or 0 (at high PVR)	↑↑	↑↑
Chronotropic effect	↑	0 or ↑	↑	↑↑	0	0
Blood pressure effect	↑	↑ (HD)	↑	0 or ↑	↓	↓
Diuretic effect	0	↑↑ (LD)	↑	0	↑	0
Recommendation class						
ESC	IIa	IIb	IIb	IIb	IIb	IIb
ACC/AHA	IIb	IIb I (CS)	I (CS)	I (CS)	Not licensed	IIb
Level of evidence	C	C	C	C	C	C
Adverse effects	Tachyarrhythmias, hypotension, headache (rarely) eosinophilic myocarditis, peripheral eosinophilia	Tachyarrhythmias, hypertension, chest pain	Tachyarrhythmias, hypertension, headache	Tachyarrhythmias, headache, anxiety, cold extremities, cerebral hemorrhage, pulmonary edema	Hypotension, atrial and ventricular tachyarrhythmias, headache, nausea	Tachyarrhythmias, hypotension, headache

HD, high dose; LD, low dose; PVR, pulmonary vascular resistances; CS, cardiogenic shock; PDE, phosphodiesterase; IV, intravenous;, ESC, European Society of Cardiology; ACC/AHA, American College of Cardiology/American Heart Association peripheral vascular resistance and BP. This agent is especially useful when combined inotropic/chronotropic and vasoconstrictor effects are urgently required. In HF patients, it is used in CS or in cardiac arrest. The beta 2/alpha 1 vascular effects of epinephrine are exerted also in the pulmonary arterial and venous vascular bed, causing increased pulmonary arterial and venous pressure through vasoconstriction and increased pulmonary blood flow. Infusion dose ranges from 0.01 μg/kg/minute to 0.03 μg/kg/minute, but as high as 0.5 μg/kg/minute may be reached. Adverse effects include myocardial ischemia, hypertension, ventricular tachyarrhythmias, pulmonary edema and cerebral hemorrhage.

Phosphodiesterase III Inhibitors

Phosphodiesterase III inhibitors exert their inotropic effect by increasing the levels of cAMP in cardiomyocytes through inhibition if its breakdown by phosphodiesterase III. PDEIs, acting through the same mechanism in vascular smooth muscle cells, cause peripheral and pulmonary vasodilatation thereby decreasing systemic arterial BP, pulmonary arterial and venous pressures and systemic and pulmonary vascular resistances (PVR). Due to the combined inotropic and vasodilator effects of PDEIs, they are considered in the group of inodilators. Because their inotropic effects is exerted through a pathway independent of beta adrenergic receptors, PDEIs are effective in patients chronically treated with beta-blockers.[5]

Milrinone

Milrinone is the PDEI that is used most commonly for cardiovascular indications. It is approved for intravenous use in the United States and Europe. Milrinone is administered as short-term treatment in patients presenting with a low cardiac output state who are not severely hypotensive [e.g., SBP >85 mmHg], especially when they were previously chronically treated with beta-blockers, since these patients have been suggested to respond better to PDEIs than to beta agonists.[5] In patients with marginal BP (e.g., 90–100 mmHg), a vasoconstrictor (e.g., norepinephrine) can be administered concomitantly. Side effects of milrinone include tachyarrhythmias and hypotension.[6] Caution is required when milrinone is administered in patients with ischemic HF, since it may increase medium-term mortality.[7] Milrinone is infused at a rate of 0.375–0.75 μg/kg/minute. Lower starting doses (0.1–0.375 μg/kg/minute) may be given in patients at increased risk for hypotension or arrhythmias. Because of the long half-life (2.5 hours) and its renal clearance, caution should be used when milrinone is administered in patients with impaired or changing renal function.

Levosimendan

Levosimendan exerts its inotropic effects through sensitization of cardiac troponin to the prevailing level of intracellular calcium. However, at high doses it also acts as a PDEI, therefore, increasing the levels of intracellular cAMP. Levosimendan also has a vasodilatory effect by opening ATP-sensitive potassium channels in the vascular smooth muscle cells. Therefore, this agent is considered in the group of inodilators. Despite the favorable results of preliminary clinical studies regarding the hemodynamic effects of levosimendan over dobutamine (LIDO)[8] and its potential survival benefit over placebo in AHF complicating acute myocardial infarction (RUSSLAN),[9] phase III trials in AHF have shown no difference between levosimendan and dobutamine in all-cause mortality at 6 months (SURVIVE),[10] while superiority over placebo in alleviating HF symptoms was compromised by a trend toward increasing all-cause mortality at 3 months postrandomization and increased rates of hypotension and ventricular arrhythmias in the REVIVE-II trial.[11] Therefore, controversy still exists regarding the role of levosimendan in AHF. Levosimendan is available for clinical use only in Europe. It is indicated for AHF patients with vital organ hypoperfusion, who do not have significant hypotension, to reverse the effect of beta-blockade if beta-blockade is thought to be contributing to hypoperfusion.[12] It is administered as an infusion at a rate of 0.05–0.2 μg/kg/minute. Adverse effects include headache, hypotension, ventricular arrhythmias, atrial fibrillation, and hypokalemia.

Newer Inotropes

Istaroxime

Istaroxime enhances cardiac contractility by inhibiting sarcolemmal sodium-potassium ATPase and stimulating sarcoplasmic reticulum calcium adenosine triphosphatase isoform 2a (SERCA2a). The first mechanism increases the levels of intracellular Ca^{2+}, thereby increasing contractility, while the latter promotes the reaccumulation of free Ca^{2+} into the sarcoplasmic reticulum stores during diastole, improving diastolic myocardial properties (lusitropy). Istaroxime has shown a significant effectiveness superiority over placebo in reducing left ventricular filling pressures (PCWP) in a dose-finding, randomized, double blind study (HORIZON-HF), with an associated rise in arterial SBP, without any adverse effects on renal function or the neurohormonal profile.[13,14] Istaroxime remains under investigation in the treatment of AHF.

Cardiac Myosin Activators

Cardiac myosin activators are novel molecules that enhance contraction by increasing the transition of the actin–myosin complex in the cardiomyocytes from a weakly to a strongly bound state and inhibit non-productive degradation of ATP.[15] By these mechanisms, the number of active cross-bridges that participate in the generation of contractile force increase during contraction, resulting in an increase in systolic ejection time, stroke volume, and fractional shortening. These effects are not accompanied by increases in heart rate or myocardial oxygen consumption, while at the cellular level, there is no increase of the intracellular cAMP or levels of free Ca^{2+}, avoiding potentially the risks of arrhythmogenesis and myocardial ischemia. Omecamtiv mecarbil was the first of these agents to be tested in clinical studies, producing increases in systolic ejection time, stroke volume, fractional shortening, and ejection fraction when administered in healthy volunteers, as well as in patients with chronic HF and reduced ejection fraction.[16,17] Phase II clinical trials are currently testing the efficacy and safety of omecamtiv mecarbil in patients with acute and chronic HF.

WHEN AND HOW TO USE INOTROPES IN AHF?

The main indication of inotropic therapy in AHF is in patients with severely reduced cardiac output that results in compromised vital organ perfusion. According to observational data from the ADHERE registry, patients with the above characteristics comprise about 10% of the total AHF population[18] and have the highest in-hospital mortality rates.[19] Therefore, short-term treatment with inotropes appears as a necessity despite the tendency of these drugs to increase adverse outcomes in AHF. The treatment goals of inotropic therapy are to stabilize patient's hemodynamic status and restore vital organ hypoperfusion. A general rule for inotropic treatment is to use them in the lowest possible doses to achieve these goals and for the shortest necessary duration of time. A proposed algorithm for the use of inotropes in the management of patients with acutely decompensated chronic HF is presented in Flowchart 1.

Acute heart failure patients that require inotropic therapy fall into one of the following categories:

- Patients with CS
- Patients with marginal BP (e.g., 85–110 mmHg) and signs of peripheral hypoperfusion, without evidence of CS.

How to Use Inotropes in Cardiogenic Shock?

Cardiogenic shock represents the most critical presentation among patients with AHF. Typically, it is defined as severe hypotension (<85 mmHg) that results from severely reduced cardiac output (CI <2.0 mL/min/m^2) leading to high intracardiac filling pressures and vital organ hypoperfusion. In CS, an inotrope (e.g., dobutamine) should be initiated immediately to stabilize patient hemodynamics and restore vital organ perfusion until a definitive therapy is planned according to the underlying cause of the shock. Usually, in CS a vasoconstrictor (such as dopamine or norepinephrine) is also required concomitantly with the inotrope in order to maintain adequate end-organ perfusion pressure. Combination of an inotrope plus a vasoconstrictor at moderate doses are preferable over any single agent at maximal doses,[20] to avoid excessive vasoconstriction that would increase left ventricular afterload and possibly lead to myocardial ischemia and also avoid the higher risk of arrhythmogenesis that is associated with maximal infusion doses. In cases where BP cannot be maintained with the combination of inotrope plus dopamine or norepinephrine, epinephrine can be used as a more potent beta 1 and alpha 1 adrenergic agonist. Mechanical circulatory support should be considered in patients unresponsive to medical therapy.

How to Use Inotropes in Patients with AHF and Peripheral Hypoperfusion without Evidence of Cardiogenic Shock

Peripheral hypoperfusion due to low cardiac output is manifested classically by hypotension. However, not always is significant hypotension present in hypoperfused patients with AHF and, the opposite, marginal BP (85–110 mmHg) does not always confirm the presence of peripheral hypoperfusion. The first scenario is encountered in patients with AHF in whom intrinsic neurohormonal activation results in clinically significant peripheral vasoconstriction, while the latter possibility is

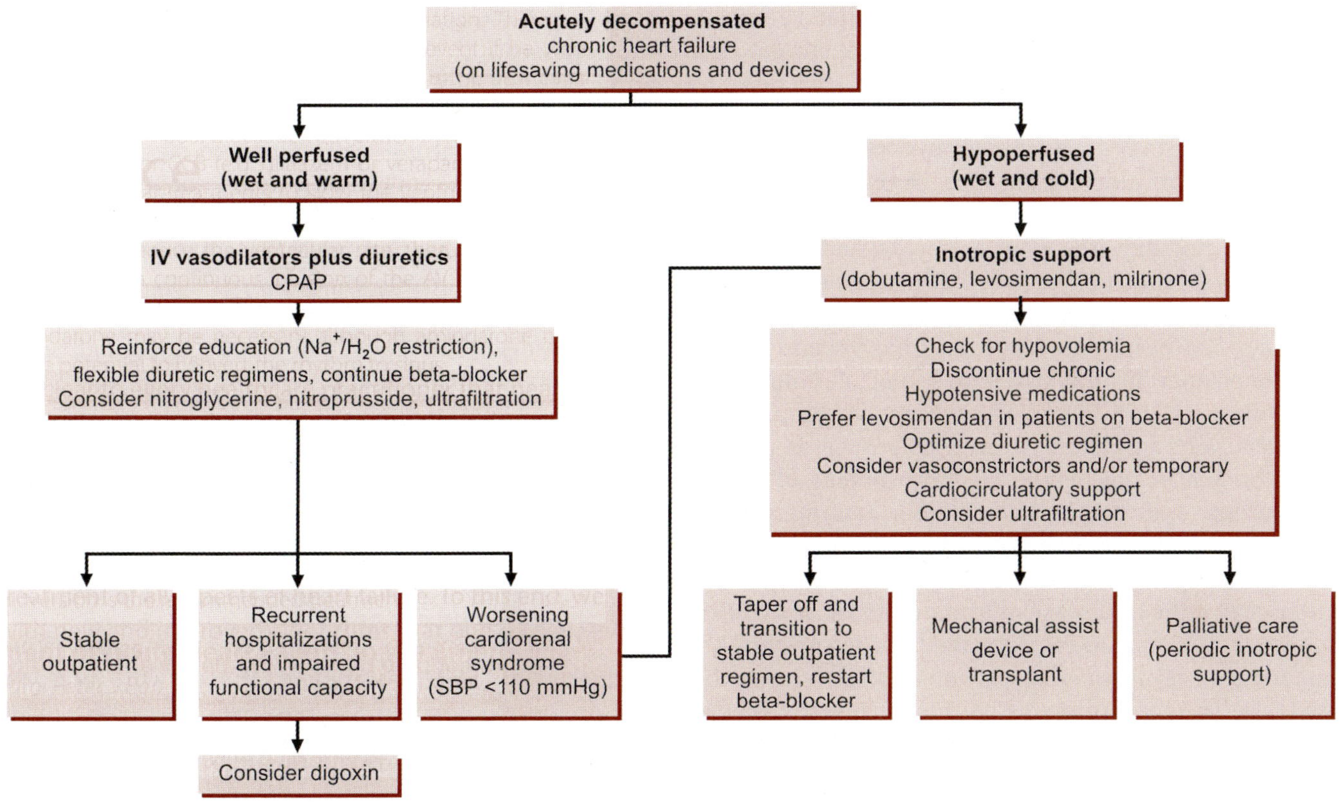

CPAP, continuous positive airway pressure; SBP, systolic blood pressure; IV, intravenous

Flowchart 1 A proposed algorithm for the use of inotropes in patients hospitalized with acutely decompensated heart failure[29]

a common case in patients with a history of chronic HF, who usually exhibit marginal arterial BP due to chronic vasodilator treatment (RAAS inhibitors/beta blockers) without displaying evidence of HF decompensation. Therefore, the clinician should search for additional clinical signs to detect hypoperfusion, including the presence of cool extremities, slowed mentation, and reduced pulse pressure. Laboratory findings indicative of peripheral hypoperfusion include worsening renal (increased blood urea nitrogen and creatinine levels) and hepatic function and hyponatremia. In such patients, an inotrope or an inodilator (milrinone or levosimendan) may be instituted to restore adequate vital organ perfusion. The choice of the specific agent depends on the clinical and hemodynamic characteristics of each patient with AHF (Table 2). Inodilators are preferred in patients who are peripherally vasoconstricted, always keeping in mind the risk for the development of significant hypotension that would necessitate initiation of an adjuvant vasoconstrictor. Inodilators are not indicated as a monotherapy in patients with SBP less than 85 mmHg. Another patient subgroup, that appears more suitable for inodilators than for beta agonists are patients with pulmonary arterial hypertension, since both

TABLE 2: Preferred inotropes in different clinical settings of acute heart failure

Clinical setting	*Agent*
Increased pulmonary artery pressure	• Levosimendan • Milrinone
Chronic beta blockade	• Levosimendan • Milrinone
Hypotension	• Dobutamine • Dopamine • Norepinephrine
Acute cardiorenal dysfunction	• Dopamine • Levosimendan • Dobutamine
Ischemic heart disease	• Levosimendan • Dobutamine

milrinone and levosimendan exert vasodilatory effects in the pulmonary arterial vasculature. Such patients are those listed for cardiac transplantation who develop significantly elevated PVR rendering them unsuitable for transplantation, in whom milrinone infusion has been effective to reduce PVR. Also, as previously noted, patients who have been on chronic beta-blockade treatment possibly respond better to levosimendan or milrinone, due to the independent mechanism of action of these agents of the beta-adrenergic receptor pathway. However, this suggestion has recently been questioned after the publication of a small, double-blind, randomized trial, the Better Effectiveness After Transition - Congestive Heart Failure (BEAT-CHF) trial that showed no difference in the degree of improvement of PCWP and cardiac index at 24 hours after treatment with levosimendan or dobutamine in 60 AHF patients who were previously on beta-blocker therapy.[21] In patients with ischemic heart disease milrinone should be avoided due to its tendency to increase medium-term mortality and instead, levosimendan or dobutamine, should be used.[22] Patients with primary renal insufficiency are better candidates for dobutamine due to its very short half-life (approximately 2 minutes) compared to milrinone (half-life of 2.5 hours) or levosimendan (half-life of the active metabolite approximately 80 hours). However, in patients with acute cardiorenal syndrome, levosimendan may be the preferable drug as there is clinical evidence that this agent exert renoprotective effects by improving renal blood flow.[23] Finally, patients with primary hepatic insufficiency are not suitable for levosimendan, because of its hepatic excretion. In contrast, patients with AHF and cardiohepatic dysfunction seem to be benefited by the use of levosimendan in comparison to dobutamine administration.[24]

Weaning of Inotropes and Inotrope Dependency

Inotropes should generally be tapered off gradually. Weaning is started as soon as adequate peripheral perfusion has been restored allowing the improvement of end-organ function, while congestion has resolved through the diuresis of excess volume. During tapering a careful concomitant adjustment of oral HF medications is necessary, which is continued after inotrope withdrawal. Patients who have received inotropes during their hospitalization should be free of such treatment for at least 48 hours before being discharged from hospital.

Most AHF patients who required treatment with inotropes can be weaned off successfully. However, in some patients, any attempt to wean off inotropic therapy precipitates symptomatic hypotension (usually SBP <80 mmHg), recurrent symptoms and signs of HF and end-organ dysfunction, such as worsening renal function. These patients are considered inotrope dependent and are maintained on inotropes for longer periods as a bridge to a definitive treatment, such as transplantation or implantation of a left ventricular assist device, or as a bridge-to-decision in those who are not yet candidates for a definitive treatment but may become so in the future. In a subset of patients who ultimately do not become candidates for any definitive therapy, inotropes may be maintained as palliative treatment to reduce the severity of HF symptoms at the end of life.

PATIENT MONITORING DURING TREATMENT WITH INOTROPIC AGENTS

Patients with AHF requiring treatment with inotropes should be admitted in an intensive care setting or at least a high dependency unit, where close monitoring is available.

ECG Monitoring

Electrocardiogram monitoring is required in all patients receiving inotropes, because of the significant risk for serious atrial and ventricular arrhythmias imposed by these agents.

Invasive Blood Pressure Monitoring

Invasive arterial BP monitoring is required in patients with CS to continuously assess their hemodynamic status and because of the potential of inotropes/vasopressor administered at moderate doses at least in such cases to induce serious hypertension or hypotension. In AHF patients who receive inotropes but are not in a shock, arterial BP can usually be monitored noninvasively, but invasive monitoring should be considered when non-responsiveness to initial therapy is observed or when there is discrepancy between patient's clinical status and the BP measurements obtained noninvasively.

Pulmonary Artery Catheter Monitoring

Pulmonary artery catheter (PAC) monitoring is not recommended routinely in patients with AHF who receive inotropes and show adequate response to the administered therapeutic regimen. However, it should be strongly considered in patients who receive inotropic therapy and:[12,25]

- Are refractory to pharmacological treatment requiring escalating doses of inotropes/vasopressors and are being considered for mechanical circulatory support
- Become apparently inotrope dependent after initial clinical improvement
- In whom there is uncertainty regarding ventricular filling pressures, cardiac output and vascular tone
- Are considered for transplantation or implantation of a left ventricular assist device, as part of the necessary initial evaluation.

CONCLUSION

Use of inotropes still remains an option for the management of acute and advanced HF patients with low output state and peripheral hypoperfusion. These drugs improve symptoms but can increase mortality rates. Thus, on the basis of the available evidence, these agents can be used only as a temporary treatment of AHF exacerbations with stringent criteria, resistant to intravenous vasodilators and/or diuretics when SBP is 100–120 mmHg or as a first-line treatment in patients with worsening of chronic cardiac failure and low SBP (<100 mmHg). The calcium sensitizer levosimendan, is a new cardiac enhancer that seems to be more effective than classical inotropes in improving cardiac mechanical efficiency and reducing congestion without causing cardiomyocyte death or increasing myocardial oxygen uptake. Recent randomized trials showed that levosimendan is not superior to placebo or dobutamine in improving 1 month and 6-month mortality, although it caused a greater reduction of neurohormonal response. Levosimendan should be used as a first-line inotrope in acute or advanced HF patients with low output state syndrome on chronic beta-blocker therapy. Investigational cardiac enhancers, such as cardiac myosin activators and istaroxime (targeting novel pathophysiologic concepts) are promising treatment approaches without significant adverse effects and ongoing trials will define their clinical efficacy and safety.

REFERENCES

1. Filippatos G, Zannad F. An introduction to acute heart failure syndromes: definition and classification. Heart Fail Rev. 2007;12(2):87-90.
2. Triposkiadis F, Parissis JT, Starling RC, et al. Current drugs and medical treatment algorithms in the management of acute decompensated heart failure. Expert Opin Investig Drugs. 2009;18(6):695-707.
3. De Luca L, Fonarow GC, Adams KF, et al. Acute heart failure syndromes: clinical scenarios and pathophysiologic targets for therapy. Heart Fail Rev. 2007;12(2):97-104.
4. Bellomo R, Chapman M, Finfer S, et al. Low-dose dopamine in patients with early renal dysfunction: a placebo-controlled randomised trial. Australian and New Zealand Intensive Care Society (ANZICS) Clinical Trials Group. Lancet. 2000;356(9248):2139-43.
5. Lowes BD, Tsvetkova T, Eichhorn EJ, et al. Milrinone versus dobutamine in heart failure subjects treated chronically with carvedilol. Int J Cardiol. 2001;81(2-3):141-9.
6. Cuffe MS, Califf RM, Adams KF, et al. Short-term intravenous milrinone for acute exacerbation of chronic heart failure: a randomized controlled trial. JAMA. 2002;287(12):1541-7.
7. Felker GM, Leimberger JD, Califf RM, et al. Risk stratification after hospitalization for decompensated heart failure. J Card Fail. 2004;10(6):460-6.
8. Follath F, Cleland JG, Just H, et al. Efficacy and safety of intravenous levosimendan compared with dobutamine in severe low-output heart failure (the LIDO study): a randomised double-blind trial. Lancet. 2002;360(9328):196-202.
9. Moiseyev VS, Poder P, Andrejevs N, et al. Safety and efficacy of a novel calcium sensitizer, levosimendan, in patients with left ventricular failure due to an acute myocardial infarction. A randomized, placebo-controlled, double-blind study (RUSSLAN). Eur Heart J. 2002;23(18):1422-32.
10. Mebazaa A, Nieminen MS, Packer M, et al. Levosimendan vs dobutamine for patients with acute decompensated heart failure: the SURVIVE Randomized Trial. JAMA. 2007;297(17):1883-91.
11. Cleland JG, Freemantle N, Coletta AP, et al. Clinical trials update from the American Heart Association: REPAIR-AMI, ASTAMI, JELIS, MEGA, REVIVE-II, SURVIVE, and PROACTIVE. Eur J Heart Fail. 2006;8(1):105-10.
12. McMurray JJ, Adamopoulos S, Anker SD, et al. ESC Guidelines for the diagnosis and treatment of acute and chronic heart failure 2012: the Task Force for the Diagnosis and Treatment of Acute and Chronic Heart Failure 2012 of the European Society of Cardiology. Developed in collaboration with the Heart Failure Association (HFA) of the ESC. Eur Heart J. 2012;33(14):1787-847.
13. Gheorghiade M, Blair JE, Filippatos GS, et al. Hemodynamic, echocardiographic, and neurohormonal effects of istaroxime, a novel intravenous inotropic and lusitropic agent: a randomized controlled trial in patients hospitalized with heart failure. J Am Coll Cardiol. 2008;51(23):2276-85.
14. Shah SJ, Blair JE, Filippatos GS, et al. Effects of istaroxime on diastolic stiffness in acute heart failure syndromes: results from the hemodynamic, echocardiographic, and neurohormonal effects of istaroxime, a novel intravenous inotropic and lusitropic agent: a randomized controlled trial in patients hospitalized with heart failure (HORIZON-HF) trial. Am Heart J. 2009;157(6):1035-41.
15. Malik FI, Hartman JJ, Elias KA, et al. Cardiac myosin activation: a potential therapeutic approach for systolic heart failure. Science. 2011;331(6023):1439-43.
16. Teerlink JR, Clarke CP, Saikali KG, et al. Dose-dependent augmentation of cardiac systolic function with the selective cardiac myosin activator, omecamtiv mecarbil: a first-in-man study. Lancet. 2011;378(9792):667-75.
17. Cleland JG, Teerlink JR, Senior R, et al. The effects of the cardiac myosin activator, omecamtiv mecarbil, on cardiac function in systolic heart failure: a double-blind, placebo-controlled, crossover, dose-ranging phase 2 trial. Lancet. 2011;378(9792):676-83.
18. Abraham WT, Adams KF, Fonarow GC, et al. In-hospital mortality in patients with acute decompensated heart failure requiring intravenous

vasoactive medications: an analysis from the Acute Decompensated Heart Failure National Registry (ADHERE). J Am Coll Cardiol. 2005; 46(1):57-64.
19. Fonarow GC, Adams KF, Abraham WT, et al. Risk stratification for in-hospital mortality in acutely decompensated heart failure: classification and regression tree analysis. JAMA. 2005;293(5):572-80.
20. Richard C, Ricome JL, Rimailho A, et al. Combined hemodynamic effects of dopamine and dobutamine in cardiogenic shock. Circulation. 1983;67(3):620-6.
21. Bergh CH, Andersson B, Dahlstrom U, et al. Intravenous levosimendan vs. dobutamine in acute decompensated heart failure patients on beta-blockers. Eur J Heart Fail. 2010;12(4):404-10.
22. Felker GM, Benza RL, Chandler AB, et al. Heart failure etiology and response to milrinone in decompensated heart failure: results from the OPTIME-CHF study. J Am Coll Cardiol. 2003;41(6):997-1003.
23. Rafouli-Stergiou P, Parissis JT, Anastasiou-Nana M. Inotropes for the management of acute heart failure patients with renal dysfunction. Still an option? Expert Opin Pharmacother. 2012;13(18):2637-47.
24. Nikolaou M, Parissis J, Yilmaz MB, et al. Liver function abnormalities, clinical profile, and outcome in acute decompensated heart failure. Eur Heart J. 2013;34(10):742-9.
25. Hunt SA, Abraham WT, Chin MH, et al. 2009 Focused update incorporated into the ACC/AHA 2005 Guidelines for the Diagnosis and Management of Heart Failure in Adults A Report of the American College of Cardiology Foundation/American Heart Association Task Force on Practice Guidelines Developed in Collaboration with the International Society for Heart and Lung Transplantation. J Am Coll Cardiol. 2009;53(15): e1-90.
26. Parissis JT, Farmakis D, Nieminen M. Classical inotropes and new cardiac enhancers. Heart Fail Rev. 2007;12(2):149-56.
27. Opie LH, Gersh BJ. Drugs for the heart, 7th edition. Philadelphia, PA: Saunders; 2009.
28. Parissis JT, Rafouli-Stergiou P, Stasinos V, et al. Inotropes in cardiac patients: update 2011. Curr Opin Crit Care. 2010;16(5):432-41.
29. Goldhaber JI, Hamilton MA. Role of inotropic agents in the treatment of heart failure. Circulation. 2010;121(14):1655-60.

Chapter 17

New Cardiovascular Disease Biomarkers in Hospital Medicine: Neutrophil Gelatinase-associated Lipocalin

Jeffrey Chan, Alan S Maisel

ABSTRACT

Neutrophil gelatinase-associated lipocalin (NGAL) has emerged as one of the most attractive and reliable biomarkers for the diagnosis and risk stratification of patients suffering from heart disease, especially with concomitant renal dysfunction. Recent research has demonstrated the potential of NGAL as a cardiac biomarker linking it to inflammatory response and atherosclerotic risk factors. More importantly, this increasingly strong correlation has led to further studies that have demonstrated its relationship to the presence, severity, and prognosis of multiple cardiovascular diseases. NGAL has repeatedly demonstrated clinical utility in three primary areas: (i) the prediction of the severity and outcome of acute decompensated heart failure (HF), (ii) the detection of kidney injury in HF, and (iii) prediction of the degree of atherosclerosis and inflammation in coronary artery disease. This chapter has been written to highlight to medical practitioners these potential scenarios and settings for which NGAL has been shown to be beneficial and why NGAL coexists among today's new biomarkers that demonstrate diagnostic and prognostic utility in risk-stratifying patients with heart disease in the hospital setting.

INTRODUCTION

In the continually expanding field of biomarker research, neutrophil gelatinase-associated lipocalin (NGAL) has emerged as one of the most attractive and reliable biomarkers for the diagnosis and risk stratification of patients suffering from heart disease, especially with concomitant renal dysfunction. Recent research has demonstrated the potential of NGAL as a cardiac biomarker linking it to inflammatory response and atherosclerotic risk factors. More importantly, this increasingly strong correlation has led to further studies that have demonstrated its relationship to the presence, severity, and prognosis of multiple cardiovascular diseases. For instance, NGAL levels have been shown to correspond to both the development and severity of coronary artery disease.[1] Additionally, among patients who have experienced an acute myocardial infarction (MI), NGAL levels have been shown to be increased and correlated with subsequent mortality and cardiovascular outcomes.[2-4] For these very reasons, this chapter has been written to highlight to medical practitioners the potential scenarios and settings for which NGAL has been shown to be beneficial and why NGAL coexists among today's new biomarkers that demonstrate diagnostic and prognostic utility in risk-stratifying patients with heart disease in the hospital setting.

PHYSIOLOGIC INTERPLAY

Structurally, NGAL is a 26 kD glycoprotein belonging to the lipocalin family of proteins.[5-7] It is a beta-barreled structure with hydrogen ligands through its core and is located in neutrophilic granules and released in response to acute injury and inflammation.[5,8,9] Once released into circulation, NGAL functions as an iron-binding siderophore and an immune modulator as it facilitates cellular apoptosis. Essentially, it is an iron-carrying lipocalin that initiates a mesenchymal to epithelial change resulting in the development of renal epithelial tubules and nephrons.[10,11] Yet, beyond its structure, the essence of NGAL's utility lies in its role in the pathogenesis of inflammation. Inflammation plays a critical role in the development and disruption of atheromatous plaques by inducing the release of inflammatory mediators that inhibit smooth muscle growth, half collagen production, and promote matrix degradation via matrix metalloproteinase-9 (MMP-9).[12,13] NGAL inhibits MMP-9 inactivation, prolonging its proteinase activity, leading to further plaque instability, propensity for thrombus formation, which altogether increase the likelihood of a MI (Fig. 1). Not surprisingly, elevated NGAL levels have been consistently observed in patient with acute post-MI heart failure for almost 64 days after the occurrence of the initial myocardial infarct. Along this same line of reasoning, serum NGAL levels undoubtedly correlate with the degree of clinical and cardiovascular neurohormonal deterioration as well as patient's post-MI undergo ventricular remodeling and subsequent left ventricular dysfunction that precipitates HF. In fact, high NGAL levels have demonstrated a high negative predictive value (97.2%) in patient with unstable angina and 98.6% in patients with acute coronary syndrome (ACS).[14]

ESTABLISHED AREAS OF CLINICAL APPLICATION AND UTILITY

In its current state, NGAL has repeatedly demonstrated clinical utility in three primary areas: (i) the prediction of the severity and outcome of acute decompensated HF, (ii) the detection of kidney injury in HF, and (iii) prediction of the degree of atherosclerosis and inflammation in coronary artery disease (Box 1). NGAL demonstrated its utility as a marker in predicting the severity and outcomes in patients presenting with acute decompensated HF via the result of the multicenter NGAL EvaLuation Along with B-type NaTriuretic Peptide in acutely decompensated heart failure (GALLANT) trial, which showed that NGAL levels in conjunction with B-type natriuretic peptide (BNP) levels at hospital discharge served as accurate markers for adverse outcomes in patients with acutely destabilized heart failure (ADHF).[15] Patients with a discharge diagnosis of acute decompensated HF with NGAL levels greater than 134 ng/mL have generally demonstrated more HF-related adverse outcomes in 30 days. For today's practitioner, utilizing NGAL in conjunction with the traditional BNP provides a potent tool in the diagnosis and prognosis of patients presents with acute decompensated HF while helping with their proper management as well. With regards to its second area of established clinical utility, NGAL has long been known by nephrologists as a marker of acute kidney injury (AKI). It has established utility in detecting kidney

Box 1: Established clinical applications

- Prediction of severity and outcomes in acutely destabilized heart failure
- Detection of kidney injury in heart failure
- Detection of atherosclerosis and inflammation in coronary artery disease

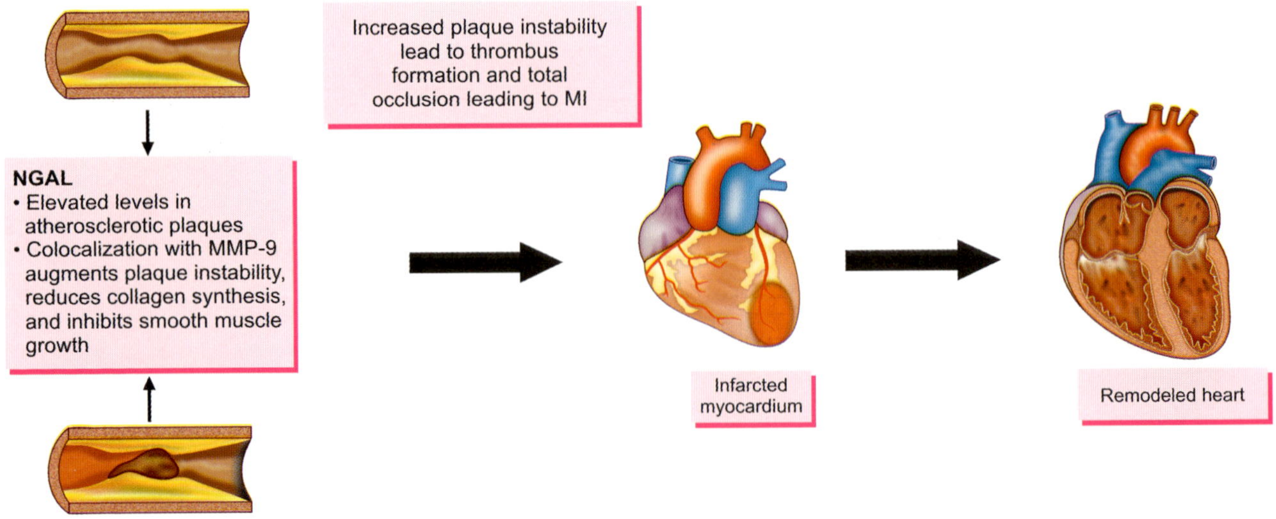

NGAL, neutrophil gelatinase-associated lipocalin; MMP-9, matrix metalloproteinase-9; MI, myocardial infarction

Fig. 1 Neutrophil gelatinase-associated lipocalin augments the inflammatory process by forming a stable dimeric complex with matrix degradation proteins and increasing its proteolytic activity leading to plaque disruption and progression to myocardial infarction injury in patient with HF. NGAL can be used to predict the development of cardiorenal syndrome type 1 within 48–72 hours with a sensitivity of 100% and specificity of 86.7% when using a cutoff value of 170 ng/mL.[16] In making diagnoses, it should be noted that NGAL can be obtained in both blood and urine, with urine NGAL levels equally shown to be just as reliable. In fact, urine NGAL levels have been shown to be just as reliable as serum NGAL as an early marker for diagnosing AKI in patients with ACS or HF undergoing coronary angiography, with a predictive power superior to the traditionally used markers of cystatin C and interleukin 18.[17] Lastly, NGAL's role in predicting the severity of inflammation and atherosclerosis has also been well established by virtue of its role as a marker of neutrophil activation, which play a key role in the inflammatory processes involved in cardiac remodeling as already explained in the introduction.

POTENTIAL AVENUES FOR FUTURE APPLICATION IN MEDICAL MANAGEMENT

By virtue of its role in neutrophil mobilization and thus its physiologic correlation with atherosclerosis and inflammation, NGAL remains an attractive candidate as a biomarker for a multitude of additional processes in cardiovascular disease and medical management that are still currently undergoing active investigation before routine implementation into clinical practice. Recent work has shed light on the potential for serum NGAL levels to predict short-term prognosis in patient with acute HF.[18] Thus far, studies have suggested that NGAL levels greater than 167.5 ng/mL may also hold utility in predicting morbidity and mortality within 3 months after admission for acute HF. Table 1 illustrates a general approach to how NGAL levels can be utilized in patient management in a clinical setting. For serum NGAL levels less than 100 ng/mL, routine HF management can be continued as there is unlikely to be any underlying renal injury. For levels between 100 ng/mL and 300 ng/mL, patients are at higher risk for impending AKI and thus nephrotoxic pharmaceuticals should be withheld, including angiotensin-converting enzyme (ACE) inhibitors, angiotensin-receptor blockers, contrast-requiring imaging, and nonsteroidal anti-inflammatory agents. More importantly, more precaution must be taken with the titration of diuretics for patients in this category. Patients with serum NGAL levels greater than 300 ng/mL should be taken most seriously as they are at risk for dialysis and even death; the patient should be admitted to the intensive care unit (ICU) for closer monitoring and consideration for ultrafiltration should be initiated.

TABLE 1: Management based on serum neutrophil gelatinase-associated lipocalin levels

NGAL level	Interpretation	Management
<100 ng/mL	No renal injury	Routine care
100–300 ng/mL	High risk for AKI	• Hold ACE/ARB • Hold aldosterone blocker • Avoid contrast • Avoid NSAIDs • Hold • Nephrotoxic agents • Conservative diuretics
>300 ng/mL	High-risk for AKI Dialysis and death	• ICU admission • Consideradation of ultrafiltration

NGAL, neutrophil gelatinase-associated lipocalin; AKI, acute kidney injury; ACE, angiotensin-converting enzyme; ARB, angiotensin receptor blocker; ICU, intensive care unit

Neutrophil gelatinase-associated lipocalin levels should be monitored in conjunction with BNP levels as optimal patient outcomes are achieved when a combination of NGAL levels less than 100 ng/mL and BNP levels less than 300 is achieved.[19] Titration of diuretics based on BNP levels will not be covered in this chapter. Utilizing both NGAL and BNP levels as an aid in achieving euvolemia helps in avoiding renal dysfunction while managing the patient's HF.

FUTURE DIRECTION

Outside the realm of cardiomyopathy, active scientific effort has also been directed on determining the potential of NGAL in differentiating early on high from low-risk patients presenting with ACS and HF to determine who would benefit from additional mechanical and pharmacological therapy during and after primary percutaneous coronary interventions (PCIs) and angiography. Ongoing metanalyses are actively investigating the potential of including NGAL as an additional component of a multimarker approach [other markers being N-terminal pro-brain natriuretic peptide (NT-proBNP), C-reactive protein (CRP), estimated glomerular filtration rate (eGFR), etc.] to allow for the calculation of a single multimarker risk score that could potentially allow for a fast and early assessment of baseline cardiovascular mortality/morbidity risk to optimize the use of adjunctive therapies prior to and after invasive cardiovascular intervention to further improve outcomes. Likewise, with regards to discharging patients, effort is also currently being directed on the potential applications NGAL holds with regards to assessing the adequacy and safety of discharging patient from the hospital after receiving treatment. More specifically, there exists much optimism in work currently evaluating the utility of obtaining NGAL levels on discharge to identify renal injury that has not yet manifested itself with elevated creatinine levels to allow for early detection of renal dysfunction, which would allow for more appropriate adjustment of discharge doses of potentially nephrotoxic cardiac medications.[15] From a broader perspective, NGAL levels at discharge could potentially serve the purpose of risk stratification of cardiac outcomes after discharge, which would allow for appropriate adjustments in follow-up frequency and outpatient diuretics.

APPLICABLE POPULATIONS

The populations that would benefit most from serum/urine NGAL measurement currently stands to include only those patient populations thus far studied in current literature. Adults with chronic HF, moderate-to-severe disease as rated by New York Heart Association (NYHA) class association, diuretic use, anemia, and generally of older ages currently appear to be the most ideal patients for whom NGAL measurements are indicated.

CONCLUSION

Neutrophil gelatinase-associated lipocalin has emerged as one of the most attractive and reliable biomarkers for the diagnosis and risk stratification of patients suffering from heart disease, especially with concomitant renal dysfunction. NGAL has demonstrated clinical utility in three primary areas: (i) the prediction of the severity and outcome of acute decompensated HF, (ii) the detection of kidney injury in HF, and (iii) prediction of the degree of atherosclerosis and inflammation in coronary artery disease. NGAL levels should be monitored in conjunction with BNP levels as optimal patient outcomes are achieved when a combination of NGAL levels less than 100 ng/mL and BNP levels less than 300 is achieved. Utilizing both NGAL and BNP levels as an aid in achieving euvolemia helps in avoiding renal dysfunction while managing the patient's HF. For these reasons, NGAL coexists among today's new biomarkers that demonstrate diagnostic and prognostic utility in risk stratifying patients with heart disease in the hospital setting.

REFERENCES

1. Zografos T, Haliassos A, Korovesis S, et al. Association of neutrophil gelatinase-associated lipocalin with the severity of coronary artery disease. Am J Cardiol. 2009;104:917-20.
2. Hemdahl AL, Gabrielsen A, Zhu C, et al. Expression of neutrophil gelatinase-associated lipocalin in atherosclerosis and myocardial infarction. Arterioscler Thromb Vasc Biol. 2006;26:136-42.
3. Lindberg S, Pedersen SH, Mogelvang R, et al. Prognostic utility of neutrophil gelatinase-associated lipocalin in predicting mortality and cardiovascular events in patients with ST-segment elevation myocardial infarction treated with primary percutaneous coronary intervention. J Am Coll Cardiol. 2012;60:339-45.
4. Sahinarslan A, Kocaman SA, Bas D, et al. Plasma neutrophil gelatinase-associated lipocalin levels in acute myocardial infarction and stable coronary artery disease. Coron Artery Dis. 2011;22:333-8.
5. Mishra J, Mori K, Ma Q. Amelioration of ischemic acute renal injury by neutrophil gelatinase-associated lipocalin. J Am Soc Nephrol. 2004;15:3073-82.
6. Mishra J, Ma Q, Prada A, et al. Identification of NGAL as a novel early urinary marker for ischemic renal injury. J Am Soc Nephrol. 2003;14:2534-43.
7. Kjeldsen L, Johnsen AH, Sengeløv H, et al. Isolation and primary structure of NGAL, a novel protein associated with human neutrophil gelatinase. J Biol Chem. 1993;268:10425-32.
8. Miethke M, Skerra A. Neutrophil gelatinase-associated lipocalin expresses antimicrobial activity by interfering with L-norepinephrine-mediated bacterial acquisition. Antimicrob Agents Chemother. 2010;54:1580-9.
9. Flower DR. The lipocalin protein family: structure and function. Biochem J 1996;318:1-14.
10. Mori K, Leet HT, Rapoport D, et al. Endocytic delivery of lipocalin-siderophore-iron complex rescues the kidney from ischemia-reperfusion injury. J Clin Invest. 2005;115:610-21.
11. Yang J, Goetz D, Li JY. An iron delivery pathway mediated by a lipocalin. Mol Cell. 2002;10:1045-56.
12. Hannson GK, Hellstrand M, Rymo L, et al. Interferon (IFN) gamma inhibits both proliferation and expression of differentiation-specific alpha-smooth muscle actin in arterial smooth muscle cells. J Exp Med. 1989;170:1595-608.
13. Yan L, Borregaard N, Kjeldsen L, et al. The high molecular weight urinary matrix metalloproteinase (MMP) activity is a complex of gelatinase B/MMP-9 activity by NGAL. J Biol Chem. 2001;276:37258-65.
14. Kafkas T, Matthew J, Yang J, et al. Sensitivity and specificity of a single emergency department measurement of urinary neutrophil gelatinase-associated lipocalin for diagnosing acute kidney injury. Ann Intern Med. 2008;148:810-9.
15. Maisel AS, Mueller C, Fitzgerald RL, et al. Prognostic utility of plasma neutrophil gelatinase-associated lipocalin in patients with acute heart failure: the NGAL evaluation along with B-type natriuretic peptide in acutely decompensated heart failure (GALLANT) trial. Eur J Heart Fail. 2011;13:846-51.
16. Alvelos M, Pimental R, Pinho E, et al. Neutrophil gelatinase-associated lipocalin in the diagnosis of type 1 cardio-renal syndrome in the general ward. Clin J Am Soc Nephrol. 2011;6:476-81.
17. Torregrosa I, Montoliu C, Urios A, et al. Early biomarkers of acute kidney failure after heart angiography or heart surgery in patients with acute coronary syndrome or acute heart failure. Nefrologia. 2012;32:44-52.
18. Alvelos M, Lourenco P, Dias C, et al. Prognostic value of neutrophil gelatinase-associated lipocalin in acute heart failure. Int J Cardiol. 2013;165:51-5.
19. Maisel AS, Mueller C, Fitzgerald R, et al. Prognostic utility of plasma neutrophil gelatinase-associated lipocalin in patients with acute heart failure: the NGAL Evaluation Along with B-type Natriuretic Peptide in acutely decompensated heart failure (GALLANT) Trial. Eur J Heart Fail. 2011;13:846-51.

Chapter 18

Practical Approach to Hyponatremia in Heart Failure

Hirsch S Mehta, Rajeev C Mohan, J Thomas Heywood

ABSTRACT

Hyponatremia is simultaneously common and overlooked in the heart failure (HF) population. Though frequently from abnormal fluid status, the mere presence of hyponatremia has prognostic implications in the treatment and future outcomes of HF patients. Identification and treatment of sodium disturbances do not have to be complicated. Here, we briefly examine the pathophysiology of hyponatremia focusing on vasopressin. Additionally, key trials from both the inpatient and outpatient settings are reviewed. Finally, a simplified approach to evaluation and treatment, complemented by tables featuring stepwise algorithms and common clinical scenarios are highlighted. These are culminated with case studies at the end of the chapter to help reinforce the topics covered.

INTRODUCTION

Hyponatremia is defined as a serum sodium below 136 mmol/L (1 mEq/L Na = 1 mmol/L).[1] It can be seen regardless of volume status but is most commonly dilutional, thus, associated with increased total body volume.

In dilutional hyponatremia, water is inappropriately reabsorbed resulting in a decreased sodium concentration even when total body sodium is elevated. This type of hyponatremia is encountered in patients with congestive heart failure (HF), cirrhosis, nephrotic syndrome, renal failure, and pregnancy. We have focused our discussion on hypotonic, hypoosmolar hyponatremia in the setting of HF.

Mechanoreceptors present in the left ventricle, carotid sinus, aortic arch, and afferent renal arterioles play an important role in the regulation of serum sodium. In patients with HF, the activation of these mechanoreceptors causes increased sympathetic tone and stimulation of the renin-angiotensin-aldosterone system (RAAS).[2,3] The increase in sympathetic tone persists despite increased total body fluid, facilitating sodium and water retention.

Clinical manifestations of hypotonic hyponatremia are mainly those of central nervous system (CNS) abnormalities. They are more profound when the serum sodium levels are lower or when levels fall acutely.

Patients with mild hyponatremia can be classified as having a serum sodium level between 131 mmol/L and 135 mmol/L. Moderate hyponatremia is seen between levels of 125 mmol/L and 130 mmol/L. Patients may be asymptomatic or present with headache, nausea, vomiting, muscle cramping, disorientation, lack of coordination, lethargy, restlessness and depressed reflexes.[1]

Severe hyponatremia is defined as a serum sodium level below 125 mmol/L. Surprisingly, some patients with severe hyponatremia remain relatively asymptomatic, particularly when the onset is slow. However, profound, rapidly developing hyponatremia can be life threatening. Clinical sequelae include seizure, coma, cerebral edema, intracranial hypertension, brainstem herniation, brain damage, respiratory arrest, and death.[1] Prompt recognition and frequent monitoring are crucial as early treatment portends a more favorable prognosis.

MECHANISM

Role of Vasopressin

Regulation of total body water is directed by the hypothalamus, which controls thirst, and the secretion of arginine vasopressin (AVP) from the posterior pituitary gland. AVPs primary functions include renal free water reabsorption, regulation of serum osmolality and blood volume, and increasing peripheral vascular resistance. Additionally, it also indirectly affects myocardial contractile function.[4]

Arginine vasopressin mediates its actions by three major receptors: (i) V1a receptors are found on vascular smooth muscle, platelets, and endometrium. Respectively, they are responsible for vasoconstriction and myocardial hypertrophy, platelet aggregation, and uterine contraction, (ii) V1b receptors are responsible for release of adrenocorticotropic hormone (ACTH) from the anterior pituitary, (iii) V2 receptors are found in the renal collecting duct where they are responsible for free water resorption via aquaporins and in vascular endothelium where they release both von Willebrand factor and factor VII.

Increased secretion of AVP can occur two ways. Pressure receptors in blood vessels, particularly baroreceptors in carotid arteries, release AVP in response to decreased mechanical stimulation causing reduced plasma volume. This is referred to as nonosmotic release of vasopressin. Secretion of AVP in response to increased plasma osmotic pressure is mediated by osmoreceptors in the hypothalamus and is referred to as osmotic release of AVP.[5]

Small changes in serum osmolality prompt changes in levels of serum AVP via a reflex arc aimed at maintaining salt and water homeostasis.[4] Under usual circumstances, AVP release is prompted by a change in plasma tonicity, depletion of plasma volume or reduction of blood pressure.[6] Changes in plasma volume and blood pressure prompt arterial receptors to trigger the release of AVP from the nonosmotic pathway. Among other factors, edematous states also tend to shift regulation toward nonosmotic regulation.[6] This pathway is a more potent form of AVP regulation.

The primary mechanism of hyponatremia in hospitalized adults is AVP release via the nonosmotic pathway. When AVP is released, diuresis is inhibited by interactions with aquaporins in the collecting duct. Aquaporins are proteins present in all cell membranes that regulate the flow of water into and out of cells. The collecting duct accounts for approximately 5% of the body's reabsorption of both sodium and water. However, it can adapt to resorb up to 25% of filtered water in times of dehydration. Specifically in the collecting duct, aquaporin V2 is crucial for water reabsorption in response to AVP.[7] During times where AVP is abundant, aquaporins allow for robust reabsorption of water, and diuresis is inhibited.

Vasopressin and Heart Failure

Correlation between elevated plasma values of vasopressin with HF and LV dysfunction have been shown in several studies.[8,9] Substudies of the SOLVD trial showed that even asymptomatic patients with LV dysfunction had higher levels of vasopressin compared to controls.[10]

Vasopressin also possesses hemodynamic effects in the management of HF. In HF patients, vasopressin is known to increase systemic vascular resistance and pulmonary capillary wedge pressure via interactions with V1a receptors. Through this same mechanism, stroke volume and cardiac output show a dose-dependent decrease in relation to levels of vasopressin.[11]

Vasopressin directly effects salt and water balance via interactions with aquaporins and V2 receptors in the collecting duct. This is done via increased expression of aquaporin-2 (AQP-2), which is inserted to cell membranes in the collecting duct. This facilitates free water absorption and an eventual decrease in serum sodium levels.[6]

Increased levels of vasopressin retard the excretion of free water (without solute) in HF patients.[6,12] It is on this premise that blocking the aquaporin V2 receptor leads to aquaresis. This has been proven to occur in a dose related fashion, where antagonism of the V2 receptor leads to increased solute-free water excretion, leading to a rise in serum sodium and osmolality in certain hypervolemic and euvolemic patients, including those with HF.[13]

Advanced HF patients are at risk for hyponatremia not only from mechanisms of water retention inherent to the disease process, but also by aggressive diuresis leading to intravascular volume depletion despite an elevated total body fluid status. Diuretics cause a mechanistic water retention pathway similar to the inherent HF disease process.

Thiazide diuretics are regarded as more potent than loop diuretics. Retrospective analysis have shown that greater than 90% of diuretic induced hyponatremia in a hospitalized population can be attributed to thiazide diuretics, with greater than 95% of these being within recommended dosages.[14]

PREVALENCE AND PROGNOSIS

Hyponatremia (without hyperglycemia) has been associated with a poorer prognosis in HF patients. This has been proven in both inpatient and outpatient settings and applies to those with preserved and depressed LV function.[15] Hyponatremia is both an independent predictor of increased rehospitalization rates as well as mortality. In cohort analysis following HF patients with hyponatremia up to 7 years post-index hospitalization, uncorrected hyponatremia remains the most significant factor for out of hospital mortality. This risk is reduced with correction of serum sodium levels.[16] Retrospective analysis of greater than 4,000 hospitalized HF patients shows a 50% increase in 30-day all-cause mortality for hyponatremic patients compared to those with normal serum sodium levels.[17] Out of hospital decreases in serum sodium levels in HF patients after hospital discharge is also found to be an independent predictor of readmission.[18]

Hyponatremia upon admission has been shown to be one of the five strongest predictors of 60-day mortality, as shown from a risk-stratification model from the outcomes of a prospective trial of intravenous milrinone for exacerbations of chronic heart failure (OPTIME-CHF).[19] This study also showed that the degree of hyponatremia correlated to length of stay, with patients in the lowest quartile of serum sodium having a twofold higher length of stay and increased 60-day mortality compared to those in higher quartiles. Additionally, the lowest quartile of patients with hyponatremia only had a 38% rate of normalizing serum sodium by discharge. These patients had an 18% 60-day mortality compared to 11% in those whose sodium normalized prior to leaving the hospital.[20] This finding was reiterated when examining patients in the ACTIV-CHF trial, where patients with depressed serum sodium had a threefold increase in 60-day mortality compared to HF patients with normal serum sodium levels. However, improvement in sodium levels of greater than or equal to 2 mEq/L during hospitalization was associated with only a 16% 60-day mortality compared to 30% for those with no improvement.[21]

Inpatient Trials

Recently, treatment with vasopressin antagonists has been extensively studied in various populations of HF patients with hyponatremia. The sentinel study with regards to vasopressin antagonist therapy in HF was the SALT trial.[22] In that study, fluid overloaded patients with hyponatremia, whether from HF or cirrhosis, were randomized to oral tolvaptan versus placebo, showing improvement in serum sodium concentrations in the tolvaptan arm at both 4 and 30 days after randomization.[22] The ACTIV in HF trial examined the effects of tolvaptan in a double-blinded fashion amongst hospitalized patients with HF and hyponatremia. Though body weight decreased and serum sodium improved, there was no appreciable change in blood urea nitrogen, serum creatinine, or serum potassium levels.[21] Subgroup analysis of the efficacy of vasopressin antagonism in heart failure outcome study with tolvaptan (EVEREST) trial, which examined a single dose of tolvaptan, showed favorable results in various measures of HF such as dyspnea, edema and weight. However, no changes in morbidity related to HF or all-cause mortality was seen with treatment of hyponatremia with tolvaptan.[23]

Outpatient Trials

The treatment of hyponatremia in stable HF patients has also been well studied. Due to the reduced acuity of outpatients, the majority of these trials too look at therapy with oral vasopressin antagonists. Earlier studies with conivaptan in Class III HF patients treated in a double blinded placebo controlled fashion saw no change in overall functional capacity, exercise tolerance or quality of life with drug treatment.[24]

More recent trials with tolvaptan have focused on less ill patients, including class II and III patients. Udelson et al. showed single dose therapy of tolvaptan compared with placebo showed decrease in body weight, increased volume of diuresis, and marked improvement in serum sodium levels without effects on potassium.[25] Tolvaptan has also shown in smaller trials to mechanistically induce a diuresis similar to furosemide, while unlike loop diuretics, having no decrease in renal blood flow with therapy.[26] In addition, the physiologic benefits are also seen at the level of the kidneys. The measuring effects on intima-media thickness: an evaluation of rosuvastatin (METEOR) trial examined the effects of tolvaptan on LV function and remodeling. After 54 weeks of therapy, tolvaptan proved to have no beneficial or adverse effect on LV remodeling, without significant change in LV end-diastolic volume index compared to controls.[27]

EVALUATION AND TREATMENT

The presence of hyponatremia in HF is a poor prognostic marker. It is associated with increased morbidity and mortality. Treatment of hyponatremia begins with optimizing therapy for congestive HF. Because of its association with disease progression and increased mortality, recognition and treatment of hyponatremia is an important component in the overall management of HF patients (Boxes 1 and 2).

Although hyponatremia is common amongst HF patients, it is important to rule out non-heart failure causes of low serum sodium. Endocrine disorders, such as syndrome of inappropriate antidiuretic hormone (SIADH), adrenal insufficiency, and hypothyroidism can all-cause hyponatremia. Women of childbearing age should be evaluated for pregnancy and a complete history, including diet, fluid intake, and illicit substances should be questioned, as all can contribute to low serum sodium levels.

Even without symptoms, significant hyponatremia in HF warrants treatment. In the outpatient setting, this begins by optimizing volume status. Hyponatremia with volume depletion simply requires holding diuretics and saline resuscitation. This scenario is less common.

More commonly, hyponatremia is dilutional and seen with hypervolemia. In this scenario, diuretics need to be increased and fluid status optimized. Increased oral consumption of fluids is a common cause of depressed sodium. Fluid restriction between 1,200 to 1,500 mL/day should be implemented in HF patients with hyponatremia.[2] In addition to correcting volume status, it is important to examine complete serum chemistries and correct all metabolic disorders. Hyponatremia can also be caused by hyperglycemia. In this scenario, normalizing blood glucose improves serum sodium levels. Hypokalemia and hypomagnesemia can also be seen in conjunction with low serum sodium, and repleting these electrolytes are necessary in the management of hyponatremia.

Every patient evaluation for hyponatremia should include careful medicine reconciliation. It is important to remove any medications contributing to hyponatremia (Box 3). Thiazide diuretics commonly worsen hyponatremia. Replacing thiazide diuretics with loop diuretics can improve hyponatremia.

Box 1: Approach to evaluating hyponatremia

- Thorough clinical history
  - Fluid intake
  - Dietary solute intake
  - Symptoms of hyponatremia
  - Screening for non-HF causes of hyponatremia
    - Cirrhosis
    - SIADH
    - Hypothyroidism
    - Adrenal insufficiency
    - Pregnancy
    - Reconcile all medications and supplements
- Establish volume status
  - Clinical examination
  - Noninvasive evaluation (echocardiography)
- Identify other electrolyte disorders:
  - Hypokalemia
  - Hypomagnesemia
  - Hyperglycemia

Box 2: Stepwise approach to treatment of hyponatremia in heart failure

Outpatient therapy

- Titrate diuretics/establish euvolemia
- Fluid restriction
- Correct all other electrolyte/metabolic disorders
- Discontinue any medications contributing to low serum sodium, e.g., Thiazide diuretics
- Optimize heart failure medications
  - Beta blockers
  - ACE inhibitors/ARB
  - Aldosterone antagonists
- Cardiac resynchronization therapy/optimization in appropriate candidates
- Consider advanced therapy
  - LVAD

Inpatient management

- Initiate vasopressin antagonists with close monitoring of serum sodium
  - Tolvaptan
  - Conivaptan
- Inotropic therapy (temporary) in certain patients
- Consider hypertonic saline infusion in patients who are refractory to treatment or who are severely symptomatic (i.e., seizure, mental status changes)
- Evaluate for definitive therapy
  - Ventricular assist device as bridge to decision or destination therapy
  - Cardiac transplantation
  - Hospice

Box 3: Medications that can exacerbate hyponatremia

- Diuretics
  - Loop diureitcs
    - Furosemide
    - Bumetanide
    - Torsemide
    - Ethacrinic acid
  - Thiazide diuretics
    - Hydrochlorothiazide
    - Chlorthalidone
    - Metolazone
- Antidepressants
  - Selective serotonin-reuptake inhibitors
  - Tricyclic antidepressants
    - Amitriptaline
    - Desipramine
  - Monoamine oxidase inhibitors
  - Buproprion
  - Duloxetine
- Antipsychotic drugs
  - Carbamazepine
  - Oxcarbazepine
  - Sodium valproate
  - Lamotrigine
- Antineoplastic agents
  - Vinca alkaloids
    - Vincristine
    - Vinblastine
  - Platinum compounds
    - Cisplatin
    - Carboplatin
  - Alkylating agents
    - Cyclophosphamide
    - Melphalan
    - Ifosamide
  - Other
    - Methotrexate
    - Interferon alpha, gamma
    - Levamisole
    - Pentostatin
    - Monoclonal antibodies
- Painkillers
  - Opiates
  - Nonsteroidal anti-inflammatory drugs
  - Acetaminophen
- ADH analogues
  - DDAVP
  - Oxytosin
- Antihypertensives
  - ACE inhibitors
  - Amlodipine
- Antibiotics
  - Trimethoprim-sulfamethoxazole
  - Ciprofloxacin
  - Sulbactam
  - Rifabutin
- Antiarrhythmic drugs
  - Amiodarone
  - Propafenone
- Miscellaneous
  - 3,4, Methylenedioxymethamphetamine (ecstacy)
  - Intravenous immune globulin
  - Theophyline
  - Proton-pump inhibitors
  - Bromocriptine

Severe hyponatremia is a marker for poor prognosis. Optimization of HF medications should be done. Maximizing beta blockers, ACE inhibitors, ARBs and aldosterone antagonists (given normal potassium and createnine levels) should be considered in patients who present with low serum sodium. ACE inhibitors have been shown to directly increase serum sodium levels. In addition to medications, advanced HF therapies should be considered in patients who have hyponatremia as a result of HF. Those with QRS duration of greater than 120 ms and a left bundle branch morphology on electrocardiography should be offered cardiac resynchronization therapy.

Patients with symptomatic or acute, severe hyponatremia require hospitalization. Correcting hyponatremia requires close monitoring of serum sodium, as levels should not increase by greater than 0.5 mmol/L/hour (<12 mEq/hour) to minimize the risk of osmotic demyelination.[28] Inpatient treatment of hypontremia involves many of the same principles as outpatient management. However, despite diuretics and titration of medicines, hyponatremia may still persist. In such patients, more aggressive therapies, such as hypertonic saline infusion or vasopressin antagonists should be considered. In an HF population, hypertonic saline infusion becomes problematic due to the increased volume and solute administered. Because of this, vasopressin antagonists, such as vaptan drugs, are a more reasonable treatment approach.

Two major vaptan drugs approved for clinical use are conivaptan, which is selective for V1a and V2 receptors, and tolvaptan, which has its effect only on V2 receptors found in the renal collecting duct. While conivaptan can be taken both orally and intravenously, the more selective tolvaptan is only available in an oral form.[29]

Both conivaptan and tolvaptan produce increased urine output and improve serum sodium levels. In HF patients, most trials show improvement in subjective and objective signs of congestion. Still, no independent benefit with regards to mortality or rehospitalization has been seen as a result of vaptan therapy amongst HF patients.[29]

Vaptan therapy in HF patients should be used in cases of symptomatic hyponatremia with concentrations less than 130 mmol/L or in those patients with concentrations less than 125 mmol/L regardless of signs or symptoms of hyponatremia. It should only be considered after conservative measures, such as fluid restriction and intravenous loop diuretics have been maximized and are refractory. Because of its selective nature to V2 and robust oral bioavailability, tolvaptan is preferred as a first line agent over conivaptan.

The starting dose for tolvaptan is 15 mg daily. Once therapy is initiated, patients should not be fluid restricted and oral hydration limits should be liberalized due to a potent aquaresis that occurs with tolvaptan.[30] The dose can be doubled daily until a desired response is achieved. The maximum suggested dose for tolvaptan is 60 mg daily. Once tolvaptan therapy has started, serum sodium should initially be checked every 6–8 hours for the first day, and can be checked once or twice daily after sodium levels and drug dosages have stabilized.

Some patients may require chronic vaptan therapy to control hyponatremia as an outpatient. This cohort includes stage IV patients whose HF is advanced and the presence of persistent electrolyte abnormalities should be considered a marker for end stage disease. In addition to evaluating such patients for advanced stage D therapies, such as ventricular assist device or transplantation, chronic vaptan therapy may be required as an outpatient to keep serum sodium levels normalized. This should only be done after therapy is initiated and a safe dose is identified during hospitalization. Patients should have twice weekly metabolic panel evaluations while on tolvaptan and frequent clinic visits to ensure fluid status and medications are optimized. Often the medication can be stopped as HF treatment is optimized.

CASE STUDIES

Case 1: Symptomatic Hypervolemic Hyponatremia

Mrs S is a 77-year-old female with severe aortic stenosis with prior bioprosthetic valve replacement and coronary artery bypass grafting 8 years ago. She has an ischemic cardiomyopathy, ejection fraction of 29%, permanent atrial fibrillation, type II diabetes mellitus and was admitted to the hospital for angina, presyncope, and fatigue.

Upon admission she had a serum sodium level of 122 mmol/L, potassium of 5.1 mmol/L, blood urea nitrogen of 41 mg/dL, and creatinine of 1.2 mg/dL. She was treated with 40 mg of IV furosemide after which a 2L diuresis was achieved. Despite this, serum sodium remained 125 mmol/L. Tolvaptan 30 mg was administered after fluid restriction was removed, and continuous infusion of furosemide at 5 mg/hour was started. Within 12 hours, the patient had an additional 2.5 L diuresis with rise in serum sodium to 129 mmol/L. The patient was continued on 30 mg daily tolvaptan and IV furosemide infusion for 48 hours.

Overall, a 6 kg diuresis was achieved with tolvaptan and furosemide combination therapy over 72 hours. Tolvaptan was discontinued and the patient was then transitioned to oral furosemide. Upon discharge, the patient was euvolemic with serum sodium of 138 mmol/L.

Case 2: Hyponatremia in Stage D Heart Failure

Mr B is a 67-year-old male with nonischemic cardiomyopathy, ejection fraction of 26%, type II diabetes and atrial fibrillation. He has a history of recurrent HF admissions for fluid overload and hyponatremia. Two weeks post-hospital discharge he presented to clinic with fatigue and weakness. Due to gradual hypotension, beta blocker, ACE inhibitor and loop diuretic were all recently reduced. On examination, he was hypervolemic and admitted for diuresis.

On admission his serum sodium was 120 mmol/L. His potassium was 4.3 mmol/L, blood urea nitrogen was 101 mg/dL, and creatinine was 2.5 mg/dL. Given his new renal dysfunction, presumed to be type 1 cardiorenal syndrome, he was started on dobutamine, after which his renal function improved. However, his serum sodium remained between 121 mmol/L and 126 mmol/L.

A right heart catheterization revealed pulmonary capillary wedge pressure of 26 mmHg and a cardiac index of 1.32 L/min/m^2. Given his volume overload as well as poor systolic function he was started on a furosemide infusion and milrinone in addition to dobutamine.

After 36 hours, his sodium increased to 128 mmol/L. His volume status and blood pressure improved, allowing for the reinitiation of beta blocker and aldosterone antagonist.

With persistent hyponatremia despite correction of volume status and HF optimization, he was started on tolvaptan. Initially a 15 mg dose was given. Serum sodium was monitored every 8 hours. After 24 hours, no change in serum sodium was appreciated, and tolvaptan dose was increased to 30 mg. With this sodium improved from 126 to 133 mmol/L over the course of 24 hours.

Despite clinical improvement, normalization of electrolytes and improved volume status, the patient remained dependent on dobutamine and milrinone infusions. He later received a left ventricular assist device, after which he was discharged from the hospital within 14 days with normal volume status and electrolyte levels.

CONCLUSION

Hyponatremia in HF patients is a negative prognostic marker associated with a high mortality and rehospitalization rate. Prompt recognition can have significant effects toward improving outcomes in this population, as shown by various large studies. Mechanistically, high levels of vasopressin are responsible for inappropriate natriuresis despite fluid overload, resulting in low serum sodium levels. Treatment centers on reversing this cycle with fluid restriction, diuresis, and AVP suppression with vaptan therapy. Though most patients can have hyponatremia corrected during a hospital stay, stage D patients may require chronic treatment for low serum sodium while awaiting advanced therapies. However, a keen clinical eye, prompt recognition, evaluation, and treatment can have large prognostic implications in treating not only electrolyte disturbances, but overall HF as well.

REFERENCES

1. Adrogue HJ, Madias NE. Hyponatremia. N Engl J Med. 2000;342:1581-9.
2. De Luca L, Klein L, Udelson JE, et al. Hyponatremia in patients with heart failure. Am J Cardiol. 2005;96(12A):19-23.
3. Schrier RW, Abraham WT. Hormones and hemodynamics in heart failure. N Engl J Med. 1999;341:577-85.
4. Wong LL, Verbalis JG. Systemic diseases associated with diseases of water homeostasis. Endocrinol Metab Clin North Am. 2002;31:121-40.
5. Schrier RW, Berl T. Nonosmolar factors affecting renal water excretion (two parts). N Engl J Med. 1975;292:81-8 and 141-5.
6. Finley JJ IV, Konstam MA, Udelson JE. Arginine vasopressin antagonists for the treatment of heart failure and hyponatremia. Circulation. 2008;118:410-21.
7. Agre P. The aquaporin water channels. Proc Am Thorac Soc. 2006;3(1):5-13.
8. Szatalowicz VL, Arnold PE, Chaimovitz C, et al. Radioimmunoassay of plasma arginine vasopressin in hyponatremic patients with congestive heart failure. N Engl J Med. 1981;305:263-6.
9. Goldsmith SR, Francis GS, Cowley AW, et al. Increased plasma arginine vasopressin levels in patients with congestive heart failure. J Am Coll Cardiol. 1983;1:1385-90.
10. Francis GS, Benedict C, Johnstone DE, et al. Comparison of neuroendocrine activation in patients with left ventricular dysfunction with and without congestive heart failure: a substudy of the studies of left ventricular dysfunction (SOLVD). Circulation. 1990;82:1724-9.
11. Goldsmith SR, Francis GS, Cowley AW, et al. Hemodynamic effects of infused arginine vasopressin in congestive heart failure. J Am Coll Cardiol. 1986;8:779-83.
12. Kalra PR, Anker SD, Coats AJ. Water and sodium regulation in chronic heart failure: the role of natriuretic peptides and vasopressin. Cardiovasc Res. 2001;51:495-509.
13. Udelson JE, Smith WB, Hendrix GH, et al. Acute hemodynamic effects of conivaptan, a dual V1A and V2 vasopressin receptor antagonist in patients with advanced heart failure. Circulation. 2001;104:2417-23.
14. Sonnenblick M, Friedlander Y, Rosin AJ. Diuretic-induced severe hyponatremia review and analysis of 129 reported patients. Chest. 1993;103:601-6.
15. Rusinaru D, Tribouilloy C, Berry C, et al. Relationship of serum sodium concentration to mortality in a wide spectrum of heart failure patients with preserved and with reduced ejection fraction: an individual patient data meta-analysis: Meta-Analysis Global Group in Chronic heart failure (MAGGIC). Eur J Heart Fail. 2012;14(10):1139-46.
16. Tribouilloy C, Buiciuc O, Leborgne L, et al. Relation of serum sodium level to long-term outcome after a first episode of heart failure: a prospective 7-year study. Int J Cardiol. 2010;140:309-14.
17. Lee DS, Austin PC, Rouleau JL, et al. Predicting mortality among patients hospitalized for heart failure: derivation and validation of a clinical model. JAMA. 2003;290(19):2581-7.
18. Rich MW, Beckham V, Wittenberg C, et al. A Multidisciplinary intervention to prevent the readmission of elderly patients with congestive heart failure. N Engl J Med. 1995;333:1190-5.
19. Felker GM, Leimberger JD, Califf RM, et al. Risk stratification after hospitalization for decompensated heart failure. J Card Fail. 2004;10:460-6.
20. Klein L, O'Connor CM, Leimberger JD, et al. Lower serum sodium is associated with increased short-term mortality in hospitalized patients with worsening heart failure: results from the OPTIME-CHF study. Circulation. 2005;111:2454-60.
21. Gheorghiade M, Gattis WA, O'Connor CM, et al. Effects of tolvaptan, a vasopressin antagonist, in patients hospitalized with worsening heart failure: a randomized control trial. JAMA. 2004;291:1963-71.
22. Schrier RW, Gross P, Gheorghiade M, et al. Tolvaptan, a selective oral vasopressin V2-receptor antagonist, for hyponatremia. N Engl J Med. 2006;355(20):2099-112.
23. Konstam MA, Gheorghiade M, Burnett JC, et al. Effects of oral tolvaptan in patients hospitalized for worsening heart failure: the EVEREST Outcome Trial. JAMA. 2007;297(12):1319-31.
24. Russell SD, Adams KF, Shaw JP, et al. Results of a twelve week double-blind, placebo-controlled, multicenter study of oral conivaptan to assess functional capacity in patients with class III chronic heart failure. J Card Fail. 2003;9:S60.

25. Udelson JE, Orlandi C, O'Brien T, et al. Vasopressin receptor blockade in patients with congestive heart failure: results from a placebo controlled, randomized study comparing the effects of tolvaptan, furosemide, and their combination. J Am Coll Cardiol. 2002;39:156A.
26. Costello-Boerrigter LC, Smith WB, Boerrigter G, et al. Vasopressin-2-receptor antagonism augments water excretion without changes in renal hemodynamics or sodium and potassium excretion in human heart failure. Am J Physiol Renal Physiol. 2006;290:F273-8.
27. Udelson JE, McGrew FA, Flores E, et al. Multicenter, randomized, double-blind, placebo-controlled study of the effect of oral tolvaptan on left ventricular dilation and function in patients with heart failure and systolic dysfunction. J Am Coll Cardiol. 2007;49:2151-9.
28. Sterns RH, Cappuccio JD, Silver SM, et al. Neurologic sequelae after treatment of severe hyponatremia: a multicenter perspective. J Am Soc Nephrol. 1994;4(8):1522-30.
29. Robertson GL. Vaptans for the treatment of hyponatremia. Nat Rev Endocrin. 2011;7:151-61.
30. Jao JT, Chiong JR. Hyponatremia in acute decompensated heart failure: mechanisms, prognosis and treatment options. Clin Cardiol. 2010;33(11): 666-71.

Chapter 19

Heart Failure and Acute Coronary Syndrome

Jeffrey Chan, Kevin S Shah, Alan S Maisel

ABSTRACT

The most common cause of chronic heart failure (CHF) is coronary artery disease (CAD). Acute coronary syndrome (ACS) itself is noted to be a significant cause of acute decompensated heart failure (HF) as well, with CAD, hypertension and atrial fibrillation continually identified as the most common underlying etiologies of new acute decompensated HF. The fact that patients with HF and CAD hold a considerably worse prognosis than those with only HF highlights the importance of recognizing the dual interplay of CAD and HF. Prognosis of patients with HF and CAD is considerably worse than that of patients without coronary disease and is related to the angiographic severity of coronary disease. Patients with a history of HF should thus always be closely screened for ACS risk factors. The evaluation for ACS will involve history and assessment of risk factors, physical examination, laboratory work and risk stratification via imaging. Systematic evaluation for CAD is an essential part of the evaluation of patients with newly diagnosed or CHF.

INTRODUCTION

The most common cause of chronic heart failure (CHF) is coronary artery disease (CAD).[1] In fact, in over 13 HF treatment trials reported in the New England Journal of Medicine over the last decade, CAD has been identified as the underlying etiology of HF in nearly 70% of patients included in these studies.[2-14] The actual prevalence of CAD in patients with HF is most likely even greater as the presence of CAD is not always explored in a systematic manner in many clinical studies. Data from large databases including the Acute Decompensated Heart Failure National Registry (ADHERE) of 267 American hospitals totaling 105,388 patients hospitalized with acute decompensated HF have demonstrated that 57% of these patients had CAD, 31% with prior myocardial infarctions (MIs), 17% with prior strokes and 18% with peripheral vascular disease.[15] Similarly, data derived from the Assessment of Treatment with Lisinopril and Survival (ATLAS) trial which looked into the circumstances of death in patients with CHF, investigators identified preexisting ischemic heart disease as a significant marker of increased risk of all-cause mortality and cardiovascular death in patients with CHF.[16] Additionally, moving beyond patients with CHF, ACS itself is noted to be a significant cause of acute decompensated HF as well, with CAD, hypertension and atrial fibrillation continually identified as the most common underlying etiologies of new acute decompensated HF.[17] Ultimately, the fact that patients with HF and CAD hold a considerably worse prognosis than those with only HF highlights the importance of recognizing the dual interplay of CAD and HF. Prognosis of patients with HF and CAD is considerably worse than that of patients without coronary disease and is related to the angiographic severity of coronary disease.[18] That being said, a systematic evaluation for CAD is an essential part of the evaluation of patients with newly diagnosed or CHF.

PATHOPHYSIOLOGY

The various mechanisms by which CAD contributes to HF are both complex and multifactorial. Underlying CAD increases one's likelihood of an ensuing MI. The associated loss of myocytes from these cardiac events, development of fibrosis and compensatory left ventricular (LV) remodeling via neurohormonal activation, all contribute to the development of HF via further deterioration of any remaining viable myocardium.[19] Cardiac ischemia itself also directly plays a role in the pathophysiological link between CAD and HF by inducing the release of endothelin, a powerful stimulator of myocyte hypertrophy and myocardial fibrosis. Alternatively, CAD additionally contributes to HF via well-established pathways involving myocardial stunning and myocardial hibernation. Episodes of transient but severe ischemia often cause prolonged systolic dysfunction that persist after the ischemic insult itself has resolved, worsening LV dysfunction. Likewise, reduced myocardial blood flow often leads to sustained cellular viability of cardiac tissue but insufficient contractility as a compensatory response of the myocardium to reduce its oxygen demands in the setting of reduced oxygen supply.[17] Though a protective mechanism, this decrease in contractility; however, ultimately worsens overall LV dysfunction.

CLINICAL APPROACH TO ACUTE CORONARY SYNDROME IN HEART FAILURE

History and Physical

The evaluation for CAD in patients with HF follows the same approach for general screening in patient's initially presenting with symptoms concerning for ACS, beginning with a thorough history and a detailed physical examination. Essential features of the history include an accurate inquiry into prior histories or current presentations of chest discomfort, including the severity, frequency, location, radiation, quality, alleviating and aggravating factors and duration of any of these symptoms. The history and physical examination findings should be assessed in the context of the overall clinical status of the patient. Typical angina is described as pain that is substernal, occurs on exertion, and is relieved with rest. In patients with a reported history of CAD, an accurate characterization of the quality and frequency of any prior chest pain episodes is essential in determining whether a change in the angina pattern has occurred [i.e., a patient with chronic stable angina now has unstable angina (UA)] or if a noncardiac origin of pain is now present (i.e., a patient with chronic stable angina now with simply musculoskeletal pain).

In all patients with HF, cardiovascular risk factors should always be reviewed. Patients with a known diagnosis of CHF will likely have medical history that puts them at increased risk for CAD. Risk factors include a history of hypertension, hyperlipidemia, obesity, diabetes mellitus, cigarette smoking and a family history of CAD (i.e., a first degree male relative with a myocardial infarction or sudden death occurring before 55 years of age or a first-degree female relative with these events occurring before 65 years of age). Additional factors that should be assessed, though uncommon, due to their contribution to ischemic cardiomyopathy include prior radiation therapy, drug use (cocaine and amphetamines), and the presence of systemic diseases associated with coronary arteritis (lupus erythematosus, polyarteritis nodosum or rheumatoid arthritis). The physical examination in patients with ACS frequently is normal. Especially concerning physical findings include a new murmur concerning for mitral regurgitation, hypotension, pulmonary rales, a new third heart sound (S3 gallop) and jugular venous distention. Chest wall tenderness reduces the likelihood of ACS. Patients with decompensated HF likely have preexisting examination findings, including pulmonary rales, jugular venous distension, and S3 gallop.

Biomarkers

Laboratory testing, specifically for biomarkers, is critical and challenging in HF patients presenting with ACS. We will specifically focus on cardiac biomarkers, troponin and the natriuretic peptides (NPs). Theoretically, the NPs are markers of HF status while troponin is a marker of cardiac myocyte injury. However, the comorbidity of CHF confounds interpretation of the laboratory data in the setting of ACS. Troponins (T, I, and C) are found in cardiac and skeletal muscle. Subtypes T and I are specific for cardiac muscle and are known as cardiac troponins. Historically, in the setting of ACS, a "positive" troponin test has been based on the 99th percentile rule. However, this cutoff does not imply that 1% of the normal population has active myocardial necrosis; this cutoff relies on, once again, a high pretest probability of ACS.[20] Interpretation of troponin results is dependent on the assay used at the institution, as assays are being developed with higher and higher levels of sensitivity. While improving clinical sensitivity for the diagnosis of MI, the increased analytic sensitivity has come at the cost of reduced specificity. This reduced specificity can confound interpretation of the assay. The interpretation of troponin levels in the setting of CHF becomes even more confounded as many patients have troponin levels elevated at baseline.

These markers represent ongoing injury from multiple processes. Theories for the origin of troponin in CHF include myocardial strain, apoptosis from failing hearts and troponin degradation products from proteolysis. The significance of elevated troponin includes an association with decreased LV ejection fraction and poor prognosis in HF. The short-term risk of adverse clinical outcomes in patients with ACS complicated by HF is directly proportional to the level of troponin elevation. Knowing a patient's "baseline" troponin level is crucial and the trends in the setting of possible ACS are more important as the leakage of enzymes may be from coronary plaque rupture causing myocardial necrosis, versus ongoing leakage from a failing heart. Routine assessment of troponin concentrations in CHF patients is not warranted, but in patients with the possibility of an acute coronary syndrome, it is critical.[21-23]

The natriuretic peptides [B-type natriuretic peptide (BNP) and pro-B-type natriuretic peptide (NT-proBNP)], have played a pivotal role in the diagnosis and prognosis of patients with CHF. Their functions are physiological in response to ventricular wall stretch, dilatation and pressure. They serve to counterregulate the renin–angiotensin–aldosterone system via natriuresis, diuresis and vasodilation. Multiple studies have demonstrated their ability to help diagnose HF in patients presenting with acute dyspnea. Furthermore, NPs have been shown to correlate with HF stage and accurately prognosticate the same patients. Their role in ACS are not as well elucidated, as they are in patients with HF. BNP concentration rises rapidly over the first 24 hours after MI and then tends to stabilize; patients with a large infarct may have a second peak approximately 5 days later. When measured 1–7 days after MI; elevation of BNP identifies patients at risk for LV dysfunction, HF and death. Here, as in CHF, the prognostic value of BNP seems to be greater than (but complementary to) that of left ventricular ejection fraction (LVEF). However, at this time, there is no recommendation for routine BNP testing in patients with ACS.[24,25]

Screening

As depicted in Flowchart 1, the process of screening for CAD/ACS in patients with HF begins with an assessment of the patient's likelihood of CAD. This assessment is based on the patient's history and cardiovascular risk factors as mentioned earlier in this section. Patients at low risk for CAD based on initial assessment do not require further workup. However, patients deemed as moderate risk for having underlying CAD, should be further evaluated with a baseline electrocardiogram (ECG). The approach to picking a stress test for evaluation of CAD involves a linear line of questioning, including why am I ordering this test (typically to rule out CAD), can the patient exercise, is the resting ECG normal, does body habitus pose problems to imaging and cost-effectiveness of the testing. Generally speaking, in patients with newly diagnosed HF a search for ischemic heart disease as the cause with stress testing is appropriate, presuming angiography has not been performed. Those with normal ECGs and with the capacity to safely engage in physical activity should undergo further evaluation with a stress ECG, with positively testing patients subsequently referred for a computed tomographic coronary angiogram. It should be noted that the predictive value of the ECG depends on the baseline risk (pretest probability) for CAD in a given patients and patients with HF tend to be higher risk. Patients demonstrating an abnormal ECG (i.e., signs of current ischemia, prior ischemia, new axis deviation, hypertrophy, rhythm blocks) and with a capacity to safely engage in exercise should be further evaluated with an exercise imaging stress test; patients with equivocal results and an unclear diagnosis of CAD should undergo a computed tomographic coronary angiogram as well. It should also be noted that severe HF is an absolute contraindication to exercise stress testing. Moderate risk patients demonstrating an abnormal ECG and unable to safely engage in exercise should be further evaluated for CAD with a pharmacologic stress test; if unable to tolerate such a test, these patients should directly undergo a computed tomographic coronary angiogram. HF patients deemed to be at high risk for underlying CAD should be immediately optimized with empiric therapy for their suspected CAD (therapy described later in this chapter) while being prepped for a computer tomographic coronary angiogram. In both medium risk and high risk patients undergoing a coronary angiogram, patients should subsequently be further stratified based upon their coronary angiogram results. Patients with normal coronary arteries as evidence on their angiogram require only outpatient management of their CAD risk factors. On the other hand, patients with demonstrated atherosclerosis on angiogram, but less than 50% stenosis, require actual pharmaceutical medical therapy for treatment of their underlying CAD. Patients with demonstrated atherosclerosis on angiogram, with more than 50% stenosis, should be subcategorized into two further patient groups: those with evidence of significant ischemia and those with evidence of only mild or trace

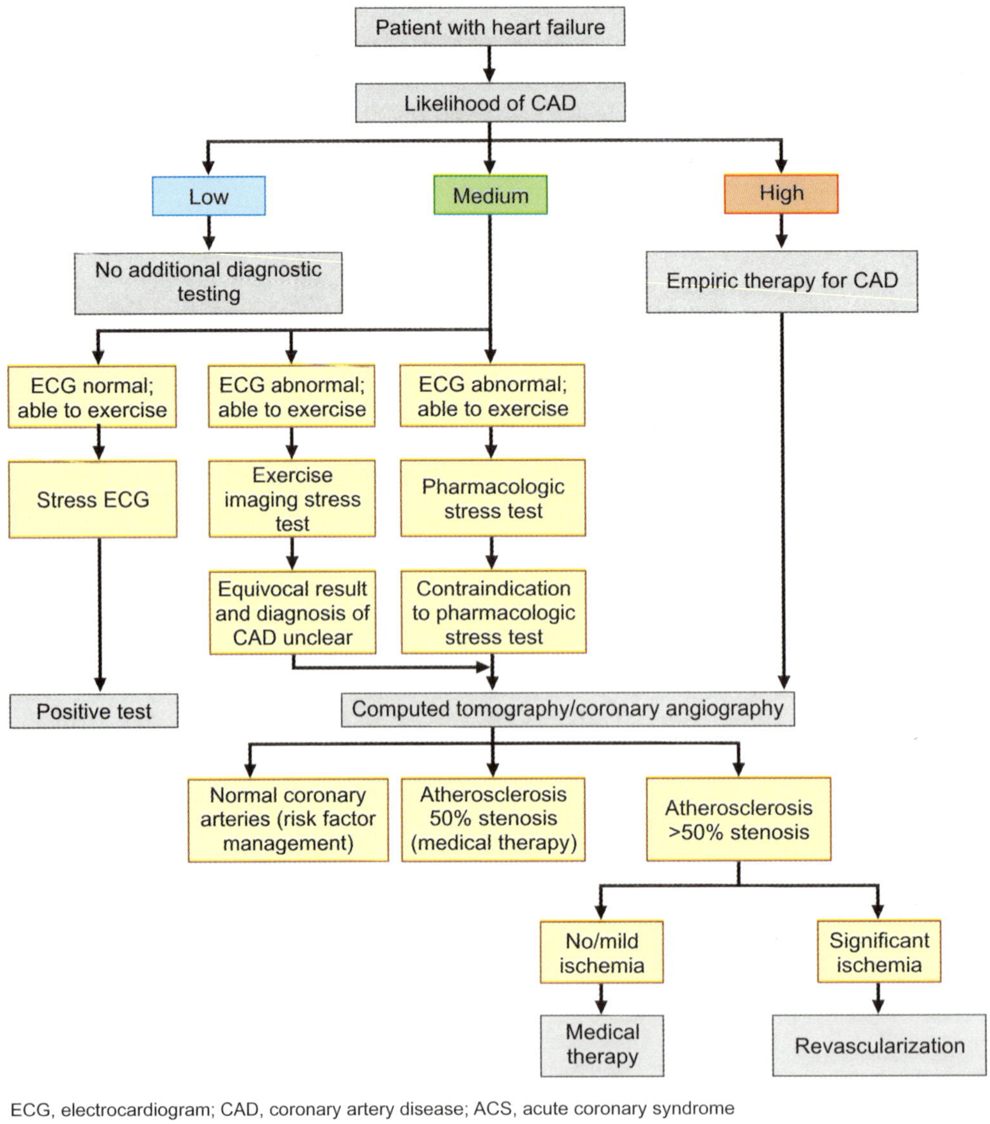

Flowchart 1 Algorithmic approach to screen for underlying coronary artery disease/acute coronary syndrome in patients with already established heart failure

ischemia. Patients with significant ischemia should undergo coronary revascularization, whereas those with only trace or mild evidence should be sufficiently treated if given medical therapy alone.

This general algorithmic approach to assess for underlying CAD should always be used alongside gold standard approaches for diagnosing HF. Ischemic cardiomyopathy contributes to a significant portion of both new onset and chronic ongoing HF, and failing to provide an accurate evaluation for its presence compromises long-term patient care.

TREATMENT OF ACUTE CORONARY SYNDROME IN HEART FAILURE

ST-elevation Myocardial Infarction

Primary treatment of ACS involves categorizing patients into the category of UA or non-ST elevation myocardial infarction (NSTEMI) versus ST-elevation myocardial infarction (STEMI). STEMI is defined as ST-segment elevations of 1 mm (0.1 mV) in two anatomically contiguous leads or 2 mm (0.2 mV) in two contiguous precordial leads, or new left bundle branch block and presentation consistent with ACS.[26,27] Initial interventions for patients with ACS include assessing airway/breathing/circulation and providing oxygen. Initial pharmacotherapy includes aspirin, treatment of angina symptoms with sublingual nitroglycerin, followed by morphine sulfate depending on institutional preference or policy. If signs or symptoms of left HF are present, afterload reduction with sublingual nitroglycerin and/or loop diuretic should be considered. Beta-blocker therapy should be initiated as long as no contraindications are present [chronic obstructive pulmonary disease (COPD) or asthma, cardiogenic shock, hypotension, symptomatic bradycardia, second- or third-degree heart block or decompensated HF is present]. Also, early delivery of statin therapy should be started preferably before percutaneous coronary intervention (PCI).[28]

The acute management of STEMI typically involves the selection of reperfusion therapy (PCI versus fibrinolytic therapy). PCI via cardiac catheterization is ideally performed within 90 minutes of patient's arrival to a hospital with capabilities. Thrombolytic therapy is indicated in the treatment of STEMI if it can be administered within 12 hours of onset of symptoms, patient eligibility based on specific inclusion or exclusion criteria, and if primary PCI is unavailable. Aside from reperfusion therapy, antiplatelet and anticoagulant therapies are essential in the management of STEMI. Antiplatelet therapy (after administration of aspirin) includes clopidogrel, ticagrelor or prasugrel, depending on the reperfusion strategy. Anticoagulation, whether via unfractionated heparin, low molecular weight heparin, direct thrombin inhibitor, and/or glycoprotein (GP) IIb/IIIa inhibitor is also indicated in the management of STEMI. However, the selection of the specific agent is beyond the scope of this chapter.

Unstable Angina/Non-ST Elevation Myocardial Infarction

With respect to UA/NSTEMI, the specific definition of UA is angina which occurs at rest, or new onset angina that limits activity, or increasing angina that is more frequent, longer duration or occurs with less exertion. NSTEMI is distinguished by the presence of elevated markers of myocardial damage.[29] Deciding on which strategy to pursue is primarily based on early invasive interventions in patients who are hemodynamically unstable, have refractory angina or have high thrombolysis in myocardial infarction (TIMI) scores (Table 1). Patients are considered to be at low risk with a score of 0–2; intermediate risk with a score of 3–4; and high risk with a score of 5–7. As a patient's TIMI score increases, so does the risk of mortality and future ischemic events. Initial management is similar to STEMI including oxygen, sublingual nitroglycerin, morphine (depending on institutional policy), beta-blocker therapy and statin therapy. Calcium channel blocker can be used as adjunctive therapy for relief of angina. Antiplatelet therapy includes aspirin and a P2Y12 receptor antagonist (ticagrelor, prasugrel, clopidogrel) should be given to all patients with NSTEMI. Decisions between antiplatelet therapies are made primarily based on risk of bleeding and cost to patient. Decision with respect to use of a GP IIb/IIIa inhibitor (eptifibatide, tirofiban, abciximab) will be determined based on which approach is being pursued. All UA/NSTEMI patients should also receive anticoagulation therapy. Indications to start heparin in intermediate or high-risk UA are listed in Box 1. Bivalirudin or unfractionated heparin

TABLE 1: Thrombolysis in myocardial infarction score for unstable angina (UA)/non-ST elevation myocardial infarction

Parameters	*Points*
Historical	
Age >65 years	1
>3 CAD risk factors (family history, HTN, cholesterol, DM, active smoker)	1
Known CAD (stenosis >50%)	1
ASA use in past 7 days	1
Presentation	
Recent (≤24 hours) severe angina	1
Cardiac marker elevation	1
ST deviation >0.5 mm	1

CAD, coronary artery disease; HTN, hypertension; DM, diabetes mellitus; ASA, acetylsalicylic acid (Aspirin)

Box 1: When to start heparin in patient with unstable angina (who is at high risk)

- Electrocardiographic changes, such as ST segment changes >1 mm or T-wave changes
- Ongoing chest pain >20 minutes
- Angina with new pulmonary edema, S3, rales, worsening mitral regurgitation or hypotension

should be used in patients undergoing an early invasive strategy while patients on track for a conservative approach, fondaparinux or enoxaparin should be given over unfractionated heparin or bivalirudin. In addition to antiplatelet and anticoagulation, all UA/NSTEMI patients should receive beta blockers, angiotensin-converting enzyme (ACE) inhibitor, aldosterone antagonist (acute MI and LVEF <40%). Selection of a management strategy for UA/NSTEMI is often made based on a patient's TIMI score. Patients with high and intermediate risk scores (3 and greater) benefit from an early invasive strategy (immediate coronary arteriography and revascularization). Patients with lower scores can undergo a conservative approach.

Discharge planning in patients with HF and ACS includes a thorough assessment of cardiac function via echocardiography, possible stress testing, and medications, including anti-ischemic, antiremodeling and antiplatelet therapy. Assessment of ejection fraction should be done in all post-STEMI patients. Stress testing should be considered in those who have undergone partial revascularization or no revascularization. Antiplatelet therapy, including aspirin should be given to all patients after myocardial infarction, while dual antiplatelet therapy (clopidogrel and other P2Y12 receptor antagonists) decision making will vary depending on stent deployment and type of stent.[30] All patients after STEMI should be on ACE inhibitor and beta-blocker therapy (as all patients with CHF, regardless of ejection fraction). These therapies should be started early, within 48 hours of hospitalization. In addition, patients on both ACE inhibitor and beta blocker with ejection fraction less than or equal to 40% should be started on aldosterone antagonist therapy to improve ventricular remodeling. Statin therapy should also be instituted prior to discharge. Treatment goals as an outpatient will include low-density lipoprotein (LDL) less than 70 mg/dL, blood pressure less than 140/90 mmHg, cessation of smoking, hemoglobin A1c (HgA1c) less than 7%, physical activity 30–60 minutes daily and body mass index (BMI) 21–25 kg/m^2.

Patients with a history of HF should be closely screened for ACS risk factors. The evaluation for ACS will involve history and assessment of risk factors, physical examination, laboratory work and risk stratification via imaging. Ultimately, the management of ACS has little variation in the setting of concomitant HF and its mainstays remain revascularization therapy and medical management (Box 2).

Box 2: Medications indicated in acute coronary syndrome

Anti-ischemic
- Nitroglycerin
- Morphine sulfate
- Beta blocker*
- Nondihydropyridine calcium channel blocker
- ACE inhibitor*

Antiplatelet
- Aspirin
- Clopidogrel
- P2Y12 ADP receptor antagonists
- GP IIB/IIIA inhibitors

Anticoagulant
- Unfractionated heparin
- Low molecular weight heparin
- Direct thrombin inhibitors
- Factor Xa inhibitors

Lipid-lowering therapy
- Statin

*Indicated in congestive heart failure
ACE, angiotensin converting enzyme; P2Y12, purinergic receptor p2y, G-protein coupled, 12; ADP, adenosine diphosphate; GP, glycoprotein

CONCLUSION

Patients with HF and CAD hold a considerably worse prognosis than those with only HF. As such, it is incredibly important to recognize the dual interplay of CAD and HF. Ischemic cardiomyopathy contributes to a significant portion of both new onset and chronic ongoing HF and failing to provide an accurate evaluation for its presence compromises long-term patient care. That being said, a systematic evaluation for CAD is an essential part of the evaluation of patients with newly diagnosed or CHF. Patients with a history of HF should be closely screened for ACS risk factors. The evaluation for ACS will involve history and assessment of risk factors, physical examination, laboratory work and risk stratification via imaging. Discharge planning in patients with HF and ACS includes a thorough assessment of:

- Cardiac function via echocardiography
- Possible stress testing
- Medications, including anti-ischemic, antiremodeling
- Antiplatelet therapy.

Ultimately, the management of ACS has little variation in the setting of concomitant HF and its mainstays remain revascularization therapy and medical management.

REFERENCES

1. Bourassa MG, Gurne´ O, Bangdiwala SI, et al. Natural history and patterns of current practice in heart failure. The Studies of Left Ventricular Dysfunction (SOLVD) Investigators. J Am Coll Cardiol. 1993;22(4 Suppl A):14A-19A.
2. Cohn JN, Archibald DG, Ziesche S, et al. Effect of vasodilator therapy on mortality in chronic congestive heart failure: results of a Veterans Administration Cooperative Study. N Engl J Med. 1986;314(24):1547-52.
3. The CONSENSUS Trial Study Group. Effects of enalapril on mortality in severe congestive heart failure. Results of the Cooperative North Scandinavian Enalapril Survival Study (CONSENSUS). The CONSENSUS Trial Study Group. N Engl J Med. 1987;316(23):1429-35.
4. DiBianco R, Shabetai R, Kostuk W, et al. A comparison of oral milrinone, digoxin, and their combination in the treatment of patients with chronic heart failure. N Engl J Med. 1989;320(11):677-83.
5. The SOLVD Investigators. Effect of enalapril on survival in patients with reduced left ventricular ejection fractions and congestive heart failure. N Engl J Med. 1991;325(5):293-302.
6. Cohn JN, Johnson G, Ziesche S, et al. A comparison of enalapril with hydralazine-isosorbide dinitrate in the treatment of chronic congestive heart failure. N Engl J Med. 1991;325(5):303-10.
7. Packer M, Carver JR, Rodeheffer RJ, et al. Effect of oral milrinone on mortality in severe chronic heart failure. The PROMISE Study Research Group. N Engl J Med. 1991;325(21):1468-75.
8. The SOLVD Investigators. Effect of enalapril on mortality and the development of heart failure in asymptomatic patients with reduced left ventricular ejection fractions. N Engl J Med. 1992;327(10):685-91.
9. Packer M, Gheorghiade M, Young JB, et al. Withdrawal of digoxin from patients with chronic heart failure treated with angiotensin-converting-enzyme inhibitors. RADIANCE Study. N Engl J Med. 1993;329(1):1-7.
10. Feldman AM, Bristow MR, Parmley WW, et al. Effects of vesnarinone on morbidity and mortality in patients with heart failure. Vesnarinone Study Group. N Engl J Med. 1993;329(3):149-55.
11. Singh SN, Fletcher RD, Fisher SG, et al. Amiodarone in patients with congestive heart failure and asymptomatic ventricular arrhythmia. Survival Trial of Antiarrhythmic Therapy in Congestive Heart Failure. N Engl J Med. 1995;333(2):77-82.
12. Packer M, Bristow MR, Cohn JN, et al. The effect of carvedilol on morbidity and mortality in patients with chronic heart failure. U.S. Carvedilol Heart Failure Study Group. N Engl J Med. 1996;334(21):1349-55.
13. Packer M, O'Connor CM, Ghali JK, et al. Effect of amlodipine on morbidity and mortality in severe chronic heart failure. Prospective Randomized Amlodipine Survival Evaluation Study Group. N Engl J Med. 1996;335(15):1107-14.
14. The Digitalis Investigation Group. The effect of digoxin on mortality and morbidity in patients with heart failure. N Engl J Med. 1997;336(8):525-33.
15. Fonarow GC, ADHERE Scientific Advisory Committee. The Acute Decompensated Heart Failure National Registry (ADHERE): opportunities to improve care of patients hospitalized with acute decompensated heart failure. Rev Cardiovasc Med. 2003;4(Suppl 7):S21-30.
16. Poole-Wilson PA, Uretsky BF, Thygesen K, et al. Mode of death in heart failure: findings from the ATLAS trial. Heart. 2003;89(1):42-8.
17. Gheorghiade M, Bonow RO. Chronic heart failure in the United States: a manifestation of coronary artery disease. Circulation. 1998;97(3):282-9.
18. Bart BA, Shaw LK, McCants CB, et al. The clinical and angiographic diagnosis of ischemic cardiomyopathy: a need to reassess our diagnostic criteria. Circulation. 1996;94(Suppl I):I-338.
19. Kruger D, Sheikhzadeh A, Giannitisis E, et al. Cardiac release and kinetics of endothelin after severe short-lasting myocardial ischemia. J Am Coll Cardiol. 1997;30(4):942-6.
20. Mahajan VS, Jarolim P. How to interpret elevated cardiac troponin levels. Circulation. 2011;124(21):2350-4.
21. Potluri S, Ventura HO, Mulumudi M, et al. Cardiac troponin levels in heart failure. Cardiol Rev. 2004;12(1):21-5.
22. Wang TJ. Significance of circulating troponins in heart failure: if these walls could talk. Circulation. 2007;116(11):1217-20.
23. Peacock WF, De Marco T, Fonarow GC, et al. Cardiac troponin and outcome in acute heart failure. N Engl J Med. 2008;358(20):2117-26.
24. Larsen AI, Dickstein K. BNP in acute coronary syndromes: the heart expresses its suffering. Eur Heart J. 2004;25(15):1284-6.
25. de Lemos JA, Morrow DA. Brain natriuretic peptide measurement in acute coronary syndromes. Circulation. 2002;106(23):2868-70.
26. O'Gara PT, Kushner FG, Ascheim DD, et al. 2013 ACCF/AHA guideline for the management of ST-elevation myocardial infarction: a report of the American College of Cardiology Foundation/American Heart Association Task Force on Practice Guidelines. Circulation. 2013;127(4):e362-425.
27. Tatum JL, Jesse RL, Kontos MC, et al. Comprehensive strategy for the evaluation and triage of the chest pain patient. Ann Emerg Med. 1997;29(1):116-25.
28. Anderson JL, Adams CD, Antman EM, et al. ACC/AHA 2007 guidelines for the management of patients with unstable angina/non-ST-elevation myocardial infarction: a report of the American College of Cardiology/American Heart Association Task Force on Practice Guidelines (Writing Committee to revise the 2002 Guidelines for the Management of Patients with Unstable Angina/Non-ST-Elevation Myocardial Infarction): developed in collaboration with the American College of Emergency Physicians, the Society for Cardiovascular Angiography and Interventions, and the Society of Thoracic Surgeons endorsed by the American Association of Cardiovascular and Pulmonary Rehabilitation and the Society for Academic Emergency Medicine. J Am Coll Cardiol. 2007;50(7):e1-e157.
29. Braunwald E. Application of current guidelines to the management of unstable angina and non-ST-elevation myocardial infarction. Circulation. 2003;108(16 Suppl 1):III28-37.
30. 2012 Writing Committee Members, Jneid H, Anderson JL, et al. 2012 ACCF/AHA focused update of the guideline for the management of patients with unstable angina/Non-ST-elevation myocardial infarction (updating the 2007 guideline and replacing the 2011 focused update): a report of the American College of Cardiology Foundation/American Heart Association Task Force on practice guidelines. Circulation. 2012;126(7): 875-910.

Chapter 20

The ABCs of Isolated Venovenous Ultrafiltration in Fluid-overloaded Heart Failure Patients

Maria R Costanzo, Connie Huberty, Jennifer LaCorte

ABSTRACT

Pulmonary and systemic congestion, occurring in the majority of patients with acutely decompensated heart failure (ADHF), results in unfavorable cardiorenal interactions, which are associated with increased morbidity and mortality. Loop diuretics, used in nearly 90% of congested patients, result in the production of hypotonic urine and neurohormonal activation. In contrast, ultrafiltration (UF) removes isotonic fluid without increasing renin secretion within the kidney. The contradictory results of studies evaluating the effects of UF in fluid-overloaded heart failure patients highlight the importance of selecting patients appropriate for this therapy and of choosing fluid removal rates based upon individual patients' clinical characteristics. Although contemporary devices make UF feasible at most hospitals and in less acute care settings, the successful use of this therapy hinges upon the creation of a program, which fulfills specific requirements. These include identification and active involvement of a physician champion, assembly of a multidisciplinary core clinical team, development of comprehensive order sets, establishment of optimal vascular access, and meticulous management of anticoagulation. Additionally, in-depth knowledge of the structure and function of the UF device is essential for the optimal delivery of this therapy.

INTRODUCTION

It is estimated that at least 70% of patients hospitalized with ADHF have pulmonary and/or venous congestion.[1,2] Among these hypervolemic patients, cardiac output (CO) is normal or decreased in approximately 50% and 20%, respectively. Congestion with preserved CO may result in increased renal venous pressure and impaired renal autoregulation, whereas congestion with reduced CO may be associated with both increased renal venous pressure and decreased renal blood flow.[3] These renal effects of hemodynamic abnormalities contribute to the impairment of kidney function observed in at least 30% of ADHF patients.[4] Therefore it is not surprising that ADHF patients with congestion (defined by the presence of dyspnea, jugular vein distention and edema) which persists after initial hospital therapy, have a twofold increase in their 60-day mortality compared to patients without congestion.[5] Loop diuretics are used to reduce congestion in approximately 90% of ADHF patients. These drugs inhibit the $Na^{+}2Cl^{-}K^{+}$ cotransporter, NKCC2, which is expressed in the thick ascending limb of the loop of Henle of the nephron. This cotransporter is also responsible for the sensing of sodium in the macula densa, which is located at the end of the thick ascending limb. By inhibiting sodium transport to the macula densa, loop diuretics create a situation analogous to low sodium delivery to the macula densa, thus, eliciting its secretion of renin.[3,6] Thus, the very mechanism of action of loop diuretics results in stimulation of renin release and activation of the renin-angiotensin-aldosterone system (RAAS), a pivotal driver of heart failure development and progression. Data from the Diuretic Optimization Strategies Evaluation (DOSE) trial show that 42% of ADHF patients reached the composite end point of death, rehospitalization or emergency room visit at 60 days regardless of whether loop diuretics were administered at low versus high dose or by bolus injection versus continuous infusion.[7] Compared to the low-dose group, the high-dose group included a higher percentage of patients developing acute kidney injury (AKI) defined as a rise in serum creatinine (sCr) greater than or equal to 0.3 mg/dL (23% vs 14%; p = 0.04). This finding suggests that high dose loop diuretics could be counterproductive from a renal standpoint. The results of several other prospective and observational studies in ADHF patients suggest that there is an association between use of high diuretic doses and increased risk of unfavorable renal outcomes.[8-11] In addition, the use in ADHF patients of intravenous (IV) loop diuretics in combination with arginine vasopressin or adenosine A_1 receptor antagonists have failed to improve inpatient mortality or reduce rehospitalization rates.[12,13] However, the question of whether high diuretic doses are the cause of worsening renal function or are a marker of more severe underlying cardiorenal disease remains unanswered.[14]

These outcomes highlight the fact that there are unmet therapeutic needs for a subset of ADHF patients at risk of developing the acute cardiorenal syndrome (CRS) type 1, and justify the interest in exploring the role that alternative methods of fluid removal, such as isolated venovenous UF, in this population.[14]

ULTRAFILTRATION: THE PROCESS

The process of UF consists of the production of plasma water from whole blood across a semipermeable membrane (hemofilter) in response to a transmembrane pressure gradient.[15] The pressure gradient across hemofilters is generated by the classic Starling forces (hydrostatic pressures in the blood and in the filtrate compartments and the oncotic pressure generated by plasma proteins). With venovenous UF hydrostatic pressure is generated by an extracorporeal pump plus the siphoning effect of suction occurring in the UF compartment. The sum of these pressures constitutes the transmembrane pressure gradient which drives plasma water through the hemofilter exactly as Starling forces operate in a capillary bed.[15]

DIFFERENTIAL MECHANISMS OF FLUID REMOVAL BY DIURETICS AND ULTRAFILTRATION

To understand the differential effects that diuretics and UF may have on hemodynamic and neurohormonal abnormalities occurring in heart failure, it is critical to recognize the distinctive characteristics of fluid removal with these two therapies (Table 1). The fluid removed with diuretics has a sodium concentration lower than that of the plasma. Edema in fluid-overloaded heart failure patients is isotonic, and therefore, edematous patients with normal serum sodium levels have significantly increased total body sodium. Because loop diuretics can inhibit reabsorption of only 25% of the filtered sodium, the loop diuretic-induced elimination of hypotonic urine will decrease excess total body water while only partially reducing excess total body sodium. In contrast, the ultrafiltrate is essentially isosmotic and isonatremic compared with plasma. Therefore, whereas approximately 150 mmoL of sodium are removed with each liter of ultrafiltrate, the sodium present in the urine of loop diuretics-treated heart failure (HF) patients rarely exceeds 100 mmoL. Thus for any amount of fluid withdrawn, more sodium can be removed with UF than with diuretics.[14,15] With diuretics intravascular volume contraction is unpredictable and, as described earlier, inhibition of sodium chloride uptake in the macula densa, coupled with augmented release of prostacyclin, enhances renal secretion of renin.[3,14,15] These effects augment neurohormonal activation which, in turn, promotes sodium and water retention ultimately reducing diuretics' ability to relieve the signs and symptoms of circulatory congestion.[16,17] In contrast, UF neither stimulates macula densa-mediated neurohormonal activation nor does it produce prolonged intravascular volume contraction if fluid is removed from the blood at the same rate at which fluid is reabsorbed from the edematous interstitium into the vascular compartment.[18] Thus, with appropriate UF rates, the extracellular fluid gradually refills the intravascular space and blood volume is maintained. If UF rate is too high, blood volume may decrease because intravascular volume depletion exceeds reabsorption of

TABLE 1: Differences between loop diuretics and ultrafiltration

Loop diuretics	*Ultrafiltration*
Elimination of hypotonic urine	Removal of isotonic plasma water
Development of diuretic resistance and lack of dosing guidelines	Precise control of rate and amount of fluid removal
Reduced glomerular filtration rate	Unchanged glomerular filtration rate
Direct neurohormonal activation	No direct neurohormonal activation
Electrolyte abnormalities	No effect on plasma concentration of electrolytes

fluid from the interstitium into the vascular space. Thus, the three key factors for the removal of an adequate amount of fluid without hemodynamic compromise or worsening renal function include accurate determination of the amount of fluid to be removed, optimization of fluid removal rate and maintenance of circulating blood volume.[15] The hematocrit (Hct) is the ratio of the volume occupied by packed red blood cells to the volume of the whole blood. Since red cell mass does not change in the short-term unless there is bleeding or administration of blood products, changes in Hct reflect changes in plasma volume, and therefore, they can be used to estimate changes in intravascular volume. Relative increases in Hct indicate volume contraction.[19] Hematocrit sensors can be incorporated in UF devices for continuous estimation of blood volume. This equipment can be programmed so that fluid removal is stopped if the increase in Hct exceeds the threshold established by the treating physician (typically 3–7%) and resumed when the Hct value falls below the prespecified limit, indicating an adequate refilling of the intravascular volume from the interstitial space.

The implementation of UF in ADHF patients has been facilitated by the introduction of simplified devices, which permit performance of UF with peripheral venous access, adjustable blood flows, and small extracorporeal blood volumes, making UF feasible at most hospitals and in less acute care settings.[20] Additional information on the components and function of a contemporary UF device and on the use of the Hct sensor is provided later in the chapter.

PILOT STUDIES OF ULTRAFILTRATION IN FLUID-OVERLOADED HEART FAILURE PATIENTS

In the United States, most studies of UF in ADHF patients have employed the Aquadex System 100 peripheral venovenous system (Gambro UF Solutions, Minneapolis, MN) (Fig. 1). In 2002, this device was approved by the Food and Drug Administration for clinical use based on the results of the Simple Access Fluid Extraction (SAFE) trial.[20] This study showed that in 21 fluid-overloaded ADHF patients the removal of an average of 2,600 mL of ultrafiltrate during an 8-hour treatment period resulted in a mean weight loss of approximately 3 kg without changes in heart rate, blood pressure, sCr and electrolytes or the occurrence of major adverse events. A subsequent study investigated whether UF begun within 12 hours of admission safely restores euvolemia, permits discharge in less than or equal to 3 days and prevents 90-day rehospitalization in 20 ADHF patients with diuretic resistance (defined as sCr ≥1.5 mg/dL combined with daily oral furosemide doses ≥80 mg or equivalent doses of other loop diuretics).[23] More than one dose of IV loop diuretic was prohibited prior to initiation of UF. An average of 8,654 ± 4,205 mL were removed with 2.6 ± 1.2 8-hour UF courses. Twelve patients (60%) were discharged in less than or equal to 3 days. One patient was readmitted in 30 and two patients in 90 days. Improvement in weight, quality of life and B-type natriuretic peptide (BNP) levels were observed after UF and persisted at 30 and 90 days. Blood pressure, renal function, and medications were unchanged.[23] Of note, in seven patients with hyponatremia (serum sodium ≤135 mg/dL), normalization of serum sodium occurred at discharge and persisted at 90 days. Because ultrafiltrate is isotonic with plasma, the rise in serum sodium cannot be due to direct effects of UF, but it may be related to lesser neurohormonal activation, as indicated by the drop in plasma BNP levels.[24]

The results of this study suggest that in ADHF patients with fluid overload and diuretic resistance, UF initiated before therapy with IV loop diuretics effectively and safely decreases length of hospitalization and readmissions with clinical benefits still present at 90 days.[23]

These favorable outcomes may be due to the fact that fluid removal by UF occurred before neurohormonal stimulation by IV loop diuretics. Indeed the favorable hemodynamic, neurohormonal, and ventilatory responses produced by hemofiltration in eight clinically stable HF patients did not occur in eight matched subjects treated with IV furosemide to achieve equivalent fluid removal.[24] In the latter group, norepinephrine, plasma renin activity and aldosterone concentrations remained elevated above pretreatment values for several days. In contrast, in hemofiltration-treated patients a sustained decrease in neurohormonal levels began 48 hours after therapy and was still detectable at 90 days.[24] Pulmonary congestion and functional measures were significantly improved at 48 hours only in the hemofiltration-treated patients. The diverging neurohumoral responses elicited by hemofiltration and IV furosemide may be related to a lesser stimulation of renin secretion by extracorporeal fluid removal compared to loop diuretics, as described earlier.[24] The results of another pilot trial, the Relief of Acutely Fluid-Overloaded Patients with Decompensated Congestive Heart Failure (RAPID-CHF) trial, showed that, compared to the usual care group, UF-treated patients had greater net fluid loss at 24 and 48 hours ($p < 0.05$) and greater 48 hours improvement in dyspnea ($p = 0.039$) and other heart failure symptoms ($p = 0.023$). Renal function,

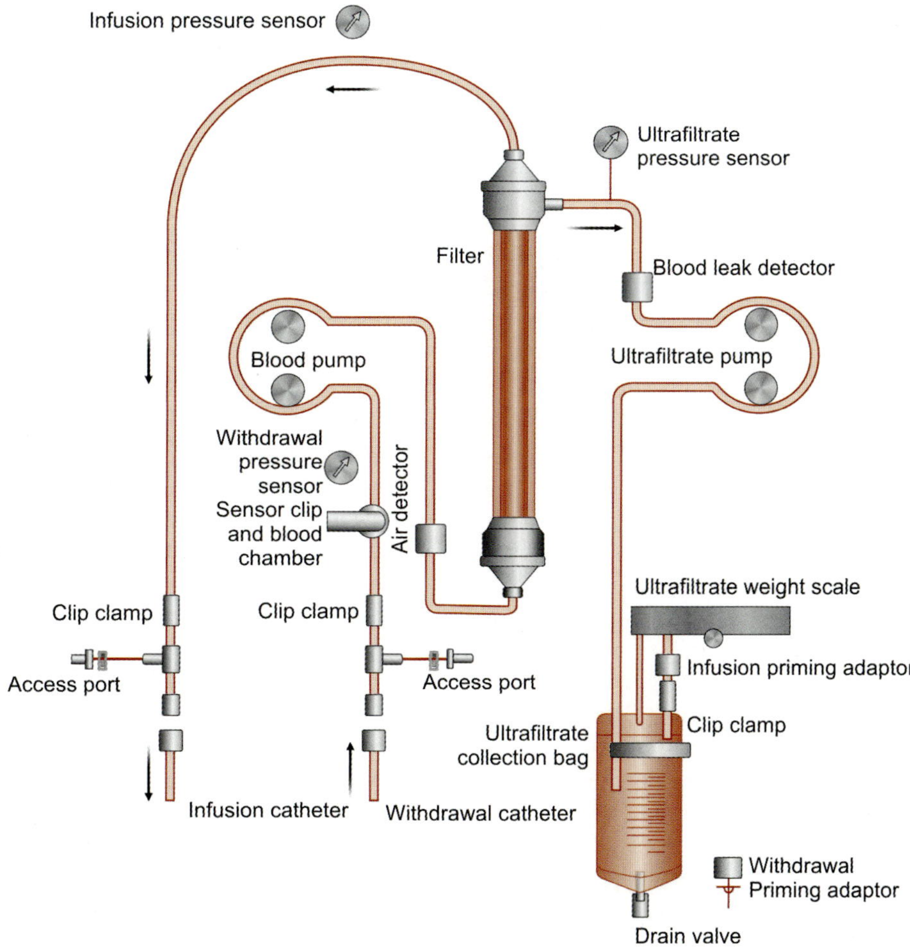

Fig. 1 The Aquadex System 100 peripheral venovenous system (Gambro UF Solutions, Minneapolis, MN). The device consists of a console, an extracorporeal blood pump, and venous catheters. The console controls blood removal rates and extracts ultrafiltrate at a user-set maximum rate. Blood is withdrawn from a vein through the withdrawal catheter. Tubing connects the withdrawal catheter to the blood pump. Blood passes through the withdrawal pressure sensor just before it enters the blood pump tubing loop. After exiting the blood pump, blood passes through the air detector and enters the hemofilter. Blood enters the filter through a port on the bottom, exits through the port at the top of the filter, and passes through the infusion pressure sensor before returning to the patient. Inside the hemofilter, there is a bundle of hollow fibers. Ultrafiltrate sequentially passes through the ultrafiltrate pressure sensor, the ultrafiltrate pump, and the collecting bag that is suspended from the weight scale. A hematocrit sensor is located on the withdrawal line

electrolytes, heart rate, systolic blood pressure and duration of the index hospitalization were similar in UF and usual care groups.

As in the previous study, effective removal of excess fluid and clinical improvement were observed with early initiation of UF, before further elevation of sCr levels resulting from the administration of large IV loop diuretic doses.[8-11,23-25]

The results of UF therapy in 11 patients described by the investigators as having "very advanced, diuretic resistant heart failure" provide important lessons on the appropriate utilization of UF in ADHF patients.[26] The study population had a pretreatment sCr of 2.2 mg/dL, mean estimated glomerular filtration rate (eGFR) of 38 mL/min (with 6/11 having eGFR below 30 mL/min) and included nine patients (82%) with documented right ventricular (RV) dysfunction. Pre-UF, therapy included a mean daily IV furosemide dose of 258 mg, additional metolazone in seven patients (64%) as well as nesiritide and dopamine, each given to four patients. The study objective to remove four liters of fluid with each 8-hour UF course was achieved in 13/32 treatments (41%). Five patients (45%) experienced an increase in sCr greater than 0.3 mg/dL and five patients ultimately required hemodialysis (HD).

The 55% 6-month mortality in this population is identical to that of the medical therapy arm of the Randomized Evaluation of Mechanical Assistance for the Treatment of Congestive Heart Failure (REMATCH) trial, the highest mortality ever reported in a heart failure clinical trial.[27] Thus the lessons emerging from this single center case series can be summarized as follows: (i) because UF does not improve the outcomes of patients with end-stage heart failure, its use is not recommended in this patient population, (ii) overly aggressive UF in heart failure patients with RV dysfunction can rapidly decrease renal perfusion pressure and lead to dialysis dependence,[26,28,29] (iii) use of high doses of IV loop diuretics before UF, by intensifying neurohormonal activation may predispose the kidney to injury by subsequent additional fluid removal with UF.

RANDOMIZED CONTROLLED CLINICAL TRIALS OF ULTRAFILTRATION IN FLUID-OVERLOADED HEART FAILURE PATIENTS

The Ultrafiltration versus Intravenous Diuretics for Patients Hospitalized for Acute Decompensated Heart Failure (UNLOAD) trial compared the safety and efficacy of an early strategy of UF versus standard IV diuretic therapy in ADHF patients with more than or equal to two unquestionable signs of congestion. Treatment assignment had to occur within 24 hours of hospital admission in patients who had received no more than two IV loop diuretic doses before randomization.[30] Two hundred patients (63 ± 15 years; 69% men; 71% ejection fraction, ≤40%) were randomized to UF or IV diuretics. At 48 hours, weight (5.0 ± 3.1 kg vs 3.1 ± 3.5 kg; p = 0.001) and net fluid loss (4.6 L vs 3.3 L; p = 0.001) were greater in the UF group.[30] Dyspnea was similarly improved in the two groups. At 90 days, the UF group had fewer patients rehospitalized for heart failure (18% vs 32%; p = 0.037), and unscheduled visits for worsening heart failure (21% vs 44%; p = 0.009). The length of the index hospitalization was similar in the two groups owing to factors other than patients' response to therapy, including diagnostic and therapeutic procedures, comorbidities, patients' placement, and lack of uniform discharge criteria.[31] Changes in sCr were similar in the two groups throughout the study. The percentage of patients with increases in sCr levels greater than 0.3 mg/dL was similar in the UF and standard care group at 24 hours (14.4% vs 7.7%; p = 0.528), at 48 hours (26.5% vs 20.3%; p = 0.430), and throughout the 90 day follow-up period.[30] Drops in serum potassium less than 3.5 mEq/L were fewer in the UF than in the diuretic group (1% vs 12%; p = 0.018). Hypotension was rare in both groups.[30] Complications specifically related to UF included clotting of five filters, one catheter infection and the requirement for hemodialysis in one patient deemed to have congestion refractory to UF.[30]

The limitations of the UNLOAD trial, such as the lack of fluid removal targets and economic analysis, do not negate the main findings of the UNLOAD trial: an early strategy of UF, initiated before the administration of high-dose IV diuretics in fluid-overloaded ADHF patients effectively reduces congestion and is associated with fewer 90-day heart failure-related rehospitalizations. The outcomes of the 100 patients treated with UF were compared to those of the 100 control group subjects, divided according to whether IV diuretics were given by continuous infusion (n = 32) or bolus injections (n = 68).[32] Despite similar amounts of fluid removed by UF and continuous IV diuretic infusion, at 90 days rehospitalizations plus unscheduled visits for HF/patient (rehospitalization equivalents) were fewer in the UF than in continuous IV diuretic infusion group (p = 0.016)[32] (Fig. 2). The simultaneous reduction of total body sodium and excess fluid by UF may be more effective than removal of hypotonic fluid by diuretics or free water by vasopressin V2 receptor blockers.[12,33] Alternatively, prehospitalization diuretic use itself may limit the natriuresis induced by IV loop diuretics.[34]

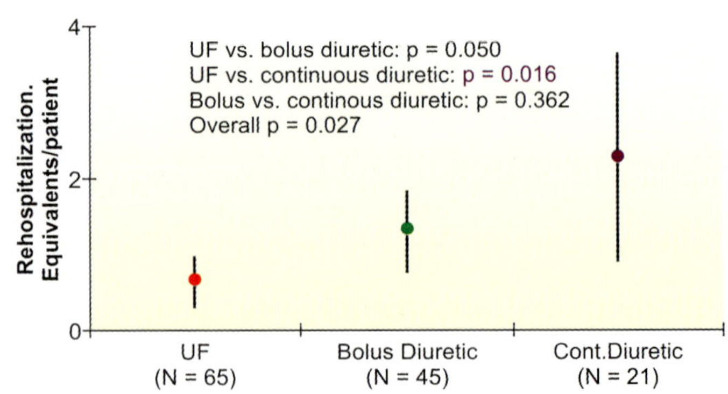

UF, ultrafiltration; IV, intravenous; CI, cardiac index

Fig. 2 Mean rehospitalization equivalents (rehospitalization + unscheduled office and emergency department visits for heart failure) in the ultrafiltration (red circle), intravenous (IV) bolus diuretic (green circle), and IV continuous diuretic (blue circle) groups; p values are for the comparison between ultrafiltration and IV bolus diuretic, ultrafiltration and IV continuous diuretic, IV bolus diuretic, and IV continuous diuretic. Error bars indicate 95% CI

Source: Adapte from Costanzo MR, Saltzberg MT, Jessup M, et al. Ultrafiltration is associated with fewer rehospitalizations than continuous diuretic infusion in patients with decompensated heart failure: results from UNLOAD. *J Card Fail*. 2010;16(4):277-84, *with permission*

The increased amounts of sodium and water reabsorbed by the kidney as a result of enhanced systemic and intrarenal neurohormonal activity predominantly fill the compliant venous circulation, increasing CVP. Transmission of venous congestion to the renal veins further impairs GFR.[35-37] If fluid is removed by UF at rates that do not exceed the interstitial fluid mobilization (plasma refill) rate of 14–15 mL/minute, CVP may be lowered without the neurohormonal activation which unavoidably occurs when IV loop diuretics limit sodium transport to the macula densa.[36,37]

In sharp contrast with the UNLOAD trial, which compared an early strategy of UF versus IV loop diuretics, the recently published Cardiorenal Rescue Study in Acute Decompensated Heart Failure (CARRESS-HF) trial compared the effects of a fixed 200 mL/hour UF rate, with those of stepped pharmacologic therapy (SPT) (inclusive of adjustable IV loop diuretic doses, thiazide diuretics, vasodilators, and inotropes) in ADHF patients demonstrating an increase in sCr greater than 0.3 mg/dL in response to escalating doses of diuretics.[38] Thus, at randomization, all subjects fulfilled the criteria for having the CRS type 1. The primary end point of CARRESS-HF was the bivariate change from baseline in sCr level and body weight at 96 hours postrandomization.[39] In the CARRESS-HF population, UF was inferior to SPT for the primary endpoint, due primarily to an increase in sCr level in the UF group (+ 0.23 ± 0.70 mg/dL for UF vs -0.04 ± 0.53 mg/dL for SPT; $p = 0.003$) without significant differences between groups in weight loss (-5.5 ± 5.1 kg for UF vs 5.7 ± 3.9 kg for SPT; $p = 0.58$). Furthermore, a higher percentage of patients in the UF group than in the SPT group had serious adverse events (72% vs 57%, $p = 0.03$), attributable mainly to higher incidences of kidney failure, bleeding events, and catheter-related complications.[38] The design and results of CARRESS-HF merit thorough discussion. In ADHF patients, transient increases in sCr may not necessarily reflect AKI or unfavorable long-term outcomes. Recent analyses have shown that hemoconcentration resulting from aggressive decongestion is associated with worsening renal function but lower 180-day mortality and all-cause 30-day rehospitalizations.[40,41] Data from UNLOAD also show that, regardless of assignment to UF or IV diuretics groups, the patients who had the greatest increases in sCr during treatment had the fewest heart failure-related hospitalizations at 90 days (Costanzo MR, personal communication). Finally in the DOSE trial greater worsening of renal function in the high dose diuretic group did not result in increased cardiovascular events. Taken together, these findings suggest that transient small increases in sCr resulting from decongestive therapies are not predictive of adverse long-term outcomes and may at times reflect fluid removal from the intravascular compartment that exceeds the rate of plasma refill. In the CARRESS-HF trial is that the rate of fluid removal was mandated to be the same (200 mL/hour) in all patients assigned to the UF arm. While this fluid removal rate may be inadequate for some patients, it may be excessively fast for patients with a lower blood pressure and/or right ventricular (RV) dysfunction who are at higher risk of worsening renal function from intravascular volume depletion.[26,42,43] In addition, clinical experience shows that, regardless of decongestive therapy, removal of fluid must be guided by careful assessment of individual patients' blood pressure, renal function variables, body mass, and urine output. In the CARRESS trial the SPT group was treated according to a complex algorithm for ongoing adjustments of IV diuretic doses, use of thiazide diuretics, vasodilators and inotropic drugs based on the individual patient's blood pressure and urine output.[39] The patients in the UF group were not given the benefit of adjustable therapy. This is achievable because, as previously stated, contemporary UF devices are equipped with Hct sensors for the estimation of blood volume. Thus thresholds of Hct changes can be set for each patient such that the pace of fluid removal does not exceed the capillary refill rate and intravascular volume depletion is avoided.[44]

In the CARRESS-HF trial vasoactive drugs could not be used in the UF group unless deemed necessary for rescue therapy. In contrast, inotropes which were included in the SPT algorithm were used in 12% of SPT patients before the 96-hour assessment and may have minimized worsening renal function due to hypotension.[38]

It should also be noted that 39% of the patients assigned to the UF arm of CARRESS-HF also received IV diuretics before the 96-hour assessment, suggesting that the greater rise in sCr observed in this group cannot be attributed solely to mechanical fluid removal.

The CARRESS-HF investigators do not provide information on whether the duration of the increase in sCr level by at least 0.3 mg/dL, required for enrollment in the trial, was similar in the two groups. Data on this variable are valuable, given the large body of experimental and clinical evidence that both severity and duration of underlying renal dysfunction are key risk factors for the development of AKI.[45]

Thus, CARRESS-HF was not a prevention trial, but a treatment trial of the CRS type 1. Recent data suggest that worsening renal function during treatment of ADHF may indicate underlying impairment of renal reserve rather than a consequence of treatment.[46] In fact the prognosis of the CARRESS-HF population was poor regardless of fluid removal method or degree of weight loss, as shown by the findings that only 10% of the patients were adequately decongested at 96 hours and more than one-third died or were readmitted for ADHF within 60 days of the index hospitalization.[38,46]

SELECTION OF POTENTIAL CANDIDATES FOR ULTRAFILTRATION

The contradictory effects of UF as a method of decongestion in ADHF patients underscore the main challenges for the use of this therapy, which include the selection of patients most likely to benefit from UF, the amount of fluid to be removed and the choice of monitoring methods.

European and North American practice guidelines state that UF is reasonable for patients with refractory congestion not responding to medical therapy.[1,47,48] The American Heart Association (AHA)/American College of Cardiology (ACC) guidelines recommend that an inadequate response to an initial dose of IV loop diuretic be treated with an increased dose of the same drug. If this measure is not effective, invasive hemodynamic assessment is recommended. Objective evidence of persistent congestion can then be treated with the addition of a thiazide diuretic (metolazone or IV chlorothiazide) or an aldosterone antagonist or the use of continuous IV infusion of a loop diuretic. If all of these measures fail, UF can be considered.[47] Although these recommendations do not specify whether changes in renal function variables should influence the choice of therapy, the degree of resistance to medical therapy that should be demonstrated before consideration of UF is startlingly comparable to the refractoriness to therapy required for enrollment in the CARRESS-HF trial. However, the unfavorable outcomes in this patient population which are in sharp contrast to the sustained benefits observed in the UNLOAD trial suggest that initiation of UF in ADHF patients before they fail high-dose IV diuretics may be a more effective and safer approach.[23,25,26,30,32,38,42-44]

Given the cost and potential complications of UF, not all ADHF patients are candidates for this therapy. Patients with new onset heart failure and not previously treated with diuretics, usually have a brisk diuresis with IV diuretics, and therefore these drugs should be used instead of or before UF is considered. A more challenging clinical question is which patients who develop ADHF despite daily oral diuretic therapy should be considered for early UF rather than IV diuretics.

Among 15 patients with ADHF who first received IV diuretics and were subsequently treated with UF due to unresolved fluid overload, the urine sodium concentration in response to IV furosemide given before initiation of UF was significantly less and more variable between patients than the sodium concentration in the ultrafiltrate after 8 hours of UF (60 ± 47 mmoL/L vs 134 ± 8.0 mmoL/L; $p = 0.000025$).[33] In this study, the lack of correlation between urinary sodium concentration and baseline renal function highlights the difficulty in predicting the natriuretic response of individual patients to a given dose of IV diuretic. Although intuitively UF may be particularly effective in patients who exhibit a poor natriuretic response to a dose of IV loop diuretics, this hypothesis should be tested in prospective randomized clinical trials.

A recent consensus statement proposes that congestion be graded according to a combination of clinical and laboratory parameters. The expert consensus suggests that a congestion grade greater than 12 together with low urine output (<1,000 mL/24 hours) should trigger consideration of extracorporeal fluid removal because patients with this degree of congestion are more likely to have diuretic resistance.[49] This recommendation, however, has not been tested in prospective controlled trials.

FLUID REMOVAL TARGETS AND MONITORING OF ULTRAFILTRATION THERAPY

The safety and efficacy of UF depend upon the ability to remove fluid without causing hypotension and/or AKI. To avoid hemodynamic instability occurring when refilling of the intravascular space from the interstitium cannot keep pace with the reduction in intravascular volume resulting from fluid withdrawal, it is recommended that UF be initially prescribed at low rates (100–200 mL/hour). After assessment of the hemodynamic response to UF, higher fluid removal rates can be tried in the absence of symptomatic hypotension and/or worsening renal function.[44] Rates of UF exceeding 250 mL/hour are no longer recommended in patients with ADHF. Patients with predominantly right sided HF or patients with HF and preserved systolic function are exquisitely susceptible to intravascular volume depletion and may only tolerate UF rates less than or equal to 150 mL/hour.[44] Clinical experience has also shown that extracorporeal fluid removal is better tolerated when conducted with low UF rates over extended periods of time (>8 hours and up to 72 hours). Unfortunately, in most published studies, UF has been used for less than or equal to 40 hours. Thus, the benefits of UF initiated before the onset of the CRS type 1 and performed with low fluid removal rates for more than 40 hours must be evaluated in controlled clinical trials. In patients being treated with UF, fluid removal can be slowed or stopped for transient episodes of hypotension and worsening renal function and resumed after hemodynamic stabilization if the patient's congestion is incompletely resolved.

A frequently used practical approach is to estimate fluid excess by comparing the patient's current weight with that measured in the absence of signs and symptoms of congestion, and remove at least 60–80% of this excess fluid without causing hemodynamic instability or worsening renal function. It is reasonable to define resolution of congestion as a jugular venous pressure ≤8 cm, absence of pulmonary rales and trace or no edema.[44]

Given the experimental and clinical evidence that increased CVP is the key hemodynamic abnormality leading to worsening renal function in patients with congestive heart failure, it may be reasonable to guide UF therapy according to the direct measurement or estimation of CVP. Indeed a small but well-conducted study has shown that in patients with heart failure UF can reduce CVP independently from changes in CO and, unlike IV diuretics, without significant neurohormonal activation.[18] Larger prospective controlled clinical trials are needed to determine if CVP, rather than other clinical or hemodynamic variables, should be used to establish fluid removal targets in ADHF patients. Ultrasonography may permit to noninvasively estimate CVP with the assessment of the respiratory excursions of the diameter of the inferior vena cava (IVC). The IVC is a compliant vessel that is less collapsible with hypervolemia and more collapsible with hypovolemia. It also expands and contracts during inspiration and expiration. The IVC caval index (IVC-CI) is the difference of the IVC diameters during maximal expiration and inspiration divided by the IVC diameter during maximal expiration. In fluid-overloaded states the IVC-CI approaches 0, whereas in volume-depleted states the IVC-CI approaches 1. One study of intensive care unit (ICU) patients undergoing continuous invasive monitoring of the CVP, showed a moderate correlation ($r = -0.31$) of IVC-CI with CVP.[50] The advantages of ultrasonography are that it is a noninvasive method which can be performed at the bedside, it does not expose the patient to radiation, and it is inexpensive. However, the reliability of ultrasonography is strictly dependent upon the skill of the operator and the respiratory effort of the patient.[50]

Blood Volume Estimation

If fluid removal by UF is within the plasma refill rate (PRR), pre- and posttreatment Hct values should be similar. Several online Hct sensors permit continuous estimation of blood volume and relative blood volume changes during UF. These sensors can be programmed so that fluid removal is stopped if the increase in Hct exceeds the threshold set by the treating physician (3–7%) and resumed when the Hct value falls below the prespecified limit, which indicates that adequate refilling of the intravascular volume from the interstitial space has occurred.[19] However, because multiple factors, including change in body position, can significantly alter hematocrit values, physical and laboratory assessments are also considered to determine the appropriate rates of UF and the amount of fluid that should be removed. The technical aspect of Hct sensors used to estimate changes in blood volume during UF are described later in the chapter.

Biomarkers

Natriuretic peptide (NP) levels are widely used in the diagnosis, treatment, and prognostic assessment of patients with heart failure.[51] Theoretically, the NP level of a patient with ADHF is the sum of two components, the baseline (dry) NP level, measured in the absence of signs and symptoms of congestion, plus the NP level occurring from acute pressure and volume overload (wet), both of which vary within the same individual over time.[52] Studies in ADHF patients have shown that while a drop in NP level in response to treatment provides useful information, the final (discharge) NP level seems to be the most accurate predictor of death or rehospitalization. Specifically, B-type natriuretic peptide (BNP) levels <350–400 pg/mL or N-terminal-proBNP (NT-proBNP) levels <4,000 pg/mL, especially if associated with clinical evidence of optivolemia, predict favorable outcomes.[53-55] Although attractive, the approach of targeting fluid removal by UF to achieve these NP levels has not been prospectively evaluated. As previously noted, AKI may occur in ADHF patients as a result of excessively aggressive diuresis or fast UF rates (CRS type 1). Awareness of this potentially serious complication of fluid removal therapies has spurred interest in new AKI biomarkers, such as neutrophil gelatinase associated lipocalin (NGAL) and kidney injury molecule (KIM-1).[21] Because these biomarkers become abnormal earlier than sCr, AKI can be detected earlier and further renal damage due to overly aggressive fluid removal by UF can be prevented. Assessment of serial changes of NGAL levels during UF may help prevent the development of the CRS type 1 resulting from excessive fluid removal.[55]

Bioimpedance Vector Analysis

Bioimpedance vector analysis (BIVA) is based on the principle that whole body impedance to an alternating current results from the electrical characteristics of the complex network of resistive and capacitive conductors arranged in parallel and in series within living soft tissues. These electrical characteristics are influenced by the amount of intra- and extracellular fluid.[56] Measurements can be made *in vivo* with the application of relatively high frequency alternating microcurrents (most commonly at 50 kHz) using a well-established system in which two pairs of electrodes are placed on the wrist and ankles to obtain total body measures (Cardio-EFG, EFG-Dublin, Ireland). Graphically, impedance (Z), resistance (Rz), reactance (Xc), and phase angle are displayed and can provide data indicative of total body water (TBW) and cellular health.[56] Corrected by height (H), BIVA measurements are highly correlated to with TBW ($r = 0.996$).[57] Data on age, gender and H of 1,800 Caucasian subjects was used to develop nomograms of resistance and reactance which permit to determine whether a subject is euvolemic, dehydrated or fluid-overloaded.[58] In healthy subjects average resistance and reactance are, respectively, approximately 300 Ω/m and 30 Ω/m. Tolerance ellipses can be drawn corresponding to the median, 75th and 95th percentiles of the impedance vector distribution calculated from the reference healthy subjects. Plotting Rz/H and Xc/H measurements on the tolerance ellipses (which reflect the population's percentile distributions) permits to determine if a subject is in a state of normal hydration.[56] Vectors above and below the minor axis of the ellipses indicate, respectively, that less (dehydration) and more (overhydration) water is present relative to cell mass in the tissues in which bioimpedance is being measured. Thus progressive shortening and downsloping of the bioimpedance vector over successive measurements indicates that progressive fluid accumulation is occurring. Conversely, a progressive lengthening and steepening of the bioimpedance vector indicates that the proportion of water in the tissues being evaluated is decreasing.[56] Data from BIVA can be translated into a nomogram indicative of whether a patient is normally hydrated, hyperhydrated or dehydrated. The latter two classes can be further subdivided into mild, moderate or severe volume abnormalities. Results from recent studies evaluated the sensitivity and specificity of BIVA in the assessment of fluid volume status in heart failure patients and used the results in combination with BNP levels to establish criteria for hospital discharge.[59,60] In addition, studies in overhydrated critically ill patients have confirmed the reliability of this parameter to guide UF and target overall volume of fluid removal.[61] It is therefore attractive to envision the use of BIVA to determine the fluid status of ADHF patients before initiation of UF and then employment of serial BIVA measurements to guide the amount and rate of fluid removal by UF, so that resolution of congestion does not occur at the expense of reductions in renal blood flow and perfusion pressure sufficiently severe to cause AKI (CRS type 1).[62] An example of how sequential BIVA measurements can be used to guide UF therapy is shown in Figure 3. Although the BIVA system is not yet approved for clinical use in the US, at several European centers BIVA has been used in conjunction with estimates of blood volume, because the former estimates the amount of fluid to be removed whereas the latter can help decide the rate of fluid removal.[62,63] The fact that multiple variables are needed to assess a patient's fluid status and establish fluid removal targets, is supported by the results of a recent study in which serial BNP and BIVA measurements were performed in 300 ADHF patients from the time of hospital admission to discharge.[60] Therapy was titrated to achieve, whenever possible, a BNP value below 250 pg/mL. Subjects were divided according to whether the target BNP was achieved early (15.3%), later after aggressive diuretic therapy (18.7%) or not reached by the time of discharge (66%). Perhaps the most important finding of the study is that 72% of patients with BNP levels persistently above 250 pg/mL even after aggressive diuresis, had discharge BIVA measurements consistent with normal hydration.[60] These patients have "dry" BNP levels so that titration of fluid removal therapy to lower BNP levels without concomitant knowledge of fluid status may lead to volume depletion and AKI (CRS type 1).[60]

Accuracy of bioimpedance measures can be reduced by many factors, including diaphoresis, hirsutism, incorrect placement of the electrodes, cutaneous alterations (such as ulcers, wounds etc.), or improper electrical grounding.

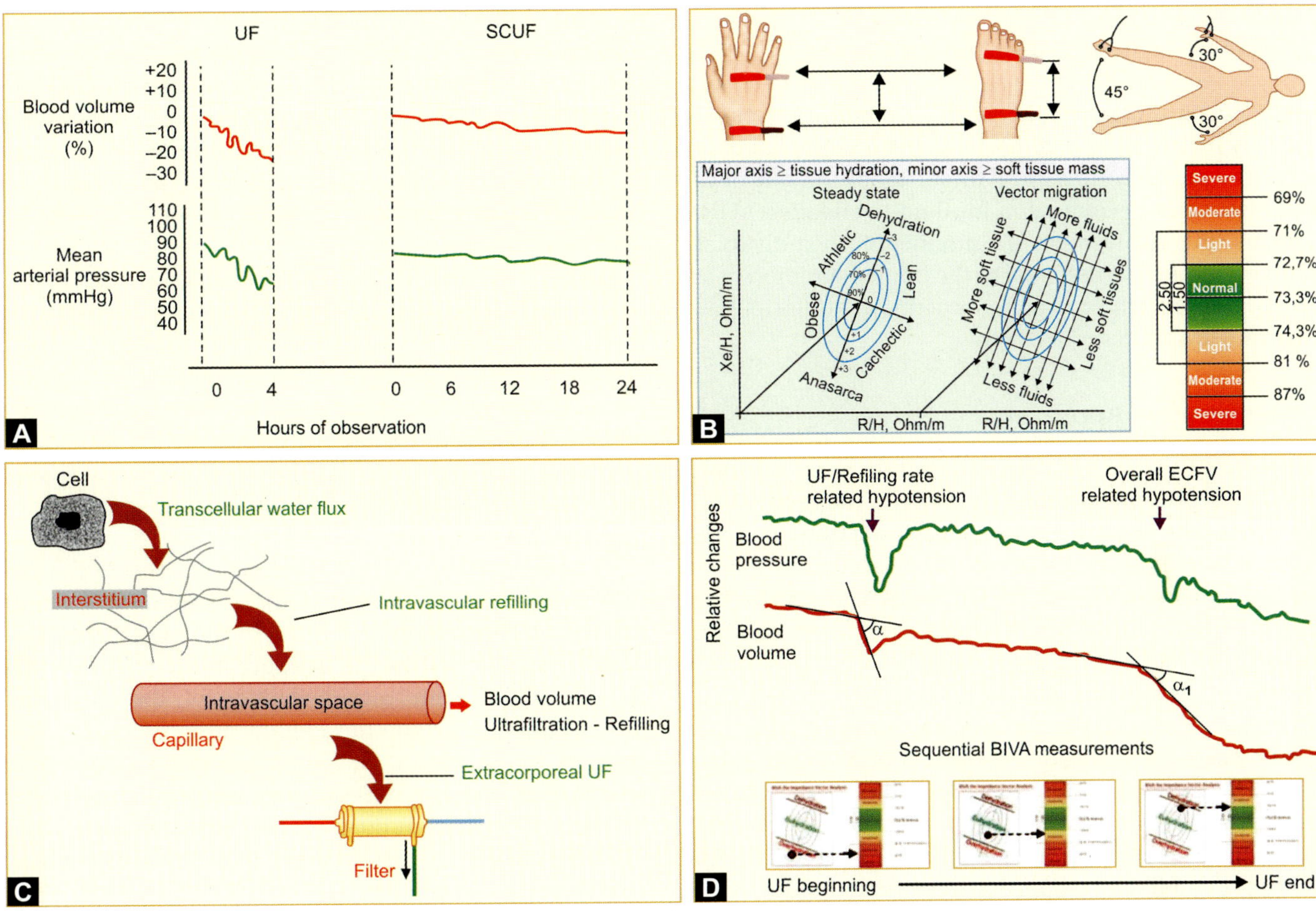

UF, ultrafiltration; SCUF, slow continuous ultrafiltration; ECFV, extracellular fluid volume; R/H, resistance/height; BIVA, bioimpedance vector analysis; CO, cardiac output

Fig. 3 A, Comparison of patients treated in with intermittent ultrafiltration and slow continuous ultrafiltration. Fluid removal without significant changes in blood volume is associated with a stable mean arterial blood pressure; **B,** Positioning of electrodes for noninvasive bioelectrical impedance vectorial analysis (BIVA). Measurement of reactance, resistance, and phase angle allow positioning of the resulting vector in the ellipse, which indicates the nutritional status and the hydration status of the patient. Vector migration along the two main axes denotes changes in hydration and nutritional status. Data from BIVA can be visually presented as a nomogram of percent total body water indicating whether a patient is normally hydrated, hyperhydrated, or dehydrated; **C,** Fluid is removed by ultrafiltration in the filter. The fluid removed is plasma water from the intravascular space. Because of oncotic forces, intravascular refilling occurs from the interstitium which is in equilibrium with the intracellular fluid compartment. These fluid shifts require time, intact capillary and cellular membranes and adequate CO. If ultrafiltration is too fast or too much, blood volume depletion exceeds plasma refill rate, resulting in hypotension, and worsening of renal function; **D,** Evaluation of blood pressure and blood volume graphs shows two situations which may occur during ultrafiltration: in the first case ultrafiltration rate is too fast, blood volume decrease rapidly (alpha angle) and hypotension occurs even if the patient is overhydrated, as documented by the bioimpedance vector analysis; in the second instance, both ultrafiltration rate and amount are excessive and exceed the amount of fluid removal required in the patient. Intravascular refilling from the interstitial space does not occur because the patient is already dehydrated, as indicated by the upward migration of the bioimpedance vector to the top of the nomogram) and a progressive drop in blood pressure occurs.

Source: Adapted from Costanzo MR, Cozzolino M, Aspromonte N, et al. Extracorporeal ultrafiltration in heart failure and cardio-renal syndromes. *Semin Nephrol*. 2012;32(1):100-11, *with permission*

BUILDING BLOCKS OF A SUCCESSFUL ULTRAFILTRATION THERAPY PROGRAM

At most institutions initiation of an UF therapy program is typically proposed by a clinician, either a physician or an advanced practice nurse, who understands the role of UF as a method of decongestion for fluid-overloaded ADHF patients. The involvement of a number of key individuals and departments is essential to the implementation of an UF program and the components of this multidisciplinary effort are briefly described below.

Administrative Approval

Support of the hospital's administration is garnered through a presentation of the potential benefits of UF therapy for the institution which may result from potential reductions in hospital length of stay, heart failure-related readmissions and costs.[23,30,32] At many centers the first step to obtain administrative support is to discuss the program outline with the institution's board (Heart Failure or Cardiology Advisory Council) charged with overseeing the initiation of new cardiac programs. The next logical step is to earn the support of the institution's financial officers, as equipment expenditures may require a capital budget request. To achieve this goal it is essential to develop a document which itemizes the costs of the UF device, hemofilters, supplies, disposables, equipment maintenance and initial staff training. Other costs related to the performance of UF therapy include program development, funding of the clinical team charged with obtaining vascular access and ongoing staff training. Once administrative approval is attained for the initiation of UF at the institution, clinical leaders are designated to develop the program.

Key Personnel and Procedures

A decade of experience in the development of UF programs has shown that several factors are essential to the success of the therapy. These include active physician involvement, a dedicated on-site clinical support person, development of comprehensive order sets, establishment of optimal vascular access, and meticulous management of anticoagulation.

Role of Physicians

A physician champion, typically a cardiologist or nephrologist, is essential to implementation of a UF program. Physician involvement in initiation and management of UF therapy is highly variable between institutions. In some centers UF is managed solely by either cardiologists or nephrologists, whereas other institutions require the collaborative effort of physicians in both specialties. Ultimately, a model of care, which is in keeping with the culture of the institution has the greatest likelihood of success.

Staff physicians should be educated about the basic principles of UF and process of therapy delivery at their institution, to enable informed decisions when considering UF for volume-overloaded, diuretic resistant patients. Physicians who can potentially refer patients to the UF program include cardiologists, nephrologists, primary care physicians, hospitalists, intensivists, cardiovascular surgeons, and emergency department physicians.

Upon initiation of a UF program, prescription of therapy should be delegated to a limited number of physicians with unique expertise in the management of ADHF patients and in the conduct of mechanical fluid removal. The main responsibilities of the physician prescribing UF include the identification of appropriate patients, completion of standing orders regarding selection of venous access, anticoagulation protocols, fluid removal rates, duration of UF, acceptable threshold of Hct change, and assessment of whether treatment goals have been achieved.

Role of the Ultrafiltration Clinical Specialist

A dedicated on-site clinical support person should be chosen to implement the UF program and oversee the process of care from establishment of vascular access to discontinuation of therapy, discharge planning and subsequent patient follow-up. The clinical specialist should ideally be an advanced practice nurse, either clinical nurse specialist or nurse practitioner, with a cardiology or critical care background and a desire to improve heart failure outcomes. A registered nurse with advanced skills in heart failure has also been successfully utilized at some institutions.

The roles of the clinical specialist are multifaceted and critically important to the success of a UF program. These duties include program development, interactions with the manufacturer of the UF equipment, assistance with process issues and communication with multiple departments, design of a curriculum for initial and ongoing staff education and assessment of competency, oversight of staff training provided by the manufacturer's clinical experts, troubleshooting of UF therapy issues and delivery of care and education to patients and their families.[64,65] Additionally, the clinical specialist should work closely with the physician champion and members of other appropriate departments in the development of patient selection criteria and standard UF orders, ongoing evaluation and refinement of the UF program and assessment of and response to outcome data.[64,65]

Role of Other Hospital Departments

A successful UF initiative employs the multidisciplinary efforts of a variety of departments in program development and implementation. Multiple meetings are often necessary to design the program and resolve process issues. Individuals and departments that should be involved in the design of the workflow of an UF program include (i) managers, clinical educators, and nursing staff of the hospital unit(s) designated to deliver UF therapy; (ii) admitting department regarding placement of patients in the appropriate hospital unit; (iii) teams skilled in the placement of peripherally inserted UF catheters; (iv) interventional radiology department if the patient requires placement of the UF catheter in a central vein; (v) laboratory department to develop a process for timely reporting of laboratory results pertaining to anticoagulation, renal function and electrolyte balance; (vi) pharmacy for the development of anticoagulation protocols and delivery of medications; (vii) biomedical engineering department for care and maintenance of the UF pumps; (viii) billing and coding departments to create the necessary treatment and procedural codes to ensure accurate billing and thus maximize reimbursement; (ix) purchasing department to develop a process for ordering materials and supplies, including catheters for vascular access, dressing supplies, and UF circuits; (x) policies and procedures committees and other hospital or cardiology specific committees or advisory boards for the oversight of UF protocols and order sets as well as ongoing evaluation of the UF program.[64,65]

Choice of Location for the Delivery of Ultrafiltration Therapy

As previously noted contemporary UF devices are portable, require only low blood flows for effective fluid removal and thus permit delivery of therapy with a peripheral venous access. These characteristics allow UF therapy to be implemented at most hospitals and in less acute care settings, such as telemetry units.[20] Although the recommended nurse to patient ratio during UF therapy is 1:4, lower ratios can be utilized during program initiation to allow for nursing staff training and development of competency with UF therapy. In some institutions, a UF therapy program is initiated in the intensive care unit and later transitioned to a telemetry unit when familiarity with the therapy is attained and the process is well established.[64,65]

Although UF is generally performed in the hospital settings describe above, this therapy can also be delivered in postcardiovascular surgery units, cardiac transplantation units, emergency departments, and, in some cases, in outpatient heart failure treatment clinics.

Development of Order Sets for the Delivery of Ultrafiltration Therapy

A comprehensive standing order set is essential for the success of UF therapy. Although individual institutions' policies vary with respect to the items that must be included in standard order sets, it is recommended that patient selection criteria, choice of vascular access selection, and guidelines for UF circuit maintenance be included in nursing policies and clinical protocols. An example of a comprehensive UF orders set, which can be tailored to individual institutions' requirements, is shown in Box 1.

Training of Nursing Staff in the Delivery of Ultrafiltration Therapy

The nurse assigned to a given patient is ultimately responsible for the actual performance of UF therapy. Early in the development of a UF program, a decision must be made on which staff nurses should be trained to deliver UF therapy. Generally, a core group of nurses are educated to develop and refine the process. This initial group typically consists of highly experienced nurses with advanced skills in patient assessment and enthusiasm for learning and implementing new therapies. Once the UF program is established, additional nurses can be trained while the original nursing group functions as a resource for assisting and mentoring the newly educated individuals.[66]

To initiate training, a clinical expert of the UF device's manufacturer can be called upon to facilitate educational sessions and hands-on training in the actual performance of UF therapy. Education may be provided in a variety of formats, including classroom lecture, self-directed computer-based learning, hands-on manipulation of the

Box 1: Heart failure ultrafiltration therapy orders#

Physician consultation

Cardiology consultation Nephrology consultation	Dietary consultation for low sodium dietary instruction Social services consultation for home needs Heart failure education

Nursing orders
- Accurate daily standing weights
- Strict intake and output
- 1,500 mL fluid restriction
- 1,500 mg sodium diet
- Activity: up to chair twice daily during treatment
- Patient may walk short distances and work with physical therapy if venous access is not compromised

Laboratory
- CMP, CBC, BNP, PTT, PT/INR prior to first treatment
- BMP, CBC daily while on ultrafiltration
- PTT baseline before heparin started, 4 hours after initial maintenance drip, then every 12 hours and as per adjustment scale while on heparin infusion
- PT/INR daily if on coumadin

Medications
- Discontinue all diuretics and electrolyte supplements for the duration of ultrafiltration therapy
- Avoid all nonsteroidal antiinflammatory drugs
- Hold dabigatran or rivaroxaban while patient is on heparin therapy

Venous access
- Obtain consent for venous access
- CHF 6 French dual lumen peripheral extended length catheter (cdELC) placed mid-bicep in basilic or
- 7–8 French dual lumen central line (dual 14 gauge or dual 16 gauge)
- 8.5 French quadruple lumen central line
- Central line flush and care per hospital policy

Anticoagulation
- Anticoagulation to begin 30 minutes prior to ultrafiltration therapy if heparin bolus is administered; or 60 minutes prior to therapy if heparin bolus is not indicated
- Confirm that patient does not have a history of allergy or sensitivity to heparin
- For heparin-induced thrombocytopenia patients, initiate argatroban Protocol and notify physician
- No heparin bolus if patient is on coumadin and INR greater than or equal to 1.8
- No heparin bolus if patient is on dabigatran or (rivaroxaban)
- Discontinue heparin at the end of therapy unless otherwise indicated
- Calculate and administer initial heparin bolus†
  70 units times__________kg (patient weight) = __________units (MAX Bolus = 7,000 units) round to nearest 100 units
- Calculate and begin heparin infusion: heparin 25,000 units in 250 mL D5W (100 units/mL)[2]
  15 units times _________ kg (patient weight) = __________units/hour (MAX initial rate = 1,500 units/hour) round to nearest 100 units

Contd...

Contd...

- Administer sliding scale heparin infusion adjustment[2]

PTT result	50–74 kg	75–99 kg	Greater than or equal to 100 kg	Next PTT
Less than 53	Bolus: 30 units times ____kg =_____(round to nearest 100 units) then increase infusion dose100 units/hour	Bolus: 30 units times ____kg =_____(round to nearest 100 units) then increase infusion dose150 units/hour	Bolus: 30 units times ___kg =_____(round to nearest 100 units) then increase infusion dose 200 units/hour	6 hours
54–64	Increase infusion dose100 units/hour	Increase infusion dose150 units/hour	Increase infusion dose 200 units/hour	6 hours
65–104	No change	No change	No change	12 hours
105–126	Decrease infusion dose 100 units/hour	Decrease infusion dose 150 units/hour	Decrease infusion dose 200 units/hour	6 hours
Greater than 126	Hold infusion for 60 minutes then decrease previous infusion dose 200 units/hour	Hold infusion for 60 minutes then decrease previous infusion dose 250 units/hour	Hold infusion for 60 minutes then decrease previous infusion dose 300 units/hour	6 hours

Treatment

- Prime blood circuit and tubing with 1 liter 0.9% normal saline
- Ultrafiltration rate _____ mL per hour for _____ hours or until _____ liters of ultrafiltrate removed

*UF removal rates greater than 250 mL/hour are no longer recommended

**For patients with volume sensitive states (right ventricular failure, pulmonary distress, hepatic disease, cardiogenic shock) consider lower UF rates of 50–150 mL/hour

Vital signs

- Vital signs every 30 minutes times 2 at the start of treatment, then every 2 hours for the remainder of treatment and PRN for patient status changes

Hematocrit sensor:

Begin ultrafiltration therapy and allow machine to run for 30 minutes to establish a baseline hematocrit value. After baselining is complete, set the hematocrit limit

- Accept default limit (–5%) or
- Set limit to ____% (range 0–7%)

Physician notification

- Monitor patient for signs of hypovolemia, hypotension and treatment complications (SBP less than 90 mmHg, heart rate greater than 130 BPM, cardiac arrhythmias, altered mental status, excessive bleeding from venous access site, or signs or symptoms of infection and notify prescribing physician or on-call physician
- If SBP less than 90 mmHg or heart rate greater than 130 BPM, decrease UF rate by 50% and notify physician
- If the Hct limit is repeatedly exceeded and the patient is otherwise stable and obviously fluid-overloaded, notify the prescribing physician for further orders

________________ ________________

Physician Signature **Date and Time**

[#] Note: This is a sample UF order set based on use of the Aquadex™ FlexFlow fluid removal system (Gambro UF Solutions Inc. Brooklyn Park, MN, USA).

[†] For educational purposes, this heparin protocol is based upon facility protocols, and aPTT ranges correlate with an antifactor Xa range of 0.3–0.7 U/mL.

CMP, complete metabolic profile; CBC, complete blood count; BNP, B-type natriuretic peptide; PTT, partial thromboplastin time; PT/INR, prothrombin time and international normalized ratio; BMP, blood metabolic profile; HIT, heparin-induced thrombocytopenia; PRN, pro re nata; SBP, systolic blood pressure; BPM, beats per minute; Hct, hematocrit; UF, ultrafiltration; CHF, congestive heart failure equipment through repeated demonstrations, formal and informal discussion and bedside mentoring.[67] These methods allow the designated nursing staff to become comfortable with the technology and eventually develop competence with the therapy.[65] Key components of nurse clinicians education should include information on the causes of fluid overload and diuretic refractoriness in ADHF patients, explanation of the process of UF, guidance to the selection of patients likely to benefit from UF therapy, description of the rationale and components of UF order sets, vascular access and anticoagulation requirements, choices of device blood flows and UF rates, guidance for patient assessment and monitoring and instruction on when to notify the prescribing physician regarding issues arising during UF therapy. In addition nurses assigned to deliver UF therapy should become proficient in gathering the UF pump and supplies, loading and priming the UF circuit, correct use of the Hct sensor for blood volume estimation, troubleshooting alarm conditions of the UF device and identifying criteria for the discontinuation of UF therapy. Instruction on these topics should not be limited to the time of initiation of a UF program, but it should rather become an essential component of ongoing clinical education of the nursing staff.[64] At most centers offering UF therapy, competencies on the delivery of this treatment are incorporated into the nursing staff's annual clinical education.

IMPORTANT CONSIDERATIONS REGARDING ULTRAFILTRATION THERAPY

Understanding the Function of a Device for Isolated Venovenous Ultrafiltration

Knowledge of the structure and function of UF device is essential for optimal delivery of this therapy. A schematic representation of a UF device is shown in Figure 1.

The term "circuit" refers to the tubing, hemofilter, and pump cartridges. The blood pump is a peristaltic rotary pump situated on the front face of the device's console.[67] The rotary action of the pump compresses the circuit tubing, generating a negative pressure that withdraws the blood from the patient. The pump rotation speed determines how quickly the blood circulates through the tubing. Once the blood passes through the pump, it is propelled into the hemofilter. Blood enters the hemofilter through a port at the bottom and exits through the port at the top. The structure of the hemofilter permits separation of the ultrafiltrate—water and electrolytes—from the patient's blood. The hemofilter consists of a bundle of hollow polysulfone fibers which have tiny pores within their wall. These pores allow smaller molecules, such as water and electrolytes, to pass through the hemofilter but block the passage of larger blood components, such as blood cells and proteins. As the ultrafiltrate is pulled from the blood by the UF pump, it fills the space between the fibers inside the filter case and exits the filter through a port near the top of the filter case, separate from the blood. The ultrafiltrate pump is a peristaltic rotary pump situated on the right side of the console. The rotary action of the pump compresses the circuit tubing, generating a negative pressure that extracts ultrafiltrate—water and electrolytes—from the blood. The pump rotation speed determines how quickly ultrafiltrate is removed from the patient's blood. Once the ultrafiltrate passes through the pump, it fills a collection bag, whereas the hemoconcentrated blood is returned to the patient.[67]

The UF device continuously receives input from three pressure sensors (blood withdrawal, blood infusion, and ultrafiltrate) integrated into the circuit. Disconnection of the pressure sensors or acute pressure changes indicative of occlusions in the circuit trigger system alarms, so that the problem can be immediately addressed and corrected. In addition, UF devices are equipped with an air detector which turns off the motor of both blood and UF pumps if an air bubble passes through the blood tubing.

Most contemporary UF devices also include a nonreusable data key, which holds information unique to a specific circuit (usage time, blood flow, UF rates, withdrawal, infusion and ultrafiltrate pressures and alarms). During therapy the data are continuously communicated to the console and stored in the console's memory.[68]

Venous Access

A reliably stable blood flow is critically important for optimal mechanical fluid removal, and therefore, establishment of an appropriate venous access is essential to the success of UF therapy.[69] With contemporary UF devices, venous access may be attained either peripherally or centrally, and it does not require the large bore catheters needed for other renal replacement therapies. Access attained via a peripheral entry site is preferred because it diminishes the risk of catheter-related complications and infections associated with central venous approaches.[66] Peripheral venous access can be established by a peripherally inserted central catheter (PICC) team, IV therapy teams or by a cardiologist or interventional radiologist. The peripheral catheter recommended for the Aquadex™ Flex Flow device (Gambro UF Solutions Inc., Brooklyn Park, MN) is a 6 French coiled dual lumen extended length catheter (cdELC) produced by the device's manufacturer. This catheter is usually placed in the basilic vein, at the level of the medial portion of the bicep muscle. The therapists who obtain vascular access employ techniques detailed in current protocol guidelines after receiving education specific to the cdELC.[70,71] Evaluation of venous anatomy is essential to achieve peripheral vascular access for UF.[72] Prior to catheter placement, the basilic vein diameter can be measured by ultrasound. For accurate measurements application of a tourniquet or blood pressure cuff to the forearm should be avoided because these instruments can increase the basilic vein diameter by as much as 0.7 mm and 0.9 mm, respectively, resulting in overestimation of vein size.[73] The desired cross-sectional vein diameter should be at least 4 mm, equivalent to a 12 French catheter lumen. The importance of this recommendation is underscored by the observation that a 6 French object (2 mm) placed in a 4 mm tube reduces downstream flow by 80%, whereas the same object placed in a 3.5 mm tube reduces downstream flow by 92%.[72]

Traditional PICC lines are not recommended due to the catheters' length and narrow bore as well as their flexible material which may result in excessive kinking leading to unwanted termination of UF therapy. Additionally, IV catheters with bores larger than 6 French are not recommended for peripheral access and are not needed due to the low blood flows employed by isolated venovenous UF devices, such as the Aquadex™ Flex Flow System. Certain patient characteristics may limit peripheral vascular access including small, tortuous or stenotic veins, poor circulation, obesity with large upper arm circumference, or an exceptional degree of fluid overload. When peripheral access is unachievable or contra-indicated, central venous access can be utilized. Central venous catheters, most commonly inserted in the internal jugular vein, can be placed by appropriately trained cardiologists or interventional radiologists, either at the bedside or in catheterization suites. Hospital policies for central venous line insertion should be followed. The minimum catheter lumen size for central venous access is 14–16 gauge. Recommended catheters for central venous access include a 7 or 8 French dual lumen or an 8.5 French quadruple lumen central venous catheter. At some institutions temporary dialysis catheters have also been utilized to deliver UF therapy. Regardless of whether a peripheral or central venous access is utilized, the institutional policies regarding anchoring and flushing of the catheter, and site dressing and care should be meticulously followed.

ANTICOAGULATION DURING ULTRAFILTRATION THERAPY

Clinical experience with venovenous UF indicates that preservation of catheter patency and prevention of filter thrombosis may be enhanced by the administration of parenteral anticoagulation. Therefore, UF may not be indicated for patients with contraindications to anticoagulation, such as a high risk for bleeding events. In such patients, performing UF without anticoagulation has been attempted, but may present challenges in achieving a desirable therapy outcome. Unfractionated heparin is the anticoagulant used in the vast majority of cases. In patients with heparin-induced thrombocytopenia (HIT), direct thrombin inhibitors may be considered as alternative agents.[62] Based on clinical experience, low-molecular-weight heparin delivered via subcutaneous injection does not effectively prevent filter clotting, and, if used for anticoagulation prior to UF therapy should be discontinued and substituted with IV heparin during mechanical fluid removal.

To reduce the incidence of filter and venous catheter thrombosis, therapeutic anticoagulation should be maintained throughout the duration of therapy. Anticoagulation goals correspond to either an antifactor Xa range of 0.3–0.7 U/mL or the equivalent activated partial thromboplastin time (aPTT) range. It should be noted that the therapeutic aPTT range can vary significantly among testing facilities due to the wide variety of testing agents used to procure and analyze blood samples.

Regardless of the testing method employed, antifactor Xa and/or aPTT should be monitored 6 hours after the initiation of IV heparin, and every 6–12 hours, thereafter, to maintain therapeutic anticoagulation throughout the duration of UF therapy.[74]

In patients fully anticoagulated on warfarin, rivaroxaban, or dabigatran, omission of an IV heparin bolus before initiation of a continuous IV infusion occurs at the discretion of the prescriber and based upon the anticoagulation protocols of the institution. Anticoagulation with IV heparin should be done according to the recommendations issued in clinical practice guidelines on the use of this drug.[74,75] Importantly, clinical experience has shown significant reductions in peripheral venous catheter or filter clotting if IV heparin is initiated at least 30 minutes prior to UF therapy when a heparin bolus is used, and at least 60 minutes before treatment if a heparin bolus is omitted. Continuation of warfarin during UF should be determined on an individual patient basis.[64] In contrast, rivaroxaban and dabigatran should be held during UF and resumed upon completion of therapy according to the practice guideline recommendations on the conversion from heparin to the appropriate doses of oral anticoagulants.[74,75]

CONSIDERATIONS ON THE MONITORING OF ULTRAFILTRATION THERAPY

Essential components of the management of patients undergoing UF include routine measurement of vital signs, with a special focus on blood pressure and heart rate, daily measurement of laboratory values, including Hct, blood urea nitrogen (BUN), sCr and appropriate biomarkers (as outlined in the standing orders shown in Box 1), electrocardiogram (ECG) monitoring for the early detection of arrhythmias, and compulsive measurement of daily fluid intake and output.

As discussed earlier in the chapter, the safety and efficacy of UF hinge upon the ability to remove fluid without causing hypotension and/or acute renal injury. Therefore, the amount and rate of fluid removal by UF should be clearly established on the basis individual patients' characteristics, including degree of pulmonary and systemic congestion, baseline blood pressure and renal function values. In addition risk of intravascular volume depletion should be carefully assessed on a case by case basis, particularly in patients with volume sensitive states, such as right heart failure, pulmonary arterial hypertension, hepatic disease, or cardiogenic shock.[29] Fluid removal rates with the Aquadex™ FlexFlow device range between 0 mL/hour and 500 mL/hour. However, fluid removal rates faster than 250 mL/hour are no longer recommended. Further, reduction of UF rates below 150 mL/hour should be considered in patients at high risk for intravascular volume depletion.[44]

In each patient, the relief of congestion by UF therapy without causing hemodynamic and renal complications is strictly dependent upon the ability to remove ultrafiltrate from the plasma at the same rate at which interstitial fluid is reabsorbed into the intravascular space (PRR).[19,62] Because there are no clinically available methods to directly measure PRR, changes in blood volume during UF can be estimated with the assessment of changes in Hct values, as outlined earlier in the chapter.[66] In contemporary UF devices Hct sensors can be placed within the circuit (proximally to UF pump) for continuous estimation of blood volume changes during UF therapy. The physician prescribing UF therapy establishes the threshold of Hct change believed to be acceptable in individual patients (typical range is between 0% and 7%). When the sensor detects that the predetermined limit of Hct change is reached, fluid removal is automatically stopped, whereas the blood pump will continue to operate to preserve filter patency.[68] Production of ultrafiltrate will automatically resume when the Hct value drops below the threshold set by the treating physician.

It is important to point out that estimation of blood volume using the Hct sensor should be used in conjunction with, and not as a substitute for, careful clinical and laboratory assessment.

If in a patient undergoing UF, changes in Hct repeatedly exceed the limit set by the treating physician, signs of volume depletion should be immediately investigated. In some patients, invasive hemodynamic assessment may be necessary if Hct values rise above the established threshold despite the persistence of signs and symptoms of fluid overload.[18,62] It must be stressed that hemodynamic instability will occur if UF rates are too fast or if UF is allowed to continue beyond the achievement of the fluid removal goals set before initiation of therapy.[62,65]

TECHNICAL ASPECTS OF HEMATOCRIT MONITORING

During UF therapy, blood passes through a small chamber integrated into the withdrawal line of the circuit, proximal to the blood pump. A sensor which uses infrared technology can measure changes in Hct in real time.[19] The Hct sensor can either be attached with a clip to the blood chamber on the blood circuit or placed in its docking station at the rear of the console.[68] Although intuitive, it is important to point out that only when attached to the blood chamber does the sensor measure the Hct in the blood withdrawn from the patient. Placement of the sensor in the docking station in the back of the console disables Hct monitoring and a message to this effect is displayed on the screen of the console. The first time the Hct sensor is placed on the blood chamber, the device will initiate a 10–20 minutes process to establish the value of the baseline Hct.[68] Upon completion of this process, the treating physician has the choice of either accepting the default increase in Hct of 5% or establishing a different limit of Hct change as the threshold at which fluid withdrawal is halted. As long as the Hct value measured by the sensor is below the set limit, fluid removal continues at the rate set by the treating physician. For example, if a patient's baseline Hct is 40% and a maximum blood volume depletion of 5% is deemed acceptable, the Hct value above which fluid withdrawal is halted is 42%, as per the formula:

$$(0.05 \times 40) + 40 = 42\%.$$

If the Hct measured by the sensor exceeds 42%, indicating that the patient's blood volume is reduced by more than 5%, the UF pump will stop fluid removal until the measured Hct declines below the set limit, whereas the blood pump will continue to function to prevent circuit clotting. It is important to note that, due to different measuring techniques, the Hct value obtained by the sensor may only be correlated, but not identical to that measured in the laboratory.[76]

NOTIFICATION OF THE PHYSICIAN PRESCRIBING ULTRAFILTRATION THERAPY

Clear guidelines should be established regarding notification of the treating physician by the nurse assigned to a patient receiving UF therapy. Appropriate instances in which the treating physician should be contacted include all the changes in a patient's condition that may warrant adjustment of fluid removal rates, discontinuation of UF or catheter-related complications.[64,65] These events include the detection of hypotension, tachycardia, cardiac arrhythmias, frequent rise of the Hct above the established limit, finding of abnormal laboratory results, excessive bleeding from the venous access site, appearance of signs or symptoms of infection and the occurrence of filter clotting.

DISCONTINUATION OF ULTRAFILTRATION THERAPY

Each institution offering UF therapy to ADHF patients should clearly outline the conditions under which the patient is deemed to have achieved the fluid removal goals established before initiation of therapy. Examples of these circumstances include resolution of pulmonary and systemic congestion, as defined earlier in the chapter, attainment of dry weight and increases in Hct and sCr levels considered as unacceptable by the treating physician.

CONCLUSION

For more than a century, sodium has been recognized as the major determinant of extracellular fluid volume in HF. Therefore, excess total body sodium should be the principal target for the therapy of patients hospitalized for worsening symptoms and signs of congestion. Loop diuretics, although often effective in removing reduced sodium concentrations in urine, are inherently incapable of consistently reducing total body sodium. Indeed, despite the nearly universal use of loop diuretics, death and rehospitalization rates for ADHF patients remain unacceptably high. Because of its mechanism, UF predictably reduces total body sodium. However, safe and effective decongestion by UF requires both careful selection of candidates for the therapy and fine-tuning of fluid removal rates according to each patient's hemodynamics and renal function. The unfavorable outcomes of the CARRESS-HF trial are a reminder. Fluid removal rates should be based upon each patient's clinical characteristics.

Conversely, the sustained benefits observed in the UNLOAD trial indicate that initiation of UF in ADHF patients before they fail high-dose IV diuretics is a safer and more effective strategy. The ongoing Aquapheresis versus Intravenous Diuretics and Hospitalizations for Heart Failure (AVOID-HF) trial (NCT01474200), with more than 800 ADHF subjects being enrolled at 40 US centers, will determine if a strategy of early UF, initiated before the onset of the CRS type 1, reduces heart failure-related hospitalizations more than IV diuretics.

While the AVOID-HF will further define the role of isolated venovenous UF in ADHF patients, clinical experience accumulated over the past decade shows that the successful use of this therapy hinges upon the creation of a program in which several key requirements are met. These include identification and active involvement of a physician champion, assembly of a multidisciplinary core clinical team, acquisition of in-depth knowledge of the structure and function of the UF device, development of comprehensive order sets, establishment of optimal vascular access, and meticulous management of anticoagulation.

REFERENCES

1. Dickstein K, Cohen-Solal A, Filippatos G, et al. ESC Guidelines for the diagnosis and treatment of acute and chronic heart failure 2008: the Task Force for the Diagnosis and Treatment of Acute and Chronic Heart Failure 2008 of the European Society of Cardiology. Developed in collaboration with the Heart Failure Association of the ESC (HFA) and endorsed by the European Society of Intensive Care Medicine (ESICM). Eur Heart J. 2008;29(19):2388-442.
2. Nohria A, Tsang SW, Fang JC, et al. Clinical assessment identifies hemodynamic profiles that predict outcomes in patients admitted with heart failure. J Am Coll Cardiol. 2003;41(10):1797-804.
3. Bram B, Cupples WA, Joles JA, et al. Systemic arterial and venous determinants of renal hemodynamics in congestive heart failure. Heart Fail Rev. 2012;17(2):161-75.

4. Heywood JT, Fonarow GC, Costanzo MR, et al. High prevalence of renal dysfunction and its impact on outcome in 118,465 patients hospitalized with acute decompensated heart failure: a report from the ADHERE database. J Card Fail. 2007;13(6):422-30.
5. Gheorghiade M, Gattis WA, O'Connor CM, et al. Effects of tolvaptan, a vasopressin antagonist, in patients hospitalized with worsening heart failure: a randomized controlled trial. JAMA. 2004;291(16):1963-71.
6. Schlatter E, Salomonsson M, Persson AE, et al. Macula densa cells sense luminal NaCl concentration via furosemide sensitive Na+2Cl-K+ cotransport. Pflugers Arch. 1989;414(3):286-90.
7. Felker GM, Lee KL, Bull DA, et al. Diuretic Strategies in patients with acute decompensated heart failure. New Engl J Med. 2011;364(9):797-805.
8. Butler J, Forman DE, Abraham WT, et al. Relationship between heart failure treatment and development of worsening renal function among hospitalized heart failure patients. Am Heart J. 2004;147(2):331-8.
9. Hasselblad V, Gattis Stough W, Shah MR, et al. Relation between dose of loop diuretics and outcomes in a heart failure population: results of the ESCAPE Trial. Eur J Heart Fail. 2007;9(10):1064-9.
10. Peacock WF, Costanzo MR, De Marco T, et al. Impact of intravenous loop diuretics on outcomes of patients hospitalized with acute decompensated heart failure: insights from the ADHERE registry. Cardiology. 2009;113(1): 12-9.
11. Metra M, Nodari S, Parrinello G, et al. Worsening renal function in patients hospitalised for acute heart failure: clinical implications and prognostic significance. Eur J Heart Fail. 2008:10(2):188-95.
12. Konstam MA, Gheorghiade M, Burnett JC Jr, et al. Effects of oral tolvaptan in patients hospitalized for worsening heart failure: the EVEREST Outcome Trial. JAMA. 2007;297(12):1319-31.
13. Massie BM, O'Connor CM, Metra M, et al. Rolofylline, an adenosine A1-receptor antagonist, in acute heart failure. New Engl J Med. 2010; 363(15):1419-28.
14. Costanzo MR, Jessup M. Treatment of congestion in heart failure with diuretics and extracorporeal therapies: effects on symptoms, renal function, and prognosis. Heart Fail Rev. 2012;17(2):313-24.
15. Ronco C, Ricci Z, Bellomo R, et al. Extracorporeal ultrafiltration for the treatment of overhydration and congestive heart failure. Cardiology. 2001;96(3-4):155-68.
16. Schrier RW, Abraham WT. Hormones and hemodynamics in heart failure. N Engl J Med. 1999;341(8):577-85.
17. Ellison DH, Velazquez H, Wright FS. Adaptation of the distal convoluted tubule of the rat. Structural and functional effects of dietary salt intake and chronic diuretic infusion. J Clin Invest. 1989;83(1):113-26.
18. Marenzi G, Lauri G, Grazi M, et al. Circulatory response to fluid overload removal by extracorporeal ultrafiltration in refractory congestive heart failure. J Am Coll Cardiol. 2001;38(4):963-8.
19. Ronco C, Brendolan A, Bellomo R. Online monitoring in continuous renal replacement therapies. Kidney Int Suppl. 1999;(72):S8-14.
20. Jaski BE, Ha J, Denys BG, et al. Peripherally inserted veno-venous ultrafiltration for rapid treatment of volume overloaded patients. J Card Fail. 2003;9(3):227-31.
21. Ronco C, Haapio M, House AA, et al. Cardiorenal syndrome. J Am Coll Cardiol. 2008;52(19):1527-39.
22. Kellum JA, Bellomo R, Ronco C. Acute Dialysis Quality Initiative (ADQI): methodology. Int J Artif Organs. 2008;31(2):90-3.
23. Costanzo MR, Saltzberg M, O'Sullivan J, et al. Early ultrafiltration in patients with decompensated heart failure and diuretic resistance. J Am Coll Cardiol. 2005;46(11):2047-51.
24. Agostoni P, Marenzi G, Lauri G, et al. Sustained improvement in functional capacity after removal of body fluid with isolated ultrafiltration in chronic cardiac insufficiency: failure of furosemide to provide the same result. Am J Med. 1994;96(3):191-9.
25. Bart BA, Boyle A, Bank AJ, et al. Ultrafiltration versus usual care for hospitalized patients with heart failure: the Relief for Acutely Fluid-Overloaded Patients with Decompensated Congestive Heart Failure (RAPID-CHF) trial. J Am Coll Cardiol. 2005;46(11):2043-6.
26. Liang KV, Hiniker AR, Wiliams AW, et al. Use of a novel ultrafiltration device as a treatment strategy for diuretic resistant, refractory heart failure: initial clinical experience in a single center. J Card Fail. 2006;12(9):707-14.
27. Rose EA, Gelijns AC, Moskowitz AJ, et al. Long-term use of a left ventricular assist device for end-stage heart failure. N Engl J Med. 2001;345(20):1435-43.
28. Cipolla CM, Grazi S, Rimondini A, et al. Changes in circulating norepinephrine with hemofiltration in advanced congestive heart failure. Am J Cardiol. 1990;66(12):987-94.
29. Marenzi G, Grazi S, Giraldi F, et al. Interrelation of humoral factors, hemodynamics, and fluid and salt metabolism in congestive heart failure: effects of extracorporeal ultrafiltration. Am J Med. 1993;94(1):49-56.
30. Costanzo MR, Guglin ME, Saltzberg MT, et al. Ultrafiltration versus intravenous diuretics for patients hospitalized for acute decompensated heart failure. J Am Coll Cardiol. 2007;49(6):675-83.
31. Elkayam U, Hatamizadeh P, Janmohamed M. The challenge of correcting volume overload in hospitalized patients with decompensated heart failure. J Am Coll Cardiol. 2007;49(6):684-6.
32. Costanzo MR, Saltzberg MT, Jessup M, et al. Ultrafiltration is associated with fewer rehospitalizations than continuous diuretic infusion in patients with decompensated heart failure: results from UNLOAD. J Card Fail. 2010;16(4):277-84.
33. Ali SS, Olinger CC, Sobotka PA, et al. Loop diuretics can cause clinical natriuretic failure: a prescription for volume expansion. Congest Heart Fail. 2009;15(1):1-4.
34. Abdallah JG, Schreier RW, Edelstein C, et al. Loop diuretic infusion increases thiazide-sensitive Na(+)/Cl(-)-cotransporter abundance: role of aldosterone. J Am Soc Nephrol. 2001;12(7):1335-41.
35. Mullens W, Abrahams Z, Francis GS, et al. Importance of venous congestion for worsening of renal function in advanced decompensated heart failure. J Am Coll Cardiol. 2009;53(7):589-96.
36. Jessup M, Costanzo MR. The cardiorenal syndrome: do we need a change of strategy or a change of tactics? J Am Coll Cardiol. 2009;53(7):597-9.
37. Ross EA. Congestive renal failure: the pathophysiology and treatment of renal venous hypertension. J Card Fail. 2012;18(12):930-8.
38. Bart BA, Goldsmith SR, Lee KL, et al. Ultrafiltration in decompensated heart failure with cardiorenal syndrome. New Engl J Med. 2012:367(24):2296-304.
39. Bart BA, Goldsmith SR, Lee KL et al. Cardiorenal rescue study in acute decompensated heart failure: rationale and design of CARRESS-HF, for the Heart Failure Clinical Research Network. J Card Fail. 2012;18(3):176-82.
40. Testani JM, Chen J, McCauley BD, et al. Potential effects of aggressive decongestion during the treatment of decompensated heart failure on renal function and survival. Circulation. 2010;122(3):265-72.
41. Bartone C, Saghir S, Menon SG, et al. Comparison of ultrafiltration, nesiritide, and usual care in acute decompensated heart failure. Congest Heart Fail. 2008;14(6):298-301.
42. Patarroyo M, Wehbe E, Hanna M, et al. Cardiorenal outcomes after slow continuous ultrafiltration therapy in refractory patients with advanced decompensated heart failure. J Am Coll Cardiol. 2012;60(19):1906-12.
43. Dev S, Shirolkar SC, Stevens SR, et al. Reduction in body weight but worsening renal function with late ultrafiltration for treatment of acute decompensated heart failure. Cardiology. 2012;123(3):145-53.

44. Costanzo MR, Ronco C. Isolated ultrafiltration in heart failure patients. Curr Cardiol Rep. 2012;14(3):254-64.
45. Singh P, Rifkin DE, Blantz RC. Chronic kidney disease: an inherent risk factor for acute kidney injury? Clin J Am Soc Nephrol. 2010;5(9):1690-5.
46. Tang WH. Reconsidering ultrafiltration in the acute cardiorenal syndrome. N Engl J Med. 2012;367(24):2351-2.
47. Jessup M, Abraham WT, Casey DE, et al. 2009 focused update: ACCF/AHA Guidelines for the Diagnosis and Management of Heart Failure in Adults: a report of the American College of Cardiology Foundation/American Heart Association Task Force on Practice Guidelines: developed in collaboration with the International Society for Heart and Lung Transplantation. Circulation. 2009;119(14):1977-2016.
48. Howlett JG, McKelvie RS, Costigan J, et al. The 2010 Canadian Cardiovascular Society guidelines for the diagnosis and management of heart failure update: Heart failure in ethnic minority populations, heart failure and pregnancy, disease management, and quality improvement/assurance programs. Can J Cardiol. 2010;26(4):185-202.
49. Gheorghiade M, Follath F, Ponikowski P, et al. Assessing and grading congestion in acute heart failure: a scientific statement from the acute heart failure committee of the heart failure association of the European Society of Cardiology and endorsed by the European Society of Intensive Care Medicine. Eur J Heart Fail. 2010;12(5):423-33.
50. Stawicki SP, Braslow BM, Panebianco NL, et al. Intensivist use of hand-carried ultrasonography to measure IVC collapsibility in estimating intravascular volume status: correlation with CVP. J Am Coll Surg. 2009;209(1):55-61.
51. Maisel AS, Krishnaswamy P, Nowak RM, et al. Rapid measurement of B-Type natriuretic peptide in the emergency diagnosis of heart failure. N Engl J Med. 2002;347(3):161-7.
52. Maisel AS. Use of BNP levels in monitoring hospitalized heart failure patients with heart failure. Heart Fail Rev. 2003;8(4):339-44.
53. Bettencourt P, Ferreira S, Azevedo A, et al. Preliminary data on the potential usefulness of B-type natriuretic peptide levels in predicting outcome after hospital discharge in patients with heart failure. Am J Med. 2002;113(3):215-9.
54. Maisel A, Mueller C, Adams K Jr, et al. State of the art: using natriuretic peptide levels in clinical practice. Eur J Heart Fail. 2008;10(9):824-39.
55. Haapio M, House AA, de Cal M, et al. Heart-kidney biomarkers in patients undergoing cardiac stress testing. Int J Nephrol. 2010;2011:425923.
56. Piccoli A, Nigelli S, Caberlotto A, et al. Bivariate normal values of the bioelectrical impedance vector in adult and elderly populations. Am J Clin Nutr. 1995;61(2):269-70.
57. Kushner RF, Schoeller DA, Fjeld CR, et al. Is the impedance index (ht2/R) significant in predicting total body water? Am J Clin Nutr. 1992;56(5):835-9.
58. Piccoli A. Whole body—single frequency bioimpedance. Contrib Nephrol. 2005;149:150-61.
59. Aspromonte N, Cruz DN, Valle R, et al. Management and monitoring of haemodynamic complications in acute heart failure. Heart Fail Rev. 2011;16(6):575-81.
60. Valle R, Aspromonte N, Milani L, et al. Optimizing fluid management in patients with acute decompensated heart failure (ADHF): the emerging role of combined measurement of body hydration status and brain natriuretic peptide (BNP) levels. Heart Fail Rev. 2011;16(6):519-29.
61. House AA, Haapio M, Lentini P, et al. Volume assessment in mechanically ventilated critical care patients using bioimpedance vectorial analysis, brain natriuretic Peptide, and central venous pressure. Int J Nephrol. 2010;2011:413760.
62. Costanzo MR, Cozzolino M, Aspromonte N, et al. Extracorporeal ultrafiltration in heart failure and cardio-renal syndromes. Semin Nephrol. 2012;32(1):100-11.
63. Ronco C., Kaushik M, Valle R, et al. Diagnosis and management of fluid overload in heart failure and the cardio-renal syndrome: the "5B" approach. Semin Nephrol. 2012;32(1):129-141.
64. Peterangelo M. Incorporating aquapheresis into the hospital setting: a practical approach. Prog Cardiovasc Nurs. 2008;23(4):168-72.
65. Walsh CT, Wagemester D. Peripheral ultrafiltration for patients with volume overload: a center's 4-year experience. Crit Care Nurs Q. 2007;30(4):329-36.
66. Dahle TG, Sobotka PA, Boyle AJ. A practical guide for ultrafiltration in acute decompensated heart failure. Congest Heart Fail. 2008;14(2):83-8.
67. Nalesso F, Garzotto F, Ronco C. Technical aspects of extracorporeal ultrafiltration: mechanisms, monitoring and dedicated technology. Contrib Nephrol. 2010;164:199-208.
68. Gambro UF Solutions Inc. Aquadex TM flex flow fluid removal system user's guide AW0021: Rev Q 4/12
69. Draftz M. (2007). Ultrafiltration: A New Challenge for Vascular Access Specialists. [Online] Available from http://www.sciencedirect.com/science/article/pii/S155288550770346X?np=y. [Accessed December, 2013].
70. Infusion Nursing Standards of Practice. J Infus Nurs. 2011:34(1s);s1-108. http://www.americannursetoday.com/Article.aspx?id=10634
71. O'Grady NP, Alexander M, Burns LA, et al. Summary of recommendations: Guidelines for the Prevention of Intravascular Catheter-related Infections. Clin Infect Dis. 2011;52(9):1087-99.
72. Nifong TP, McDevitt TJ. The effect of catheter to vein ratio on blood flow rates in a simulated model of peripherally inserted central venous catheters. Chest. 2011;140(1):48-53.
73. Mahler SA, Massey G, Meskill L, et al. Can we make the basilic vein larger? Maneuvers to facilitate ultrasound guided peripheral intravenous access: a prospective cross-sectional study. Int J Emerg Med. 2011; 4:53.
74. Hirsch J, Bauer KA, Donati MB, et al. Parenteral anticoagulants: American College of Chest Physicians Evidence-Based Clinical Practice Guidelines (8th Edition). Chest. 2008;133(6 Suppl):141S-159S.
75. Cushman M, Lim W, Zakai NA. (2011). 2011 Clinical Practice Guide on Anticoagulant Dosing and Management of Anticoagulant-Associated Bleeding Complications in Adults. [online] Available from http://www.hematology.org/practice/guidelines/7243.aspx. [Accessed November, 2013]
76. Steuer RR, Bell DA, Barrett LL. Optical measurement of hematocrit and other biological constituents in renal therapy. Adv Ren Replace Ther. 1999;6(3):217-24.

Chapter 21

Who Should Receive a Pulmonary Artery Catheter

Robert T Cole, Javed Butler

ABSTRACT

Since the development of the bedside flotation catheter in 1970, the pulmonary artery catheter (PAC) has been an invaluable tool in the evaluation and treatment of patients with critical illness, including shock, sepsis, respiratory failure, pulmonary hypertension (HTN) and heart failure (HF). Yet, the bulk of available data from randomized controlled trials (RCTs) suggest that there is no benefit to the use of PACs in these populations; in fact, in many cases, their use may result in harm. However, there has only been one such RCT in the HF population, and this trial excluded the very patients most likely to benefit from this procedure. Clearly, there are a number of clinical scenarios in which HF patients may benefit from hemodynamic assessment with a PAC, including those with cardiogenic shock, unexplained hypotension, unexplained renal failure, and those who do not respond appropriately to standard therapies, to name a few. Both the Heart Failure Society of America (HFSA) and the American College of Cardiology (ACC)/American Heart Association (AHA) have proposed recommendations on the appropriate use of PACs. The judicious use of the PAC will undoubtedly continue to provide critical, timely information to HF clinicians, particularly when used in patients with advanced disease.

INTRODUCTION

Perhaps no diagnostic tool has been as vital to our understanding of cardiac physiology and pathophysiology as the pulmonary artery catheter (PAC); yet, there continues to be considerable controversy over its clinical utility. This is particularly true in patients with HF. While randomized controlled trials (RCTs) of the PAC may have resulted in neutral effect on outcomes, clinically the usefulness of PAC in advanced HF patients cannot be denied. In this chapter, we will review the history of the PAC with special emphasis on the HF patient, the available literature on the PAC and the common indications for PAC placement in HF patients.

HISTORICAL PERSPECTIVE

The origin of the PAC finds its roots in an operating room in Eberswalde, Germany, where Werner Forssmann first inserted a 65 cm ureteral catheter into his own right atrium via an antecubital vein approach.[1] His pioneering self-experimentation laid the foundation for the rapidly expanding field of "angiocardiography". Decades of ensuing research and technological advances led to our current understanding of cardiac physiology and pathophysiology. However, it was not until the creation of the small, balloon-tipped flotation catheter by Drs Swan and Ganz in 1970 that the use of the PAC became widespread.[2] For the first time, a PAC could be placed safely at the bedside without the use of fluoroscopy, and it could provide immediate clinical information in critically ill patients.

By the 1990s, the PAC found widespread use in most intensive care units (ICUs), with as many as 40% of patients having a PAC placed within 24 hours of admission.[3] While there was initially little data to support or refute the common use of this diagnostic tool, it provided invaluable information in patients presenting with acute myocardial infarction (AMI), shock, severe HF, acute respiratory distress syndrome (ARDS) and

TABLE 1: Randomized controlled trials of pulmonary artery catheters

RCT	*Year*	*N value*	*Clinical indication/study*	*Outcomes studied*	*Conclusion*
Rhodes et al.[16]	2002	201	Critically ill patients	Survival at 28 days Length of stay Organ dysfunction	No difference in outcomes between PAC and non-PAC groups
Sandham et al.[12]	2003	1994	Elderly, high-risk surgical patients requiring intensive care unit stay after urgent or elective surgery	In-hospital survival Survival at 6 and 12 months In-hospital morbidity (MI, PE, CHF, PNA, arrhytmia, etc.)	No difference in outcomes between PAC and non-PAC groups Higher rates of PE in PAC group
Richard et al.[13]	2003	676	Patients with shock, ARDS, or both	Survival at 28 days Survival at 14 and 90 days Organ dysfunction at 14 days Vasoactive agents and renal support at 14 days Hospital, ICU, and ventilator-free days at 28 days	No difference outcomes between PAC and non-PAC groups
Harvey et al.[14] (PAC-Man trial)	2005	1014	Critically ill patients	In-hospital survival Adverse events	No difference in outcomes between PAC and non-PAC groups
Binanay et al.[15] (ESCAPE trial)	2005	433	Advanced heart failure patients	Days alive out of hospital at 6 months Exercise, biochemical, QOL, and echo changes	No difference in outcomes between PAC and non-PAC groups
Wheeler et al.[17] (NHLBI ARDS-Network trial)	2006	1000	ARDS patients PAC vs central venous access	Survival at 60 days Organ dysfucntion	No difference in outcomes between PAC and non-PAC groups Twice as many catheter-related complications in PAC group

RCT, randomized controlled trial; PAC, pulmonary artery catheter; MI, myocardial infarction; PE, pulmonary embolism; CHF, congestive heart failure; ICU, intensive care unit; QOL, quality of life; ARDS, acute respiratory distress syndrome; PAC-Man trial, pulmonary artery catheters in management of patients in intensive care; ESCAPE, Evaluation Study of Congestive Heart Failure and Pulmonary Artery Catheterization Effectiveness; NHLBI, National Heart, Lung, and Blood Institute

pulmonary HTN.[4] However, as with any new technology, overuse, and in cases by inexperienced operators, led to adverse events, including death. One early study, for example, cited a 4% risk of PAC-related mortality when used in patients with pulmonary edema of unclear etiology.[5] Such adverse outcomes in the absence of a RCT data demonstrating the benefit of PACs led many to call for a "moratorium" on their use.[6-9] Several observational studies emerged suggesting that the routine use of PACs resulted in either neutral or negative outcomes compared to standard therapy alone.[3,10,11] The growing concerns over the safety of PACs eventually led to a number of RCTs to truly assess the efficacy of PACs in a variety of clinical scenarios.[12-17] None of these RCTs showed a benefit to the use of PAC-guided therapy in patients with critical illness, shock, ARDS, or HF (Table 1).

Subsequently, the use of PACs in the ICU has declined substantially over the last 10–15 years. For example, between the years of 1993 and 2004, the number of PACs declined from 5.66 to 1.99 per 1,000 hospital admissions, a 65% relative reduction.[18] This was found to be true regardless of diagnosis at the time of admission (Fig. 1), although the greatest decrease in PAC use was seen in AMI patients (81% reduction). The use of PACs in patients admitted with HF also fell by 65% during the same time period.

PULMONARY ARTERY CATHETER USE IN HEART FAILURE

Since the development of the bedside flotation catheter in 1970, the PAC has been an invaluable tool in the

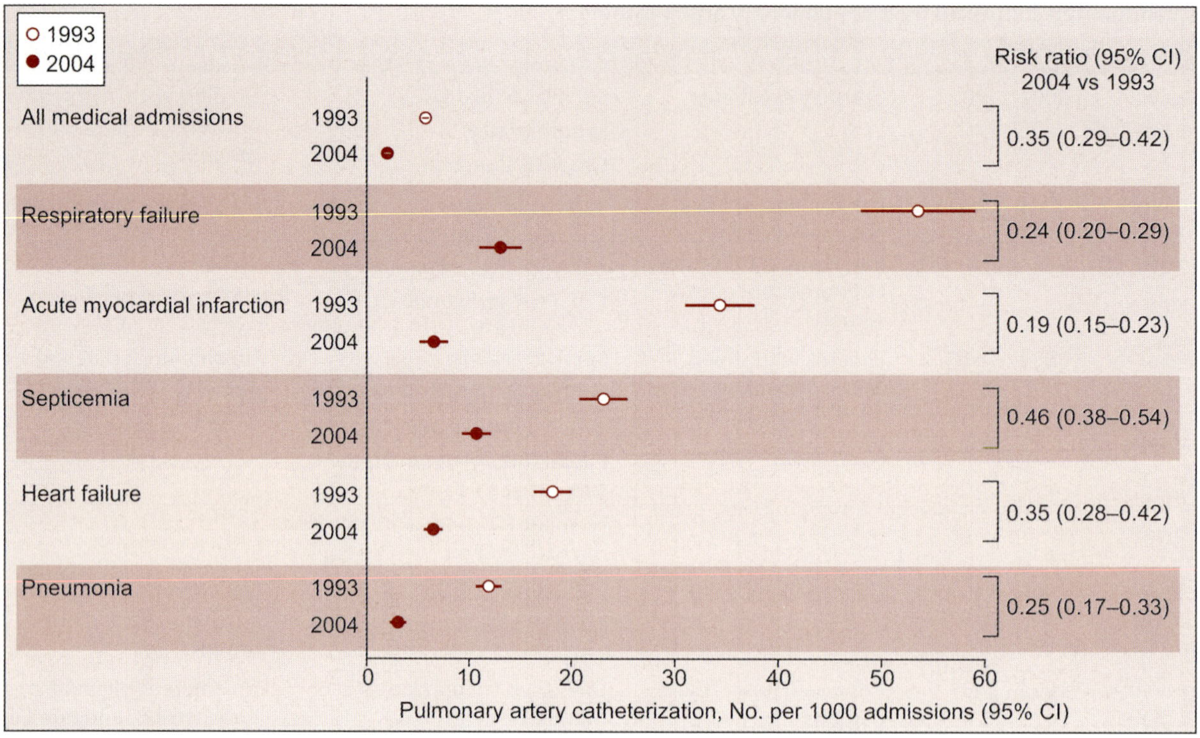

CI, confidence interval

Fig. 1 Differences in pulmonary artery catheter (PAC) use from 1993 to 2004. The use of PAC declined substantially from 1993 to 2004 in a variety of clinical settings. On average, there was a 65% relative reduction in their use during this time period[18]

evaluation and treatment of patients with HF, especially those with severe disease. Early studies suggested that patients with the most severe derangements in filling pressures and systemic vascular resistance (SVR) had the worst outcomes.[19,20] In light of these findings, the PAC was subsequently used to "tailor" hemodynamics in HF patients with advanced disease. In the "tailored therapy" paradigm, patients receive a PAC to facilitate rapid titration of intravenous vasodilators, most commonly sodium nitroprusside, toward prespecified hemodynamic goals [pulmonary capillary wedge pressure (PCWP) <16 mmHg, right atrial pressure (RAP) <8 mmHg and SVR <1,200 dynes sec cm^{-5}].[21] Upon achieving the optimal hemodynamics, nitroprusside was weaned while oral vasodilators (e.g., captopril, hydralazine and isosorbide dinitrate) were uptitrated to maintain similar hemodynamics. Employment of this strategy resulted in improvement in symptoms, increased exercise capacity,[22,23] reduction in neurohormonal activation[24] and allowed for the safe discharge of patients referred for urgent transplantation.[25] Importantly, those who were poor responders to tailored therapy had worse survival at 1 year (38% vs 83%, $p = 0.001$).[26]

While these earlier data on the use of the PAC to tailor therapy in HF showed great promise, the results were based on observational studies. In addition, these studies were undertaken in an era during which therapy for HF did not routinely include therapies like beta blockers, which have dramatically changed the landscape of HF treatment and prognosis. In 2005, the ESCAPE (Evaluation Study of Congestive Heart Failure and Pulmonary Artery Catheterization Effectiveness) investigators published the first RCT of PACs in HF.[15] This landmark trial randomized advanced HF patients to therapy guided by a PAC or by clinical assessment. A total of 433 patients from 26 centers in the United States and Canada were included. Only patients with severe, symptomatic HF were included [mean ejection fraction 19%, systolic blood pressure (SBP) 106 mmHg], but there were several notable exclusion criteria. In particular, the trial did not include patients deemed sick enough to warrant placement of a PAC by the treating physician. Other exclusions included patients with a serum creatinine (sCr) greater than 3.5 mg/dL, any prior use of dobutamine or dopamine at doses greater than 3 μg/kg/minute, or the use of milrinone during the concurrent hospitalization. Thus, the sickest HF patients were not in this trial. The results of ESCAPE showed that there was no difference between the two arms in the primary outcome of days alive out the hospital (Fig. 2). In addition, there was no difference in time to death or hospitalization, death, or total days hospitalized. A number of secondary outcomes were also neutral, including natriuretic peptide levels and functional assessments. The number of adverse events was greater in the PAC group, although there was no increase in mortality associated with PAC use as described in earlier studies.

The authors of the ESCAPE trial concluded that the use of a PAC was not warranted in the routine treatment of advanced hospitalized HF patients. Unfortunately, this result is commonly misinterpreted to mean that PACs are not useful in HF patients. As noted previously, the sickest patients and those who required a PAC clinically were excluded from ESCAPE. Despite the neutral outcomes in ESCAPE, PAC remains an invaluable diagnostic tool in a number of clinical scenarios, including HF patients with cardiogenic shock, hypotension, or those who worsen despite standard therapy, etc.

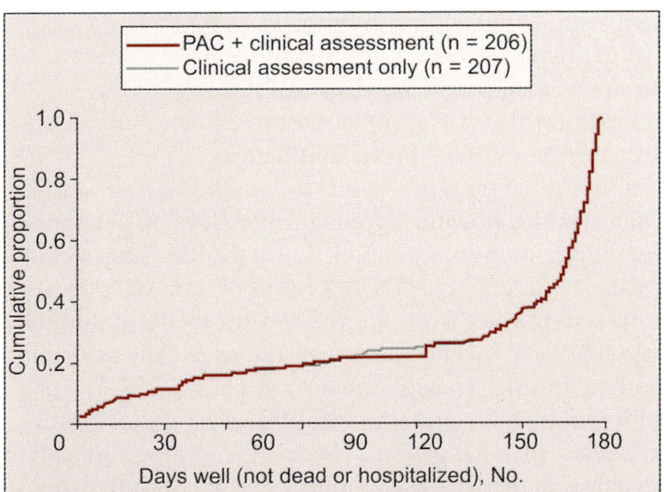

Cumulative proportion of patients contributing each possible numeric outcome for the number of days neither follow-up. Patients at the far left side of the curve represent early deaths, while those counted as 180 days survived for 6 months without rehospitalization. The curves for the treatment groups, pulmonary artery catheter plus clinical assessment and clinical assessment only are superimposed.

PAC, pulmonary artery catheter

Fig. 2 Primary outcome in the Evaluation Study of Congestive Heart Failure and Pulmonary Artery Catheterization Effectiveness (ESCAPE) trial. The primary outcome of days alive out of the hospital was not different in advanced heart failure patients randomized to pulmonary artery catheter guided therapy compared to clinical assessment[15]

COMMON INDICATIONS

While clearly not every patient with HF needs a PAC, there are a number of scenarios when PAC placement may be particularly helpful (Table 2).

Cardiogenic Shock

Patients admitted with decompensated HF and evidence of end-organ malperfusion (rising sCr, poor urine output, altered mental status, lactic acidosis, etc.) may benefit from the placement of a PAC to help facilitate the most appropriate therapeutic interventions, including inotropic support, intravenous vasodilators, or intra-aortic balloon pump (IABP).

Acutely Decompensated Heart Failure Not Responding to Standard Therapy

Some patients, particularly those with advanced disease, will worsen clinically despite appropriate therapy. A full hemodynamic assessment with a PAC may unveil unexpected abnormalities in cardiac index (CI), filling pressures and vascular resistance that are not readily apparent by bedside assessment. Many long-standing HF patients are ambulatory and functional despite a significantly reduced CI, e.g., less than 2.0 L/minutes/m^2 and decompensation may lead to even lower values that may not be clinically evident. In addition, some patients may have discordant elevations in left- and right-sided filling pressures, which may lead to inappropriate under- or overdiuresis.

Acutely Decompensated Heart Failure and Worsening Renal Function

The etiologies of worsening renal function (WRF) in acute decompensated heart failure (ADHF) are many, and include elevations in RAP (renal vein congestion), volume depletion and overdiuresis, underperfusion due to low CI or high SVR, overvasodilation, medication-related [angiotensin-converting enzyme inhibitors (ACEIs)], interstitial nephritis (from sulfa-based diuretics) and concomitant infections. The cause of WRF, especially in the setting of appropriate therapy for ADHF, can sometimes be difficult to decipher. The use of a PAC in some circumstances may unmask alterations in

TABLE 2: Clinical uses of pulmonary artery catheter in heart failure patients

Clinical conditions	*Utility*
Cardiogenic shock	Assess hemodynamics Initiate/titrate inotropic, vasodilator, vasopressor, or IABP support
ADHF not responding to therapy	May reveal unexpected hemodynamic abnormalities to facilltate appropriate interventions
ADHF and worsening renal function	Assess for etiology of WRF, including low CI, high SVR, low SVR, elevated RA pressure
ADHF and hypotension	Assess for over-vasodilation, low CI, volume depletion, etc.
Pretransplant evalution	Risk stratify patients with most severe hemodynamic derangements Identify pulmonary HTN (especially severe, irreversible) Identify need for inotropes, etc.
Assess reversibility of pulmonary HTN	Vasodialator challenge (iNO, nitroprusside, adenosine, etc.) to assess for reversibility in pretransplant patients with high transpulmonary gradient
Pre-LVAD evalution	Assess degree of RV dysfunction, (RAP, RVISWI, RA/PCWP ratio) and pulmonary HTN
Post-LVAD troubleshooting	Assess RV function, etiology of low pump flows, hypotension, worsening renal function, worsening CHF, etc. LVAD weaning protocols in patients who recover LV function
Maintenance of UNOS IA status	To meet "inotrope criteria" for IA listing, a PAC is required in the absence of contraindication

PAC, pulmonary artery catheter; HF, heart failure; ADHF, acutely decompensated heart failure; IABP, intra-aortic balloon pump; WRF, worsening renal function; CI, cardiac index; SVR, systemic vascular resistance; HTN, hypertension; iNO, inhaled nitric oxide; LVAD, left ventricular assist device; RV, right ventricular; RAP, right atrial pressure; RVSWI, right ventricular stroke work index; PCWP, pulmonary capillary wedge pressure; CHF, congestive heart failure; LV, left ventricular; UNOS 1A, United Network for Organ Sharing 1A

physiology that can help elucidate the cause of WRF and allow for appropriate intervention.

Acutely Decompensated Heart Failure and Hypotension

Similar to WRF, there are also many causes of hypotension in ADHF, including low cardiac output and cardiogenic shock, overdiuresis, smoldering sepsis/infection, medication-induced (ACEIs) and "pseudosepsis" or overvasodilation. When the source of hypotension is not obvious, the use of a PAC can allow for a full assessment of CI and SVR, and therefore, appropriate intervention to reverse the process.

Pretransplant Evaluation

A full hemodynamic assessment is recommended as part of any pretransplant evaluation, and can help to risk-stratify patients based on the severity of their hemodynamic derangements. PAC may also uncover unexpected pulmonary HTN, which, if severe enough and irreversible, may preclude successful transplantation (see below the topic of Pulmonary Vasodilator Challenge).

Pulmonary Vasodilator Challenge

Many patients with advanced HF develop significant secondary pulmonary HTN.[27] In the earliest stages of this process, pulmonary HTN is a result of passive congestive forces translated from the left atrium to the pulmonary vascular bed. This passive congestion is usually associated with a normal transpulmonary gradient (TPG = mean pulmonary artery pressure " PCWP) of less than 12 mmHg. However, in some patients chronic congestion can lead to reactive changes in the pulmonary circulation and therefore an elevated TPG (>12 mmHg). Ultimately, some will develop irreversible anatomical changes in the pulmonary vasculature and potentially irreversible pulmonary HTN that is well out of proportion to the elevated left-sided filling pressures. Fixed pulmonary HTN with a markedly elevated TPG is associated with poor outcomes after heart transplantation due to right ventricular failure (RVF).[28,29] Thus, it is important to assess for the degree of pulmonary HTN with a PAC prior to transplant, and to assess for reversibility in patients with a high TPG. A number of reversibility protocols have been developed that utilize a variety of pulmonary vasodilators, including sodium nitroprusside, adenosine and inhaled nitric oxide.

Left Ventricular Assist Device Candidacy Evaluation

One of the most devastating complications of left ventricular assist device (LVAD) placement is the development of RVF in the postoperative period. A number of RVF risk scores, echocardiographic parameters, hemodynamic parameters and laboratory values (bilirubin, sCr, etc.) have been used to try to predict RVF, but with little success. From a hemodynamic perspective, there are several parameters that have been associated with an increased risk of RVF. These include the right ventricular stroke work index (RVSWI), RAP, and RAP to PCWP ratio (RAP/PCWP). In the HeartMate II bridge-to-transplant trial, RAP greater than 15 mmHg and RVSWI less than 300 mmHg × mL/m^2 were predictors of postoperative RVF, while a RAP/PCWP ratio of greater than 0.63 was predictive in multivariate analysis as well.[30] Patients exhibiting significant RVF preoperatively should undergo "tailored" optimization of right ventricular (RV) hemodynamics with volume removal, inotropic support, or IABP as indicated prior to LVAD placement.[31]

Troubleshooting Left Ventricular Assist Device Patients

The current continuous-flow LVAD devices are not without significant complications, including pump thrombosis. These devices will display estimated cardiac output or "flow", but these values are not true, direct measurements of cardiac output. It can sometimes be challenging to troubleshoot LVAD patients with worsening HF, low pump flows, hypotension, or WRF. In these circumstances, PAC placement may help facilitate appropriate interventions. In addition, a PAC may be used as a part of weaning protocols in patients who have significant left ventricular (LV) recovery.

Maintenance of United Network for Organ Sharing 1A Status

A number of criteria must be met in order for a patient to be considered clinically sick enough to warrant urgent listing for heart transplantation as a United Network for Organ Sharing (UNOS) 1A status. To be listed under

TABLE 3: Practice guidelines (HFSA and ACC/AHA) recommendations

HFSA recommendations on PAC	*ACC/AHA recommendations on PAC*

• The routine use of invasive hemodynamic monitoring in patients with ADHF in not recommended
• Invasive hemodynamic monitoring should be considered in a patient:
  ○ who is refractory to initial therapy
  ○ whose volume status and filling pressures are unclear
  ○ who has clinically significant hypotension (typically SBP <80 mmHg) or worsening renal function during therapy and
  ○ in whom documentation of an adequate hemodynamic response to the inotropic agent is necessary when choronic outpatient infusion is being considered
	Class I
	Invasive hemodynamic monitoring should be performed to guide therapy in patients who are in respiratory distress or with clinical evidence of impaired perfusion in whom the adequacy or excess of intracardiac filling pressures cannot be determined from clinical assessment
	Class IIA
	Invasive hemodynamic monitoring can be useful for carefully selected patients with acute HF who have persistent symptoms despite empiric adjustment of standard therapies, and
	a. whose fluid status, perfusion, or systemic or pulmonary vascular resistances are uncertain,
	b. whose systolic pressure remains low or is associated with symptoms, despite initial therapy,
	c. whose renal function is worsening with therapy,
	d. who require parenteral vasoactive agents, or
	e. who may need consideration for advanced device therapy or transplantation
	Class III
	Routine use of invasive hemodynamic monitoring in normotensive patients with acutely decompensated HF and congestion with symptomatic response to diuretics and vasodilators is not recommended

HFSA, Heart Failure Society of America; PAC, pulmonary artery catheter; ACC, American College of Cardiology; AHA, American Heart Association; ADHF, acutely decompensated heart failure; SBP, systolic blood pressure; HF, heart failure "inotrope criteria", patients must have a PAC in place, and require a substantial degree of inotropic support, defined as milrinone at doses of 0.5 μg/kg/minutes or higher, dobutamine at doses of 7.5 μg/kg/minutes or higher, or some combination of two inotropes.

GUIDELINES RECOMMENDATIONS

Both the ACC/AHA and the HFSA HF practice guidelines give recommendations for appropriate use of PACs (Table 3).[32,33]

CONCLUSION

Despite the controversy surrounding the use of PACs in a variety of clinical settings, their utility in advanced HF is evident. In the only RCT of PACs in HF, the routine use of invasive hemodynamics did not improve outcomes compared to clinical assessment. However, this trial excluded the sickest HF patients, in particular those who clinically needed a PAC. Thus, the trial does not apply to the many clinical scenarios discussed above. PACs remain an invaluable tool in the management of these advanced, complex, and often critically ill patients.

REFERENCES

1. Forssmann-Falck R. Werner Forssmann: a pioneer of cardiology. Am J Cardiol. 1997;79(5):651-60.
2. Swan HJ, Ganz W, Forrester J, et al. Catheterization of the heart in man with use of a flow-directed balloon-tipped catheter. N Engl J Med. 1970;283(9):447-51.
3. Connors AF, Speroff T, Dawson NV, et al. The effectiveness of right heart catheterization in the initial care of critically ill patients. SUPPORT Investigators. JAMA. 1996;276(11):889-97.
4. Chatterjee K. The Swan-Ganz catheters: past, present, and future. A viewpoint. Circulation. 2009;119(1):147-52.
5. Fein AM, Goldberg SK, Walkenstein MD, et al. Is pulmonary artery catheterization necessary for the diagnosis of pulmonary edema? Am Rev Respir Dis. 1984;129(6):1006-9.
6. Robin ED. Death by pulmonary artery flow-directed catheter. Time for a moratorium? Chest. 1987;92(4):727-31.
7. Dalen JE, Bone RC. Is it time to pull the pulmonary artery catheter? JAMA. 1996;276(11):916-8.
8. Dalen JE. The pulmonary artery catheter-friend, foe, or accomplice? JAMA. 2001;286(3):348-50.
9. Rose H, Venn R. Recently published papers: dying Swans and other stories. Crit Care. 2006;10(4):152.
10. Gore JM, Goldberg RJ, Spodick DH, et al. A community-wide assessment of the use of pulmonary artery catheters in patients with acute myocardial infarction. Chest. 1987;92(4):721-7.
11. Zion MM, Balkin J, Rosenmann D, et al. Use of pulmonary artery catheters in patients with acute myocardial infarction. Analysis of experience in 5,841 patients in the SPRINT Registry. SPRINT Study Group. Chest. 1990;98(6):1331-5.
12. Sandham JD, Hull RD, Brant RF, et al. A randomized, controlled trial of the use of pulmonary-artery catheters in high-risk surgical patients. N Engl J Med. 2003;348(1):5-14.
13. Richard C, Warszawski J, Anguel N, et al. Early use of the pulmonary artery catheter and outcomes in patients with shock and acute respiratory distress syndrome: a randomized controlled trial. JAMA. 2003;290(20):2713-20.
14. Harvey S, Harrison DA, Singer M, et al. Assessment of the clinical effectiveness of pulmonary artery catheters in management of patients in intensive care (PAC-Man): a randomised controlled trial. Lancet. 2005;366(9484):472-7.
15. Binanay C, Califf RM, Hasselblad V, et al. Evaluation study of congestive heart failure and pulmonary artery catheterization effectiveness: the ESCAPE trial. JAMA. 2005;294(13):1625-33.
16. Rhodes A, Cusack RJ, Newman PJ, et al. A randomised, controlled trial of the pulmonary artery catheter in critically ill patients. Intensive Care Med. 2002;28(3):256-64.
17. National Heart, Lung, and Blood Institute Acute Respiratory Distress Syndrome (ARDS) Clinical Trials Network, Wheeler AP, Bernard GR, et al. Pulmonary-artery versus central venous catheter to guide treatment of acute lung injury. N Engl J Med. 2006;354(21):2213-24.
18. Wiener RS, Welch HG. Trends in the use of the pulmonary artery catheter in the United States, 1993-2004. JAMA. 2007;298(4):423-9.
19. Franciosa JA, Wilen M, Ziesche S, et al. Survival in men with severe chronic left ventricular failure due to either coronary heart disease or idiopathic dilated cardiomyopathy. Am J Cardiol. 1983;51(5):831-6.
20. Unverferth DV, Magorien RD, Moeschberger ML, et al. Factors influencing the one-year mortality of dilated cardiomyopathy. Am J Cardiol. 1984; 54(1):147-52.
21. Stevenson LW, Tillisch JH. Maintenance of cardiac output with normal filling pressures in patients with dilated heart failure. Circulation. 1986; 74(6):1303-8.
22. Stevenson LW, Sietsema K, Tillisch JH, et al. Exercise capacity for survivors of cardiac transplantation or sustained medical therapy for stable heart failure. Circulation. 1990;81(1):78-85.
23. Stevenson LW, Steimle AE, Fonarow G, et al. Improvement in exercise capacity of candidates awaiting heart transplantation. J Am Coll Cardiol. 1995;25(1):163-70.
24. Johnson W, Omland T, Hall C, et al. Neurohormonal activation rapidly decreases after intravenous therapy with diuretics and vasodilators for class IV heart failure. J Am Coll Cardiol. 2002;39(10):1623-9.
25. Stevenson LW, Dracup KA, Tillisch JH. Efficacy of medical therapy tailored for severe congestive heart failure in patients transferred for urgent cardiac transplantation. Am J Cardiol. 1989;63(7):461-4.
26. Stevenson LW, Tillisch JH, Hamilton M, et al. Importance of hemodynamic response to therapy in predicting survival with ejection fraction less than or equal to 20% secondary to ischemic or nonischemic dilated cardiomyopathy. Am J Cardiol. 1990;66(19):1348-54.
27. Guazzi M, Borlaug BA. Pulmonary hypertension due to left heart disease. Circulation. 2012;126(8):975-90.
28. Erickson KW, Costanzo-Nordin MR, O'Sullivan EJ, et al. Influence of preoperative transpulmonary gradient on late mortality after orthotopic heart transplantation. J Heart Transplant. 1990;9(5):526-37.
29. Costard-Jackle A, Fowler MB. Influence of preoperative pulmonary artery pressure on mortality after heart transplantation: testing of potential reversibility of pulmonary hypertension with nitroprusside is useful in defining a high risk group. J Am Coll Cardiol. 1992;19(1):48-54.
30. Kormos RL, Teuteberg JJ, Pagani FD, et al. Right ventricular failure in patients with the HeartMate II continuous-flow left ventricular assist device: incidence, risk factors, and effect on outcomes. J Thoracic Cardiovasc Surg. 2010;139(5):1316-24.
31. Slaughter MS, Pagani FD, Rogers JG, et al. Clinical management of continuous-flow left ventricular assist devices in advanced heart failure. J Heart Lung Transplant. 2010;29(4 Suppl):S1-39.
32. Heart Failure Society of a. Executive summary: HFSA 2006 Comprehensive Heart Failure Practice Guideline. J Cardiac Fail. 2006;12(1):10-38.
33. Hunt SA, Abraham WT, Chin MH, et al. 2009 focused update incorporated into the ACC/AHA 2005 Guidelines for the Diagnosis and Management of Heart Failure in Adults. Circulation. 2009;119(14):e391-479.

3

SECTION

Chronic Heart Failure in the Outpatient Setting

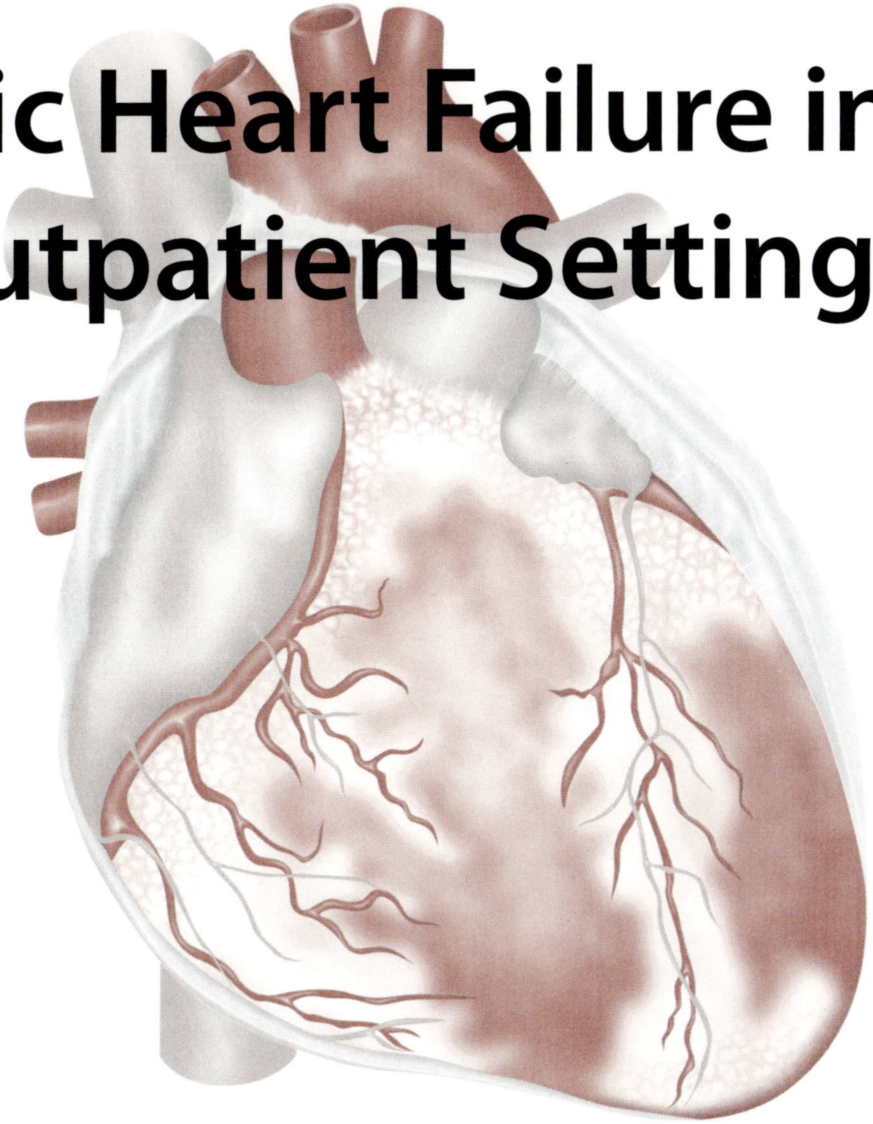

Chapter 22

Outpatient Follow-up—What Should We Monitor

Tina Baykaner, Yu Xie, Michelle Schlueter, Barry Greenberg

ABSTRACT

The majority of care for heart failure (HF) patients takes place in the outpatient setting. The major goals of outpatient follow-up are to relieve symptoms and to reduce morbidity and mortality. Establishing a database about the patient, which includes information about the cause of HF, severity and prognosis, presence of comorbidities, and challenges to treatment is essential for devising and successfully implementing a therapeutic strategy. Information from the patient's interval history and current physical examination along with laboratory examinations and other diagnostic tests is used to assess the patient and inform decisions about optimizing therapy in the outpatient setting. At our medical center, the visit involves input from several members of a multidisciplinary team that is comprised of HF physicians, pharmacists, and advanced practice nurses. Education of the patient and family members involved in their care is stressed during these visits, and efforts are made to uncover potential impediments to the patient's ability to adhere to the medical regimen. The frequency, duration, and focus of each visit are tailored to the patients' specific needs in regards to their disease course. More recently, follow-up care between visits has begun to utilize remote contact (e.g., telephonic or computer-based) between the patient and the medical team and/or homecare services as a means of providing increased surveillance and in order to prevent episodes of decompensation.

GOALS OF OUTPATIENT FOLLOW-UP OF THE HEART FAILURE PATIENT

Introduction

The majority of care of HF patients takes place in the outpatient setting, providing a crucial opportunity for healthcare providers to focus on both immediate- and long-term management. Outpatient clinic visits should address a very specific set of goals and objectives. When this is accomplished successfully, there is evidence of improved patient outcomes, including decreases in risk of mortality and hospitalization as well as improvements in symptoms and quality of life.[1,2] In this chapter, we will discuss the short- and long-term goals of outpatient follow-up of HF patients and how the clinic visit can be directed toward implementing strategies that help improve outcomes. We intend to describe how our practice is set up and to share our experience in achieving management goals in the outpatient setting.

Immediate Goals

Improving Symptoms

Patients often endorse symptoms, including shortness of breath (either at rest or during exercise), cough, orthopnea, paroxysmal-nocturnal dyspnea, decreased exercise capacity, lower extremity edema, abdominal or scrotal swelling, and weight gain. None of these, however, is specific to HF and if the goal of providing relief of symptoms is to be accomplished, the patients' complaints must be viewed from a broad perspective that encompasses the impact of other medical conditions as well as the patients' motivation and capacity. Patients often minimize symptoms, so it is not always sufficient to accept "carte blanche" what the patient states without probing further into the situation. For instance, in assessing exercise capacity, asking the patients how their performance compares to either a point in time when they were doing well or to that of their peer group often provides great insight into whether or not the patients have regressed from their own baseline. Similarly, asking the patient's "significant other" to confirm (or more often refute!), the patient's description of their exercise capacity often reveals that the limitation is far greater than what the patient describes.

In addition to having the patients describe their symptoms, several tests can be used to assess their functional status. These include the 6-minute walk test (6MWT) and cardiopulmonary exercise stress testing. These tests not only help determine the cause of the patient's symptoms and better classify functional capacity, but also provide important prognostic information.[3,4] We employ such tests when there is a need to get an independent measure of the patient's functional capacity when there is a discrepancy between the patient's history and other measures of the severity of HF. These tests also help determine whether to move toward advanced care options, such as mechanical circulatory support or transplantation and to determine the exercise prescription or the patient's ability to return to work.[5,6]

Optimizing Pharmacological Therapy and Determining the Need for Devices

- Management of congestion: Patients often present with symptoms of volume overload, and the uses of loop diuretics, dietary salt restriction, and long-acting nitrates are usually effective in providing symptomatic relief. Presumably, this approach also reduces the risk of hospitalization, but there is little evidence that loop diuretics improve the survival of HF patients. The dose of diuretics should be adjusted to achieve the "dry weight" of a patient. Defining the goal dry weight, however, can be a challenge, especially in newly diagnosed patients, or in patients losing or gaining weight due to dietary reasons or other illnesses. In our clinic, we aim to involve the patients in determining their own volume status by measuring daily weights, and self-adjusting their diuretic regimen according to a sliding scale that is carefully described and reinforced to the patient during the clinic visit. In most cases, we recommend uptitrating the dose of loop diuretic or adding thiazide diuretic or metolazone when the weight increase is 3 pounds or more over a given period of time, although there is considerably variability in this parameter. We have found that the addition of a second diuretic in addition to a loop diuretic, however, may be associated with more profound diuresis than anticipated and is often associated with development of significant hyponatremia or hypokalemia. Thus, we reserve this approach for truly refractory patients and provide more intense surveillance of electrolytes and renal function when this approach is taken, particularly when therapy is first initiated. When appropriate, we also devise plans for reducing the dose of diuretics based on the patient's ability to monitor their weight at home in order to avoid overdiuresis
- Optimizing therapy with neurohormonal blocking agents and vasodilators in patients with HF and reduced ejection fraction (EF) (HFrEF): For HFrEF patients, neurohormonal blocking agents are used to improve symptoms as well as the natural history of the disease. The additions of beta blockers, angiotensin-converting enzyme inhibitors (ACEIs) or angiotensin receptor blockers (ARBs), and aldosterone antagonists[7-10] to the medical regimen all have been shown to reduce morbidity and mortality across a wide range of HFrEF patients. Thus, initiation and/or uptitration of these drugs to optimal target doses (defined as those used in clinical trials) is an important component of the outpatient visit. Patients who do not tolerate ACEI or ARB therapy or whose renal function precludes their use may benefit from a combination of hydralazine and nitrates. Of note is the fact that the addition of a fixed dose combination of these vasodilators to African American patients who were already receiving neurohormonal blocking agents has been shown to improve survival as well as quality of life.[11]

An individual patient's ability to tolerate these medications is highly variable due to side effects, such as hypotension, fatigue or worsening renal function so that careful monitoring including periodic assessment of electrolytes and renal function in the clinic setting is required. In general, neurohormonal blocking agents are started or increased individually to avoid side effects or adverse consequences that may be additive (e.g., increased potassium with ACEIs or ARBs and aldosterone antagonists). Whereas, ACEIs, ARBs, aldosterone antagonists, and vasodilators can be uptitrated over a relatively short period of time, beta-blockers need to be advanced more cautiously with a doubling of the dose recommended no more frequently than every 2 weeks until the target is reached. With initiation and uptitration of beta blockers, patients may experience worsening symptoms, including fatigue and increased congestion. Patients are advised to watch for these symptoms and to alert the clinic if they persist more than a few days or are progressive or severe. Although patients are also advised to monitor their blood pressures, hypotension in the absence of any related symptoms rarely requires lowering the dosage of neurohormonal blocking agents unless the blood pressure is extremely low or there is evidence of a negative impact of the low pressure on organ perfusion or function

- Determining the need for further therapy with devices: For HFrEF patients who have reached the optimal (or maximal tolerated) doses of neurohormonal blocking medications, cardiac function should be re-evaluated after 3–6 months. If the patient remains symptomatic and EF is less than or equal to 35%, referral for implantable cardioverter defibrillator (ICD) placement for primary prevention of sudden cardiac death should be considered. Patients with prolonged QRS duration may also further benefit from cardiac resynchronization therapy (CRT) in addition to ICD placement.[12-14] For patients who have biventricular pacemakers, appropriate follow-up should be ensured as outpatient for optimization of device parameters
- Managing patients with HF with preserved EF (HFpEF): The medical management of HFpEF patients is largely directed toward treating symptoms by managing volume status and congestion, and preventing episodes of decompensation. Diuretics and nitrates are the most commonly used drugs for controlling symptoms. In HFpEF patients, it is important to identify the underlying etiology for exacerbations. Optimal control of blood pressure in hypertensive patients, rate or rhythm control in patients with atrial fibrillation or flutter and preventing episodes of myocardial ischemia are among measures to help improve symptoms in patients with preserved EF.

Understanding the Etiology

Determining the etiology of HF often influences further management decisions. Thus, for patients with newly diagnosed HF (as well as for those with chronic HF in whom the etiology has not been clearly established), determining the underlying cause of cardiac dysfunction is an important immediate goal in the outpatient setting. While a detailed description of how this is accomplished is beyond the scope of the present chapter, in general the workup is oriented toward defining whether the patient is suffering from HFrEF or HFpEF and differentiating ischemic from nonischemic causes of HF. If HF is due to a nonischemic cause, further evaluation to determine as best as possible the nature of the disease is warranted. Unusual causes of HF, such as infiltrative diseases of the heart or myocarditis, should be considered in the differential and there are often clues in the patient's history, physical or routine laboratory tests that point the workup in a particular direction.

Determining Risk for Adverse Events

- Review of major risk factors for unfavorable clinical course: Worsening chronic HF is the major reason and accounts for 75% of HF hospitalizations.[15] An additional 23% are due to new onset HF while the remainder can be attributed to advanced or end-stage HF. In HFrEF patients, early hospital readmissions are often due to worsening HF, whereas later hospital readmissions are more often due to comorbidities. Conversely, in patients with HFpEF, comorbidities play a more important role in hospital readmissions throughout the course. Nonetheless, the 60–90-day survival for posthospital discharge is similar among patients with HFrEF and HFpEF.[16] These data alert us to the fact that there are both cardiac and noncardiac triggers and risk factors that are associated with hospitalization and that both need to be considered when the patient is seen in the outpatient setting
- Easily accessible risk factors can be used to determine risk of patients post discharge following HF hospitalization. As opposed to low cardiac output, elevated pulmonary capillary wedge pressure (PCWP) has been noted to be associated with worse outcomes post discharge.[17] Although right heart catheterization is not routinely performed in this population, information obtained from the history and physical examination regarding the persistence of signs and/or symptoms of congestion at the time of hospital discharge has been associated with an unfavorable clinical course, including increased long-term mortality.[18] Predischarge brain natriuretic peptide (BNP) levels,[19] worsening renal function during the period of hospitalization (defined as a change in Cr ≥25% and/or ≥0.3 mg/dL),[19,20] persistent hyponatremia[21] and low blood pressure[22] also can be used to define high-risk patients. We have also noted that patients who are frail[23] or who have poor social support[24] tend to

do poorly post hospitalization. Referral of patients who are identified as being at increased risk to a multidisciplinary outpatient HF team is often quite helpful in improving the clinical course

- Use of risk scores: Several modalities exist for evaluation and calculating risk of future events such as the Seattle Heart Failure Model[25] and Heart Failure Survival Score.[26] Monitoring for change in risk score can serve as an objective finding for clinicians that can help direct therapy. Changes in survival with treatment can also be used to motivate patients who do not adhere to the medical regimen.

Identifying Comorbidities and Impediments to Therapy

Comorbidities strongly influence the clinical course of HF patients. Many of the diseases that predispose a patient to developing HF, such as diabetes, atherosclerosis, hypertension, hyperlipidemia, morbid obesity, heavy tobacco and alcohol use, also put the patients at risk for involvement of other organs, especially kidney, liver and lung. Disease in other organs both interacts with and may adversely affect cardiac function as well as limit use of effective therapies. Coexisting kidney disease, in particular, impacts management of HF and may greatly limit therapeutic options. Therefore, as we evaluate our patient primarily for congestive heart failure (CHF), it is important to also pay attention to the presence of comorbidities and to address them as completely as possible.

Of particular note is the fact that obstructive sleep apnea (OSA) or central sleep apnea (CSA) occurs in up to 50% of CHF patients, and yet, it often goes undiagnosed.[27] Symptoms include daytime somnolence, snoring, multiple night awakenings with/without remembrance and physical examination findings include thick neck circumference and obesity. Often patients are not aware of apneic episodes while asleep. A thorough history from the patient's sleep partner can be very helpful. Although the treatment of OSA can improve EF, reduce the level of pulmonary hypertension, and decrease the prevalence of atrial fibrillation episodes, the impact of therapy on mortality is uncertain.[28-31]

In addition to the physiological factors mentioned above, it is also important to consider psychosocial barriers that may affect clinical outcomes. These include the patient's psychological state, presence and severity of depression, economic status, and the social support system that is available to help the patient.

Long-term Goals

Improve Natural History

The "iceberg phenomenon" is a frequently used analogy to describe the relatively smaller portion of severely symptomatic patients with late stage C or D HF versus the much larger proportion of patients who have mild or even no HF symptoms. While patients with severe HF require a disproportionally large percentage of clinical and hospital resources, one of the key goals of the outpatient follow-up of HF patients is to identify individuals who would benefit from therapy that can significantly limit disease progression and reduce the risk of future events. For all HF patients, the major objectives of the follow-up are to risk stratify them to determine the likelihood of decompensation and risk of future events and to initiate and optimize an appropriate treatment regimen in order to improve the natural history of the disease. As noted in the initial portion of the chapter, there is good evidence that optimal treatment for HF patients can favorably affect long-term outcome.

Prevent Readmission

Heart failure is one of the most important causes of hospitalization in the US and is the number one expense for Medicare.[32] Despite improvement in hospital mortality and mean length of stay, readmission rate and posthospital mortality rates remain unacceptably high following a HF hospitalization. According to the Organized Program to Initiate Lifesaving Treatment in Hospitalized Patients with Heart Failure (OPTIMIZE-HF) study, postdischarge mortality is 9% and readmission rate is 30%[33] within the first 60–90 days. Furthermore, many patients never reach their previous functional level and cardiac function posthospital discharge. Therefore, one of the overall goals of outpatient follow-up for these patients is to decrease or prevent hospital admission, restore them to previous functional status and decrease mortality.

In addition to the factors outlined in the first section of the chapter, other potentially treatable causes of re-admission have been identified. For instance, medication noncompliance accounts for 24% of the causes of hospital admission, dietary noncompliance accounts for an additional 24%, followed by 19% due to failure to seek care, and 16% due to inappropriate pharmacological treatment.[34] Other triggers for decompensation include recurring myocardial ischemia, poorly controlled blood pressure, arrhythmias [particularly atrial fibrillation, medications that depress cardiac function, such as calcium channel blocker (CCB) or nonsteroidal anti-inflammatory drugs (NSAIDs)], intercurrent infection, worsening kidney or liver function and other comorbidities.[35,36]

Multidisciplinary HF clinics only account for a small proportion of the outpatient HF clinic care received by patients. There is evidence that this approach is associated with better implementation of evidence-based therapy, greater relief of HF symptoms and improved functional capacity, better quality of life, and a reduction in the hospital readmission rate and total medical cost for HF patients.[37] Patients most likely to benefit from referral to a multidisciplinary HF clinic are those judged to be at high risk based on characteristics described in the initial section of the chapter as well as by persistent New York Heart Association (NYHA) Class III/IV symptoms, repetitive hospitalizations, multiple comorbid conditions, active depression, cognitive impairment, and history of medication and/or dietary nonadherence.

Hospital readmission rates are the highest in the immediate postdischarge period, where the patient is most vulnerable to medication errors, changes in diet and compliance, and decreased monitoring. This is a crucial time to establish close HF clinic follow-up and minimize hospital readmission and decompensation of HF.

COMPONENTS OF THE FOLLOW-UP CLINIC VISIT

How is the Visit Constructed?

The frequency and duration of outpatient visits vary according to individual patient needs. Patients whose condition is tenuous and those who need to be educated about their condition may need to be seen as frequently as every week until their course stabilizes. Patients who are doing well on optimal therapy can be seen far less frequently than this and intervals between clinic visits may extend out to 3 or 6 months. Factors that determine the frequency of follow-up include disease severity, risk for future events, comorbidities, need for titrating medications, including optimization of the dose of neurohormonal blocking agents, patient reliability, and the functionality of the patient. Distance from the clinic and the patients' support network also influence how often they can be seen back in clinic.

As a patient's clinical course varies, the frequency of follow-up should be adjusted accordingly. For those patients with a recent HF exacerbation, particularly if it required emergent outpatient treatment or hospitalization, early follow-up evaluation is indicated. There is evidence that early posthospital discharge follow-up within a 7–10-day period is associated with a reduced rate of rehospitalization.[38] We have found that an early postdischarge visit is required to determine the adequacy of treatment, possible medication errors, the patients understanding of the medical plan and other issues that must be addressed in order to circumvent a recurrent episode of decompensation that will require repeat hospitalization.

The duration of the outpatient visit also varies. Patients new to our system are allocated 40–60 minutes, a time that allows the patient to be seen by several members of the team including a HF physician, a Pharm D, and an advanced practice nurse. Individuals who are seen in follow-up after a prolonged interval may also require an extended clinic visit in order to ascertain a full understanding of the interval history and to update the patient on the status of their disease. It is ideal to have family members join the patient for these lengthier clinic visits, particularly when discussions regarding disease status, prognosis, or major changes in therapy are planned.

Overview of the Visit

The components of an outpatient follow-up visit are summarized in Box 1. The visit should focus on detecting changes in the signs and symptoms of HF that auger impending decompensation or a complication due to HF therapy itself (e.g., worsening renal function due to excessive diuresis). This involves systematic monitoring of the patient's functional status, medications, laboratory values, dietary compliance and other common symptoms of HF as well as an assessment of the side effects of the medical regimen.

Box 1: Major components to evaluate during outpatient visit

- Symptoms of congestion
- Symptoms of poor perfusion
- Presence and change in the status of comorbid conditions (e.g., arrhythmias, hypertension, diabetes mellitus, chronic kidney disease)
- Medication and diet compliance
- Exercise regimen
- Changes in social support

Treatment Team

The life cycle of the HF patient extends from the treatment of acute episodes of decompensation requiring hospitalization to chronic management in the outpatient setting. Patients are often trapped in a "revolving door" of frequent hospitalizations due to inadequate treatment, guidance and follow-up. Moreover, the complicated medical care of HF is often fragmented involving multiple caregivers in both the in- and outpatient setting. This scenario provides the rationale for the use of an integrated multidisciplinary team to treat HF patients. In our hospital, the core team includes physicians specializing in HF, nurse practitioners, registered nurses (RNs) and pharmacists. Social workers and case managers are often consulted, particularly when patients are physically debilitated, lack full financial and social support or are unfamiliar with navigating the complex maze of social services and insurance requirements that characterize our healthcare system. Access to dieticians, primary care physicians and specialists in other disciplines may also be required. In addition to seeing a patient in the clinic, a fully integrated multidisciplinary team can provide advice and counseling during between-visit phone calls, identify medication user errors, and help the patient find insurance coverage and social support that may be lacking.

Patient Assessment

Obtaining a thorough past medical history, including major illnesses, past surgeries and previous hospitalizations is crucial information during the initial outpatient clinic visit. The presence of comorbidities affects the prognosis and medication choice, and warrants a detailed discussion with the patient and reviewing prior medical records.

A detailed social history can help reveal the underlying etiology of HF and identify factors that make successful treatment problematic. It is advised to assess use of tobacco, alcohol and other illicit drugs (both at present and in the past) in detail at the initial visit, and to revisit these issues at future visits whenever there is a suspicion that they may be impacting the clinical course. Exploring the dietary habits and salt intake of patients may reveal why a patient is not responding to medical treatment. Obtaining a thorough family history may guide further diagnostic evaluation and, in selected cases, lead to genetic testing.

An assessment of prior medication regimens and related side effects or patient intolerance of certain medications helps provide direction for the current and future medical therapy. Reviewing interval hospital admissions for HF exacerbations and inpatient interventions is essential in pinpointing the exacerbating factors and incorporating information about the patient's condition that will help determine treatment options.

A carefully performed physical examination can provide important information immediately and at virtually no cost. The general appearance of the patient often reveals the severity of the HF as well as coexisting conditions (both medical and social) that will impact management. Cardiac cachexia is a manifestation of advanced HF, while confusion, mental obtundation and cold extremities suggest reduced cardiac output. The appearance of dyspnea when the patient moves to the examining table or lies down on it is often an indication of severe congestion. Patients' hygiene is an indicator of their general adherence to health measures, and characteristic olfactory evidence of cigarette smoking or alcohol consumption may provide targets for education and/or counseling.

Assessing the volume status of a patient is a core function of the clinic visit. Evidence of a rapid increase in body weight is often an indication that the patient is retaining fluid. In our experience, however, some patients demonstrate remarkable ability to gain substantial amounts of tissue or nonwater weight between visits. Also, the presence of HF induced cachexia may counterbalance the effect of fluid retention on body weight so that the absence of an increase in weight is not always an indication that the patient is not congested. Thus, other physical findings should be used to determine the patient's volume status. Measurement of jugular venous pressure (JVP) remains the most helpful physical finding for assessing the volume status of the patient. The presence of hepatojugular reflux (elicited by applying gentle pressure to the right upper quadrant of the patient's abdomen) often helps when venous pulsations are obscure or there is borderline elevation of the neck veins. The presence of an S3 gallop is often an indicator of volume overload, although it is not a particularly sensitive finding. More importantly, both the third heart sound and elevated jugular pressure provide prognostic information among patients with left ventricular dysfunction.[39] While the absence of rales does not rule out volume overload, particularly in patients with long-standing HF who develop compensatory changes in the lymphatic system of the lungs, their presence usually indicates pulmonary congestion provided that conditions, such as pneumonia, bronchiectasis, etc. are not present.

Peripheral edema is a classical manifestation of congestion in the HF patient and it is often one of the first signs that alerts the patient that their condition is worsening. It is, however, important to consider peripheral edema in the context of other physical findings, and not to treat with increasing doses of diuretics unless there is evidence of elevated filling pressures as indicated by an elevated JVP or pulmonary congestion. It is not uncommon for patients to have no evidence of lower extremity edema, but to accumulate excess water as ascites or scrotal edema.

Although signs of low cardiac output usually occur in patients who are also volume-overloaded, it may be present in those who are euvolemic or hypovolemic. Hypotension, compensatory tachycardia, cool skin, slow capillary refill time, cyanosis, narrowed pulse pressure, pulsus alternans and poor cognition are among signs of poor perfusion, and they usually indicate the presence of severe heart failure.

In addition to assessing volume status and perfusion, physical examination could yield further information, such as cardiomegaly by palpating a laterally displaced apical impulse and the presence of regurgitant murmurs suggesting mitral or tricuspid valvular dysfunction. Auscultation of new or changing murmurs often warrants an echocardiogram, and auscultation of an irregular or a rapid rhythm would require an electrocardiogram (ECG) in clinic to evaluate for arrhythmias.

Laboratory Findings

Results from laboratory studies are an important component of the outpatient visit. We generally obtain a basic metabolic panel within a week or two following initiation or change in dosage of diuretics, ACE inhibitors, ARBs or aldosterone antagonists. For patients on a stable medical regimen, a chemistry panel is advised every 6 months to reassess electrolytes and renal function, although it is prudent to obtain this more often in patients who have had problems with worsening of renal function or electrolyte abnormalities in the past.

Measurement of the natriuretic peptides BNP and N-terminal proBNP (NT-BNP) are helpful in determining whether shortness of breath in the emergency department is due to HF or some other cause. Such differentiation is often helpful in the outpatient setting when the etiology of shortness of breath is unclear, or physical assessment of volume status is ambiguous. Levels of natriuretic peptides, troponin and other biomarkers also provide prognostic information.[40,41] The natriuretic peptides are also being used to help guide and drive therapy for HF[42,43] although whether or not they improve long-term outcomes remains uncertain.

Imaging and Other Studies

An ECG is advised in all patients who present with new onset HF. It is also obtained periodically during follow-up in the outpatient clinic whenever there is an indication that there might have been a change that could further influence management decisions. In patients with systolic dysfunction, the ECG is also useful in determining if there is an intraventricular conduction defect present that would make the patient a candidate for CRT.

All HF patients should have a baseline transthoracic echocardiogram (TTE) to evaluate ventricular systolic and diastolic function, size of all four of the cardiac chambers, the presence of hypertrophy and valve structure and function. The TTE can also provide information about intracardiac filling pressures and the patient's volume status. Results of the echocardiogram often guide us toward the underlying etiology of HF, with global hypokinesis suggesting nonischemic etiologies and regional wall motion abnormalities suggesting that ischemic disease may be present. A repeat TTE is only needed if there is a suspected change in the cardiac function, or if it would further guide management options. Guidelines suggest repeating an echocardiogram in 3–6 months after a new diagnosis of HF with reduced EF to reassess EF, and to consider the need for device placement.[44]

Patient and Caregiver Education

One of the most common reasons for clinical deterioration and hospitalization of HF patients is poor self care. As such, education and counseling are the foundation to help patients manage themselves at home. Since HF patients may have cognitive or functional impairment or other learning barriers, providers must actively engage the appropriate caregiver or family member in the teaching session as well. Heart failure education should include education on medications, activity and exercise, the need to follow a low sodium diet, instruction on daily weight monitoring, a prescription for fluid restriction, and training on how to recognize worsening symptoms.

Education should be done by members of the multidisciplinary team, including physicians, advanced practice nurses, home health nurses, pharmacists, and dieticians. Video and reading materials should be used

Box 2: Universal health literacy principles

- Simple words (1–2 syllables)
- Short and simple sentences
- Short paragraphs (1 topic)
- Plain language
- Reading level of 6th grade or below
- Headings and subheadings
- Lots of white space
- Highlighted or bolded key information
- Visuals and graphics

Box 3: Teach-back method concepts

- Use plain language
- Speak slowly
- Use short sentences
- Avoid yes/no questions
- Segment education (2–3 concepts per session)
- Check understanding
- Alter strategy if needed

to supplement the teaching sessions. Limited health literacy is common among patients and caregivers and many have difficulty processing and understanding basic health information. To involve patients in their own care, we have to ensure they can read, understand, and act on the information relevant to their care. Patient education materials should be written using universal health literacy principles listed in Box 2.

Teaching should be done frequently and throughout multiple encounters with the patient. After each learning session, assessment of understanding should be performed. One strategy to assess understanding of the concepts taught is to employ the teach-back method. The teach-back method ensures the patient understands the material and can explain in his or her own words the concepts taught. Components of the teach-back method are listed in Box 3.

Monitoring Devices

Most ICD devices currently have an integrated thoracic impedance sensor function to monitor patients' volume status. This data regarding the volume status of patients could be a valuable addition to the physical examination findings, or to remote monitoring of patients, but such monitoring impedance data and guiding management of HF through monitoring of the impedance data has not shown any benefit in clinical outcomes or the rate of hospitalizations.[45,46]

With current advances in technology, wireless implantable hemodynamic monitoring devices (pulmonary artery pressure sensors) are available and are shown to decrease HF related hospital admissions in patients with NYHA class III symptoms in recent studies.[47,48]

Given the importance of hypervolemia in HF related events, monitoring of weight and HF specific symptoms as a surrogate for fluid status received considerable attention. The data regarding structured phone calls or remote telemonitoring of weight, heart rate and blood pressure have shown mixed results in several randomized clinical trials.[49]

Follow-up Between Outpatient Visits

Although regular structured telephone calls and telemonitoring has not been shown conclusively to benefit HF patients, we have found that contact with patients via phone in between clinic visits can be beneficial for selected patients, especially within the immediate postdischarge period. For those patients who require frequent follow-up after hospitalization and have issues with access to care due to resources, geographic or physical barriers or are tenuous, this can be a viable and sometimes only option to prevent clinical deterioration in the interim. Telephone calls can be done by RNs, nurse practitioners, pharmacists and/or others on the multidisciplinary team. Patients are often called on to report vital signs, weight and symptoms and make medication adjustments as necessary. The clinician can also use this opportunity to reinforce education (diet, nutrition, symptom management) or instructions that were given in clinic. Patients should also be given the HF clinic number and encouraged to report signs and symptoms of worsening HF.

CONCLUSION

Heart failure is one of the most common discharge diagnoses in the US, and outpatient follow-up of patients with HF plays a critical role in disease management. A multidisciplinary approach can significantly improve the patient's condition and lead to improvements in both short- and long-term outcomes. These benefits are achieved not only through optimizing use of pharmacological and device therapies, but also through patient and family counseling, dietary assessment and education about the disease and the various therapies that are used to treat it.

REFERENCES

1. Kasper EK, Gerstenblith G, Hefter G, et al. A randomized trial of the efficacy of multidisciplinary care in heart failure outpatients at high risk of hospital readmission. J Am Coll Cardiol. 2002;39(3):471-80.
2. McAlister FA, Stewart S, Ferrua S, et al. Multidisciplinary strategies for the management of heart failure patients at high risk for admission: a systematic review of randomized trials. J Am Coll Cardiol. 2004;44(4):810-9.
3. Bittner V, Weiner DH, Yusuf S, et al. Prediction of mortality and morbidity with a 6-minute walk test in patients with left ventricular dysfunction. SOLVD Investigators. JAMA. 1993;270(14):1702-7.
4. Mancini DM, Eisen H, Kussmaul W, et al. Value of peak exercise oxygen consumption for optimal timing of cardiac transplantation in ambulatory patients with heart failure. Circulation. 1991;83(3):778-86.
5. Osada N, Chaitman BR, Miller LW, et al. Cardiopulmonary exercise testing identifies low risk patients with heart failure and severely impaired exercise capacity considered for heart transplantation. J Am Coll Cardiol. 1998;31(3):577-82.
6. Balady GJ, Arena R, Sietsema K, et al. Clinician's Guide to cardiopulmonary exercise testing in adults: a scientific statement from the American Heart Association. Circulation. 2010;122(2):191-225.
7. Packer M, Coats AJ, Fowler MB, et al. Effect of carvedilol on survival in severe chronic heart failure. N Engl J Med. 2001;344(22):1651-8.
8. Effect of enalapril on survival in patients with reduced left ventricular ejection fractions and congestive heart failure. The SOLVD Investigators. N Engl J Med. 1991;325(5):293-302.
9. Granger CB, McMurray JJ, Yusuf S, et al. Effects of candesartan in patients with chronic heart failure and reduced left-ventricular systolic function intolerant to angiotensin-converting-enzyme inhibitors: the CHARM-Alternative trial. Lancet. 2003;362(9386):772-6.
10. Pitt B, Zannad F, Remme WJ, et al. The effect of spironolactone on morbidity and mortality in patients with severe heart failure. Randomized Aldactone Evaluation Study Investigators. N Engl J Med. 1999;341(10):709-17.
11. Taylor AL, Ziesche S, Yancy C, et al. Combination of isosorbide dinitrate and hydralazine in blacks with heart failure. N Engl J Med. 2004;351(20):2049-57.
12. Moss AJ, Hall WJ, Cannom DS, et al. Cardiac-resynchronization therapy for the prevention of heart-failure events. N Engl J Med. 2009;361(14):1329-38.
13. Tang AS, Wells GA, Talajic M, et al. Cardiac-resynchronization therapy for mild-to-moderate heart failure. N Engl J Med. 2010;363(25):2385-95.
14. Bristow MR, Saxon LA, Boehmer J, et al. Cardiac-resynchronization therapy with or without an implantable defibrillator in advanced chronic heart failure. N Engl J Med. 2004;350(21):2140-50.
15. Fonarow GC. The Acute Decompensated Heart Failure National Registry (ADHERE): opportunities to improve care of patients hospitalized with acute decompensated heart failure. Rev Cardiovasc Med. 2003;4 Suppl 7:S21-30.
16. Fonarow GC, Stough WG, Abraham WT, et al. Characteristics, treatments, and outcomes of patients with preserved systolic function hospitalized for heart failure: a report from the OPTIMIZE-HF Registry. J Am Coll Cardiol. 2007;50(8):768-77.
17. Fonarow GC. The treatment targets in acute decompensated heart failure. Rev Cardiovasc Med. 2001;2 Suppl 2:S7-12.
18. Lucas C, Johnson W, Hamilton MA, et al. Freedom from congestion predicts good survival despite previous class IV symptoms of heart failure. Am Heart J. 2000;140(6):840-7.
19. Logeart D, Thabut G, Jourdain P, et al. Predischarge B-type natriuretic peptide assay for identifying patients at high risk of re-admission after decompensated heart failure. J Am Coll Cardiol. 2004;43(4):635-41.
20. Metra M, Ponikowski P, Dickstein K, et al. Advanced chronic heart failure: A position statement from the Study Group on Advanced Heart Failure of the Heart Failure Association of the European Society of Cardiology. Eur J Heart Fail. 2007;9(6-7):684-94.
21. Lee WH, Packer M. Prognostic importance of serum sodium concentration and its modification by converting-enzyme inhibition in patients with severe chronic heart failure. Circulation. 1986;73(2):257-67.
22. Gheorghiade M, Abraham WT, Albert NM, et al. Systolic blood pressure at admission, clinical characteristics, and outcomes in patients hospitalized with acute heart failure. JAMA. 2006;296(18):2217-26.
23. Cacciatore F, Abete P, Mazzella F, et al. Frailty predicts long-term mortality in elderly subjects with chronic heart failure. Eur J Clin Invest. 2005;35(12):723-30.
24. Krumholz HM, Butler J, Miller J, et al. Prognostic importance of emotional support for elderly patients hospitalized with heart failure. Circulation. 1998;97(10):958-64.
25. Levy WC, Mozaffarian D, Linker DT, et al. The Seattle Heart Failure Model: prediction of survival in heart failure. Circulation. 2006;113(11):1424-33.
26. Aaronson KD, Schwartz JS, Chen TM, et al. Development and prospective validation of a clinical index to predict survival in ambulatory patients referred for cardiac transplant evaluation. Circulation. 1997;95(12):2660-7.
27. Javaheri S, Parker TJ, Liming JD, et al. Sleep apnea in 81 ambulatory male patients with stable heart failure. Types and their prevalences, consequences, and presentations. Circulation. 1998;97(21):2154-9.
28. Bradley TD, Floras JS. Sleep apnea and heart failure: Part I: obstructive sleep apnea. Circulation. 2003;107(12):1671-8.
29. Bradley TD, Floras JS. Sleep apnea and heart failure: Part II: central sleep apnea. Circulation. 2003;107(13):1822-6.
30. Javaheri S. Central sleep apnea-hypopnea syndrome in heart failure: prevalence, impact, and treatment. Sleep. 1996;19(10 Suppl):S229-31.
31. Wang H, Parker JD, Newton GE, et al. Influence of obstructive sleep apnea on mortality in patients with heart failure. J Am Coll Cardiol. 2007;49(15):1625-31.
32. Roger VL, Go AS, Lloyd-Jones DM, et al. Heart disease and stroke statistics—2012 update: a report from the American Heart Association. Circulation. 2012;125(1):e2-e220.
33. Fonarow GC, Abraham WT, Albert NM, et al. Influence of a performance-improvement initiative on quality of care for patients hospitalized with heart failure: results of the Organized Program to Initiate Lifesaving Treatment in Hospitalized Patients With Heart Failure (OPTIMIZE-HF). Arch Intern Med. 2007;167(14):1493-502.
34. Vinson JM, Rich MW, Sperry JC, et al. Early readmission of elderly patients with congestive heart failure. J Am Geriatr Soc. 1990;38(12):1290-5.
35. Tsuyuki RT, McKelvie RS, Arnold JM, et al. Acute precipitants of congestive heart failure exacerbations. Arch Intern Med. 2001;161(19):2337-42.
36. Fonarow GC, Abraham WT, Albert NM, et al. Factors identified as precipitating hospital admissions for heart failure and clinical outcomes: findings from OPTIMIZE-HF. Arch Intern Med. 2008;168(8):847-54.
37. Moser DK, Mann DL. Improving outcomes in heart failure: It's not unusual beyond usual care. Circulation. 2002;105(24):2810-2.
38. Hernandez AF, Greiner MA, Fonarow GC, et al. Relationship between early physician follow-up and 30-day readmission among Medicare beneficiaries hospitalized for heart failure. JAMA. 2010;303(17):1716-22.
39. Drazner MH, Rame JE, Dries DL. Third heart sound and elevated jugular venous pressure as markers of the subsequent development of heart failure in patients with asymptomatic left ventricular dysfunction. Am J Med. 2003;114(6):431-7.

40. Latini R, Masson S, Anand IS, et al. Prognostic value of very low plasma concentrations of troponin T in patients with stable chronic heart failure. Circulation. 2007;116(11):1242-9.
41. Tsutamoto T, Wada A, Maeda K, et al. Attenuation of compensation of endogenous cardiac natriuretic peptide system in chronic heart failure: prognostic role of plasma brain natriuretic peptide concentration in patients with chronic symptomatic left ventricular dysfunction. Circulation. 1997;96(2):509-16.
42. Januzzi JL Jr, Rehman SU, Mohammed AA, et al. Use of amino-terminal pro-B-type natriuretic peptide to guide outpatient therapy of patients with chronic left ventricular systolic dysfunction. J Am Coll Cardiol. 2011;58(18):1881-9.
43. Jourdain P, Jondeau G, Funck F, et al. Plasma brain natriuretic peptide-guided therapy to improve outcome in heart failure: the STARS-BNP Multicenter Study. J Am Coll Cardiol. 2007;49(16):1733-9.
44. Epstein AE, DiMarco JP, Ellenbogen KA, et al. ACC/AHA/HRS 2008 Guidelines for Device-Based Therapy of Cardiac Rhythm Abnormalities: a report of the American College of Cardiology/American Heart Association Task Force on Practice Guidelines (Writing Committee to Revise the ACC/AHA/NASPE 2002 Guideline Update for Implantation of Cardiac Pacemakers and Antiarrhythmia Devices) developed in collaboration with the American Association for Thoracic Surgery and Society of Thoracic Surgeons. J Am Coll Cardiol. 2008;51(21):e1-62.
45. van Veldhuisen DJ, Braunschweig F, Conraads V, et al. Intrathoracic impedance monitoring, audible patient alerts, and outcome in patients with heart failure. Circulation. 2011;124(16):1719-26.
46. Conraads VM, Tavazzi L, Santini M, et al. Sensitivity and positive predictive value of implantable intrathoracic impedance monitoring as a predictor of heart failure hospitalizations: the SENSE-HF trial. Eur Heart J. 2011;32(18):2266-73.
47. Abraham WT, Adamson PB, Bourge RC, et al. Wireless pulmonary artery haemodynamic monitoring in chronic heart failure: a randomised controlled trial. Lancet. 2011;377(9766):658-66.
48. Bourge RC, Abraham WT, Adamson PB, et al. Randomized controlled trial of an implantable continuous hemodynamic monitor in patients with advanced heart failure: the COMPASS-HF study. J Am Coll Cardiol. 2008;51(11):1073-9.
49. Desai AS. Home monitoring heart failure care does not improve patient outcomes: looking beyond telephone-based disease management. Circulation. 2012;125(6):828-36.

Chapter 23

Echocardiography: Getting It Right

Daniel G Blanchard

ABSTRACT

Echocardiography is the most commonly used cardiac imaging technique and is extremely useful in multiple clinical settings, including heart failure, coronary heart disease, valvular heart disease pericardial disease and cardiomyopathy. Echocardiography can also be used to estimate left ventricular (LV) filling pressure and pulmonary artery pressure. This chapter discusses the various clinical uses of echocardiography today.

INTRODUCTION

Echocardiography is the second most commonly performed cardiac test, behind only electrocardiography. Compared to other cardiac imaging techniques, such as computed tomography and magnetic resonance imaging, echocardiography has the advantages of portability, rapid image acquisition, no ionizing radiation, and lower cost.[1] Echocardiograms should not be performed on everyone; however, it is important to understand when echocardiographic studies are the most helpful. This chapter will discuss the utility of echocardiography and the specific clinical scenarios where it is most useful for good patient care.

HEMODYNAMIC INSTABILITY/SHOCK

Let us start with the most frightening clinical scenario: a patient with unstable vital signs and frank hypotension. Sometimes, the physical examination, chest X-ray, and laboratory results are enough to make an accurate diagnosis but definitely not always. Echocardiography can be enormously helpful in assessing several critical parameters in a patient with shock.

Ventricular Systolic Function

A normal or hyperdynamic left ventricular (LV) ejection fraction (EF) would strongly suggest that the shock is not cardiogenic but rather septic, hypovolemic, or vasodilatory. On the other hand, a depressed LV EF does not conclusively mean the shock is cardiogenic, but it dramatically increases the odds of it (especially if the LV dysfunction is new). Echocardiography can also assess right ventricular (RV) function. If RV function is depressed in the setting of shock, one should strongly consider a large pulmonary embolus or RV infarction.

Valvular Function

One of the strengths of echocardiography is the assessment of cardiac valves. In most settings, echocardiography can diagnose severe valve dysfunction (e.g., severe aortic and mitral regurgitation and/or stenosis). A sudden onset of hemodynamic instability is more likely due to acute aortic or mitral regurgitation, as valvular stenosis is a more gradual process. Color Doppler imaging is diagnostic in most cases, but transesophageal echocardiography (TEE, discussed later) is occasionally necessary.

Regional Wall Motion Abnormalities

Echocardiography can be used to estimate LV EF, but can also identify regional abnormalities of LV function which occur in myocardial infarction (MI). In cases of acute MI, non-affected areas of the LV often become hyperdynamic to maintain a near-normal EF. Echocardiography can detect regional abnormalities, which may lead to shock (MI with ventricular septal rupture, inferior MI with severe mitral regurgitation and LV free-wall rupture). Intravenous injection of echocardiography contrast (Optison, Definity) is often helpful, as the contrast opacifies the LV cavity and makes the wall motion abnormalities more apparent.

Estimation of Intracardiac Pressures

First, echocardiography can estimate right atrial (central venous) pressure. This is done by evaluating the diameter of the inferior vena cava (IVC) and its response to inspiration. Normally, the IVC diameter is less than 2 cm, and it collapses greater than 50% with inspiration (this occurs because intrathoracic pressure drops during inspiration and "sucks" blood from the abdomen into the heart). In this case, right atrial pressure is not greater than 5 mmHg. If the IVC is dilated but its diameter still decreases greater than 50% with inspiration, the right atrial pressure is likely around 10 mmHg. However, when the IVC is markedly dilated and decreases in diameter during inspiration by less than 10%, the right atrial pressure is probably in the range of 15–20 mmHg. Unfortunately, this method does not work in an intubated patient, as the positive-pressure ventilation prevents the normal decrease in IVC diameter with inspiration.

Pulmonary artery pressure can be estimated using the modified Bernoulli equation. This states that the pressure in the right ventricle is directly related to the velocity of tricuspid regurgitation (TR) blood flow. Most people have mild TR, and the velocity of this flow can be measured with Doppler echocardiography. Using an analogy of a garden hose nozzle, the velocity of water through the nozzle increases exponentially as the pressure within the hose increases. It turns out that the pressure gradient across the tricuspid valve (the "nozzle") is equal to four times the velocity of the tricuspid regurgitant velocity squared, plus the right atrial pressure. If there is no pulmonic stenosis, then the RV systolic pressure is essentially the same as the systolic pulmonary artery pressure:

Systolic pulmonary artery pressure = $4 \times (\text{TR velocity})^2$ + right atrial pressure

When the TR velocity exceeds 3 m/s, pulmonary hypertension is usually present.

Finally, Doppler echocardiography can help estimate LV filling pressure. This is not an exact scientific method, but it is still very useful. This topic is discussed below under the heading Heart Failure. Suffice it to say that diastolic flow patterns through the mitral valve and pulmonary veins can distinguish patients with normal versus high LV filling pressures.

HEART FAILURE

As mentioned above, LVEF can be accurately estimated in the great majority of patients presenting with dyspnea and possible congestive heart failure (CHF).[2] The presence, severity and anatomical distribution of LV hypertrophy can also be assessed with echocardiography. In the last few years, there has been a growing appreciation that heart failure can occur in patients with preserved LV systolic function [heart failure with preserved ejection fraction (HF-pEF)] as well as those with reduced systolic function [heart failure with reduced ejection fraction (HF-rEF)]. Patients in the first group tend to have more diastolic abnormalities, and have increased LV filling pressures despite normal LV EF. HF-pEF may occur in the settings of long-term hypertension, aortic or mitral valvular disease, myocardial fibrosis, infiltrative cardiomyopathy, or pericardial constriction.

Diastolic function is a very important parameter assessed by echocardiography. In a normal individual, about two-thirds of LV filling occurs early during diastole (the early rapid filling or "E" wave), and one-third during late diastole (the atrial contraction or "A" wave). Similarly, the majority of flow from the pulmonary vein into the left atrium occurs during diastole (the "D" wave), and less during ventricular systole (the "S" wave). As humans age, the normally rapid myocardial relaxation phase after systole gradually slows. By the sixth decade, most people develop a pattern of mild diastolic dysfunction (also called "abnormal relaxation"), where the transmitral E wave velocity is less than that of the A wave (and the pulmonary venous S wave becomes greater than the D wave). Though technically abnormal, this change in diastolic filling is expected with aging, and predicts a *normal* mean LV diastolic pressure.

In patients with HF-pEF, moderate-to-severe diastolic LV dysfunction is often present. In these cases, the transmitral E velocity is greater than the A velocity, but the pulmonary venous S velocity is less than the D velocity. In addition, the mitral annular diastolic velocity (e′) is also markedly reduced. The reader is referred to the article by DeMaria for a more complete discussion of the Doppler evaluation of diastolic function.[1] If CHF is suspected and LV EF is normal, it is important to check the left atrial size. Enlargement of the left atrium strongly suggests elevated LV diastolic pressure and therefore HF-pEF. Finally, if LV EF is normal in a patient presenting with CHF, consider asking for a specialized Doppler examination to rule out pericardial constriction.

ISCHEMIC HEART DISEASE

Chronic

As mentioned above, echocardiography can detect regional wall motion abnormalities that are signs of old MIs, and can estimate overall LV EF.

Acute

When a patient presents with an obvious acute ST-elevation MI, he or she should be transferred to the catheterization laboratory immediately for direct revascularization. However, clinical presentations of possible acute myocardial ischemia are not always obvious. For example, patients with left bundle branch block, old LV aneurysm, or preexisting ST-T wave abnormalities may present with chest pain, and in these cases, the electrocardiogram may not be diagnostic of an MI—even though one is occurring. Echocardiography is particularly useful in these settings, as the finding of a new LV wall motion abnormality will direct the care toward acute intervention. On the other hand, unchanged or normal LV systolic function is reassuring and suggests that a more conservative medical approach is appropriate. In addition, echocardiography can evaluate RV systolic function. This is especially important in cases of inferior MI, as RV involvement portends a worse prognosis and, therefore, should be treated quickly and aggressively.

VALVULAR HEART DISEASE

Two-dimensional (2-D) echocardiography is extremely useful for diagnosing valvular disease (including aortic and mitral stenosis, mitral valve prolapse, etc.), but Doppler echocardiography is necessary to estimate its severity.[3] Doppler echocardiography measures velocity of blood within the heart and vasculature. Color Doppler (where different shades of color representing different blood velocities are superimposed on a 2D image) can quickly screen for the presence of valvular regurgitation.

Echocardiography is reasonably quantitative in the evaluation of stenotic lesions but is only semiquantitative for evaluating regurgitant lesions. In the case of aortic stenosis, the *continuity equation* is used:

$$A_1 \times V_1 = A_2 \times V_2$$

where A_1 and V_1 are the cross-sectional area of and maximum systolic velocity through the LV outflow tract, and V_2 is the maximum velocity through the aortic valve. These three variables can be measured with echocardiography and then used to solve for aortic valve area. The accuracy of the continuity equation measurements is relatively good, though not perfect. If the severity of the echocardiography measurements is not consistent with the clinical findings, then TEE or cardiac catheterization may be necessary.

Mitral stenosis is quantified using the *pressure half-time* method, which measures how quickly the pressure gradient between the left atrium and left ventricle decreases during diastole. If the gradient decreases quickly between the two chambers, then the stenosis is relatively mild; if the gradient decreases slowly, the stenosis is more severe. The overall accuracy of the pressure half-time method is also relatively good, although it becomes inaccurate temporarily after percutaneous mitral valvuloplasty.

The quantification of valvular regurgitation is sometimes difficult. Color Doppler is an essential part of the examination and, in general, shows larger and larger color "jets" in the left atrium and right atrium as mitral regurgitation and TR (respectively) worsen. The same is true for color jets in the left ventricle as aortic regurgitation worsens. However, regurgitant jets are not always central and may be quite eccentric. In these cases, the jet may be "wall-hugging" and lead to underestimation of the regurgitation severity. More recently, the size of the color jet *proximal* to the valve has been used to estimate severity with some success. Doppler echocardiography measurements can also be used to calculate the "effective regurgitant orifice" (ERO) size. Unfortunately, this method uses several assumptions that are often incorrect. For cases of mitral regurgitation, an ERO of less than 0.2 cm^2 is generally mild, while approximately 0.4 cm^2 is more likely moderate and approximately 0.6 cm^2 is usually severe. In cases of aortic regurgitation, the pressure half-time method can also be used. If the pressure gradient between the aorta and the left ventricle decreases quickly, the aortic regurgitation is likely severe. A pressure half-time less than 250 milliseconds almost always signifies severe aortic regurgitation.

In the setting of positive blood cultures and possible infective endocarditis, transthoracic echocardiography (TTE) should be ordered. Echocardiography is reasonably sensitive for detecting valvular vegetations, and is especially good at diagnosing regurgitation due to infective destruction of the valve leaflets. However, TTE is not very accurate in visualizing valvular abscesses and small vegetations. So, if endocarditis is strongly suspected (persistent fevers and multiple positive blood cultures), a TEE should be ordered. TEE has a much greater diagnostic accuracy that regular echocardiography, especially in detecting valvular abscesses. This is important because a valvular abscess generally means that antibiotic treatment alone will be unsuccessful and that surgery will be required.[4]

Echocardiography can help evaluate the function of both bioprosthetic and mechanical prosthetic heart valves. Doppler echocardiography can estimate mean gradients through prosthetic valves and thereby screen for valve stenosis or dysfunction. Because prosthetic valves (especially mechanical valves) block ultrasound waves and cause "shadowing" posterior to the valve, TEE may be necessary to evaluate a prosthesis more completely (to check for valvular vegetations or abscesses in cases of suspected endocarditis).

PERICARDIAL DISEASE

Acute Pericarditis

The diagnosis of pericarditis is a clinical one, based on history, physical examination, and the electrocardiogram. An echocardiography should be ordered for all patients thought to have pericarditis (to make sure they do not have cardiac tamponade), but the *absence of an effusion does not rule out pericarditis.* It is important to remember that even raging pericarditis can be present without a pericardial effusion.[5]

Pericardial Effusion

Echocardiography is extremely accurate in detecting pericardial effusions, anywhere from trivial to huge in size. Small pericardial effusions tend to be posterior, especially if the patient is supine. Larger effusions can be circumferential or loculated, and may contain clot, fibrinous strands, or tumor. Purulent effusions tend to be loculated. This distinction between loculated and nonloculated effusions is clinically important, as loculated effusions are harder to drain completely via pericardiocentesis. In these cases, surgical drainage/debridement and creation of a pericardial window may be required.

Cardiac Tamponade

The three main findings in tamponade are: (i) hypotension, (ii) elevated central venous pressure, and (iii) pulsus paradoxus. Unfortunately, none of these findings are specific for tamponade (including pulsus paradoxus, which can occur in other conditions, such as status asthmaticus). Echocardiography now plays a major in the diagnosis of cardiac tamponade. Although a number of findings have been reported over the last several years, the most important echocardiography findings in tamponade are:

- *Distension of the inferior vena cava*: This is a nonspecific finding but, in the presence of a moderate-to-large pericardial effusion, denotes elevated central venous pressure
- *Diastolic compression of the right ventricle*: There is enhanced ventricular interdependence in cardiac tamponade. In severe cases, the overall volume of the entire heart remains constant throughout the cardiac cycle. Thus, when the LV increases in size during diastole, the RV is compressed. On echocardiography, the RV free wall "buckles" transiently in early diastole. This finding is more specific for cardiac tamponade
- *Abnormal mitral inflow Doppler echocardiography pattern*: This finding is the most specific of the three. During normal inspiration, venous return increases more on the right side of the heart than the left. This leads to a mild (<10%) increase in peak transtricuspid blood flow velocity and a reciprocal mild decrease in transmitral blood flow velocity. As mentioned, ventricular interdependence is enhanced in tamponade. As the heart is abnormally compressed, any increase in filling and enlargement of the RV during inspiration leads to a decrease in LV size and diastolic filling. Several important studies have shown that a *respiratory variation in mitral "E" velocity of greater than 25%* strongly suggests cardiac tamponade when a pericardial effusion is present.

Pericardial Constriction

Constrictive pericarditis is relatively uncommon, but in affected patients, the diagnosis is often missed for many years. Patients with this disorder usually do not have significant pericardial effusions, but the pericardium gradually constricts down onto the heart and leads to elevated RV and LV diastolic pressures. The hemodynamics are similar to those of cardiac tamponade in several ways, and both IVC dilation and jugular venous distention are often present. Importantly, abnormal variation in mitral inflow also occurs. So, if a patient presents with heart failure but normal ventricular systolic function and greater than 25% variation in mitral inflow velocity with respiration, pericardial constriction may well be the correct diagnosis.

CARDIOMYOPATHIES

There are three basic forms of primary cardiomyopathies: (i) dilated, (ii) restrictive, and (iii) hypertrophic.[6] Echocardiography is useful—though not always diagnostic—in distinguishing these various forms. Patients with dilated cardiomyopathy (DCM) usually have global LV enlargement with global systolic dysfunction. This may affect both ventricles. Moderate-to-severe diastolic dysfunction is also frequently seen. By definition, significant coronary artery disease is not present. Regional LV dysfunction argues for ischemic heart disease, but this is not 100% specific.

Restrictive cardiomyopathy can be completely idiopathic, but is most commonly caused by infiltrative processes, such as amyloidosis, sarcoidosis, and hemochromatosis. Echocardiographic evaluation often shows increased LV wall thickness, valvular thickening, marked biatrial enlargement, and moderate-to-severe LV diastolic dysfunction. Magnetic resonance imaging is particularly useful in confirming a diagnosis of amyloidosis. Severe diastolic dysfunction by echocardiography is an accurate sign of poor prognosis in these patients.

In the setting of hypertrophic cardiomyopathy (HCM), echocardiography can detect asymmetric septal hypertrophy, one of the cardinal findings of HCM. In cases of obstructive HCM, echocardiography can identify systolic anterior motion (SAM) of the mitral valve leaflet (which causes outflow tract obstruction), elevated late systolic blood flow velocity through the LV outflow tract, and late systolic partial closure of the aortic valve. Taken together, the presence of all these findings are diagnostic of obstructive HCM is the majority of cases.

RIGHT HEART DISEASE

As mentioned, echocardiography is reasonably good at detecting right heart enlargement and RV dysfunction. Doppler echocardiography is excellent in estimating RV and pulmonary artery systolic pressure, and color Doppler imaging can assess severity of tricuspid and pulmonic regurgitation. Echocardiography is indicated in cases of pulmonary embolism, and residual thrombi are occasionally seen in the right atrium or ventricle: this finding often requires thrombolysis to prevent further massive pulmonary embolus. In cases of severe pulmonary hypertension, the RV is markedly enlarged, and the interventricular septum is flattened by the high RV pressure. By measuring peak TR velocity, echocardiography can assess the responses to treatment for pulmonary hypertension.

TRANSESOPHAGEAL ECHOCARDIOGRAPHY

Transesophageal echocardiography provides outstanding close-up images of the heart, from a posterior-anterior perspective rather than the opposite with TTE. Without going into extensive detail, when should a TEE be ordered?

- *Suboptimal TTE images*: If the surface images are poor and cardiac imaging is essential, TEE can help
- *Suspected endocarditis*: If endocarditis is strongly suspected (positive blood cultures and persistent fevers) but TTE is unrevealing, TEE should be performed
- *Staphylococcus aureus bacteremia*: If this occurs in the absence of an identified source, TEE is indicated to rule out endocarditis and intracardiac abscess
- *Inadequate response to treatment for endocarditis*: If a patient with endocarditis does not defervesce quickly or clear blood cultures with appropriate antibiotic treatment, TEE is indicated to rule out an intracardiac abscess
- *Valvular heart disease*: In certain cases, severity of valvular disease may be difficult to ascertain with TTE. TEE is often very useful in determining the degree of mitral, aortic and TR. TEE can also assess whether patients with mitral regurgitation are good versus poor candidates for valve repair.
- *Source of embolus*: In many cases, the source of stroke/systemic embolism is obvious (e.g., a 75-year-old woman with chronic atrial fibrillation and a new stroke), but in other cases, the source is unclear (e.g., a 35-year-old male with no known thrombotic risk factors). In these cases, TEE can be very useful

to check for unusual sources of cardiogenic emboli, including patent foramen ovale, benign cardiac tumors (e.g., myxoma and papillary fibroelastoma) and left atrial appendage thrombus.

REFERENCES

1. DeMaria AN, Blanchard DG. Echocardiography. In: Fuster V, Walsh RA, Harrington RA (Eds). Hurst's The Heart, 13th edition. New York, USA: McGraw-Hill Professional; 2010. pp. 411-89.
2. Jessup M, Abraham WT, Casey DE, et al. 2009 Focused Update: ACCF/AHA Guidelines for the Diagnosis and Management of Heart Failure in Adults: A Report of the American College of Cardiology Foundation/American Heart Association Task Force on Practice Guidelines developed in collaboration with the International Society for Heart and Lung Transplantation. Circulation. 2009;119:1977-2016.
3. Bonow RO, Carabello BA, Chatterjee K, et al. 2008 focused update incorporated into the ACC/AHA 2006 guidelines for the management of patients with valvular heart disease: a report of the American College of Cardiology/American Heart Association Task Force on Practice Guidelines (Writing Committee to revise the 1998 guidelines for the management of patients with valvular heart disease). Endorsed by the Society of Cardiovascular Anesthesiologists, Society for Cardiovascular Angiography and Interventions, and Society of Thoracic Surgeons. J Am Coll Cardiol. 2008;52(13):e1-142.
4. Hoen B, Duval X. Clinical practice. Infective endocarditis. N Engl J Med. 2013;368(15):1425-33.
5. Khandaer MH, Espinosa RE, Nishimura RA, et al. Pericardial disease: diagnosis and management. Mayo Clin Proc. 2010;85(6):572-93.
6. Maron BJ. Contemporary insights and strategies for risk stratification and prevention of sudden death in hypertrophic cardiomyopathy. Circulation. 2010;121(3):445-56.

Chapter 24

A Practical Guide for Reducing Readmissions in Heart Failure

Eugene C DePasquale, Gregg C Fonarow

ABSTRACT

Heart failure is a significant and growing public health problem resulting in substantial morbidity, mortality, and healthcare expenditures. Despite improvements in reducing mortality in this population, rates of readmission continue to increase approaching 30% within 60–90 days of discharge. Reducing preventable readmission in heart failure is a national focus but very challenging. Strategies to prevent readmissions are critical not only for the patient, but also for institutions, as significant financial penalties are being levied through the Hospital Readmissions Reduction Program of the Centers for Medicare and Medicaid Services (CMS). Significant opportunities exist to improve the quality of care, care transitions, and outcomes for patients hospitalized with heart failure. Certain practical strategies and programs have been successful in identifying patients at higher risk for rehospitalization and reducing rehospitalization in heart failure. Additional approaches and strategies are needed to reduce preventable rehospitalizations in the first 30 days and beyond as well as improve survival.

INTRODUCTION

Heart failure is a significant and growing public health problem, with a prevalence of 5.7 million cases in the United States alone, associated with high morbidity and mortality. In addition, there are high healthcare expenditures with substantial admissions and readmissions for heart failure occurring annually accounting for a large portion of the estimated $44.6 billion spent on heart failure hospitalizations annually in the United States. Despite improvements in reducing mortality in this population, rates of readmission continue to increase approaching 30% within 60–90 days of discharge.[1] Strategies to prevent readmissions are critical not only for the patient, but also for institutions, as significant financial penalties are being levied through the Hospital Readmissions Reduction Program of the Centers for Medicare and Medicaid Services (CMS).[2]

SCOPE OF THE PROBLEM

The epidemic of heart failure continues to grow with 5.7 million individuals in the United States and 15 million Europeans with this condition [as per data from European Society of Cardiology (ESC)].[1,3] It is projected that there will be an additional 3 million people with heart failure in the United States by 2030, a 25% increase in prevalence from 2010. The complex interplay between physiological, psychological, social and healthcare system issues makes the management of this chronic disease challenging. The annual number of heart failure hospitalizations have increased over the past decades from approximately 800,000 and peaking at over 1 million as primary diagnosis.[1] More recently, there has been a trend toward decreased admission rates for heart failure as the primary discharge diagnosis among Medicare beneficiaries.[4] In 2006, the hospitalization rate in the United States amongst those over the age of 64 years was 23 per 1,000 for men and 20 per 1,000 for women, showing heart failure as the leading cause of hospital admissions in this age range.[5]

Despite the apparent reduction in heart failure admissions amongst the Medicare population, heart failure readmissions have not decreased and may have increased during the same period of time.[4] Additionally, approximately 25% of those hospitalized for heart failure will be readmitted within 30 days postdischarge and 30%, within 60–90 days.[6,7] Data of Medicare beneficiaries hospitalized from 2005–2008 failed to show a strong correlation of risk-standardized rehospitalization rates and mortality rates, suggesting that the factors that may be important for mortality are not necessarily as the same as those defining readmission risk.[8] Readmission risk is high within the following 30 days, with a majority of readmissions following a heart failure hospitalization due to other causes.[9]

Strategies aimed at reducing hospitalizations in patients with heart failure include optimization of evidence-based drug and device therapies, treating comorbidities, addressing the etiology of the heart failure and improving management of care (Box 1). While there is considerable evidence establishing the efficacy of these therapies in reducing mortality and hospitalizations in patients with heart failure and reduced ejection fraction, therapy is empiric for heart failure with preserved ejection fraction stemming from a dearth of evidence with recent negative studies examining the aldosterone blockade[10] and 5-phosphodiesterase inhibition,[11] which is concerning in light of the fact that this condition accounts for roughly half of readmissions.[12]

Box 1: Practical strategies for reducing readmission in heart failure

- Identify key precipitating factors for hospitalization and rehospitalization, and address prior to discharge
- Optimize evidence-based heart failure medication and device therapy
- Provide predischarge heart failure patient education by trained educators
- Begin comprehensive discharge planning right away
- Schedule early postdischarge physician follow-up
- For higher risk patients, refer to comprehensive heart failure disease management programs
- When appropriate consider palliative care services
- Systems of care approaches (Get with the guidelines—Heart Failure, Hospital to Home)

CHALLENGES

Patient factors, provider and health system factors, and the postdischarge environment can all impact the probability of readmission of patients with heart failure (Fig. 1).[13] There are a variety of challenges in mitigating the risk of early readmission after a heart failure hospitalization.

Socioeconomic Factors

Socioeconomic factors have a significant impact on adherence to medical therapies as well as to ability to comply with the overall care plan. Every effort should be made to minimize the impact of these factors. Patients should be routinely asked whether they can afford their medications and physicians should know the costs of common medications and make efforts to reduce the financial burden these therapies can have on patients. Medication cost is a major barrier to adherence.[14] The main three classes of medications these patients receive are all available in generic form. Major retailers are now offering these medications at significantly reduced prices. Every effort should be made to select therapies that patients can afford.

These barriers also extend to behavioral change. It may be difficult for patients with financial limitations to avoid low cost sodium-rich food if the healthier alternative is more expensive or to purchase a weight scale.

Therapy-related Factors

Medication side effects are a significant barrier as well to adherence. It is important to inform patients of the common adverse side effects to expect from heart failure medications. It is also important to educate the patient on the importance of these medications and the potential benefits they may experience.[14] The number of medications is a barrier as well and once-a-day formulations may enhance patient adherence.

Challenges to Adherence

Health literacy, the ability for an individual to understand and process of basic health information to make informed health decisions, can be a significant challenge to adherence. A retrospective cohort study (n = 2,156) conducted at Kaiser Permanente Colorado demonstrated that low health literacy was independently associated with higher mortality [unadjusted rate, 17.6% vs 6.3%; adjusted hazard ratio, 1.97; confidence interval (CI) = 1.3–2.97],

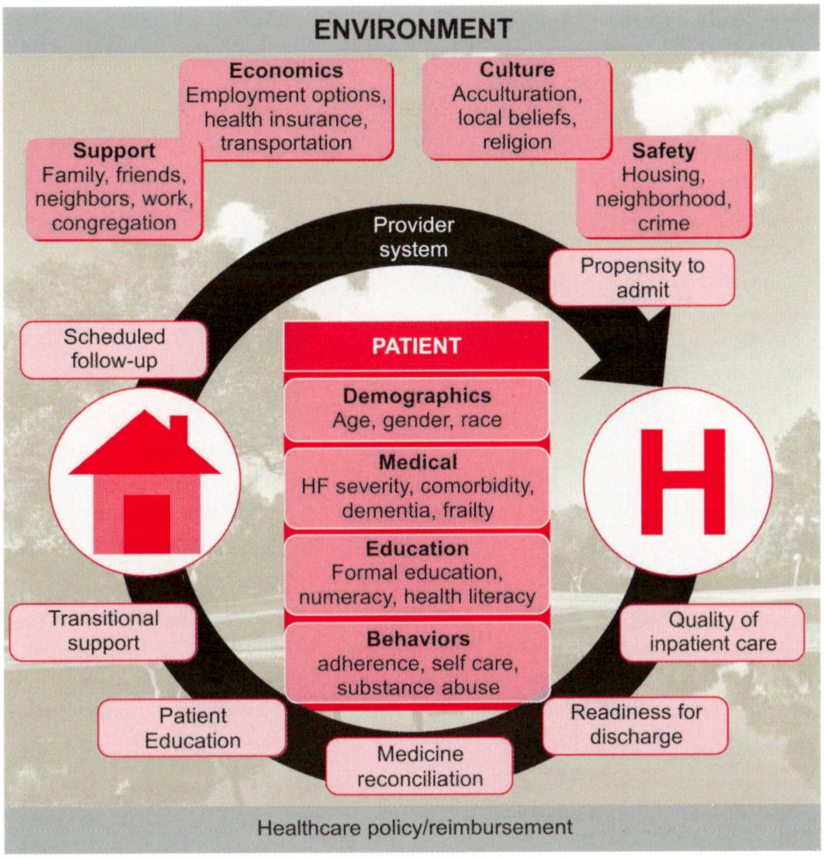

H, hospital

Fig. 1 Conceptual model for heart failure readmission

Source: Adapted from Hersh AM, Masoudi FA, Allen LA. Postdischarge environment following heart failure hospitalization: expanding the view of hospital readmission. *J Am Heart Assoc*. 2013;2(2):e000116. *with permission*

but not hospitalization. Patients with low health literacy were older, of lower socioeconomic status, less likely to have at least a high school education, and had higher rates of comorbidities.[15] Recognition of health literacy is important as targeting education to a patient's health literacy level has been demonstrated to reduce the risk of hospitalization or death.[16]

Multiple chronic illnesses can have additional impact on patients with respect to physical, cognitive, and functional challenges. When coupled with the realities of dealing with multiple comorbidities (i.e., multiple clinicians, conflicting recommendations, large medication lists), this can severely limit adherence to medical and behavioral therapies. The impact of multiple comorbidities is not well studied as randomized controlled trials typically exclude these patients.

Depression and anxiety are common amongst patients with heart failure.[17] These conditions can impair adherence with effects on cognition, function, motivation, social support, and engagement.[18] In a study of 522 patients with heart failure, it was demonstrated that patients with depression and heart failure have higher rates of medication nonadherence.[19] In another study of 958 patients with heart failure, severe depressive symptoms were associated with a greater than 40% higher risk for heart failure readmission or death.[20] Screening tools for depression have been validated and are available.[21] Screening for depression may be important given the significant deleterious impact this condition has with respect to mortality and readmission in heart failure.

STRATEGIES FOR REDUCING READMISSIONS: SUCCESS AND FAILURE

Disease management programs have been created to provide a multidisciplinary framework for patients with a chronic condition, such as heart failure. This framework helps provide for the development of an individualized plan to provide education and support for patients as well as coordinating care amongst the healthcare providers and patients. The American Heart Association Taxonomy Writing Group suggests that these programs include multidisciplinary care (including physicians, nurses, social workers and others), use of evidence-based practice guidelines, frequent contact with providers, comprehensive patient education, discharge and early postdischarge support, process, and outcomes measurement.[22]

Heart Failure Education

A number of randomized controlled trials have been performed to evaluate the impact of discharge support in reducing rehospitalization. A meta-analysis of 18 randomized controlled trials (n = 3,304) of comprehensive discharge planning and postdischarge support found a significant reduction in all-cause readmissions [risk ratio (RR) = 0.75, 95% CI = 0.64–0.88).[23] Some of these interventions included heart failure education. In a smaller randomized controlled trial of 223 patients, the importance of the addition of a 1-hour nurse-educator delivered teaching session at the time of discharge was established and demonstrated improved clinical outcomes and reduced readmissions 180 days following discharge. In addition, this intervention resulted in cost savings of an estimated $2,823 per patient.[24]

Multidisciplinary Teams

Complex medical and socioeconomic factors contribute to high readmission rates necessitating a team approach. The management of each patient is determined by the goals of care, socioeconomic circumstances, educational background, and support network. Palliative options should be addressed in those with end-stage heart failure. The importance of providing both affordable medications and providing an achievable diet should not be overlooked.

An integrated team approach, including the patient, primary care physician, hospital physician, cardiologist, other specialty physicians, nurse, pharmacist, family, social worker, and health education provides important contributions to aiding efforts to reduce rehospitalizations. A randomized controlled trial (n = 1,306) studying the effect of a nurse-directed multidisciplinary intervention (comprehensive education, prescribed diet, social service consultation, planning for early discharge, medication reconciliation and intensive follow-up) on readmission rates within 90 days, quality of life and cost of care for high-risk patients 70 years of age or older hospitalized for heart failure demonstrated improvements in each of these components.[25]

Meta-analyses have typically divided heart failure management strategies into broad categories: multidisciplinary follow-up (home or clinic), primarily self-care and those restricted to telephone support. This may not be helpful as most approaches include an array of these methods.

Strategies incorporating either home or clinic multidisciplinary follow-up led to reduced heart failure hospitalization, all-cause hospitalizations and mortality. This was demonstrated in a meta-analysis examining 29 trials (n = 5,039). Approaches that included specialized multidisciplinary team follow-up led to reduced mortality (RR = 0.75, 95% CI = 0.59–0.96), reduced hospitalizations for heart failure (RR = 0.74, 95% CI = 0.63–0.87) and all-cause hospitalizations (RR = 0.81, 95% CI = 0.71–0.92). The majority of the trials analyzed examining cost-effectiveness demonstrated cost-saving.[26]

Structured Telephone Support

Approaches studying structured telephone support involving direct calls to patients have demonstrated reduced heart failure hospitalizations. There have been mixed results with reduction in all-cause hospitalization or mortality. In a meta-analysis conducted by McAlister et al. strategies employing telephone contact to their primary care physician reduced heart failure hospitalizations (RR = 0.75, 95% CI = 0.57–0.99), though did not reduce mortality or all-cause hospitalizations. However, subsequent meta-analyses have demonstrated not only reduced heart failure hospitalizations, but also reduction in all-cause mortality as well.[26]

Patient Self Care

Self-care strategies with limited follow-up have also been employed. In a meta-analysis (n = 857), strategies were used to teach patients to monitor their condition and to recognize when to seek medical assistance. Education typically included information about the signs and symptoms of heart failure, importance of daily weights, dietary restrictions and adherence to the medication regimen. These self-care strategies reduced heart failure readmissions (RR = 0.44, 95% CI = 0.27–0.71) and all-cause hospital readmissions (RR = 0.59,

95% CI = 0.44–0.80). However, no significant effect on mortality was observed.[27]

Transitions of Care and Early Postdischarge Follow-up

The period immediately following discharge is a high-risk period following a heart failure hospitalization discharge. Retrospective analysis of the Efficacy of Vasopressin Antagonism in Heart Failure Outcome Study with Tolvaptan (EVEREST) trial (n = 4,133), which randomized patients hospitalized for worsening heart failure with ejection fraction less than or equal to 40% to tolvaptan or placebo in addition to standard therapy, demonstrated that early mortality and rehospitalization was preceded by significant worsening of clinical signs and symptoms (i.e., orthopnea, low systolic blood pressure, higher heart rate), laboratory values (i.e., low serum sodium, decreased renal function, lower albumin levels) and neurohormonal parameters (increased levels of aldosterone and arginine vasopressin).[28]

These factors illustrate the importance of transitions of care upon discharge. Rich et al. demonstrated the importance of a multidisciplinary team in a previously discussed trial. In addition, their interventions included home-care services and individualized home visits with telephone follow-up.[25]

The early postdischarge visit has been demonstrated to decrease the risk of readmission in observational data. An observational analysis of 30,136 patients aged 65 years or older participating in the Organized Program to Initiate Lifesaving Treatment in Hospitalized Patients with Heart Failure (OPTIMIZE-HF) and the Get With the Guideline-Heart Failure quality improvement program described patterns of follow up after heart failure hospitalization and association with readmission rates. There was considerable variation in hospital-level rates of early outpatient postdischarge follow-up. The median percentage of patients who had early follow-up, defined as an appointment in 7 days or less, was 38.3%. Patients discharged from hospitals with higher early follow-up rates had a lower risk of 30-day readmission. However, patients at hospitals in the lowest quartile of early postdischarge follow-up (hospitals where it was less likely to have follow up within 7 days), had an approximately 3% higher readmission rate at 30-days.[29]

The usefulness of early postdischarge appointments may depend on the quality of care at the visit. The type of transitional care was studied in 10,599 patients with heart failure evaluated at emergency departments in Ontario, Canada (2004-7). In this study, the patients were subdivided into four groups according to their postdischarge care: no physician visit, primary care only, cardiologist only and collaborative care (including primary care and cardiologist). Patients treated with a collaborative approach were more likely to undergo evidence-based assessments and therapies. In addition, collaborative care was associated with reduced mortality more so than primary care alone as well as no physician follow-up. Results were also similar for composite endpoints of death, emergency department visits, and heart failure rehospitalizations.[30]

Postdischarge assessment should ideally assess volume status, review, adjust and add evidence-based medications, plan additional studies and incorporate patient education. However, this approach may not be feasible for the multitude of patients hospitalized for heart failure and ideally should be focused on those of the highest risk of cardiac events. Predictors of post-discharge events include low systolic blood pressure,[31,32] prolonged QRS duration,[33] renal dysfunction,[34] elevated natriuretic peptide level,[35] galectin-3,[36] hyponatremia,[37] and other comorbidities.[38] In addition, length of stay and the number of readmissions are major prognostic variables.[39] Further study is warranted to define the patient population most likely to benefit from these interventions given the increased attention to resource utilization.

Observational studies of general medicine patients have not demonstrated that prompt communication with outpatient clinicians, whether through direct communication or receipt of a discharge summary within 2 weeks, results in reduced readmissions.[40,41] However, while no benefit was observed, these were not randomized controlled studies. The question is raised as to whether these interventions would make a difference depending on patient complexity or the quality of the discharge summary.

Transitional care strategies should include comprehensive discharge support with early post-discharge follow-up. A comprehensive approach facilitating the transition from inpatient to discharge follow-up incorporating patient education, medication reconciliation, care coordination, guideline-based care and early postdischarge follow-up is more likely to succeed than approaches focused on one aspect of the process. Strategies aimed solely at process-based performance measures may not be successful. A large observational study of 16,791 patients hospitalized with heart failure at 150 hospitals failed to show a relationship with meeting the CMS requirement for discharge instructions and readmissions at 1 year.[42]

Medication Reconciliation

Medication reconciliation is critical not only to ensure that patients are discharged with appropriate therapies, but also to prevent medication errors. Therapies such as nonsteroidal anti-inflammatory drugs or nasal congestants should be avoided in patients with heart failure. Education and reconciliation are simple approaches to prevent heart failure patients taking these potentially harmful medications.[43]

Congestion Management

It is important to prevent clinical and subclinical congestion to reduce rehospitalization rates.[44] Sodium restriction is critically important in the postdischarge period to control fluid management. Loop diuretic therapy is the mainstay of congestion management, with novel therapies, such as vasopressin antagonists, adenosine-blocking agents, and ultrafiltration yielding mixed results or being untested.[45] Diuretic therapy may worsen renal function during hospitalization. However, this may be transient and not represent kidney injury and should not prevent aggressive diuresis.[34] Angiotensin-converting enzyme (ACE) inhibitors or angiotensin receptor blocker (ARB) may worsen renal function despite demonstrating mortality benefits and should be used if appropriate.[46]

During hospitalization, the majority of patients will have significant improvement in clinical congestion, however, may have persistence of subclinical congestion. Elevated natriuretic peptide levels are a poor prognostic feature at the time of discharge and may warrant further evaluation.[28] Initial and maintenance diuretic dosing should be guided by blood pressure measurement (supine and orthostatic) and renal function.[47] Metolazone may be used as an adjunctive therapy for those unresponsive to initial therapy. However, this carries a significant risk of hyponatremia and other electrolyte abnormalities. Aldosterone antagonists may be beneficial at reducing congestions and have been demonstrated to significantly reduce early hospitalization rates.[48,49] Tolvaptan, a vasopressin antagonist, may be helpful in patients with hyponatremia, relative hypotension and/or impaired renal function; however, the long-term effects of this agent were neutral in the overall hospitalized with heart failure population and the efficacy in patients with hyponatremia require further study.[50,51]

Use of Evidence-based Therapies

While national trends are improving there is a gap between guideline recommendations and actual clinical practice. Performance measures have been established to address this gap. However, these measures may be insufficient to improve postdischarge outcomes of such a complex medical condition.[52,53] It is well established that patients with systolic heart failure should receive recommended doses of beta blockers,[54,55] ACE inhibitors/ARBs,[56-58] and aldosterone antagonists.[49,59] Despite this, a recent study demonstrated that less than one-third of eligible patients hospitalized with heart failure received aldosterone antagonists, though this may be related to renal function and serum potassium level. The OPTIMIZE-HF registry demonstrated that adherence to guideline therapies resulted in reduced readmissions.[60] Despite representing roughly half of the heart failure population, data regarding therapies for heart failure with preserved ejection fraction are limited. Hydralazine and nitrate therapy is recommended for African Americans with heart failure and reduced ejection fraction.[61] Guideline-directed medical therapies have also proven to be highly cost-effective or cost-saving. A study examining the incremental cost-effectiveness ratios of ACE inhibitors, beta blockers and aldosterone antagonists demonstrated that the greatest gains in quality-adjusted life-years occurred when all three guideline-directed therapies were provided.[62]

In addition, revascularization candidates should be identified. Moreover, device therapies should be discussed with appropriate candidates meeting criteria for implantable cardiac defibrillators or cardiac resynchronization therapies.[63] Digoxin, which has hemodynamic, neurohormonal and electrophysiological effects, may be beneficial in heart failure patients.[64,65] Recent reanalysis of the Digitalis Investigation Group Trial demonstrated the digoxin reduces 30-day all-cause hospital admission in ambulatory older patients with chronic systolic heart failure.[66] Further study of digoxin is warranted as the effects of digoxin in a modern population or effects on readmissions have not been examined.

Optimization of Medications

Optimization of heart failure therapies is critical. The clinical status of the patient should be continuously reassessed and every attempt should be made to reach target doses of ACE inhibitors/ARBs, beta blockers and aldosterone antagonists[67] used in clinical trials, if clinically indicated. It should not be assumed that smaller doses are as effective as this has not been studied. Often these interventions can be made not only through a clinical visit, but also through other forms of direct communication. The use of guideline-directed therapies has shown to improve mortality, reduce readmissions and result in cost-savings.[62]

Telemonitoring

Telemonitoring is a form of chronic disease management where patients are given equipment, such as scales and blood pressure monitors to obtain clinical data at home. These data are typically remotely transmitted to care providers at regular intervals (i.e., daily or intermittently) to allow close assessment of the clinical status of patients without need for office or home visits. Initial meta-analyses (23 randomized controlled trials and 9 observational studies; total n = 5,792) demonstrated reduced all-cause mortality and heart failure readmissions. However, the included trials were of low-to-moderate quality with small numbers of patients.[68-70] Since these analyses, two large trials have been reported. The Telemonitoring to Improve Heart Failure Outcomes (Tele-HF) trial (n = 1,653) randomized patients to telemonitoring using an automated telephone-based system collecting daily information (symptoms, weight) or usual care. The primary endpoint was readmission for any reason or all-cause mortality at 180 days with a secondary endpoint of heart failure readmission. This trial was largely negative with no significant differences between the two groups.[71] The Telemedical Interventional Monitoring in Heart Failure (TIM-HF) trial (n = 710), conducted in Germany, also found no difference in mortality or the composite secondary endpoint of heart failure hospitalization or cardiovascular death.[72] The lack of benefit may not completely preclude the role of telemonitoring as an intervention. It is possible that the appropriate markers were not followed (i.e., weight or symptoms). In addition, the telemonitoring system may have been underused as in the Tele-HF trial; only 55% of patients were making three calls weekly by week 26 and only 86% making any calls.[71] Combined with other interventions this approach may have promise.

Advanced Monitoring Approaches

Implantable systems for chronic monitoring of intracardiac and pulmonary artery pressures have been developed to aid in the management of heart failure with the aim of preventing readmissions. The CardioMEMS Heart Sensor Allows Monitoring of Pressure to Improve Outcomes in New York Heart Association (NYHA) class III Heart Failure Patients (CHAMPION) trial assessed whether this intervention showed merit in NYHA class III patients. The primary endpoint was the rate of heart failure-related hospitalizations at 6 months. The study demonstrated significant 37% reduction in readmissions with the wireless implantable hemodynamic monitoring system (84 hospitalizations, n = 270) compared to the control group (120 hospitalizations, n = 280). Freedom from device-related complications was 98.6%.[73] However, this device has not been approved by the Food and Drug Administration (FDA) following reanalysis of the data and questions regarding subgroup populations (i.e., treatment effect was shown in men, but not women) and study conduct.[74] Implantable wireless hemodynamic monitoring may have merit; however, in light of recent findings of the FDA another trial may be needed.

Use of Cardiac Resynchronization Therapy

In addition to medical therapy, some patients with heart failure benefit from simultaneous pacing of both ventricles or cardiac resynchronization therapy (CRT) with the rationale that ventricular dyssynchrony can impair further a failing ventricle. CRT may help improve performance and reverse ventricular remodeling. CRT is currently recommended for heart failure patients who are NYHA class II–IV with severe systolic dysfunction and intraventricular conduction delay (i.e., QRS ≥120 msec), with the greatest benefit in patients with left bundle branch block.[75] In the Comparison of Medical Therapy, Pacing and Defibrillation in Heart Failure (COMPANION) trial, 1,520 patients with advanced heart failure were assigned in a 1:2:2 ratio to optimal medical therapy, optimal medical therapy plus CRT or CRT with defibrillator. This study demonstrated that the use of CRT was associated with significant reduction in the combined risk of death or all-cause hospitalizations. Compared with optimal medical therapy, CRT was associated with a 21–25% reduction in all-cause readmissions and a 41–44% reduction in heart failure readmissions per patient-year of follow up. CRT should be considered for heart failure patients meeting criteria for CRT. This study demonstrates the added benefit of this intervention in not only reducing mortality, but also in reducing readmissions.[76]

ADDITIONAL RESOURCES

Hospital to Home

The hospital to home (H2H; h2hquality.org) initiative, led by the American College of Cardiology and the Institute for Healthcare improvement, is a national quality improvement campaign to reduce cardiovascular-related readmissions and improve transitions home for patients hospitalized with cardiovascular disease. This initiative provides tools and webinars to better address readmissions and transitions of care. It also provides a mechanism to learn from other institutions.

Target: Heart Failure

Target: Heart Failure is an endeavor by the American Heart Association to help hospitals improve transition from inpatient to outpatient care and help reduce readmission through a number of resources including educational tools (i.e., Get With The Guidelines-Heart Failure),[77] prevention programs, quality initiatives and outcome-based programs.

FUTURE DIRECTIONS

Despite advances in the management of heart failure, high hospital readmission rates continue to persist. Early assessment postdischarge of clinical condition as well as monitoring signs and symptoms of congestion are critical. However, the whole patient should be considered and not solely the congestive symptoms to prevent not only readmissions, but also mortality as well. Establishing a comprehensive system incorporating patient education, assessment of patient resources, multidisciplinary care, mechanisms for continuous communication between patients and providers (i.e., direct telephone communication), and continuous assessment of the patient for congestive signs and symptoms as well as ensuring the use of guideline-based therapies are all critical for the success of the patient. Heart failure patients with preserved ejection fraction represent roughly half of readmissions and for whom evidence-based therapies are lacking and sorely needed. It remains to be seen how measures aimed at reducing 30-day readmission rates will impact survival and other patient-centered outcomes. Long-term follow-up from registry and trial data are needed to better understand the mechanisms leading to readmission to identify interventions that can prevent this and lead to improved outcomes. Many patients with symptomatic heart failure may not warrant acute intervention beyond decongestive therapies and the question is raised whether admission is really necessary? Observation unit management may be a beneficial alternative for low-to-intermediate risk patients with heart failure potentially leading to unnecessary admissions and reducing readmissions. Whether observation units for heart failure are comparable or superior to current approaches is unknown and warrants a randomized clinical trial.[78,79]

CONCLUSION

Significant opportunities exist to improve the quality of care, care transitions and outcomes for patients hospitalized with heart failure. Reducing preventable readmission in heart failure is a national focus but very challenging. Some practical strategies and programs have been successful in reducing 30-day rehospitalization in heart failure. However new approaches and strategies are needed to reduce preventable rehospitalizations in the first 30 days and beyond as well as improve survival. Reducing readmissions is a worthwhile and achievable endeavor; however, it will require the coordination of resources of all levels and further research into effective strategies to improve this outcome.

REFERENCES

1. Go AS, Mozaffarian D, Roger VL, et al. Executive summary: heart disease and stroke statistics—2013 update: a report from the American Heart Association. Circulation. 2013;127(1):143-52.
2. Joynt KE, Jha AK. A path forward on Medicare readmissions. N Engl J Med. 2013;368(13):1175-7.
3. Dickstein K, Cohen-Solal A, Filippatos G, et al. ESC Guidelines for the diagnosis and treatment of acute and chronic heart failure 2008: the Task Force for the Diagnosis and Treatment of Acute and Chronic Heart Failure 2008 of the European Society of Cardiology. Developed in collaboration with the Heart Failure Association of the ESC (HFA) and endorsed by the European Society of Intensive Care Medicine (ESICM). Eur Heart J. 2008;29(19):2388-442.
4. Chen J, Normand SL, Wang Y, et al. National and regional trends in heart failure hospitalization and mortality rates for Medicare beneficiaries, 1998-2008. JAMA. 2011;306(15):1669-78.
5. Liu L. Changes in cardiovascular hospitalization and comorbidity of heart failure in the United States: findings from the National Hospital Discharge Surveys 1980-2006. Int J Cardiol. 2011;149(1):39-45.
6. Fonarow GC, Stough WG, Abraham WT, et al. Characteristics, treatments, and outcomes of patients with preserved systolic function hospitalized for heart failure: a report from the OPTIMIZE-HF Registry. J Am Coll Cardiol. 2007;50(8):786-77.
7. Jencks SF, Williams MV, Coleman EA. Rehospitalizations among patients in the Medicare fee-for-service program. N Engl J Med. 2009;360(14):1418-28.

8. Krumholz HM, Lin Z, Keenan PS, et al. Relationship between hospital readmission and mortality rates for patients hospitalized with acute myocardial infarction, heart failure, or pneumonia. JAMA. 2013;309(6):587-93.
9. Dharmarajan K, Hsieh AF, Lin Z, et al. Diagnoses and timing of 30-day readmissions after hospitalization for heart failure, acute myocardial infarction, or pneumonia. JAMA. 2013;309(4):355-63.
10. Edelmann F, Wachter R, Schmidt AG, et al. effect of spironolactone on diastolic function and exercise capacity in patients with heart failure with preserved ejection fraction: the Aldo-DHF Randomized controlled trial. JAMA. 2013;309(8):781-91.
11. Redfield MM, Chen HH, Borlaug BA, et al. Effect of phosphodiesterase-5 inhibition on exercise capacity and clinical status in heart failure with preserved ejection fraction: a randomized clinical trial. JAMA. 2013;309(12):1268-77.
12. Steinberg BA, Zhao X, Heidenreich PA, et al. Trends in patients hospitalized with heart failure and preserved left ventricular ejection fraction: prevalence, therapies, and outcomes. Circulation. 2012;126(1):65-75.
13. Hersh AM, Masoudi FA, Allen LA. Postdischarge environment following heart failure hospitalization: expanding the view of hospital readmission. J Am Heart Assoc. 2013;2(2):e000116.
14. Wu JR, Moser DK, Lennie TA, et al. Medication adherence in patients who have heart failure: a review of the literature. Nurs Clin North Am. 2008;43(1):133-53.
15. Peterson PN, Shetterly SM, Clarke CL, et al. Health literacy and outcomes among patients with heart failure. JAMA. 2011;305(16):1695-701.
16. DeWalt DA, Malone RM, Bryant ME, et al. A heart failure self-management program for patients of all literacy levels: a randomized, controlled trial [ISRCTN11535170]. BMC Health Serv Res. 2006;6:30.
17. Haworth JE, Moniz-Cook E, Clark AL, et al. Prevalence and predictors of anxiety and depression in a sample of chronic heart failure patients with left ventricular systolic dysfunction. Eur J Heart Fail. 2005;7(5):803-8.
18. Riegel B, Moser DK, Anker SD, et al. State of the science: promoting self-care in persons with heart failure: a scientific statement from the American Heart Association. Circulation. 2009;120(12):1141-63.
19. Morgan AL, Masoudi FA, Havranek EP, et al. Difficulty in taking medications, depression, and health status in heart failure patients. J Card Fail. 2006;12(1):54-60.
20. Lesman-Leegte I, van Veldhuisen DJ, Hillege HL, et al. Depressive symptoms and outcomes in patients with heart failure: data from the COACH study. Eur J Heart Fail. 2009;11(12):1202-7.
21. Löwe B, Kroenke K, Gräfe K. Detecting and monitoring depression with a two-item questionnaire (PHQ-2). J Psychosom Res. 2005;58(2):163-71.
22. Krumholz HM, Currie PM, Riegel B, et al. A taxonomy for disease management: a scientific statement from the American Heart Association Disease Management Taxonomy Writing Group. Circulation. 2006;114(13):1432-45.
23. Phillips CO, Wright SM, Kern DE, et al. Comprehensive discharge planning with postdischarge support for older patients with congestive heart failure: a meta-analysis. JAMA. 2004;291(11):1358-67.
24. Koelling TM, Johnson ML, Cody RJ, et al. Discharge education improves clinical outcomes in patients with chronic heart failure. Circulation. 2005;111(2):179-85.
25. Rich MW, Beckham V, Wittenberg C, et al. A multidisciplinary intervention to prevent the readmission of elderly patients with congestive heart failure. N Engl J Med. 1995;333(18):1190-5.
26. McAlister FA, Stewart S, Ferrua S, et al. Multidisciplinary strategies for the management of heart failure patients at high risk for admission: a systematic review of randomized trials. J Am Coll Cardiol. 2004;44(4):810-9.
27. Jovicic A, Holroyd-Leduc JM, Straus SE. Effects of self-management intervention on health outcomes of patients with heart failure: a systematic review of randomized controlled trials. BMC Cardiovasc Disord. 2006;6:43.
28. Gheorghiade MM, Pang PS, Ambrosy AP, et al. A comprehensive, longitudinal description of the in-hospital and post-discharge clinical, laboratory, and neurohormonal course of patients with heart failure who die or are re-hospitalized within 90 days: analysis from the EVEREST trial. Heart Fail Rev. 2012;17:485-509.
29. Hernandez AF, Greiner MA, Fonarow GC, et al. Relationship between early physician follow-up and 30-day readmission among Medicare beneficiaries hospitalized for heart failure. JAMA. 2010;303(17):1716-22.
30. Lee DS, Stukel TA, Austin PC, et al. Improved outcomes with early collaborative care of ambulatory heart failure patients discharged from the emergency department. Circulation. 2010;122(18):1806-14.
31. Gheorghiade M, Abraham WT, Albert NM, et al. Systolic blood pressure at admission, clinical characteristics, and outcomes in patients hospitalized with acute heart failure. JAMA. 2006;296(18):2217-26.
32. O'Connor CM, Abraham WT, Albert NM, et al. Predictors of mortality after discharge in patients hospitalized with heart failure: an analysis from the Organized Program to Initiate Lifesaving Treatment in Hospitalized Patients with Heart Failure (OPTIMIZE-HF). Am Heart J. 2008;156(4): 662-73.
33. Wang NC, Maggioni AP, Konstam MA, et al. Clinical implications of QRS duration in patients hospitalized with worsening heart failure and reduced left ventricular ejection fraction. JAMA. 2008;299(22):2656-66.
34. Blair JE, Pang PS, Schrier RW, et al. Changes in renal function during hospitalization and soon after discharge in patients admitted for worsening heart failure in the placebo group of the EVEREST trial. Eur Heart J. 2011; 32:2563-72.
35. Shah AN, Nodari S, Gheorghiade M. Biomarkers in acute heart failure syndromes - are they fulfilling their promise? Cardiology. 2011;120(1): 19-21.
36. van der Velde AR, Gullestad L, Ueland T, et al. Prognostic value of changes in galectin-3 levels over time in patients with heart failure: data from CORONA and COACH. Circ Heart Fail. 2013;6(2):219-26.
37. Gheorghiade M, Abraham WT, Albert NM, et al. Relationship between admission serum sodium concentration and clinical outcomes in patients hospitalized for heart failure: an analysis from the OPTIMIZE-HF registry. Eur Heart J. 2007;28(8):980-8.
38. Mentz RJ, Fiuzat M, Wojdyla DM, et al. Clinical characteristics and outcomes of hospitalized heart failure patients with systolic dysfunction and chronic obstructive pulmonary disease: findings from OPTIMIZE-HF. Eur J Heart Fail. 2012;14(4):395-403.
39. Solomon SD, Dobson J, Pocock S, et al. Influence of nonfatal hospitalization for heart failure on subsequent mortality in patients with chronic heart failure. Circulation. 2007;116(13):1482-7.
40. Hansen LO, Strater AA, Smith LL, et al. Hospital discharge documentation and risk of rehospitalisation. BMJ Qual Saf. 2011;20(9):773-8.
41. Bell CM, Schnipper JL, Auerbach AD, et al. Association of communication between hospital-based physicians and primary care providers with patient outcomes. J Gen Intern Med. 2009;24(3):381-6.
42. Patterson ME, Hernandez AF, Hammill BG, et al. Process of care performance measures and long-term outcomes in patients hospitalized with heart failure. Med Care. 2010;48(3):210-6.
43. Wiggins BS, Rodgers JE, DiDomenico RJ, et al. Discharge counseling for patients with heart failure or myocardial infarction: a best practices model developed by members of the American College of Clinical Pharmacy's Cardiology Practice and Research Network based on the Hospital to Home (H2H) Initiative. Pharmacotherapy. 2013;33(5):558-80.
44. Gheorghiade M, Follath F, Ponikowski P, et al. Assessing and grading congestion in acute heart failure: a scientific statement from the acute heart failure committee of the heart failure association of the European

Society of Cardiology and endorsed by the European Society of Intensive Care Medicine. Eur J Heart Fail. 2010;12(5):423-33.
45. Goldsmith SR, Brandimarte F, Gheorghiade M. Congestion as a therapeutic target in acute heart failure syndromes. Prog Cardiovasc Dis. 2010;52(5):383-92.
46. Valika AA, Gheorghiade M. Ace inhibitor therapy for heart failure in patients with impaired renal function: a review of the literature. Heart Fail Rev. 2013;18(2):135-40.
47. Felker GM, Lee KL, Bull DA, et al. Diuretic strategies in patients with acute decompensated heart failure. N Engl J Med. 2011;364(9):797-805.
48. Schrier RW, Gheorghiade M. Challenge of rehospitalizations for heart failure: potential of natriuretic doses of mineralocorticoid receptor antagonists. Am Heart J. 2011;161(2):221-3.
49. Zannad F, McMurray JJ, Krum H, et al. Eplerenone in patients with systolic heart failure and mild symptoms. N Engl J Med. 2011;364:11-21.
50. Gheorghiade M, Konstam MA, Burnett JC, et al. Short-term clinical effects of tolvaptan, an oral vasopressin antagonist, in patients hospitalized for heart failure: the EVEREST Clinical Status Trials. JAMA. 2007;297(12):1332-43.
51. Schrier RW, Gross P, Gheorghiade M, et al. Tolvaptan, a selective oral vasopressin V2-receptor antagonist, for hyponatremia. N Engl J Med. 2006;355(20):2099-112.
52. Fonarow GC, Abraham WT, Albert NM, et al. Association between performance measures and clinical outcomes for patients hospitalized with heart failure. JAMA. 2007;297(1):61-70.
53. Hernandez AF, Fonarow GC, Liang L, et al. The need for multiple measures of hospital quality: results from the Get with the Guidelines-Heart Failure Registry of the American Heart Association. Circulation. 2011;124(6):712-9.
54. Cleland JG, McGowan J, Clark A, et al. The evidence for beta blockers in heart failure. BMJ. 1999;318(7187):824-5.
55. Packer M, Coats AJ, Fowler MB, et al. Effect of carvedilol on survival in severe chronic heart failure. N Engl J Med. 2001;344(22):1651-8.
56. Effect of enalapril on mortality and the development of heart failure in asymptomatic patients with reduced left ventricular ejection fractions. The SOLVD Investigators. N Engl J Med. 1992;327(10):685-91.
57. Jong P, Demers C, McKelvie RS, et al. Angiotensin receptor blockers in heart failure: meta-analysis of randomized controlled trials. J Am Coll Cardiol. 2002;39(3):463-70.
58. Pitt B, Poole-Wilson PA, Segal R, et al. Effect of losartan compared with captopril on mortality in patients with symptomatic heart failure: randomised trial—the Losartan Heart Failure Survival Study ELITE II. Lancet. 2000;355(9215):1582-7.
59. Albert NM, Yancy CW, Liang L, et al. Use of aldosterone antagonists in heart failure. JAMA. 2009;302(15):1658-65.
60. Fonarow GC, Abraham WT, Albert NM, et al. Influence of a performance-improvement initiative on quality of care for patients hospitalized with heart failure: results of the Organized Program to Initiate Lifesaving Treatment in Hospitalized Patients With Heart Failure (OPTIMIZE-HF). Arch Intern Med. 2007;167(14):1493-502.
61. Taylor AL, Ziesche S, Yancy C, et al. Combination of isosorbide dinitrate and hydralazine in blacks with heart failure. N Engl J Med. 2004;351(20): 2049-57.
62. Banka G, Heidenreich PA, Fonarow GC. Incremental cost-effectiveness of guideline-directed medical therapies for heart failure. J Am Coll Cardiol. 2013;61(13):1440-6.
63. Hunt SA, Abraham WT, Chin MH, et al. 2009 focused update incorporated into the ACC/AHA 2005 Guidelines for the Diagnosis and Management of Heart Failure in Adults: a report of the American College of Cardiology Foundation/American Heart Association Task Force on Practice Guidelines: developed in collaboration with the International Society for Heart and Lung Transplantation. Circulation. 2009;119(14):e391-479.
64. Digitalis Investigation Group. The effect of digoxin on mortality and morbidity in patients with heart failure. N Engl J Med. 1997;336(8):525-33.
65. Ahmed A, Rich MW, Fleg JL, et al. Effects of digoxin on morbidity and mortality in diastolic heart failure: the ancillary digitalis investigation group trial. Circulation. 2006;114(5):397-403.
66. Bourge RC, Fleg JL, Fonarow GC, et al. Digoxin reduces 30-day all-cause hospital admission in older patients with chronic systolic heart failure. Am J Med. 2013;126(8):701-8.
67. Hernandez AF, Mi X, Hammill BG, et al. Associations between aldosterone antagonist therapy and risks of mortality and readmission among patients with heart failure and reduced ejection fraction. JAMA. 2012;308(20):2097-107.
68. Inglis SC, Clark RA, McAlister FA, et al. Structured telephone support or telemonitoring programmes for patients with chronic heart failure. Cochrane Database Syst Rev. 2010;(8):CD007228.
69. Clark RA, Inglis SC, McAlister FA, et al. Telemonitoring or structured telephone support programmes for patients with chronic heart failure: systematic review and meta-analysis. BMJ. 2007;334(7600):942.
70. Polisena J, Tran K, Cimon K, et al. Home telemonitoring for congestive heart failure: a systematic review and meta-analysis. J Telemed Telecare. 2010;16(2):68-76.
71. Chaudhry SI, Mattera JA, Curtis JP, et al. Telemonitoring in patients with heart failure. N Engl J Med. 2010;363(24):2301-9.
72. Koehler FF, Winkler SS, Schieber MM, et al. Telemedical Interventional Monitoring in Heart Failure (TIM-HF), a randomized, controlled intervention trial investigating the impact of telemedicine on mortality in ambulatory patients with heart failure: study design. Eur J Heart Fail. 2010;12:1354-62.
73. Abraham WT, Adamson PB, Bourge RC, et al. Wireless pulmonary artery haemodynamic monitoring in chronic heart failure: a randomised controlled trial. Lancet. 2011;377(9766):658-66.
74. Loh JP, Barbash IM, Waksman R. Overview of the 2011 Food and Drug Administration Circulatory System Devices Panel of the Medical Devices Advisory Committee Meeting on the CardioMEMS Champion Heart Failure Monitoring System. J Am Coll Cardiol. 2013;61(15):1571-6.
75. Epstein AE, DiMarco JP, Ellenbogen KA, et al. 2012 ACCF/AHA/HRS focused update incorporated into the ACCF/AHA/HRS 2008 guidelines for device-based therapy of cardiac rhythm abnormalities: a report of the American College of Cardiology Foundation/American Heart Association Task Force on Practice Guidelines and the Heart Rhythm Society. J Am Coll Cardiol. 2013;61(3):e6-75.
76. Anand IS, Carson P, Galle E, et al. Cardiac resynchronization therapy reduces the risk of hospitalizations in patients with advanced heart failure: results from the Comparison of Medical Therapy, Pacing and Defibrillation in Heart Failure (COMPANION) Trial. Circulation. 2009;119:909-11.
77. Kociol RD, Peterson ED, Hammill BG, et al. National survey of hospital strategies to reduce heart failure readmissions: findings from the Get With the Guidelines-Heart Failure registry. Circ Heart Fail. 2012;5(6):680-7.
78. Collins SP, Pang PS, Fonarow GC, et al. Is hospital admission for heart failure really necessary?: the role of the emergency department and observation unit in preventing hospitalization and rehospitalization. J Am Coll Cardiol. 2013;61(2):121-6.
79. Peacock WF, Braunwald E, Abraham W, et al. National Heart, Lung, and Blood Institute working group on emergency department management of acute heart failure: research challenges and opportunities. J Am Coll Cardiol. 2010;56(5):343-51.

Chapter 25

Initiation of Angiotensin-converting Enzyme Inhibitors and Beta Blockers in Heart Failure: Putting Evidence into Practice

Jeffrey Chan, Alan S Maisel

ABSTRACT

A remarkable number of randomized double-blinded clinical trials have been conducted on patients with heart failure (HF), in which clinically important outcome measures, including death, composites of death, and relevant nonfatal events have been measured alongside the effect of various treatment options. However, the actual uptake of these evidence-based treatments into real clinical practice has been variable despite the continual publication of relevant clinical trials in various medical journals and the summation of their findings in various pertinent guidelines. The clinical short-term and long-term benefits of beta blockers and angiotensin-converting enzyme inhibitors (ACEIs) in patients with HF are well known. However, underprescribing and underdosing of these proven beneficial medications is a persistent problem. This chapter's concise clinical recommendations for administering these two clinically proven medical therapies provide the clear framework for easily implementing ACEIs and beta blockers effectively in HF.

INTRODUCTION

A remarkable number of randomized double-blinded clinical trials have been conducted on patients with heart failure (HF), in which clinically important outcome measures including death, composites of death, and relevant nonfatal events have been measured alongside the effect of various treatment options. As a result, there is now significant evidence for the efficacy and implementation of a considerable body of medical treatments for HF.[1-7] However, the actual uptake of these evidence-based treatments into real clinical practice has been variable despite the continual publication of relevant clinical trials in various medical journals and the summation of their findings in various pertinent guidelines.[8-17] This, in turn, has resulted in HF patients being denied the benefit of proven treatments that have been shown to increase both their length and quality of life.[18-21] Therefore, this chapter serves the purpose of providing practical guidance on the appropriate and safe use of treatments of proven benefit in the management of patients with HF.

In this chapter, we focus specifically on the initiation of angiotensin-converting enzyme inhibitors (ACEIs) and beta blockers in patients with HF. ACEIs were in fact among the first new treatments introduced in the management of HF. Interestingly, many clinical surveys that have been conducted across various clinical settings have demonstrated that a substantial portion of patients who should have been treated with an ACEI never actually were, both in outpatient and inpatient medical settings.[22,23] Additionally, the doses utilized by practitioners were found to often be lower than the recommended doses that had been shown to improve survival.[24-29] Beta blockers were the next class of agents shown to demonstrate clinically utility in patients with HF. At least four large randomized clinical trials between 1999 and 2001 demonstrated that the addition of a beta blocker to standard treatment with a diuretic and ACEI led to increased survival, reduced hospital admissions and improvement in quality of life in patients with HF.[4,6,7,9,10] As in the case with ACEIs, similar issues with translating trial findings to actual practice also emerged, depriving patients access to treatments of proven benefit.

It is this very ongoing phenomenon of undertreatment and underdosing of both ACEI and beta blockers that we hope to rectify in this chapter by specifying the benefits of treatment, suitable candidates for treatment, and appropriate dosing strategies for both beta blockers and ACEI in patients with HF. More importantly, our practical recommendations in this chapter are not meant to replace existing guidelines, but rather to complement them and offer a clear manner in implementing them.

GENERAL FOUR-STEP APPROACH TO MEDICATION INITIATION

Assuming the diagnosis of HF has been made and that diuretics have been initiated to treat symptoms and signs of sodium and water retention, the general approach in initiating ACEIs and beta blockers follows a four-step process. The first step involves the already mentioned task of establishing a clinical diagnosis of HF and initiating appropriate diuretic treatment (details on diuretics are not addressed in this chapter). The second step involves verifying the presence of left ventricular dysfunction (typically defined as an ejection fraction <0.4) via echocardiography, radionuclide ventriculography, radiological left ventricular angiography, or cardiac magnetic resonance imaging as part of routine standard of care. The third step, and the topic of this chapter, is the initiation of first-line therapy for all patients with HF due to left ventricular dysfunction, namely an ACEI and a beta blocker unless contraindications are present. ACEI generally should be initiated first at a low dose and quickly followed by a beta blocker once the patient is considered no longer decompensated. The dosage of the ACEI should be uptitrated slowly with a goal of titrating to the target doses shown to yield clinical benefit in clinical trials. The same approach applies to beta blockers as well, starting at a low dose and gradually titrating upward to target goals proven in studies to demonstrate clinical benefit. In situations where the ACEI is not tolerated, such as situations of coughing, angiotensin receptor blockers (ARB) should be utilized. The last step in this general approach to HF management involves the implementation of additional pharmacologic therapy for patients with persisting signs and symptoms of HF, specifically the use of spironolactone in patients with New York Heart Association (NYHA) class III/IV after optimization of ACEIs and beta blockers and the addition of eplerenone in situations where unpleasant antiandrogenic side effects of spironolactone become too bothersome. A triple treatment strategy of combining an ARB with spironolactone on top of the usual ACEI and beta blocker has not been shown to add additional clinical benefit in current studies and is, therefore, not recommended. Specific recommendations on initiating ARBs will not be the focus of this chapter. Lastly, among this category of additional pharmacologic therapy, digoxin should be considered for use, as it has been shown to reduce hospital admissions.

APPROACH TO INITIATE ANGIOTENSIN-CONVERTING ENZYME INHIBITOR IN HEART FAILURE

The justification for initiating ACEI in patients with HF stems from a multitude of studies supporting their use. The CONSENSUS I (Cooperative North Scandinavian Enalapril Survival Study I) and SOLVD-T (treatment arm of the Studies of Left Ventricular Dysfunction) clinical trials alongside multiple meta-analyses demonstrated that ACEIs increased survival, reduced hospital admissions and improved NYHA class and quality of life in patients with all grades of symptomatic HF.[1,2] In fact, the ATLAS trial extended the applicability of these findings by demonstrating that higher doses of ACEI further reduced the composite endpoint of death and hospital admissions. Along similar lines, ACEIs have also been shown to delay and prevent the development of symptomatic HF in patients with asymptomatic left ventricular dysfunction as well. These findings form the foundation for the indications for ACEIs as summarized in Box 1.

Box 1: Indications and contraindications for angiotensin-converting enzyme inhibitors in heart failure

Indications

- Potentially all patients with heart failure
- First-line treatment in NYHA II-IV
- Beneficial in asymptomatic LVSD (NYHA I)

Contraindications

- History of angioedema
- Bilateral renal artery stenosis

Cautions

- Hyperkalemia
- Cr >2.5 mg/dL
- Symptomatic or severe asymptomatic hypotension (SBP <90 mmHg)

NYHA, New York Heart Association; LVSD, left ventricular systolic dysfunction; Cr, creatinine; SBP, systolic blood pressure

Absolute contraindications that must be considered prior to starting ACEI include prior history of angioedema and known bilateral renal artery stenosis. General precaution should also be taken if the patient presents with a history of significant hyperkalemia [potassium (K) >5.0 mmol/L], significant renal dysfunction [serum creatinine (Cr) >2.5 mg/dL] and either symptomatic or severe asymptomatic hypotension [systolic blood pressure (SBP) <90 mmHg].

Specific ACEIs that should be utilized in patient with HF are outlined in Table 1. The general strategy regarding their initiation is to start at a low dose (doses specified in Table 1) and double the dose at 2 week intervals till the optimum target dose is achieved (target doses also listed in Table 1). Blood pressure and blood chemistry, specifically the blood urea nitrogen, serum creatinine, and serum potassium levels should be monitored 1–2 weeks following initiation of ACEI and additionally monitored again 1–2 weeks after the final titration dose adjustment. Embedded within this scheduled blood chemistry monitoring is having an appropriate plan of action ready for common anticipated issues that are encountered when starting patients on ACEIs. Asymptomatic hypotension generally does not warrant any change in therapy. Symptomatic hypotension, however, should prompt consideration of decreasing the patient's diuretic dose, if there are no signs or symptoms of volume overload or congestion, or reconsideration of the use of nitrates and calcium-channel blockers and other vasodilators if the patient complains of dizziness, lightheadedness, or confusion. Worsening renal function is a common anticipated problem that also accompanies that initiation of ACEIs. In fact, a small rise in urea, creatinine and potassium is to be expected after initiation of an ACEI; if the increase is small, no interventions are necessary. More specifically, an increase in creatinine up to 50% above baseline or 3 mg/dL (whichever is smaller) is acceptable. An increase in serum potassium to less than 5.5 mmol/L is acceptable as well. In situations where the increase in creatinine or potassium exceeds those aforementioned boundaries, the dose of the ACEI should be halved and repeat blood chemistries should be assessed in 1–2 weeks after the dosage adjustment.

TABLE 1: Angiotensin-converting enzyme inhibitors and proper dosing

ACEIs	*Starting dose*	*Target dose*
Captopril	6.25 mg TID	50 mg TID
Enalapril	2.5 mg BID	10–20 mg BID
Lisinopril	2.5–5 mg QD	20–35 mg QD
Ramipril	2.5 mg QD	10 mg QD
Trandolapril	0.5 mg QD	4 mg QD

ACEIs, angiotensin-converting enzyme inhibitors; TID, thrice a day; BID, twice a day; QD, every day

Compliance with treatment regiments can be markedly enhanced with appropriate education of the patients regarding the importance, indications and risks of treatment. Patients should be informed that symptoms generally improve only after a few weeks to a few months after treatment initiation. They should be advised to report primarily principal adverse side effects, including dizziness, symptomatic hypotension, and cough and to avoid nonsteroidal anti-inflammatory drugs (NSAIDs) not prescribed by a physician and salt substitutes high in potassium to avoid hyperkalemia.

APPROACH TO INITIATE BETA BLOCKERS IN HEART FAILURE

As with ACEIs, the justification for initiating beta blockers in patients with HF also stems from a multitude of evidence-based clinical studies. Several major randomized controlled clinical trials [US Carvedilol heart failure Program (USCP), Carvedilol Prospective Randomized Cumulative Survival (COPERNICUS), Cardiac Insufficiency Bisoprolol Study II (CIBIS II), the Metoprolol Controlled Release (CR)/Extended Release (XL) Randomized Intervention Trial in chronic Heart Failure (MERIT-HF)] have convincingly demonstrated that specific beta blockers increase survival, reduce hospital admissions and improve NYHA class and quality of life in patients with stable mild and moderate HF and even in some patients with severe HF.[5,6] The indications for beta blocker therapy are outlined clearly in Box 2.

Box 2: Indications and contraindications for beta blockers in heart failure

Indications

- Potentially all patients with stable mild/moderate HF
- First-line treatment (in addition to ACEIs) in NYHA II-III HF

Contraindications

- Asthma

Cautions

- NYHA IV HF
- Heart block/heart rate <60 beats per minute
- Persisting sign of volume overload
- Current exacerbation of HF

NYHA, New York Heart Association; ACEIs, angiotensin-converting enzyme inhibitors; HF, heart failure

TABLE 2: Beta blockers and proper dosing

Beta blockers	*Starting dose*	*Target dose*
Bisoprolol	1.25 mg QD	10 mg QD
Carvedilol	3.125 mg BID	25–50 mg BID
Metoprolol CR/XL	1.25–25 mg QD	200 mg QD
Nebivolol	1.25 mg QD	10 mg QD

CR, controlled release; XL, extended release; QD, every day; BID, twice a day

The primary absolute contraindication to initiating beta blocker therapy is asthma. However, general care and precaution should still also be taken before initiating beta blockers in patients with severe NYHA IV HF, ongoing or recent (<4 weeks) congestive heart failure (CHF) exacerbation, heart block, bradycardia, persisting signs of congestion and hypotension (SBP <90 mmHg). In these particular cases, collaboration with a specialist prior to initiating beta blocker treatment is recommended.

Specific beta blockers that should be considered for patients with HF are tabulated in Table 2. As with ACEI, the listed beta blockers should be started at low doses as listed in the Table 2, with a goal of doubling the dose at 2 week intervals till the target dose shown to yield clinical benefit is achieved. Vital signs, including heart rate, blood pressure, volume status and body weight should be closely monitored. As with ACEIs, blood chemistry should also be checked 1–2 weeks after starting the treatment, and again 1–2 weeks immediately after making the final titration changes in dose. To optimize adherence to these particular approaches, the patient should always be well informed of the reasoning behind such management plans, specifically the intention and anticipated benefits. Patient should understand that beta blockers are initiated to improve symptoms and prevent worsening HF. However, symptomatic improvement may not develop immediately, often taking 3–6 months or longer at times. Patients should be advised to immediately report any worsening dyspnea, fatigue, however, should not decrease their beta blocker dose without consulting their physician. If increasing volume status is observed, diuretic dosing should be increased or the beta blocker dose should be halved if increased dieresis does not result in improvement. Increased fatigue or bradycardia should be managed with a reduction in the beta blocker dose as well. With regards to anticipated issues with blood pressure management, asymptomatic hypotension does not warrant any change in the beta blocker dose; symptomatic hypotension, in conjunction with euvolemic volume status, warrants consideration for reducing the patient's diuretic or ACEI dose.

CONCLUSION

The clinical short-term and long-term benefit of beta blockers and ACEI in patients with HF is well known. However, underprescribing and underdosing of these proven beneficial medications is a persistent problem. Whether underprescribing or underdosing, the common sequela of patients not receiving treatment that can reduce mortality and morbidity adversely affects not only individual patient care, but also more globally, healthcare as a whole by burdening the medical system with repeated hospital admissions that are entirely avoidable. This chapter's concise clinical recommendations for administering clinically proven medical therapies provides the clear framework for easily implementing proven evidence-based therapies appropriately and effectively.

REFERENCES

1. Effects of enalapril on mortality in severe congestive heart failure. Results of the Cooperative North Scandinavian Enalapril Survival Study (CONSENSUS). The CONSENSUS Trial Study Group. N Engl J Med. 1987;316(23):1429-35.
2. Effects of enalapril on survival in patients with reduced left ventricular ejection fractions and congestive heart failure. The SOLVD Investigators. N Engl J Med. 1991;325(5):293-302.
3. Packer M, Bristow MR, Cohn JN, et al. The effect of carvediolol on morbidity and mortality in patients with chronic heart failure. U.S. Carvedilol Heart Failure Study Group. N Engl J Med 1996;334(21):1349-55.
4. Digitalis Investigation Group. The effect of digoxin on mortality and morbidity in patients with heart failure. N Engl J Med. 1997;336(8):525-33.
5. The Cardiac Insufficiency Bisoprolol Study II (CIBIS-II): a randomized trial. Lancet. 1999;353(9146):9-13.
6. Effect of metoprolol CR/XL in chronic heart failure: Metoprolol CR/XL Randomized Intervention Trial in Congestive Heart Failure (MERIT-HF). Lancet. 1999;353(9169):2001-7.
7. Pitt B, Zannad F, Remme WJ, et al. The effect of spironolactone on morbidity and mortality in patients with severe heart failure. Randomized Aldactone Evaluation Study Investigators. N Engl J Med. 1999;341(10):709-17.
8. Konstam MA, Dracup K, Baker DW, et al. Heart failure: evaluation and care of patients with left ventricular systolic dysfunction. J Card Fail. 1995;1(2):183-7
9. McMurray J, Gyarfas I, Wenger NK, et al. Concise guide to the management of heart failure. Am J Geriatr Cardiol. 1996;5:13-30.
10. The National Heart Foundation of New Zealand, Cardiac Society of Australia and New Zealand, the Royal New Zealand College of General Practitioners Working Party. New Zealand guidelines for management of chronic heart failure. NZ Med J. 1997;110:99-107.
11. Heart Failure Society of America (HFS) practice guidelines. HFSA guidelines for management of patients with heart failure caused by left ventricular systolic dysfunction—pharmacological approaches. J Card Fail. 1999;5(4):357-82.
12. Hoppe UC, Erdmann E, Kommission Klinische Kardiologie. Guidelines for the treatment of chronic heart failure. Issued by the executive committee of the German society of cardiology—heart and circulation research,

compiled on behalf of the commission of clinical cardiology in cooperative with pharmaceutic commission of the German physicians' association. Z Kardiol. 2001;90:218-37.

13. Krum H, Jelinek MV, Stewart S, et al. 2011 update to National Heart Foundation of Australia and Cardiac Society of Australia and New Zealand Guidelines for the prevention, detection and management of chronic heart failure in Australia, 2006. Med J Aust. 2011;194(8):405-9.
14. Hunt SA, Baker DW, Chin MH, et al. ACC/AHA guidelines for the evaluation and management of chronic heart failure in the adult: executive summary. A report of the American College of Cardiology/American Heart Association Task Force on Practice Guidelines (Committee to Revise the 1995 Guidelines for the Evaluation and Management of Heart Failure). J Am Coll Cardiol. 2001;104:2996-3007.
15. Liu P, Arnold JM, Belenkie I, et al. Canadian Cardiovascular Society. The 2002/3 Canadian Cardiovascular Society consensus guideline update for the diagnosis and management of heart failure. Can J Cardiol. 2003;19:347-56.
16. National Institute for Health and Clinical Excellence. (2010). Chronic heart failure: Management of chronic heart failure in adults in primary and secondary care. NICE clinical guideline 108. [online] Available from www.nice.org.uk/nicemedia/live/13099/50517/50517.pdf. [Accessed December, 2013].
17. Mosterd WL, Rosier PF. Guideline 'chronic heart failure'. Tijdschr Geneeskd. 2004;148:609-14.
18. Bungard TJ, McAlister FA, Johnson JA, et al. Underutilization of ACE inhibitors in patients with congestive heart failure. Drugs. 2001;61(14): 2021-33.
19. Hobbs FD, Jones MI, Allan TF, et al. European survey of primary care physician perceptions on heart failure diagnosis and management (Euro-HF). Eur Heart J. 2000;21(22):1877-87.
20. Cleland JG, Cohen-Solal A, Aguilar JC, et al. Management of heart failure in primary care (the IMPROVEMENT of Heart Failure Programme): an international survey. Lancet. 2002;360(9346):1631-9.
21. Komajda M, Follath F, Swedberg K, et al. The EuroHeart Failure Survey programme—a survey on the quality of care among patients with heart failure in Europe. Part 2: treatment. Eur Heart J. 2003;24(5):464-74.
22. Mair FS, Crowley TS, Bundred PE. Prevalence, aetiology and management of heart failure in general practice. Br J Gen Pract. 1996;46(403):77-9.
23. Houghton AR, Cowley AJ. Why are angiotensin converting enzyme inhibitors underutilized in the treatment of heart failure by general practitioners? Int J Cardiol. 1997;59(1):7-10.
24. Boyles PJ, Peterson GM, Bleasel MD, et al. Undertreatment of congestive heart failure in an Australian setting. J Clin Pharm Ther. 2004;29(1): 15-22.
25. Masoudi FA, Rathore SS, Wang Y, et al. National patterns of use and effectiveness of angiotensin-converting enzyme inhibitors in older patients with heart failure and left ventricular systolic dysfunction. Circulation. 2004;110(6):724-31.
26. Muntwyler J, Cohen-Solal A, Freemantle N, et al. Relation of sex, age and concomitant diseases to drug prescription for heart failure in primary care in Europe. Eur J Heart Fail. 2004;6(5):663-8.
27. Murphy NF, Simpson CR, McAlister FA, et al. National survey of the prevalence, incidence, primary care burden, and treatment of heart failure in Scotland. Heart. 2004;90(10):1129-36.
28. Roman-Sanchez P, Conthe P, Garcia-Alegria J, et al. Factors influencing medical treatment of heart failure patients in Spanish internal medicine departments: a national survey. QJM. 2005;98(2):127-38.
29. Krum H, Tonkin AM, Currie R, et al. Chronic heart failure in Australian general practice. The Cardiac Awareness Survey and Evaluation (CASE) Study. Med J Aust. 2001;174(9):439-44.

Chapter 26

Mineralocorticoid Receptor Antagonists in Patients with Heart Failure and a Reduced Left Ventricular Ejection Fraction: How to Do It Right

Bertram Pitt

ABSTRACT

Evidence from prospective double-blind randomized trials, including Randomized Aldactone Evaluation Study (RALES), Eplerenone Post-Acute Myocardial Infarction Heart Failure Efficacy and Survival Study (EPHESUS) and Eplerenone in Mild Patients Hospitalization and Survival Study in Heart Failure (EMPHASIS-HF) in patients with heart failure and a reduced left ventricular ejection fraction (HFREF) provides the basis for current guideline recommendations in the United States (US), Europe, and many parts of the world recommending mineralocorticoid-receptor antagonists (MRAs) as a class 1 indication. Despite this evidence and guideline recommendations, there remains an underuse of MRAs in patients with HFREF, in part due to the fear of inducing hyperkalemia and/or renal failure. Recommendations for serial monitoring of serum potassium (K), renal function and for adjusting the dose of the MRA accordingly along with suggestions regarding which MRA to choose and potential new strategies to further reduce these risks reviewed in this chapter should minimize these risks, and allow more optimum use of MRAs in patients with HFREF with a consequent reduction in cardiovascular (CV) mortality, hospitalizations for HF, and therefore, healthcare costs.

INTRODUCTION

Evidences from prospective randomized double-blind randomized trials in patients with severe chronic heart failure (HF) and a reduced left ventricular ejection fraction (REF), such as Randomized Aldactone Evaluation Study (RALES);[1] heart failure with reduced ejection fraction (HFREF) with mild symptoms, such as Eplerenone in Mild Patients Hospitalization And Survival Study in Heart Failure (EMPHASIS-HF)[2] and HFREF early post-myocardial infarction (MI) such as Eplerenone Post-Acute Myocardial Infarction Heart Failure Efficacy and Survival Study (EPHESUS)[3] have shown that a mineralocorticoid receptor antagonist (MRA) when added to standard therapy for HF, including an angiotensin-converting enzyme inhibitor (ACEI) or angiotensin receptor blocking agent (ARB) and/or a beta-adrenergic-blocking agent (BB) significantly reduces the combined endpoint of cardiovascular (CV) mortality and hospitalizations for HF as well as total mortality and total hospitalizations. These results have resulted in a class 1 indication for the use of a MRA, either spironolactone 12.5–50 mg/day or eplerenone 25–50 mg/day in patients with chronic HFREF and HFREF post-MI in both US and European guidelines.[4-6] These results are supported by a recent meta-analysis of randomized trials evaluating the use of an MRA and other blockers of the renin–angiotensin–aldosterone system (RAAS) in patients with HFREF suggesting that in patients with HFREF on an ACEI, there is more benefit from adding an MRA than an ARB.[7] The design and results of these prospective double-blind randomized CV outcome trials are relatively well known and will be only briefly summarized here along with the background information leading to the use of these drugs to reduce CV mortality in patients with HFREF.

BACKGROUND INFORMATION FOR THE USE OF A MINERALOCORTICOID RECEPTOR ANTAGONIST IN PATIENTS WITH HEART FAILURE WITH REDUCED EJECTION FRACTION

Spironolactone, a steroidal MRA, has been known to be an effective potassium (K^+) sparring diuretic for over 50 years. Doses of 100–200 mg/day had been shown to be effective in overcoming diuretic resistance in patients with HF[8,9] and doses of up to 400 mg/day are used in the treatment of ascites. Its use, however, in the US, where it has long been generic, and in many other parts of the world, was relatively minimal due to the focus in the 1980s and 1990s on the efficacy of branded ACEIs, ARBs and BBs. However, in the early 1980s, Stassen et al.[10] had shown in patients with essential hypertension that while an ACEI, such as captopril, could inhibit the production of angiotensin II (ATII) and the stimulation of the AT II type 1 receptor (AT1R), which in part results in the adrenal release of aldosterone that while aldosterone release from the adrenal gland was initially suppressed over several months there was an increase in aldosterone levels back to or above baseline levels prior to administration of an ACEI, despite its continued administration ("aldosterone escape"). This knowledge prompted the design and initiation of the RALES dose finding trial.[11] In this study, patients with chronic HFREF were randomized to placebo or increasing doses of spironolactone from 12.5 to 75 mg/day on top of standard therapy for HF. Efficacy was assessed by monitoring the increase in serum aldosterone levels, indicating blockade of the mitral regurgitation (MR) and the decrease in atrial natriuretic peptide (ANP) levels, indicating a reduction in atrial tension. Safety was assessed by the level of serum potassium (K^+) increase and the incidence of hyperkalemia (HK) (serum K^+ >5.5 mEq/L). Although a dose of spironolactone of 75 mg/day was found to be the most effective dose, it was associated with a clinically significant increase in serum K^+. A dose of 25 mg/day was also thought to be effective in comparison to placebo as evidenced by an increase in serum aldosterone and a decrease in ANP levels but in contrast to a dose of 75 mg/day was associated with only a mild increase in serum K^+ levels. It was, therefore, reasoned that while 75 mg/day might be more effective than 25 mg/day, it would be associated with a significant increase in the incidence of HK and, therefore, patient drop outs, which in a large scale double blind randomized trial using an "intent to treat" analysis would have made it difficult to determine the potential benefit of spironolactone. An initial dose of spironolactone 25 mg/day was therefore chosen for evaluation in the RALES study with the possibility of up titration to 50 mg/day after 1 month if there was evidence of progressive HF and the serum K^+ remained less than 5.0 mEq/L or down titration to 12.5 mg/day at any time if the serum K^+ rose above 5.5 mEq/L.

Prior to the time the RALES study was initiated, there was a report that spironolactone inhibited reactive myocardial and perivascular collagen formation following experimental myocardial injury.[12] Although these results have subsequently been confirmed by several investigators and shown to be of importance, at the time the RALES study was initiated, they were unconfirmed and their implications under appreciated. Subsequently, MRAs have been shown to prevent ventricular and perivascular remodeling and fibrosis; reduce oxidative stress, inflammatory cytokine activation and apoptosis; improve endothelial function and nitric oxide availability; and reduce norepinephrine release, ventricular and atrial arrhythmias, including atrial fibrillation, sudden cardiac death, death due to progressive HF, hospitalizations for HF and renal injury.[13,14]

Patients in the RALES study[1] were included with a history of severe HFREF, New York Heart Association (NYHA) class IV within the 6 months prior to randomization but could have been in NYHA class III or IV at the time of randomization to placebo or spironolactone 12.5–50 mg/day on top of standard therapy for HF. Patients with a serum K^+ more than 5.0 mEq/L and/or a serum creatinine more than 2.5 mg/dL at baseline were excluded. The study was prematurely stopped on the advice of the data safety monitoring committee due to the finding of a 30% reduction in total mortality in patients randomized to spironolactone after a mean follow-up of 24 months. This reduction in total mortality as well as a reduction in hospitalizations for HF was associated with a 3% increased incidence of HK (serum K^+ >5.5 mEq/L). There were, however, no deaths attributable to HK in patients randomized to spironolactone. Although the presence of concomitant chronic kidney disease (CKD) was shown to be a predictor for the development of HK both in those patients randomized to placebo and spironolactone, a recent analysis of the RALES study has shown that the beneficial effects of spironolactone on mortality was greater in those patients with CKD than in those without CKD.[15] Also of interest was the finding that patients randomized to spironolactone had a significant reduction in the incidence of hypokalemia (serum K^+ <3.5 mEq/L). While these results suggested an important benefit of spironolactone in addition to standard therapy for HF many clinicians remained skeptical due to the fact that BBs had been shown to be of benefit in reducing CV mortality and hospitalizations for HF in patients with severe HF, but only 10% of patients in the study were on a BB at the time of randomization. At the time the RALES study[1] was initiated, BBs had not however been shown to be safe or effective in patients with severe HFREF. A second study EPHESUS[3] was therefore initiated in patients with HFREF post-MI using the second generation MRA eplerenone. Eplerenone had been shown to be a more specific blocker of the MR than spironolactone, which also blocks androgen and progesterone receptors accounting for its well-known side effects of breast pain, gynecomastia and impotence in males as well as menstrual irregularities and hirsutism in premenstrual females. Patients in EPHESUS[3] with clinical evidence of HFREF post-MI and/or type 2 diabetes mellitus were randomized to eplerenone 25–50 mg/day or placebo in addition to standard therapy between 3 days and 14 days post-MI. At the end of the study after a mean follow-up of 16 months, it was found that patients randomized to eplerenone had a significant 15% reduction in total mortality as well as a significant reduction in the combined endpoint of CV death and hospitalization for HF. Also of interest was the finding of a significant decrease in total mortality, mainly due to a reduction in sudden cardiac death (SCD) within 30 days postrandomization.[16] These beneficial results were associated with a 1.4% increase in the incidence of HK in comparison to patients randomized to placebo. However, as in the RALES study,[1] there were no deaths attributable to HK in patients randomized to eplerenone. Also of interest was the finding that patients randomized to eplerenone did not have a significant increase in the incidence of the sexual side effects seen in previous studies with spironolactone, attesting to the specificity of eplerenone relative to spironolactone for the MR. Of importance was the fact that in contrast to the RALES study[1] that 75% of patients in EPHESUS[3] were on a BB and more than 85% on an ACEI or ARB at the time of randomization. An analysis of the results showed that eplerenone reduced total mortality even in patients on optimum therapy for HF post-MI including an aspirin, reperfusion, a statin, ACEI or ARB, and a BB. Of interest, a subsequent analysis of EPHESUS[17] has shown that the major benefit of eplerenone on mortality in patients with HFREF post-MI occurs when it is administered relatively early post-MI (3–7 days) and that there is relatively little benefit on mortality when it is delayed after 7 days post-MI. A study by Hyashi et al.[18] has shown that administration of a MRA on day 1 post-MI in patients undergoing percutaneous revascularization was safe and effective in reducing ventricular remodeling and collagen formation. In the recent Reduction of Heart Failure Morbidity in Patients with Acute ST-elevation Myocardial Infarction (REMINDER)[19] study, eplerenone was administered in the early hours post-ST-elevation MI (STEMI) in patients without HF starting with a dose of 25 mg/day which could subsequently be up titrated to 50 mg/day. In this study, eplerenone was shown to be effective in reducing a combined endpoint, mainly driven by a reduction in B-type natriuretic peptide (BNP) or N-terminal pro-B-type natriuretic peptide (NT-proBNP) as well as evidence of a progressive decrease in left ventricle (LV) function and/or the development of HF. Most importantly, eplerenone was safe and well tolerated. This is of importance since in many of these patients eplerenone was administered before the results of serum K^+, and renal function were available. On the basis of the results of EPHESUS,[3,17] the study by Hyashi et al.,[18] and the REMINDER study[19] it would appear to be safe to administer eplerenone on day 1 post-MI in patients with evidence of HF and or a REF (≤40%). Further prospective studies will, however, be required to confirm this recommendation.

The EPHESUS study[3] was followed by the EMPHASIS-HF[2] study in which patients with chronic HFREF and mild symptoms (NYHA class II) who either were hospitalized for HF within the 6 months prior to randomization and/or who had an elevation in BNP or NT-proBNP levels were randomized to placebo or eplerenone 25–50 mg/day which could be increased to 50 mg/day after 1 month if the serum K^+ was less than 5.0 mEq/L. As in RALES[1] the study was prematurely stopped on the advice of the data safety monitoring committee due to a significant reduction in total mortality. There was also a significant 37% decrease in the incidence of the primary combined endpoint of CV mortality and hospitalization for HF as well as total hospitalizations in patients randomized to eplerenone. In EMPHASIS-HF, more than 90% of patients at baseline were on an ACEI or ARB and more than 85% on a BB. The benefits of eplerenone were seen in all of the prespecified subgroups. These beneficial effects, as in the prior RALES[1] and EPHESUS trials,[3] were associated with a significant 4.3% increase in the incidence of HK. However, as in RALES[1] and EPHESUS,[3] there were no deaths attributable to HK in patients randomized to eplerenone. There was also no significant increase in the incidence of patients stopping study drug or developing renal failure. There was, however, a significant decrease in the incidence of hypokalemia (serum K^+ <3.5 mEq/L).

Of great interest was the finding that the incidence of new onset atrial fibrillation was also significantly reduced in patients randomized to eplerenone. The proposed mechanisms for this reduction in the incidence of atrial fibrillation include a reduction in atrial fibrosis, an improvement in atrial function and a decrease in atrial oxidative stress and inflammatory cytokine activation. While the primary endpoint was the time to CV death or hospitalization for HF, it was of special interest to find that the incidences of repeat hospitalizations for HF were significantly reduced by 47%. Given the costs associated with hospitalization for HF these findings have important implications for future healthcare costs.

Despite the evidence cited above and the designation in both US and European guidelines[4-6] that the use of a MRA in patients with chronic HFREF and HFREF post-MI is a class 1 indication the use of a MRA in patients with chronic HFREF remains suboptimal in comparison to the use of an ACEI or ARB and or a BB. For example, approximately one-third of patients who qualify for an MRA according to current guidelines for chronic HFREF in the US received a MRA.[20] It is likely that the percent of patients receiving an MRA for chronic HFREF has increased over the past few years but still remains suboptimal. The situation in patients with HFREF post-MI in whom the use of a MRA is also a class 1 indication is even more remarkable in that only 2–3% of those eligible to receive an MRA according to current guidelines in the US actually receive an MRA.[21] This apparent under use of an MRA in patients with chronic HFREF and especially in patients with HFREF post-MI provides a challenge and an opportunity to further reduce CV mortality, hospitalizations for HF and therefore healthcare costs potentially greater than that predicted by new drugs or devices under current investigation.

The reasons for the apparent underuse of MRAs in patients with HFREF are not entirely clear but likely include the fear of inducing HK and, therefore, SCD; the inconvenience and cost associated with serial monitoring of serum K^+ and renal function as well as recent reports from registry data suggesting that MRAs may not be effective in reducing CV mortality and hospitalizations for HF. The fear of inducing HK and therefore SCD in large part stems from the report by Jurlink et al.[22] from Canada shortly after publication of the RALES[1] results in which they found a significant increase in the incidence of hospitalizations for HK in patients using spironolactone form HF. A critical review of the data of Jurlink et al.[22] as well as data from several smaller studies suggests that the increase in HK observed in these studies was in part due to the use of higher doses of spironolactone than had been used in the RALES trial (12.5–50 mg/day); the inclusion of older patients than included in the RALES study with a relatively high incidence of concomitant CKD. In RALES patients with a serum creatinine more than 2.5 mg/dL as well as those with a serum K^+ more than 5.0 mEq/L were excluded. However, in the elderly the use of serum creatinine as a guide to renal function may underestimate glomerular filtration rate (GFR) such that patients with severe CKD and an estimated GFR (eGFR) less than 30 mL/minute/1.73 m^2 may have been given spironolactone. In some current guidelines and in the EMPHASIS-HF trial[2] patients are excluded with an eGFR less than 30 mL/minute/1.73 m^2. A recent analysis of EMPHASIS-HF in the subset of patients with CKD (eGFR <60 mL/minute/1.73 m^2), diabetes mellitus (DM) and/or age ≥75 years using this exclusion and a serum K^+ >5.0 mEq/L has found that even in these high risk subgroups, the safety of eplerenone 25–50 mg/day was excellent and not significantly different from those patients without these high-risk factors.[23] While there was a significant increase in the incidence of HK (serum K^+ >5.5 mEq/L) in EMPHASIS-HF[2] overall and in these high risk subgroups there was as mentioned above not a single death attributable to HK in patients randomized to a MRA in either RALES,[1] EPHESUS[3] or EMPHASIS-HF.[2] More experience in patients more than 75 years of age will however be required. It would therefore be prudent to reduce the starting dose of a MRA in these patients similar to those patients with CKD. While there is patient inconvenience and increased costs associated with serial monitoring of serum K^+ and renal function it should be pointed out that that this is more than balanced by the significant reduction in total mortality, hospitalizations for HF and total hospitalizations. Clinicians should not hesitate to monitor international normalized ratio (INR) in a patient with atrial fibrillation receiving Coumadin nor should they hesitate to monitor serum K^+ and renal function in those patients eligible to receive a MRA for HFREF. In patients with an eGFR more than or equal to 50 mL/minute/1.73 m^2 serum K^+ and renal function should be measured before instituting therapy with a MRA, such as spironolactone 25 mg/day or eplerenone 25 mg/day. These measurements should then be repeated approximately 1 week and 1 month after starting therapy and then again at routine follow-up visits every 4 months. At any time the serum K^+ is more than 5.5 mEq/L the MRA should be withheld for at least 72 hours and restarted at one-half the prior dose with a subsequent repeat check of serum K^+ within 1 week. The finding of a serum K^+ more than or equal to 6.0 mEq/L on a nonhemolyzed blood sample at any time should prompt immediate withdrawal of the MRA unless a precipitating factor can be found such as the use of a K^+ supplement, nonsteroidal anti-inflammatory drug (NSAID), use of a salt substitute containing K^+, and/or dietary indiscretion involving foods with a high K^+ content, such as tomatoes or watermelons. All patients considered for a MRA should undergo dietary counseling with careful review of high K^+ containing foods. If at any time electrolyte imbalance is suspected, such as with episodes of vomiting or diarrhea, the serum K^+ and renal function should be rechecked and the MRA withheld if the serum K^+ is more than 5.0 mEq/L. In those patients with an eGFR less than 50 and more than or equal to 30 mL/minute/1.73 m^2, it would be appropriate to monitor serum K^+ and renal function more closely. In these patients spironolactone should be started at a dose of 25 mg every other day or preferably, due to its shorter half-life and lesser affinity to the MR, eplerenone 12.5 mg/day with monitoring of serum K^+ and renal function at 72 hours, 1 week, 2 weeks, 1 month and every 3 months after starting a MRA. While the risk of HK is greater in those patients with an eGFR less than 50 mL/minute/1.73 m^2 it should be pointed out that a recent analysis of the RALES data has suggested that the benefit of spironolactone was even greater in those with CKD than in those without it.[23] Given the fact that CKD is a major risk factor for death and hospitalization for HF in patients with HFREF, these are the very patients in which every effort should be made to administer a MRA in patients eligible according to current guidelines. Another reason for the underuse of MRAs in patients with HFREF may relate to many clinicians extrapolating the results with spironolactone in RALES[1] in patients with severe HFREF to those with chronic HFREF and mild symptoms such as in EMPHASIS-HF,[2] those with HFREF post-MI, such as in EPHESUS[3] and in those with an acute STEMI without HF, such as in REMINDER[19] in which eplerenone 25–50 mg/day was found to be effective and safe. The safety results in REMINDER[18] in which eplerenone 25 mg was administered on day 1 of an acute STEMI often without a baseline measurement of serum K^+ are particularly reassuring. As mentioned above, based upon the results of the major randomized trials of MRAs in patients with HFREF current guidelines[4-6] recommend the use of a MRA in patients reflecting the inclusion and exclusion criteria of these trials. In general current guidelines do not however strongly recommend the use of spironolactone only in patients with severe HFREF as studied in RALES[1] but rather suggest the use of either spironolactone or eplerenone in both severe HF as well as HFREF with mild symptoms and HFREF post-MI in which eplerenone was the agent shown to be effective and safe in these studies.[2,3] While spironolactone 12.5–50 mg/day is an effective MRA, as evidenced by the results in RALES,[1] it should be pointed out that spironolactone is more tightly bound to the MR than eplerenone such that approximately 25 mg/day of spironolactone is equivalent to 50 mg/day of eplerenone. Spironolactone, due to its active metabolite canrenoate also has a much longer half-life than eplerenone[24] such that it can be postulated that if a patient develops HK while on spironolactone, it would take a considerably longer time to reduce this risk than in a patient on eplerenone. While spironolactone is considerably less expensive than eplerenone, due to the relatively high costs involved in the synthesis of eplerenone, in the long run eplerenone may be more cost effective if it is better tolerated than spironolactone. The induction of HK and/or the fear of inducing HK resulting in the withholding of a MRA in eligible patients with HFREF would place the patient at increased risk for both death and repeated hospitalization for HF, which in the long run could be far more costly than the cost of eplerenone. Another explanation for the relatively low use of MRAs in patients with HFREF may relate to the findings in some registry studies that the use of a MRA, mainly spironolactone, was not associated with a reduction in death or hospitalizations for HF.[25] One should however be skeptical of evidence from registry studies that contradict the results of large scale prospective randomized studies that have been critically reviewed and included in major guidelines due to the fact that registry data may be confounded by indication. For example, in registry data, evaluating the use of MRAs it is likely that patients selected to receive a MRA had more severe HF than those who did not receive them. While techniques, such as propensity matching can minimize several differences in baseline characteristics, they cannot entirely eliminate them. Clinicians should rely upon the results of well-designed prospective randomized trials that have been critically reviewed and incorporated in major guidelines rather than registry data with their inherent limitations in comparison to randomized studies. While further studies are required to determine the efficacy of a MRA in the early hours post-MI without HF on the basis of current evidence, the results of EPHESUS[3] and that of Hyashi et al.[18] it would appear to be safe to administer eplerenone at a dose of 25 mg on day 1 post-MI in patients with evidence of HF. The extrapolation of the results of RALES[1] in which spironolactone was initiated at a dose of 25 mg/day to the early post-MI period in which eplerenone 25 mg/day has been shown to be safe[19] might lead to an increased risk of HK in the early hours post-MI due to the relatively greater potency of spironolactone 25 mg and its longer half-life[24] and might therefore lead to the conclusion that a MRA would not be safe or well tolerated early post-MI. While in general it is prudent to use the drug and the dosing strategy tested in the pivotal large scale randomized trials responsible for drug approval current evidence would suggest the following (Box 1): In patients with HFREF and an eGFR more than 50 mL/minute/1.73 m^2 without DM or other major risk factors for HK, especially in postmenopausal woman, initiation of MRA therapy with spironolactone 25 mg/day, in large part due to its lower cost, appears to be appropriate. While eplerenone is generic in the US and will soon be generic in many parts of the world, its cost will likely remain considerably higher than those associated with the use of spironolactone due to the relatively higher costs involved in its synthesis. However, in patients with HFREF at increased risk for HK, such as those with CKD, DM, the use of K^+-sparring drugs, the very old and in those patients who cannot adhere to a low K^+ diet, I would favor initiating MRA therapy with eplerenone 12.5–25 mg/day. It should, however, be emphasized that these are my personal recommendations and as mentioned above current guidelines in general support the use of either spironolactone of eplerenone in approved indications.

Box 1: Mineralocorticoid receptor antagonists in patients with heart failure with reduced ejection fraction: the guidelines to patient selection and dosing*

Patient selection

- Stable with chronic HFREF or HFREF early post-MI
- On standard guideline recommended therapy, including an ACEI or ARB and a BB if tolerated
- Serum K^+ less than 5.0 mmol/L, eGFR more than or equal to 30 mL/minute/1.73 m^2

Patient initial dosing

- Patients with an eGFR more than 50 mL/minute/1.73 m^2 and those less than 75 years of age
  - Start with spironolactone 25 mg/day, especially in those with severe chronic HFREF, or eplerenone 25 mg/day and up titrate at 1 month if serum K^+ is less than 5.0 mmol/L
- Patients with an eGFR less than 50 mL/minute/1.73 m^2 and those more than 75 years of age
  - Start with eplerenone 12.5 mg/day and up titrate at 1 month if serum K^+ is less than 5.0 mmol/L

*Check the text of this paper for further details regarding dosing and serial monitoring of serum K^+ and renal function as well as latest applicable HF guidelines before initiating dosing with a MRA.

HFREF, heart failure with reduced ejection fraction; MI, myocardial infarction; ACEI, angiotensin-converting enzyme inhibitor; ARB, angiotensin receptor-blocking agent; BB, beta-adrenergic-blocking agent; HF, heart failure; MRA, mineralocorticoid receptor antagonist; eGFR, estimated glomerular filtration rate

There are some potential advances that might modify the recommendations for the use of MRAs in patients with HFREF in the near future. First, a new K^+ binding polymer RLY 5016 has been suggested to prevent the development of HK in patients with HFREF given 25 mg of spironolactone, which was subsequently up titrated to 50 mg who either did not tolerate a RAAS inhibitor or BB and/or who had CKD.[26] RLY 5016 is currently undergoing evaluation in a large scale randomized study in patients with CKD +/– HF and evidence of HK (serum K^+ more than or equal to 5.1 mEq/L, but has not yet been approved for clinical use by either the Food and Drug Administration (FDA) or European Medicines Agency (EMA). The second potential advance is the introduction of new nonsteroidal MRAs, such as BAY 94-8862. In a recent study, BAY 94-8862,[27] at doses of 2.5–10 mg/day were compared to placebo using a double blind randomized strategy and also compared to spironolactone 25–50 mg using an open label randomized strategy in patients with HFREF + CKD. BAY 94-8862 was shown to be effective in blocking the MR as evidenced by a significant decrease in BNP and NT-proBNP levels, a decrease in urinary albuminuria, and an increase in serum aldosterone levels, reflecting blockade of the MR in comparison to placebo. In comparison to spironolactone 25–50 mg BAY 94-8862 was found to be at least as effective as evidenced by a similar reduction in BNP, NT-proBNP levels and albuminuria but with a significantly lesser increase in serum K^+ and incidence of HK. The reduction in systolic blood pressure was however significantly greater with spironolactone than with BAY 94-8862. This lesser degree of blood pressure reduction with BAY 94-8862 might be an advantage in patients with HFREF and concomitant vascular disease who are prone to myocardial, cerebral and/or renal ischemia. On the other hand, it might be a disadvantage in patients with HFREF and concomitant hypertension. BAY 94-8862 is currently undergoing further prospective evaluation in patients with HFREF + CKD in comparison to placebo and eplerenone 25–50 mg/day. While its long-term efficacy and safety remain to be evaluated in further large scale prospective double blind randomized studies, it would appear that the promise exists for reducing the incidence of HK associated with the use of an MRA in patients with HFREF and CKD. However, in the interim the evidence currently available as detailed in both US and European guidelines[4-6] and reviewed above should prompt an increased use of either spironolactone or eplerenone in patients with chronic HFREF and HFREF post-MI. The benefits of applying this strategy to eligible patients with HFREF on CV mortality, hospitalizations for HF and therefore healthcare costs is likely to be as great or greater than that achieved by several newer drugs for HFREF currently under investigation.

REFERENCES

1. Pitt B, Zannad F, Remme WJ, et al. The effect of spironolactone on morbidity and mortality in patients with severe heart failure. Randomized Aldactone Evaluation Study Investigators. N Engl J Med. 1999;341(10):709-17.
2. Zannad F, McMurray JJ, Krum H, et al. Eplerenone in patients with systolic heart failure and mild symptoms. N Engl J Med. 2011;364(1):11-21.
3. Pitt B, Remme W, Zannad F, et al. Eplerenone, a selective aldosterone blocker, in patients with left ventricular dysfunction after myocardial infarction. N Engl J Med. 2003;348(14):1309-21.
4. Bonow RO, Ganiats TG, Beam CT, et al. ACCF/AHA/AMA-PCPI 2011 performance measures for adults with heart failure: a report of the American College of Cardiology Foundation/American Heart Association Task Force on Performance Measures and the American Medical Association-Physician Consortium for Performance Improvement. Circulation. 2012;125(19):2382-401.
5. Jessup M, Abraham WT, Casey DE, et al. 2009 focused update: ACCF/AHA Guidelines for the Diagnosis and Management of Heart Failure in Adults: a report of the American College of Cardiology Foundation/American Heart Association Task Force on Practice Guidelines: developed in collaboration with the International Society for Heart and Lung Transplantation. Circulation. 2009;119(14):1977-2016.
6. McMurray JJ, Adamopoulos S, Anker SD, et al. ESC Guidelines for the diagnosis and treatment of acute and chronic heart failure 2012: The Task Force for the Diagnosis and Treatment of Acute and Chronic Heart Failure 2012 of the European Society of Cardiology. Developed in collaboration with the Heart Failure Association (HFA) of the ESC. Eur Heart J. 2012;33(14):1787-847.
7. Bangalore S, Kumar S, Messerli FH. When conventional heart failure therapy is not enough: angiotensin receptor blocker, direct renin inhibitor, or aldosterone antagonist? Congest Heart Fail. 2013;19(3):107-15.
8. van Vliet AA, Donker AJ, Nauta JJ, et al. Spironolactone in congestive heart failure refractory to high-dose loop diuretic and low-dose angiotensin-converting enzyme inhibitor. Am J Cardiol. 1993;71(3):21A-28A.
9. Hensen J, Abraham WT, Durr JA, et al. Aldosterone in congestive heart failure: analysis of determinants and role in sodium retention. Am J Nephrol. 1991;11(6):441-6.
10. Staessen J, Lijnen P, Fagard R, et al. Rise in plasma concentration of aldosterone during long-term angiotensin II suppression. J Endocrinol. 1981;91(3):457-65.
11. Effectiveness of spironolactone added to an angiotensin-converting enzyme inhibitor and a loop diuretic for severe chronic congestive heart failure (the Randomized Aldactone Evaluation Study [RALES]). Am J Cardiol. 1996;78(8):902-7.
12. Brilla CG, Matsubara LS, Weber KT. Anti-aldosterone treatment and the prevention of myocardial fibrosis in primary and secondary hyperaldosteronism. J Mol Cell Cardiol. 1993;25(5):563-75.
13. Struthers AD, Unger T. Physiology of aldosterone and pharmacology of aldosterone blockers. 2011;13SuppB:B27-30.
14. Ma T, Szeto CC. Mineralocorticoid receptor antagonist for renal protection. Ren Fail. 2012;34(6):810-7.
15. Vardeny O, Wu DH, Desai A, et al. Influence of baseline and worsening renal function on efficacy of spironolactone in patients With severe heart failure: insights from RALES (Randomized Aldactone Evaluation Study). J Am Coll Cardiol. 2012;60(20):2082-9.
16. Pitt B, White H, Nicolau J, et al. Eplerenone reduces mortality 30 days after randomization following acute myocardial infarction in patients with left ventricular systolic dysfunction and heart failure. J Am Coll Cardiol. 2005;46(3):425-31.
17. Adamopoulos C, Ahmed A, Fay R, et al. Timing of eplerenone initiation and outcomes in patients with heart failure after acute myocardial infarction complicated by left ventricular systolic dysfunction: insights from the EPHESUS trial. Eur J Heart Fail. 2009;11(11):1099-105.
18. Hayashi M, Tsutamoto T, Wada A, et al. Immediate administration of mineralocorticoid receptor antagonist spironolactone prevents post-infarct left ventricular remodeling associated with suppression of a marker of myocardial collagen synthesis in patients with first anterior acute myocardial infarction. Circulation. 2003;107(20):2559-65.
19. Montalescot G, Zannad F, Lopez dSE, et al. Early administration of eplerenone in patients with acute myocardial infarction without heart failure: Results of the randomized, double-blind, placebo-controlled reminder trial. Am Coll Cardiol. 2013. (In Press).
20. Albert NM, Yancy CW, Liang L, et al. Use of aldosterone antagonists in heart failure. JAMA. 2009;302(15):1658-65.
21. Rassi AN, Cavender MA, Fonarow GC, et al. Temporal trends and predictors in the use of aldosterone antagonists post-acute myocardial infarction. J Am Coll Cardiol. 2013;61(1):35-40.
22. Juurlink DN, Mamdani MM, Lee DS, et al. Rates of hyperkalemia after publication of the Randomized Aldactone Evaluation Study. N Engl J Med. 2004;351(6):543-51.
23. Eschalier R, McMurray JJ, Swedberg K, et al. Safety and efficacy of eplerenone in patients at high risk for hyperkalemia and/or worsening renal function: analyses of the EMPHASIS-HF study subgroups (Eplerenone in Mild Patients Hospitalization And Survival Study in Heart Failure). J Am Coll Cardiol. 2013:62(17):1585-93.
24. Struthers A, Krum H, Williams GH. A comparison of the aldosterone-blocking agents eplerenone and spironolactone. Clin Cardiol. 2008;31(4):153-8.
25. Hernandez AF, Mi X, Hammill BG, et al. Associations between aldosterone antagonist therapy and risks of mortality and readmission among patients with heart failure and reduced ejection fraction. JAMA. 2012;308(20):2097-107.
26. Pitt B, Anker SD, Bushinsky DA, et al. Evaluation of the efficacy and safety of RLY5016, a polymeric potassium binder, in a double-blind, placebo-controlled study in patients with chronic heart failure (the PEARL-HF) trial. Eur Heart J. 2011;32(7):820-8.
27. Pitt B, Kober L, Ponikowski P, et al. Safety and tolerability of the novel non-steroidal mineralocorticoid receptor antagonist BAY 94-8862 in patients with chronic heart failure and mild or moderate chronic kidney disease: a randomized, double-blind trial. Eur Heart J. 2013;34(31):2453-63.

Chapter 27

Atrial Fibrillation Done Right

Amir A Schricker, David E Krummen

ABSTRACT

Atrial fibrillation (AF) is frequently encountered in heart failure patients. It has a broad range of clinical presentations, and thus accurate diagnosis is essential. Successful AF therapy includes preventing thromboembolism with appropriate anticoagulation, controlling the heart rate, and in symptomatic patients attempting to maintain sinus rhythm via either pharmacologic or nonpharmacologic therapies. With appropriate management, the risks of stroke, congestive heart failure (CHF) and death may be significantly reduced and the quality of life improved. This chapter discusses the diagnosis, workup and management of AF, based on current guidelines and clinical experience.

INTRODUCTION

Atrial fibrillation (AF) is frequently encountered in clinical practice. Debilitating symptoms, frequent recurrences and suboptimal therapy can cause AF to be a frustrating experience for patients and caregivers alike. However, directing therapy according to evidence-based principles can significantly improve the quality of care: (i) prevention of thromboembolism according to CHA_2DS_2–VASc score (Table 1), (ii) appropriate heart rate control (based on the recent guidelines, as discussed in Table 2), and (iii) maintenance of sinus rhythm if significant symptoms are present after achieving adequate rate control. This chapter discusses the diagnosis, evaluation, and management of AF based upon current guidelines by American and European societies, and clinical experience.

EPIDEMIOLOGY

Atrial fibrillation is the most common sustained arrhythmia, occurring in approximately 1% of the population and increasing steadily with age. The risk of AF reaches almost 10% in patients over the age of 80 years.[1] AF is uncommon in childhood but increases to approximately 6% in those older than 65 years. The true prevalence of AF, however, is unknown as AF is often asymptomatic.[2] AF, although in general not dangerous acutely (except in the presence of a rapidly-conducting accessory pathway), is associated with increased risks of stroke, heart failure, hospitalization, dementia, and premature death.[3] Mortality rates in AF patients are higher than those in sinus rhythm.[4]

TABLE 1: Components of the CHA_2DS_2–VASc scoring system

	Condition	*Points*
C	Congestive heart failure (or left ventricular systolic dysfunction)	1
H	Hypertension or treated hypertension on medications	1
A_2	Age ≥75 years	2
D	Diabetes mellitus	1
S_2	Prior stroke or transient ischemic attack	2
V	Vascular disease (peripheral artery disease)	1
A	Age 65–74 years	1
Sc	Sex category (i.e., female gender)	1

Source: Adapted from references 7 and 10.

Risk factors for AF include transient reversible causes and underlying heart disease. Transient causes include thyrotoxicosis, alcohol ingestion, acute myocardial infarction (MI), recent cardiac surgery, pericarditis and pulmonary disease. Obstructive sleep apnea is also being increasingly recognized as an independent risk factor for AF.[5] Underlying heart disease is a significant risk factor for the development of AF. Acute AF often develops during acute MI in up to 10% of patients, and in postcardiac surgery patients in up to 50%. CHF is also associated with AF, as approximately 40% of patients with CHF develop AF. Furthermore, advanced age, hypertension, and ischemic heart disease are also well-established risk factors.

Several groups have attempted to develop a risk score to predict an individual's risk of developing AF. A recent study incorporated age, sex, blood pressure, treatment for hypertension, PR interval, cardiac murmur, body mass index, and heart failure.[6]

CLASSIFICATION

Many terms have been used to classify AF. Current guidelines propose the following classification scheme for AF:[7]

- First-detected AF: The term to describe AF at first diagnosis.
- Paroxysmal AF: Recurrent AF episodes that terminate spontaneously in 7 days or less.
- Persistent AF: Characterized as AF with episodes that last longer than 7 days and typically require pharmacologic or electrical cardioversion to restore sinus rhythm.
- Longstanding AF: Refers to AF that has lasted for 1 year or more.
- Permanent AF: AF in which cardioversion has failed, or AF patients in whom sinus rhythm restoration is no longer pursued or deemed futile.

This classification scheme applies to recurrent episodes of AF lasting more than 30 seconds that are unrelated to reversible causes.

CLINICAL PRESENTATION

Atrial fibrillation can be asymptomatic or symptomatic. Up to 90% of paroxysmal AF episodes may not be symptomatic, even with rapid heart rates. A significant proportion with asymptomatic AF may present with stroke as their first symptom. Symptoms due to AF vary and are often due to the degree of heart rate elevation. Common symptoms include palpitations, tachycardia, shortness of breath, weakness and fatigue. Less commonly patients may present with chest pain or syncope.

CLINICAL EVALUATION

History and Physical Examination

A complete history and physical examination is an essential part of the workup of patients with AF. Important aspects of the patient's history include the timeline of symptoms, frequency duration, severity of AF episodes, and precipitating factors. Additionally, a detailed history of the patient's past medical problems, including cardiovascular disease, hypertension, diabetes, history of stroke and presence of vascular disease are important for decisions regarding anticoagulation.

A complete physical examination, including a detailed cardiac examination should be performed in all patients. Aspect to note include vital signs (in particular during AF), presence of valvular disease and evidence of heart failure.

Laboratory Tests

Comprehensive baseline laboratory testing should be performed to assess for electrolyte abnormalities, renal dysfunction, and other potentially reversible causes. Tests should include a chemistry panel with renal function, complete blood count, and thyroid function panel.

Electrocardiogram

Electrocardiogram (ECG) is an essential tool in the diagnosis and management of AF, which is characterized by an absence of clear P waves, a coarse and undulating baseline, and an irregularly irregular RR interval. An example of ECG showing AF is shown in Figure 1. AF needs to be distinguished from sinus rhythm with frequent premature atrial complexes, multifocal atrial tachycardia and atrial flutter with variable atrioventricular (AV) block.

Other important electrocardiographic information includes evidence of prior MI, left ventricular hypertrophy (LVH), Wolff-Parkinson-White (WPW) syndrome and evidence for pericarditis, all of which are associated with AF.

Echocardiogram

A transthoracic echocardiogram is performed to assess for structural disease, including cardiomyopathy and

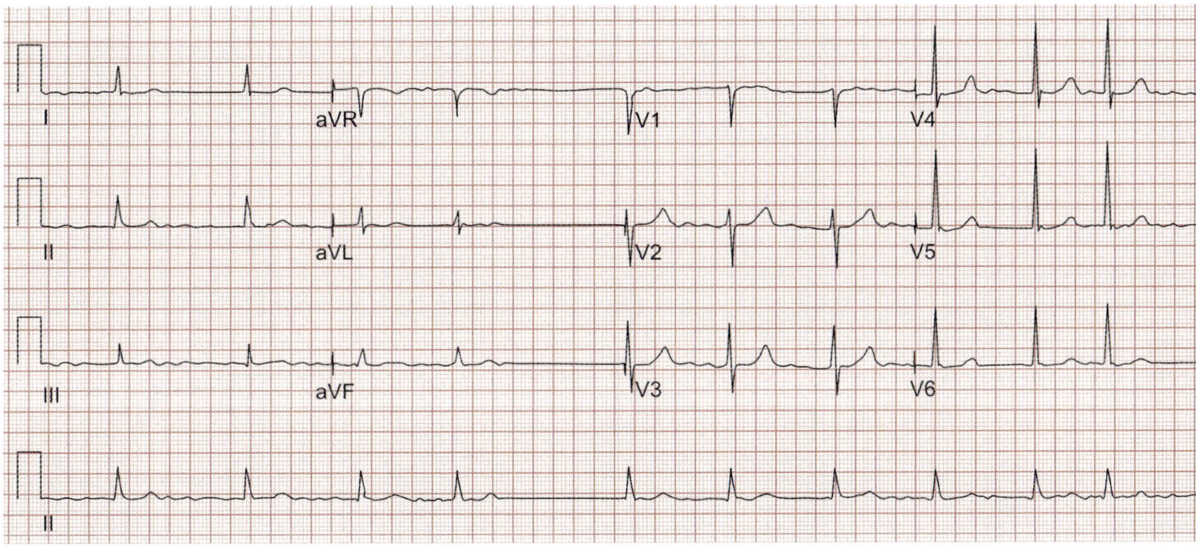

Fig. 1 Electrocardiogram showing atrial fibrillation. Note the lack of P-waves and irregularly irregular rhythm

valvular disease. Left ventricular (LV) wall thickness should also be noted if antiarrhythmic medications are being considered, as LVH is a contraindication to class I agents. Additionally, a transesophageal echocardiogram (TEE) may be necessary to assess for a left atrial appendage thrombus, if cardioversion is considered.

TREATMENT

The treatment of any unstable AF patient—one who is very symptomatic or hemodynamically unstable—is immediate direct-current cardioversion (DCCV). For patients who are tolerant of AF, the three central goals of AF management are: (i) anticoagulation for prevention of systemic embolization, (ii) control of ventricular heart rate, and (iii) restoring sinus rhythm if symptoms are present.

An important decision in the management of AF is the long-term treatment strategy for the patient. In general, there are two management strategies: rate control and rhythm control. Notably, several large studies compared the rate and rhythm control strategies, and neither was associated with a significant difference in long arm morbidity and mortality.[8]

Anticoagulation

All patients, regardless of management strategy, require protection from systemic embolization. Current guidelines[7,9,10] recommend the use of the CHA_2DS_2-VASc scoring system to assess for risk of systemic embolization (Table 1).

Patients whose CHA_2DS_2-VASc score is greater than or equal to 2 require long-term oral anticoagulation (OAC). Traditionally, the vitamin K antagonist warfarin is initiated [with a goal international normalized ratio (INR) of 2.0–3.0]. More recently, newer agents have been introduced and include direct thrombin inhibitors, such as dabigatran, and factor Xa inhibitors, such as rivaroxaban and apixaban. For new-onset AF, current guidelines recommend that patients who have been in AF for longer than 48 hours be anticoagulated.

Patients with a score of zero may be managed with aspirin therapy alone. Patients whose score is one may be treated with either aspirin or OAC therapy.

Ventricular Rate Control

For asymptomatic patients, it is appropriate to proceed with the rate control strategy. The strategy consists of anticoagulation and medications to control ventricular heart rate. Since patients with AF typically present with elevated heart rates, therapy entails drugs that slow conduction through the AV node, such as beta blockers or calcium-channel blockers. Digoxin may be used in combination with these agents for additional rate control. Table 2 summarizes rate-control medications.

Results from the Rate Control Efficacy in Permanent Atrial Fibrillation (RACE II) trial[11] have redefined rate-control targets for AF, to less than 110 beats per minute

TABLE 2: Medications to achieve ventricular rate control in atrial fibrillation (AF)

Drugs	*Intravenous doses*	*Oral maintenance doses*
Beta blockers		
Metoprolol	2.5–5 mg bolus every 5 minutes, up to three doses	25–100 mg BID (metoprolol succinate ER: 50–200 mg daily)
Esmolol	Bolus: 500 µg/kg Continuous: 50–200 µg/kg/minute	N/A
Carvedilol	N/A	3.125–25 mg BID (up to 50 mg BID if >85 kg)
Calcium-channel blockers		
Diltiazem	Bolus: 0.25 mg/kg (average 20 mg) every 5 minutes Continuous: 5–15 mg/hour	120–480 mg daily
Verapamil	0.075–0.15 mg/kg	120–480 mg daily (slow-release available)
Digitalis		
Digoxin	Load: 500 µg, followed every 6 hours by 250 µg twice (adjust based on renal function)	0.125–0.375 µg daily
Other		
Amiodarone	150 mg over 10 minutes, then 0.5–1 mg/minute	200 mg daily

BID, twice a day; ER, extended-release; N/A, not applicable

Source: Adapted from references 7 and 10.

(bpm). Lenient rate control to less than or equal to 110 bpm is as effective clinically as the traditional and strict rate-control goal of less than or equal to 80 bpm. If palpitations and other symptoms of tachycardia persist; however, more aggressive heart rate control is required.

For symptomatic and refractory AF where ventricular rate is unable to be controlled, one option is AV node ablation followed by implantation of a permanent pacemaker. Long-term anticoagulation is required in these patients.

Restoring and Maintaining Sinus Rhythm

For persistent AF patients, typically at least one attempt to restore sinus rhythm is made. This may be accomplished by achieving therapeutic anticoagulation for 3 weeks and then performing cardioversion. Alternatively, if cardioversion cannot be delayed, a TEE may be performed to rule out a left atrial appendage thrombus, and if a thrombus is not present cardioversion may be performed at that time. Flowchart 1 provides an overview of the cardioversion decision process.

Otherwise, for patients with significant symptoms due to AF, a rhythm control strategy is appropriate. In this strategy, the patient is placed on appropriate anticoagulation and attempts are made to restore and maintain sinus rhythm, either via cardioversion (pharmacologic or DC) or ablation. Although several older studies have shown no benefit to the rhythm control strategy,[8] more recent studies have shown benefit in younger, healthier patients with significant symptoms.[12]

Direct-current Cardioversion

Direct-current cardioversion is effective greater than 75% of the time, with increased chances of success depending on the duration of AF and the size of the left atrium. The success rate is approximately 90% when AF duration is less than 1 year, compared to 50% when AF has been present for more than 5 years. As stated above, a common strategy involves achieving adequate anticoagulation for 3 weeks prior to cardioversion. An alternative is to perform a TEE prior to cardioversion to verify the absence of left atrial appendage thrombus.

Antiarrhythmic Medications

Antiarrhythmic medications are typically administered by a cardiologist or electrophysiologist, as the side effects and safety profile require close supervision.[13] Some options are described here.

Class IC antiarrhythmic drugs: Therapy with class IC antiarrhythmic agents is associated with increased mortality in patients with underlying cardiovascular disease, as shown in the Cardiac Arrhythmia Suppression Trial (CAST) trial.[14] However, in patients without structural or ischemic heart disease, these agents may be safely used to prevent AF. Most commonly used examples

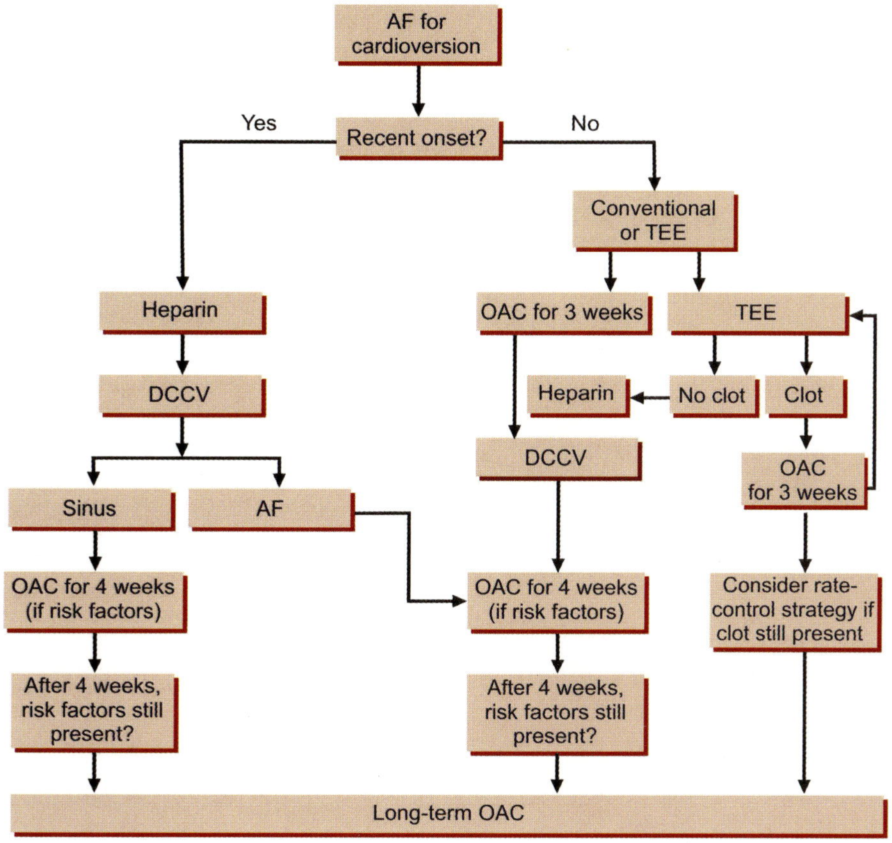

AF, atrial fibrillation; DCCV, direct-current cardioversion; OAC, oral anticoagulation; TEE, transesophageal echocardiogram

Flowchart 1 An overview to guide cardioversion of hemodynamically stable atrial fibrillation

from this antiarrhythmic class include flecainide and propafenone.

Class III antiarrhythmic drugs: The major action of these drugs is to prolong refractoriness in cardiac tissue. Sotalol and dofetilide may be safely used in patients with CHF. However, patients must be closely monitored during initiation of these medications and dofetilide must be administered in hospital for the first five doses to observe for QTc prolongation. Amiodarone is the most effective antiarrhythmic drug, but also has significant side effects. Dronedarone is the newest of the class III agents; unlike amiodarone and dofetilide, dronedarone is contraindicated in patients with CHF.

Although effective, we frequently avoid long-term therapy with amiodarone in younger patients when possible due to often-irreversible side effects. Instead, we use Vaughn–Williams class IC and III drugs, as indicated in Flowchart 2.

Catheter Ablation

Ablation is typically reserved for symptomatic patients who have failed one or more antiarrhythmic drugs. Ablation is most commonly performed by an electrophysiologist, but also may be performed by a cardiothoracic surgeon during concomitant open-heart surgery, such as valve replacement or coronary artery bypass grafting.

Traditionally, the goals of the ablation procedure are to electrically isolate the pulmonary veins, as the pulmonary veins have been identified as the source of AF-triggering ectopy in some patients. However, more recent data suggest that localized sources, such as electrical rotors and focal drivers, sustain AF and may be successfully targeted to improve ablation success.[15] Figures 2A and B show an example of a left atrial rotor, which was successfully ablated, resulting in restoration of sinus rhythm.

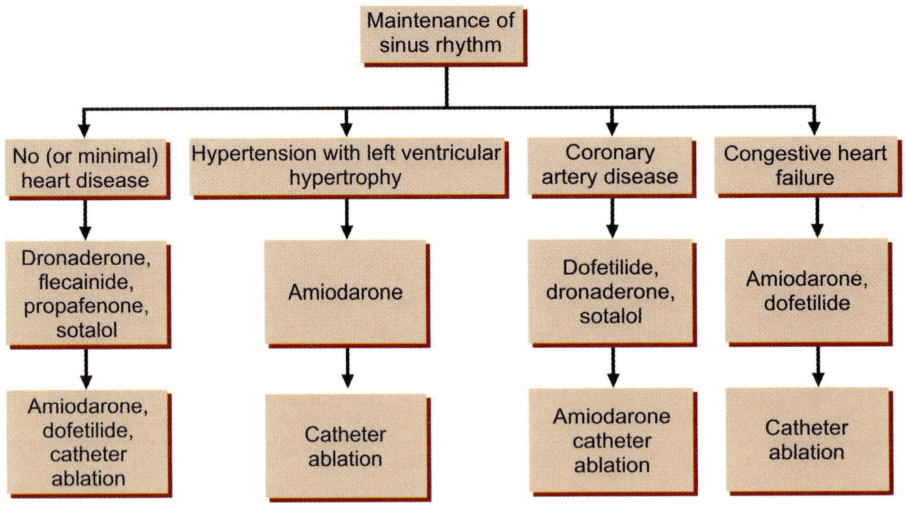

Flowchart 2 Antiarrhythmic flowchart based upon concomitant heart disease

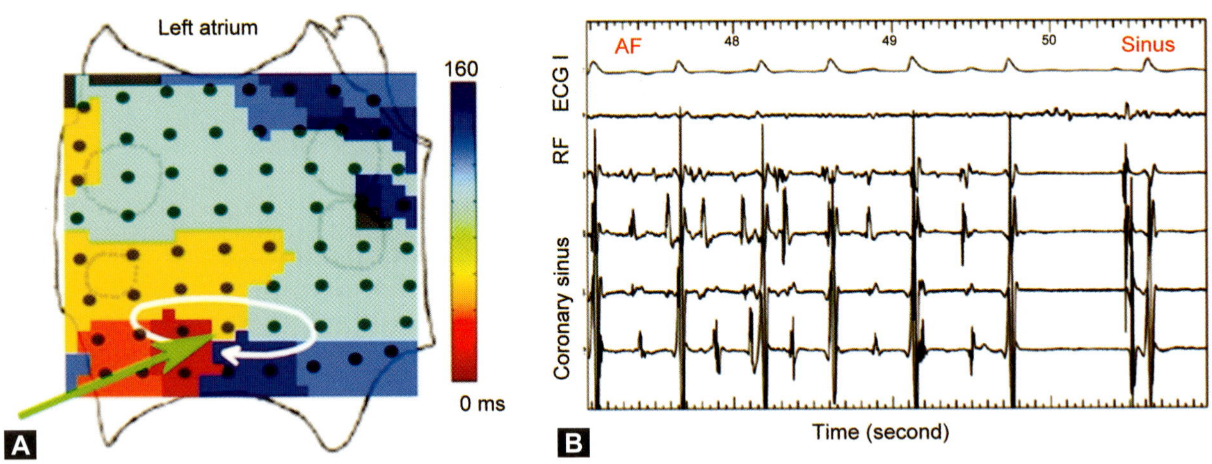

AF, atrial fibrillation; RF, radiofrequency; ECG, electrocardiogram

Figs 2A and B Isochronal representation (A) of left atrial electrical activation during atrial fibrillation, showing a clockwise rotor (white circular arrow). Focal ablation at the site indicated by the green arrow terminated atrial fibrillation to sinus rhythm (B). The patient remains atrial fibrillation-free on follow-up

ATRIAL FIBRILLATION AND HEART FAILURE

Given the focus of this textbook on CHF, we wanted to specifically address this important subgroup of patients with AF.

Overall, patients with CHF should receive the same care for AF as patients without CHF. However, there are important caveats to keep in mind:

- Typically, beta blockers are recommended as first-line therapy for rate control, as patients with heart failure require this medication for long-term management. Digoxin should be strongly considered if a second agent is needed
- Antiarrhythmic therapy for CHF patients is predominantly limited to dofetilide, amiodarone and occasionally sotalol. Dofetilide requires inpatient administration, but has a low long-term side effect profile. Amiodarone is highly effective, but cumulative toxicity and recent reports showing increased hazard with amiodarone therapy[16] limit the long-term appeal of this medication
- Patients who fail medical rate control may be candidates for AV node ablation and biventricular pacing
- Although ablation therapy is less likely to be effective in patients with heart failure, successful ablation may help improve LV function.[17]

SPECIAL SITUATION

Occasionally, AF occurs in conjunction with an accessory pathway, which presents an increased risk of sudden death to the patient. In the setting of preexcited AF, therapy should begin with an antiarrhythmic drug, such as intravenous (IV) procainamide or ibutilide rather than a pure AV nodal blocking agent, which may paradoxically increase the ventricular rate and lead to ventricular fibrillation. Such patients should also be referred for electrophysiology evaluation and possible electrophysiology study and ablation of the accessory pathway.

PROGNOSIS

Patient with AF are at a significantly increased risk of stroke, CHF and mortality. However, appropriate rate control and anticoagulation significantly reduces these complications. In patients with significant symptoms despite adequate rate control, restoration of sinus rhythm improves quality of life.

CONCLUSION

In this chapter, we have attempted to provide a broad overview of AF management. For issues not addressed in this work, readers are advised to consult the excellent AF guidelines by Fuster,[18] Wann,[19] and Camm.[7]

REFERENCES

1. Go AS, Hylek EM, Phillips KA, et al. Prevalence of diagnosed atrial fibrillation in adults: national implications for rhythm management and stroke prevention: the AnTicoagulation and Risk Factors in Atrial Fibrillation (ATRIA) Study. JAMA. 2001;285(18):2370-5.
2. Lim HS, Lip GY. Asymptomatic atrial fibrillation on device interrogation. J Cardiovasc Electrophysiol. 2008;19(8):891-3.
3. Miyasaka Y, Barnes ME, Gersh BJ, et al. Secular trends in incidence of atrial fibrillation in Olmsted County, Minnesota, 1980 to 2000, and implications on the projections for future prevalence. Circulation. 2006;114(2):119-25.
4. Crandall MA, Horne BD, Day JD, et al. Atrial fibrillation significantly increases total mortality and stroke risk beyond that conveyed by the $CHADS_2$ risk factors. Pacing Clin Electrophysiol. 2009;32(8):981-6.
5. Gami AS, Hodge DO, Herges RM, et al. Obstructive sleep apnea, obesity, and the risk of incident atrial fibrillation. J Am Coll Cardiol. 2007;49(5):565-71.
6. Schnabel RB, Sullivan LM, Levy D, et al. Development of a risk score for atrial fibrillation (Framingham Heart Study): a community-based cohort study. Lancet. 2009;373(9665):739-45.
7. European Heart Rhythm Association; European Association for Cardio-Thoracic Surgery, Camm AJ, et al. Guidelines for the management of atrial fibrillation: the Task Force for the Management of Atrial Fibrillation of the European Society of Cardiology (ESC). European Heart J. 2010; 31(19):2369-429.
8. Wyse DG, Waldo AL, DiMarco JP, et al. A comparison of rate control and rhythm control in patients with atrial fibrillation. N Engl J Med. 2002; 347(23):1825-33.
9. Calkins H, Kuck KH, Cappato R, et al. 2012 HRS/EHRA/ECAS expert consensus statement on catheter and surgical ablation of atrial fibrillation: recommendations for patient selection, procedural techniques, patient management and follow-up, definitions, endpoints, and research trial design: a report of the Heart Rhythm Society (HRS) Task Force on Catheter and Surgical Ablation of Atrial Fibrillation. Developed in partnership with the European Heart Rhythm Association (EHRA), a registered branch of the European Society of Cardiology (ESC) and the European Cardiac Arrhythmia Society (ECAS); and in collaboration with the American College of Cardiology (ACC), American Heart Association (AHA), the Asia Pacific Heart Rhythm Society (APHRS), and the Society of Thoracic Surgeons (STS). Endorsed by the governing bodies of the American College of Cardiology Foundation, the American Heart Association, the European Cardiac Arrhythmia Society, the European Heart Rhythm Association, the Society of Thoracic Surgeons, the Asia Pacific Heart Rhythm Society, and the Heart Rhythm Society. Heart Rhythm. 2012;9:632-696.e21.
10. European Heart Rhythm A, Heart Rhythm S, Fuster V, et al. ACC/AHA/ESC 2006 guidelines for the management of patients with atrial fibrillation—executive summary: a report of the American College of Cardiology/American Heart Association Task Force on Practice Guidelines and the European Society of Cardiology Committee for Practice Guidelines (Writing Committee to Revise the 2001 Guidelines for the Management of Patients With Atrial Fibrillation). J Am Coll Cardiol. 2006;48:854-906.
11. Van Gelder IC, Groenveld HF, Crijns HJ, et al. Lenient versus strict rate control in patients with atrial fibrillation. N Engl J Med. 2010;362(15):1363-73.
12. Ogawa S, Yamashita T, Yamazaki T, et al. Optimal treatment strategy for patients with paroxysmal atrial fibrillation: J-RHYTHM Study. Circulation. 2009;73(2):242-8.
13. Brunton LL, Chabner B, Knollmann BC. Goodman & Gilman's The Pharmacological Basis of Therapeutics, 12th edition. New York, USA: McGraw-Hill Professional; 2011.
14. Pratt CM, Moye LA. The cardiac arrhythmia suppression trial. Casting suppression in a different light. Circulation. 1995;91(1):245-7.
15. Narayan SM, Krummen DE, Shivkumar K, et al. Treatment of atrial fibrillation by the ablation of localized sources: CONFIRM (Conventional Ablation for Atrial Fibrillation With or Without Focal Impulse and Rotor Modulation) trial. J Am Coll Cardiol. 2012;60(7):628-36.
16. Saksena S, Slee A, Waldo AL, et al. Cardiovascular outcomes in the AFFIRM Trial (Atrial Fibrillation Follow-Up Investigation of Rhythm Management). An assessment of individual antiarrhythmic drug therapies compared with rate control with propensity score-matched analyses. J Am Coll Cardiol. 2011;58(19):1975-85.
17. Hsu LF, Jais P, Sanders P, et al. Catheter ablation for atrial fibrillation in congestive heart failure. N Engl J Med. 2004;351(23):2373-83.
18. Fuster V, Ryden LE, Cannom DS, et al. ACC/AHA/ESC 2006 Guidelines for the Management of Patients with Atrial Fibrillation: a report of the American College of Cardiology/American Heart Association Task Force on Practice Guidelines and the European Society of Cardiology Committee for Practice Guidelines (Writing Committee to Revise the 2001 Guidelines for the Management of Patients With Atrial Fibrillation): developed in collaboration with the European Heart Rhythm Association and the Heart Rhythm Society. Circulation. 2006;114:e257-354.
19. Wann LS, Curtis AB, January CT, et al. 2011 ACCF/AHA/HRS focused update on the management of patients with atrial fibrillation (updating the 2006 guideline): a report of the American College of Cardiology Foundation/American Heart Association Task Force on Practice Guidelines. Circulation. 2011;123(1):104-23.

Chapter 28

Ventricular Tachycardia Done Right

Gautam G Lalani, David E Krummen

ABSTRACT

Ventricular tachycardia (VT) is a life-threatening arrhythmia frequently seen in heart failure patients. Initial management is directed at termination of VT and arrhythmia suppression. Next, a thorough evaluation is required to determine the etiology of the arrhythmia. Modern, long-term management may include antiarrhythmic medications, ablation, and implantable cardioverter-defibrillator therapy, and frequently requires consultation with an electrophysiologist. Tailored therapies for specific types of VT are also discussed. The overall goal of this chapter is to assist the clinician in providing timely guideline-directed therapy to positively impact patient outcomes.

INTRODUCTION

Ventricular tachycardia (VT) is a common, life-threatening arrhythmia with a high prevalence in patients with heart failure. Because of the high risk of morbidity and mortality, rapid identification and initiation of proper management are of paramount importance. For VT survivors, a thorough patient evaluation is essential to determine the specific etiology. Fortunately, advances in both short- and long-term therapies for VT can significantly improve patient survival. In this chapter we will discuss the clinical presentation, evaluation, workup, and management of VT based upon current guidelines and clinical experience.

EPIDEMIOLOGY

In the United States, approximately 450,000 cases of sudden cardiac death (SCD) occur annually, the majority of which are due to ventricular arrhythmias. A number of predisposing factors have been identified which significantly increase an individual's risk of VT. Such factors include hypertrophic cardiomyopathy (HCM), ischemic or dilated cardiomyopathy, infiltrative cardiomyopathy, cardiac sarcoidosis, and arrhythmic right-ventricular cardiomyopathy/dysplasia (ARVC/D). Other etiologies include inherited channelopathies, such as long QT syndrome (LQTS), short QT syndrome (SQTS), Brugada syndrome, and catecholaminergic polymorphic VT (CPVT). Unfortunately, the majority of arrhythmias continue to occur in patients not identified by current criteria.[1]

CLINICAL PRESENTATION

The presentation of VT can vary from mildly symptomatic to syncope and SCD, and depends on the characteristics of the tachycardia such as rate, duration, and extent of structural or ischemic heart disease. Episodes can be nonsustained VT (NSVT; <30 seconds), sustained with hemodynamic stability, or unstable potentially resulting in severe palpitations, chest pain, syncope, and arrest. Electrical storm, defined as three or more episodes of VT occurring within 24 hours, is a severe presentation of VT with a poor prognosis.

CLINICAL EVALUATION

History and Physical Examination

A thorough history and physical examination are essential in the workup of patients with ventricular arrhythmias. Important elements include frequency and duration of episodes, precipitating factors, and severity of symptoms—particularly symptoms suggesting hemodynamic instability, such as syncope or presyncope. Pertinent past medical problems include history of coronary heart disease or prior myocardial infarction, prior cardiac procedures or surgery, congestive heart failure (CHF), and associated risk factors, such as hypertension and diabetes mellitus. Family members should also be screened for syncope, SCD, and inherited syndromes associated with VT/ventricular fibrillation (VF), such as LQTS, SQTS, HCM, ARVC/D, CPVT or Brugada syndrome.

A complete physical examination, including vital signs, with thorough cardiac assessment should also be performed. Particular attention should be given to signs of heart failure, including assessment for cardiac enlargement, a positive S4, jugular venous distension, pulmonary rales, and lower extremity edema.

Laboratory Testing

Comprehensive metabolic testing should be performed at baseline to assess for electrolyte abnormalities, renal dysfunction, liver dysfunction, and thyroid abnormalities. Additionally, biomarkers should be drawn to evaluate for myocardial infarction and ventricular overload.

Electrocardiogram

The electrocardiogram (ECG) is the most important tool in establishing the diagnosis of VT. The diagnosis of VT requires three or more consecutive ventricular beats which exceeds an average rate of 100 beats per minute (bpm).

The ECG during VT may show a single QRS morphology (monomorphic VT) or may continuously change over time (polymorphic VT). For monomorphic VT, an important aspect of ECG interpretation is differentiating the arrhythmia from other wide complex tachycardias (WCTs) such as supraventricular tachycardias (SVTs) with aberrant conduction and antidromic atrioventricular (AV) reentrant tachycardia. One of the hallmarks of VT is the evidence of independent atrial and ventricular activation (AV dissociation), which can have one of several manifestations: lack of a fixed A-V relationship, fusion beats or capture beats (Fig. 1).

However, there can be 1:1 retrograde ventricular-atrial conduction or no discernable P-waves during rapid tachycardia, which makes the diagnosis more difficult. Several algorithms have been developed to assist in the differentiation between VT and SVT with aberrancy (Flowchart 1), including the Brugada[2] and aVR[3] criteria.

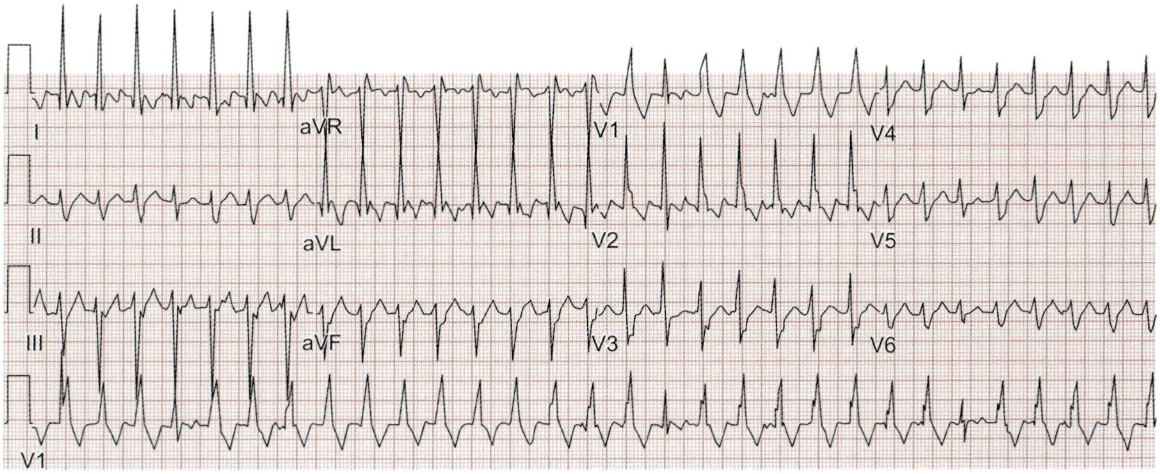

Fig. 1 Ventricular tachycardia (VT) with capture beats. Complexes 4, 17, and 25 are narrower than others, and represent capture beats, consistent with atrioventricular dissociation and VT in this wide complex tachycardia in a patient with severe palpitations and presyncope. Due to the morphology and axis of the VT, fascicular VT (discussed later) was suspected, and VT was successfully suppressed with verapamil

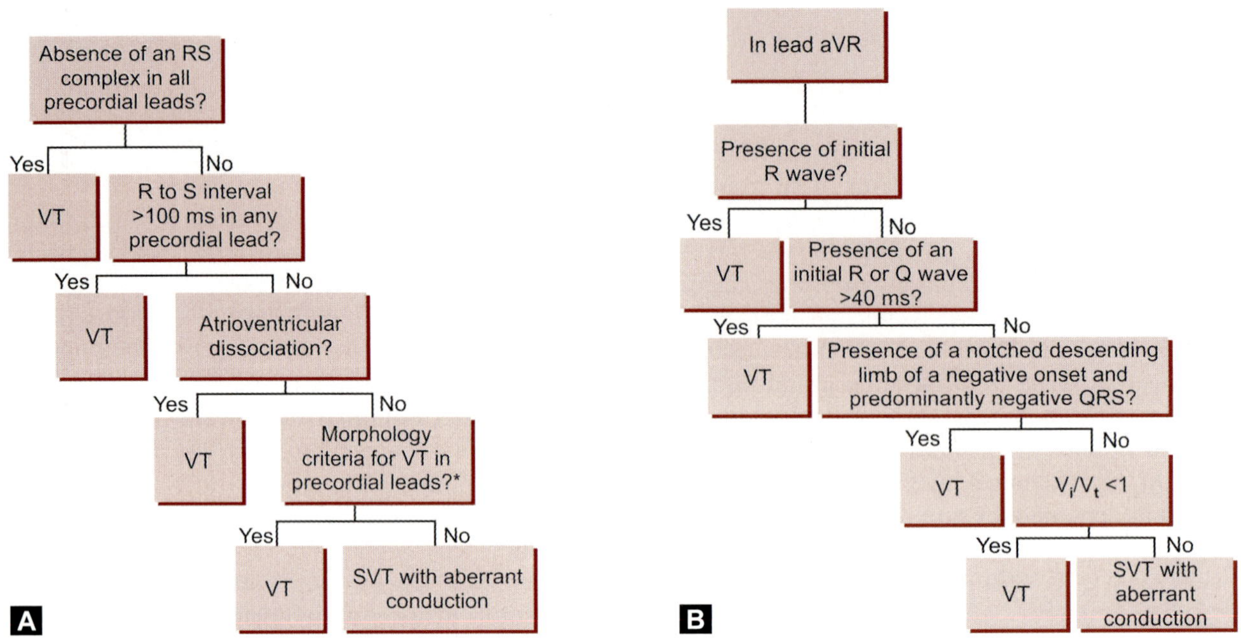

*Refer to reference 2 for complete morphology criteria
VT, ventricular tachycardia; SVT, supraventricular tachycardia

Flowchart 1 **A,** The Brugada criteria has a stepwise approach to the assessment of wide complex tachycardia (WCT). If any of the criteria are satisfied, ventricular tachycardia (VT) is diagnosed; **B,** The *aVR* criteria utilizes only lead aVR in a sequential approach to differentiate WCT

Source: **A,** Adapted from Brugada P, Brugada J, Mont L, et al. A new approach to the differential diagnosis of a regular tachycardia with a wide QRS complex. *Circulation*. 1991;83(5):1649-59, *with permission*. **B,** Adapted from Vereckei A, Duray G, Szénási G, et al. New algorithm using only lead aVR for differential diagnosis of wide QRS complex tachycardia. *Heart Rhythm*. 2008;5(1):89-98, *with permission*

The ECG should also be evaluated for the potential etiology of VT including ischemia, electrolyte abnormalities, prior infarcts, abnormal QT intervals, epsilon waves, and J-point elevation.

Imaging

A transthoracic echocardiogram is essential in the evaluation for structural heart disease, including assessment of left ventricular (LV) function, hypertrophy, and signs of cardiomyopathy. Computed tomography and cardiac magnetic resonance imaging may provide information about ventricular size and scar distribution. Cardiac magnetic resonance imaging may also be useful in the evaluation of ARVC/D or HCM.

Ischemic Evaluation

An ischemic etiology of VT should always be considered. If suspicion remains high, patients should undergo ischemic evaluation, either by perfusion imaging, or more commonly by coronary angiography. Identified ischemia may then be referred for potential revascularization.

TREATMENT

Acute

In the acute setting of sustained VT, the most important determinant of treatment strategy is patient stability. In stable patients, initial medical therapy strategy should be implemented. In contrast, if there is any evidence of hemodynamic instability, patient should proceed directly to direct-current (DC) cardioversion, which can be followed with an antiarrhythmic medication to prevent recurrence (Flowchart 2).

In the hemodynamically stable setting, amiodarone and procainamide are often first-line medical therapy for VT conversion.[4] Amiodarone is the most commonly used antiarrhythmic medication in this setting and is usually administered as a 150 mg intravenous (IV) bolus over 10 minutes, followed by a continuous infusion over

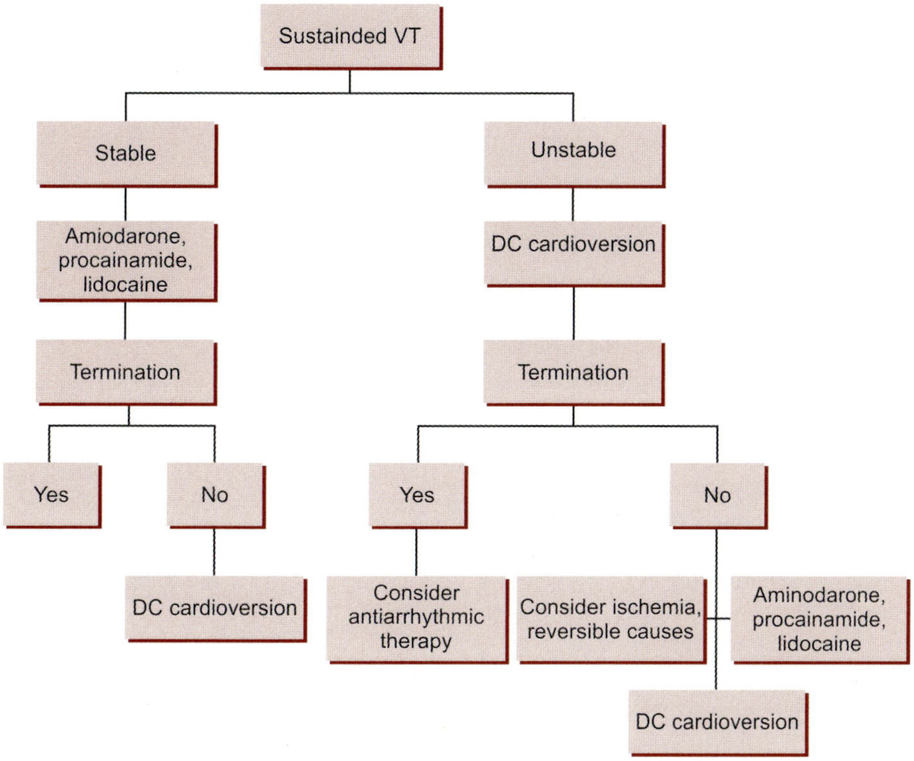

VT, ventricular tachycardia; DC cardioversion, direct-current cardioversion

Flowchart 2 Stepwise approach to the acute treatment of sustained ventricular tachycardia

the next 24 hours. Procainamide is also very effective, but has recently become more difficult to obtain in the United States and should be used cautiously in patients with severe CHF or renal dysfunction. Lidocaine can also be effective, often as an adjunctive agent in refractory VT, particularly in the setting of ischemia given its enhanced efficacy in underperfused tissue.

If medication is ineffective in terminating the VT, DC cardioversion should be applied to convert the patient into normal rhythm. Synchronized shock at 200 joules with biphasic waveform is the usual starting energy. Although lower energy is often effective, we must consider the risks and discomfort of multiple shocks delivered if initial attempts are unsuccessful.

Patients with incessant VT/VF or VT storm should be evaluated promptly for ischemia and may need additional mechanical circulatory support.

Tailored Acute Medical Therapy for Specific Types of Ventricular Tachycardia

- Patients with fascicular VT (Fig. 1), characterized by right bundle branch block (RBBB) and a superior axis, may be particularly responsive to verapamil
- In electrical storm associated with inferolateral early repolarization or LQTS, isoproterenol can be used for VT/VF suppression and prevention of recurrence[5]
- Transvenous pacing at higher rates can also be effective in suppressing VT/VF recurrence in LQTS.

Ablation in the acute setting: Patients in electrical storm who fail medical management may be taken to emergency ablation in experienced centers.

Once the patient has been stabilized, a complete evaluation as listed above should be performed in order to determine the presence of any reversible causes. Identified reversible causes should be promptly treated.

Chronic

Long-term treatment strategies are directed at preventing arrhythmic recurrence, and are largely dependent on the presence or absence of structural heart disease.

Absence of Structural Heart Disease

In the absence of structural heart disease, treatment should be focused at VT suppression, and medical therapy is often the first line of therapy. Although not technically VT, a high burden of premature ventricular contractions (PVCs) (>15,000 PVCs per 24 hours) may be a risk factor for the development of cardiomyopathy,[6] and should be considered for suppressive therapy as well. Beta blockers are typically used as first-line agents in this setting. If ineffective, sotalol, dofetilide, and amiodarone may be considered.

Sotalol and dofetilide require baseline renal function assessment and monitoring for QTc prolongation, both at initiation and at regular follow-up. In addition, amiodarone requires baseline and yearly thyroid function, liver function, pulmonary function and ophthalmologic testing to monitor for side effects.

Tailored Chronic Medical Therapy for Specific Types of Ventricular Tachycardia

- Verapamil may be considered for long-term suppression of fascicular VT in patients in whom ablation is not an option or is not desired
- Recently, quinidine (class IA) has been shown to be useful in patients with early repolarization syndrome.[5]

Frequently, idiopathic VT subtypes such as left or right ventricular outflow tract VTs are amenable to ablation, which may be considered early in the treatment strategy. A cardiac electrophysiology consultation should be obtained for a detailed discussion of all treatment options.

Presence of Structural Heart Disease

The presence NSVT/VF in the setting of structural heart disease [ejection fraction (EF) <40%] is associated with a high risk of mortality, and patients should be considered for implantable cardioverter-defibrillator (ICD) therapy[7] for primary prevention of SCD.[8,9] For secondary prevention of sustained VT in patients with structural ischemic heart disease, ICD therapy has been shown to be superior to medical therapy,[10-12] with the greatest benefit in the patients with depressed left ventricular ejection fraction (LVEF).[7,13-15]

Although effective, ICD therapy itself has adverse effects on patients' psychologic and physical health, and patients with recurrent ICD shocks benefit from suppression of their ventricular arrhythmias with antiarrhythmics or ablation.[16] Specifically, beta blockers, sotalol, dofetilide, and amiodarone are commonly used in this setting, tailored to patients' response, tolerance, and side effects. Sotalol in particular should be used with caution in patients with depressed LV function.

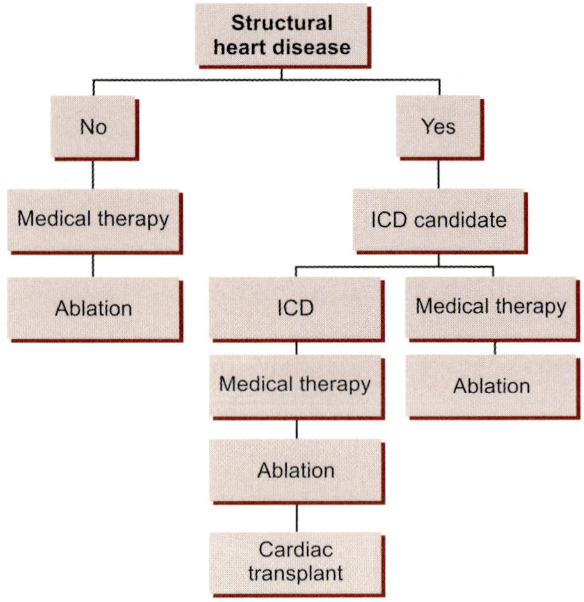

ICD, implantable cardioverter-defibrillator

Flowchart 3 Treatment of chronic ventricular tachycardia is based largely upon the presence or absence of structural heart disease

Patients who are not responsive to medical therapy or ablation with frequent ventricular arrhythmias should be considered for sympathectomy[17] or cardiac transplant (Flowchart 3).

Ablation in the chronic management of VT: Studies have shown the utility of ablation for the chronic management of VT,[16] including reducing appropriate ICD shocks. Consultation with electrophysiologist is recommended to allow a thorough discussion with the patient of all the risks, benefits, and probability of success in each case.

PROGNOSIS

The prognosis for patients with ventricular arrhythmias is dependent upon both the specific etiology and the presence of structural heart disease. For patients with idiopathic VT and normal ventricular function, the prognosis is relatively benign. In contrast, patients with inherited channelopathies such as LQTS, or those with VT and structural heart disease, may be at higher risk and require further stratification and ICD implantation, based upon current guidelines.[8,9]

CONCLUSION

The presentation of VT can vary from asymptomatic, nonsustained episodes to unstable events precipitating

VF. Initial evaluation should focus on hemodynamic stability, with immediate intervention in unstable patients. Once suppressed, further diagnostics are required for determining the correct identification of the arrhythmia and etiology. Long-term management is directed at both arrhythmia elimination via antiarrhythmic drugs or ablation, and risk reduction with ICD implantation, as required. With the advent of advanced electrophysiology care, timely initiation of optimal management has the potential to dramatically improve the survival of patients with VT.

REFERENCES

1. Myerburg RJ, Mitrani R, Interian A, et al. Interpretation of outcomes of antiarrhythmic clinical trials: design features and population impact. Circulation. 1998;97(15):1514-21.
2. Brugada P, Brugada J, Mont L, et al. A new approach to the differential diagnosis of a regular tachycardia with a wide QRS complex. Circulation. 1991;83(5):1649-59.
3. Vereckei A, Duray G, Szénási G, et al. New algorithm using only lead aVR for differential diagnosis of wide QRS complex tachycardia. Heart Rhythm. 2008;5(1):89-98.
4. Zipes DP, Camm AJ, Borggrefe M, et al. ACC/AHA/ESC 2006 guidelines for management of patients with ventricular arrhythmias and the prevention of sudden cardiac death: a report of the American College of Cardiology/ American Heart Association Task Force and the European Society of Cardiology Committee for Practice Guidelines (writing committee to develop Guidelines for Management of Patients with Ventricular Arrhythmias and the Prevention of Sudden Cardiac Death): developed in collaboration with the European Heart Rhythm Association and the Heart Rhythm Society. Circulation. 2006;114(10):e385-484.
5. Haissaguerre M, Sacher F, Nogami A, et al. Characteristics of recurrent ventricular fibrillation associated with inferolateral early repolarization role of drug therapy. J Am Coll Cardiol. 2009;53(7):612-9.
6. Baman TS, Lange DC, Ilg KJ, et al. Relationship between burden of premature ventricular complexes and left ventricular function. Heart Rhythm. 2010;7(7):865-9.
7. Buxton AE, Lee KL, Fisher JD, et al. A randomized study of the prevention of sudden death in patients with coronary artery disease. Multicenter Unsustained Tachycardia Trial Investigators. N Engl J Med. 1999;341(25):1882-90.
8. Epstein AE, DiMarco JP, Ellenbogen KA, et al. ACC/AHA/HRS 2008 Guidelines for Device-Based Therapy of Cardiac Rhythm Abnormalities: a report of the American College of Cardiology/American Heart Association Task Force on Practice Guidelines (Writing Committee to Revise the ACC/AHA/NASPE 2002 Guideline Update for Implantation of Cardiac Pacemakers and Antiarrhythmia Devices): developed in collaboration with the American Association for Thoracic Surgery and Society of Thoracic Surgeons. Circulation. 2008;117(21):e350-408.
9. Epstein AE, DiMarco JP, Ellenbogen KA, et al. 2012 ACCF/AHA/HRS focused update incorporated into the ACCF/AHA/HRS 2008 guidelines for device-based therapy of cardiac rhythm abnormalities: a report of the American College of Cardiology Foundation/American Heart Association Task Force on Practice Guidelines and the Heart Rhythm Society. Circulation. 2013;127:e283-352.
10. Siebels J, Cappato R, Rüppel R, et al. Preliminary results of the Cardiac Arrest Study Hamburg (CASH). CASH Investigators. Am J Cardiol. 1993;72(16):109F-113F.
11. Connolly SJ, Gent M, Roberts RS, et al. Canadian Implantable Defibrillator Study (CIDS): study design and organization. CIDS Co-Investigators. Am J Cardiol. 1993;72(16):103F-108F.
12. A comparison of antiarrhythmic-drug therapy with implantable defibrillators in patients resuscitated from near-fatal ventricular arrhythmias. The Antiarrhythmics versus Implantable Defibrillators (AVID) Investigators. N Engl J Med. 1997;337(22):1576-83.
13. Moss AJ, Zareba W, Hall WJ, et al. Prophylactic implantation of a defibrillator in patients with myocardial infarction and reduced ejection fraction. N Engl J Med. 2002;346(12):877-83.
14. Kadish A, Dyer A, Daubert JP, et al. Prophylactic defibrillator implantation in patients with nonischemic dilated cardiomyopathy. N Engl J Med. 2004;350(21):2151-8.
15. Bardy GH, Lee KL, Mark DB, et al. Amiodarone or an implantable cardioverter-defibrillator for congestive heart failure. N Engl J Med. 2005;352(3):225-37.
16. Reddy VY, Reynolds MR, Neuzil P, et al. Prophylactic catheter ablation for the prevention of defibrillator therapy. N Engl J Med. 2007;357(26):2657-65.
17. Hayase J, Patel J, Narayan SM, et al. Percutaneous stellate ganglion block suppressing VT and VF in a patient refractory to VT ablation. J Cardiovasc Electrophysiol. 2013;24(8):926-8.

Chapter 29

Issues in Anticoagulation

Christos Dresios, Gregory YH Lip

ABSTRACT

In heart failure (HF), thromboembolic events are associated with increased morbidity and mortality. Atrial fibrillation complicating HF significantly increases the risk of stroke and the use of anticoagulation is well established. However, anticoagulation potentially could also be considered in certain subgroups of patients with HF in sinus rhythm (SR), e.g., the presence of HF with decreased ejection fraction and previous thromboembolism, newly diagnosed intracardiac thrombus and right HF with pulmonary hypertension.

There is lack of evidence to support the routine use of aspirin as thromboprophylaxis in patients with HF who are in SR. Moreover coadministration of oral anticoagulant with antiplatelet agent should be avoided in patients with chronic (>12 months after an acute event) coronary or other arterial disease, due to the high risk of major bleeding. Finally, the patient should always be actively involved in the decision-making process. Indeed, patient values and preferences should always be taken into consideration when balancing the risk of thromboembolism against bleeding.

INTRODUCTION

Heart failure (HF) represents a devastating clinical disorder that despite significant advances in medical treatment is associated with a high morbidity and mortality of greater than 30% in patients with severe HF. HF constitutes a major and fast growing public health issue that acquired epidemic proportion and represents an important economic burden on public health systems worldwide.

EPIDEMIOLOGY AND PATHOPHYSIOLOGY: A BRIEF OVERVIEW

It is estimated that 1–2% of the adult population in industrialized countries suffers from HF.[1] Irrespective of the definition used, both incidence and prevalence of HF increases significantly with age.[2] The prevalence of HF rises to greater than or equal to 10% among adults aged 70 years and older.[3] There is no evidence of specific gender differences in the incidence and prevalence of HF. In the Framingham study, the five-year risk of developing HF among white adults aged 40 years is approximately 0.1–0.2%.[4]

In USA, HF accounts for 34% of cardiovascular-related deaths and represents the most frequent cause of hospitalization in elderly patients.[5] Of note, HF has been associated with an increased risk of stroke and thromboembolism.[6] Indeed, retrospective analyses of data from large studies revealed that stroke rates ranged from 1.2–1.8 per 100 patient-years in the populations included in these studies.[7-10] On reviewing the pathophysiological aspects, many predisposing factors to HF and themselves associated with increased thromboembolic risk, and in addition to HF, may contribute to render HF patients vulnerable to thromboembolic episodes.[11]

Pathophysiologically, several mechanisms operating in HF lead to the establishment of the well-recognized prerequisites of thrombogenesis, which represent the components of the Virchow's classic triad.

These are summarized as follows:

- Increased coagulability

- Impaired blood flow
- Vascular abnormalities.

A low cardiac output and dilatation of cardiac chambers may promote intracardiac stasis and lead to an increased propensity toward the formation of intracardiac thrombi and consequently to thromboembolism. Furthermore, systolic dysfunction predisposes to thromboembolism not only by altering the rheological characteristics of the blood but also by causing abnormalities in platelet function and hemostasis.[12-15] The reduced ventricular ejection fraction in conjunction with reduced physical activity and peripheral edema leads also to the increased risk of the development of venous thrombi. Finally, endothelial damage or dysfunction is evident in HF. Specifically, vascular dysfunction and endothelium-derived nitric oxide (NO) availability represent prominent pathophysiological factors that lead to the development of the prothrombotic state in HF patients.[16]

In short, the establishment of such a prothrombotic state in the setting of HF predisposes to the increased risk of stroke and thromboembolism in the setting of HF.[17]

WHAT IS THE ROLE OF ANTICOAGULATION IN HEART FAILURE?

Heart failure patients represent a heterogeneous group of patients with difference not only regarding etiology and prognosis but also in the risk of stroke. In the wider HF population, there are groups of HF patients with certain characteristics that confer an increased risk of stroke and thromboembolic episodes, such as atrial fibrillation (AF). In this setting, the role of long-term oral anticoagulation is well established.

HEART FAILURE AND ATRIAL FIBRILLATION

Atrial fibrillation constitutes an important risk factor that contributes to the development of stroke and thromboembolic complications in HF patients. Indeed AF is the most common arrhythmia in HF, and AF is present in approximately one-third of HF patients. Nonetheless, the prevalence of AF increases with increasing HF severity, being as high as 50% in New York Heart Association (NYHA) class IV patients. Various cardiac functional and structural abnormalities constitute a substrate for the development to the arrhythmia.[18,19]

Conversely, symptomatic HF (NYHA classes II–IV) is present in 30–40% of AF patients. Thus, there is a close and intimate relationship between HF and AF. Indeed, HF not only represents a cause of the arrhythmia due to increased atrial pressure and volume overload but also can be a consequence of AF. Taking into consideration the reciprocal relation between HF and AF, it has been suggested that the hypercoagulable state in the context of incident HF could be attributed to unrecognized episodes of silent AF; thus, the presence of AF in this setting could support not only the high risk of thromboembolic complications but also could represent the etiologic basis of the episodes of incident HF and episodes of decompensation.[20,21] When both clinical conditions coexist the risk of thromboembolic episodes is substantially increased and long-term prognosis is worse.[22]

The risk for stroke and thromboembolism in AF patients is not homogenous and is dependent upon the presence of specific risk factors. The risk of stroke in AF patients is a continuum, and the current guidelines recognize the need to be more inclusive of common stroke risk factors. The European Society of Cardiology (ESC) recommends use of the CHA_2DS_2-VASc score in its most recent AF and HF guidelines (Table 1).[23-25]

Heart failure represents the "C" in the CHA_2DS_2-VASc and older $CHADS_2$ stroke risk stratification scores. Specifically, the "C" criterion refers to systolic HF [e.g., moderate-to-severe systolic left ventricular (LV) dysfunction on echocardiography] or recent decompensated HF (e.g., requiring hospitalization). In the latter patients, thromboembolism is increased, irrespective of ejection fraction.[26]

Based on the ESC guidelines, patients with a CHA_2DS_2-VASc score greater than or equal to 2 are recommended oral anticoagulant therapy (class I, level of evidence A). In patients with a CHA_2DS_2-VASc score of 1, oral anticoagulant therapy should also be considered, based

TABLE 1: The CHA_2DS_2-VASc score

Risk factor	*Score*
Congestive cardiac failure	1
Hypertension	1
Age ≥75 years	2
Diabetes mellitus	1
Stroke/transient ischemic attack/ thromboembolism	2
Vascular disease	1
Age 65–74 years	1
Female sex	1
Maximum score	9

TABLE 2: Hypertension, abnormal renal and liver function, stroke, bleeding history or predisposition, labile international normalized ratio, elderly, drugs/alcohol (HAS–BLED) score for the evaluation of the bleeding risk

Letter	*Clinical characteristics*	*Points assigned*
H	Hypertension, i.e., uncontrolled blood pressure	1
A	Abnormal renal and liver function	1 or 2
S	Stroke	1
B	Bleeding	1
L	Labile international normalized ratios (only applies if a patient is on warfarin)	1
E	Elderly (age >65 years, frail condition)	1
D	Drugs or alcohol	1 or 2
		Maximum 9 points

upon an assessment of the risk of bleeding complications and patient preferences (class IIa, level of evidence A).

Before initiating anticoagulation in AF patients at high risk for stroke, individual assessment of the bleeding risk should be considered. In order to evaluate reliably the individual risk of bleeding, the 2012 ESC HF and AF guidelines both recommend use of the hypertension, abnormal renal and liver function, stroke, bleeding history or predisposition, labile international normalized ratio, elderly, drugs/alcohol (HAS–BLED) score[27] (Table 2).

Atrial fibrillation patients with a HAS–BLED score of greater than or equal to 3 are at high risk, but a high HAS–BLED score *per se* is not to be used to stop oral anticoagulation but to "flag up" those at risk for regular review and follow-up as well as to correct reversible risk factors for bleeding, e.g., uncontrolled blood pressure (BP), labile international normalized ratios (INRs), etc.

Thus, both ischemic and bleeding risk should always be taken into consideration on individual basis in order to strike the right balance between protection against ischemic stroke and avoidance of hemorrhagic complications. Indeed, the net clinical benefit balancing ischemic stroke against serious bleeding is usually in favor of oral anticoagulation, with the exception of those at lowest risk, i.e., CHA_2DS_2-VASc score equal to zero.[28,29]

Oral Anticoagulation: What are the Options?

Oral anticoagulation (OAC) is recommended as thromboprophylaxis for patients with AF in the presence of HF. OAC use can be as vitamin K antagonists [(VKAs), e.g., warfarin] or one of the novel OACs. The latter fall into two broad categories: the oral direct thrombin inhibitors (e.g., dabigatran) and the oral factor Xa inhibitors (e.g., rivaroxaban, apixaban).

Vitamin K Antagonists

The VKAs work by inhibition of VKA dependent coagulation factors, factors II, VII, IX, and X. The use of warfarin in AF patients reduces the risk of stroke by 64% and all-cause mortality by 26%, compared to placebo/control.

Although warfarin is recognized as a highly effective anticoagulant drug presents certain pharmacological limitations and drawbacks. Specifically, its narrow therapeutic window multiple food and drug interactions, and considerable variability in dose and metabolism within/between patients represent major clinical concerns that have led to its underuse in clinical practice.[30] Another issue that has been raised concerns with warfarin is the high rates of its discontinuation.[31,32] Commonly, quality of anticoagulation control is suboptimal, as represented by the time in therapeutic range (TTR), and if the average TTR is less than 65%, the outcomes with regard to stroke and bleeding with the VKAs are increased.[33]

Novel Anticoagulant Agents

The pharmacological limitations of warfarin prompted the development of novel oral anticoagulants (NOACs) that have more favorable pharmacological characteristics and safety-efficacy profile. One of the major advantages of NOACs is that there is no need for routine coagulation monitoring. In addition, the NOACs are generally well-tolerated drugs and are associated with few known drug interactions. The pharmacokinetic and pharmacodynamic characteristics of NOACs are depicted in Table 3.

Thus, the use of NOACs has been approved by regulatory bodies, such as the Food and Drug Administration (FDA) and the European Medicines Agency (EMA) and, currently, represents a reliable alternative to the VKAs for the protection against thromboembolism.

In patients with severe renal impairment, NOACs exhibit prolonged excretion rates and their use in this setting raise serious safety concerns, particularly with dabigatran. Indeed the 2012 ESC guidelines recommend that the use of NOACs is contraindicated in patients with severe renal dysfunction [creatinine clearance (CrCl) <30 mL/minute]. Thus warfarin still remains the treatment

TABLE 3: Pharmacokinetic and pharmacodynamic characteristics of three novel oral anticoagulants

	Apixaban	*Rivaroxaban*	*Dabigatran*
Bioavailability (%)	50	60–80	6
C_{max}	3 hours	3 hours	3 hours
Half-life	9–14 hours	5–13 hours	12–17 hours
Elimination	27% renal 73% hepatic	33% renal active 33% renal inactive 33% hepatic	80% renal 20% hepatic
Dose	5 mg BID	20 mg OD	150 mg BID/110 mg in renal impairment
Monitoring	No	No	No
Interactions	CYP3A4 P-gp	CYP3A4 P-gp	P-gp

BID, twice daily; OD, once daily; CYP3A4, cytochrome P450-3A4; P-gp, P-glycoprotein 1

of choice for patients with a creatinine clearance close to or less than 30 mL/min. It is very important that all patients that are considered candidates for treatment with NOACs should undergo thorough assessment of their renal function (by CrCl). Thereafter, renal function should be regularly evaluated.

Based on the results of the Randomized Evaluation of Long-term anticoagulant therapy (RE-LY) trial dabigatran was the first NOAC drug to be approved.[38] Approximately 30% of patients that were included in RE-LY study had symptoms of HF. Dabigatran 150 mg BID is the default dose, with the 110 mg BID dose being recommended for:

- Age greater than 80 years
- CrCl 30–50 mL/minute and a high risk of bleeding, including elderly patients
- Concomitant use of P-glycoprotein inducers or inhibitors
- High risk of bleeding complications (HAS-BLED ≥3).

Based on the Rivaroxaban Reduced Stroke and Systemic Embolism Compared with Warfarin in Nonvalvular Atrial Fibrillation (ROCKET AF) trial, the oral factor Xa inhibitor, rivaroxaban, has been also approved for prevention of first and recurrent stroke in patients with nonvalvular AF.[34] Rivaroxaban is the only FDA approved anticoagulant agent in AF with the advantage to be administered once daily. The ROCKET AF trial showed that rivaroxaban is no inferior to warfarin for the prevention of stroke or systemic. Notably, 60% of patients included in ROCKET trial had symptomatic HF. In patients with moderate renal impairment, rivaroxaban is recommended at the dose of 15 mg once daily.

Box 1: Summary of potential limitations of new anticoagulants

- No known antidote
- Long-term safety profile is not established
- Absence of well-established tests to monitor anticoagulant effect
- Preoperative management of patients on novel anticoagulants is not well consolidated
- Cost-effectiveness compared to warfarin is remained to be clarified in patients with very well controlled international normalized ratio

Based on the findings of the apixaban for reduction in stroke and other thromboembolic events (ARISTOTLE) and the apixaban versus acetylsalicylic acid to prevent stroke in atrial fibrillation patients who have failed or are unsuitable for vitamin K antagonist treatment (AVERROES) trials, apixaban has been recently approved.[35,36] In ARISTOTLE, apixaban was superior to warfarin for both efficacy and safety but there was also a significant reduction in mortality. In AVERROES trial, apixaban was superior to aspirin for stroke prevention, and major bleeding (and intracranial bleeding) was not significantly different between apixaban and aspirin. Apixaban is currently recommended at the dose of 5 mg twice daily in patients with nonvalvular AF patients who have one or more risk factors. The dosing scheme should be reduced to 2.5 mg BID in patients with 2 of the following risk factors: serum creatinine greater than or equal to 1.5 mg/dL, age greater than or equal to 80 years or body weight less than or equal to 60 kg.

Nonetheless, the NOACs have also certain limitations and drawbacks (Box 1). In particular, there are no established agents to reverse their anticoagulant effects. There are also no well-established tests to monitor anticoagulant effect, which may deprive physicians of the ability to evaluate patient compliance. In certain clinical situations, the assessment of the anticoagulant effect of NOACs is of importance, as in the case of bleeding complications or clinical situations, such as hemorrhage or in surgical emergencies. Common tests, such as the activated partial thromboplastin time (aPTT) and prothrombin time (PT) are useful to ascertain the presence of anticoagulant effects in a patient taking dabigatran or rivaroxaban, respectively but, in any case are not considered accurate enough for understanding

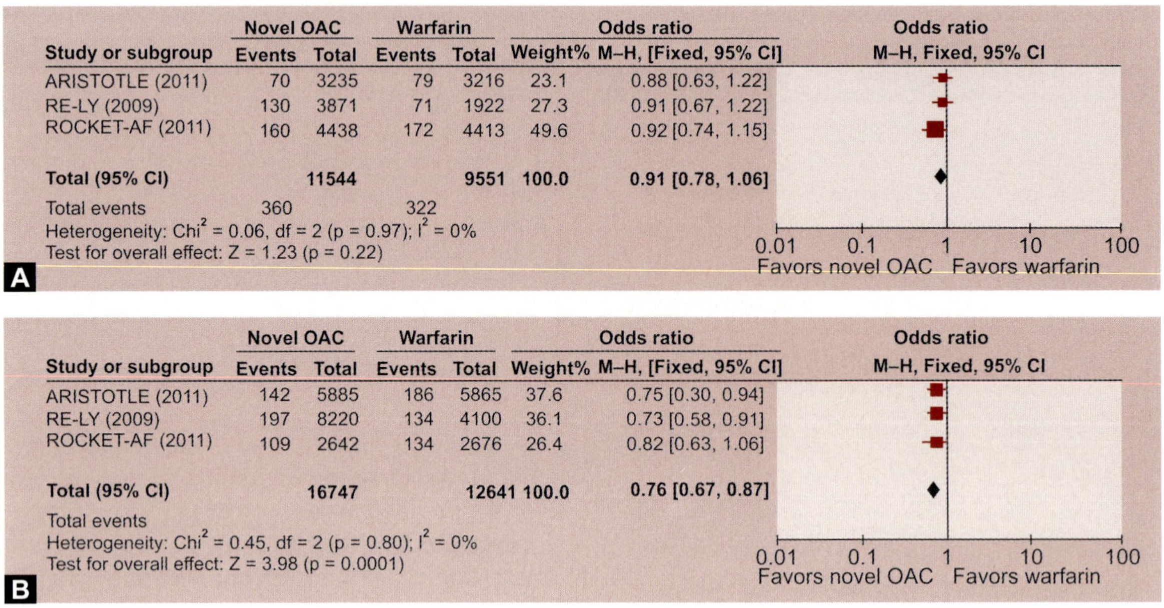

ROCKET AF, Rivaroxaban Reduced Stroke and Systemic Embolism Compared with Warfarin in Nonvalvular Atrial Fibrillation; ARISTOTLE, apixaban for reduction in stroke and other thromboembolic events; RE-LY, Randomized Evaluation of Long-term anticoagulant therapy; df, degrees of freedom; M–H, Mantel–Haenszel; OAC, oral anticoagulant; Z, Z-score; CI, confidence interval

Fig. 1 Comparison of new oral anticoagulants and warfarin for patients **A,** with heart failure and **B,** without heart failure

anticoagulation intensity nor dose amendments. Finally, long-term safety data are currently lacking regarding the use of NOACs.

What is the Evidence for Novel Oral Anticoagulants in Patients with Atrial Fibrillation and Heart Failure?

Within the large AF clinical trials of the NOACs, a significant proportion had symptomatic HF or evidence of impaired cardiac function. A recent crude meta-analysis of the data from recent trials comparing warfarin against the NOACs demonstrates that for patients without HF, the NOACs are superior to warfarin: odds ratio (OR) = 0.76; 95% confidence interval (CI) = 0.67–0.87; $p < 0.0001$ (Fig. 1).[37] The NOACs were not significantly different to warfarin among patients with evidence of HF: OR = 0.91; 95% CI = 0.78–1.06; p = 0.22.

ANTICOAGULATION THERAPY IN HEART FAILURE WITH SINUS RHYTHM

As mentioned above, HF *per se* is associated with a prothrombotic state that is associated with high risk of stroke and thromboembolic events. Indeed, stroke represents an important cause of morbidity and mortality, and HF has long been implicated as a risk factor. Overall, the risk of stroke in HF patients is high and potentially it could be related to low left ventricular ejection fraction (LVEF).[38] For example, the risk of stroke has been estimated at 1% per annum in mild to moderate HF in sinus rhythm (SR), and up to 4% in severe HF.

Taking into consideration that the risk of stroke in the general population is almost 0.5% and that the absolute annual risk of stroke in AF patients is around 5%, depending on the presence (or absence) of risk factors, the issue of antithrombotic treatment in HF patients is of crucial importance.

The risk of stroke and thromboembolism is also not uniform, and changes over time. For example, evidence provided from the Rotterdam study suggests that the risk of stroke was significantly higher 30 days after diagnosis of HF. The risk gradually reduced over the following period, and become nonsignificant at 6 months after diagnosis.[39] Similarly, in the Danish Diet, Cancer and Health study, the presence of incident HF represented a prominent risk factor for stroke and death; with the risk bring considerably higher in the initial 30 days after diagnosis of HF.[40] In general, newly diagnosed patients with HF appear to have increased risk of thrombo-embolic complications and high mortality rates[41-43] (Table 4).

TABLE 4: Epidemiological cohort studies

Study	*Participants*	*Follow-up*	*Risk of stroke*
Rotterdam study[39]	7,546	10 years	More than five-fold increased risk of ischemic stroke in the first month after diagnosis of HF compared with no HF diagnosis
Diet, Cancer, and Health cohort study[40]	57,053 in the cohort (1,239 patients with incident)	>6 months	Higher rate of death and stroke (ischemic or hemorrhagic) in the initial 30 days following the diagnosis of incident HF
Framingham heart study[47]	5,209 included in the original cohort	24 years	The risk of stroke resulted to be 4.1% per year for men and 2.8% per year for women with HF
Population-based study from Rochester[43]	1,111	5 years	The risk of death after first stroke was 7% ± 0.7% at 7 days, 14% ± 1.0% at 30 days, 27% ± 1.3% at 1 year and 53% ± 1.5% at 5 yearsThe risk of stroke recurrence after first cerebral infarction was 2% ± 0.4% at 7 days, 4% ± 0.6% at 30 days, 12% ± 1.1% at 1 year, and 29% ± 1.7% at 5 years

HF, heart failure

In addition, evidence provided from an analysis of 516 deaths in a community long-term study comparing HF patients with LV dysfunction versus those with preserved LV function showed that prognosis was very much related to LV function. Indeed, the sudden death rate was higher in the first group of patients (21% versus 16%, respectively).[44] Moreover, population-based studies revealed that the rate of stroke recurrence and the mortality after stroke are higher among HF patients.[45,46] In the Framingham heart study, the risk of stroke was 4.1% per year for men and 2.8% per year for women with HF. However, it should be taken into consideration that many HF patients, included in this study, may also suffer from AF which may be "silent".[47]

Whilst there is less robust evidence that support that HF is an independent risk factor for the development of venous thromboembolism (VTE), there are studies that correlate closely HF with increased risk of VTE. Of note, low ejection fraction (EF) has been a major predisposing factor associated with the risk of VTE.[48] In particular, the risk of VTE in presence of HF appears to be higher in patients with EF less than 20%.[49] Furthermore, relative immobility in patients with severe HF contributes significantly to the risk of deep vein thrombosis (DVT) and consequently to the risk of pulmonary embolism (PE).

Additionally, the incidence of LV thrombus formation is higher in HF patients especially in the subset of patients with low EF. For example, older echocardiographic and autopsy studies revealed that the incidence of intracavitary thrombus in HF patients reaches up to 50%.[50-53] More recent studies do not confirm these data, reporting lower but still significantly high rates of LV thrombus formation.[51,54-56]

Given the high prevalence of HF and the likelihood of thromboembolic complications, defining the role of OAC in the setting of HF represents an essential clinical issue with potentially important implications in clinical practice. Several studies have supported the role of anticoagulation in HF patients revealing its beneficial effects in the reduction of the risk of thromboembolic events and death. Nevertheless, these studies were fraught with limitation given the fact that many patients that have been included in these trials had comorbities that themselves are correlated with increased risk of thromboembolic events (e.g., AF, significant valvular heart disease, etc.).[57-59]

Cross-sectional Studies

Evidence provided from small observational studies carried out three decades ago proposed that anticoagulant therapy have significant protective effects in preventing thromboembolic events in HF patients.[60,61] Of note, these studies included patients with nonischemic cardiomyopathy. Other studies included patients with either ischemic or nonischemic cardiomyopathy.[50,52,54,55,62]

One study which included patients with either ischemic or nonischemic cardiomyopathy awaiting cardiac transplantation did not reveal a considerable difference in regard to the rate of thromboembolism in the group of patients (37%) receiving (nonrandomized) warfarin therapy.[54] Additionally, retrospective studies have demonstrated that in HF patients with severe LV dysfunction the risk of stroke is increased (Table 5). Again, some of these studies included patients with AF. Thus

TABLE 5: Thromboembolic events in observational case–control studies of patients with heart failure

Study	Patients	Diagnosis	Atrial fibrillation	Ejection fraction	Anticoagulation	Thromboembolic events
Kyrle[61]	38	DCM	NA	NA	100%	44.7% before initiation of OA treatment. No thromboembolic events occurred during the period of OA therapy
Falk[67]	25	DCM	0%	NA	0%	7.8%
Fuster[50]	106	DCM	23%	NA	NA	3.5%
Gottdiener	123	DCM ICM	NA	27%	NA	5.7%
Ciaccheri[63]	126	DCM	0%	NA	0%	1.4%
Sharma	144	DCM ICM	NA	27%	57%	12.5%
Diaz[64]	169	DCM	20%	NA	20%	5.6%
Natterson[54]	224	DCM ICM	19%	20%	37%	3.2%
Katz[52]	264	DCM ICM	13%	27%	13%	1.7%
Cioffi[55]	406	DCM ICM	16%	23%	48%	1.7%

OA, oral anticoagulants; NA: not available; ICM, ischemic cardiomyopathy; DCM, dilated cardiomyopathy

it could be inferred that AF could account for both the increased risk of thromboembolic events and the benefit conferred by the anticoagulant therapy in this population of patients.

Post Hoc Analyses of Clinical Trials

Valuable data in relation to the clinical assessment of thromboembolic risk in HF patients is provided from retrospective analyses of large trials, that include Vasodilator-Heart Failure Trial (V-HeFT), Studies of Left Ventricular Dysfunction (SOLVD), Survival and Ventricular Enlargement (SAVE) and Sudden Cardiac Death in Heart Failure Trial (SCD-HeFT)[7,8,15] (Table 6). An important limitation in these retrospectives studies is that it is unknown to what extent other comorbidities (e.g., AF) has affected the risk of thromboembolic events in this population.

Low left ventricular ejection fraction (LVEF) represents also prominent risk factor that correlates with high thromboembolic risk. In the SAVE trial, for example, that assessed patients after myocardial infarction (MI) with LV systolic dysfunction, a reduced ejection fraction and greater age were both identified as independent risk factors of stroke.[17] The risk of stroke appeared to be inversely related to LVEF, whereby in patients with EF less than 28%, there was a two-fold increase of risk of stroke in comparison to patients with a LVEF greater than 28%.

In the SOLVD trial, there were gender differences in the risk of stroke in the population with low EF in SR, whereby low EF had a significantly greater impact on the risk of thromboembolic events in women compared to men.[7] Notably, women presented a 53% increased risk of thromboembolic events for every 10% decline in EF. The overall annual incidence of thromboembolic events, including stroke, pulmonary and peripheral arterial embolism, was 2.4% in women and 1.8% in men ($P = 0.04$).[65] This difference was mainly attributed to a higher rate of pulmonary emboli in women (24%) in comparison to men (14%) ($P = 0.01$).[7]

In a post hoc analyses of HF randomized trials that included the SOLVED and V-HeFT I and II studies, either anticoagulant or antiplatelet therapy did not result to confer explicit benefits in terms of survival or in reduction of the risk of VTE risk.[9,51,65,72-74] However, trials that enrolled post-MI patients provided some evidence that the use of either anticoagulant or antiplatelet agents confers significant benefits. For example, in the SAVE trial, there was significant reduction in the rate of stroke

TABLE 6: Retrospective analyses of large trials

Study	*Patients*	*Follow-up (months)*	*Atrial fibrillation*	*Anticoagulation*	*Cerebrovascular accident (% per year)*	*Systemic thrombo-embolic events (% per year)*
V-HeFT-I	642	44	15%	19%	1.8	2.5
V-HeFT-II	840	53	15%	21%	1.8	2.3
SCD-HeFT	2,114	44	0	46%	2.6	1
SAVE	2,231	100	Not available	28%	1.5	NA
SOLVD	6,797	79	6%	28%	1.1	1.6

V-HeFT, Vasodilator-Heart Failure Trial; SCD-HeFT, Sudden Cardiac Death in Heart Failure Trial; SAVE, Survival and Ventricular Enlargement; SOLVD, Studies of Left Ventricular Dysfunction

in patients receiving warfarin. Similarly, aspirin use was associated with a significant trend toward the reduction of the incidence of stroke in post-MI patients, and the benefits were accentuated in patients with severe LV dysfunction (EF <28%).[66]

In the SOLVD trial, the use anticoagulant therapy appeared to be associated with a decrease in sudden cardiovascular death and all-cause death which notably were unrelated to the reduction in the thromboembolic events.[8] In the V-HeFT I trial, anticoagulation treatment did not differ for the rates of thromboembolism compared to no antithrombotic therapy.[9] Unexpectedly, in the V-HeFT II trial, patients receiving anticoagulation treatment had a higher rate of thromboembolic events compared to those not on antithrombotic therapy.[9] In the SAVE study, warfarin compared to no antithrombotic therapy was very effective in reducing stroke risk, but no comparable data are available relation to the use of warfarin and aspirin. Similarly, a retrospective analysis of evidence provided from PROMISE study revealed that warfarin conferred significant benefit in terms of reduction of stroke risk. This benefit was observed only in HF patients with severe LV dysfunction.[67]

An important finding of concern emerged from retrospective analyses of the SOLVD and Cooperative New Scandinavian Enalapril Survival Study II (CONSENSUS II) studies. In these studies, it was revealed that aspirin led to the reduction of the benefits conferred by the use of angiotensin-converting enzyme (ACE) inhibitors.[65,68] In both studies, the relative risk reduction in mortality attributed to enalapril appeared to decrease in the group of patients receiving aspirin. Since both ACE inhibitors and aspirin are often used concomitantly in this finding, raised concerns in regard to the influence of aspirin in the clinical outcomes in HF patients.

The debate in regard to the potential interaction between ACE inhibitors and aspirin has been also fueled by other analysis that support the argument that a clinically significant interaction exists between aspirin and ACE inhibitors in HF patients.[69,70] One retrospective analysis of the Global Utilization of Streptokinase and TPA for Occluded Arteries (GUSTO-1) trial revealed that patients receiving both aspirin and an ACE inhibitor had a higher mortality rate.[71] An observational study which included over 7,000 patients from 103 Canadian hospitals concluded that aspirin did not attenuate the benefits conferred by the use of ACE inhibitors.[72] In a retrospective analysis of the Benzafibrate Infarction Prevention (BIP) trial, aspirin was also proven to be effective in patients with coronary artery disease treated with ACE inhibitors.[73] Notwithstanding, further research is required in order to elucidate the putative interaction, if any, between the ACE inhibitors and aspirin therapy.

Factors Influencing Thromboembolism in Heart Failure

Heart Failure Etiology

In V-HeFT and SOLVD studies in which warfarin was ineffective against stroke and thromboembolic events, 70–80% of the patients that were included were diagnosed to have HF of attributed to coronary heart disease.[9,65]

However, in studies that have included patients with chronic HF of different origins, the etiology of HF did not appear to affect the incidences of the thromboembolic events.[80-82] For example, the EPICAL (Epidémiologie de l'Insuffisance Cardiaque Avancée en Lorraine) study, which included patients with severe HF mainly of nonischemic etiology suggested that anticoagulant therapy was significantly effective in protecting against thromboembolic events.[74] Despite conflicting evidence, the effectiveness of anticoagulant therapy could be related to the etiology of HF since patients with nonischemic

HF may be at higher risk of stroke and thromboembolic events.

Left Ventricular Aneurysm

Left ventricular aneurysms represent a complication of MI that may be an important cause of morbidity and mortality. Despite the advances in the treatment approach of patients with MI, aneurysm formation occurs in up to 15% of patients with Q-wave MI.[69] With a ventricular aneurysm, areas of rheological abnormalities in conjunction with the loss of normal endocardium which is replaced by interstitial fibrotic tissue create sites where mural thrombosis could take place. Thus, up to 50% of the LV aneurysms are complicated with the formation of mural thrombus.[75,76]

The presence of a LV aneurysm, which is complicated with thrombus increases significantly the risk of thromboembolic events in the first 3 months following acute MI, and the benefits conferred by anticoagulation therapy is well established.[77-79]

On the other hand, there is insufficient evidence to support that the thromboembolic risk associated with the presence of ventricular aneurysm in patients with chronic HF is high enough to justify the routine use of anticoagulant therapy.[80,81] Evidence provided from older studies suggests that the risk of thromboembolic complications in the setting of chronic LV aneurysm is considerably lower compared to the acute phase after MI.[84] Retrospective analysis of previous studies revealed that the risk of systemic embolization in patients with chronic LV aneurysm and LV thrombus resulted similar to that associated with the presence of LV thrombus without aneurysm.[71,78]

Left Ventricular Thrombus

One important factor that has been proposed to increase the risk for thromboembolism is the presence of LV thrombus, especially in patients with acute MI.[66,77,79,82,83]

On the other hand, the prognostic impact of LV thrombi in patients with chronic HF has not been clearly established. Accordingly, there is insufficient evidence that support the effectiveness of anticoagulation in the setting of the prevention of thromboembolism. Thus, some studies support the presence of clots in LV with the risk of embolic events, but other studies do not confirm these results.[55,67,84]

The potential of embolic risk associated with the presence of intracavitary thrombi seems to vary and appear to be related to certain echocardiographic characteristics, for example, whereby mobile and protruding thrombi are related to higher risk of embolic events.[55,66,85-87] Conversely, thrombus with flat morphology are associated with lower embolic risk.[81,88] The quantification of the risk of stroke is also limited from diagnostic accuracy of image evaluation techniques.[89]

Effect of Mitral Regurgitation

In a study that included HF with low EF, severe mitral regurgitation may reduce the risk of thromboembolic events, raising the possibility that regurgitation abolishes one of the three components of Virchow's triad, namely the stasis of blood.[60,90]

Other Comorbidities

The predictive impact of a previous embolic event represents a controversial issue. Post hoc analysis of large studies, such as V-HeFT I and II studies, which included patients either in SR or with AF found that previous stroke increased the risk of a new cerebrovascular accident.[9] The SOLVD trial suggested that presence of a previous embolic event had prognostic impact regarding a new embolic event and notably, the prognostic value was associated with gender differences, whereby only men with SR at the time of randomization were affected from a history of an embolic event.[7]

Role of Antithrombotic Therapy in Heart Failure Patients in Sinus Rhythm

Contemporary trials have investigated the use of antithrombotic therapy in HF are shown in Table 7.

The Warfarin/Aspirin Study in Heart Failure (WASH) trial included 279 patients, and was designed to compare warfarin, aspirin and no antithrombotic therapy in relation to the rate of all-cause death, non-fatal MI and cerebrovascular accident (CVA).[91] There was no difference between the three arms studied, for the primary outcome (death, nonfatal myocardial infarction, or nonfatal stroke), but warfarin was superior to aspirin in relation for the reduction of stroke rates. On the other hand, bleeding complications requiring blood transfusion (despite being infrequent) were higher in patients assigned to receive warfarin compared with all other treatment groups.

The Heart Failure Long-Term Antithrombotic Study (HELAS) included 197 patients and compared oral anticoagulants with aspirin and placebo in HF patients

TABLE 7: Contemporary randomized controlled trials of antithrombotic therapy in heart failure

	WASH 2004	*HELAS 2006*	*WATCH 2010*	*WARCEF 2012*
Patients (n)	279	197	1,587	2,305
Characteristics	LVEF ≤35%	LVEF <35% NYHA II–IV	LVEF ≤35% NYHA II–IV	LVEF <35%
Follow-up (mean)	27 ±1 months	18.5–21.9 months	21 months	42.1 months
Intervention	No therapy, aspirin (300 mg), warfarin	Warfarin versus aspirin (325 mg) for ICM (115 mg), warfarin or placebo for DCM (82 mg)	Warfarin versus aspirin (162 mg) versus clopidogrel (75 mg)	Warfarin versus aspirin (325 mg)
Primary outcome	Death, non-fatal MI, non-fatal stroke	Death, MI, peripheral/ pulmonary embolism, non-fatal stroke, re-hospitalization (including HF), exacerbation of HF	All-cause mortality, non-fatal MI, non-fatal stroke	First to occur of death, ischemic stroke, or intracerebral hemorrhage
Results	Primary outcome (%): 26 No med, 32 Aspirin, 26 Warfarin (NS)HF Hospitalization (%): 48, 64, 47 (P = 0.04) Major bleeds: NS	Primary outcome (%): NSHF Hospitalization (%): NS Major bleeds: only inwarfarin groups	Primary outcome (%): 20.7 Aspirin, 21.6 Clopidogrel, 19.6 Warfarin (NS) Stroke (%): 2.3, 2.3, 0.6 (P = 0.016) HF Hospitalization (%): 22.2, 18.5, 16.5 (P = 0.0186, aspirin versus warfarin). Major bleeds (%): 3.6, 2.1,5.2 (P = 0.007)	Primary outcome (%): 27.5 Aspirin, 26.4 Warfarin (NS) Ischemic stroke (%): 4.7 Aspirin, 2.5 Warfarin (P = 0.005) Major bleeds (%): 2.7 Aspirin, 5.8 Warfarin (P = 0.001)

WASH, Warfarin/Aspirin Study in Heart failure; HELAS, Heart failure Long-term Antithrombotic study; WATCH, Warfarin and Antiplatelet Therapy in Chronic Heart Failure trial; NS: Non-significant; WARCEF, Warfarin versus Aspirin in Reduced Cardiac Ejection Fraction trial; LVEF, left ventricular ejection fraction; NYHA, New York Heart Association; ICM, ischemic cardiomyopathy; DCM, dilated cardiomyopathy; MI, myocardial infarction; HF, heart failure

with SR.[92] Patients with ischemic HF were assigned to receive warfarin or aspirin, whilst patients with nonischemic cardiomyopathy group were assigned to receive warfarin or placebo. There was an overall neutral effect on mortality between warfarin and aspirin. Additionally, stroke rate turned out to be lower in the group receiving warfarin, but at the cost of increased major hemorrhage. The study results did not show any significant differences between the three groups in regard to the combined primary endpoint (stroke, PE, MI, hospitalization, death).

The Warfarin and Antiplatelet Therapy in Chronic Heart Failure (WATCH) study included 1,587 patients and evaluated the rate of death, nonfatal stroke and nonfatal MI patients who were assigned to receive warfarin aspirin or clopidogrel.[93] Despite being terminated early owing to limitations in the recruitment process, this study found no difference in the primary endpoint between the treatment arms, but suggested that warfarin was superior to either aspirin or clopidogrel in preventing ischemic stroke but at the cost of increased major hemorrhagic complications. Furthermore, the use of aspirin was associated with increase of hospitalization rate for HF exacerbation. Notably, the WATCH study did not assigned patients to antithrombotic therapy and consequently the efficacy *per se* of the different antithrombotic strategies compared to placebo/control has not been evaluated.

The Warfarin versus Aspirin in Reduced Cardiac Ejection Fraction (WARCEF) trial was a large double-blind, double-dummy randomized trial that aimed at comparing the effectiveness of warfarin and antiplatelet therapy.[9,78] After a mean follow-up of 42.1 months, there was no difference between aspirin and warfarin for the primary (first to occur of death, ischemic stroke or intracerebral hemorrhage) and secondary endpoint (first to occur of death, ischemic stroke or intracerebral hemorrhage intracranial hemorrhage, HF hospitalization and MI). Of the secondary endpoints, warfarin was proven to be superior to aspirin in regard to ischemic stroke prevention [0.72% versus 1.36% per year; hazard ratio (HR) = 0.52; 95% CI = 0.33–0.82; P = 0.005], but at the cost of higher rates of major bleeding. In contrast to previous studies, WARCEF trial did not find an increase in HF hospitalizations with aspirin compared to warfarin. Additionally, in a time-varying analysis, it was proven that after 4 or more years of treatment warfarin was slightly superior to aspirin for primary endpoints. As far as the main secondary endpoint is concerned, there was no marked difference seen between the two treatment arms. Major hemorrhage was significantly higher in the group of warfarin. Also, there were no significant differences in intracerebral or intracranial hemorrhage between the two treatment strategies.

Recent meta-analysis of WASH, HELAS, WATCH, and WARCEF trials showed that in HF patients with LV dysfunction and SR, the use of warfarin compared to aspirin is associated with significant relative risk reduction (RRR) in all stroke that is comparable to the benefit conferred by warfarin in the setting of in nonvalvular AF patients.[94,95] In relation to MI, a small difference was demonstrated in favor of warfarin [risk ratio (RR) = 0.87], but no difference in mortality between the different therapeutic approaches was seen.[96]

The benefit conferred in terms of ischemic stroke reduction by warfarin was offset by an increase in the incidence of major bleeding, mainly gastrointestinal. Of note, the rate of intracranial hemorrhage was very low. Thus, protective effects conferred by warfarin against ischemic stroke outweigh the risk of intracranial hemorrhage. This meta-analysis found no significant difference in hospitalizations between patients receiving aspirin and warfarin, in contrast to the WARCEF trial.

In another recent meta-analysis of WASH, HELAS, WATCH, and WARCEF trials, OAC therapy did not demonstrate better efficacy-safety profile compared to antiplatelet treatment in HF patients in SR. Warfarin and aspirin seem to be similar in reducing mortality. Specifically, warfarin was associated with reduced rate of ischemic stroke but at the cost of increased major bleeding events. In this meta-analysis, warfarin and aspirin appeared to be similar in reducing mortality.[97] Of note in a recent systematic review and meta-analysis of randomized trials comparing warfarin and aspirin found a nonsignificant propensity toward an increase in major bleeding risk in patients assigned to receive warfarin [odds ratio (OR) 1.27; 95% CI 0.83–1.94].[98]

These results are also confirmed by other similar meta-analysis, which addressed the issue of the proper antithrombotic strategy in HF patients in SR. These meta-analyses concluded that warfarin compared to aspirin was associated with reduction in the risk of stroke, a neutral effect on mortality rate, and an increase in major hemorrhage.[79,84,99,100]

In summary, there is lack of hard evidence regarding the advantages of anticoagulant therapy over antiplatelet agents in HF patients in SR. The analysis of the results derived from 4 studies that have addressed the role of antithrombotic therapy in HF (WASH, HELAS, WATCH and WARCEF trials) all show that warfarin was better than aspirin as far as the risk of stroke is concerned. Despite the use of warfarin was associated with increase in major hemorrhage without significant differences regarding intracerebral or intracranial hemorrhage. In addition to that, no benefit in terms of mortality was conferred with the use of warfarin in relation to aspirin. At present, there is also no evidence from long-term randomized controlled trials (RCTs) to recommend use of aspirin to prevent thromboembolic complications in patients with HF in SR.

The identification of the high-risk group in which the benefits in terms of stroke mortality and morbidity could outweigh the risk of major bleeding may be difficult. Thus, both the choice whether to administrate antithrombotic therapy and the selection of the antithrombotic strategy should be assessed on individual basis. Development of risk stratification schemes that could assist to the identification of patients at high risk that could benefit from antithrombotic therapy would be useful. In addition to that, patient values and preferences should be taken into consideration in the design of the treatment strategy. Indeed, patients should be actively involved in the clinical decision making process and influence the final therapeutic approach. Additionally, another important aspect that remains to be elucidated is the role of the NOACs in the setting of HF in SR.

In the broader HF population, there are certain groups of patients in which the risk of stroke and other thromboembolic events is considered to be very high and, consequently, justify the use of anticoagulant therapy. According to the American College of Cardiology/American Heart Association (ACC/AHA) 2009 guidelines,[101] given the absence of supportive data in favor of the use of anticoagulant therapy in patients with HF with SR, anticoagulation with warfarin is most warranted in patients with HF who have either experienced a previous embolic event or suffer from AF (class I, level of evidence A). The use of anticoagulation should also be considered in patients with underlying disorders that may be associated with an increased thromboembolic risk (e.g., amyloidosis, LV noncompaction) and in patients with familial dilated cardiomyopathy and a history of thromboembolism in first-degree relatives (class IIb, level of evidence B).

Heart Failure Society of America (HFSA)[102] has issued independent guidelines that address anticoagulation in patients with chronic HF. Specifically, treatment with warfarin is recommended for all patients with HF and chronic or documented AF (strength of evidence A) or a history of systemic or pulmonary emboli, including stroke or transient ischemic attack (strength of evidence C), unless contraindicated. It is recommended that patients with symptomatic or asymptomatic ischemic cardiomyopathy and documented recent large anterior MI or recent MI with documented LV thrombus be treated with warfarin for the initial 3 months post-MI (strength of evidence B) unless contraindicated. Other patients with ischemic or nonischemic cardiomyopathy and LV thrombus should be considered for chronic anticoagulation, depending on the characteristics of the thrombus, such as its size, mobility and degree of calcification (strength of evidence C).

According to ESC guidelines for the diagnosis and treatment of acute and chronic HF in 2008, anticoagulant therapy is recommended in patients with HF and AF without contraindications to anticoagulation (class of recommendation I, level of evidence A).[18] Anticoagulation is also recommended in patients with intracardiac thrombus detected by imaging or evidence of systemic embolism (class of recommendation I, level of evidence C).

In the 2012 ESC guidelines for the diagnosis and treatment of acute and chronic HF, the routine use of anticoagulant therapy in HF patients in SR is not recommended.

Clinical guidelines on HF and the associated recommendations on antithrombotic therapy are summarized in Box 2.

Box 2: Synopsis of clinical guidelines regarding the use of anticoagulation in heart failure patients in sinus rhythm

ESC 2008

Oral anticoagulation (OAC) is strongly recommended in patients that present intracardiac thrombus or evidence of systemic thromboembolism (class IC).

ESC 2012

No recommendation provided regarding the use of OAC in HF patients in sinus rhythm

HFSA 2010

- The use of OAC is recommended in patients with previous thromboembolic events
- The use of OAC is recommended in patients with that suffer from ischemic cardiomyopathy and large anterior MI, or when LV thrombus has been identified in the setting of a recent MI (for 3 months post-MI)
- The use of OAC should also be considered in other cases of cardiomyopathy associated with the presence of LV thrombus in relation to the characteristics of the thrombus in the imaging tests
- The use of OAC in patients with dilated cardiomyopathy and low EF (≤35%) is less well established

ACC/AHA 2009

- OAC is recommended in patients with a history of previous thromboembolic event
- OAC should be considered in patients with high thrombo-embolic risk (e.g., amyloidosis or LV noncompaction) and in those who suffer from familial dilated cardiomyopathy and a history of thromboembolism in first-degree relatives.

ESC, European Society of Cardiology; HF, heart failure; HFSA, Heart Failure Society of America; MI, myocardial infarction; LV, left ventricular; EF, ejection fraction; ACC/AHA, American College of Cardiology/ American Heart Association

Specific Populations

The presence of a mobile and protruding thrombus in the left ventricle clearly justifies OAC. Ventricular thrombi develop more frequently at the level of LV apex in patients who have experienced previous acute myocardial infarction. In this setting, patients should receive anticoagulation therapy for at least 3 months aiming at decreasing the risk of thromboembolic events.

Additionally, HF patients who suffer from some types of valvular heart disease are also at increased risk of developing intracardiac thrombi. Although the incidence of rheumatic heart disease has been significantly reduced, especially in the Western world, rheumatic heart disease still represents an important risk factor for thromboembolic events, particularly in developing countries.[103-108]

Patients with mechanical valves are at increased risk of thromboembolic events. Thus, antithrombotic management should include not only the use of antithrombotic drugs but also effective control of modifiable risk factors for embolic events. According to the 2012 ESC guidelines, patients implanted with mechanical valves need permanent OAC (class I, level of evidence B).[109] Of note, even with the use of warfarin, the risk of thromboembolic is estimated to be 1–2% per year.[110-114] Moreover, there is some (weak) evidence in favor of the use of low-dose aspirin in patients with a mechanical prosthesis who have experienced previous thromboembolic event despite adequate INR (class IIa, level of evidence C). Bioprosthetic valves are associated with a lower risk of stroke, and according to the 2012 ESC guidelines on the management of valvular heart disease, OAC is indicated for the first 3 months after implantation of a mitral or tricuspid bioprosthesis (class IIa, level of evidence C). OAC is also indicated for the first 3 months after mitral valve repair (class IIa, level of evidence C). Aspirin should be considered for the first 3 months after implantation of an aortic bioprosthesis (class IIa, level of evidence C).[109] On the other hand, lifelong oral anticoagulation is recommended for patients with bioprosthesis with underlying comorbidities associated high risk of stroke (like AF) (class I, level of evidence C).

Heart failure patients in SR with a history of previous thromboembolic events represent another clinical scenario in which OAC treatment should also be considered. In these patients, anticoagulation could confer some benefits reducing the risk of a new episode of stroke. The use of anticoagulant therapy in patients with a history of diseases that promote the risk of thromboembolic events (e.g., amyloidosis) and in patients suffering from familial dilated cardiomyopathy with history of previous venous thromboembolism in first-degree relatives is not well established.

In addition, patients with right HF with pulmonary hypertension (PH) represent a population that anticoagulant therapy may potentially be considered.[115] However, further research is required in order to elucidate the role of oral anticoagulation in this setting. Such patients with PH have a higher risk of developing thromboembolic complications due to abnormalities in coagulation implicated in the pathophysiology of pulmonary arterial hypertension (PAH) as well as other risk factors for thromboembolic events, such as HF and immobility. Currently, OAC is recommended only in patients with idiopathic pulmonary arterial hypertension (IPAH), heritable PAH and secondary drug-induced PAH.[116,117]

Another group of HF patients whose management is a challenging task is represented by those with end stage HF patients. In the last few years, great advances have been made not only in the field of the cardiac resynchronization therapy with the implantation of biventricular pacemakers, but also in the prevention of sudden death with the implantation of implantable cardioverter-defibrillators (ICDs). An important issue that is frequently raised in the management of anti-coagulated HF patients is the necessity of interruption of anticoagulation when patients undergo pacemaker or ICD implantation. Indeed, the periprocedural approach in this setting represents a clinical issue in which best clinical practice is not yet well established.

Transition of their warfarin to heparin in anticipation of these procedures is very common in clinical practice. On the other hand, many centers undertake these procedures whilst on therapeutic INR. Nevertheless, the clinical decision whether to discontinue oral anticoagulation therapy in anticipation of interventional procedures has represented a controversial issue. More recent studies that support implantation of pacemakers and ICDs in patients at moderate-to-high thromboembolism risk whilst under therapeutic anticoagulation.[118] Also, a recent study shows that interruption of anticoagulant therapy without bridging with heparin, seems to result in increased risk of thromboembolic events, whilst interruption of warfarin under overlapping anticoagulant therapy appear increase the risk of bleeding complications.[119]

In the last few years, advances have also been made in the field of mechanical circulatory support, and currently, left ventricular assist devise (LVAD) have created expectations for many patients with severe HF. Indeed, LVADs are now approved for bridge patients. Despite technological improvements in regard to the design of the assist systems the implementation of mechanical circulatory support (MCS), these appear to predispose increased risk of stroke and thromboembolic events.[120] The major risk factors for the establishment of the hypercoagulable state in this setting are the direct contact between blood elements and the surfaces of the implanted devise the rheological abnormalities promoted by the LVAD function and the blood stasis in the native heart.[121] The rate of thromboembolic events varies from 5–50% in relation to the different LVAD types and to the anticoagulation strategies used.[122]

CONCLUSION

It is well recognized that in HF, thromboembolic events are associated with increased morbidity and mortality. Whilst anticoagulation treatment carries an intrinsic risk of bleeding complications, its routine use in patients with HF with SR is not currently evidence based. AF complicating HF significantly increases, the risk of stroke, and the use of anticoagulation is well-established. However, anticoagulation potentially could also be considered in certain subgroups of patients with HF in SR; for example, the presence of HF with decreased EF and previous thromboembolism, newly diagnosed intracardiac thrombus and right HF with PH may potentially justify the use of OAC.

Despite the fact that aspirin is proven to be very effective in certain groups of patients such as those who suffer from coronary artery disease, there is lack of evidence to support its routine use, as thromboprophylaxis in patients with HF who are in SR. Moreover, coadministration of OAC with antiplatelet agent should be avoided in patients with chronic (>12 months after an acute event) coronary or other arterial disease, due to the high risk of major bleeding. Particular emphasis should be placed on the management of the modifiable risk factors, which results in the beneficial modification of the individual ischemic and bleeding risk profile. Finally, the patient should always be actively involved in the decision making process. Indeed, it is of crucial importance that patient's values and preferences should always be taken into consideration when balancing the risk of thromboembolism against bleeding.

REFERENCES

1. McMurray JJ, Adamopoulos S, Anker SD, et al. ESC Guidelines for the diagnosis and treatment of acute and chronic heart failure 2012: The Task Force for the Diagnosis and Treatment of Acute and Chronic Heart Failure 2012 of the European Society of Cardiology. Developed in collaboration with the Heart Failure Association (HFA) of the ESC. Eur Heart J. 2012;33(14):1787-847.
2. Bleumink GS, Knetsch AM, Sturkenboom MC, et al. Quantifying the heart failure epidemic: prevalence, incidence rate, lifetime risk and prognosis of heart failure The Rotterdam Study. Eur Heart J. 2004;25(18):1614-9.
3. Mosterd A, Hoes AW. Clinical epidemiology of heart failure. Heart. 2007;93(9):1137-46.
4. Lloyd-Jones DM, Larson MG, Leip EP, et al. Lifetime risk for developing congestive heart failure: the Framingham Heart Study. Circulation. 2002;106(24):3068-72.
5. Roger VL, Go AS, Lloyd-Jones DM, et al. Heart disease and stroke statistics—2011 update: a report from the American Heart Association. Circulation. 2011;123(4):e18-e209.
6. Beemath A, Stein PD, Skaf E, et al. Risk of venous thromboembolism in patients hospitalized with heart failure. Am J Cardiol. 2006;98(6):793-5.
7. Dries DL, Rosenberg YD, Waclawiw MA, et al. Ejection fraction and risk of thromboembolic events in patients with systolic dysfunction and sinus rhythm: evidence for gender differences in the studies of left ventricular dysfunction trials. J Am Coll Cardiol. 1997;29(5):1074-80.
8. Loh E, Sutton MS, Wun CC, et al. Ventricular dysfunction and the risk of stroke after myocardial infarction. N Engl J Med. 1997;336(4):251-7.
9. Dunkman WB, Johnson GR, Carson PE, et al. Incidence of thromboembolic events in congestive heart failure. The V-HeFT VA Cooperative Studies Group. Circulation. 1993;87(6 Suppl):VI94-101.
10. Freudenberger RS, Hellkamp AS, Halperin JL, et al. Risk of thromboembolism in heart failure: an analysis from the Sudden Cardiac Death in Heart Failure Trial (SCD-HeFT).Circulation. 2007;115(20):2637-41.
11. Lip GY, Gibbs CR. Does heart failure confer a hypercoagulable state? Virchow's triad revisited. J Am Coll Cardiol. 1999;33(5):1424-6.
12. Sbarouni E, Bradshaw A, Andreotti F, et al. Relationship between hemostatic abnormalities and neuroendocrine activity in heart failure. Am Heart J. 1994;127(3):607-12.
13. Lip GYH, Lowe GDO, Metcalfe MJ, et al. Effects of warfarin therapy on plasma fibrinogen, von Willebrand factor and fibrin D-dimer in left ventricular dysfunction secondary to coronary artery disease with and without aneurysms. Am J Cardiol. 1995;76(7):453-8.
14. Jafri SM, Ozawa T, Mammen E, et al. Platelet function, thrombin and fibrinolytic activity in patients with heart failure. Eur Heart J. 1993;14(2): 205-12.
15. Jafri SM, Mammen EF, Masura J, et al. Effects of warfarin on markers of hypercoagulability in patients with heart failure. Am Heart J. 1997;134(1):27-36.
16. Kubo SH, Rector TS, Bank AJ, et al. Endothelium-dependent vasodilatation is attenuated in patients with heart failure. Circulation. 1991; 84(4):1589-96.
17. Witt BJ, Gami AS, Ballman KV, et al. The incidence of ischemic stroke in chronic heart failure: a meta-analysis. J Card Fail. 2007;13(6):489-96.
18. Dickstein K, Cohen-Solal A, Filippatos G, et al. ESC Guidelines for the diagnosis and treatment of acute and chronic heart failure 2008: the Task Force for the Diagnosis and Treatment of Acute and Chronic Heart Failure 2008 of the European Society of Cardiology. Developed in collaboration with the Heart Failure Association of the ESC (HFA) and endorsed by the European Society of Intensive Care Medicine (ESICM). Eur Heart J. 2008;29(19):2388-442.
19. Bertini M, Borleffs CJ, Delgado V, et al. Prediction of atrial fibrillation in patients with implantable cardioverter-defibrillator and heart failure. Eur J Heart Fail. 2010;12(10):1101-10.
20. Deedwania PC, Lardizabal JA. Atrial fibrillation in heart failure: a comprehensive review. Am J Med. 2010;123(3):198-204.
21. Hart RG, Pearce LA, Aguilar MI. Meta-analysis: antithrombotic therapy to prevent stroke in patients who have nonvalvular atrial fibrillation. Ann Intern Med. 2007;146(12):857-67.
22. Bettari L, Fiuzat M, Becker R, et al. Thromboembolism and antithrombotic therapy in patients with heart failure in sinus rhythm: current status and future directions. Circ Heart Fail. 2011;4(3):361-8.
23. Lip GY, Halperin JL. Improving stroke risk stratification in atrial fibrillation. Am J Med. 2010;123(6):484-8.
24. Lip GY, Nieuwlaat R, Pisters R, et al. Refining clinical risk stratification for predicting stroke and thromboembolism in atrial fibrillation using a novel risk factor-based approach: the euro heart survey on atrial fibrillation. Chest. 2010;137(2):263-72.
25. European Heart Rhythm Association, European Association for Cardio-Thoracic Surgery, Camm AJ, et al. Guidelines for the management of atrial fibrillation: the Task Force for the Management of Atrial Fibrillation of the European Society of Cardiology (ESC). Europace. 2010;12(10):1360-420.
26. Banerjee A, Taillandier S, Olesen JB, et al. Ejection fraction and outcomes in patients with atrial fibrillation and heart failure: the Loire Valley Atrial Fibrillation Project. Eur J Heart Fail. 2012;14(3):295-301.
27. Heit JA, Silverstein MD, Mohr DN, et al. Risk factors for deep vein thrombosis and pulmonary embolism: a population-based case-control study. Arch Intern Med. 2000;160(6):809-15.
28. Olesen JB, Lip GY, Lindhardsen J, et al. Risks of thromboembolism and bleeding with thromboprophylaxis in patients with atrial fibrillation: A net clinical benefit analysis using a 'real world' nationwide cohort study. Thromb Haemost. 2011;106(4):739-49.
29. Friberg L, Rosenqvist M, Lip GY. Net clinical benefit of warfarin in patients with atrial fibrillation: a report from the Swedish atrial fibrillation cohort study. Circulation. 2012;125(19):2298-307.

30. Bungard TJ, Ghali WA, Teo KK, et al. Why do patients with atrial fibrillation not receive warfarin? Arch Intern Med. 2000;160(1):41-46.
31. Birman-Deych E, Radford MJ, Nilasena DS, et al. Use and effectiveness of warfarin in Medicare beneficiaries with atrial fibrillation. Stroke. 2006;37(4):1070-4.
32. Hylek EM, Evans-Molina C, Shea C, et al. Major hemorrhage and tolerability of warfarin in the first year of therapy among elderly patients with atrial fibrillation. Circulation. 2007;115(21):2689-96.
33. Gallagher AM, Setakis E, Plumb JM, et al. Risks of stroke and mortality associated with suboptimal anticoagulation in atrial fibrillation patients. Thromb Haemost. 2011;106(5):968-77.
34. Patel MR, Mahaffey KW, Garg J, et al. Rivaroxaban versus warfarin in nonvalvular atrial fibrillation. N Engl J Med. 2011;365(10):883-91.
35. Granger CB, Alexander JH, McMurray JJ, et al. Apixaban versus warfarin in patients with atrial fibrillation. N Engl J Med. 2011;365(11):981-92.
36. Connolly SJ, Eikelboom J, Joyner C, et al. Apixaban in patients with atrial fibrillation. N Engl J Med. 2011;364(9):806-17.
37. Ahmad Y, Lip GY, Apostolakis S. New oral anticoagulants for stroke prevention in atrial fibrillation: impact of gender, heart failure, diabetes mellitus and paroxysmal atrial fibrillation. Expert Rev Cardiovasc Ther. 10(12):1471-80.
38. Freudenberger RS, Schumaecker MM, Homma S. What is the appropriate approach to prevention of thromboembolism in heart failure? Thromb Haemost. 2010;103(3):489-95.
39. Alberts VP, Bos MJ, Koudstaal P, et al. Heart failure and the risk of stroke: the Rotterdam Study. Eur J Epidemiol. 2010;25(11):807-12.
40. Lip GY, Rasmussen LH, Skjøth F, et al. Stroke and mortality in patients with incident heart failure: the Diet, Cancer and Health (DCH) cohort study. BMJ Open. 2012;2(4).
41. Szummer KE, Solomon SD, Velazquez EJ, et al. Heart failure on admission and the risk of stroke following acute myocardial infarction: the VALIANT registry. Eur Heart J. 2005;26(20):2114-9.
42. Wolf PA, Kannel WB, McNamara PM. Occult impaired cardiac function, congestive heart failure, and risk of thrombotic stroke: the Framingham Study. Neurology. 1970;20(4):373.
43. Witt BJ, Brown RD, Jacobsen SJ, et al. Ischemic stroke after heart failure: a community-based study. Am Heart J. 2006;152(1):102-9.
44. Grigorian-Shamagian L, Otero Raviña F, Abu Assi E, et al. Why and when do patients with heart failure and normal left ventricular ejection fraction die? Analysis of >600 deaths in a community long-term study. Am Heart J. 2008;156(6):1184-90.
45. Petty GW, Brown RD, Whisnant JP, et al. Survival and recurrence after first cerebral infarction: a population-based study in Rochester, Minnesota, 1975 through 1989. Neurology. 1998;50(1):208-16.
46. Sacco RL, Shi T, Zamanillo MC, et al. Predictors of mortality and recurrence after hospitalized cerebral infarction in an urban community: the Northern Manhattan Stroke Study. Neurology. 1994;44(4):626-34.
47. Kannel WB, Wolf PA, Verter J. Manifestations of coronary disease predisposing to stroke. The Framingham Study. JAMA. 1983;250(21):2942-6.
48. Howell MD, Geraci JM, Knowlton AA. Congestive heart failure and outpatient risk of venous thromboembolism: a retrospective, case-control study. J Clin Epidemiol. 2001;54(8):810-6.
49. Darze ES, Latado AL, Guimarães AG, et al. Incidence and clinical predictors of pulmonary embolism in severe heart failure patients admitted to a coronary care unit. Chest. 2005;128(4):2576-80.
50. Gottdiener JS, Gay JA, VanVoorhees L, et al. Frequency and embolic potential of left ventricular thrombus in dilated cardiomyopathy: assessment by 2-dimensional echocardiography. Am J Cardiol. 1983;52(10):1281-5.
51. Falk RH, Foster E, Coats MH. Ventricular thrombi and thromboembolism in dilated cardiomyopathy: a prospective follow-up study. Am Heart J. 1992;123(1):136-42.
52. Katz SD, Marantz PR, Biasucci L, et al. Low incidence of stroke in ambulatory patients with heart failure: a prospective study. Am Heart J. 1993;126(1):141-6.
53. Roberts WC, Ferrans VJ. Pathologic anatomy of the cardiomyopathies. Idiopathic dilated and hypertrophic types, infiltrative types, and endomyocardial disease with and without eosinophilia. Human Pathol. 1975;6(3):287-342.
54. Natterson PD, Stevenson WG, Saxon LA, et al. Risk of arterial embolization in 224 patients awaiting cardiac transplantation. Am Heart J. 1995;129(3):564-70.
55. Cioffi G, Pozzoli M, Forni G, et al. Systemic thromboembolism in chronic heart failure. A prospective study in 406 patients. Eur Heart J. 1996;17(9):1381-9.
56. Jugdutt BI, Sivaram CA. Prospective two-dimensional echocardiographic evaluation of left ventricular thrombus and embolism after acute myocardial infarction. J Am Coll Cardiol. 1989;13(3):554-64.
57. Anderson GM, Hull E. The effects of dicumarol upon the mortality and incidence of thromboembolic complications in congestive heart failure. Am Heart J. 1950;39(5):697-702.
58. Griffith GC, Stragnell R, Levinson DC, et al. A study of the beneficial effects of anticoagulant therapy in congestive heart failure. Ann Intern Med. 1952;37(5):867-87.
59. Harvey WP, Finch CA. Dicumarol prophylaxis of thromboembolic disease in congestive heart failure. N Engl J Med. 1950;242(6):208-11.
60. Fuster V, Gersh BJ, Giuliani ER, et al. The natural history of idiopathic dilated cardiomyopathy. Am J Cardiol. 1981;47(3):525-31.
61. Kyrle PA, Korninger C, Gössinger H, et al. Prevention of arterial and pulmonary embolism by oral anticoagulants in patients with dilated cardiomyopathy. Thromb Haemost. 1985;54(2):521-3.
62. Sharma ND, McCullough PA, Philbin EF, et al. Left ventricular thrombus and subsequent thromboembolism in patients with severe systolic dysfunction. Chest. 2000;117(2):314-20.
63. Ciaccheri M, Castelli G, Cecchi F, et al. Lack of correlation between intracavitary thrombosis detected by cross sectional echocardiography and systemic emboli in patients with dilated cardiomyopathy. Br Heart J. 1989;62(1):26-9.
64. Diaz RA, Obasohan A, Oakley CM. Prediction of outcome in dilated cardiomyopathy. Br Heart J. 1987;58(4):393-9.
65. Al-Khadra AS, Salem DN, Rand WM, et al. Warfarin anticoagulation and survival: a cohort analysis from the Studies of Left Ventricular Dysfunction. J Am Coll Cardiol. 1998;31(4):749-53.
66. Stratton JR, Resnick AD. Increased embolic risk in patients with leftventricular thrombi. Circulation. 1987;75(5):1004-11.
67. Falk RH, Pollak A, Tandon PK, et al. The effect of warfarin on prevalence of stroke in patients with severe heart failure. J Am Coll Cardiol. 1993;21:218.
68. Nguyen KN, Aursnes I, Kjekshus J. Interaction between enalapril and aspirin on mortality after acute myocardial infarction: subgroup analysis of the Cooperative New Scandinavian Enalapril Survival Study II (CONSENSUS II). Am J Cardiol. 1997;79(2):115-19.
69. Teo KK, Yusuf S, Pfeffer M, et al. Effects of long-term treatment with angiotensin-converting-enzyme inhibitors in the presence or absence of aspirin: a systematic review. Lancet. 2002;360(9339):1037-43.
70. Latini R, Tognoni G, Maggioni AP, et al. Clinical effects of early angiotensin-converting enzyme inhibitor treatment for acute myocardial infarction are similar in the presence and absence of aspirin: systematic overview of individual data from 96,712 randomized patients. Angiotensin-converting Enzyme Inhibitor Myocardial Infarction Collaborative Group. J Am Coll Cardiol. 2000;35(7):1801-7.
71. Peterson J, Topol EJ, Sapp SK, et al. Evaluation of the effects of aspirin combined with angiotensin converting enzyme inhibitors in patients with coronary artery disease. Am J Med. 2000;109(5):371-77.

72. McAlister FA, Ghali WA, Gong Y, et al. Aspirin use and outcomes in a community-based cohort of 7352 patients discharged after first hospitalization for heart failure. Circulation. 2006;113(22):2572-78.
73. Leor J, Reicher-Reiss H, Goldbourt U, et al. Aspirin and mortality in patients treated with angiotensin-converting enzyme inhibitors. J Am Coll Cardiol. 1999;33(7):1920-25.
74. Echemann M, Alla F, Briancon S, et al. Antithrombotic therapy is associated with better survival in patients with severe heart failure and left ventricular systolic dysfunction (EPICAL study). Eur J Heart Fail. 2002;4(5):647-54.
75. Favoloro RG, Effler DB, Groves LK, et al. Ventricular aneurysm: clinical experience. Ann Thorac Surg. 1968;6(3):227-43.
76. Loop FD, Effler DB, Navia JA, et al. Aneurysm of the left ventricle: survival and results of a 10-year surgical experience. Ann Surg. 1973;178(4): 399-404.
77. Vaitkus PT. Left ventricular mural thrombus and the risk of embolic stroke after acute myocardial infarction. J Cardiovasc Risk. 1995;2(2):103-6.
78. Stratton JR. Left ventricular thrombosis and systemic emboli in myocardial infarction and cardiomyopathy. In: Colman RW, Hirsh J, Marder VJ, et al. (Eds). Haemostasis and Thrombosis. Philadelphia: Lippincott Williams & Wilkins; 2001. pp.1325-38.
79. Keren A, Goldberg S, Gottlieb S, et al. Natural history of left ventricular thrombi: their appearance and resolution in the posthospitalization period of acute myocardial infarction. J Am Coll Cardiol. 1990;15(4):790-800.
80. Lapeyre AC, Steele PM, Kazmier FJ, et al. Systemic embolization in chronic left ventricular aneurysm: incidence and the role of anticoagulation. J Am Coll Cardiol. 1985;6(3):534-38.
81. Cabin HS, Roberts WC. Left ventricular aneurysm, intraaneurysmal thrombus and systemic embolus in coronary heart disease. Chest. 1980; 77(5):586-90.
82. Vaitkus PT, Barnathan ES. Embolic potential, prevention and management of mural thrombus complicating anterior myocardial infarction: a meta-analysis. J Am Coll Cardiol. 1993;22(4):1004-9.
83. Visser CA, Kan G, Meltzer RS, et al. Embolic potential of left ventricular thrombus after myocardial infarction: a two-dimensional echocardiographic study of 119 patients. J Am Coll Cardiol. 1985;5(6):1276-80.
84. Crawford TC, Smith WT, Velazquez EJ, et al. Prognostic usefulness of left ventricular thrombus by echocardiography in dilated cardiomyopathy in predicting stroke, transient ischemic attack, and death. Am J Cardiol. 2004;93(4):500-3.
85. Domenicucci S, Chiarella F, Bellotti P, et al. Long-term prospective assessment of left ventricular thrombus in anterior wall acute myocardial infarction and implications for a rational approach to embolic risk. Am J Cardiol. 1999;83(4):519-24.
86. Haugland JM, Asinger RW, Mikell FL, et al. Embolic potential of left ventricular thrombi detected by two-dimensional echocardiography. Circulation. 1984;70(4):588-98.
87. Reeder GS, Lengyel M, Tajik AJ, et al. Mural thrombi in left ventricular aneurysm: incidence, role of angiography, and relation between anticoagulation and embolization. Mayo Clin Proc. 1981;56(2):77-81.
88. Katz SD. Left ventricular thrombus and the incidence of thromboembolism in patients with congestive heart failure: can clinical factors identify patients at increased risk? J Cardiovasc Risk. 1995;2(2):97-102.
89. Schmidt R, Fazekas F, Offenbacher H, et al. Brain magnetic resonance imaging and neuropsychological evaluation of patients with idiopathic dilated cardiomyopathy. Stroke. 1991;22(2):195-9.
90. Kalaria VG, Passannante MR, Shah T, et al. Effect of mitral regurgitation on left ventricular thrombus formation in dilated cardiomyopathy. Am Heart J. 1998;135(2 Pt 1):215-20.
91. Cleland JG, Findlay I, Jafri S, et al. The Warfarin/Aspirin Study in Heart Failure (WASH): a randomized trial comparing antithrombotic strategies for patients with heart failure. Am Heart J. 2004;148(1):157-64.
92. Cokkinos DV, Haralabopoulos GC, Kostis JB, et al. Efficacy of antithrombotic therapy in chronic heart failure: the HELAS study. Eur J Heart Fail. 2006;8(4):428-32.
93. Massie BM, Collins JF, Ammon SE, et al. Randomized trial of warfarin, aspirin, and clopidogrel in patients with chronic heart failure: the Warfarin and Antiplatelet Therapy in Chronic Heart Failure (WATCH) trial. Circulation. 2009;119(12):1616-24.
94. Homma S, Thompson JL, Pullicino PM, et al. Warfarin and aspirin in patients with heart failure and sinus rhythm. N Engl J Med. 2012;366(20):1859-69.
95. Aguilar MI, Hart R, Pearce LA. Oral anticoagulants versus antiplatelet therapy for preventing stroke in patients with non-valvular atrial fibrillation and no history of stroke or transient ischemic attacks. Cochrane Database Syst Rev. 2007;(3):CD006186.
96. Hopper I, Skiba M, Krum H. Updated meta-analysis on antithrombotic therapy in patients with heart failure and sinus rhythm. Eur J Heart Fail. 2013;15(1):69-78.
97. Rengo G, Pagano G, Squizzato A, et al. Oral anticoagulation therapy in heart failure patients in sinus rhythm: a systematic review and meta-analysis. PLoS One. 2013;8(1):e52952.
98. Warkentin AE, Donadini MP, Spencer FA, et al. Bleeding risk in randomized controlled trials comparing warfarin and aspirin: a systematic review and meta-analysis. J Thromb Haemost. 2012;10(4):512-20.
99. Kumar G, Goyal MK. Warfarin versus Aspirin for Prevention of Stroke in Heart Failure: A Meta-analysis of Randomized Controlled Clinical Trials. J Stroke Cerebrovasc Dis. 2012;22(8):1279-87.
100. Lee M, Saver JL, Hong KS, et al. Risk-benefit profile of warfarin vs. aspirin in patients with heart failure and sinus rhythm: a meta-analysis. Circ Heart Fail. 2013;6(2):287-92.
101. Hunt SA, Abraham WT, Chin MH, et al. 2009 Focused update incorporated into the ACC/AHA 2005 Guidelines for the Diagnosis and Management of Heart Failure in Adults. A Report of the American College of Cardiology Foundation/American Heart Association Task Force on Practice Guidelines Developed in Collaboration With the International Society for Heart and Lung Transplantation. J Am Coll Cardiol. 2009;53(15):e1-90.
102. Heart Failure Society of America, Lindenfeld J, Albert NM, et al. HFSA 2010 Comprehensive Heart Failure Practice Guideline. J Card Fail. 2010;16(6):e1-194.
103. Wang D, Liu M, Hao Z, et al. Features of acute ischemic stroke with rheumatic heart disease in a hospitalized Chinese population. Stroke. 2012;43(11):2853-7.
104. Ghandehari K, Izadi-Mood Z. Etiology of young adult onset brain infarction in Iran. Arch Iran Med. 2006;9(3):240-3.
105. Constante Sotelo JL, Mendez Dominguez A. Rheumatic heart disease: cause of cerebrovascular disease at the National Institute of Cardiology "Ignacio Chavez". Arch Cardiol Mex. 2006;76(1):47-51.
106. Chockalingam A, Gnanavelu G, Elangovan S, et al. Clinical spectrum of chronic rheumatic heart disease in India. J Heart Valve Dis. 2003;12(5): 577-81.
107. Srinivasan K. Ischemic cerebrovascular disease in the young: Two common causes in India. Stroke. 1984;15(4):733-5.
108. Grunkemeier GL, Li HH, Naftel DC, et al. Long-term performance of heart valve prostheses. Curr Probl Cardiol 2000;25:73–154.
109. Vahanian A, Alfieri O, Andreotti F, et al. Guidelines on the management of valvular heart disease (version 2012): the Joint Task Force on the Management of Valvular Heart Disease of the European Society of Cardiology (ESC) and the European Association for Cardio-Thoracic Surgery (EACTS). Eur Heart J. 2012;33(19):2451-2496.
110. O'Brien MF, Stafford EG, Gardner MA, et al. Allograft aortic valve replacement: long-term follow-up. Ann Thorac Surg. 1995;60(2 Suppl):S65-70.
111. Vongpatanasin W, Hillis LD, Lange RA. Prosthetic heart valves. N Engl J Med 1996;335(6):407-16.

112. Hammermeister K, Sethi GK, Henderson WG, et al. Outcomes 15 years after valve replacement with a mechanical versus a bioprosthetic valve: final report of the Veterans Affairs randomized trial. J Am Coll Cardiol. 2000;36(4):1152-8.
113. Bloomfield P, Wheatley DJ, Prescott RJ, et al. Twelve-year comparison of a Bjork-Shiley mechanical heart valve with porcine bioprostheses. N Engl J Med. 1991;324(9):573-9.
114. Cobanoglu A, Fessler CL, Guvendik L, et al. Aortic valve replacement with the Starr-Edwards prosthesis: a comparison of the first and second decades of follow-up. Ann Thorac Surg. 1988;45(3):248-52.
115. Lip GY, Ponikowski P, Andreotti F, et al. Thrombo-embolism and antithrombotic therapy for heart failure in sinus rhythm. A joint consensus document from the ESC Heart Failure Association and the ESC Working Group on Thrombosis. Eur J Heart Fail. 2012;14(7):681-95.
116. Rich S, Kaufmann E, Levy PS. The effect of high doses of calcium-channel blockers on survival in primary pulmonary hypertension. N Engl J Med. 1992;327(2):76-81.
117. Fuster V, Steele PM, Edwards WD, et al. Primary pulmonary hypertension: natural history and the importance of thrombosis. Circulation. 1984;70(4): 580-7.
118. Cano O, Munoz B, Tejada D, et al. Evaluation of a new standardized protocol for the perioperative management of chronically anticoagulated patients receiving implantable cardiac arrhythmia devices. Heart Rhythm. 2012;9(3):361-7.
119. Ahmed I, Gertner E, Nelson WB, et al. Continuing warfarin therapy is superior to interrupting warfarin with or without bridging anticoagulation therapy in patients undergoing pacemaker and defibrillator implantation. Heart Rhythm. 2010;7(6):745-9.
120. Lazar RM, Shapiro PA, Jaski BE, et al. Neurological events during long-term mechanical circulatory support for heart failure: the Randomized Evaluation of Mechanical Assistance for the Treatment of Congestive Heart Failure (REMATCH) experience. Circulation. 2004;109(20): 2423-7.
121. Charron M, Follansbee W, Ziady GM, et al. Assessment of biventricular cardiac function in patients with a Novacor left ventricular assist device. J Heart Lung Transplant. 1994;13(2):263-7.
122. Rose EA, Gelijns AC, Moskowitz AJ, et al. Long-term use of a left ventricular assist device for end-stage heart failure. N Engl J Med. 2001; 345(20):1435-43.

Chapter 30

Management of the Patient with Heart Failure with Preserved Ejection Fraction

Alan S Maisel, Gerasimos S Filippatos, Kevin S Shah, Jeffrey Chan

ABSTRACT

Patients of heart failure with preserved ejection fraction (HFPEF) constitute roughly 30–55% of the total heart failure patients. The pathogenesis of HFPEF is complex and is affected by multiple comorbidities, including diastolic dysfunction, hypertension, obesity, diabetes mellitus, and chronic obstructive pulmonary disease, all contributing to a proinflammatory state. Diagnosis of HFPEF relies on assessment for clinical signs and symptoms of heart failure, such as dyspnea, reduced exercise capacity, orthopnea, edema, and subsequently, verifying the presence of a preserved left ventricular ejection fraction via an echocardiogram. Mainstays in the treatment of HFPEF include blood pressure monitoring, low sodium diet, and diuresis to improve signs and symptoms of volume overload. Beta blockers should be used to control comorbidities, such as tachyarrhythmias and hypertension. Angiotensin-converting enzyme inhibitors and angiotensin receptor blockers have not demonstrated mortality benefit but have shown a moderate impact in preventing admissions for congestive heart failure among patients with HFPEF. In future, novel therapies may include anti-inflammatories, antianginals, and heart rate control through devices.

INTRODUCTION

Patients of heart failure with preserved ejection fraction (HFPEF) constitute a large proportion of heart failure patients. In fact, epidemiologic studies have shown that roughly 30-55% of heart failure patients with acute decompensation have in fact normal or near normal left ventricular (LV) function.[1-5] HFPEF has emerged as the predominant, form of heart failure in the elderly and in women, and may, in fact, eventually emerge as the predominant form of heart failure in the general population as well.[6] Yet, despite this growing prevalence, HFPEF has been largely understudied because of the difficulty in its diagnosis and lack of clarity in the management, as guidelines are still currently being discussed and modified. In the past, HFPEF was frequently referred to as "diastolic" heart failure as opposed to "systolic" heart failure, which corresponded with heart failure with reduced ejection fraction (HFREF). However, because diastolic LV dysfunction was also observed in patients with reduced left ventricular ejection fractions (LVEFs), the term "diastolic" heart failure was eventually replaced by HFPEF.[7]

Heart failure with preserved EF has been defined, according to Framingham criteria, as heart failure with a LVEF greater than 45% and the absence of mitral stenosis, pericardial disease, or noncardiac causes of dyspnea, edema, and fatigue.[8,9] It is a broad classification that essentially encompasses patients with LV diastolic heart failure and preserved EF.[10,11]

PATHOPHYSIOLOGY

Though similar in many ways to HFREF, HFPEF demonstrates a variety of distinct disease characteristics that uniquely distinguish it. Patients with HFPEF generally exhibit a concentric pattern of LV remodeling, normal or near-normal end-diastolic volume, increased wall thickness, and a high ratio of mass to volume with a high ratio of wall thickness to chamber radius. Alongside these hemodynamic characteristics, certain cellular processes also stand out as defining features. Cardiomyocytes often exhibit an increased diameter, and collagen content and changes in calcium homeostasis contribute to impaired cardiomyocyte relaxation and increased stiffness.[12] This stiff ventricle is the driving force behind much of the signs and symptoms demonstrated in HFPEF exacerbations.

The actual pathogenesis of HFPEF, however, is far more complex and currently embedded in a broad spectrum of interrelated diseases and comorbidities. Hypertension is believed to be the main foundation from which the majority of cardiovascular changes occur that ultimately lead to HFPEF. In fact, compared to healthy patients, those with HFPEF have been noted to have markedly increased rest brachial pulse pressure and systolic blood pressure.[13] In theory, prolonged elevations in blood pressure would facilitate microvascular remodeling that would in time induce arterial stiffness and thus a decreased ability of the vasculature to accommodate large volumes of blood ejected from the LV. The resulting increased systolic blood pressure and LV afterload ultimately induce compensatory processes of myocardial hypertrophy, increased myocardial oxygen consumption and LV hypertrophy that perpetuate an ongoing cycle of organ damage and progressively worsening heart failure.[14] Whether patients develop diastolic or systolic dysfunction remains a poorly understood phenomenon. Other theories behind HFPEF include the thought that comorbidities, such as obesity, diabetes mellitus, chronic obstructive pulmonary disease (COPD) contribute to a proinflammatory state.[15] This state may also lead to endothelial inflammation and downstream hypertrophy and fibrosis of cardiomyocytes. Figure 1 demonstrates multiple comorbidities and their interplay with the development of HFPEF.

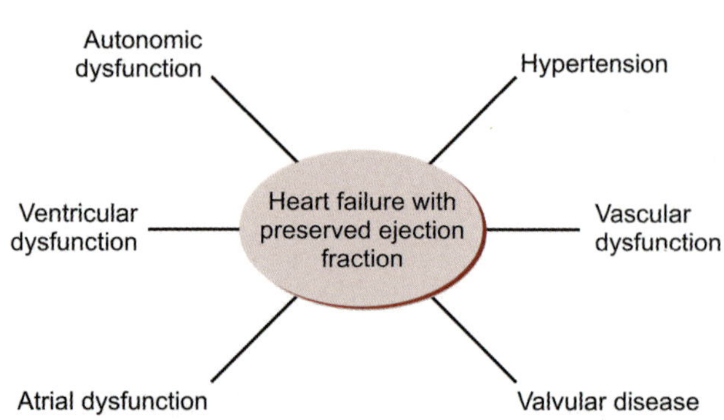

Fig. 1 Comorbidities associated with heart failure with preserved ejection fraction

DIAGNOSIS

In general, the process of diagnosing HFPEF is a two-step process. The first step should be to verify the presence of clinical signs and symptoms of heart failure, such as dyspnea, reduced exercise capacity, orthopnea, edema, or ascites. The second step focuses on verifying the presence of a preserved LVEF via an echocardiogram.[10] Particular emphasis however should initially be placed on appropriately diagnosing heart failure in general and excluding other explanations for the observed clinical symptoms as other conditions, including obesity, respiratory disease, and myocardial ischemia can present similarly to heart failure. Once these alternative diagnoses have been ruled out, a diagnosis of HFPEF can then be presumed in patients with symptoms of heart failure, normal LVEF, and no valvular abnormalities.[11] According to the Heart Failure Society of America (HFSA) guidelines, patients with HFPEF should then be further characterized in order to distinguish between the various types of cardiac disorders, including hypertensive hypertrophic heart disease, ischemic heart failure, infiltrative cardiomyopathy, familial hypertrophic cardiomyopathy, pericardial constriction, high cardiac output state, and right ventricular dysfunction. However, for purposes of clarity, the general approach described above for making the official diagnosis of HFPEF in accordance with European Society of Cardiology (ESC) guidelines is illustrated in Box 1.

While the approach described above appears quite simplistic, the actual details of diagnosing HFPEF with regard to echocardiography are much more intricate. Four sets of guidelines for the diagnosis of HFPEF have been published in current studies.[16-18] They all require the simultaneous presence of signs/symptoms of heart failure, evidence of normal systolic LV function, and evidence of diastolic LV dysfunction or surrogate markers of diastolic LV dysfunction [LV hypertrophy, left atrial (LA) enlargement, atrial fibrillation] or

Box 1: Diagnosis of heart failure with preserved ejection fraction

Diagnostic criteria for heart failure with preserved ejection fraction (all four must be met):

1. Symptoms of heart failure
2. Signs typical of heart failure
3. Normal or mildly reduced left ventricular ejection fraction and left ventricular not dilated
4. Relevant structural heart failure

elevated plasma natriuretic peptide levels. The various guidelines include the Working Group on Myocardial Function of the ESC, the National Heart, Lung, and Blood Institute (NHLBI) Framingham Heart Study and the Lahey Clinic. The fourth set of guidelines, which is the selected approach in this chapter, comes from the Heart Failure and Echocardiography Associations of the ESC.[19] In accordance to this last set of guidelines, the diagnosis of HFPEF requires signs or symptoms of heart failure and the following echocardiographic findings: a LVEF greater than 50%, a left ventricular end diastolic volume index (LVEDVI) less than 97 mL/m^2, evidence of diastolic LV dysfunction, left ventricular end-diastolic pressure (LVEDP) greater than 16 mmHg, pulmonary capillary wedge pressure greater than 12 mmHg, and/or early mitral valve flow velocity to early tissue Doppler (TD) lengthening velocity ratio greater than 15 if there is sufficient evidence of diastolic LV dysfunction and greater than 8 if there is supportive evidence with natriuretic peptides [B-type natriuretic peptides (BNP) >200 pg/mL]; also, a mitral flow velocity Doppler signal demonstrating a ratio of the early to late mitral flow velocity [early mitral inflow velocity/early mitral annular tissue Doppler velocity (E/E2)] less than 0.5 cm/s, and a pulmonary vein flow velocity signal showing a duration of reverse pulmonary vein atrial systole flow. A detailed flowsheet illustrating this guideline is depicted in Flowchart 1.[19]

The use of cardiac biomarkers in the diagnosis of HFPEF remains controversial. While BNP or N-terminal proBNP (NT-proBNP) levels have been firmly established

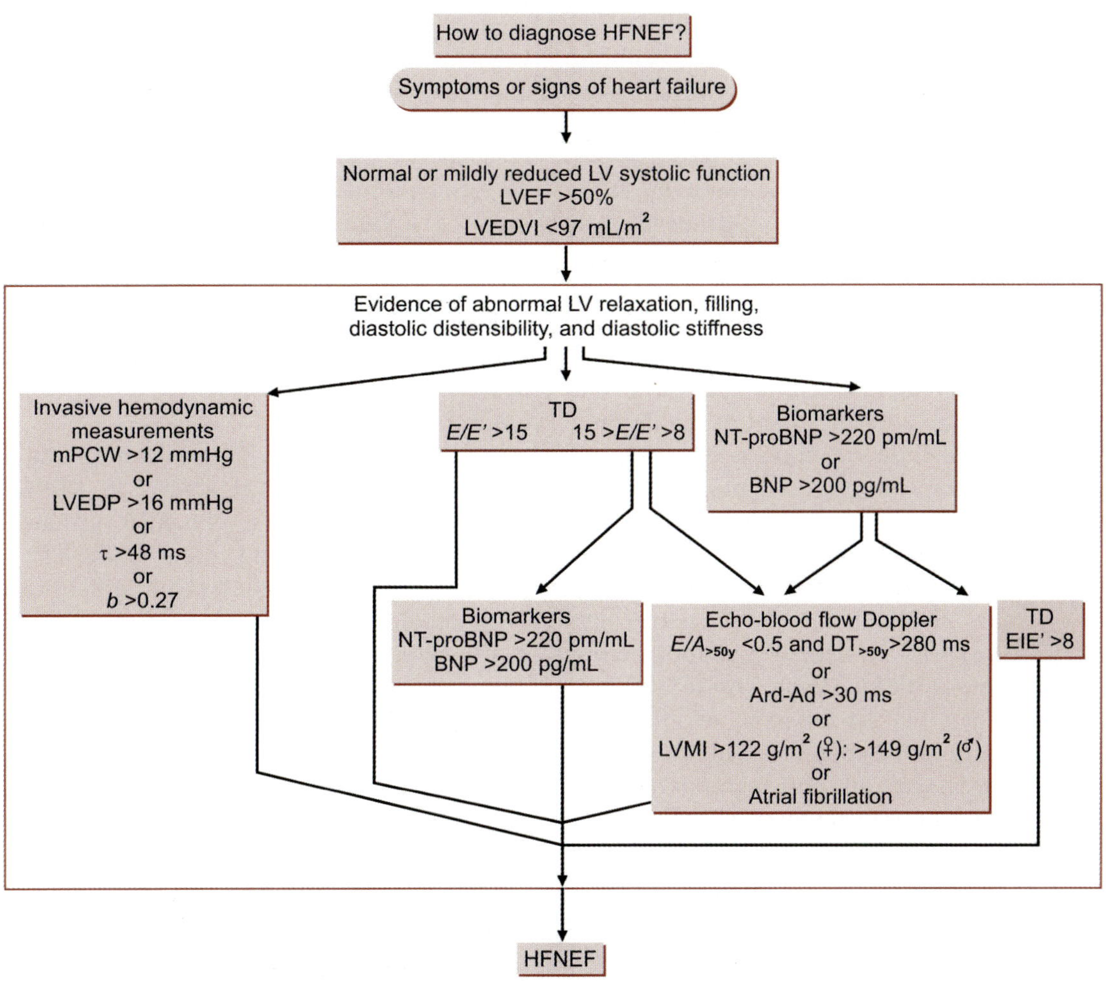

HFNEF, heart failure with a normal ejection fraction; LV, left ventricular; LVEF, left ventricular ejection fraction; LVEDVI, left ventricular end diastolic volume index; mPCW, mean pulmonary capillary wedge pressure; LVEDP, left ventricular end diastolic pressure; TD, tissue Doppler; BNP, B-type natriuretic peptide; NT-proBNP, N-terminal proBNP; E, early mitral inflow velocity; E', early mitral annular tissue Doppler velocity; LVMI, left ventricular mass index; τ, time constant for relaxation

Flowchart 1 Diagnosis of heart failure with preserved ejection fraction (HFPEF) incorporating echocardiography and biomarkers as markers of heart failure, the use of such markers to specifically identify HFPEF is less clear. In the current guideline for diagnosing HFPEF, an NT-proBNP greater than 220 pg/mL or a BNP greater than 200 pg/mL are factored into the algorithm for making the diagnosis. In current literature, levels of NT-proBNP and BNP are known to be higher in patients with HFPEF than normal, but lower than in patients with HFREF.[20-22] Exact cutoffs to help the diagnosis of HFPEF have yet to be determined, but will likely play a pivotal role as the diagnosis of HFPEF is further refined in the future.

TREATMENT

The management of HFPEF has been extremely challenging primarily due to very limited clinical trial data thus far. The current heart failure guidelines[10] recommend blood pressure monitoring, low sodium diet and diuresis to improve signs and symptoms of volume overload. The primary approach to management of HFPEF involves symptomatic relief of dyspnea and clinical volume overload with aggressive use of diuretics. In the inpatient setting, intravenous (IV) loop diuretics are the preferred agent of choice. Evidence has demonstrated that diuretic therapy improves symptoms and quality of life in HFPEF.[23] Similarly to HFREF, goals of diuresis include symptomatic relief of dyspnea/congestion and return to baseline dry weight. Low sodium diet and blood pressure management are also important in the chronic management to prevent fluid retention and worsening of diastolic dysfunction in the case of chronic elevated blood pressure.

Beta blockers, in multiple large scale randomized controlled trials, have demonstrated mortality benefit in chronic systolic heart failure.[24-30] Specifically, most benefit is found with carvedilol and long-acting metoprolol. However, no trials have yet to show a mortality benefit for beta-blocker use in acute or chronic HFPEF. Despite no mortality benefit, beta blockers have shown ability to slow heart rate and regression of LV hypertrophy, and even improvement of LV filling and relaxation on echocardiogram.[31] Currently, beta blockers should be used in HFPEF to control comorbidities, such as tachyarrhythmias and hypertension.

Angiotensin-converting enzyme inhibitors (ACEIs) and angiotensin receptor blockers (ARBs) have also demonstrated a significant mortality benefit in multiple large trials in patients with HFREF. Three large trials have not yielded similar results in the HFPEF patient population. The Candesartan in Heart Failure Assessment of Reduction in Mortality and Morbidity (CHARM)-preserved trial demonstrated a moderate impact in preventing admissions for congestive heart failure (CHF) among patients with HFPEF.[32] The ACEI perindopril has also shown a similar ability prevent readmissions, but fell short of a mortality benefit in HFPEF.[33] The ARB irbesartan was also trialed against placebo in against patients with HFPEF (EF >45%) and there was no benefit in mortality, heart failure death or rehospitalization.[34] In HFPEF thus far, the large trials have shown that ACEIs and ARBs as a whole have not been able to show the mortality benefit as seen in patients with HFREF.

Alternative pharmacological approaches to HFPEF have been studied with similarly negative results. The calcium-channel blocker verapamil has demonstrated improvement of exercise capacity in small studies.[35] Digoxin has also shown no morbidity or mortality benefit.[36] Retrospective data has shown some mortality benefit in HFPEF.[37] One novel therapy has yielded recent positive results with respect to symptomatic relief in decompensated HFPEF. This is serelaxin, a recombinant drug of human relaxin 2. In patients with HFPEF randomized to serelaxin administration, significant improvement in symptoms of dyspnea was observed in one trial. Once again, no mortality benefit was seen. However, this is a novel drug and future trials utilizing it in acute and chronic heart failure will be developed in the future.[38]

In conclusion, no single therapy has proven to demonstrate a mortality benefit in HFPEF. However, diuretics, beta blockers, ACE/ARB all have small roles in terms of improving other indicators of disease (Flowchart 2). In patients with other indications for these medications (i.e., tachyarrhythmias, hypertension in the setting of diabetes mellitus), institution of these medications is still warranted to help with management of comorbidities that are integral players in the pathophysiology of HFPEF.

PROGNOSIS

The overall prognosis of HFPEF has somewhat conflicting data. Some studies have shown a 5-year survival rate after a first episode of 43% with similar mortality rates as in HFREF.[39] Other meta-analyses have shown that mortality among patients with HFPEF was half that observed in those with HFREF.[40] Once again, comorbidities are numerous amongst these populations, and it can be difficult to discern what disease entity is the major player

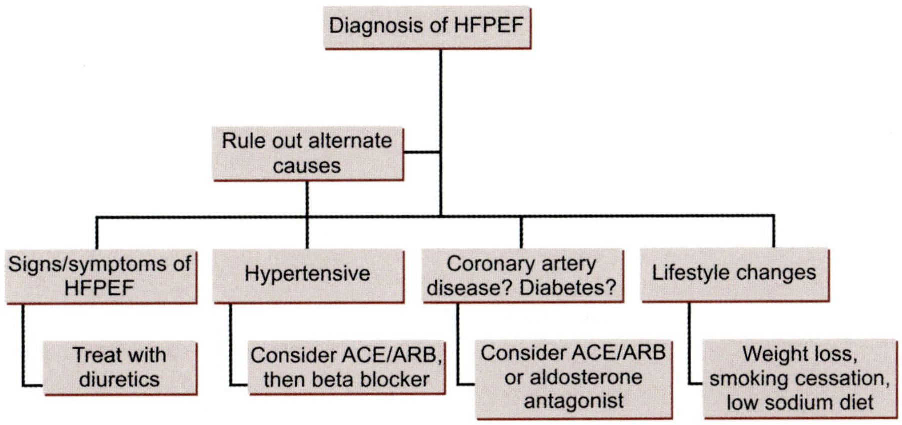

HFPEF, heart failure with preserved ejection fraction; ACE, angiotensin-converting enzyme; ARB, angiotensin receptor blocker

Flowchart 2 Treatment of heart failure with preserved ejection fraction

in terms of mortality. Nevertheless, heart failure in general portends a poor prognosis, regardless of EF.

FUTURE DIRECTIONS

The future direction of HFPEF management includes multiple novel therapies targeting different pathophysiologic mechanisms. Therapies, such as ranolazine (an antianginal), phosphodiesterase-5 inhibitors, xanthine-oxidase inhibitors (anti-inflammatories) and heart rate control through devices are all being considered. Promising basic science research has shown a role for these therapies in HFPEF, but translation to clinical results are yet to be seen.

CONCLUSION

In conclusion, HFPEF is a common subtype of CHF. HFPEF is difficult to diagnose and associated with multiple comorbidities. Approach to the management of HFPEF has not demonstrated as many therapies with as strong mortality benefits as in HFREF, but treatment of comorbidities and management of symptoms are current recommendations to help improve outcomes and quality of life in those suffering with this prevalent condition.

REFERENCES

1. Bhatia RS, Tu JV, Lee DS, et al. Outcome of heart failure with preserved ejection fraction in a population-based study. N Engl J Med. 2006;355(3):260-9.
2. Bursi F, Weston SA, Redfield MM, et al. Systolic and diastolic heart failure in the community. JAMA. 2006;296(18):2209-16.
3. Cleland JG, Swedberg K, Follath F, et al. The EuroHeart Failure survey programme—a survey on the quality of care among patients with heart failure in Europe. Part 1: patient characteristics and diagnosis. Eur Heart J. 2003;24(5):442-63.
4. Hogg K, Swedberg K, McMurray J. Heart failure with preserved left ventricular systolic function; epidemiology, clinical characteristics, and prognosis. J Am Coll Cardiol. 2004;43(3):317-27.
5. Owan TE, Hodge DO, Herges RM, et al. Trends in prevalence and outcome of heart failure with preserved ejection fraction. N Engl J Med. 2006;355(3):251-9.
6. Masoudi FA, Havranek EP, Smith G, et al. Gender, age, and heart failure with preserved left ventricular systolic function. J Am Coll Cardiol. 2003;41(2):217-23.
7. McMurray J, Pfeffer MA. New therapeutic options in congestive heart failure: Part II. Circulation. 2002;105(18):2223-8.
8. Gutierrez C, Blanchard DG. Diastolic heart failure: challenges of diagnosis and treatment. Am Fam Physician. 2004;69(11):2609-16.
9. Zile MR, Baicu CF, Bonnema DD. Diastolic heart failure: definitions and terminology. Prog Cardiovasc Dis. 2005;47(5):307-13.
10. Heart Failure Society of America, Lindenfeld J, Albert NM, et al. HFSA 2010 Comprehensive Heart Failure Practice Guideline. J Card Fail. 2010; 16(6):e1-194.
11. Hunt SA, Abraham WT, Chin MH, et al. ACCDAHA 2005 Guideline Update for the Diagnosis and Management of Chronic Heart Failure in the Adult: a report of the American College of Cardiology/American Heart Association Task Force on Practice Guidelines (Writing Committee to Update the 2001 Guidelines for the Evaluation and Management of Heart Failure): developed in collaboration with the American College of Chest Physicians and the International Society for Heart and Lung Transplantation: endorsed by the Heart Rhythm Society. Circulation. 2005;112(12):e154-235.
12. Chatterjee K, Massie B. Systolic and diastolic heart failure: differences and similarities. J Card Fail. 2007;13(7):569-76.
13. Hundley WG, Kitzman DW, Morgan TM, et al. Cardiac cycle-dependent changes in aortic area and distensibility are reduced in older patients with isolated diastolic heart failure and correlate with exercise intolerance. J Am Coll Cardiol. 2001;38(3):796-802.
14. Vasan RS, Levy D. The role of hypertension in the pathogenesis of heart failure. A clinical mechanistic overview. Arch Intern Med. 1996;156(16): 1789-96.

15. Paulus WJ, Tschöpe C. A novel paradigm for heart failure with preserved ejection fraction: Comorbidities drive myocardial dysfunction and remodeling through coronary microvascular endothelial inflammation. Am Coll Cardiol. 2013;62(4):263-71.
16. Paulus WJ. How to diagnose diastolic heart failure. European Study Group on Diastolic Heart Failure. Eur Heart J. 1998;19:990-1003.
17. Vasan RS, Levy D. Defining diastolic heart failure: a call for standardized diagnostic criteria. Circulation. 2000;101(17):2118-21.
18. Yturralde RF, Gaasch WH. Diagnostic criteria for diastolic heart failure. Prog Cardiovasc Dis. 2005;47(5):314-9.
19. Oghlakian GO, Sipahi I, Fang JC. Treatment of heart failure with preserved ejection fraction: have we been pursuing the wrong paradigm? Mayo Clin Proc. 2011;86(6):531-9.
20. McMurray J, Carson PE, Komajda M, et al. Heart failure with preserved ejection fraction: clinical characteristics of 4133 patients enrolled in the I-PRESERVE trial. Eur J Heart Fail. 2008;10(2):149-56.
21. Carson P, Massie BM, McKelvie R, et al. The irbesartan in heart failure with preserved systolic function (I-PRESERVE) trial: rationale and design. J Card Fail. 2005;11(8):576-85.
22. van Veldhuisen DJ, Linssen GC, Jaarsma T, et al. B-type natriuretic peptide and prognosis in heart failure patients with preserved and reduced ejection fraction. J Am Coll Cardiol. 2013;61(14):1498-506.
23. Yip GW, Wang M, Wang T, et al. The Hong Kong diastolic heart failure study: a randomised controlled trial of diuretics, irbesartan and ramipril on quality of life, exercise capacity, left ventricular global and regional function in heart failure with a normal ejection fraction. Heart. 2008; 94(5):573-80.
24. Heidenreich PA, Lee TT, Massie BM. Effect of beta-blockade on mortality in patients with heart failure: a meta-analysis of randomized clinical trials. J Am Coll Cardiol. 1997;30(1):27-34.
25. Lechat P, Packer M, Chalon S, et al. Clinical effects of beta-adrenergic blockade in chronic heart failure: a meta-analysis of double-blind, placebo-controlled, randomized trials. Circulation. 1998;98(12):1184-91.
26. The Cardiac Insufficiency Bisoprolol Study II (CIBIS-II): a randomised trial. Lancet. 1999;353(9146):9-13.
27. Effect of metoprolol CR/XL in chronic heart failure: Metoprolol CR/XL Randomised Intervention Trial in Congestive Heart Failure (MERIT-HF). Lancet. 1999;353(9169):2001-7.
28. Packer M, Bristow MR, Cohn JN, et al. The effect of carvedilol on morbidity and mortality in patients with chronic heart failure. U.S. Carvedilol Heart Failure Study Group. N Engl J Med. 1996;334(21):1349-55.
29. Packer M, Fowler MB, Roecker EB, et al. Effect of carvedilol on the morbidity of patients with severe chronic heart failure: results of the carvedilol prospective randomized cumulative survival (COPERNICUS) study. Circulation. 2002;106(17):2194-9.
30. Flather MD, Shibata MC, Coats AJ, et al. Randomized trial to determine the effect of nebivolol on mortality and cardiovascular hospital admission in elderly patients with heart failure (SENIORS). Eur Heart J. 2005;26(3): 215-25.
31. Bergström A, Andersson B, Edner M, et al. Effect of carvedilol on diastolic function in patients with diastolic heart failure and preserved systolic function. Results of the Swedish Doppler-echocardiographic study (SWEDIC). Eur J Heart Fail. 2004;6(4):453-61.
32. Yusuf S, Pfeffer MA, Swedberg K, et al. Effects of candesartan in patients with chronic heart failure and preserved left-ventricular ejection fraction: the CHARM-Preserved Trial. Lancet. 2003;362(9386): 777-81.
33. Cleland JG, Tendera M, Adamus J, et al. The perindopril in elderly people with chronic heart failure (PEP-CHF) study. Eur Heart J. 2006;27(19): 2338-45.
34. Massie BM, Carson PE, McMurray JJ, et al. Irbesartan in patients with heart failure and preserved ejection fraction. N Engl J Med. 2008;359(23): 2456-67.
35. Setaro JF, Zaret BL, Schulman DS, et al. Usefulness of verapamil for congestive heart failure associated with abnormal left ventricular diastolic filling and normal left ventricular systolic performance. Am J Cardiol. 1990;66(12):981-6.
36. Ahmed J, Rich MW, Flegl JL, et al. Effects of digoxin on morbidity and mortality of diastolic heart failure: the Ancillary Digitalis Investigation Group trial. Circulation. 2006;114(5):397-403.
37. Tehrani F, Morrissey R, Phan A, et al. Statin therapy in patients with diastolic heart failure. Clin Cardiol. 2010;33(4):E1-5.
38. Teerlink JR, Cotter G, Davison BA, et al. Serelaxin, recombinant human relaxin-2, for treatment of acute heart failure (RELAX-AHF): a randomised, placebo-controlled trial. Lancet. 2013;381(9860):29-39.
39. Tribouilloy C, Rusinaru D, Mahjoub H, et al. Prognosis of heart failure with preserved ejection fraction: a 5 year prospective population-based study. Eur Heart J. 2008;29(3):339-47.
40. Somaratne JB, Berry C, McMurray JJ, et al. The prognostic significance of heart failure with preserved left ventricular ejection fraction: a literature-based meta-analysis. Eur J Heart Fail. 2009;11(9):855-62.

Chapter 31

Implantable Cardioverter-defibrillator and Cardiac Resynchronization Therapy in Heart Failure Patients: How to Choose the Right Device for the Right Patients

Khwaja S Alim, Erik A Green

ABSTRACT

There have been continuing and expanding indications for device therapy in patients with heart failure (HF). Patients with HF are at an increased risk for sudden cardiac death (SCD), and many clinical trials conducted over the last 2 decades have shown the value of implantable cardioverter-defibrillators (ICDs) in the prevention of SCD. Several landmark studies like Multicenter Automatic Defibrillator Implantation Trial II (MADIT II) and Defibrillators in Nonischemic Cardiomyopathy Treatment Evaluation (DEFINITE) trial, to name a few, have laid the foundation for indications for automatic ICD placement.

In a selected group of patients with conduction abnormalities, cardiac resynchronization therapy (CRT) has demonstrated improved functional capacity, reversed remodeling as well as improved survival. The patients who benefit the most from CRT are those with a wide QRS (>150 ms), left ventricular ejection fraction less than 35% and patients with New York Heart Association (NYHA) HF class III and ambulatory class IV.

As the number of patients with cardiac implantable electronic devices increases and our understanding of HF and HF therapy develops and grows, the indications of ICD and CRT therapy are continuously being modified.

INTRODUCTION

There have been continuing and expanding indications for device therapy in patients with heart failure (HF). Patients with HF are at an increased risk for sudden cardiac death (SCD) and many clinical trials conducted over the last 2 decades have shown the value of implantable cardioverter defibrillators (ICDs) in the prevention of SCD. Many HF patients can also develop cardiac conduction system abnormalities, such as left bundle branch block (LBBB). In such patients, cardiac resynchronization therapy (CRT) has demonstrated improved functional capacity, reversed remodeling, as well as improved survival.

As the number of patients with cardiac implantable electronic devices (CIED) increases and our understanding of HF and HF therapy develops and grows, the indications of ICD and CRT therapy are continuously being modified. Findings from recent clinical studies have prompted a recent update in CIED guidelines, on one hand widening indications to include New York Heart Association (NYHA) II patients but on the other hand also recognizing that some patients respond better to CRT therapy depending on QRS width. There are also areas where CIED is less well established or questionable, such as early after a myocardial infarction (MI) or in the new onset dilated cardiomyopathy (DCM) patient. This chapter will focus on an up-to-date understanding of device therapy in HF patients; key clinical trials will be discussed and guidelines on choosing between ICD and CRT for a range of HF patients will be presented.

INDICATIONS FOR IMPLANTABLE CARDIOVERTER DEFIBRILLATORS

Over the last several years, there have been several remarkable studies which paved the pathway for the current recommendations for ICD placement. Some of these landmark studies are discussed below.

Multicenter Automatic Defibrillator Implantation Trial II[1]

In Multicenter Automatic Defibrillator Implantation Trial II (MADIT II) study, 1,232 patients were included. They were over 1 month post-MI and had left ventricular ejection fraction (LVEF) less than or equal to 30%. They were randomized to ICD (n = 742) or medical therapy (n = 490). There was a 6% absolute and 31% relative-risk reduction in all-cause mortality with ICD therapy (p = 0.016) when compared to the medical therapy.

Comparison of Medical Therapy, Pacing, and Defibrillation in Heart Failure Trial[2]

In Comparison of Medical Therapy, Pacing, and Defibrillation in Heart Failure (COMPANION) trial, 1,520 patients with NYHA class III or IV HF were enrolled. The inclusion criteria was ischemic cardiomyopathy (ICM) or nonischemic cardiomyopathy (NICM) and QRS of at least 120 ms. They were randomized to optimal pharmacological therapy (OPT) alone or in combination with CRT with either a pacemaker (CRT-P) or pacemaker-defibrillator (CRT-D). Both device arms significantly reduced combined risk of all-cause hospitalization and all-cause mortality by approximately 20% compared with OPT. On further analysis, CRT-D had reduction in mortality by 36% when compared with OPT (p = 0.003). There was insufficient evidence to conclude that CRT-P was inferior to CRT-D.

Defibrillators in Nonischemic Cardiomyopathy Treatment Evaluation Trial[3]

In Defibrillators in Nonischemic Cardiomyopathy Treatment Evaluation (DEFINITE) trial, 458 patients were studied. The inclusion criteria was NYHA class I–III, with NICM, LVEF less than or equal to 36% and premature ventricular contractions (>10 per hour) or nonsustained ventricular tachycardia (NSVT). They were randomized to standard medical therapy (SMT) alone or in combination with single-chamber ICD. There was a strong trend toward reduction in all-cause mortality with ICD therapy, although it was not statistically significant (p = 0.08).

Sudden Death in Heart Failure Trial[4]

In Sudden Cardiac Death in Heart Failure (SCD-HeFT) study, 2,521 patients were enrolled. The inclusion criteria was NYHA class II or III HF with ICM, or NICM and LVEF less than or equal to 35%. They were randomized to conventional therapy for HF plus placebo; conventional therapy for HF plus amiodarone; or conventional therapy for HF plus conservatively programmed shock-only single lead ICD. There was no survival benefit with amiodarone therapy, but there was 23% reduction in overall mortality with ICD therapy.

On the basis of these studies, the recommendations for ICD placement are described in Table 1.

All primary SCD prevention ICD recommendations apply only to patients who are receiving optimal medical therapy, and have reasonable expectation of survival with good functional capacity for more than 1 year.

INDICATIONS FOR IMPLANTABLE CARDIOVERTER-DEFIBRILLATORS IN HYPERTROPHIC CARDIOMYOPATHY

Hypertrophic cardiomyopathy (HCM) is the disease of the myocardium in which a portion of the myocardium is hypertrophied. This disease is infamously known to cause sudden death in otherwise healthy young athletic individuals, who are at the prime of their respective athletic performance. Younger people are likely to have a more severe form of this disease.[5-7]

A multicenter registry study was performed called: ICDs and prevention of SCD in HCM.[8] This study included 506 unrelated patients with HCM who had implanted ICDs. These patients were at high risk for SCD due to established criteria (family history of SCD, septal thickness ≥30 mm, NSVT, syncope). Mean patient age was 42 years [standard deviation (SD) = 17] and 87% had no or only mild limiting symptoms. In the secondary prevention group, the appropriate ICD discharge rates were 11% per year compared to 4% per year for the primary prevention group. For primary prevention group, 35% of patients with appropriate ICD interventions had undergone implantation for only one risk factor.

Hence, the SCD risk stratification-recommendations are as follows.

CLASS I

- All patients with HCM should undergo comprehensive SCD risk stratification at initial evaluation to determine the presence of the following (*Level of Evidence: B*):
    - A personal history for VF, sustained VT, or SCD events, including appropriate ICD therapy for ventricular tachyarrhythmias

TABLE 1: Recommendations for implantable cardioverter defibrillator placement

Recommendation	*Medical conditions*
IA	• Patients who are survivors of cardiac arrest due to VF or hemodynamically unstable sustained VT after evaluation to define the cause of the event and to exclude any completely reversible causes • Patients with LVEF ≤35% due to prior MI who are at least 40 days post-MI and are in NYHA functional class II or III • Patients with LV dysfunction due to prior MI who are at least 40 days post-MI, have an LVEF ≤30%, and are in NYHA functional class I
IB	• Patients with structural heart disease and spontaneous sustained VT, whether hemodynamically stable or unstable • Patients with syncope of undetermined origin with clinically relevant, hemodynamically significant sustained VT or VF induced at electrophysiological study • Patients with nonischemic DCM who have an LVEF ≤35% and who are in NYHA functional class II or III • Patients with nonsustained ventricular tachycardia due to prior MI, LVEF ≤40%, and inducible VF or sustained VT at electrophysiological study
IIaB	• ICD implantation is reasonable to reduce SCD in patients with long-QT syndrome who are experiencing syncope and/or VT while receiving beta blockers
IIaC	• ICD implantation is reasonable for patients with unexplained syncope, significant LV dysfunction and nonischemic DCM • ICD implantation is reasonable for patients with sustained VT and normal or near-normal ventricular function • ICD implantation is reasonable for patients with hypertrophic cardiomyopathy (HCM) who have one or more major risk factors for SCD • ICD implantation is reasonable for the prevention of SCD in patients with arrhythmogenic right ventricular dysplasia (ARVD)/cardiomyopathy (CMP) who have one or more risk factors for SCD • ICD implantation is reasonable for nonhospitalized patients awaiting transplantation • ICD implantation is reasonable for patients with Brugada syndrome who have had syncope • ICD implantation is reasonable for patients with Brugada syndrome who have documented VT that has not resulted in cardiac arrest • ICD implantation is reasonable for patients with catecholaminergic polymorphic VT who have syncope and/or documented sustained VT while receiving beta blockers • ICD implantation is reasonable for patients with cardiac sarcoidosis, giant cell myocarditis, or Chagas' disease
IIbB	• ICD therapy may be considered for patients with long-QT syndrome and risk factors for SCD
IIbC	• ICD therapy may be considered in patients with nonischemic heart disease who have an LVEF ≤35% and who are in NYHA functional class I • ICD therapy may be considered in patients with syncope and advanced structural heart disease in whom thorough invasive and noninvasive investigations have failed to define a cause • ICD therapy may be considered in patients with a familial cardiomyopathy associated with sudden death • ICD therapy may be considered in patients with LV noncompaction

VF, ventricular fibrillation; VT, ventricular tachycardia; LVEF, left ventricular ejection fraction; MI, myocardial infarction; NYHA, New York Heart Association; LV, left ventricular; DCM, dilated cardiomyopathy; ICD, implantable cardioverter defibrillator; SCD, sudden cardiac death

- ○ A family history for SCD events, including appropriate ICD therapy for ventricular tachyarrhythmias
- ○ Unexplained syncope
- ○ Documented NSVT defined as 3 or more beats at greater than or equal to 120 beats per minutes (bpm) on ambulatory (Holter) echocardiography (ECG)
- ○ Maximal left ventricular (LV) wall thickness greater than or equal to 30 mm.

CLASS IIA

- It is reasonable to assess blood pressure response during exercise as part of SCD risk stratification in patients with HCM (*Level of Evidence: B*)

- Sudden cardiac death risk stratification is reasonable on a periodic basis (every 12–24 months) for patients with HCM who have not undergone ICD implantation but would otherwise be eligible in the event that risk factors are identified (12–24 months).

CLASS III

- Invasive electrophysiologic testing as routine SCD risk stratification for patients with HCM should not be performed

CARDIAC RESYNCHRONIZATION THERAPY

Cardiac resynchronization therapy is another marvel of modern day medicine, which has transformed the treatment of HF. In an appropriately selected patient, it improves exercise capacity as measured by VO_2 (maximal oxygen consumption) uptake, LVEF, NYHA class, and overall mortality benefit.

Biventricular pacing (VP) has been found to be superior to right VP in patients with atrioventricular (AV) block and LV systolic dysfunction with NYHA class I, II, or III HF.[9] The beneficial impact of CRT comes from the ability of combined right ventricular and left VP with the goal to restore both inter- and intraventricular synchrony toward normal. This results not only in the improvement of the LV geometry, but also in the mechanical function, contractility and performance.[10] Subsequently this positive remolding causes reduction in the LV size, which in turn causes improvement in the mitral regurgitation (if present).[10] Patients who benefit the most are those with a wide QRS (>150 ms), LVEF less than 35% and patients with NYHA HF class III and ambulatory class IV[11,12] (Flowchart 1).

According to the combined cardiac resynchronization and implantable cardioversion defibrillation in advanced chronic HF: the Multicenter InSync ICD Randomized Clinical Evaluation (MIRACLE ICD) trial,[13] CRT improved quality of life, functional status and exercise capacity

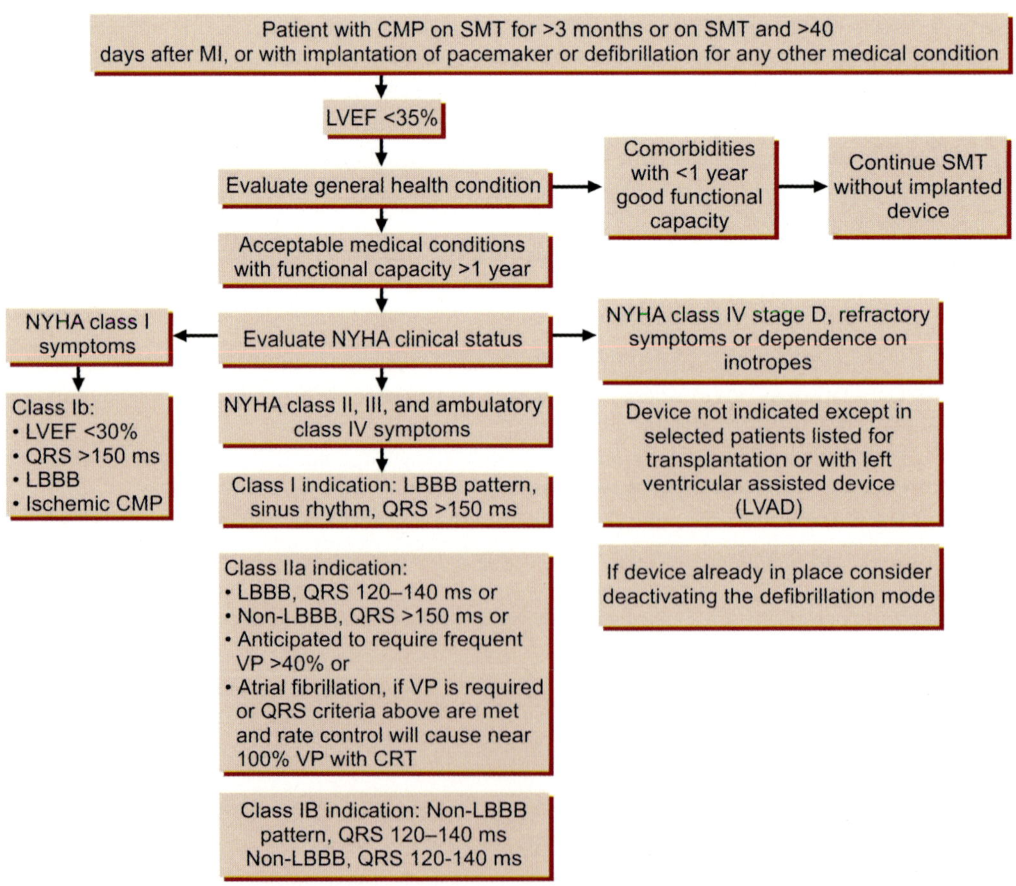

CMP, cardiomyopathy; MI, myocardial infarction; LVEF, left ventricular ejection fraction; NYHA, New York Heart Association; LBBB, left bundle branch block; CRT, cardiac resynchronization therapy; VP, ventricular pacing; SMT, standard medical therapy

Flowchart 1 Algorithm for the indications for cardiac resynchronization therapy

TABLE 2: The recommendation for cardiac resynchronization therapy

Recommendation	*Medical condition*
IA	• CRT is indicated for patients who have LVEF ≤35%, sinus rhythm, LBBB with a QRS duration ≥150 ms and New York Heart Association (NYHA) class II, III, or ambulatory IV symptoms on GDMT
IB	• *Level of Evidence: B* for NYHA class II
IIaA	• CRT can be useful for patients who have LVEF ≤35%, sinus rhythm, a non-LBBB pattern with a QRS duration ≥150 ms and NYHA class III/ambulatory class IV symptoms on GDMT[3]
IIaB	• CRT can be useful for patients who have LVEF ≤35%, sinus rhythm, LBBB with a QRS duration 120–149 ms and NYHA class II, III, or ambulatory IV symptoms on GDMT • CRT can be useful in patients with atrial fibrillation and LVEF ≤35% on GDMT if: ○ The patient requires ventricular pacing (VP) or otherwise meets CRT criteria ○ Atrioventricular nodal ablation or pharmacologic rate control will allow near 100% VP with CRT
IIaC	• CRT can be useful for patients on GDMT who have LVEF ≤35% and are undergoing new or replacement device placement with anticipated requirement for significant (>40%) VP
IIbB	• CRT may be considered for patients who have LVEF ≤35%, sinus rhythm, a non-LBBB pattern with QRS duration 120–149 ms, and NYHA class III/ambulatory class IV on GDMT[2] • CRT may be considered for patients who have LVEF ≤35%, sinus rhythm, a non-LBBB pattern with a QRS duration ≥150 ms, and NYHA class II symptoms on GDMT
IIbC	• CRT may be considered for patients who have LVEF ≤30%, ischemic etiology of heart failure, sinus rhythm, LBBB with a QRS duration of ≥150 ms, and NYHA class I symptoms on GDMT
IIIB	• CRT is not recommended for patients with NYHA class I or II symptoms and non-LBBB pattern with QRS duration <150 ms
IIIC	• CRT is not indicated for patients whose comorbidities and/or frailty limit survival with good functional capacity to <1 year

CRT, cardiac resynchronization therapy; LBBB, left bundle branch block; NYHA, New York Heart Association; GDMT, guideline-directed medical therapy; LVEF, left ventricular ejection fraction

in patients with moderate-to-severe HF, who had a wide QRS interval, and suffered from life-threatening arrhythmias. These improvements occurred when the patients continued to receive underlying appropriate medical management without proarrhythmia or compromised ICD function. In another study, the baseline LV dyssynchrony was not predictive of ventricular tachycardia (VT)/ventricular fibrillation (VF)/death or VT/VF in mild HF patients with or without LBBB. But, CRT-induced improvement of LV dyssynchrony was found to be associated with significant reduction of ventricular arrhythmias in patients with LBBB.[14]

On the basis of several other studies, the recommendation for CRT is given in Table 2.

In some recent studies, slow VT episodes have been found to be predictive of subsequent fast VT/VF. Slow VT and fast VT/V episodes in CRT-D patients are associated with an increased risk of subsequent HF or death. Hence, CRT-D-treated LBBB patients with slow VTs may have a significantly higher risk of mortality.[15] Further studies have to be done to validate this finding.

ACKNOWLEDGMENT

Special thanks to Professor Ulrika Birgersdotter-Green for her immense guidance in writing this highly technical chapter.

REFERENCES

1. Moss AJ, Zareba W, Hall WJ, et al. Prophylactic implantation of a defibrillator in patients with myocardial infarction and reduced ejection fraction. N Engl J Med. 2002;346(12):877-83.
2. Bristow MR, Saxon LA, Boehmer J, et al. Cardiac-resynchronization therapy with or without an implantable defibrillator in advanced chronic heart failure. N Engl J Med. 2004;350:2140-50.
3. Kadish A, Dyer A, Daubert JP, et al. Prophylactic defibrillator implantation in patients with nonischemic dilated cardiomyopathy. N Engl J Med. 2004;350(21):2151-8.
4. Bardy GH, Lee KL, Mark DB, et al. Amiodarone or an implantable cardioverter-defibrillator for congestive heart failure. N Engl J Med. 2005;352(3):225-37.
5. Richardson P, McKenna W, Bristow M, et al. Report of the 1995 World Health Organization/International Society and Federation of Cardiology Task Force on the Definition and Classification of cardiomyopathies. Circulation. 1996;93(5):841-2.

6. Maron BJ. Hypertrophic cardiomyopathy: a systemic review. JAMA. 2002;287(10):1308-20.
7. Sherrid MV, Chaudhry FA, Swistel DG. Obstructive hypertrophic cardiomyopathy: echocardiography, pathophysiology, and the continuing evolution of surgery for obstruction. Ann Thorac Surg. 2003;75(2):620-32.
8. Maron BJ, Spirito P, Shen WK, et al. Implantable cardioverter-defibrillators and prevention of sudden cardiac death in hypertrophic cardiomyopathy. JAMA. 2007;298(4):405-12.
9. Curtis AB, Worley SJ, Adamson PB, et al. Biventricular pacing for atrioventricular block and systolic dysfunction. N Eng J Med. 2013;368(17):1585-93.
10. António N, Teixeira R, Coelho L, et al. Identification of 'super-responders' to cardiac resynchronization therapy: the importance of symptom duration and left ventricular geometry. Europace. 2009;11(3):343-9.
11. Bristow MR, Saxon LA, Boehmer J, et al. Cardiac-resynchronization therapy with or without an implantable defibrillator in advanced chronic heart failure. N Engl J Med. 2004;350(21):2140-50.
12. Cleland JG, Daubert JC, Erdmann E, et al. The effect of cardiac resynchronization on morbidity and mortality in heart failure. N Engl J Med. 2005;352(15):1539-49.
13. Young JB, Abraham WT, Smith AL, et al. Combined cardiac resynchronization and implantable cardioversion defibrillation in advanced chronic heart failure: the MIRACLE ICD Trial. JAMA. 2003;289(20):2685-94.
14. Kutyifa V, Pouleur AC, Knappe D, et al. Dyssynchrony and the risk of ventricular arrhythmias. JACC Cardiovasc Imaging. 2013;6(4):432-44.
15. Kutyifa V, Klein HU, Wang PJ, et al. Clinical significance of ventricular tachyarrhythmias in patients treated with CRT-D. Heart Rhythm. 2013;10(7):943-50.

Chapter 32

Clinical Decision-making in the Outpatient Setting: The Use of Galectin-3

Allart R van der Velde, Wouter C Meijers, Rudolf A de Boer

ABSTRACT

Galectin-3 is involved in inflammatory and fibrotic processes and is secreted into the circulation. As such, galectin-3 is a new biomarker for risk prediction and stratification in heart failure (HF). Several clinical observations have been made showing that galectin-3 is a strong and independent predictor for adverse outcome in acute and ambulatory HF patients. Also, in the general population, it has been shown that increased galectin-3 is associated with increased risk for new onset HF. Serial measurements of galectin-3 add incremental prognostic power. The interpretation of the biomarker galectin-3 should take into consideration other analytes, including N-terminal pro-B-type natriuretic peptide (NT-proBNP) and serum creatinine. Analyses from drug studies have suggested that galectin-3 might be helpful to guide therapy. Next to its function as a biomarker, galectin-3 targeted therapy, such as mineralocorticoid receptor antagonists (MRAs), might be a promising approach to target galectin-3 mediated fibrosis. In this chapter, we propose a new algorithm for the use of galectin-3 in clinical decision-making.

USEFULNESS OF GALECTIN-3 IN PROGNOSTICATION AND GUIDANCE OF HEART FAILURE TREATMENT

Prognostic Value in Chronic Heart Failure

Galectin-3 has recently emerged as a novel independent predictor of mortality in patients with chronic heart failure (HF).[1] Galectin-3 is a galactosidase binding lectin that is secreted by macrophages and other inflammatory cells in the interstitial space of the heart and many other organs. It has a pivotal role in cardiac fibrosis and the remodeling process. As such, circulating (plasma or serum) galectin-3 is believed to reflect matrix turnover and progressive cardiac remodeling. Higher levels of galectin-3 are associated with most common cardiovascular (CV) risk factors, both in HF and the general population,[2,3] including age, sex and renal (dys)function.[4] In (severe) chronic HF, galectin-3 predicts prognosis independent from N-terminal pro-B-type natriuretic peptide (NT-proBNP) levels,[4] and was shown to be associated with left ventricular remodeling determined by serial echocardiography—patients in whom the left ventricular end-diastolic volume decreased over time had significant lower levels of galectin-3 at entry.[5] Other studies confirmed that high levels of galectin-3 are associated with all-cause mortality[6] and renal dysfunction.[7,8] However, galectin-3 is not elevated (cutoff value: 17.8 ng/mL) in all patients with HF. It has consistently been observed, that approximately 40–60% of all patients have high galectin-3 levels, which represents the most severe HF patients.[9] Furthermore, galectin-3 is a relatively stable marker. Mechanical circulatory support devices, that unload the heart, do not alter galectin-3 level, or other markers that are related to fibrosis, while, e.g., natriuretic peptides are substantially decreased by mechanical unloading.[10] The observation that galectin-3 levels are independent from loading conditions is supported by the fact that patients admitted with acute decompensated HF have similarly increased galectin-3 compared with chronic stable HF patients.[8] While increased galectin-3 is associated with adverse long-term CV outcomes, it does predict response to cardiac resynchronization therapy (CRT). Cardiac resynchronization therapy did not decrease serum concentrations of extracellular matrix markers, including galectin-3.[11]

Prognostic Value in Acute Heart Failure

N-terminal pro-B-type natriuretic peptide was superior to both apelin and galectin-3 for proper diagnosis of (acute) HF in acutely dyspneic patients. However, galectin-3 was shown to be the superior independent predictor of 60-day mortality. Interestingly, the combination of elevated galectin-3 and NT-proBNP was even an even better predictor of mortality.[12]

Nowadays, almost 50% of all patients admitted with acute HF suffer from HF with preserved ejection fraction (HFPEF). An identical increase in plasma galectin-3 levels in patients presenting with acute HF turned out to confer a much stronger incremental risk for experiencing the primary outcome in patients with HFPEF in comparison with patients with HF with reduced ejection fraction (HFREF). Although absolute galectin-3 levels did not differ between these patient groups, the difference in prognostic consequences warrants further study.[13] Supportive evidence was obtained from a substudy from the ProBNP investigation of dyspnea in the emergency department study (PRIDE), where echocardiographic markers of diastolic function (E/Ea ratio) showed significant relationships with higher galectin-3 levels.[14] These observations are consistent with a potential role for galectin-3 in mediating cardiac stiffness (thereby impeding diastolic filling) and potentially worsening renal function. Furthermore, galectin-3 is significantly correlated with serum markers of cardiac extracellular matrix turnover in HF patients.[15]

Prognostic Value in Acute Coronary Syndrome

Patients developing HF after an acute coronary syndrome have higher baseline galectin-3 values. Patients with baseline galectin-3 above the median have an odds ratio of 2.1 (95% CI 1.2–3.6, $p = 0.01$). In this patient cohort, galectin-3 showed a graded relationship with the risk of developing HF.[16]

Prognostic Value in the Community

Galectin-3 correlates with a wide range of risk factors of CV disease, including age, sex, blood pressure, serum lipids, body mass index, renal function and NT-proBNP. There is a particularly strong association between galectin-3 and age and the interaction between age and galectin-3 is a confounder of the relation between galectin-3 and outcome. Furthermore, it was observed that female subjects have higher median galectin-3 levels and galectin-3 levels in women more strongly correlate with risk factors of CV disease. After correction for classical CV risk factors (smoking, blood pressure, cholesterol, and diabetes), galectin-3 independently predicts all-cause mortality.[2] This was confirmed in the Framingham Heart Study. Here was also found that higher concentrations of galectin-3 were associated with an increased risk for adverse outcome, including mortality and new onset HF.[3]

Prognostic Value of Serial Measurements

In general, the dynamics of biomarkers are of interest since changes over time may signify disease progression or regression. Several recent reports indicated that follow-up measurements of galectin-3 may be useful in stratification of high risk patients and add to the prognostic power. In two large cohorts of patients with chronic and acute HF, repeated measurements of galectin-3 level provided important and significant prognostic value in identifying HF patients at elevated risk for subsequent HF morbidity and mortality. A first study [which was a substudy of the Controlled Rosuvastatin in Multinational Study in Heart Failure (CORONA) and Coordinating Study Evaluating Outcomes of Advising and Counseling in Heart Failure (COACH) studies] showed that patients whose galectin-3 increases by more than 15% (compared to baseline level, repeat measure after 3–6 months) had a 50% higher relative risk of adverse event, compared with those whose galectin-3 stays within +/– 15% of the baseline value, independent of age, gender, diabetes, left ventricular ejection fraction (LVEF), renal function, medication [beta-blocker, angiotensin-converting enzyme inhibitors (ACEI), angiotensin-receptor blocker (ARB)] and NT-proBNP.[17] This was confirmed in a substudy from the Valsartan Heart Failure Trial (Val-HeFT trial). In this study it was found that galectin-3 levels were elevated in approximately 40% of the patients, which comprised the more severe HF patients. In this cohort, an increase over time of galectin-3 was independently associated with higher risk for mortality.[9]

GALECTIN-3: ITS POTENTIAL USE IN CLINICAL DECISION-MAKING

Interference/Confounders

In the use of galectin-3 in clinical decision-making, there are a few very well-established confounders that have to be taken into account. Clinical factors associated with elevated galectin-3 were identified by linear regression modeling in the general population[2] and HF.[18] Among them we will discuss some of the most important factors: NT-proBNP and estimated glomerular filtration rate (eGFR) since these factors are generally acknowledged as important prognosticators in HF.

N-Terminal Pro-B-type Natriuretic Peptide

In several acute and chronic HF patients cohorts, it was shown that galectin-3 is independently associated with mortality, also after adjustment for baseline NT-proBNP.[4,13] However, other studies with chronic HF patients showed that galectin-3 was a significant predictor of outcome, but after adjustment of NT-proBNP, this association did not persist. Maybe the markedly "healthier" population—median galectin-3 level was 14.0 ng/mL—has contributed to this difference compared with other HF studies.[18] But recently, these results were confirmed in the CORONA trial. Addition of NT-proBNP to the statistical model attenuated the association with between galectin-3 and outcome and this was no longer significant.[19] These results suggest that the usefulness for galectin-3 as a biomarker to guide clinical practice should be considered carefully.

In a first attempt to use galectin-3 in our outpatient clinic, we measured galectin-3 in 33 patients with stable chronic HF (mean eGFR was 53.2% ± 22.3, mean LVEF was 33.0% ± 11.5) and all patients were treated with optimal HF medication. Analysis of this small cohort of chronic HF patients (n = 33), showed a significant relation between galectin-3 and NT-proBNP (Pearson coefficient 0.41, P < 0.01. The cutoff value of 17.8 ng/mL of galectin-3 is depicted as a red line in Figure 1). However, when we consider the plot that displays this association, we noted that a substantial proportion of the patients has a relatively low NT-proBNP, while galectin-3 was increased (red circle). This may indicate that a set of patients exists that may effectively been unloaded, as suggested by relatively low NT-proBNP levels, while galectin-3 was very high, which may indicate a tendency towards fast progression of HF.

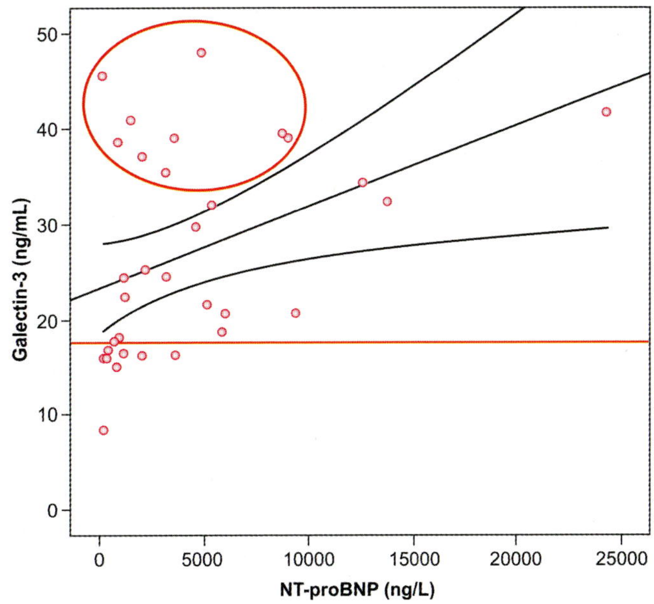

NT-proBNP, N-terminal pro-B-type natriuretic peptide

Fig. 1 Scatter plot (95% CI) showing a significant correlation between galectin-3 and NT-proBNP

Estimated Glomerular Filtration Rate

Renal dysfunction is an established determinant of outcome in HF.[20] Most of the studies up to date have shown that galectin-3 is an independent predictor for outcome, also after correcting for eGFR.[4,7,12] In all patient cohorts, an inverse relationship between eGFR and galectin-3 has been observed. This may lead to the thought that high levels of galectin-3 are the result of renal dysfunction. So does galectin-3 really predict for outcome "independently", or is this the result of renal impairment? It is indeed correct that eGFR shows a very clear correlation with galectin-3, regardless of the severity of HF or the type of HF.[8] In patients with chronic HF, eGFR even accounts for 20% of the total variability in galectin-3 levels.[9] The inverse relation between galectin-3 and eGFR is surprisingly not affected by the presence or absence of clinical HF. Moreover, galectin-3 levels in patients with HF with preserved ejection fraction compared to patients with HF with reduced ejection fraction are not different.[8,13] The intimate relation between galectin-3 and renal function should be taken into account for proper interpretation of galectin-3 levels in a clinical setting.

Again, in our small cohort of chronic HF patients (n = 33), a significant correlation between galectin-3 and eGFR was found (Fig. 2: Pearson coefficient: 0.658,

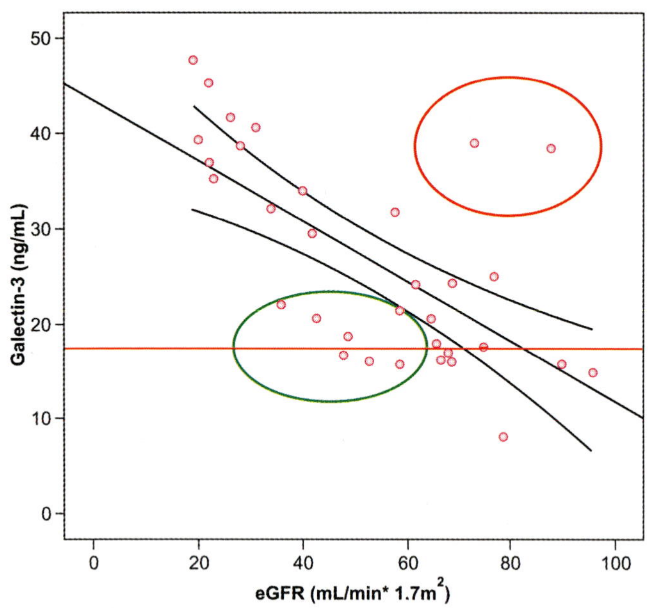

eGFR, estimated glomerular filtration rate

Fig. 2 Scatter plot showing a significant correlation between galectin-3 and eGFR

P < 0.001). As with NT-proBNP, we observed that a (small) subset of patients has clearly elevated galectin-3 levels, despite normal eGFR (red circle). Interestingly, there seems to be patients with clearly decreased renal function (eGFR <60 mL/minute) that have relative low galectin-3 levels (green circle). These two groups of patients are of particular interest, since there seems to exist a dissociation between eGFR and galectin-3 levels.

GALECTIN-3 TO GUIDE THERAPY: INTERACTION BETWEEN EVIDENCE-BASED HEART FAILURE DRUGS AND GALECTIN-3

Angiotensin-converting Enzyme Inhibitors

Little is known about the effect of ACEI on galectin-3. Preclinical research showed that N-acetyl-seryl-aspartyl-lysyl-proline (ac-SDKP) was able to attenuate the profibrotic effects of galectin-3. Since ACEI increase the circulating levels of ac-SDKP, it may be argued that ACEI could attenuate the effects of galectin-3 via ac-SDKP accumulation, but clinical data are lacking to prove this hypothesis. Future research should elucidate this interesting hypothesis.[21]

Angiotensin-receptor Blocker

The well-established ARB, valsartan, is of beneficial effect in patients with HF, but only those with low galectin-3 and not in those with higher levels of galectin-3.[9] In the group of patients with low galectin-3, valsartan resulted in a significant 44% reduction in HF hospitalizations. Patients with high galectin-3 levels did not benefit from the use of valsartan. These findings might suggest that the use of ARBs in patients with high galectin-3 levels, and therefore more severe HF, is not beneficial to patients and withdrawal of ARBs in this patient group may therefore be considered.[9]

Statins

It is already known that statins have a beneficial effect in HF patients with low values of NT-proBNP.[22] This suggested that statins only exerted effect in patients with less advanced stages of HF. Recently it was discovered in the same study—Controlled Rosuvastatin in Multinational Study in Heart Failure trial (CORONA)—that the same applies to the fibrosis marker galectin-3. It was found that only patients with relatively low galectin-3 levels (<19 ng/mL) benefited from statin therapy. Since it is thought that statins may influence the anti-inflammatory effect of the cytokine network these results may be found conflicting because galectin-3 is also known to be promoting inflammation. This suggests that statins may exert its effect on inflammation via different pathways.[23]

Mineralocorticoid Receptor Antagonists

The effect of mineralocorticoid receptor antagonists (MRAs) on galectin-3 has not been studied extensively, but might be very promising. Recent preclinical research showed that aldosterone-induced vascular fibrosis is galectin-3 dependent. Since MRAs have their effect on the mineralcorticoid (aldosterone) receptor, it is expected that MRAs will also affect galectin-3 levels. Interestingly, both the use of the MRA spironolactone and the galectin-3 inhibitor modified citrus pectin (MCP) inhibited aldosterone-induced fibrosis via galectin-3.

It would be of great interest to study the effect of MRA in patients with elevated levels of galectin-3 since we hypothesize that they will probably have more galectin-3-induced fibrosis.[24]

Cardiac Resynchronization Therapy

In patients with HF, CRT has shown to improve symptoms and reduces morbidity and mortality rates.[25] It is believed that the success rate of CRT depends on the amount of fibrosis. However, galectin-3 does not predict response to CRT. Cardiac resynchronization therapy does not favorably affect serum concentrations of galectin-3 or other markers of extracellular matrix.[11] The Multicenter Automatic Defibrillator Implantation Trial with Cardiac Resynchronization Therapy [MADIT-CRT] study showed that CRT was beneficial in patients with low and high galectin-3. But the absolute benefit of CRT was twice in the high galectin-3 group compared with the low galectin-3 group, because the event rate was higher in the group with elevated levels of galectin-3. These study results can be used to prioritize patients eligible for CRT treatment.[26]

GALECTIN-3 IN CLINICAL DECISION-MAKING: A PROPOSED ALGORITHM

In our view, plasma galectin-3 provides solid information on the severity of HF and its prognosis on middle- and long-term. We have created an algorithm how to use galectin-3 in clinical decision-making (Flowchart 1).

Initial galectin-3 sampling will result in HF patients with low versus high galectin-3 levels. Of note, NT-proBNP levels will often be available and galectin-3 and NT-proBNP levels are complementary in many patients.

Patients with low levels may be followed less intensely. We advice to repeat galectin-3 sampling after 3–6 months, as an increase in galectin-3 puts patients in a category with less favorable prognosis. From post hoc analyses in Val-HeFt and CORONA, it may be considered to continue ARBs and statins in HF patients with low galectin-3 levels.

If galectin-3 levels are increased we advice to take eGFR into account. Patients with low eGFR and high galectin-3 levels have the worst prognosis, and should be closely monitored, possibly by a multidisciplinary team, including a nephrologist. Patients with relatively preserved eGFR and high galectin-3 should be treated with maximum antifibrotic drug regimen, including ACEI and MRA. Physicians should actively search for other causes of increased galectin-3, including renal disease, liver disease, and cancer.

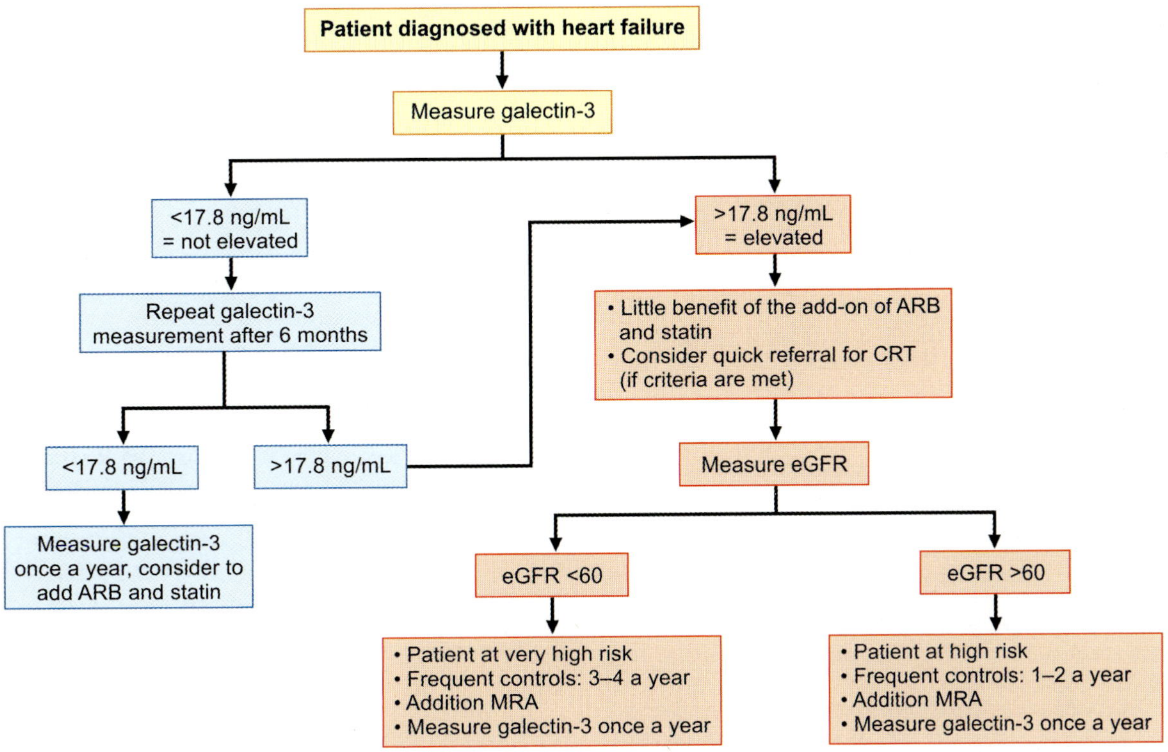

NT-proBNP, N-terminal pro-B-type natriuretic peptide; ARB, angiotensin-receptor blocker; CRT, cardiac resynchronization therapy; eGFR, estimated glomerular filtration rate; MRA, mineralocorticoid receptor antagonist

Flowchart 1 Proposed algorithm of galectin-3 guided clinical decision-making. Measurements of galectin-3 would be additional, next to already established risk indicators like age and NT-proBNP

Caveats and Limitations

Currently, no prospective data are available to support the standard use of galectin-3. However, given the dismal prognosis of HF we believe we should intensify our efforts to properly prognosticate and treat HF patients. The precise role for galectin-3 will emerge in the coming years but we hypothesize galectin-3 will be helpful in this respect.

CONCLUSION

Galectin-3 is a strong predictor for outcome in HF and may help to guide therapy, but confounders have to be taken into account. Galectin-3 targeted therapy appears a feasible approach that could prevent galectin-3 and aldosterone-centered fibrosis and development of HF.

Conflict of Interest

A Rogier van der Velde and Wouter C Meijers have no conflicts of interest.

Rudolf A de Boer has received research grants from Abbott, BG Medicine and Netherlands Organisation for Scientific Research, VIDI grant (No. 917.13.350); consultancy and/or speaker fees from Abbott, AstraZeneca, Biomérieux, BG Medicine, Pfizer, Baxter, and Novartis; and ownership interest in Pectacea."

REFERENCES

1. de Boer RA, Voors AA, Muntendam P, et al. Galectin-3: a novel mediator of heart failure development and progression. Eur J Heart Fail. 2009;11(9):811-7.
2. de Boer RA, van Veldhuisen DJ, Gansevoort RT, et al. The fibrosis marker galectin-3 and outcome in the general population. J Intern Med. 2012;272(1):55-64.
3. Ho JE, Liu C, Lyass A, et al. Galectin-3, a marker of cardiac fibrosis, predicts incident heart failure in the community. J Am Coll Cardiol. 2012;60(14):1249-56.
4. Lok DJ, Van Der Meer P, de la Porte PW, et al. Prognostic value of galectin-3, a novel marker of fibrosis, in patients with chronic heart failure: data from the DEAL-HF study. Clin Res Cardiol. 2010;99(5):323-8.
5. Lok DJ, Lok SI, Bruggink-Andre de la Porte PW, et al. Galectin-3 is an independent marker for ventricular remodeling and mortality in patients with chronic heart failure. Clin Res Cardiol. 2013;102(2):103-10.
6. Ueland T, Aukrust P, Broch K, et al. Galectin-3 in heart failure: high levels are associated with all-cause mortality. Int J Cardiol. 2011;150(3):361-4.
7. Tang WH, Shrestha K, Shao Z, et al. Usefulness of plasma galectin-3 levels in systolic heart failure to predict renal insufficiency and survival. Am J Cardiol. 2011;108(3):385-90.
8. Gopal DM, Kommineni M, Ayalon N, et al. Relationship of plasma galectin-3 to renal function in patients with heart failure: effects of clinical status, pathophysiology of heart failure, and presence or absence of heart failure. J Am Heart Assoc. 2012;1(5):e000760.
9. Anand IS, Rector TS, Kuskowski M, et al. Baseline and serial measurements of galectin-3 in patients with heart failure: relationship to prognosis and effect of treatment with valsartan in the Val-HeFT. Eur J Heart Fail. 2013;15(5):511-8.
10. Milting H, Ellinghaus P, Seewald M, et al. Plasma biomarkers of myocardial fibrosis and remodeling in terminal heart failure patients supported by mechanical circulatory support devices. J Heart Lung Transplant. 2008; 27(6):589-96.
11. Lopez-Andres N, Rossignol P, Iraqi W, et al. Association of galectin-3 and fibrosis markers with long-term cardiovascular outcomes in patients with heart failure, left ventricular dysfunction, and dyssynchrony: insights from the CARE-HF (Cardiac Resynchronization in Heart Failure) trial. Eur J Heart Fail. 2012;14(1):74-81.
12. van Kimmenade RR, Januzzi JL Jr, Ellinor PT, et al. Utility of amino-terminal pro-brain natriuretic peptide, galectin-3, and apelin for the evaluation of patients with acute heart failure. J Am Coll Cardiol. 2006;48(6):1217-24.
13. de Boer RA, Lok DJ, Jaarsma T, et al. Predictive value of plasma galectin-3 levels in heart failure with reduced and preserved ejection fraction. Ann Med. 2011;43(1):60-8.
14. Shah RV, Chen-Tournoux AA, Picard MH, et al. Galectin-3, cardiac structure and function, and long-term mortality in patients with acutely decompensated heart failure. Eur J Heart Fail. 2010;12(8):826-32.
15. Lin YH, Lin LY, Wu YW, et al. The relationship between serum galectin-3 and serum markers of cardiac extracellular matrix turnover in heart failure patients. Clin Chim Acta. 2009;409(1-2):96-9.
16. Grandin EW, Jarolim P, Murphy SA, et al. Galectin-3 and the development of heart failure after acute coronary syndrome: pilot experience from PROVE IT-TIMI 22. Clin Chem. 2012;58(1):267-73.
17. van der Velde AR, Gullestad L, Ueland T, et al. Prognostic value of changes in galectin-3 levels over time in patients with heart failure: data from CORONA and COACH. Circ Heart Fail. 2013;6(2):219-26.
18. Felker GM, Fiuzat M, Shaw LK, et al. Galectin-3 in ambulatory patients with heart failure: results from the HF-ACTION study. 2012;5(1):72-8.
19. Gullestad L, Ueland T, Kjekshus J, et al. Galectin-3 predicts response to statin therapy in the Controlled Rosuvastatin Multinational Trial in Heart Failure (CORONA). Eur Heart J 2012;33(18):2290-6.
20. Hillege HL, Girbes AR, de Kam PJ, et al. Renal function, neurohormonal activation, and survival in patients with chronic heart failure. Circulation. 2000;102(2):203-10.
21. Liu YH, D'Ambrosio M, Liao TD, et al. N-acetyl-seryl-aspartyl-lysyl-proline prevents cardiac remodeling and dysfunction induced by galectin-3, a mammalian adhesion/growth-regulatory lectin. Am J Physiol Heart Circ Physiol. 2009;296(2):H404-12.
22. Cleland JG, McMurray JJ, Kjekshus J, et al. Plasma concentration of amino-terminal pro-brain natriuretic peptide in chronic heart failure: prediction of cardiovascular events and interaction with the effects of rosuvastatin: a report from CORONA (Controlled Rosuvastatin Multinational Trial in Heart Failure). J Am Coll Cardiol. 2009;54(20):1850-9.
23. Gullestad L, Ueland T, Kjekshus J, et al. The predictive value of galectin-3 for mortality and cardiovascular events in the Controlled Rosuvastatin Multinational Trial in Heart Failure (CORONA). Am Heart J. 2012;164(6): 878-83.
24. Calvier L, Miana M, Reboul P, et al. Galectin-3 mediates aldosterone-induced vascular fibrosis. Arterioscler Thromb Vasc Biol. 2013;33(1):67-75.
25. Cleland JG, Daubert JC, Erdmann E, et al. The effect of cardiac resynchronization on morbidity and mortality in heart failure. N Engl J Med. 2005;352(15):1539-49.
26. Stein KM. (2012). Galectin-3 as an aid in prioritizing candidates for CRT treatment—Results of the MADIT-CRT Study. Abstract ESC 2012. [online] Available from investor.bg-medicine.com/releasedetail.cfm?ReleaseID=659292. [Accessed December, 2013].

Chapter 33

Guiding Heart Failure Care with Natriuretic Peptides

James L Januzzi Jr

ABSTRACT

The use of B-type natriuretic peptide (BNP) and its N-terminal prohormone of brain natriuretic peptide (NT-proBNP) has revolutionized the diagnostic and prognostic evaluation of patients with heart failure (HF). Additionally, trends in both BNP and NT-proBNP over time yield incremental prognostic information compared to single measurements. Therapies with benefits for patients with HF tend to lower BNP and NT-proBNP concentrations in parallel with their benefits. This has led to the use of these peptides for monitoring therapy. Beyond this application, a growing interest has developed toward applying knowledge of BNP or NT-proBNP concentrations in therapeutic decision-making for patients with HF. Specifically, the goal of so-called "guided" therapy is not only to titrate HF drugs based on symptoms and signs, but also adjusting therapies to also achieve reduction of BNP or NT-proBNP below prognostic targets. Several, generally underpowered studies have examined this approach, with mixed results. However, several studies have appeared promising, with substantial reduction in risk in some trials, and both meta-analyses and pooled individual patient data analyses have indicated value for the approach. Thus, a better understanding of the optimal means by which natriuretic peptide (NP)-guided therapy should be deployed has developed, and the approach is being analyzed in larger multicenter trials.

INTRODUCTION

There are numerous challenges to deliver optimal care to patients suffering from chronic heart failure (HF). Among the challenges faced by clinicians and patients alike is the fact that it is a major challenge to achieve an optimal medical program that simultaneously minimizes HF symptoms and potential side effects, while simultaneously achieving the prespecified guideline-derived medical therapy goal doses of these therapies. Furthermore, it may be challenging to easily identify when maximal doses of therapies are achieved: the busy clinician can easily articulate many circumstances when patients have tolerated substantial uptitration of HF therapies despite seemingly being maximized.

In order to achieve goals of therapy, frequent office visits with constant evaluation and management is most often needed; this more often than not requires great skill to recognize opportunities to titrate therapies and the acumen to implement such changes.

Despite clearly defined targets for HF care, there is a well-documented worldwide gap in adherence to HF practice guidelines,[1] with eligible patients going undertreated, and missed opportunities to optimize care frequently present. Higher-risk patients are often missed as being at higher likelihood for complications, so such treatment gaps have even greater ramification. This has led to a considerable focus on methods to: identify those patients in need of therapy titration and stratify risk in an objective manner, in order to better deliver care to those patients at the highest risk for an adverse outcome. Very few tools for this application exist—indeed, beyond clinical judgment the everyday clinician has very few easily-obtainable, inexpensive and widely available ways to support their judgment to manage their patients with chronic HF. Several emerging options for objective evaluation of the patient with HF have been investigated, including invasively placed hemodynamic monitoring devices and noninvasive hemodynamic and impedance monitors. However, each of these options have issues, including cost, the need for invasive placement, and lack of data supporting their use.

One intriguing option to guide the care of the patient with HF is the use of biomarkers to assist in therapeutic decision making. This approach is attractive, given the wide availability, low cost, easy measurement and noninvasive nature of biomarkers. Indeed, the natriuretic peptides (NPs), B-type natriuretic peptide (BNP) and its amino terminal pro-peptide equivalent [N-terminal prohormone of brain natriuretic peptide (NT-proBNP)] have been shown to provide easily obtainable and meaningful prognostic information in chronic HF, which is linked directly to the biology of the diagnosis, and additive to other objective means to assess risk. Both NPs appear not only able to identify those at higher risk for adverse outcome, but their results interact with HF therapies such that their serial measurement may also inform success or failure of HF therapy changes. This therefore allows for BNP or NT-proBNP to act as targets for HF care, much as serum cholesterol is in a patient with hyperlipidemia.

In order to better understand the potential role of BNP or NT-proBNP for guiding chronic HF management, it is necessary to review several important topics, including factors influencing their concentrations, as well as how to interpret the prognostic information informed by their levels. This will be followed by a review of studies examining biomarker "guided" therapy, an interpretation of their results, and recommendations for application of BNP or NT-proBNP for HF care.

INTERPRETATION OF NATRIURETIC PEPTIDE VALUES IN AMBULATORY HEART FAILURE

Triggers of B-type Natriuretic Peptide or N-terminal Prohormone of Brain Natriuretic Peptide Release

The topic of NP release in patients with chronic HF is extensive, and exceeds the scope of this chapter; however, a review of certain concepts is worthwhile.

Physiologically, it is reasonable to consider the concentration of either BNP or NT-proBNP as being a sum total of two separate triggers: volume status and cardiac structure and function.

TABLE 1: Cardiac abnormalities associated with elevation of B-type natriuretic peptide or N-terminal prohormone of brain natriuretic peptide

Characteristic	
Myocardial processes	• Systolic dysfunction • Diastolic dysfunction • Fibrosis/scar • Hypertrophy • Infiltrative diseases
Valvular abnormalities	• Mitral stenosis, regurgitation • Aortic stenosis, regurgitation • Tricuspid regurgitation • Pulmonic stenosis
Cardiac chamber size	• Ventricular enlargement • Atrial enlargement
Filling pressures	• Atrial, ventricular • Pulmonary
Ischemic heart disease	• Coronary artery ischemia
Heart rhythm abnormalities	• Atrial fibrillation, flutter
Pericardial diseases	• Constriction, tamponade
Congenital abnormalities	• Shunts, stenotic lesions

It is well established that myocardial stretch consequent to volume status is an important trigger for release of NPs, and when interpreting the results for either BNP or NT-proBNP, clinicians should remember that a significant percentage of their release is triggered by filling pressures, particularly when very high values for either peptide are present (BNP >500 pg/mL, NT-proBNP >5,000 pg/mL). Importantly, however, it is well-established that filling pressures are only one trigger for BNP or NT-proBNP secretion. Of the wide variety of structural and functional cardiac abnormalities leading to the release of BNP or NT-proBNP (Table 1), each has significant prognostic importance and potential therapeutic interventions exist for their management; this begins to delineate how a clinician might specifically intervene in the context of an elevation of NP concentration. For example, abnormalities of left ventricular systolic function might be addressed with vasodilators or mineralocorticoid receptor antagonist (MRA) therapy, while heart rhythm abnormalities might better addressed with beta (β) blockers (BB).

How to Measure Natriuretic Peptides for Prognosis in Ambulatory Heart Failure

Both BNP and NT-proBNP represent the biomarker "gold standard" for prognostication in chronic HF, identifying risk across a wide range of adverse outcomes in HF, from pump complications to heart rhythm abnormalities.[2] While a single measurement of BNP or NT-proBNP provides useful prognostic data for such adverse outcomes, it is well established that serial measurement provides incrementally unique information.[3-5] Indeed, compared to a single point measurement, addition of subsequent measurement of BNP or NT-proBNP allows for the identification of changes in risk over time: some patients have a falling NP, which predicts a lower risk than a baseline value might suggest, while others develop a rising pattern, which predicts a higher likelihood for impending complications (Fig. 1).

The link between temporal trends in NP concentrations and outcome is quite important, as it implies the potential value of BNP or NT-proBNP for "monitoring" patients at each office visit. Indeed, recent guidelines imply the importance of serial measurement of BNP or NT-proBNP for this indication.[6]

Logically, one recognizes the importance of a stable NP concentration to identify those patients who are less likely to suffer progressive HF. For example, in the context of a low BNP or NT-proBNP and no change in clinical status, a low-risk situation is present, and as such standard imaging follow-up might be delayed or deferred as suggested.[5] In contrast, in those with a high or changing concentration, complications are more likely, and more careful monitoring would be recommended, with consideration for therapy adjustments.

Very importantly, the prognostic thresholds of BNP or NT-proBNP for adverse outcomes of all types have been identified, and while they are slightly different based on the outcome in question (such as pump events versus arrhythmia), in general, they tend to be lower than those values seen in patients with acutely decompensated HF.[3,7] For BNP, as indicated by Masson et al., it would appear that a concentration of approximately 125 pg/mL represents the point of increase in risk, while for NT-proBNP, repeated studies have more solidly established the value at 1,000 pg/mL. Above these risk thresholds, one may see a higher risk for adverse outcome directly proportional to the concentration of BNP or NT-proBNP, while below these levels the risk tends to be considerably lower.

Following extensive therapy titration and optimization of volume status, their BNP or NT-proBNP result may be considered the "dry" value. This "dry" NP value—ostensibly the best NP result a patient can reach—may be then used to assess risk for mortality and morbidity; if still elevated above prognostic thresholds, this finding is of considerable importance.

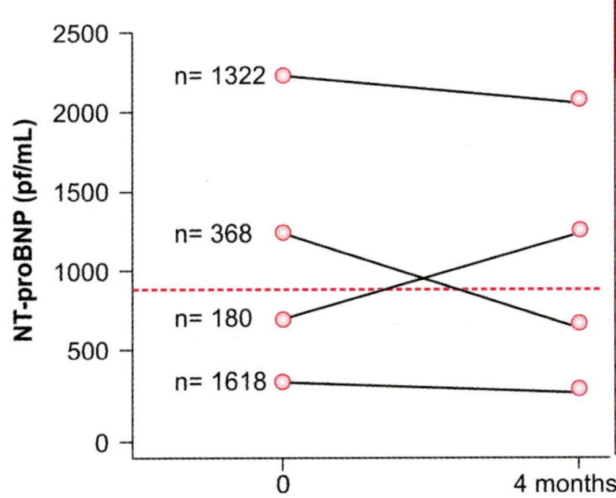

	Mortality (%)	Hospitalization for HF (%)
High→High	25.6	26.8
Low→High	17.2	21.1
High→Low	13.6	10.1
Low→Low	8.6	6.7

HF, heart failure; NT-proBNP, N-terminal prohormone of brain natriuretic peptide

Fig. 1 Trends in natriuretic peptide concentrations add considerably to a single value for prognostication

Source: Adapted from Masson S, Latini R, Anand IS, et al. Prognostic value of changes in N-terminal pro-brain natriuretic peptide in Val-HeFT (Valsartan Heart Failure Trial). *J Am Coll Cardiol.* 2008;52(12):997-1003, *with permission*

Interpreting B-type Natriuretic Peptide or N-terminal Prohormone of Brain Natriuretic Peptide Results in the Office: Understanding Changes in Concentrations and Timing of Measurement

When measuring biomarkers, it is common to see a rise and/or fall in the absence of an *obvious* pathologic process; when this change in the biomarker concentrations occurs, it is known as biological variability. In the case of NPs, biological variability is likely related to subtle changes in synthesis, as well as dynamic changes in cardiac filling pressures, pulmonary pressure, hemodynamics and changes in NP clearance, all of which may be entirely asymptomatic.

It is well established that in normal patients, the biological variability of BNP or NT-proBNP is high; this is because the values of BNP and NT-proBNP in patients unaffected by structural heart disease are very low. At these very low ranges of BNP or NT-proBNP concentrations, a substantial change must occur before a clinically relevant rise or fall may be identified; an example of such change is a 100% rise from a BNP of 10–20 pg/mL. Of course, on a clinical level, a doubling in this low range is considerably different than a doubling in the pathologic NP range that characterizes HF. Indeed, in patients suffering from HF, a biological variability of 25% for NT-proBNP and 40% for BNP is considered a substantial enough change to identify a biologically relevant shift in value.[8] Thus, a rise or fall in excess of these limits implies significant change in physiology. This point is particularly important to know when making decisions about drug therapy changes based on BNP or NT-proBNP values.

Another important topic relevant to serial testing is the amount of time after a physiologic change it takes for BNP or NT-proBNP to reach a new "steady state". While biological data are largely lacking in this regard, on a clinical level, it has been suggested that the largest prognostic value relative to changes in NT-proBNP values is observed at 2–4 weeks after a therapy change.[9] Accordingly, this identifies a timeframe when resampling may optimally occur.

Effect of Heart Failure Therapies on Natriuretic Peptide Concentrations

Therapies for HF directly affect the processes that contribute the rise of BNP or NT-proBNP; thus, it is well-established that many HF therapies lower the concentration of both BNP and NT-proBNP following their introduction or intensification (Table 2). These include, of course, loop diuretics, but also angiotensin-converting enzyme inhibitors (ACEI), angiotensin receptor blockers (ARB), ÂB, MRAs, exercise therapy and cardiac resynchronization therapy (CRT). In addition to drug therapy, BNP or NT-proBNP can also be lowered by exercise therapy and CRT, both important adjuncts to the care of the HF patient.[10]

TABLE 2: Therapies for heart failure that may lower B-type natriuretic peptide or N-terminal prohormone of brain natriuretic peptide values

Therapy	*Effect on BNP/NT-proBNP*
Diuresis (loop or thiazide)	↓
ACEI	↓
ARB	↓
β-blockers	Some transiently ↑, most ↓
MRAs	↓
Hydralazine/nitrates	↓
CRT	↓
Exercise	↓
Rate control of AF	↓

BNP, B-type natriuretic peptide; NT-proBNP, N-terminal prohormone of brain natriuretic peptide; ACEI, angiotensin-converting enzyme inhibitor; ARB, angiotensin receptor blocker; MRA, mineralocorticoid receptor antagonist; CRT, cardiac resynchronization therapy; AF, atrial fibrillation

NATRIURETIC PEPTIDES FOR GUIDING HEART FAILURE MANAGEMENT

The concept of utilizing a NP as a target for therapy was first examined more than a decade ago. In a seminal study,[11] the investigators demonstrated HF care "guided" by NT-proBNP was superior to that guided by a congestion score; in this study, efforts were made to suppress NT-proBNP values below a rather low target value were accompanied by a positive result, which sets the stage for understanding results of other trials that have followed, with various designs and target NP goals. Some of these trials have demonstrated benefit from biomarker-guided therapy[12-14] and others have not shown harm, but no benefit[15-20] (Table 3).

Before reviewing experiences gained from the studies performed, it is worthwhile to emphasize that whether positive or negative, pooled analyses of all the studies in the area (positive and negative) indicate a 20–25% adjusted reduction in mortality associated with biomarker-guided care on top of standard management,[22,23] while an

TABLE 3: Summary of biomarker-guided therapy studies

Studies/trials	*Age (years)*	*HFpEF?*	*Target natriuretic peptide (NP)?*	*Significant NP lowering?*	*More aggressive care in NP arm?*
Neutral studies					
STARBRITE[19]	60	No	BNP at hospital discharge (~ 450 pg/mL)	No	Yes
PRIMA[15]	72	Yes	NT-proBNP at hospital discharge	No	No
SIGNAL-HF[17]	78	No	NT-proBNP 50% below entry to the trial	No	No
UPSTEP[20]	71	No	BNP <150 pg/mL for <75 year old; <300 pg/mL for ≥75 years old	Not reported	No
Neutral studies with positive trends					
TIME-CHF[18]	77	No	NT-proBNP <400 pg/mL for age <75 year old and 800 pg/mL for age ≥75 year old	No	Yes
BATTLESCARRED[16]	76	Yes	NT-proBNP 1,270 pg/mL	No	Yes
Positive studies					
Troughton, et al.[11]	70	No	NT-proBNP 1,735 pg/mL	Yes	Yes
STARS-BNP[13]	65	No	BNP 100 pg/mL	Unknown	Yes
Berger et al.[12]	71	No	NT-proBNP 2,200 pg/mL	Yes	Yes
PROTECT[14,21]	63	No	NT-proBNP 1,000 pg/mL	Yes	Yes

HFpEF, heart failure with preserved ejection fraction; STARBRITE, Strategies for Tailoring Advanced Heart Failure Regimens in the Outpatient Setting: BRain NatrIuretic Peptide Versus the Clinical CongesTion ScorE study; BNP, B-type natriuretic peptide; PRIMA, Can PRo-brain-natriuretic peptide guided therapy of chronic heart failure IMprove heart fAilure morbidity and mortality study; NT-proBNP, N-terminal prohormone of brain natriuretic peptide; SIGNAL-HF, Study of NT-proBNP Guided Management of Heart Failure (Swedish Intervention study—Guidelines and NT-proBNP AnaLysis in Heart Failure); UPSTEP, Use of PeptideS in Tailoring hEart failure Project; TIME-CHF, Trial of Intensified vs Standard Medical Therapy in Elderly Patients With Congestive Heart Failure; BATTLESCARRED, NT-proBNP-Assisted Treatment To Lessen Serial Cardiac Readmissions and Death; STARS-BNP, Systolic Heart Failure Treatment Supported by BNP; PROTECT, ProBNP Outpatient Tailored Chronic HF Therapy

upcoming pooled analysis of the primary data indicate a 41% reduction in all-cause mortality in those less than 75 years of age (J Januzzi, Personal Communication).

Through the entire experience of the trials that have been executed in this area, more and more clarity is being gained about how biomarker-guided care may be of greatest value. Indeed, in retrospect, it is possible to understand why some trials failed, and others did not. With such an understanding it may be possible to inform where and how the approach may be best applied;[10,21] based on the experience gained, in order to be successful with BNP or NT-proBNP guided care.

A low natriuretic peptide target is necessary: Most of the negative trials typically chose BNP or NT-proBNP targets that were too high to improve outcomes in patients managed with guided therapy. For example, in the Strategies for Tailoring Advanced Heart Failure Regimens in the Outpatient Setting: BRain NatrIuretic Peptide Versus the Clinical CongesTion ScorE (STARBRITE) study,[19] the goal BNP value was near 450 pg/mL, with a nominal change by the end of the study (to 413 pg/mL), no different than biological variability. In addition to having inappropriately high NP targets, many negative trials, including STARBRITE, achieved no NP separation between the guided therapy and standard care arms, leaving the strategy of NP lowering untested.

Clearly, when using the approach, achievement of a proper target is necessary; notably, studies that achieved improved outcome associated with guided therapy, such as the Systolic Heart Failure Treatment Supported by BNP (STARS-BNP)[13] or ProBNP Outpatient Tailored Chronic HF Therapy (PROTECT) trial[14,24] a low target NP value was sought (BNP of 100 pg/mL and NT-proBNP of 1,000 pg/mL) and more often than not, achieved. To do so, therapy adjustments in the biomarker-guided arms were typically greater than the standard management arm.

Of note, one reason for neutral trials in this area was that the control arm received high-quality care with parallel suppression of the BNP or NT-proBNP in this arm of the study, frequently comparable to the unblinded arm.[16,20] Thus, a low posttreatment NP value is desirable, whether as a consequence of guided therapy or simply from excellent care. With this caveat in mind, in the

NT-proBNP-Assisted Treatment To Lessen Serial Cardiac Readmissions and Death (BATTLESCARRED) study, three arms were analyzed: (i) an NT-proBNP guided arm, (ii) an intensified arm treated by cardiologists, and (iii) a usual care arm. While there was no difference in mortality between the NT-proBNP guided arm and intensified treatment, a substantial reduction in mortality was noted when outcomes were compared between NT-proBNP and usual care arms, and by 3 years of follow-up, NT-proBNP guidance was the superior approach.

Beyond benefits on HF events, successful reduction in NP concentrations during HF therapy may be associated with collateral benefits on cardiac structure and function. Keeping in mind the large number of cardiac and structural correlates that determine BNP or NT-proBNP levels in HF, in one study, a strategy of aggressive NP lowering was accompanied not only by reduced cardiac events, but also substantial improvement in cardiac structure and function, with more reverse remodeling and improvements in diastolic function, pulmonary pressures, right ventricular size and function as well as less mitral regurgitation.[25]

Respect the prognostic value of BNP or NT-proBNP: A common scenario is that a patient may have an elevated BNP or NT-proBNP value, but their clinician feels "the patient is stable" and does not adjust their therapy. Experience has taught, again and again, that no matter how stable a patient with HF appears, when BNP or NT-proBNP are elevated above their prognostic threshold, a measurable and imminent risk is present. Ignoring such a powerful objective signal of risk increases the likelihood for a missed opportunity to improve outcome. Tellingly, in most of the negative trials, there was no difference in office visits between guided versus control arms,[15,17] whereas a trade-off of increased outpatient visits was seen in the successful studies. Disease management programs, with HF care delivered by nurse clinicians is one method for achieving the close follow-up that it sometimes takes to optimize care using biomarkers.[12]

It may take time and effort to lower BNP and NT-proBNP values: While the low BNP or NT-proBNP target values may seem unreachable in many patients, the successful trials of guided therapy would argue otherwise—the lesson learned is that it takes gradual drug titration and more office visits to achieve these goals. In the PROTECT study, one of the most thoroughly executed studies of NT-proBNP guided care to date, significant lowering of NT-proBNP was achieved in the biomarker-guided arm, but it required extraoffice visits compared to standard HF management.

When using biomarker-guided therapy, addition or uptitration of therapies should be based on treatment approach that reduce morbidity and mortality and done so with good clinical judgment: When titrating therapies to lower BNP or NT-proBNP in patients with left ventricular systolic dysfunction (LVSD), the approach should not be a primarily diuretic-driven strategy. While diuretics have a particularly potent effect to lower both NPs—particularly in the context of marked elevations of the biomarkers (BNP ≥500 pg/mL, NT-proBNP ≥5000 pg/mL)—titration of other agents such as vasodilators, BB, MRAs would be indicated first otherwise, as would be continuous reassessment of salt and water restriction, medication adherence, improvement of heart rhythm control for those with atrial fibrillation (AF), consideration for exercise prescription, as well as optimization of CRT.

In following this approach, studies not only suggest it is possible to improve care of patients using BNP or NT-proBNP through uptitration of agents other than loop diuretics (Fig. 2); in one study, NT-proBNP guided care allowed for the downward titration of loop diuretics,[14] a desirable outcome.

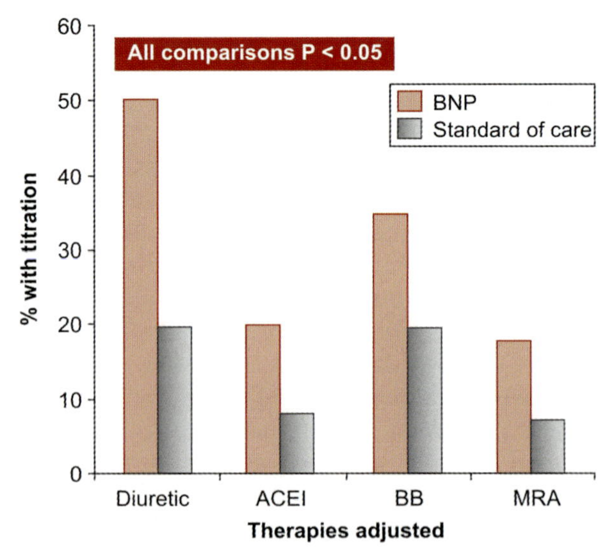

BNP, B-type natriuretic peptide; ACEI, angiotensin-converting enzyme inhibitor; BB, beta blockers; MRA, mineralocorticoid receptor antagonist

Fig. 2 Uptitration of heart failure medicines in the Systolic Heart Failure Treatment Supported by B-type Natriuretic Peptide (STARS-BNP) trial. As is the case in each biomarker-guided HF trial, BNP-guided care in this study led to significant upward adjustment of HF medicines

Source: Adapted from Jourdain P, Jondeau G, Funck F, et al. Plasma brain natriuretic peptide-guided therapy to improve outcome in heart failure: the STARS-BNP Multicenter Study. *J Am Coll Cardiol*. 2007;49(16):1733-9, *with permission*

Importantly, across all studies, BNP or NT-proBNP guided therapy did not lead to excessive risk for serious treatment-related complications consequent to mindless uptitration of therapies with subsequent therapy-related adverse outcomes; this reassures that clinicians did not use the result of the biomarker ignoring the rest of the information gained at the bedside, such as symptoms and vital signs. Thus, with confidence, it is fair to say biomarker-guided therapy does not replace clinical judgment—it supplements it.

Not all patients respond equally to biomarker-guided care: This says less about biomarker-guided HF care, and more about the varied responses patients show to therapeutic intervention in HF. Indeed, in practice, it is common to find patients in whom concentrations of BNP or NT-proBNP are lowered, but do not achieve the goal value, no matter how hard a clinician may adjust therapies. Aggregate experience would suggest that any lowering is better than no lowering at all; in two neutral trials, subjects that had a robust reduction in their NT-proBNP had improvement in outcome, despite the negative overall trial results.[15,20] Lending further support to this, in the PROTECT Study, a clear gradient of risk was present relative to achieved NT-proBNP values: that those patients achieving the target of 1,000 pg/mL had considerably lower risk than those at intermediate or higher values (Fig. 3).[26] While some patients achieved the goal value set in PROTECT and were maintained below it, others achieved the goal but only intermittently so, and others did not achieve it at all; those constantly below an NT-proBNP of 1,000 pg/mL had best outcomes, while those intermittently so had intermediate outcomes, and those with values constantly above it had the worst outcomes;[26] nonresponders also had the most deleterious ventricular remodeling.

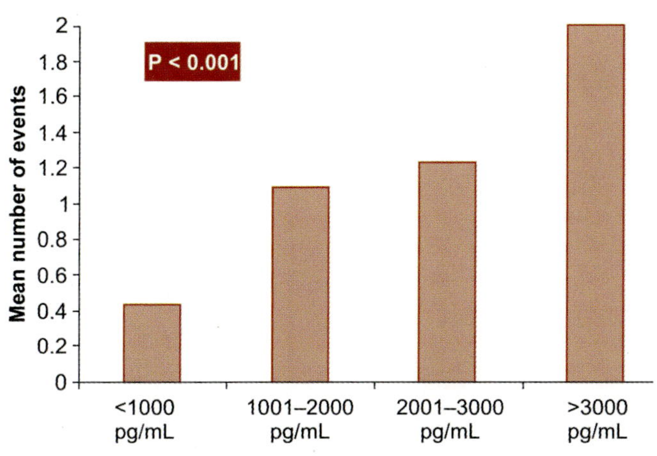

Fig. 3 Risk of adverse outcome as a function of achieved N-terminal prohormone of brain natriuretic peptide (NT-proBNP) value in the ProBNP Outpatient Tailored Chronic HF Therapy (PROTECT) study. A rising risk was observed above the target value of NT-proBNP ≤1,000 pg/mL

Source: Adapted from Januzzi JL, Rehman SU, Mohammed AA, et al. Use of amino-terminal Pro-B-type natriuretic peptide to guide outpatient therapy of patients with chronic left ventricular systolic dysfunction. *J Am Coll Cardiol*. 2011;58(18):1881-9, *with permission*

This concept of "therapeutic time in response" is very similar to that seen with respect to benefits predicted by international normalized ratio testing during vitamin K antagonist therapy,[27] where more time "in range" is associated with greater benefit, and provides a paradigm for discussing patients relative to the goal NP concentrations.

There may be specific groups that are less able to "respond" to biomarker-guided care. Based on the experiences from two of the larger studies of the approach,[16,18] a commonly held belief is that older patients benefit less than younger patients. In point of fact, this observation likely has less to do with the inadequacies of biomarker-guided therapy, and more to do with the effects of age on HF care. Intolerances to therapies are greater in older patients, and goal doses of drugs are less likely to be achieved as a consequence. Thus, compared to the younger HF patient, the elderly patient typically requires a thoroughly different approach to their management, with more gradual and careful drug titration. This is not to say that elderly patients absolutely cannot respond to biomarker-guided care; indeed, recent data from the PROTECT study would imply that elders not only responded to NT-proBNP guided care, it was the elders that had the greatest event rate reduction related to guided therapy, and drove the primary endpoint of the study[28] (Fig. 4). Presumably, the answer lays in how care is optimized in older subjects treated with guided therapy: more gradual care and careful uptitration may be needed in such patient. For example, in PROTECT, elders were seen considerably more frequently than younger patients to achieve intended biomarker reduction.

It is worth mention that in the Trial of Intensified vs Standard Medical Therapy in Elderly Patients With Congestive Heart Failure (TIME-CHF) study, a generally elderly patient population was studied; in this trial, the overall primary endpoint of all-cause death and all-cause hospitalization was not favorably affected by biomarker-guided care, but when examining secondary outcomes, such as cardiovascular (CV) death and hospitalization, a significant reduction in risk was observed.[18] The TIME-CHF investigators have recently reported that biomarker-guided care was cost-effective in the study.

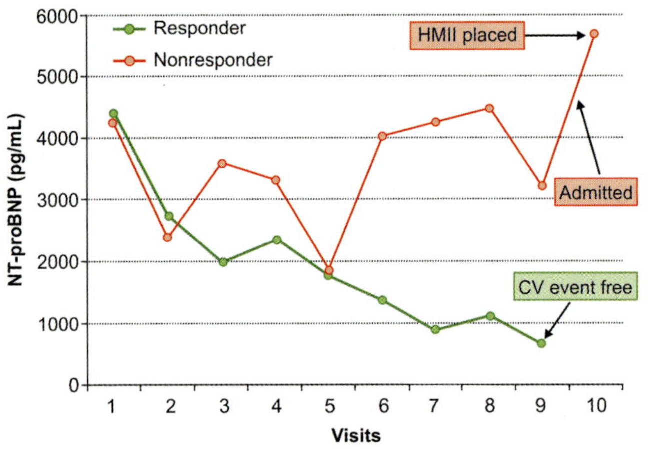

HM II, HeartMate II; CV, cardiovascular; NT-proBNP, N-terminal prohormone of brain natriuretic peptide

Fig. 4 Examples of two patients undergoing N-terminal prohormone of brain natriuretic peptide guided care in the ProBNP Outpatient Tailored Chronic Heart Failure Therapy (PROTECT) study. One patient is a nonresponder (in red), with high natriuretic peptide values and several cardiovascular events resulting in placement of a HeartMate II left ventricular assist device

Another important consideration is the effect of guided therapy on outcomes from HF due to LVSD versus heart failure with preserved ejection fraction (HFpEF). Given the lack of a clearly effective treatment strategy of care for those with HFpEF, it is reasonable to expect that guided therapy may be less effective in these patients. While clinical trials have not specifically addressed this question, those trials, including only those with LVSD have been particularly successful. This is not to say that certain patients with HFpEF may benefit from monitoring using BNP or NT-proBNP, but the fact remains that the therapeutic approach for HFpEF is unproven, and a biomarker-guided strategy for such patients is hard to articulate in a general sense.

If truly optimized, the "dry" BNP or NT-proBNP is an important data point to integrate into decision making. If a patient is truly managed as optimally as possible and still has a markedly elevated BNP or NT-proBNP, strong consideration for alternative therapeutic strategies—including invasive hemodynamic monitors, mechanical

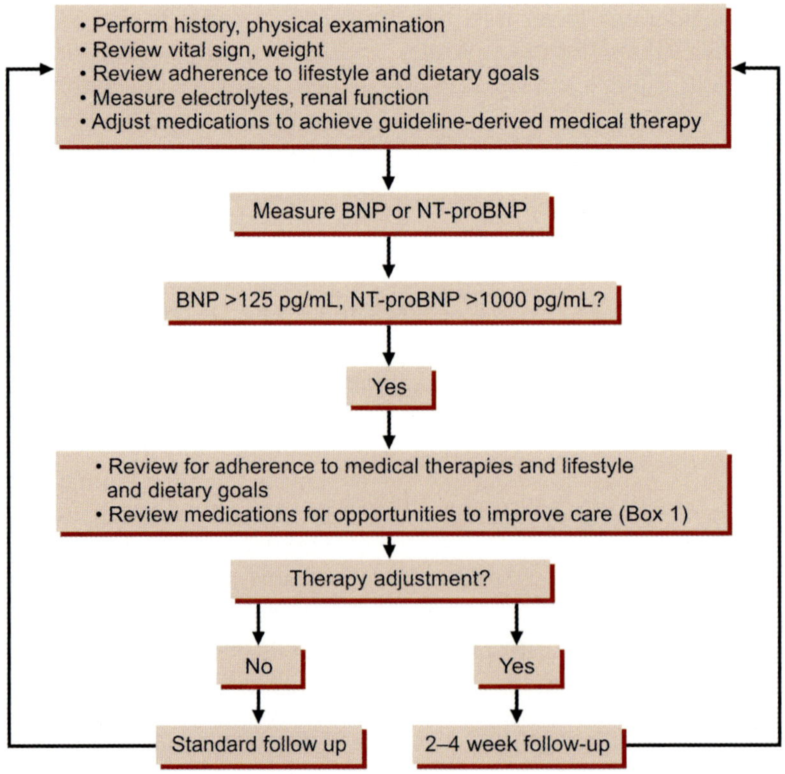

BNP, B-type natriuretic peptide; NT-proBNP, N-terminal prohormone of brain natriuretic peptide

Fig. 5 Suggested algorithm for use of biomarker-guided care in the outpatient setting; interventions as described in Box 1

Box 1: Clinical interventions to lower natriuretic peptide concentrations

- Uptitrate or add ACEI or ARB
- Uptitrate or add β-blocker (if not clinically congested)
- Uptitrate or add hydralazine/nitrates in African-American patients
- Increase loop diuretic dosage (especially if BNP >500 pg/mL or NT-proBNP >5,000 pg/mL)
- Add oral thiazide diuretic
- Add digoxin
- Consider adding ARB to ACEI (if not on MRA)
- Consider optimization of cardiac resynchronization therapy (if CRT device implanted)
- Uptitrate or add MRA if tolerated by renal function and potassium
- Consider hydralazine/nitrates in non-African-American patients
- Intensified or repeated heart failure (HF) education regarding diet, sodium restriction, etc.
- Reconsider potential indications for CRT (if not previously implanted)
- If in atrial fibrillation, maximize rate control or consider more aggressive attempts at normal sinus rhythm
- Consider exercise training or cardiac rehabilitation

ACEI, angiotensin-converting enzyme inhibitor; ARB, angiotensin receptor blocker; MRA, mineralocorticoid receptor antagonist; CRT, cardiac resynchronization therapy; AF, atrial fibrillation; BNP, B-type natriuretic peptide

support, cardiac transplantation, or palliative care initiation—would be reasonable, given the high likelihood for impending adverse outcome.

CONCLUSION

Biomarker-guided care of chronic HF using either BNP or NT-proBNP now has a sufficient evidence base to recommend its growing use. The available data would imply that when utilized in a manner consistent with successful clinical trials BNP or NT-proBNP guided care allows for safe optimization of HF therapies, and associated with significant reductions in adverse outcomes.

The potential interventions along with an algorithm for implementation of biomarker-guided care is displayed in Figure 5 and Box 1.

REFERENCES

1. Fonarow GC, Albert NM, Curtis AB, et al. Improving evidence-based care for heart failure in outpatient cardiology practices: primary results of the Registry to Improve the Use of Evidence-Based Heart Failure Therapies in the Outpatient Setting (IMPROVE HF). Circulation. 2010; 122(6):585-96.
2. Scott PA, Townsend PA, Ng LL, et al. Defining potential to benefit from implantable cardioverter defibrillator therapy: the role of biomarkers. Europace. 2011;13(10):1419-27.
3. Masson S, Latini R, Anand IS, et al. Prognostic value of changes in N-terminal pro-brain natriuretic peptide in Val-HeFT (Valsartan Heart Failure Trial). J Am Coll Cardiol. 2008;52(12):997-1003.
4. Cleland JG, McMurray JJ, Kjekshus J, et al. Plasma concentration of amino-terminal pro-brain natriuretic peptide in chronic heart failure: prediction of cardiovascular events and interaction with the effects of rosuvastatin: a report from CORONA (Controlled Rosuvastatin Multinational Trial in Heart Failure). J Am Coll Cardiol. 2009;54(20):1850-9.
5. Kubanek M, Goode KM, Lanska V, et al. The prognostic value of repeated measurement of N-terminal pro-B-type natriuretic peptide in patients with chronic heart failure due to left ventricular systolic dysfunction. Eur J Heart Fail. 2009;11(4):367-77.
6. McIntyre HF. Leveraging guidelines: understanding heart failure, organizing care. Commentary on the 2010 NICE chronic heart failure guideline update. Eur J Heart Fail. 2010;13(1):14-7.
7. Masson S, Latini R, Anand IS, et al. Direct comparison of B-type natriuretic peptide (BNP) and amino-terminal proBNP in a large population of patients with chronic and symptomatic heart failure: the Valsartan Heart Failure (Val-HeFT) data. Clin Chem. 2006;52(8):1528-38.
8. Araujo JP, Azevedo A, Lourenco P, et al. Intraindividual variation of amino-terminal pro-B-type natriuretic peptide levels in patients with stable heart failure. Am J Cardiol. 2006;98(9):1248-50.
9. Pascual-Figal DA, Domingo M, Casas T, et al. Usefulness of clinical and NT-proBNP monitoring for prognostic guidance in destabilized heart failure outpatients. Eur Heart J. 2008;29(8):1011-8.
10. Motiwala SR, Januzzi JL. The role of natriuretic peptides as biomarkers for guiding the management of chronic heart failure. Clin Pharmacol Ther. 2013;93(1):57-67.
11. Troughton RW, Frampton CM, Yandle TG, et al. Treatment of heart failure guided by plasma aminoterminal brain natriuretic peptide (N-BNP) concentrations. Lancet. 2000;355(9210):1126-30.
12. Berger R, Moertl D, Peter S, et al. N-terminal pro-B-type natriuretic peptide-guided, intensive patient management in addition to multidisciplinary care in chronic heart failure a 3-arm, prospective, randomized pilot study. J Am Coll Cardiol. 2010;55(7):645-53.
13. Jourdain P, Jondeau G, Funck F, et al. Plasma brain natriuretic peptide-guided therapy to improve outcome in heart failure: the STARS-BNP Multicenter Study. J Am Coll Cardiol. 2007;49(16):1733-9.
14. Januzzi JL, Rehman SU, Mohammed AA, et al. Use of amino-terminal Pro-B-type natriuretic peptide to guide outpatient therapy of patients with chronic left ventricular systolic dysfunction. J Am Coll Cardiol. 2011;58(18):1881-9.
15. Eurlings LW, van Pol PE, Kok WE, et al. Management of chronic heart failure guided by individual N-terminal pro-B-type natriuretic peptide targets: results of the PRIMA (Can PRo-brain-natriuretic peptide guided therapy of chronic heart failure IMprove heart fAilure morbidity and mortality?) study. J Am Coll Cardiol. 2010;56(25):2090-100.
16. Lainchbury JG, Troughton RW, Strangman KM, et al. N-terminal pro-B-type natriuretic peptide-guided treatment for chronic heart failure: results from the BATTLESCARRED (NT-proBNP-Assisted Treatment To Lessen Serial Cardiac Readmissions and Death) trial. J Am Coll Cardiol. 2009;55(1): 53-60.
17. Persson H, Erntell H, Eriksson B, et al. Improved pharmacological therapy of chronic heart failure in primary care: a randomized Study of NT-proBNP Guided Management of Heart Failure—SIGNAL-HF (Swedish Intervention study—Guidelines and NT-proBNP AnaLysis in Heart Failure). Eur J Heart Fail. 2010;12(12):1300-8.

18. Pfisterer M, Buser P, Rickli H, et al. BNP-guided vs symptom-guided heart failure therapy: the Trial of Intensified vs Standard Medical Therapy in Elderly Patients With Congestive Heart Failure (TIME-CHF) randomized trial. JAMA. 2009;301(4):383-92.
19. Shah MR, Califf RM, Nohria A, et al. The STARBRITE trial: a randomized, pilot study of B-type natriuretic peptide-guided therapy in patients with advanced heart failure. J Card Fail. 2011;17(8):613-21.
20. Karlström P, Alehagen U, Boman K, et al. Brain natriuretic peptide-guided treatment does not improve morbidity and mortality in extensively treated patients with chronic heart failure: responders to treatment have a significantly better outcome. Eur J Heart Fail. 2011;13(10): 1096-103.
21. Januzzi JL. Use of biomarkers to "guide" care in chronic heart failure: what have we learned (so far)? J Card Fail. 2011;17(8):622-5.
22. Felker GM, Hasselblad V, Hernandez AF, et al. Biomarker-guided therapy in chronic heart failure: a meta-analysis of randomized controlled trials. Am Heart J. 2009;158(3):422-30.
23. Porapakkham P, Porapakkham P, Zimmet H, et al. B-type natriuretic peptide-guided heart failure therapy: A meta-analysis. Arch Intern Med. 2010;170(6):507-14.
24. Bhardwaj A, Rehman SU, Mohammed A, et al. Design and methods of the Pro-B Type Natriuretic Peptide Outpatient Tailored Chronic Heart Failure Therapy (PROTECT) Study. Am Heart J. 2010;159(4):532-8.e1.
25. Weiner RB, Baggish AL, Chen-Tournoux A, et al. Improvement in structural and functional echocardiographic parameters during chronic heart failure therapy guided by natriuretic peptides: mechanistic insights from the ProBNP Outpatient Tailored Chronic Heart Failure (PROTECT) study. Eur J Heart Fail. 2013;15(3):342-51.
26. Gaggin HK, Truong QA, Rehman SU, et al. Characterization and prediction of natriuretic peptide "nonresponse" during heart failure management: results from the ProBNP Outpatient Tailored Chronic Heart Failure (PROTECT) and the NT-proBNP-Assisted Treatment to Lessen Serial Cardiac Readmissions and Death (BATTLESCARRED) study. Congest Heart Fail. 2013;19(3):135-42.
27. Cavallari LH, Limdi NA. Warfarin pharmacogenomics. Curr Opin Mol Ther. 2009;11(3):243-51.
28. Gaggin HK, Mohammed AA, Bhardwaj A, et al. Heart failure outcomes and benefits of NT-proBNP-guided management in the elderly: results from the prospective, randomized ProBNP Outpatient Tailored Chronic Heart Failure Therapy (PROTECT) study. J Card Fail. 2012;18(8):626-34.

Chapter 34

ST2: How to Really Do It Right

Lori B Daniels

ABSTRACT

ST2 is a marker of cardiomyocyte strain and is involved in the pathway leading to cardiomyocyte hypertrophy and fibrosis. Information gained from ST2 levels appears to be additive to natriuretic peptides, and is useful for prognosis in the settings of acute and chronic heart failure (HF). In both of these settings, measurement of ST2 now carries a class IIb recommendation in the recent American College of Cardiology/American Heart Association guidelines for the management of HF. Among inpatients with acute decompensated heart failure, "ST2 responders" (i.e., those whose ST2 levels fall at least 25% within 48 hours of treatment) have better outcomes than "nonresponders". In the setting of large myocardial infarctions, an ST2 level greater than 35 ng/mL may identify a subset of individuals more likely to benefit from therapy with a mineralocorticoid receptor antagonist. ST2 levels are also useful in the outpatient setting, where patients with chronic HF whose levels fail to drop by at least 25% within 2 weeks after a HF decompensation may identify a particularly high-risk subgroup who should be targeted for more aggressive medical titration and follow-up. ST2 levels may also be useful as part of a multimarker panel to identify individuals from the general population who are at high risk for development of HF and cardiovascular disease. Future studies will continue to clarify the optimal way to utilize ST2 levels in inpatient and outpatient settings, to maximize the clinical benefit for all those we treat.

INTRODUCTION

There are currently no randomized controlled trials prospectively evaluating the use of ST2, so whether the use of ST2 in any setting can truly improve outcomes is unknown. However, there is a growing body of observational studies showing consistent associations between higher ST2 levels with worse outcomes, and an emerging body of literature showing interactions between ST2 levels and specific treatments, such as aldosterone inhibitors. The following chapter, therefore, draws heavily upon the observational literature, and suggests ways, albeit currently unproven, that ST2 levels might be incorporated into clinical practice.

BACKGROUND

ST2 is a member of the interleukin (IL)-1 receptor-like family of proteins, and through alternative splicing is found in two isoforms, a membrane-bound form (ST2L) and a soluble form (sST2, hereafter denoted as ST2).[1-3] Cardiomyocytes and fibroblasts express ST2 in response to mechanical stress. The ligand for ST2 is IL-33, which is thought to protect against myocardial fibrosis, left ventricular (LV) hypertrophy and adverse cardiovascular remodeling in pressure-overload states.[4] Soluble ST2, which is the isoform measured by current assays, is thought to act as a decoy receptor. When high levels of sST2 are around, it binds IL-33 thereby leaving less IL-33 available to bind the membrane-bound ST2L. Thus, excess levels of sST2 are thought to limit activation of the beneficial cascade triggered by the IL-33/ST2L interaction.[5] Higher levels of sST2 (hereafter referred to simply as "ST2") are associated with increased myocardial fibrosis, cardiac remodeling and worse cardiovascular outcomes.[6]

HOW TO USE ST2 IN THE INPATIENT SETTING

Heart Failure

ST2 levels are prognostic in the setting of acute decompensated heart failure (ADHF), both in the emergency department (ED) and among inpatients. Among patients presenting to the ED with dyspnea, higher ST2 levels are associated with increased risk of 30-day and 1-year mortality and levels are synergistic with natriuretic peptides.[7-9] Using serial measurements of ST2 for those patients who go on to be admitted to the hospital may further refine a patient's risk category. A study out of Basel, Switzerland evaluated patients in the ED with acute dyspnea, and divided them into early "ST2 responders"—those whose ST2 levels fell by at least 25% at 48 hours—and nonresponders. In this study, being an early responder was associated with a lower risk of mortality at 1 year.[10] Similarly, a study from the Veterans Affairs San Diego Healthcare System of patients hospitalized with ADHF showed that those patients whose predischarge ST2 levels failed to drop by at least 15% compared to their admission level had a higher risk of death at 90 days.[11]

Based upon these studies and others, measurement of ST2 now carries a class IIb recommendation in recent clinical practice guideline updates from the ACC/AHA in ADHF (Level of Evidence A) and in chronic HF (Level of Evidence B).[12] A reasonable approach to patients presenting with ADHF in the ED would be to obtain an initial ST2 level in the ED or early upon admission in moderate or higher risk patients. Those patients with an ST2 level of 35 ng/mL or higher should be more closely monitored, especially if they also have elevated levels of natriuretic peptides or cardiac troponin.[13] For those who fail to show rapid clinical improvement, a second ST2 level at 48 hours or predischarge could be considered. If serial sampling shows a patient to be in a higher risk category, care should be given to ensure optimization of proven heart failure (HF) medications, with an emphasis on the inclusion of aldosterone blockers if the patient's potassium (K) level and renal function permit this. Serious consideration should also be given to following the patient very closely upon discharge, with home monitoring, phone calls, and/or an early follow-up visit.

Myocardial Infarction

ST-Elevation Myocardial Infarction

Several studies have reported an association between ST2 levels and prognosis in the setting of ST-elevation myocardial infarction (STEMI). Evaluation of data from the Thrombolysis in Myocardial Infarction (TIMI) 14 and TIMI 23 studies showed that ST2 levels peak at 12 hours after an acute MI, and higher ST2 levels were associated with a greater risk of development of new congestive HF or of death at 30 days.[14] ST2 levels above the median were also associated with increased risk of HF and cardiovascular death at 30 days in the Clopidogrel as Adjunctive Reperfusion Therapy-TIMI (CLARITY-TIMI) 28 trial, and ST2 levels improved risk stratification even in conjunction with N-terminal pro-B-type natriuretic peptide (NT-proBNP).[15] In addition to the benefit of ST2 levels early after STEMI, predischarge ST2 levels may also have prognostic value in STEMI patients. A recent study showed an association between higher predischarge ST2 levels and 30-day mortality that was independent of the Global Registry of Acute Coronary Events (GRACE) risk score and NT-proBNP levels.[16]

Baseline ST2 levels were associated with infarct size and left ventricular ejection fraction (LVEF) in a study evaluating data from the Effects of Eplerenone on Left Ventricular Remodeling Following Heart Attack (EPHESUS) trial, a study of post-MI patients (90% were STEMI's) with LV dysfunction who were randomized to either eplerenone or placebo.[6] A *post hoc* analysis from this study also suggested that baseline ST2 levels may be useful in determining which MI patients benefit most from aldosterone inhibition. Individuals with elevated ST2 levels were more likely to develop adverse ventricular remodeling, including increased LV end-systolic volume index and LV end-diastolic volume index, at 24 weeks. However, this adverse remodeling appeared to be attenuated in the group of high ST2 patients who were randomized to eplerenone, such that their LV parameters more closely matched those of patients with low ST2 levels. This study, albeit *post hoc*, sheds some light upon the potential use of ST2 levels in post-MI patients to help personalize medical therapy. Even though it has yet to be replicated prospectively, using ST2 to guide the use of aldosterone inhibitors may have a place clinically, since aldosterone inhibitors are already recommended

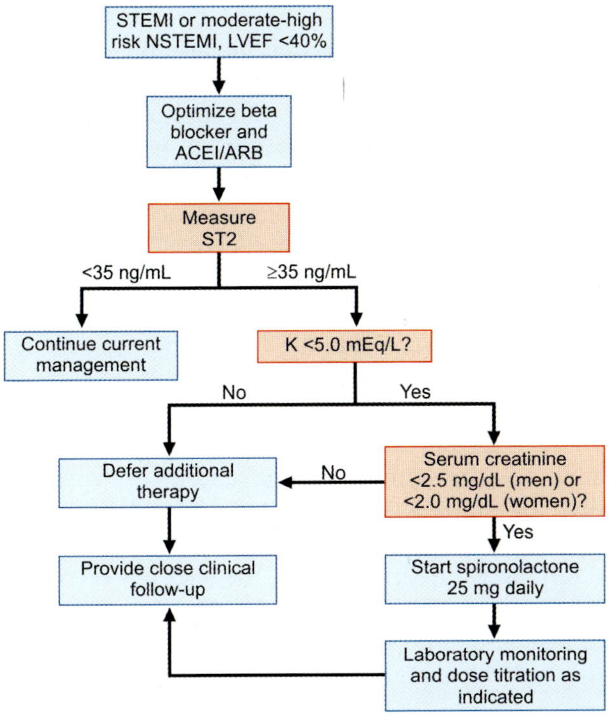

STEMI, ST-elevation myocardial infarction; NSTEMI, non-ST-elevation myocardial infarction; LVEF, left ventricular ejection fraction; ACEI, angiotensin-converting enzyme inhibitors; ARB, angiotensin receptor blocker

Flowchart 1 Algorithm for using ST2 in acute myocardial infarction patients

yet underutilized in this and other settings.[17] It may be such that an elevated ST2 level could provide that needed additional nugget of encouragement to convince physicians and patients that adding one more medication to their post-MI regimen is truly worth it. A proposed algorithm for how to use ST2 levels to help guide therapy after STEMI is shown in flowchart 1.

Non-ST-Elevation Acute Coronary Syndromes

There is less data and clinical experience with using ST2 levels in the setting of non-ST-elevation acute coronary syndrome (NSTEACS)/non-ST-elevation myocardial infarction (NSTEMI) compared with STEMI's, but for higher risk NSTEMI, the data and implications mirror those for STEMI. In fact, 10% of the patients enrolled in the EPHESUS trial, discussed above, were NSTEMI patients.[6] Other studies evaluating ST2 have generally focused on moderate- and high-risk NSTEMI patients, which make sense given the pathophysiology of ST2, whereby small/low-risk MI's are unlikely to cause marked elevation in ST2 levels. In the setting of moderate- to high-risk NSTEMI, ST2 levels do appear to be prognostic, as was shown in the Metabolic Efficiency With Ranolazine for Less Ischemia in Non-ST-Elevation Acute Coronary Syndromes-TIMI (MERLIN-TIMI) 36 trial.[18] In this study, ST2 levels over 35 ng/mL were associated with an increased risk of HF or cardiovascular death at both 30 days and 1 year. Thus, the recommendations for patients with a moderate- or high-risk MI are the same as those for STEMI (Flowchart 1). On the other hand, measurement of ST2 in the setting of unstable angina or low-risk NSTEMI is probably not warranted at this time.

HOW TO USE ST2 IN THE OUTPATIENT SETTING

Chronic Heart Failure

A number of studies have shown that higher ST2 levels are associated with worse prognosis in ambulatory patients with HF.[19-21] Although most studies have focused on patients with more severe, chronic HF, ST2 levels were also predictive of a higher risk of death at 1 year in a cohort of outpatients referred for echocardiogram for any reason.[22]

While single measurements of ST2 clearly provide prognostic information, there is growing evidence that the way to "really do it right" when it comes to outpatient monitoring of HF patients, is to follow serial levels of ST2. There is some precedent for using serial biomarkers to monitor and guide therapy in patients with chronic HF—natriuretic peptides have been used this way, and several studies have shown that this approach can lead to improved outcomes.[23-26] ST2 actually has lower biological variability than the natriuretic peptides, and may be a better marker to follow serially to guide therapy in outpatients with HF.[27] Among healthy individuals, Wu et al. showed that the long-term intraindividual variation of ST2 was only 11%. This variation, combined with the analytical variation of the assay, leads to a reference change value (RCV) of 30% for ST2, which is the amount by which the ST2 result would need to change in order to presume that the change is clinically relevant and not merely due to variation. This RCV is considerably lower than the value of approximately 100% for the natriuretic peptides, and can serve as a framework for interpreting serial ST2 levels in the outpatient setting.

Data from Wu et al. also suggest that, based upon its assay characteristics, comparing serial ST2 levels may be a better way to determine an individual patient's risk versus using a single value and comparing it to a reference ranges.[27] For example a patient whose ST2 level increases from 10 ng/mL to 20 ng/mL over several months (an increase of 100%) would be at increased risk of adverse events and likely has had progression of HF, even though both values are still within the suggested reference range for ST2.

Along these lines, a recent study of decompensated ambulatory HF patients evaluated the use of serial ST2 levels with measurements made at baseline and 2 weeks later, and found that a higher "ST2 ratio" (2 weeks/baseline) was associated with a higher risk of death, HF admission, or cardiac transplantation at 1 year, and performed better than a baseline ST2 level alone.[28] The optimal cutpoint for the ST2 ratio in this study was 0.75. Similarly, a study of patients with severe, chronic, ischemic HF showed that change in ST2 level at 2 weeks (but not baseline ST2 level) was associated with risk of mortality or need for cardiac transplant, independent of natriuretic peptides.[29] Thus, ST2 appears to be a sensitive measure of disease progression in chronic HF, even over a relatively short-time period. As such, the best way to assess risk in outpatients with HF seems to be to follow serial ST2 levels; those whose level fails to drop by at least 25% within 2 weeks after a decompensation are at higher risk (Flowchart 2).

One approach for patients with chronic, symptomatic HF after a recent acute exacerbation, especially in the setting of a reduced LVEF, is to measure a baseline ST2 level once beta-blocker, angiotensin-converting enzyme inhibitors (ACEI)/angiotensin receptor blocker (ARB), and loop diuretic therapies have been initiated. They may be especially important in individuals with persistently elevated natriuretic peptide levels, or conversely in patients who remain symptomatic despite natriuretic peptide levels that are relatively normal. If the baseline ST2 level is greater than or equal to 35 ng/mL, aldosterone inhibition with either spironolactone or eplerenone should be started unless contraindicated based upon renal function or serum potassium level. If the baseline ST2 level is less than 35 ng/mL, the level can be repeated in approximately 2 weeks. Failure to drop by at least 25% over this time period, despite adequate treatment with a beta-blocker, an ACEI or ARB, and a loop diuretic

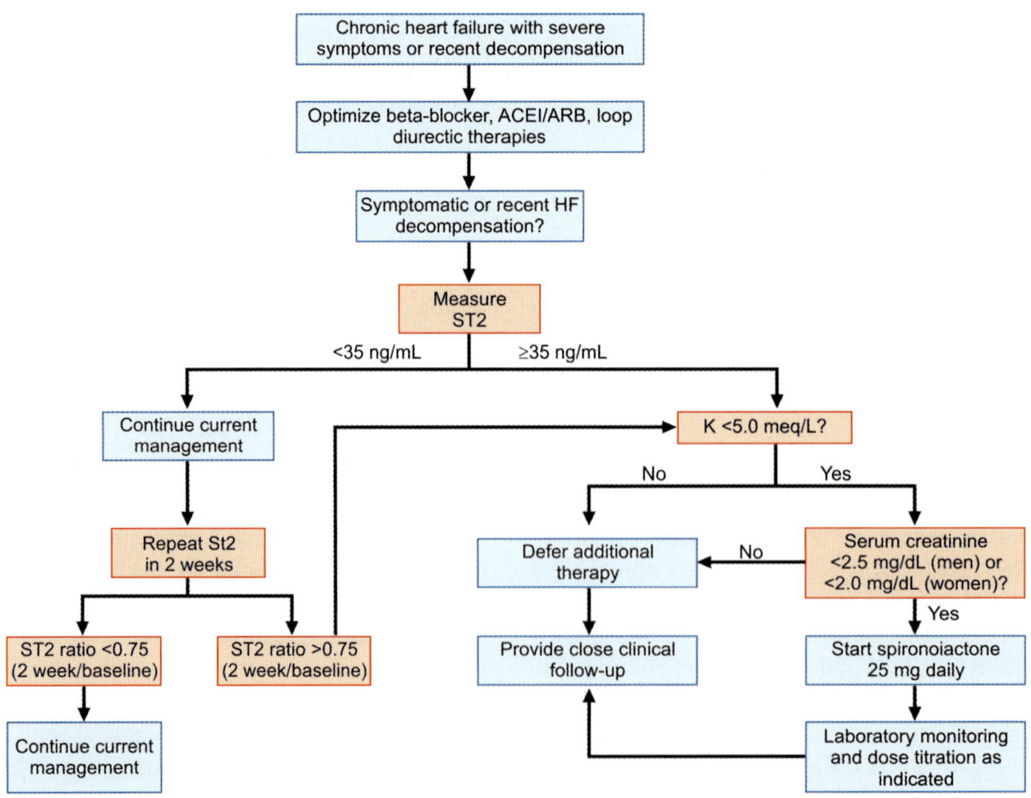

ACEI, angiotensin-converting enzyme inhibitors; ARB, angiotensin receptor blocker; HF, heart failure

Flowchart 2 Algorithm for using ST2 in chronic heart failure patients indicates a higher risk patient in whom aldosterone inhibition should also be considered, and closer clinical follow-up instituted.

Primary Prevention

Current methods of assessing cardiovascular risk in the community, which include assessment of traditional cardiovascular risk factors, can help identify a large percentage of individuals who will go on to develop cardiovascular disease, however, a significant portion still go undetected. Better ways of identifying those who are at risk could help improve preventive efforts, but how to do this remains elusive.

ST2, in conjunction with other novel cardiovascular biomarkers, may be one answer to this dilemma. Wang et al. recently reported that measurement of ST2 as part of a multimarker panel in conjunction with B-type natriuretic peptide (BNP), growth differentiation factor-15 (GDF-15), high-sensitivity troponin I, and high-sensitivity C-reactive protein (hsCRP) could help predict death, HF, and major cardiovascular events among ambulatory individuals followed for an average of 11 years.[30] As medicine moves toward a more personalized approach, it may be that using risk scores, such as this one, which incorporates markers that reflect abnormalities in several distinct pathologic pathways, can help physicians target their preventive efforts more accurately and thus more effectively.

CONCLUSION

ST2, though relatively new to the biomarker scene, has a growing body of evidence supporting its prognostic role for both inpatients and outpatients. To "really do it right", ST2 levels should be measured early in patients with STEMI or higher-risk NSTEMI to help guide therapy; on admission and, in higher risk patients, prior to discharge for patients with ADHF; and should be measured at least twice, approximately 2 weeks apart, in outpatients with symptomatic HF and a recent decompensation. ST2 levels are probably most useful in conjunction with other proven markers, such as natriuretic peptides, to identify truly high-risk patients. When ST2 levels are elevated or fail to fall by at least 25% over 2 weeks in a patient whose beta-blocker, ACEI (or ARB), and loop diuretic therapies are already apparently optimized, current data supports institution of aldosterone inhibition if renal function and serum potassium levels are acceptable. These individuals may also benefit from closer clinical follow-up. As more studies are completed in the coming years, further nuances are sure to emerge, along with new recommendations for how to tweak and optimize treatment regimens based upon ST2 levels. This is a rapidly changing field, with exciting possibilities for the continuing trend toward personalization of medical care.

REFERENCES

1. Kieser A, Goodnight J, Kölch W, et al. Identification of the primary growth response gene, ST2/T1, as a gene whose expression is differentially regulated by different protein kinase C isozymes. FEBS Lett. 1995;372(2-3): 189-93.
2. Yanagisawa K, Tsukamoto T, Takagi T, et al. Murine ST2 gene is a member of the primary response gene family induced by growth factors. FEBS Lett. 1992;302(1):51-3.
3. Tominaga S. A putative protein of a growth specific cDNA from BALB/c-3T3 cells is highly similar to the extracellular portion of mouse interleukin 1 receptor. FEBS Lett. 1989;258(2):301-4.
4. Schmitz J, Owyang A, Oldham E, et al. IL-33, an interleukin-1-like cytokine that signals via the IL-1 receptor-related protein ST2 and induces T helper type 2-associated cytokines. Immunity. 2005;23(5):479-90.
5. Sanada S, Hakuno D, Higgins LJ, et al. IL-33 and ST2 comprise a critical biomechanically induced and cardioprotective signaling system. J Clin Invest. 2007;117(6):1538-49.
6. Weir RA, Miller AM, Murphy GE, et al. Serum soluble ST2 a potential novel mediator in left ventricular and infarct remodeling after acute myocardial infarction. J Am Coll Cardiol. 2010;55(3):243-50.
7. Socrates T, deFilippi C, Reichlin T, et al. Interleukin family member ST2 and mortality in acute dyspnoea. J Intern Med. 2010;268(5):493-500.
8. Januzzi JL, Peacock WF, Maisel AS, et al. Measurement of the interleukin family member ST2 in patients with acute dyspnea: results from the PRIDE (Pro-Brain Natriuretic Peptide Investigation of Dyspnea in the Emergency Department) study. J Am Coll Cardiol. 2007;50(7):607-13.
9. Rehman SU, Mueller T, Januzzi JL. Characteristics of the novel interleukin family biomarker ST2 in patients with acute heart failure. J Am Coll Cardiol. 2008;52(18):1458-65.
10. Breidthardt T, Balmelli C, Twerenbold R, et al. Heart failure therapy induced early ST2 changes may offer long-term therapy guidance. 2013;pii: S1071-9164(13)01233-5.
11. Boisot S, Beede J, Isakson S, et al. Serial sampling of ST2 predicts 90-day mortality following destabilized heart failure. J Card Fail. 2008;14(9):732-8.
12. Yancy CW, Jessup M, Bozkurt B, et al. 2013 ACCF/AHA guideline for the management of heart failure: a report of the American College of Cardiology Foundation/American Heart Association Task Force on Practice Guidelines. J Am Coll Cardiol. 2013;62(16):e147-239.
13. Pascual-Figal DA, Manzano-Fernandez S, Boronat M, et al. Soluble ST2, high-sensitivity troponin T- and N-terminal pro-B-type natriuretic peptide: complementary role for risk stratification in acutely decompensated heart failure. Eur J Heart Fail. 2011;13(7):718-25.
14. Shimpo M, Morrow DA, Weinberg EO, et al. Serum levels of the interleukin-1 receptor family member ST2 predict mortality and clinical outcome in acute myocardial infarction. Circulation. 2004;109(18):2186-90.
15. Sabatine MS, Morrow DA, Higgins LJ, et al. Complementary roles for biomarkers of biomechanical strain ST2 and N-terminal prohormone B-type natriuretic peptide in patients with ST-elevation myocardial infarction. Circulation. 2008;117(15):1936-44.

16. Dhillon OS, Narayan HK, Khan SQ, et al. Pre-discharge risk stratification in unselected STEMI: is there a role for ST2 or its natural ligand IL-33 when compared with contemporary risk markers? Int J Cardiol. 2013;167(5):2182-8.
17. Albert NM, Yancy CW, Liang L, et al. Use of aldosterone antagonists in heart failure. JAMA. 2009;302(15):1658-65.
18. Kohli P, Bonaca MP, Kakkar R, et al. Role of ST2 in non-ST-elevation acute coronary syndrome in the MERLIN-TIMI 36 trial. Clin Chem. 2012; 58(1):257-66.
19. Broch K, Ueland T, Nymo SH, et al. Soluble ST2 is associated with adverse outcome in patients with heart failure of ischaemic aetiology. Eur J Heart Fail. 2012;14(3):268-77.
20. Ky B, French B, McCloskey K, et al. High-sensitivity ST2 for prediction of adverse outcomes in chronic heart failure. Circ Heart Fail. 2011;4(2):180-7.
21. Bayes-Genis A, de Antonio M, Galan A, et al. Combined use of high-sensitivity ST2 and NTproBNP to improve the prediction of death in heart failure. Eur J Heart Fail. 2012;14(1):32-8.
22. Daniels LB, Clopton P, Iqbal N, et al. Association of ST2 levels with cardiac structure and function and mortality in outpatients. Am Heart J. 2010;160(4):721-8.
23. Januzzi JL, Rehman SU, Mohammed AA, et al. Use of amino-terminal pro-B-type natriuretic peptide to guide outpatient therapy of patients with chronic left ventricular systolic dysfunction. J Am Coll Cardiol. 2011; 58(18):1881-9.
24. Troughton RW, Frampton CM, Yandle TG, et al. Treatment of heart failure guided by plasma aminoterminal brain natriuretic peptide (N-BNP) concentrations. Lancet. 2000;355(9210):1126-30.
25. Jourdain P, Jondeau G, Funck F, et al. Plasma brain natriuretic peptide-guided therapy to improve outcome in heart failure: the STARS-BNP Multicenter Study. J Am Coll Cardiol. 2007;49(16):1733-9.
26. Berger R, Moertl D, Peter S, et al. N-terminal pro-B-type natriuretic peptide-guided, intensive patient management in addition to multidisciplinary care in chronic heart failure a 3-arm, prospective, randomized pilot study. J Am Coll Cardiol. 2010;55(7):645-53.
27. Wu AH, Wians F, Jaffe A. Biological variation of galectin-3 and soluble ST2 for chronic heart failure: implication on interpretation of test results. Am Heart J. 2013;165(6):995-9.
28. Bayes-Genis A, Pascual-Figal D, Januzzi JL, et al. Soluble ST2 monitoring provides additional risk stratification for outpatients with decompensated heart failure. Rev Esp Cardiol. 2010;63(10):1171-8.
29. Weinberg EO, Shimpo M, Hurwitz S, et al. Identification of serum soluble ST2 receptor as a novel heart failure biomarker. Circulation. 2003;107(5):721-6.
30. Wang TJ, Wollert KC, Larson MG, et al. Prognostic utility of novel biomarkers of cardiovascular stress: the Framingham Heart Study. Circulation. 2012; 126(13):1596-604.

Chapter 35

Using Cardiac Troponin to Assist in the Management of Patients with Congestive Heart Failure—A Practical Guide

Affan Irfan, Wayne L Miller, Allan S Jaffe

ABSTRACT

Cardiac troponins (cTns) are sensitive and specific markers of cardiac injury. There is growing data that measurement will be helpful in patients with acute and/or chronic HF. Both the acute and subclinical injury in more chronic heart failure (HF) patients are easily detected with high sensitive troponin assays and there appears to be a relationship between elevations and outcomes. Unlike acute ischemic heart disease, the persistent myocyte injury in chronic HF patients not only allows assessment of prognosis but also may lead to insights that permit better selection of therapies, more facile monitoring of the response to treatment and lead to new therapies. This approach may allow physicians to screen populations at risk for HF, e.g., elderly and those on certain therapeutic cardiotoxic drugs. Combining cTn with other circulating biomarkers, most notably the natriuretic peptides are likely to be synergistic in all of these areas. Despite very convincing preliminary data, its clinical use remains ill-defined. In this chapter, we will explore how the use of cTns in patients with HF has evolved over time, and based on the available data and our clinical experience, we will make recommendations on how to use cTns clinically.

PATHOPHYSIOLOGY OF CARDIAC TROPONIN RELEASE IN PATIENTS WITH HEART FAILURE

Introduction

The cardiac troponins (cTn) regulatory complex is comprised of three proteins; cardiac cTnC (calcium-binding), cTnT (tropomyosin-binding), and cTnI (inhibitory) which regulate the calcium-mediated contractile interactions of actin and myosin. The cardiac isoforms of cTnT and cTnI are encoded by unique genes and thus are highly cardiac specific. The bulk of cTn protein is predominantly found structurally bound to other proteins intracellularly, with a small percentage more loosely bound (6–8% for cTnT and 3.5% for cTnI). This "early releasable" pool is thought to be responsible for the immediate detectable levels observed after acute cardiac injury. The release ratios (the percentage found in blood over the percentage depleted from the heart) for cTns are thought to be high.

There is controversy about whether cTn release requires death of cardiomyocytes from apoptosis and/or necrosis and/or autophagia. However, regardless of the mechanisms, ongoing cardiac injury appears to be a critical pathophysiological component in the progression of heart failure (HF). From a clinical perspective, it is impossible to distinguish one mechanism from another, and it is unclear if they have any differential impact on prognosis. Cardiac injury may be more overtly apparent in acute settings and more subtle, but just as important, in chronic HF where progressive loss of cardiomyocytes over time results in the progression of HF. The putative mechanisms for ongoing cardiac injury in HF have a multiplicity of potential causes (Fig. 1). Before cardiac cell death occurs, known problems occur in cell signaling, calcium handling, contractile protein isoform switching in myocytes and in the cytoskeleton. Damage may occur from oxidative stress, direct effects of sympathetic and renin-angiotensin system stimulation, cytokines and/or calpain-mediated stretch-induced proteolysis.

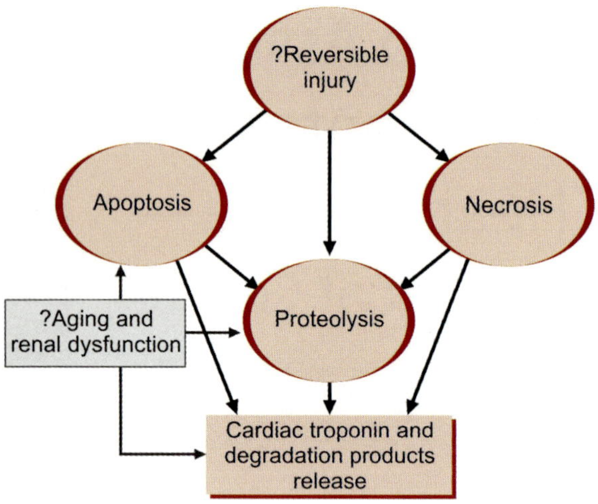

Fig. 1 Release of cardiac troponin from reversible injury, necrotic, and apoptotic myocardial cell death in heart failure

Finally, there is supply-demand imbalance in the subendocardium, which is largely dependent on left ventricular end diastolic pressure (LVEDP).

USING CARDIAC TROPONIN

In order to properly use cTn values, one must appreciate how to optimally utilize determinations. There has been great reluctance to embrace the increased sensitivity of cTn measurements because most of the elevations are not due to ischemic heart disease, as was the case in the past with creatine kinase MB (CKMB) and that provides a diagnostic challenge for clinicians. However, such an approach also obfuscates the important diagnostic and prognostic importance of the marker. Some quick rules for use include:

- The appropriate cutoff value for an abnormal cTn value is the 99th% of a upper reference limit (URL). The 99th% value represents roughly three standard deviations from the mean value and was chosen to minimize the overlap with normal subjects
- Having good precision at low levels allows for changing values to be more easily identifiable. However, having less than the recommended 10% coefficient of variation (CV) at the 99th% value does not cause false positive assessments and, as such, assays with less than ideal precision are useable unless imprecision exceeds 20%
- It is important to have some sense of the relative sensitivity of the assay that is being used in any given institution. Many assays developed years ago are still being used and there are many new very sensitive assays. Thus, the range of sensitivities in the clinical arena varies by more than a log unit. It should be recognized that many assays and especially point of care assays are egregiously insensitive and thus miss substantial numbers of elevations
- False positive and false negative results are uncommon but can occur. One should ask the laboratory to repeat values that do not fit with the clinical presentation of the patient. High values that continue over time with little change should evoke an evaluation for so-called heterophilic antibodies which is easily done by any laboratory using heterophile-blocking tubes (HBT) or with dilution studies. These problems will be more frequent with high-sensitivity assays where minor differences can be of importance
- An understanding of the range of values normally expected with any given clinical situation will help clinicians determine if consideration of other processes as well as the primary one can be helpful. For example, with chronic HF, the cTn elevations that occur tend to be modest. Thus, marked elevations should evoke additional scrutiny for other potential injurious processes
- The criteria for a changing pattern of values are unique to each assay and to the timing of the evaluations. This has not been elucidated as clearly as would be ideal in many of the publications reporting in this area. With contemporary assays (non-high sensitivity ones), analytical variation can be calculated by the laboratory to aid in this determination. We advocate that laboratory reports should include this information. With high-sensitivity assays, this determination is more complex and requires consideration of biological variation as well. More data are necessary with high-sensitivity cardiac troponin (hscTn) assays in this critical area. At present, we endorse the use of the guidelines recommended by the European Society of Cardiology (ESC) (Table 1)[1]
- Almost all high-sensitivity assays will require the use of gender specific cutoff values for the 99th% URL.

POSSIBLE MECHANISMS FOR ELEVATED CARDIAC TROPONIN IN PATIENTS WITH HEART FAILURE

A wide variety of causes can lead to cTn release in chronic and decompensated HF. Acute ischemic heart disease is a common cause of HF and thus, the concept that ongoing ischemia due to coronary artery disease could

TABLE 1: Recommended guidelines by European Society of Cardiology for the use of cardiac tropnin

- Any type of myocardial injury, not just ischemic injury, can result in release of cardiac troponin
- Cardiac troponin values should be interpreted relative to the clinical settings
- The 99th% URL is the value to consider abnormal. It should be understood that in some studies, there is some increased risk even at values below this value
- Scrutiny of the kinetics of troponin release in blood is essential to differentiate acute from chronic myocardial injury
- The interpretation of changes cannot be done in isolation from the clinical situation and particularly the timing of the event being evaluated
- If the timing of sample acquisition is consistent, laboratories can and should report changes that exceed analytic, and if relevant for very high-sensitivity assays, biological variation
- Patients with heart failure often have troponin elevations and can have a rising pattern of values. It can be difficult to distinguish these events from AMI on biochemical basis only
- Gender specific values for the 99th% URL will be necessary with high-sensitivity assays

URL, normal reference limit; AMI, acute myocardial infarction

occur is axiomatic. Such events could include both type 1 and type 2 acute myocardial infarction (AMI). Type 1 myocardial infarction (MI) is the spontaneous infarction that appears to occur due to acute plaque rupture and can manifest as ST-segment elevation myocardial infarction (STEMI) or non-STEMI. Type 2 MI encompasses other forms of ischemic cardiac injury, such as those due to hemodynamic compromise, for example due to tachycardia, hypo- or hypertension in patients with fixed coronary artery disease, events related predominantly to coronary endothelial dysfunction and/or vasospasm, and events due to severe increases in demand, such as severe tachycardia or severe hypertension. Data from EuroHeart Failure survey suggest that criteria for an acute coronary event may be present in up to 20% of acute HF patients. It is also worth appreciating that myocarditis has become a more widely recognized mimicker of acute ischemic heart disease and obviously can be the cause of or an exacerbant of HF. cTn elevations can be as high with acute myocarditis as values that are seen with STEMI or very low in patients with a less fulminant or even an indolent course. Nonetheless, having a high index of suspicion for this diagnosis is suggested.

In many, but not all studies, cTn elevations are similar between patients with ischemic and nonischemic etiologies of HF emphasizing the importance of other mechanisms and suggesting that cardiomyocyte injury may simply be a final common pathway. Acute preload-induced stretch leads to the release of cTn from cells dying eventually due to apoptosis. This may be an important mechanism in patients with HF and renal failure. In addition, there is a link between cTn release and integrin stimulation, which also may be relevant especially given the coagulation abnormalities intrinsic to both ischemic heart disease and poorly controlled HF. Recent data indicate that high intracardiac pressures (i.e., LVEDP), which reduces subendocardial blood flow at a time when oxygen demand is high leading to supply-demand imbalance, is the most important determinant of a gradient for hscTnT across the coronary sinus. Thus, although one is obligated to consider acute ischemic heart disease, whether type 1 or type 2 MI as possible etiologies of any given episode of decompensation in patients with HF, elevations of cTn, even those with a rising pattern in patients with HF do not in and of themselves mandate a diagnosis of AMI.

INITIAL CLINICAL STUDIES IN PATIENTS WITH HEART FAILURE

In 1995, Missov et al. were the first investigators to measure cTn in 11 end-stage HF patients and 11 control subjects. The initial studies measured cTnI using the first-generation assay (Sanofi Diagnostic Pasteur) that had epitopes directed towards the carboxyterminal sequence which was sensitive but had a limited window of detectability as these epitopes are cleaved rapidly in the blood. The same group then used a still more sensitive second-generation assay and measured cTnI in clinically stable patients with New York Heart Association (NYHA) Class III and IV HF (n = 35), health volunteers (n = 55) and hospitalized patients with no known cardiac disease (n = 25).[2] cTnI concentrations (mean ± standard error of mean) were more than double in HF patients (72.1 ± 15.8 pg/mL) compared to healthy (20.4 ± 3.2 pg/mL) and hospitalized control subjects (36.5 ± 5.5 pg/mL). The same cohort was also assessed with the first-generation assay and showed mean cTnI concentrations that were almost identical in all three groups. Thus, as with the initial studies, the more sensitive the cTn assay, the better the information. This trend still exists today. These results were then paralleled in another landmark study[3] by same group in 1999 with cTnT using the second-generation assay ES 300 system analyzer (Boehringer Mannheim now Roche). These preliminary data supported the hypothesis of ongoing cardiac damage in patients with HF and set the stage for the modern use of cTn in patients with HF.

The earliest evidence of association between cTn and the severity of HF was provided by Vecchia et al. using the Stratus II cTnI assay in 1997[4] in 26 consecutive inpatient and outpatient patients with nonischemic HF. Patients in the HF group with detectable cTn levels had significantly lower ejection fraction (EF), higher HF scores, worse NYHA classes, and higher mortality. Importantly, improvement in HF was associated with disappearance of detectable levels of cTnI. The prognostic value of cTnT was evaluated by Setsuta et al.[5] in chronic HF patients and yielded similar results. These studies were among the first to suggest cTns could be used to stratify patients into high- and low-risk groups for future adverse events. It also suggested for that first time that monitoring cTn might provide guidance concerning the efficacy of HF therapy. The association of cTnI and cTnT with worsening hemodynamics is also now well established. This issue was first studied in 2003 by Horwich et al. in advanced HF patients referred for cardiac transplantation.[6] Patients with detectable cTn values had significantly higher pulmonary artery and pulmonary capillary wedge pressures, lower cardiac indexes, and higher ventricular mass. Furthermore, there was a significant correlation between detectable levels of cTn and a progressive decline in EF over time.

DATA TO GUIDE USE IN PATIENTS WITH HEART FAILURE

Inpatient Use of Cardiac Troponins: Background and Recommendations

Since these early seminal descriptions, many reports have documented the substantial frequency of detectable levels of cTn and their use in the evaluation and risk stratification of patients with both ischemic and nonischemic HF. The largest data in acute decompensated HF emanated from the "Acute Decompensated Heart Failure National Registry (ADHERE)" study.[7,8] cTn I and T were measured (using several different immunoassays with varying upper reference values as measured by local laboratories) in 61,379 (cTnI) and 7,880 (cTnT) patients. The local values were considered positive in 3,253 patients (5.3%) and 1,035 patients (13.1%), respectively.[8] This is likely an underestimation given the reluctance of many clinicians to use the recommended cutoff values. Patients with elevated cTn had lower systolic blood pressures on

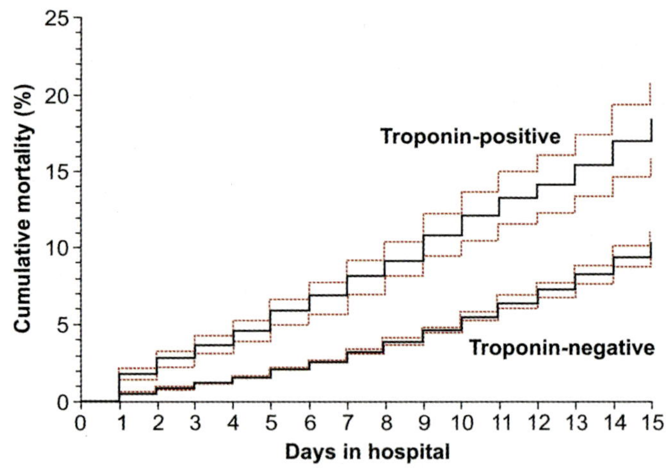

Fig. 2 Mortality according to number of days in the hospital and troponin status at presentation. P < 0.001 by the log-rank test. Dashed lines show 95% confidence intervals[7]

admission, lower EFs, and higher in-hospital mortality (8.0% vs. 2.7%, P < 0.001). The adjusted odds ratio for death in patients with an elevated cTn was 2.55 (95% confidence interval, 2.24–2.89; P < 0.001) (Fig. 2). Patients with HF of an ischemic etiology manifested similar findings to those with a nonischemic etiology for their HF, although the study was not designed to probe that question. Another report[7] from the ADHERE investigators evaluated the additive prognostic value of cTn and B-type natriuretic peptide (BNP) in more than 41,500 patients and showed that elevations of both cTnI or T and BNP were significantly associated with highest risk for mortality and that the combination was positively synergistic. Because of these types of data, cTn testing to evaluate the possibility of acute coronary syndromes precipitating HF hospitalizations was included in the 2009 American Heart Association (AHA)/American College of Cardiology (ACC) guidelines for heart failure management (Class I, Level of Evidence C).

There has been a wide range (6–80%) of reported prevalence of elevated cTn levels among patients hospitalized for HF even in those who are said to not have evidence of acute coronary syndrome. However, caution is warranted about this issue since comprehensive surveillance studies have not been done. These differences in prevalence are dependent on the selection of study patients (i.e., etiology of HF, NYHA class, EF, etc.) and also on the analytical properties of the immunoassays and their cutoff values used to define elevations. In general, most of the studies have used older generation and thus less sensitive assays for both cTnI and cTnT. In these types of studies, elevated cTn values are found in about 30–40% of acute HF patients. Invariably, these patients have an adverse prognosis. However, as seen in patients with acute coronary syndromes, when studies are done with "high sensitive" or "high sensitivity" assays, a much higher prevalence of elevated values (in the range of 80–90%) are seen. Not surprisingly, these newer assays are not only more sensitive but also provide more robust prognostic separation of patients at risk.

Serial measurements of cTn during hospitalization further assist in evaluating the severity of myocardial injury, the impact of therapy, and provide additional prognostic information in these patients. It has been suggested that targeting cTn levels would help in optimization of therapy and better salvage the myocardium at risk, but the data supporting such an approach is lacking at present. In hospital, serial measurements were first performed by the investigators of The Pilot Randomized Study of Nesiritide Versus Dobutamine in Heart Failure (PRESERVD-HF) in 2003 in 46 acute ischemic HF patients admitted for therapy.[9] The level of detection of immunoassays used was greater than 0.01 μg/L for cTnT (Roche Diagnostics) and greater than 0.03 μg/L for cTnI (Dade Stratus CS). Both cTnT and cTnI were unchanged from 0 to 32 hours, increased from 32 hours to 56 hours, then either plateaued (cTnT) or decreased to baseline levels (cTnI) through 80 hours. Thus, an increasing pattern of cTn should be expected to occur in these patients, making the distinction between acute HF and AMI potentially problematic.

Xue et al.[10] showed increased 90-day all-cause mortality and more frequent HF-related readmissions among 144 acute decompensated HF patients with a rising pattern of values and/or persistent elevations of high sensitive cTnI levels. This is the first study to use hscTn assays in the acute setting (Fig. 3). It is not clear from this report whether some or all of these patients had non-STEMI since the underlying substrate (i.e., coronary artery disease) was often present. It is, however, very likely that the finding of a rising pattern of values in HF patients will be common with hscTn assays. Unfortunately, the optimal change criteria with hscTn assays to differentiate between different causes are not yet defined. It is clear, however, that the change criteria will be assay- and population-dependent but it may or may not be similar to that derived for patients with acute ischemic heart disease.

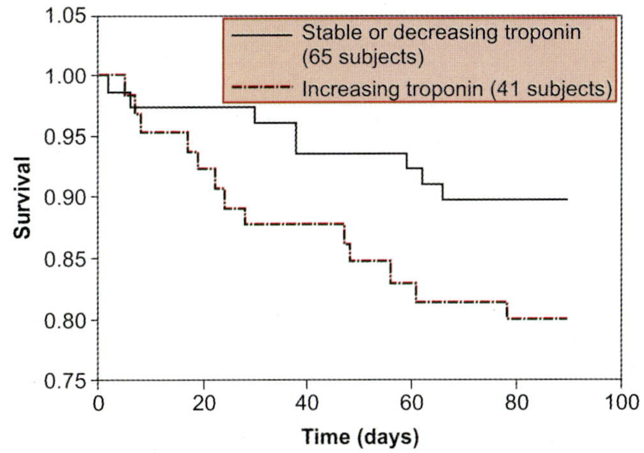

Fig. 3 Survival by increasing versus stable or decreasing troponin I. Mortality is signicantly increased in patients with increasing troponin I during serial measurements (P = 0.047, hazard ratio = 4.52)[10]

Recommendations for the Use of Cardiac Troponin in Hospitalized Patients

- Measurements of cTn are necessary whenever there is suspicion of acute ischemic heart disease
- The diagnosis of an acute ischemic event should not be made solely on the basis of cTn. cTn should be interpreted in proper clinical context
- A nonischemic etiology (e.g., tachycardia, hypotension) should be considered as a possible cause for elevated cTn values
- It is reasonable to serially measure cTn in all patients admitted with acute HF. A rising pattern and persistently elevated values are an adverse prognostic finding. However, the optimal change criteria to use or what exactly should be done to remediate this adverse prognosis has yet to be defined
- Patients with adverse prognosis, including those identified with elevated cTn, should be considered for more aggressive care and more aggressive outpatient surveillance (Flowchart 1).

Outpatient Use of Cardiac Troponins: Background and Recommendations

Elevated cTn levels have also been found in stable HF patients and seem to carry a significant independent short- and long-term high mortality risk. With high-sensitive assays, the prevalence of elevated cTn values

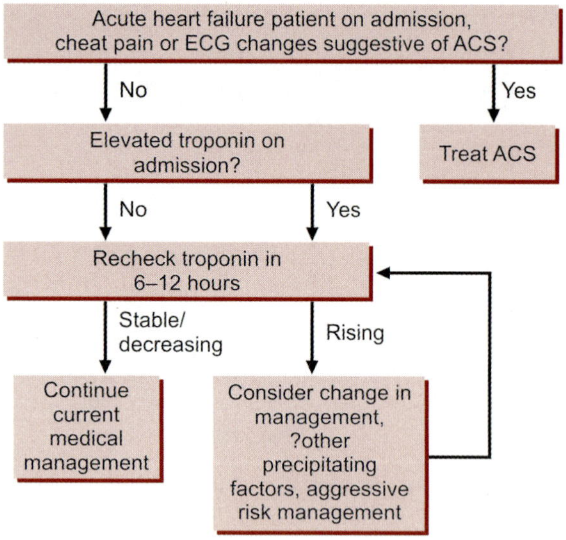

ECG, electrocardiogram; ACS, acute coronary syndrome

Flowchart 1 Clinical use of troponin testing in acute heart failure patients

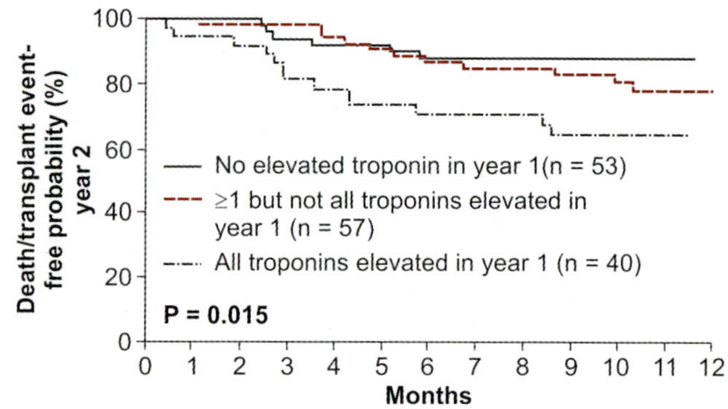

Fig. 4 Kaplan-Meier analysis of the risk of death or cardiac transplantation in year 2 based on cardiac troponin T patterns from year 1 of clinical follow-up[14]

greater than 99th percentile URL has been 50–90% compared to 10–50% with standard assays. Furthermore, similar to patients with acute decompensated HF, even low concentrations of high-sensitive cTn previously undetected by standard assays carries prognostic value in stable patients. The prognostic value of very low plasma concentrations of high-sensitive cTnT measured in patients with stable HF patients has been shown to be robust by Latini et al. from the Valsartan Heart Failure Trial (Val-HefT)[11] and others. With these hscTn assays, even deciles of risk can be determined. Like natriuretic peptides, high-sensitive cTn measurements should be considered as continuous variables across a spectrum of risk and not simply detectable or undetectable.

Serial cTn monitoring in stable patients also provides information allowing early identification of patients at risk of disease progression. This has been first demonstrated in 2003 by Ishii et al.[12] who measured cTnT with the third-generation assay and BNP in 100 consecutive HF patients at baseline (on admission) when treatment was initiated and then again after 2 months. They found significant decreases in cTn concentrations (from elevations in 60% at baseline to elevations in 35% at 2 months) together with improvement in left ventricular ejection fraction (LVEF), symptoms, and a decrease in BNP levels, suggesting the ongoing myocardial damage was at least partly suppressed by treatment. The patients with persistent elevations of cTn at 2 months were found to be at increased risk for mortality. In a 200-patient cohort study, Miller and colleagues have shown that changes in cTn but not natriuretic peptides are important predictors of prognosis. Specifically, increases in cTn predicted relatively short-term events.[13] Also persistent elevations of serial troponin in ambulatory HF patients were associated with increased risk of future events (Fig. 4).[14] It may well be that the cTn signal that occurs is similar to that seen in hospitalized patients but is less overtly symptomatic. The data suggest that cTn might be a good way to monitor patients and/or to direct therapy.[15]

With hscTn assays, these important initial observations have been confirmed. From first principle, one might expect that hscTn might be a better way to monitor patients than natriuretic peptides given it has a markedly lower biological variability. Recently, analyses from two large randomized clinical trials of 5,284 patients with chronic HF[16] seemed to confirm that speculation that changes over time (3–4 months) in the circulating levels of high-sensitive cTnT are associated with the severity and progression of HF and have a robust prognostic value (median follow-up time was >24 months). Similar results have been obtained with high-sensitive cTnI by other studies.

Recommendations for the Use of Cardiac Troponin in Outpatients with Heart Failure

- Elevated cTn values are associated with increased risk and thus such measurements are worth considering in chronic HF patients to help assess prognosis
- Specific therapeutic interventions in response to elevated cTn levels in these patients have not yet been defined

- Like natriuretic peptides, identifying a "baseline value" for cTn could help to distinguish chronic elevations from acute cardiac injury
- It is reasonable but unproven to measure cTn before and after starting medical therapy for HF management (including device therapy) to guide therapy
- Routine cTn measurements should be obtained in patients on medications known to cause cardiotoxicity (e.g., chemotherapeutic drugs) to provide early identification of patients at risk and to guide therapeutic interventions.

HEART FAILURE WITH PRESERVED SYSTOLIC FUNCTION

Even in patients with HF with preserved LVEF, elevations in cTn are prevalent and strongly associated with abnormal left ventricular (LV) relaxation, increased LV mass, and poor long-term and short-term outcomes. Recently, 500 consecutive HF patients with EF greater than or equal to 40% were reported by Perna et al.[17] cTnT measured with the third-generation immunoassay was abnormal in 44% of patients. Patients with elevated cTnT manifested lower LVEF values, higher serum creatinine values, a higher prevalence of a history of ischemic heart disease and diabetes mellitus, higher NYHA class, and higher natriuretic peptide levels. Not surprisingly, elevations were an independent factor for all-cause death and/or rehospitalization for acute HF. In another study by the same group involving 184 HF patients with normal ventricular function,[18] they observed that these patients had lower cTnT levels within 6 hours of admission compared with patients with systolic dysfunction, but cTnT values were comparable between the two groups by 24 hours.

As with HF with reduced EF (HFREF), hscTn assays are starting to be used in patients with HF and preserved EF (HFPEF). In a subgroup of 49 patients without coronary artery disease selected from 130 consecutive hospitalized patients referred to elective coronary angiography[19] hscTnT was detectable, at a level of 3.0 pg/mL or greater, in 87% patients and was greater than 99th% URL in 33%. This was in contrast with 65% detectability in patients with asymptomatic LV diastolic dysfunction group and 36% of the control subjects ($P = 0.017$). Importantly, elevations (>14 pg/mL) were found in only 15% of those with asymptomatic LV diastolic dysfunction group, and in 0% of the control group subjects ($P = 0.05$). HscTnT levels were significantly associated with the presence or more severity of diastolic dysfunction ($P < 0.001$).

Special Situations

Cardiac troponin has been used in experimental studies to evaluate not only cardiac but noncardiac medications (e.g., chemotherapeutic agents) suspected to cause cardiotoxicity and HF. Patients who, for example, receive adriamycin for the treatment of malignancy are known to manifest elevated levels of cTn, and it is that group which is most at risk for the subsequent development of HF. Similar findings have been reported with trastuzumab. Importantly, angiotensin-converting enzyme inhibitors not only reduce cTn values but reduce the propensity to the development of HF (Fig. 5).[20] Despite such convincing data with serial monitoring of cTn, we are still far from using serial cTns in daily practice for this purpose. Aarones et al.[21] have shown the ability of hscTnT to predict the response to cardiac resynchronization therapy with the lowering of values being associated with a better response, as there is not only huge variation in the interval of serial measurements in between studies but also little is known on how to decrease the risk once identified in these patients.

Studies in community populations and amongst subgroups of patients (e.g., those with chronic kidney disease) have shown strong independent associations between values of hscTnT and HF prevalence. Furthermore, several studies have observed that in select patients (e.g., the elderly) elevated hscTnT levels at baseline are independent predictors of HF (Fig. 6).[22] Furthermore, those with rising values are the ones most apt to develop HF.[20] One study[23] found hscTnT above the 99th percentile of healthy population among 36% of 470 elderly patients (age range 65–86 years) presenting with symptoms of HF. HscTnT and N-terminal pro-brain natriuretic peptide (NT-proBNP) measurements combined provided better prognostic information than using either biomarker separately in when these patients were symptomatic.

Because there are different 99% values for men and women with hscTn assays and different pathophysiologies with more HFPEF in women, it may be that women will require different cutoff values. Unfortunately, no studies specifically studying this issue have been reported. However, studies that have adjusted for age show more similar hscTn values in women than those that did not correct for age. Multivariate analyses have consistently shown only older age group and worsening renal function are correlated with hscTn levels in patients with HF and so at present, this issue remains a concern but one cannot make a data-driven recommendation.

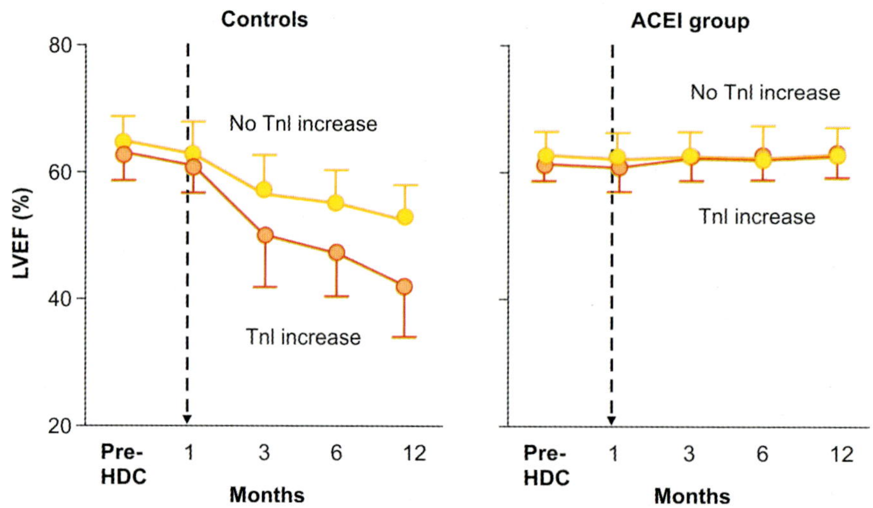

ACEI, angiotensin-converting enzyme inhibitor; LVEF, left ventricular ejection fraction; TnI, cardiac troponin I; HDC, high-dose chemotherapy

Fig. 5 Patients without elevations of cardiac troponin I did not manifest marked reductions in ejection fractions over time. Those with elevations in the control group did however. This decrease was ablated with the use of an angiotensin-converting enzyme inhibitor[20]

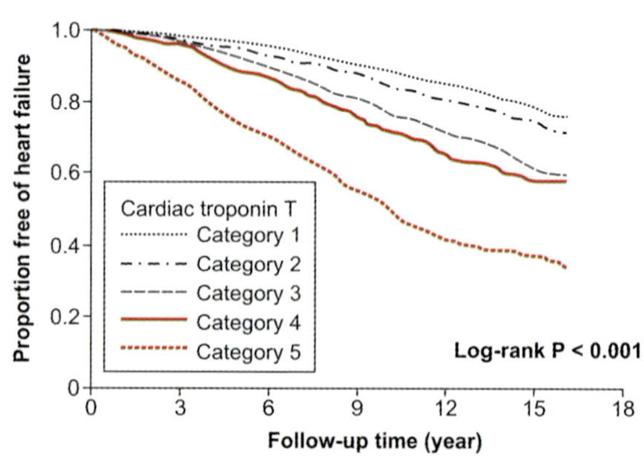

No. at risk

Category 1	1427	1380	1281	1131	956	763	461
Category 2	697	658	586	508	401	291	169
Category 3	700	642	550	435	333	231	131
Category 4	697	628	505	377	272	176	99
Category 5	700	532	357	213	119	77	36

Categories of high-sensitivity cardiac troponin T concentrations were divided into category 1 (<3.00 pg/mL), category 2 (3.00–5.44 pg/mL), category 3 (5.45–8.16 pg/mL), category 4 (8.17–12.94 pg/mL), and category 5 (>12.94 pg/mL).

Fig. 6 Kaplan-Meier curves reflecting cumulative proportion of older adults free of heart failure over time based on baseline high-sensitivity cardiac troponin T concentrations[22]

CONCLUSION

Using cTn in patients with HF is extremely attractive based on the available clinical information at present. Additional studies will be necessary to refine this ability and to develop the treatment algorithms necessary to make this a reality.

REFERENCES

1. Thygesen K, Mair J, Katus H, et al. Recommendations for the use of cardiac troponin measurement in acute cardiac care. Eur Heart J. 2010;31(18):2197-204.
2. Missov E, Calzolari C, Pau B. Circulating cardiac troponin I in severe congestive heart failure. Circulation. 1997;96(9):2953-8.
3. Missov E, Mair J. A novel biochemical approach to congestive heart failure: cardiac troponin T. Am Heart J. 1999;138(1 Pt 1):95-9.
4. La Vecchia L, Mezzena G, Ometto R, et al. Detectable serum troponin I in patients with heart failure of nonmyocardial ischemic origin. Am J Cardiol. 1997;80(1):88-90.
5. Setsuta K, Seino Y, Takahashi N, et al. Clinical significance of elevated levels of cardiac troponin T in patients with chronic heart failure. Am J Cardiol. 1999;84(5):608-11, A9.
6. Horwich TB, Patel J, MacLellan WR, et al. Cardiac troponin I is associated with impaired hemodynamics, progressive left ventricular dysfunction, and increased mortality rates in advanced heart failure. Circulation. 2003;108(7):833-8.
7. Fonarow GC, Peacock WF, Horwich TB, et al. Usefulness of B-type natriuretic peptide and cardiac troponin levels to predict in-hospital mortality from ADHERE. Am J Cardiol. 2008;101(2):231-7.
8. Peacock WF 4th, De Marco T, Fonarow GC, et al. Cardiac troponin and outcome in acute heart failure. N Engl J Med. 2008;358(20):2117-26.
9. Gheorghiade M, Gattis WA, Adams KF Jr, et al. Rationale and design of the pilot randomized study of nesiritide versus dobutamine in heart failure (PRESERVD-HF). Am Heart J. 2003;145(2 Suppl):S55-7.
10. Xue Y, Clopton P, Peacock WF, et al. Serial changes in high-sensitive troponin I predict outcome in patients with decompensated heart failure. Eur J Heart Fail. 2011;13(1):37-42.

11. Latini R, Masson S, Anand IS, et al. Prognostic value of very low plasma concentrations of troponin T in patients with stable chronic heart failure. Circulation. 2007;116(11):1242-9.
12. Ishii J, Cui W, Kitagawa F, et al. Prognostic value of combination of cardiac troponin T and B-type natriuretic peptide after initiation of treatment in patients with chronic heart failure. Clin Chem. 2003;49(12):2020-6.
13. Miller WL, Hartman KA, Burritt MF, et al. Serial biomarker measurements in ambulatory patients with chronic heart failure: the importance of change over time. Circulation. 2007;116(3):249-57.
14. Miller WL, Hartman KA, Burritt MF, et al. Profiles of serial changes in cardiac troponin T concentrations and outcome in ambulatory patients with chronic heart failure. J Am Coll Cardiol. 2009;54(18):1715-21.
15. Januzzi JL Jr, Filippatos G, Nieminen M, et al. Troponin elevation in patients with heart failure: on behalf of the third Universal Definition of Myocardial Infarction Global Task Force: Heart Failure Section. Eur Heart J. 2012;33(18):2265-71.
16. Masson S, Anand I, Favero C, et al. Serial measurement of cardiac troponin T using a highly sensitive assay in patients with chronic heart failure: data from 2 large randomized clinical trials. Circulation. 2012;125(2):280-8.
17. Perna ER, Aspromonte N, Cimbaro Canella JP, et al. Minor myocardial damage is a prevalent condition in patients with acute heart failure syndromes and preserved systolic function with long-term prognostic implications: a report from the CIAST-HF (Collaborative Italo-Argentinean Study on Cardiac Troponin T in Heart Failure) study. J Card Fail. 2012;18(11):822-30.
18. Perna ER, Macin SM, Cimbaro Canella JP, et al. Minor myocardial damage detected by troponin T is a powerful predictor of long-term prognosis in patients with acute decompensated heart failure. Int J Cardiol. 2005;99(2):253-61.
19. Dinh W, Nickl W, Futh R, et al. High sensitive troponin T and heart fatty acid binding protein: novel biomarker in heart failure with normal ejection fraction? A cross-sectional study. BMC Cardiovasc Disord. 2011;11:41.
20. Cardinale D, Colombo A, Sandri MT, et al. Prevention of high-dose chemotherapy-induced cardiotoxicity in high-risk patients by angiotensin-converting enzyme inhibition. Circulation. 2006;114(23):2474-81.
21. Aarones M, Gullestad L, Aakhus S, et al. Prognostic value of cardiac troponin T in patients with moderate to severe heart failure scheduled for cardiac resynchronization therapy. Am Heart J. 2011;161(6):1031-7.
22. de Filippi CR, de Lemos JA, Christenson RH, et al. Association of serial measures of cardiac troponin T using a sensitive assay with incident heart failure and cardiovascular mortality in older adults. JAMA. 2010;304(22):2494-502.
23. Alehagen U, Dahlstrom U, Rehfeld JF, et al. Prognostic assessment of elderly patients with symptoms of heart failure by combining high-sensitivity troponin T and N-terminal pro-B-type natriuretic peptide measurements. Clin Chem. 2010;56(11):1718-24.

Chapter 36

Biomarkers on the Horizon for Chronic Heart Failure

Christian Prinz

ABSTRACT

In patients with heart failure (HF), biomarkers like brain natriuretic peptide and N-terminal pro B-type natriuretic peptide are still the gold standard for prognostic and diagnostic information. However, biomarker testing is rapidly expanding. Biomarkers are reflecting pathophysiological events at a cellular level. New biomarkers like galectin-3, procalcitonin, and others can be used on its own or in combination in order to improve diagnostic accuracy, particularly when other clinical and diagnostic parameters seem unclear. Furthermore, it was demonstrated that monitoring biomarker levels can provide incremental information on disease progression. Therefore, future research seems required for improving diagnosis and treatment of HF patients.

INTRODUCTION

The diagnosis of chronic heart failure (CHF) is made clinically through the use of a detailed history, the physical examination, imaging studies and more recently biomarkers. Traditional biomarkers for HF, such as brain natriuretic peptide (BNP), N-terminal pro B-type natriuretic peptide (NT-proBNP) and high sensitivity troponin are currently the standards for assessing cardiac function in HF. While these markers do possess a great deal of prognostic and diagnostic information, new biomarkers have recently emerged that complement and provide additional information in the setting of CHF. This chapter aims to discuss how these newer biomarkers can be used to advance care in patients with heart disease.

TRADITIONAL BIOMARKERS

Brain Natriuretic Peptide

Brain natriuretic peptide is released by the ventricles under high pressures and significant amounts of volume stress, as in the setting of HF and HF exacerbations. BNP has been shown to increase diagnostic accuracy in this setting, providing strong negative and positive predictive values.[1] In patients presenting with shortness of breath a BNP level less than 100 pg/mL suggests that HF is unlikely, while a value of over 400 pg/mL is strongly indicative of HF.[1] When BNP values fall between these two cutoffs, further examination is required to exclude HF as the diagnosis. Thus, it can be said that BNP levels over 400 pg/mL, accompanied by physical examination findings and imaging studies, provide ample diagnostic evidence for congestive HF.

Brain natriuretic peptide also provides a great deal of prognostic information regarding patients with HF. Studies have shown that BNP levels at the time of discharge strongly correlate with mortality and hospital readmission at 6 months; it has also been demonstrated that for every 100 pg/mL increase in BNP levels, there is a 35% increased risk of death due to CHF.[2,3] This indicates that BNP levels can be used to predict which patients are at higher risk for future adverse events and thus require additional monitoring and follow-up. Additionally, BNP levels can be used as a guide for therapy, as demonstrated clearly by the Systolic Heart Failure Treatment Supported by BNP (STARS-BNP) trial.[4] It was determined that physician knowledge of patient BNP levels, along with physical examination findings, led to more optimization of medications, including the addition of angiotensin-converting enzyme (ACE) inhibitors, beta-blockers, and diuretics.[4]

B-type natriuretic peptide is currently considered the standard biomarker for HF and hypervolemia. It has diagnostic and prognostic qualities that are superior to other biomarkers presently available, and in addition, it can be used to tailor medication and guide medical management.

N-terminal Pro B-type Natriuretic Peptide

N-terminal pro B-type natriuretic peptide is the precursor to BNP and in normal patients is found at plasma levels similar to BNP. In the setting of HF like BNP, levels of NT-proBNP are highly elevated.[5] Unlike BNP diagnostic cutoffs of NT-proBNP can vary widely amongst age groups, for less than 50 years of age, 50–75 years of age, and greater than 75 years of age; they are 450 pg/mL, 900 pg/mL, and 1,800 pg/mL, respectively. Studies have shown that an NT-proBNP level lower than 125 pg/mL has a strong negative predictive value.[6] Unfortunately, NT-proBNP has been found to have a very low specificity and levels have been shown to be elevated in a variety of settings. One study demonstrated that NT-proBNP levels were elevated in patients with atrial fibrillation in the setting of preserved systolic function, while another demonstrated that patients in the intensive care unit (ICU) without acute coronary syndrome (ACS) or decompensated HF had a markedly increased level of NT-proBNP.[7,8] Thus, NT-proBNP may be highly useful in the exclusion of CHF, but it has less value as a true positive indicator of CHF.

NEW VALUABLE MARKERS

Galectin-3

Galectin-3 is a member of the lectin family of proteins and has been shown to be highly associated with fibrogenesis, and can be used as a fibrotic marker in the setting of HF.[9-11] Like many of the previous markers discussed, it has valuable prognostic values for patients with both acute and CHF. High levels of galectin-3 add to the prognostic value of subsequent HF morbidity and mortality, even to the extent that one galectin-3 measurement upon hospital admission can predict mortality out to 4 years regardless of echocardiogram findings and disease severity.[12-16]

In addition to its prognostic value, galectin-3 can also help predict which patients may rapidly progress to HF, thus aiding in risk stratification of HF patients, particularly when used in conjunction with BNP.[17] Doubling in G3 levels regardless of baseline has been shown to predict rapid progression of HF, particularly after ACS, eventually resulting in hospitalization or death.[18,19] This makes galectin-3 an ideal marker for identifying those patients that require closer follow-up and more thorough medical care. Galectin-3 can also be beneficial in determining how patients benefit from cholesterol-lowering therapy, in the Controlled Rosuvastatin Multinational Trial in Heart Failure (CORONA) trial levels of G3 helped identify those patients that would most likely benefit from treatment with statins. Galectin-3 is an attractive marker for HF in that it is able to further risk stratify patients when used with BNP, predict those patients that may rapidly progress to HF, identify those patients with likely adverse outcomes, and thereby help tailor pharmacologic therapy.

ST-2

The ST2 protein, also known as IL1RL1 (interleukin 1 receptor-like 1), is a member of the interleukin receptor family (IL-1). ST2 signaling is thought to be significant in regulating the myocardial response to overload in cardiac myocytes and stretched cardiac fibroblasts.[20-23]

A growing body of literature has emerged in the past decade indicating that ST2 is a novel biomarker in HF and that it can effectively be used to predict mortality in patients with acute and CHF. Januzzi et al. studied a group of nearly 600 patients with and without acute destabilized HF admitted into the emergency department with acute dyspnea. While ST2 concentrations did not predict HF as accurately as NT-proBNP, concentrations of ST2 were higher among patients with acute HF.[24] This indicates that ST2 can be used as an effective diagnostic biomarker of HF in conjunction with NT-proBNP.[24] Among the most striking findings in the study was the correlation between levels of ST2 and mortality risk within 1 year of the presentation of dyspnea. An ST2 level of less than 0.20 ng/mL was a strong predictor of mortality at 1 year suggesting strong prognostic value. This has been further corroborated by studies showing that elevated ST2 levels and associated changes in those levels correlate with higher mortality rates in acute and CHF.[25,26] Additional studies have shown a correlation between levels of ST2 and severity of HF, identifying ST2 as a potential resource for further risk stratification of the HF patient.[20] The recent evidence suggests that ST2 is a valuable biomarker in the prognosis, diagnosis, and risk stratification of patients with HF, and can be used to help improve medical management in those individuals.[27]

Procalcitonin

Procalcitonin is the precursor protein to calcitonin, a vital regulator of calcium homeostasis, and is released by parafollicular cells of the thyroid gland, and neuroendocrine cells of the lung and small intestine. Procalcitonin has been used as an indicator of infection, and has been shown to be helpful in determining the etiology of dyspnea in HF patients. Dyspnea is a common symptom of HF exacerbation, although many times it is unclear if hemodynamic collapse, an underlying infection, or a combination of the two is the cause of shortness of breath.

Procalcitonin has been shown to aid in the diagnosis of pneumonia in patients with acute HF exacerbation, potentially indicating if antibiotic treatment is required in these patients.[28] Additionally, procalcitonin has been shown to be predictive of infection post-cardiac surgery, with a serum concentration of greater than 10 ng/mL indicating septic shock.[29,30] Procalcitonin has been proven to be a valuable marker for determining the underlying etiology of dyspnea in the acute HF patient and can greatly aid in the management and care of these patients. It can prevent unnecessary antibiotic use, and may also indicate when additional pharmacology is needed in these patients.

Copeptin

Copeptin is the C-terminal portion of the protein pro-AVP (arginine vasopressin), the precursor to vasopressin. Because mature vasopressin is difficult to measure, copeptin is an attractive option for determining if the vasopressin system has been activated, particularly in those patients with HF. In the clinical setting, copeptin has been shown to be highly useful in adding prognostic information, optimizing medication and identifying high-risk patients with HF. Serial measurements of this peptide help predict adverse events in HF, particularly when combined with hyponatremia and adjusted for BNP and cardiac troponins.[31,32] This may help identify those patients that are at high risk for secondary complications attributed to their cardiac dysfunction.

In addition to identifying high-risk patients, copeptin has been shown to be helpful in determining various end-points for patients with cardiovascular disease. In patients with HF elevated copeptin levels were prognostic, independent of clinical variables, for an increase in 90-day all-cause mortality, hospital readmissions, and emergency department visits.[33-36] Some recent evidence even identifies copeptin as superior to BNP and NT-proBNP in predicting these outcomes, particularly after myocardial infarction.[37-41] Copeptin has also been shown to be useful in beta-blocker titration in patients with heart failure with reduced ejection fraction (HFrEF) where levels have been shown to reflect successful uptitration faster than NT-proBNP.[42] Current clinical evidence has shown that copeptin is a useful prognostic indicator in patients with HF, and as such its use should be considered in conjunction with traditional biomarkers of cardiac disease, such as BNP and troponin.

Midregional Proadrenomedullin

Midregional proadrenomedullin (MR-proADM) is the stable precursor peptide of adrenomedullin, a protein with presumed vasodilatory effects. Like many of the previous biomarkers discussed, MR-proADM has been shown to be very useful in the prognosis and risk-stratification of patients with HF. In patients presenting with shortness of breath caused by an acute HF exacerbation, plasma MR-proADM levels provided strong prognostic information for short- and long-term mortality, particularly when combined with NT-proBNP and copeptin.[43-46] Some evidence even suggests that MR-proADM may be prognostically superior to BNP and NT-proBNP in predicting mortality and morbidity, particularly in the setting of HF and an acute myocardial infarction.[47] Additional investigation of MR-proADM is required to further clarify its role in the clinical setting. However, the current research supports its use as a prognostic indicator for patients presenting with acute and CHF.[48]

High-sensitivity Cardiac Troponin

High-sensitivity cardiac troponin (hs-cTnT) is released by cardiac muscle after myocardial injury, and has been shown to be a valuable marker in the diagnosis of myocardial infarction soon after patient presentation when levels are greater than 0.01 ng/mL.[49] Recently this biomarker has also shown utility beyond the scope of myocardial infarction, particularly in the setting of HF. A recent study has demonstrated that levels of hs-cTnT correlated with cardiac dysfunction demonstrated by echocardiogram findings and high levels of natriuretic peptides. This identifies hs-cTnT as a potential diagnostic marker for patients with HF, especially when myocardial injury may be playing a role.[50,51]

As a prognosticator, hs-cTnT has also been shown to have valuable clinical utility. High levels of hs-cTnT have been shown to identify patients, with and without coronary artery disease, at risk of developing HF.[52,53] Once a HF diagnosis has been established, high levels of this biomarker have been shown to identify patients at risk for adverse cardiac events and poor outcomes.[49,54,55] Additionally, it has been shown to aid in risk stratification of HF patients, particularly when used in combination with other natriuretic peptides like NT-proBNP.[56] In correlating with disease severity hs-cTnT has been shown to be elevated along with left ventricular dysfunction, thus allowing further risk stratification and potentially aiding in medical management of HF.[51]

High-sensitivity cardiac troponin is commonly thought of as a biomarker used in the identification of myocardial injury after myocardial infarction. Although recent evidence has demonstrated that it has strong clinical use in the setting of HF. When additional information regarding cardiac dysfunction and HF is warranted hs-cTnT may prove very useful. It can aid in the risk stratification, diagnosis and prognosis of HF, and future use should be directed at incorporating this biomarker into all aspects of cardiac care, particularly in myocardial injury and cardiac dysfunction.

RENAL BIOMARKERS

Cystatin C

Cystatin C has classically been used as a marker for renal function, however recent evidence has shown that it can be used as a means of assessing cardiovascular disease. As cardiac function deteriorates, as in HF, the kidneys are often affected leading to kidney disease and injury. While many biomarkers are currently used to assess kidney function and status, high serum levels of these markers are detected only after symptoms and injury occur. Cystatin C is an emerging biomarker that has shown to be an easy estimate of renal function in the HF patient, and predicts risk of death and/or hospitalization superior to standard measures of renal function such as glomerular filtration rate and creatinine.[57-60] When assessing acute HF exacerbations cystatin C has also been shown to be superior to NT-proBNP in the assessment and prognosis of these patients.[61] Furthermore it is a strong predictor of adverse outcomes in chronic and acute HF even when renal function is preserved.[61-63] Cystatin C shows significant utility in the setting of cardiovascular disease with and without renal impairment, and can help further risk stratify, prognosticate and assess renal function in HF patients even when symptoms may not be apparent.

Neutrophil Gelatinase-associated Lipocalin

Many patients with HF suffer from secondary problems, particularly renal dysfunction. Traditionally, estimated glomerular filtration rate (eGFR) and creatinine levels have been used to assess renal function, although recently neutrophil gelatinase-associated lipocalin (NGAL) has emerged as a promising new biomarker for identifying kidney injury in the setting of HF. NGAL is a protein that has been shown to be released into the blood and urine 2 hours after renal tubular injury.[64] Thus, it is an excellent biomarker for acute kidney injury (AKI) and has been used as a diagnostic and prognostic indicator for patients with HF.

As a diagnostic tool it has been demonstrated that NGAL is elevated in patients with CHF and was associated with elevated NT-proBNP and BNP levels.[65] NGAL levels at admission are strongly correlated with mortality and AKI in patients with acute HF even when other renal parameters, such as eGFR appear normal.[66-68] Additional studies have found similar findings for patient discharge, with elevated NGAL levels strongly predicting 30-day outcomes for renal injury and cardiac events.[69] Another advantage to using NGAL as a biomarker for kidney injury in the setting of HF is that NGAL levels may rise prior to kidney injury, providing a warning for AKI.[70]

The role of NGAL as a biomarker has traditionally been reserved for nephrology, although recent evidence shows that it can be beneficial in the prognosis and diagnosis of HF and other cardiac conditions with secondary renal problems. In the setting of acute decompensated HF, NGAL levels should be attained to detect early signs of kidney injury and determine patient prognosis in the hopes of better patient management and care.

Kidney Injury Molecule-1

Kidney injury molecule-1 (KIM-1) is a transmembrane protein found in the proximal tubule, released by cells due to various renal injuries, such as acute tubular necrosis or end-stage renal failure (1-minal). KIM-1 is seen in high levels in association with other renal biomarkers of AKI such as NGAL and serum creatinine. Because KIM-1 is associated with AKI it has been identified as a potential marker for cardiorenal syndrome and thus may identify tubular injury in patients with CHF, even when kidney function and eGFR appear normal.[71,72] KIM-1 also shows utility in the administration of diuretics, where it has been shown to increase after diuretic withdrawal and as a result may identify patients that require continuing diuresis to prevent kidney injury and dysfunction.[73] KIM-1 is a new and useful biomarker in identifying AKI and diuretic administration; it should be used in the setting of HF to identify potentially dangerous renal damage secondary to cardiac dysfunction thus preventing future adverse outcomes. In the future, additional research may be able to predict renal injury in cardiac patients based off risk factors and urinary markers like KIM-1 before the renal injury augments.

OTHER BIOMARKERS

C-reactive Protein

C-reactive protein (CRP) is an acute phase plasma protein that is regularly produced by the liver.[74] During a systemic response to inflammation, CRP levels are upregulated by inflammatory cytokines such as IL-6, and tumor necrosis factor alpha.[74] In many past studies, CRP has been associated with HF disease severity and prognosis, high levels of CRP have been shown to be predictive of adverse outcomes in cardiovascular disease.[75-80]

Previous studies have demonstrated CRP's role in cardiovascular disease. One study showed that levels of CRP are elevated in both nonischemic and ischemic patients admitted with HF and levels of CRP were directly related to New York Heart Association (NYHA) class.[74,81] HF patients with elevated CRP levels were also found to be at a greater risk of hospitalization during the 18-month follow-up period when compared to patients with normal CRP levels.[74]

There is undoubtedly potential for CRP in the diagnosis, prognosis, and risk stratification in HF patients. It can be used in tandem with well-established neurohormonal markers for greater resolution of outcomes in HF patients. It has been demonstrated in a study that CRP and BNP levels combined identified a high-risk group with a tendency for poor outcome not discriminated by cardiac function.[82] There should also not be any concern regarding the measurement of CRP, which is already standardized without requiring special collection procedures. The association of CRP levels with adverse outcomes in heart disease and ease of testing make it a possible biomarker in the future for the risk stratification and therapy guidance in HF patients.[83]

Carbohydrate Antigen-125

Carbohydrate antigen-125 (CA-125) is a high molecular weight soluble glycoprotein synthesized by epithelial serosal cells.[84-86] Elevated CA-125 levels are found in ascitic, pleural, or pericardial fluid of patients with cardiac failure, correlating with NYHA stages of cardiac failure, severity of clinical symptoms and short-term prognosis.[84,87] CA-125 is currently recognized as a promising biomarker for HF.

Additionally, multiple studies have demonstrated the relation of CA-125 to HF prognosis. Serum CA-125 has been reported as an independent predictor of short-term mortality upto sixth months.[88] It has also been reported that serum levels of CA-125 are elevated in parallel to natriuretic peptides in patients with CHF adding additional prognostic information and risk stratification, particularly when used in combination with one another.[89,90] In general, serum levels of CA-125 are associated with severity of CHF and have also been shown to be an independent predictive marker for rehospitalizations.

Due to the wide availability, additional prognostic utility beyond other biomarkers and sustained changes over time, CA-125 may be useful for the diagnosis and prognosis of HF, especially when combined with natriuretic peptides values.[91,92] However, there are limitations to the use of CA-125. Studies have reported that these markers demonstrate low sensitivity and low specificity to disease.[93,94] Baseline levels also vary across age and gender, so reference limits must be established in each of these groups.[94] CA-125 demonstrates the potential to help improve risk stratification and guide therapeutic decisions in HF patients.

Growth Differentiation Factor 15

The cytokine growth differentiation biomarker-15 is a stress responsive biomarker that is important in inflammatory and apoptotic pathways.[95] While not a uniquely cardiac biomarker, it has been demonstrated to have a role in the setting of cardiovascular disease. In the setting of HF levels of growth differentiation factor 15 (GDF-15) has been shown to have strong prognostic value. In particular, it can be used to identify healthy individuals and those with acute coronary disease, who have a high likelihood of developing latent HF.[96,97] GDF-15 has also demonstrated clinical utility as a diagnostic marker for HF; particularly systolic dysfunction [heart failure with preserved ejection fraction (HFpEF)], and in some cases

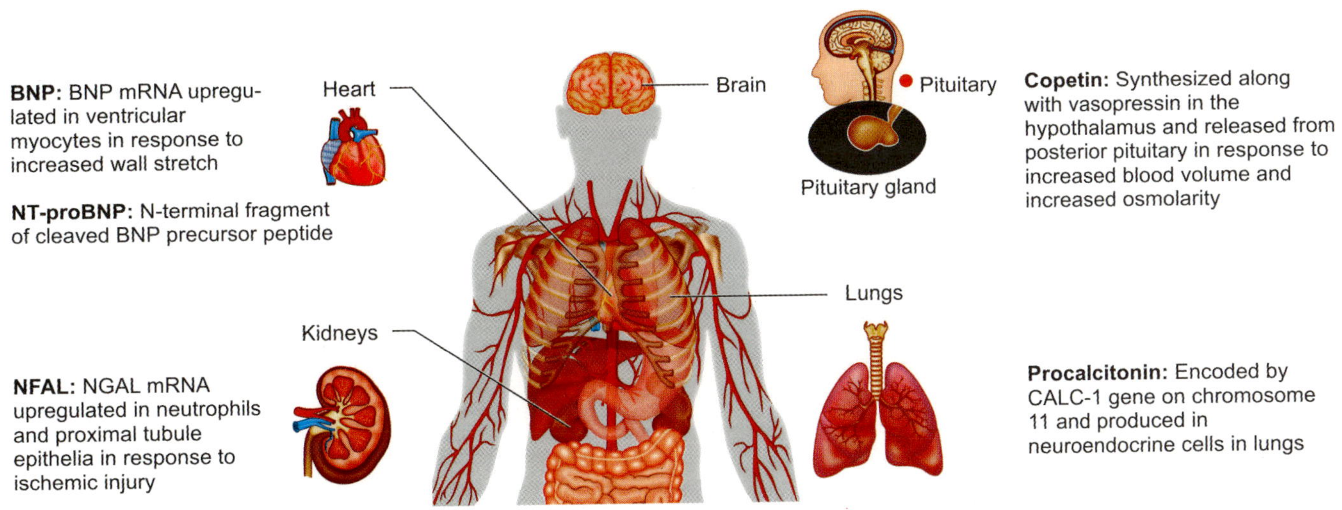

BNP, brain natriuretic peptide; mRNA, messenger ribonucleic acid; NT-proBNP, N-terminal pro-B-type natriuretic peptide; NGAL, neutrophil gelatinase-associated lipocalin

Fig. 1 The different organs of origin, clinical utility and clinical strength for each biomarker

has been shown to be superior to NT-proBNP.[98-100] Additionally, when risk-stratifying patients with HF, GDF-15 can be used to identify high-risk patients, as levels of this biomarker have been shown to correlate with worsening stages of HF.[101,102] GDF-15 shows promise as a useful biomarker in cardiovascular disease, and can be used in conjugation with other biomarkers to aid in the prognosis, diagnosis and risk stratification of HF patients.

Endothelin-1

Endothelin (ET) is a family of potent, long-acting vasoconstrictors of endothelial origin.[103,104] Cavero et al. first presented the relationship between ET and HF in a model of CHF in anesthetized canines, which showed increased circulating concentrations of ET-1.[104] Additional studies in humans have demonstrated that patients with HF had higher circulating levels of ET-1 compared to control subjects.[105-107] These same studies also showed that levels of ET-1 were directly correlated with the severity of HF and other cardiac parameters like right atrial pressure and left ventricular ejection fraction.[107] In addition to valuable diagnostic information, ET-1 has been shown to be a predictor of increased mortality. One study demonstrated that a plasma ET-1 level higher than 5 pg/mL was correlated with higher mortality rates in patients with ischemic and nonischemic cardiomyopathy.[108] ET-1 shows promise as a prognostic and diagnostic biomarker, particularly in the setting of HF, and may soon become further integrated into the clinical setting.

CONCLUSION

The utilization of biomarkers in the field of medicine is becoming increasingly more important as we transition toward preventative medicine. Ongoing research and evidence demonstrates that these markers can be used to predict poor outcomes and disease progression prior to the onset of symptoms and terminal disease. This makes their use paramount particularly in the setting of HF, where disease often progresses rapidly with high rates of morbidity and mortality. Biomarkers like BNP and NT-proBNP are still the gold standard for prognostic and diagnostic information in HF, however, other biomarkers have also been shown to be highly useful in the management, diagnosis, and treatment of this disease.[109] While further research is required to clarify their role in the clinical setting, biomarkers like NGAL, galectin-3, procalcitonin, and others can be used to aid in the diagnosis of HF patients when other parameters seem unclear (Fig. 1 and Table 1).

TABLE 1: The different organs of origin, clinical utility, and clinical strength for each biomarker previously discussed in this chapter, with four "+" signs indicating high clinical strength and one "+" sign indicating low clinical strength[109]

Biomarker	*Organ of origin*	*Clinical use*	*Clinical strength*
BNP/NT-proBNP	Heart	Hypervolemia Heart failure • Exacerbation • Diagnosis • Prognosis • Risk stratification • Guided therapy	++++
Galectin-3	Multiple	Identification of fibrosis Heart failure • Prognosis • Risk stratification • Guided therapy	+++
ST-2	Heart	Heart failure • Risk stratification • Diagnosis • Prognosis • Guided therapy	+++
Procalcitonin	Thyroid gland and small intestine	Heart failure • Identification of secondary infection/ pneumonia	+++
Copeptin	Brain	Heart failure • Prognosis	++
MR-proADM	Kidney/adrenal gland	Heart failure • Prognosis	++
High-sensitivity cardiac troponin	Heart	Myocardial injury Heart failure • Diagnosis • Prognosis • Risk stratification	+++
Cystatin C	Kidney	Assessment of renal function Heart failure • Prognosis • Risk stratification	++
NGAL	Kidney	Renal tubule Injury/acute kidney injury (AKI)	++
KIM-1	Kidney	Identification of AKI Marker for cardiorenal syndrome Identification of need for additional diuretic	++
C-reactive protein	Liver	Inflammation Heart failure • Diagnosis • Prognosis • Risk stratification	+
Carbohydrate antigen-125	Multiple	Heart failure • Prognosis • Identification of disease severity	+

Contd...

Contd...

Biomarker	*Organ of origin*	*Clinical use*	*Clinical strength*
Growth differentiation factor-15	Multiple	Heart failure • Prognosis • Diagnosis • Risk stratification	+
Endothelin	Kidney	Heart failure • Prognosis • Diagnosis	+

BNP, brain natriuretic peptide; NT-proBNP, N-terminal pro B-type natriuretic peptide; MR-proADM, midregional proadrenomedullin; NGAL, neutrophil gelatinase-associated lipocalin; KIM-1, kidney injury molecule-1

REFERENCES

1. Maisel A. B-type natriuretic peptide levels: diagnostic and prognostic in congestive heart failure: What's next? Circulation. 2002;105(20):2328-31.
2. Aspromonte N, Valle R, Peacock WF, et al. Inpatient monitoring and prognostic importance of B-type natriuretic peptide. Congest Heart Fail. 2008;14(4 Suppl 1):30-4.
3. Gopal DJ, Iqbal MN, Maisel A. Updating the role of natriuretic peptide levels in cardiovascular disease. Postgrad Med. 2011;123(6):102-13.
4. Jourdain P, Jondeau G, Funck F, et al. Plasma brain natriuretic peptide-guided therapy to improve outcome in heart failure: The STARS-BNP multicenter study. J Am Coll Cardiol. 2007;49(16):1733-9.
5. Betti I, Castelli G, Barchielli A, et al. The role of N-terminal PRO-brain natriuretic peptide and echocardiography for screening asymptomatic left ventricular dysfunction in a population at high risk for heart failure. The PROBE-HF study. J Card Fail. 2009;15(5):377-84.
6. Januzzi JL, van Kimmenade R, Lainchbury J, et al. NT-proBNP testing for diagnosis and short-term prognosis in acute destabilized heart failure: an international pooled analysis of 1256 patients: the International Collaborative of NT-proBNP study. Eur Heart J. 2006;27(3):330-7.
7. Letsas KP, Filippatos GS, Pappas LK, et al. Determinants of plasma NT-pro-BNP levels in patients with atrial fibrillation and preserved left ventricular ejection fraction. Clin Res Cardiol. 2009;98(2):101-6.
8. Shah KB, Nolan MM, Rao K, et al. The characteristics and prognostic importance of NT-ProBNP concentrations in critically ill patients. Am J Med. 2007;120(12):1071-7.
9. Sharma UC, Pokharel S, van Brakel TJ, et al. Galectin-3 marks activated macrophages in failure-prone hypertrophied hearts and contributes to cardiac dysfunction. Circulation. 2004;110(19):3121-8.
10. Liu YH, D'Ambrosio M, Liao TD, et al. N-acetyl-seryl-aspartyl-lysyl-proline prevents cardiac remodeling and dysfunction induced by galectin-3, a mammalian adhesion/growth-regulatory lectin. Am J Physiol Heart Circ Physiol. 2009;296(2):H404-12.
11. Lin YH, Lin LY, Wu YW, et al. The relationship between serum galectin-3 and serum markers of cardiac extracellular matrix turnover in heart failure patients. Clin Chim Acta. 2009;409(1-2):96-9.
12. van der Velde AR, Gullestad L, Ueland T, et al. Prognostic value of changes in galectin-3 levels over time in patients with heart failure: data from CORONA and COACH. Circ Heart Fail. 2013;6(2):219-26.
13. Ho JE, Liu C, Lyass A, et al. Galectin-3, a marker of cardiac fibrosis, predicts incident heart failure in the community. J Am Coll Cardiol. 2012;60(14):1249-56.
14. Ueland T, Aukrust P, Broch K, et al. Galectin-3 in heart failure: high levels are associated with all-cause mortality. Int J Cardiol. 2011;150(3):361-4.
15. Tang WH, Shrestha K, Shao Z, et al. Usefulness of plasma galectin-3 levels in systolic heart failure to predict renal insufficiency and survival. Am J Cardiol. 2011;108(3):385-90.
16. Shah RV, Chen-Tournoux AA, Picard MH, et al. Galectin-3, cardiac structure and function, and long-term mortality in patients with acutely decompensated heart failure. Eur J Heart Fail. 2010;12(8):826-32.
17. Fermann GJ, Lindsell CJ, Storrow AB, et al. Galectin 3 complements BNP in risk stratification in acute heart failure. Biomarkers. 2012;17(8):706-13.
18. McCullough PA, Olobatoke A, Vanhecke TE. Galectin-3: A novel blood test for the evaluation and management of patients with heart failure. Rev Cardiovasc Med. 2011;12(4):200-10.
19. Grandin EW, Jarolim P, Murphy SA, et al. Galectin-3 and the development of heart failure after acute coronary syndrome: Pilot experience from PROVE IT-TIMI 22. Clin Chem. 2012;58(1):267-73.
20. Rehman SU, Mueller T, Januzzi JL. Characteristics of the novel interleukin family biomarker ST2 in patients with acute heart failure. J Am Coll Cardiol. 2008;52(18):1458-65.
21. Shimpo M, Morrow DA, Weinberg EO, et al. Serum levels of the interleukin-1 receptor family member ST2 predict mortality and clinical outcome in acute myocardial infarction. Circulation. 2004;109(18):2186-90.
22. Sadoshima J, Izumo S. The cellular and molecular response of cardiac myocytes to mechanical stress. Annu Rev Physiol. 1997;59:551-71.
23. Manabe I, Shindo T, Nagai R. Gene expression in fibroblasts and fibrosis: Involvement in cardiac hypertrophy. Circ Res. 2002;91(12):1103-13.
24. Januzzi JL, Peacock WF, Maisel AS, et al. Measurement of the interleukin family member ST2 in patients with acute dyspnea: Results from the PRIDE (pro-brain natriuretic peptide investigation of dyspnea in the emergency department) study. J Am Coll Cardiol. 2007;50(7):607-13.
25. Boisot S, Beede J, Isakson S, et al. Serial sampling of ST2 predicts 90-day mortality following destabilized heart failure. J Card Fail. 2008;14(9):732-8.
26. Weinberg EO, Shimpo M, Hurwitz S, et al. Identification of serum soluble ST2 receptor as a novel heart failure biomarker. Circulation. 2003;107(5):721-6.
27. Taub PR, Gabbai-Saldate P, Maisel A. Biomarkers of heart failure. Congest Heart Fail. 2010;16(Suppl 1):S19-24.
28. Maisel A, Neath SX, Landsberg J, et al. Use of procalcitonin for the diagnosis of pneumonia in patients presenting with a chief complaint of dyspnoea: Results from the BACH (biomarkers in acute heart failure) trial. Eur J Heart Fail. 2012;14(3):278-86.
29. Aouifi A, Piriou V, Bastien O, et al. Usefulness of procalcitonin for diagnosis of infection in cardiac surgical patients. Crit Care Med. 2000;28(9):3171-6.
30. Brunkhorst FM. Endotoxins in chronic heart failure. Lancet. 1999; 354(9178):599-600.
31. Miller WL, Hartman KA, Grill DE, et al. Serial measurements of midregion proANP and copeptin in ambulatory patients with heart failure:

Incremental prognostic value of novel biomarkers in heart failure. Heart. 2012;98(5):389-94.
32. Miller WL, Grill DE, Struck J, et al. Association of hyponatremia and elevated copeptin with death and need for transplantation in ambulatory patients with chronic heart failure. Am J Cardiol. 2013;111(6):880-5.
33. Maisel A, Xue Y, Shah K, et al. Increased 90-day mortality in patients with acute heart failure with elevated copeptin: Secondary results from the biomarkers in acute heart failure (BACH) study. Circ Heart Fail. 2011;4(5):613-20.
34. Alehagen U, Dahlstrom U, Rehfeld JF, et al. Association of copeptin and N-terminal proBNP concentrations with risk of cardiovascular death in older patients with symptoms of heart failure. JAMA. 2011;305(20):2088-95.
35. Neuhold S, Huelsmann M, Strunk G, et al. Prognostic value of emerging neurohormones in chronic heart failure during optimization of heart failure-specific therapy. Clin Chem. 2010;56(1):121-6.
36. Balling L, Kistorp C, Schou M, et al. Plasma copeptin levels and prediction of outcome in heart failure outpatients: Relation to hyponatremia and loop diuretic doses. J Card Fail. 2012;18(5):351-8.
37. Kelly D, Squire IB, Khan SQ, et al. C-terminal provasopressin (copeptin) is associated with left ventricular dysfunction, remodeling, and clinical heart failure in survivors of myocardial infarction. J Card Fail. 2008;14(9):739-45.
38. Gegenhuber A, Struck J, Dieplinger B, et al. Comparative evaluation of B-type natriuretic peptide, mid-regional pro-A-type natriuretic peptide, mid-regional pro-adrenomedullin, and copeptin to predict 1-year mortality in patients with acute destabilized heart failure. J Card Fail. 2007;13(1):42-9.
39. Stoiser B, Mortl D, Hulsmann M, et al. Copeptin, a fragment of the vasopressin precursor, as a novel predictor of outcome in heart failure. Eur J Clin Invest. 2006;36(11):771-8.
40. Voors AA, von Haehling S, Anker SD, et al. C-terminal provasopressin (copeptin) is a strong prognostic marker in patients with heart failure after an acute myocardial infarction: Results from the OPTIMAAL study. Eur Heart J. 2009;30(10):1187-94.
41. Neuhold S, Huelsmann M, Strunk G, et al. Comparison of copeptin, B-type natriuretic peptide, and amino-terminal pro-B-type natriuretic peptide in patients with chronic heart failure: Prediction of death at different stages of the disease. J Am Coll Cardiol. 2008;52(4):266-72.
42. Loncar G, von Haehling S, Tahirovic E, et al. Effect of beta blockade on natriuretic peptides and copeptin in elderly patients with heart failure and preserved or reduced ejection fraction: Results from the CIBIS-ELD trial. Clin Biochem. 2012;45(1-2):117-22.
43. Peacock WF, Nowak R, Christenson R, et al. Short-term mortality risk in emergency department acute heart failure. Acad Emerg Med. 2011;18(9):947-58.
44. Shah RV, Truong QA, Gaggin HK, et al. Mid-regional pro-atrial natriuretic peptide and pro-adrenomedullin testing for the diagnostic and prognostic evaluation of patients with acute dyspnoea. Eur Heart J. 2012;33(17): 2197-205.
45. von Haehling S, Filippatos GS, Papassotiriou J, et al. Mid-regional pro-adrenomedullin as a novel predictor of mortality in patients with chronic heart failure. Eur J Heart Fail. 2010;12(5):484-91.
46. Maisel A, Mueller C, Nowak RM, et al. Midregion prohormone adreno-medullin and prognosis in patients presenting with acute dyspnea: Results from the BACH (biomarkers in acute heart failure) trial. J Am Coll Cardiol. 2011;58(10):1057-67.
47. Klip IT, Voors AA, Anker SD, et al. Prognostic value of mid-regional pro-adrenomedullin in patients with heart failure after an acute myocardial infarction. Heart. 2011;97(11):892-8.
48. Adlbrecht C, Hulsmann M, Strunk G, et al. Prognostic value of plasma midregional pro-adrenomedullin and C-terminal-pro-endothelin-1 in chronic heart failure outpatients. Eur J Heart Fail. 2009;11(4):361-6.
49. Barlera S, Tavazzi L, Franzosi MG, et al. Predictors of mortality in 6975 patients with chronic heart failure in the gruppo italiano per lo studio della streptochinasi nell'infarto miocardico-heart failure trial: Proposal for a nomogram. Circ Heart Fail. 2013;6(1):31-9.
50. Kusumoto A, Miyata M, Kubozono T, et al. Highly sensitive cardiac troponin T in heart failure: Comparison with echocardiographic parameters and natriuretic peptides. J Cardiol. 2012;59(2):202-8.
51. Jungbauer CG, Riedlinger J, Buchner S, et al. High-sensitive troponin T in chronic heart failure correlates with severity of symptoms, left ventricular dysfunction and prognosis independently from N-terminal pro-b-type natriuretic peptide. Clin Chem Lab Med. 2011;49(11):1899-906.
52. McQueen MJ, Kavsak PA, Xu L, et al. Predicting myocardial infarction and other serious cardiac outcomes using high-sensitivity cardiac troponin T in a high-risk stable population. Clin Biochem. 2013;46(1-2):5-9.
53. Egstrup M, Schou M, Tuxen CD, et al. Prediction of outcome by highly sensitive troponin T in outpatients with chronic systolic left ventricular heart failure. Am J Cardiol. 2012;110(4):552-7.
54. Nagarajan V, Hernandez AV, Tang WH. Prognostic value of cardiac troponin in chronic stable heart failure: A systematic review. Heart. 2012;98(24):1778-86.
55. Masson S, Anand I, Favero C, et al. Serial measurement of cardiac troponin T using a highly sensitive assay in patients with chronic heart failure: Data from 2 large randomized clinical trials. Circulation. 2012;125(2):280-8.
56. Melki D, Lind S, Agewall S, et al. Prognostic value of combining high sensitive troponin T and N-terminal pro B-type natriuretic peptide in chest pain patients with no persistent ST-elevation. Clin Chim Acta. 2012;413(9-10):933-7.
57. Manzano-Fernandez S, Januzzi JL, Boronat-Garcia M, et al. Beta-trace protein and cystatin C as predictors of long-term outcomes in patients with acute heart failure. J Am Coll Cardiol. 2011;57(7):849-58.
58. Damman K, van der Harst P, Smilde TD, et al. Use of cystatin C levels in estimating renal function and prognosis in patients with chronic systolic heart failure. Heart. 2012;98(4):319-24.
59. Campbell CY, Clarke W, Park H, et al. Usefulness of cystatin C and prognosis following admission for acute heart failure. Am J Cardiol. 2009;104(3):389-92.
60. Gao C, Zhong L, Gao Y, et al. Cystatin C levels are associated with the prognosis of systolic heart failure patients. Arch Cardiovasc Dis. 2011;104(11):565-71.
61. Perez-Calvo JI, Ruiz-Ruiz FJ, Carrasco-Sanchez FJ, et al. Prognostic value of serum cystatin C and N-terminal pro b-type natriuretic peptide in patients with acute heart failure. Eur J Intern Med. 2012;23(7):599-603.
62. Carrasco-Sanchez FJ, Galisteo-Almeda L, Paez-Rubio I, et al. Prognostic value of cystatin C on admission in heart failure with preserved ejection fraction. J Card Fail. 2011;17(1):31-8.
63. Dupont M, Wu Y, Hazen SL, et al. Cystatin C identifies patients with stable chronic heart failure at increased risk for adverse cardiovascular events. Circ Heart Fail. 2012;5(5):602-9.
64. Bennett M, Dent CL, Ma Q, et al. Urine NGAL predicts severity of acute kidney injury after cardiac surgery: A prospective study. Clin J Am Soc Nephrol. 2008;3(3):665-73.
65. Damman K, van Veldhuisen DJ, Navis G, et al. Urinary neutrophil gelatinase associated lipocalin (NGAL), a marker of tubular damage, is increased in patients with chronic heart failure. Eur J Heart Fail. 2008;10(10):997-1000.
66. Damman K, Masson S, Hillege HL, et al. Clinical outcome of renal tubular damage in chronic heart failure. Eur Heart J. 2011;32(21):2705-12.
67. Macdonald S, Arendts G, Nagree Y, et al. Neutrophil Gelatinase-Associated Lipocalin (NGAL) predicts renal injury in acute decompensated cardiac failure: a prospective observational study. BMC Cardiovasc Disord. 2012;12:8.
68. Aghel A, Shrestha K, Mullens W, et al. Serum neutrophil gelatinase-associated lipocalin (NGAL) in predicting worsening renal function in acute decompensated heart failure. J Card Fail. 2010;16(1):49-54.

69. Maisel AS, Mueller C, Fitzgerald R, et al. Prognostic utility of plasma neutrophil gelatinase-associated lipocalin in patients with acute heart failure: The NGAL EvaLuation along with B-type NaTriuretic peptide in acutely decompensated heart failure (GALLANT) trial. Eur J Heart Fail. 2011;13(8):846-51.
70. Dupont M, Shrestha K, Singh D, et al. Lack of significant renal tubular injury despite acute kidney injury in acute decompensated heart failure. Eur J Heart Fail. 2012;14(6):597-604.
71. Damman K, Masson S, Hillege HL, et al. Clinical outcome of renal tubular damage in chronic heart failure. Eur Heart J. 2011;32(21):2705-12.
72. Jungbauer CG, Birner C, Jung B, et al. Kidney injury molecule-1 and N-acetyl-beta-D-glucosaminidase in chronic heart failure: possible biomarkers of cardiorenal syndrome. Eur J Heart Fail. 2011;13(10):1104-10.
73. Damman K, Ng Kam Chuen MJ, MacFadyen RJ, et al. Volume status and diuretic therapy in systolic heart failure and the detection of early abnormalities in renal and tubular function. J Am Coll Cardiol. 2011;57(22):2233-41.
74. Alonso-Martinez JL, Llorente-Diez B, Echegaray-Agara M, et al. C-reactive protein as a predictor of improvement and readmission in heart failure. Eur J Heart Fail. 2002;4(3):331-6.
75. Gottdiener JS, Arnold AM, Aurigemma GP, et al. Predictors of congestive heart failure in the elderly: The cardiovascular health study. J Am Coll Cardiol. 2000;35(6):1628-37.
76. Elster SK, Braunwald E, Wood HF. A study of C-reactive protein in the serum of patients with congestive heart failure. Am Heart J. 1956;51(4):533-41.
77. Lassus J, Gayat E, Mueller C, et al. Incremental value of biomarkers to clinical variables for mortality prediction in acutely decompensated heart failure: the Multinational Observational Cohort on Acute Heart Failure (MOCA) study. Int J Cardiol. 2013;168(3):2186-94.
78. Berton G, Cordiano R, Palmieri R, et al. C-reactive protein in acute myocardial infarction: Association with heart failure. Am Heart J. 2003;145(6):1094-101.
79. Vasan RS, Sullivan LM, Roubenoff R, et al. Inflammatory markers and risk of heart failure in elderly subjects without prior myocardial infarction: the Framingham Heart Study. Circulation. 2003;107(11):1486-91.
80. Murray DR, Freeman GL. Proinflammatory cytokines: predictors of a failing heart? Circulation. 2003;107(11):1460-2.
81. Milo O, Cotter G, Kaluski E, et al. Comparison of inflammatory and neurohormonal activation in cardiogenic pulmonary edema secondary to ischemic versus nonischemic causes. Am J Cardiol. 2003;92(2):222-6.
82. Tanner H, Mohacsi P, Fuller-Bicer GA, et al. Cytokine activation and disease progression in patients with stable moderate chronic heart failure. J Heart Lung Transplant. 2007;26(6):622-9.
83. Adams J, Apple F. Cardiology patient page. new blood tests for detecting heart disease. Circulation. 2004;109(3):E12-4.
84. D'Aloia A, Faggiano P, Aurigemma G, et al. Serum levels of carbohydrate antigen 125 in patients with chronic heart failure: Relation to clinical severity, hemodynamic and doppler echocardiographic abnormalities, and short-term prognosis. J Am Coll Cardiol. 2003;41(10):1805-11.
85. Nagele H, Bahlo M, Klapdor R, et al. CA 125 and its relation to cardiac function. Am Heart J. 1999;137(6):1044-9.
86. Gaetje R, Winnekendonk DW, Ahr A, et al. Ovarian cancer antigen CA 125 influences adhesion of human and mammalian cell lines in vitro. Clin Exp Obstet Gynecol. 2002;29(1):34-6.
87. Kouris NT, Zacharos ID, Kontogianni DD, et al. The significance of CA125 levels in patients with chronic congestive heart failure. correlation with clinical and echocardiographic parameters. Eur J Heart Fail. 2005;7(2):199-203.
88. Kouris NT, Kontogianni DD, Papoulia EP, et al. Clinical and prognostic value of elevated CA125 levels in patients with congestive heart failure. Hellenic J Cardiol. 2006;47(5):269-74.
89. Ordu S, Ozhan H, Alemdar R, et al. Carbohydrate antigen-125 and N-terminal pro-brain natriuretic peptide levels: Compared in heart-failure prognostication. Tex Heart Inst J. 2012;39(1):30-5.
90. Nunez J, Sanchis J, Bodi V, et al. Improvement in risk stratification with the combination of the tumour marker antigen carbohydrate 125 and brain natriuretic peptide in patients with acute heart failure. Eur Heart J. 2010;31(14):1752-63.
91. Nunez J, Minana G, Gonzalez M, et al. Antigen carbohydrate 125 in heart failure: Not just a surrogate for serosal effusions? Int J Cardiol. 2011;146(3):473-4.
92. Nagele H, Bahlo M, Klapdor R, et al. Fluctuations of tumor markers in heart failure patients pre and post heart transplantation. Anticancer Res. 1999;19(4A):2531-4.
93. Sturgeon C. Practice guidelines for tumor marker use in the clinic. Clin Chem. 2002;48(8):1151-9.
94. Sikaris KA. CA125—a test with a change of heart. Heart Lung Circ. 2011;20(10):634-40.
95. Zimmers TA, Jin X, Hsiao EC, et al. Growth differentiation factor-15/ macrophage inhibitory cytokine-1 induction after kidney and lung injury. Shock. 2005;23(6):543-8.
96. Wollert KC, Kempf T. Growth differentiation factor 15 in heart failure: An update. Curr Heart Fail Rep. 2012;9(4):337-45.
97. Norozi K, Buchhorn R, Yasin A, et al. Growth differentiation factor 15: An additional diagnostic tool for the risk stratification of developing heart failure in patients with operated congenital heart defects? Am Heart J. 2011;162(1):131-5.
98. Baessler A, Strack C, Rousseva E, et al. Growth-differentiation factor-15 improves reclassification for the diagnosis of heart failure with normal ejection fraction in morbid obesity. Eur J Heart Fail. 2012;14(11):1240-8.
99. Dinh W, Futh R, Lankisch M, et al. Growth-differentiation factor-15: A novel biomarker in patients with diastolic dysfunction? Arq Bras Cardiol. 2011;97(1):65-75.
100. Stahrenberg R, Edelmann F, Mende M, et al. The novel biomarker growth differentiation factor 15 in heart failure with normal ejection fraction. Eur J Heart Fail. 2010;12(12):1309-16.
101. Anand IS, Kempf T, Rector TS, et al. Serial measurement of growth-differentiation factor-15 in heart failure: Relation to disease severity and prognosis in the valsartan heart failure trial. Circulation. 2010;122(14):1387-95.
102. Wang F, Guo Y, Yu H, et al. Growth differentiation factor 15 in different stages of heart failure: Potential screening implications. Biomarkers. 2010;15(8):671-6.
103. Cody RJ, Haas GJ, Binkley PF, et al. Plasma endothelin correlates with the extent of pulmonary hypertension in patients with chronic congestive heart failure. Circulation. 1992;85(2):504-9.
104. Cavero PG, Miller WL, Heublein DM, et al. Endothelin in experimental congestive heart failure in the anesthetized dog. Am J Physiol. 1990;259(2 Pt 2):F312-7.
105. Zolk O, Quattek J, Sitzler G, et al. Expression of endothelin-1, endothelin-converting enzyme, and endothelin receptors in chronic heart failure. Circulation. 1999;99(16):2118-23.
106. McMurray JJ, Ray SG, Abdullah I, et al. Plasma endothelin in chronic heart failure. Circulation. 1992;85(4):1374-9.
107. Pacher R, Stanek B, Hulsmann M, et al. Prognostic impact of big endothelin-1 plasma concentrations compared with invasive hemodynamic evaluation in severe heart failure. J Am Coll Cardiol. 1996;27(3):633-41.
108. Pousset F, Isnard R, Lechat P, et al. Prognostic value of plasma endothelin-1 in patients with chronic heart failure. Eur Heart J. 1997;18(2):254-8.
109. Maisel AS, Choudhary R. Biomarkers in acute heart failure—state of the art. Nat Rev Cardiol. 2012;9(8):478-90.

4

SECTION

Special Issues in Heart Failure

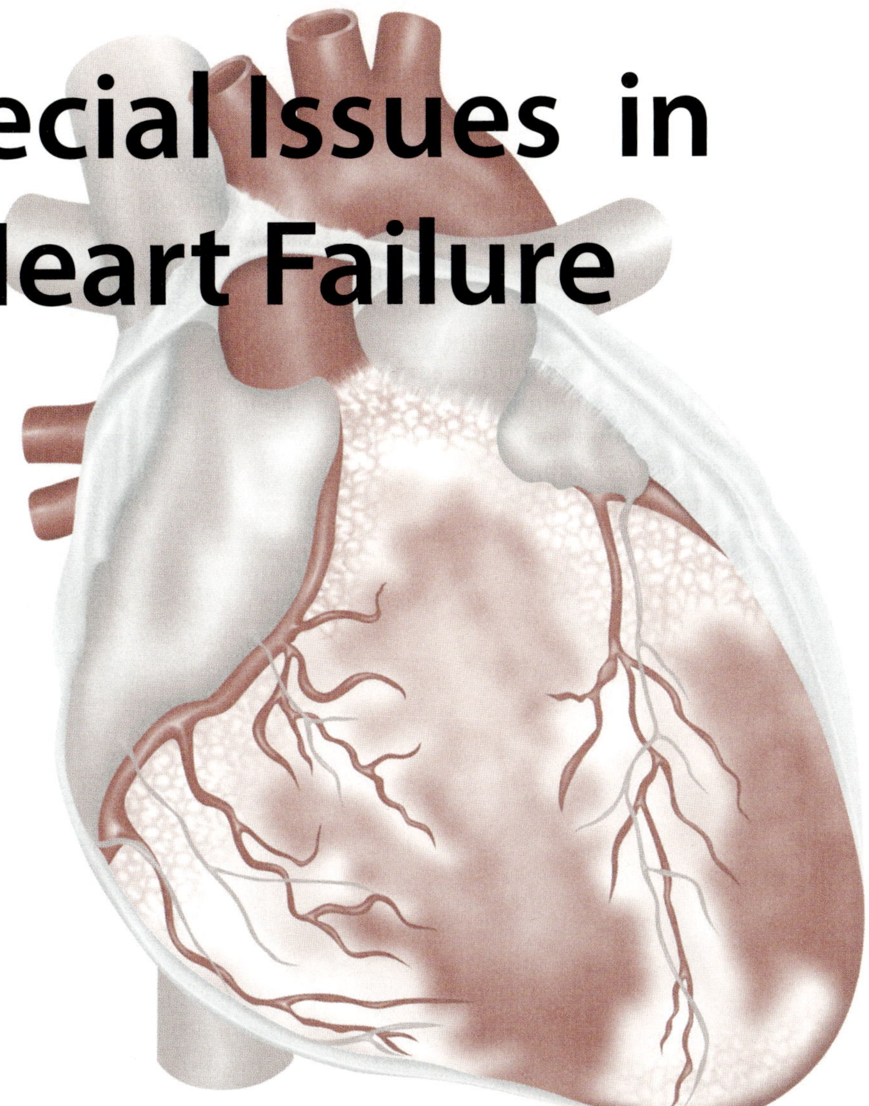

Chapter 37

Sex Differences in Heart Failure: Implications for Clinical Practice

Nancy J Gardetto, Denise D Barnard

ABSTRACT

Heart failure (HF) is one of the fastest-growing chronic cardiac conditions in the United States and throughout the world. Emerging epidemiologic data reveal that women account for a substantial portion of the growing HF epidemic, yet we do not have a clear picture of the extent or the importance of sex differences in the heterogeneous HF syndrome. Despite changing epidemiological trends and the potential growing threat to women's health, women have been poorly represented in clinical cardiovascular research trials. That said, HF research populations have included proportionately more women than most coronary heart disease trials. Until large, adequately powered, prospective research studies prove otherwise, HF guideline treatment strategies should be uniformly applied to both men and women. The aim of this chapter is to describe sex differences in HF epidemiology, risk factors, clinical characteristics, and treatment which may influence future guideline algorithms.

INTRODUCTION AND EPIDEMIOLOGIC TRENDS

Heart failure (HF) is a staggering public health problem of epidemic proportions and one of the fastest-growing chronic cardiac conditions in the United States.[1] There has been a steady rise in the incidence and prevalence of HF in recent years.[1,2] It has been hypothesized that in an aging society which has benefitted from advances in medical care of chronic diseases and enhanced survival from ischemic heart disease, HF will continue to increase as a major and costly public health problem.[2,3] Data from the National Heart, Lung, and Blood Institute (NHLBI) sponsored Framingham Heart Study (FHS) indicate that the overall prevalence rates of HF in men and women are similar, with an estimated annual incidence approaching 10 per 1,000 populations after 65 years of age.[4]

Although the incidence of HF has increased by 9% in women and 6% in men during the last 20 years, we do not have a clear picture of the extent or the importance of sex differences in people with HF.[4] This is not surprising, as the epidemiology of HF as a chronic disease is known to be complex and reflects a markedly heterogeneous clinical syndrome. Population-based cohort studies have determined epidemiological trends in HF by various methods including: hospital discharge diagnosis, retrospective medical record reviews, death certificate registration, self-report surveys, and a host of national and industry-sponsored registries. General observations described by previous HF researchers include: (1) HF is a common chronic disease in women, African Americans, and the elderly of either sex and any race; (2) HF is three times more common in people with hypertension (HTN) compared to normotensive persons; and finally (3) HF is five times greater in persons who have had a heart attack compared to persons who have not.[1,4,5] Projections of crude prevalence show that by 2030 HF will affect 3.5% of the American population, and incur nearly $78 billion in direct care costs.[2] HF has already become the leading cause of hospital admission in Medicare recipients.[1,2,5] HF hospitalization and readmission rates between men and women appear similar;[6,7] but for reasons that are unclear, survival following the diagnosis of HF has been reported to be somewhat better in women than men.[8-10] The observed favorable difference in survival may be related to sex differences in HF etiology. Although women with HF are more likely to be older at disease onset, a higher proportion of women have HF with preserved systolic function (HFPSF) and nonischemic cardiomyopathy.[11-13]

Emerging epidemiologic data reveal that women account for a substantial portion of the growing HF epidemic. The FHS demonstrated that while HF incidence remained stable over the last 30 years in men, it is increased by approximately 5% in women.[14,15] These findings were mirrored in the Olmsted County Study, which showed no significant increase in HF incidence in men, but a significant 10% increase in women since 1979.[5] Despite these changing trends and significant threat to women's health; women have been significantly underrepresented in large, multicenter clinical research trials. The population estimate of HF among women in the United States is about 50%, yet only 17–23% of participants enrolled in randomized clinical HF trials are women.[10] There has been an increased awareness of gender-specific gaps in HF pathophysiology, diagnosis and treatment strategies. Recruitment strategies targeting women are increasingly effective, as the major HF trials evaluating treatments for HF with reduced ejection fraction (HFREF) included proportionately more women than did the major coronary artery disease (CAD) trials. However, there is a clear need for balanced enrollment in HF trials and a better understanding of the biological basis for the observed variability in clinical outcomes for people with HF. The role of sex differences in HF management remains an area that requires further investigation.

HEART FAILURE ETIOLOGY AND RISK FACTOR BURDEN

Until recently, much of the epidemiological and clinical data regarding cardiovascular disease (CVD) in general and HF in particular were extrapolated to the entire population. Because of the high morbidity, poor prognosis, and substantial burden placed on the individual, family members and society, HF has figured prominently into ensuing public efforts to improve chronic illness care and outcomes. A better understanding of sex differences related to HF outcomes may help healthcare providers and researchers tailor or modify optimal therapy according to gender and guide future quality improvement efforts. Recently published studies suggest that biological variability in response to risk factors may account for observed differences in HF epidemiology, clinical characteristics, and treatment response in women compared with their male counterparts. Until prospective trial data can prove otherwise, HF treatment guidelines should be uniformly applied to both men and women.[3,15-17] The aim here is to highlight and summarize some of the differences reported in recently published research studies and pertinent reviews.

Age

Advances in revascularization for acute and chronic coronary heart disease (CHD) and better management of HTN are allowing people to live longer, thus shifting the age profile of the disease. Although the prevalence of HF increases with age for both genders, women develop HF later in life than men.[5,13,14,17-22] Table 1 provides a brief snapshot of studies cited in this chapter showing the age profile for women and men at time of HF diagnosis.[5,17-20] The fact that women are generally diagnosed with HF at an older age may be explained by the higher prevalence of the associated risk factors of HTN, left ventricular hypertrophy (LVH) and diabetes, and a lower prevalence of ischemic heart disease. As population studies do not generally distinguish variations in the HF phenotypes [HF with preserved ejection fraction (HFPEF) vs HFREF], the lifetime risk for developing HF is, therefore, equal in women and men, namely, one person in five (20%) at the age of 40 years.[1,2]

In 2010, there were 23.0 million older women and 17.5 million older men in the United States representing a sex ratio of 132 women for every 100 men.[22] The female to male sex ratio increases with age, ranging from 1.12 for the 65–69 years age-group to a high of 2.06 for persons 85 years and over. Women, therefore, will continue to comprise an increasing percentage of symptomatic HF populations. In the comprehensive treatment of the HF patient, nonpharmacologic strategies and caregiver support are important adjuncts for improving compliance and in optimizing outcomes.[3,17,18] The following statistics also suggest that adjunctive HF therapies may require

TABLE 1: Studies summarizing mean age in years at time of heart failure diagnosis

Study author (year)	*Women (years)*	*Men (years)*	*p-value*
Roger et al. (2004)[5]	79	73	<0.001
Lenzen et al. (2008)[18]	75	68	<0.001
Rathore et al. (2005)[19]	81	78	0.001
McCullough et al. (2002)[20]	74	69	<0.001
Ho et al. (1993)[21]	72	68	<0.001

a different focus in elderly populations. Older men are much more likely to be married than are older women (72% of men vs 42% of women), and 40% of older women in 2010 were widows. About 29% (11.3 million) of noninstitutionalized older persons live alone (8.1 million women, 3.2 million men), but almost half of women (47%) 75+ years of age live alone.[22]

Hypertension

Owing to its high prevalence, HTN has the greatest population-attributable risk (PAR) influence in both sexes; yet HTN appears to have different etiologic-risk profiles for HF in men and women.[16] According to Cleland et al. (2003), HTN increases the risk of developing HF by threefold in women, compared with approximately twofold in men.[23] Similarly in the FHS, investigators calculated the PAR and determined that HTN was associated with 59% of the incident of HF cases in women and 39% in men.[24] The FHS demographic was predominantly white and had an equal prevalence of HTN between both sexes (60% men, 62% women). Many additional studies have found HTN to be an important risk factor for HF in women, especially young black women with uncontrolled blood pressure. The prevalence of HTN in Afro-American and Hispanic women appears to be less age-dependent.[24,25] The significant prevalence in women over 55 years of age has been attributed to higher systolic blood pressure after menopause.[26]

Left Ventricular Hypertrophy

There is a causal association between LVH with a history of chronic HTN and/or diabetes that has been well documented as an independent precursor of HF.[13,27-31] In a multivariate analysis of data taken from the FHS, the increased risk for HF in hypertensive subjects with electrocardiographic (ECG) evidence of LVH persisted, despite adjusting for the influence of other HF risk factors.[24] Although the presence of LVH on ECG increased the HF risk more for women than men [hazard ratio (HR) 2.80 in women, 1.97 in men], the PAR was nearly equivalent with 5% for women and 4% for men. Topol first detailed sex differences in the phenotypic response of the ventricle to pressure-overload conditions in 1985, in what is classically described as a hypertensive hypertrophic cardiomyopathy of the elderly.[32] Thus, research designs that include study participants of advanced age may include a greater proportion of women with LVH, regardless of prior history of HTN and other risk factors.

The proportion of persons with HF and preserved left ventricular (LV) systolic function has increased over time due to the high prevalence of HTN, and in part due to recognition of the disorder as a clinical syndrome independent of disease etiology and physiology.[1] The literature has a variety of nomenclature for this group of patients including HF with normal ejection fraction (HFNEF), HFPSF, and the most recently adopted terminology, HFPEF. There is mounting evidence supporting a significantly higher incidence of HFPEF in women, especially the elderly.[13,18,33-36] Although the cut-off for ejection fraction (EF) varies from greater than 40% to greater than 45%, table 2 highlights a few studies that compare the incidence of HFPEF in women versus men.[25,26,33,34] It has been postulated that the higher incidence of HFPEF combined with a lower incidence of ischemic heart disease in part accounts for the superior survival after diagnosis that has been observed in women with HF.[5,11,21,27,28,37,38]

Regitz-Zagrosek et al. (2007) provides an excellent review of the literature exploring the role of gender in HFPEF. The authors suggest that some reports may have overestimated the prevalence of HFPEF by using a clinical diagnosis of HF together with documentation of normal systolic ventricular function. This is further confounded by either failure to measure diastolic functional parameters and/or by the lack of consensus on which parameters to utilize to define diastolic HF.[28] The diagnostic criteria for HFPEF and the systematic use of echocardiography in the evaluation of HF are still evolving. However flawed, when applied to all HF patients, the bulk of clinical evidence to date favors a preponderance of HFPEF among women.[13,22,27,28,33-35]

TABLE 2: Summary of studies comparing incidence of heart failure with preserved ejection fraction in women versus men*

Study author (year)	*LVEF (%)*	*Women (%)*	*Men (%)*	*Other variables*
Wong et al. (2010)[33]	>45	62	39	Age, SS, RI, anemia, AF
Nieminen et al. (2008)[34]	≥45	50	25	Multiple variables by gender*
Galvao et al. (2006)[35]	>40	58	28	Multiple variables by gender*
Lee et al. (2004)[36]	≥40	55	41	Age, HTN, RI

LVEF, left ventricular ejection fraction; SS, social support; RI, renal impairment; AF, atrial fibrillation; HTN, hypertension

*Cut-off for ejection fraction varies.

Accordingly, the established risk factors for HFPEF include, age, HTN, diabetes, obesity, and CHD as these are all known to reduce both LV and arterial compliance. There are sex-related differences in ventricular diastolic volumes and distensibility, vascular stiffness, ventricular-vascular coupling ratio, and skeletal muscle adaptations to HF.[39] These factors may explain why the perception of symptoms, such as dyspnea is greater in women than men with HF despite an equivalent or higher EF. There are a number of underlying molecular functions involved in ventricular and vascular smooth muscle relaxation that are thought to be influenced by estrogen, and a growing body of evidence suggesting that sex hormones affect components of the renin-angiotensin system (RAS) through a number of mechanisms.[28-30] This area of research needs more investigation to elucidate sex differences in the role of these molecular and hormonal events and their activity during different parts of the cardiac cycle.

Diabetes and Obesity

Diabetes and obesity both are major health risks in a majority of global populations. They affect all parts of society, adults as well as children; but represent a more severe CV risk factor in women. The probability of a diabetic patient developing HF is strongly linked to glycemic control. A study of more than 48,000 diabetic patients showed a probability of 4.3/1,000 HF cases/year with a glycated hemoglobin (HbA1c) value of less than 7% and a probability of 9.2/1,000 HF cases/year with a HbA1c value of more than 10%.[40] Although diabetes mellitus (DM) is common in both genders, it is becoming a powerful and independent risk factor for the development of HF in women as it also increases the risk of CHD and myocardial infarction (MI).[41] Even gestational diabetes is a strong predictor of the development of both HTN and diabetes later in life.

Diabetes leads to impairment of ventricular relaxation in both men and women. In the FHS, diabetes increased the prevalence of HF in men (2.4-fold) and in women (fivefold) with an even greater difference observed in women (men, fourfold; women, eightfold) who were 65 years and younger.[42] The presence of concomitant HTN and DM yields a substantial increased HF risk, especially in women.[24] This is postulated to relate to increased myocardial fibrosis and ventricular hypertrophy in diabetic women, in the absence of CHD.[43] The prevalence and severity of CV disease as well as carrying a worse prognosis are higher in diabetics versus non-diabetics, with the risk enhanced in diabetic women versus diabetic men.

Data from the Heart and Estrogen/progestin Replacement Study (HERS) reported that in the known CHD cohort the extent of glycemic control in diabetes was the strongest predictive outcome parameter with an adjusted HR of 3.1 [95% confidence interval (CI) = 2.3–4.2; $p < 0.001$].[41] In the absence of other risk factors, DM increased the annual HF incidence rate over sixfold, or to 3% per year. Concomitant diabetes and renal insufficiency increased the annual incidence to 12.5% and morbid obesity (body mass index >35 kg/m^2) increased the annual incidence to 7%.[3]

Obesity is an integral component of the metabolic syndrome and a major risk factor for diabetes in both sexes. Age, body mass index, and genetic factors play comparable risk roles in both men and women, whereas physical inactivity is more important in women.[44] The pattern of fat distribution appears to be more critical than weight by itself, in particular, central body adiposity represents a major CHD and HF risk factor.[45] The combination of obesity and hormonal disturbances in postmenopausal women seems particularly dangerous.

Obesity predisposes an individual to the toxic effects of fatty acids on the myocardium and the additional detrimental effects of cytokines and angiotensin II released by adipose tissue, thus creating the physiological mechanism by which HF develops and making obesity a substantial risk for HF in both men and women. In the FHS, the risk of HF was twice higher for the obese persons compared to subjects with normal body weight.[46]

Coronary Heart Disease

Coronary artery disease, prior MI and other forms of CHD are major risk factors for the development of HF. An estimated 82 million Americans adults (over 1 in 3) have one or more types of CHD.[1] Death rates attributed to CHD have declined, yet the burden of disease remains high. CHD accounted for 32.3% of all deaths in the U.S. in 2009.[1] The incidence, prevalence, and contribution of CHD to CV death are lower in women than men; however, this gap in women narrows with advancing age.[45] Although the incidence of MI is lower in women, especially younger women, those who sustain an MI are far more likely than their matched male counterparts to develop HF.[1,2]

While CAD is less common in women, its presence becomes such a strong risk factor that women with CAD are more likely to develop HF than are women without CAD and HTN.[12,15,29] For example, in the National

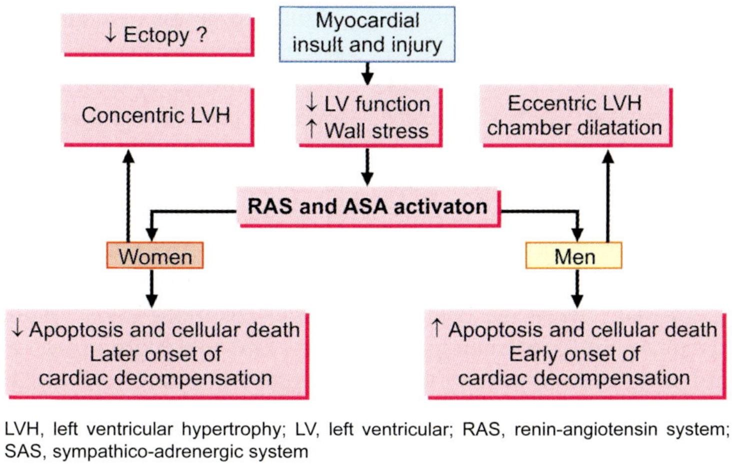

Flowchart 1 Sex differences in the pathophysiology of mechanisms of heart failure and survival[52]

Health and Nutrition Examination Survey (NHANES) I, which included 8,098 women without HF, 27% had HTN and only 3% had CAD. However, the relative risk (RR) of developing HF for women in that sample was significantly higher if they had CAD (RR = 8.16; CI = 6.75–9.8; $p < 0.0001$) than if they had HTN (RR = 1.51; 95% CI = 1.29–1.77; $p < 0.001$).[47] Diabetes and CAD are each associated with excess mortality in women with HFREF compared to men.[41] It has been well documented that an ischemic etiology for HFREF carries with it a poor prognosis for both men and women.[12] While women tend to have less ischemic causes for HF than their male counterparts, the survival advantage appears confined to women with a nonischemic etiology.[48,49]

It is important to recognize that lifetime estimates for CHD and attributable mortality can change over time and are increasing in women. A good example is the pooled analysis of survival data taken (between 1964 through 2008) from five NHLBI-funded community cohorts: FHS, Framingham Offspring Study, Atherosclerosis Risk in Communities Study, Chicago Heart Association Detection Project in Industry Study, and Cardiovascular Health Study.[50] All participants were free of CHD at baseline with risk factor data recorded (blood pressure, cholesterol, diabetes, and smoking status) and total CV deaths tracked. Lifetime risk estimates (to age 95 years) for total CV death exceeded 60% for men and 56% for women overall. Previously, lifetime risk estimates taken from the FHS cohort for CHD alone (to age 95 years) were 48% for men and 32% for women.[14,51]

Chronic ischemia with or without MI can lead to the development of systolic dysfunction as well as disturbances of ventricular relaxation. Higher rates of HFPEF in individuals with CHD risk factors but without MI may be partially due to this phenomenon.[35] Flowchart 1 illustrates a postulate of Jessup and Piña (2004) suggesting that sex-related HF survival rates can be influenced by the mechanism of myocardial injury and the adaptive and maladaptive responses to injury.[52] More focused research is needed to fully appreciate the pathophysiology of sex differences in HF and their relationship among risk factor burden and survival.

SEX DIFFERENCES IN CLINICAL PRESENTATION

Heart failure is a clinical diagnosis based on a constellation of signs and symptoms that have different characteristics in men and women.[3] Part of the difference in women is attributable to age, ventricular function, and the etiology of HF. Women tend to delay seeking care longer than men and have more advanced CAD when presenting with an acute coronary syndrome and/or MI. Women with HF not due to an ischemic substrate are more symptomatic than their male counterparts. Several studies have shown striking sex-related differences in the prevalence and severity of HF symptoms.[3,52-54] Despite having similar EF, data taken from the Studies of Left Ventricular Dysfunction (SOLVD) reported that women experienced more exertional dyspnea (58% vs 48% in men; $p < 0.001$), edema (22% vs 15% in men), and were less likely to have New York Heart Association I symptoms (6% vs 12% in men; $p < 0.001$).[53] Women also have a greater impairment of exercise capacity than men, as well as more physical signs of HF, such as an S3 gallop and jugular venous engorgement.[52,53]

The Multinational Monitoring of Trends and Determinants in Cardiovascular Disease (MONICA) study confirmed that despite comparable LVEF measurements and less ischemic heart disease women are more symptomatic than men.[54] The MONICA study investigators attributed the higher prevalence and increased symptom severity to lower threshold of pain perception and of depression among women. In a sample of Portuguese middle-aged and elderly adults, women had a higher prevalence of signs and symptoms consistent with HF.[55] In addition to female gender, older age, and obesity; depressive symptoms accounted for the largest portion of clinical symptoms suggestive of HF.[55] Depression is a very common comorbid condition in chronic diseases, such as HF and with aging. Although controversial, there is growing body of research suggesting that women with HF are more prone to somatic depression than men, and thus have higher rates of major depression.[56,57] In HF populations, major depression is associated with higher in-hospital and disease specific mortality rates, and a lower quality of life.[5,8,29,58] The interrelationship of sex with depression, age, and HF outcomes has not been prospectively studied. Demographic and social factors clearly would be confounding in this endeavor since as previously mentioned, almost half of women (47%) 75+ years of age live alone.[22]

INFLUENCE OF SEX ON BIOMARKERS

The use of biomarkers both for diagnosis and as a surrogate index of prognosis in HF patients has been a topic of great interest. The biomarkers brain natriuretic peptide (BNP) and N-terminal pro-BNP have been demonstrated to be very accurate and effective in establishing or excluding a diagnosis of HF in acute dyspnea in numerous clinical trials.[59-68] Natriuretic peptide (NP) assay results are generally reported using the same reference ranges for both males and females in healthy populations. However, it is well documented that NP values tend to increase with age, and are generally higher in women than men.[66-68]

In a study of 2,042 randomly selected residents (>44 years old) of Olmsted County, Minnesota the distribution of BNP levels using Shionogi and Biosite assays differed by age, gender and assay system.[67] BNP increased significantly with age and was higher in women among subjects without CV disease or cardiac dysfunction, and indeed, the optimal discriminatory value of BNP for detection of systolic dysfunction in this population was higher in women and older persons.[67] The magnitude of the effects of age and gender on BNP levels in this data suggests that both parameters need to be considered when interpreting BNP.[67] To further clarify the impact of age and sex on plasma NP levels, Wang et al. examined NP levels [N-terminal atrial natriuretic peptide (NT-ANP)] and BNP in a large, community-based sample of health subjects (composed of 342 men and 569 women) from the FHS.[68] Women had markedly higher NP levels (1.6-fold higher plasma BNP level) than men.[68] The strongest predictors of higher NP levels were older age and female sex, underscoring the important implications for the use of these tests in clinical practice and an ongoing need for future research.[68] Although Redeld et al. found 21% higher BNP levels in women taking hormone replacement therapy suggesting a role for female sex hormones on NP expression; the physiologic basis for sex-related differences in NP levels is unclear.[67] Other factors affecting biomarker levels include body weight versus composition relating both to muscle mass and glomerular filtration rate. NP levels are known to be lower in the obese, and higher in patients with renal insufficiency. Further investigation is required to determine what the physiological and clinical implications might be, particularly in regard to whether sex-specific reference ranges should be used in clinical practice.

Christ and colleagues compared all-cause mortality rates to BNP levels in a cohort of 190 female and 262 male patients presenting with acute dyspnea in the B-type Natriuretic Peptide for Acute Shortness of Breath Evaluation (BASEL) study.[66] The main results showed the following: (1) patients presenting with acute dyspnea displayed a higher mortality rate independent of gender; (2) BNP levels were significantly higher in the women who died compared with the men (medians of 835 pg/mL vs 459 pg/mL); and (3) women with BNP levels greater than 500 pg/mL had significantly higher mortality than men with BNP levels greater than 500 pg/mL.[66] This data is similar to other research showing that NP levels in women are in excess of NP levels in men with comparable symptoms and disease severity, and emphasizes the need for clinicians to take into consideration sex and possibly age when interpreting NP levels.

The prognostic value of biomarkers can be further increased by using a multimarker approach where each biomarker provides incremental insight into different pathophysiologic processes, such as myocyte necrosis [cardiac troponin (cTn)], inflammation (C-reactive protein), and LV overload (BNP).[69] For example,

Velagaleti et al. used a multibiomarker panel (BNP, C-reactive protein, plasminogen activator inhibitor-1, homocysteine, aldosterone-to-rennin ratio, and urinary albumin-to-creatinine ratio). Through the use of a multimarker approach, these investigators identified BNP and urinary albumin-to-creatinine ratio as important risk factors for new-onset HF.[69] Elevations in biomarkers of myocardial damage, such as cTn I and T are found in acute MI, but also in decompensated HF in the absence of acute coronary syndromes. The degree of elevation in decompensated HF provides reliable prognostic information.[70,71] At present there are no significant sex-related differences in cTn reference measurements. However, as the high sensitivity cTn assays become more widely available, the relative utility of the test in detecting CVD may reflect important differences in population cohorts, including sex.[72] Biomarkers can be effectively used in conjunction with clinical risk tools and as more date becomes available could be integrated into risk models. Refining HF prediction is a fundamental step to preventing the condition and improving HF outcomes, much more work is needed.

DETERMINING OPTIMAL HEART FAILURE THERAPY

There is ongoing debate about the reasons for observed sex-based differences in the treatment of HF. Recognition of the pathophysiologic and clinical differences between men and women with HF has led to conjecture that the clinical dose response or efficacy might differ as well. There are known sex-based differences in drug metabolism, bioavailability, pharmacokinetics, and toxicity. Most of the changes are attributed to differences in body composition, volume of distribution, and systemic clearance rates. However, women are 50–75% more likely than men to experience an adverse drug reaction. The influence of hormonal status and other sex-based influences on drug pharmacodynamics are underappreciated. Women are more prone to develop the malignant arrhythmia *torsades de pointes* when receiving medications known to prolong the QT interval.[73] Cough due to angiotensin-converting-enzyme (ACE) inhibitors is more than twice as common in women compared to men and can result in drug discontinuation. Substitution of angiotensin-receptor blockers (ARBs) for ACE inhibitors may, therefore, be more common in women compared to men, but this has not been substantiated.

Results of individual controlled clinical trials, even of standard therapeutic agents for HF with systolic dysfunction, generally are statistically inconclusive on this issue due to the smaller number of women recruited. However, data from pooled analyses improve the cumulative weight of evidence for therapeutic efficacy among women for most standard HF therapies. Recommendations made in the context of limited databases were summarized in the 2010 Heart Failure Society of America (HFSA) comprehensive practice guideline.[17] The guideline reviews of the experience of women in several large prospective mortality trials and meta-analyses. The HFSA recommends the use of both ACE inhibitors and beta-blockers in all patients with symptomatic LV dysfunction and specifically reports that women and men benet to a similar degree in reduction of mortality and mortality plus hospitalization in women. The recommendations for the use of ARBs in women have a level of evidence similar to those for men. The European and Canadian guidelines for the diagnosis and management of HF do not make any specific treatment recommendations based upon sex.

In the prevention of HF progression from the presence of asymptomatic structural heart disease (reduced EF) to an overt clinical HF syndrome, a potential difference in efficacy of ACE inhibitors between men and women in the treatment of asymptomatic LV dysfunction has been suggested. In a meta-analysis of seven major trials, men clearly have a mortality benefit when treated with ACE inhibitors for either symptomatic or asymptomatic LV systolic dysfunction.[74] A significant mortality benefit for women with asymptomatic LV dysfunction was not demonstrated (RR = 0.96; 95% CI = 0.75–1.22). However, since the ratio of RR for treatment effect between men and women did not reach statistical significance, a significant difference in therapeutic response between men and women could not be concluded.

The same meta-analysis pooled sex-specific data from four major beta-blocker trials in HFREF. The pooled studies included 2,134 women and 7,885 men. The random effects pooled estimate for the RR of mortality for women was 0.63 (95% CI = 0.44–0.91), whereas for men, the estimate was 0.66 (95% CI = 0.59–0.75). The authors did state that the most important limitation specific to their analysis was the inability to control for possible differences between subpopulations in the etiology of HF, with both women and blacks being less likely to have an ischemic etiology than white males.

Although digoxin therapy has been demonstrated to decrease HF hospitalization it has not been demonstrated to improve survival. In a *post hoc* subgroup analysis of the Digitalis Investigation Group (DIG) trial, digoxin was associated with an increased risk of death (5.8%) from any cause among women, but not men, with HF and reduced LVEF.[75] Furthermore, among women the effect of digoxin therapy was also associated with increased risk of death from worsening HF and other CV events, and a smaller reduction in rate of hospitalization for worsening HF than men.[75] However, that analysis did not account for serum potassium concentration and serum digoxin concentration differences. Another analysis of the same trial reported no excess mortality in either women or men with digoxin at serum concentrations between 0.5 mg/mL and 0.9 mg/mL, whereas the risk for mortality was greater with serum concentrations greater than or equal to 1.2 ng/mL in women.[76] This report demonstrated that digoxin levels were higher in women compared to men at any given dose presumably due to decreased lean body mass and glomerular filtration rate. Analysis of the SOLVD trials did not demonstrate an increase in mortality in women with digoxin.[53]

Although sex-specic data is not available from prospective trials on the benet of aldosterone antagonists for women with LV systolic dysfunction and symptoms of HF, adequate numbers of women were included in the large randomized, controlled trials of these agents. Subgroup analyses confirmed a therapeutic benet in women.[17]

One might expect less variability in the therapeutic approach to HF based on patient sex in HF specialty clinics, but this does not appear to be the case. In Spain, data from 4,720 patients from a registry of 62 specialty HF clinics found significant differences in pharmacological treatments utilized between men and women.[77] These differences were considered contributory to higher readmission rates for HF in women, despite similar mortality. Disparity in the application of medical therapeutics to women with HF, were consistent with those seen in other reports which the authors summarized.

Ancillary nonpharmacologic therapies are also underutilized in women with HF. Heart Failure and A Controlled Trial Investigating Outcomes of Exercise TraiNing (HF-ACTION) evaluated the impact of exercise training on clinical HF outcomes, and included the first prospectively planned analysis of the primary end-point by sex.[78] Exercise training showed significant reduction for all-cause mortality or all-cause hospitalization among female participants (HR = 0.74, 95% CI = 0.59–0.92) randomized to exercise compared to the males (0.99, 95% CI = 0.86–1.13). In HF-ACTION, suboptimal dosing of beta blockers was observed among women. In addition left bundle branch block (LBBB) was more common in women, yet the women had less biventricular pacing compared to the men.

Although controversial, there remains a lower referral rate for women with ischemic heart disease for therapeutic interventions with documented benefit. While the gender referral gap for revascularization may be dissipating in part due to improvements in technology, eligible women have fewer prophylactic internal cardiac defibrillators (ICDs) implanted than men.[79] Similarly, cardiac resynchronization therapy (CRT) is less often employed in women, yet there is evidence that women with HFREF and LBBB benefit to a greater degree than men from CRT.[80] There is a similar underrepresentation of eligible women referred for more advanced HF therapies, such as cardiac transplantation and mechanical assist devices.[81,82] In the German Heart Center Berlin heart transplant database, females donate 32% of organs and receive 18%, while males donate 68% and receive 82% of organs.

These are similar to the data available from the United Network of Organ Sharing in the United States, where females receive approximately 20% of donated hearts. In most transplant centers, the rates of acceptance for transplant and outcomes following transplantation are similar among men and women.[81] This suggests that the observed difference is due to strong referral bias, which might be overcome with community and provider education.

HEART FAILURE PREVENTION STRATEGIES

When discussing preventive strategies, it is important to recognize that sex-related differences of risk factor burden and CHD free survival change over time. In Wilkins et al. (2012), pooled analysis of survival data taken from 1964 through 2008 where all participants were free of CHD at baseline with risk factor data (blood pressure, cholesterol, diabetes and smoking status) and total CVD.[50] The overall risk for total CVD was substantially greater in individuals with greater risk factor burden and the lifetime risk still exceeded 30% in men and women with an optimal risk factor profile.[51] This highlights the large public health burden of CVD for both men and women and creates a large impetus for prevention. A discussion of the optimal sex-specific pharmacotherapy and ancillary treatment strategies for the prevention or treatment of HTN, diabetes, obesity, and CHD is beyond the scope of this discussion.

CONCLUSION AND PRACTICE IMPLICATIONS

There is a growing need for a better understanding of sex differences in the management of HF. Identifying sex differences or gender-specific clinical characteristics may help focus quality improvement efforts and guide future efforts on the formulation of specific plans for balanced recruitment of both men and women in clinical trials at a rate commensurate with the prevalence of HF. It is reasonable to postulate that a better understanding of sex differences might suggest novel approaches to early screening and prevention. Moreover, additional insight into sex differences in pathophysiologic mechanisms that lead to HF will contribute to further development of unique new therapies for this lethal disease. Finally, clinical implications of sex differences in HF may guide healthcare providers and researchers to recognize that one shoe does not fit all and catalyze implementing tailored or modified approaches to achieving optimal therapy for this prevalent syndrome, and thus further quality improvement efforts. In an aging society, we can expect to see a sustained increase in the number of new HF cases, particularly among women, favoring HFPEF as the predominant physiological phenotype.

REFERENCES

1. Roger VL, Go AS, Lloyd-Jones DM, et al. Heart disease and stroke statistics—2012 update: a report from the American Heart Association. Circulation. 2012;125(1):e2-220.
2. Heidenreich PA, Trogdon JB, Khavjou OA, et al. Forecasting the future of cardiovascular disease in the United States: a policy statement from the American Heart Association. Circulation. 2011;123(8):933-44.
3. Hunt SA, Abraham WT, Chin MH, et al. Focused update incorporated into the ACC/AHA 2005 Guidelines for the Diagnosis and Management of Heart Failure in Adults. A Report of the American College of Cardiology Foundation/American Heart Association Task Force on Practice Guidelines Developed in Collaboration with the International Society for Heart and Lung Transplantation. J Am Coll Cardiol. 2009;53(15):e1-90.
4. Lloyd-Jones DM, Larson MG, Leip EP, et al. Framingham Heart Study. Lifetime risk for developing congestive heart failure: The Framingham Heart Study. Circulation. 2002;106:3068-72.
5. Roger VL, Weston SA, Redfield MM, et al. Trends in heart failure incidence and survival in a community-based population. JAMA. 2004;292:344-50.
6. Ross JS, Chen J, Lin Z, et al. Recent national trends in readmission rates after heart failure hospitalization. Circ Heart Fail. 2010;3:97-103.
7. Lee WY, Capra AM, Jensvold NG, et al. Gender and risk of adverse outcomes in heart failure. Am J Cardiol. 2004;94:1147-52.
8. Koelling TM, Chen RS, Lubwama RN, et al. The expanding national burden of heart failure in the United States: the influence of heart failure in women. Am Heart J. 2004;147:74-8.
9. Braunstein JB, Anderson GF, Gerstenblith G, et al. Noncardiac comorbidity increases preventable hospitalizations and mortality among Medicare beneficiaries with chronic heart failure. J Am Coll Cardiol. 2003;42: 1226-33.
10. Hsich EM, Pina IL. Heart failure in women: a need for prospective data. J Am Coll Cardiol. 2009;54:491-8.
11. Hunt SA, Abraham WT, Chin MH, et al. 2009 focused update incorporated into the ACC/AHA 2005 Guidelines for the Diagnosis and Management of Heart Failure in Adults. JACC. 2009;53(15):e1-90.
12. O'Meara E, Clayton T, McEntegart MB, et al. Sex differences in clinical characteristics and prognosis in a broad spectrum of patients with heart failure: results of the Candesartan in Heart failure: Assessment of Reduction in Mortality and morbidity (CHARM) program. Circulation. 2007; 115:3111-20.
13. Masoudi FA, Havranek EP, Smith G, et al. Gender, age, and heart failure with preserved left ventricular systolic function. J Am Coll Cardiol. 2003; 41(2):217-23.
14. Levy D, Kenchaiah S, Larson MG, et al. Long-term trends in the incidence of and survival with heart failure. N Engl J Med. 2002;347(18):1397-402.
15. Barnard DD. Heart failure in women. Curr Cardio Rep. 2005;7(3):159-63.
16. Shah RU, Klein L, Lloyd-Jones DM. Heart failure in women: epidemiology, biology and treatment. Womens Health (Lond Engl). 2009;5(5):517-27.
17. Heart Failure Society of America, Lindenfeld J, Albert NM, et al. HFSA 2010 Comprehensive Heart Failure Practice Guideline. J Card Fail. 2010;16(6):e1-194.
18. Lenzen MJ, Rosengren A, Scholte op Reimer WJ, et al. Management of patients with heart failure in clinical practice: differences between men and women. Heart. 2008;94(3):e10.
19. Rathore SS, Floody JM, Wang Y, et al. Sex, quality of care, and outcomes of elderly patients hospitalized with heart failure: findings from the National Heart Failure Project. Am Heart J. 2005;149(1):121-8.
20. McCullough PA, Philbin EF, Spertus JA, et al. Confirmation of a heart failure epidemic: findings from the Resource Utilization Among Congestive Heart Failure (REACH) study. J Am Coll Cardiol. 2002;39(1):60-9.
21. Ho KK, Anderson KM, Kannel WB, et al. Survival after the onset of congestive heart failure in Framingham Heart Study subjects. Circulation. 1993;88(1):107-15.
22. Administration on Aging US Department of Health and Human Services. (2011). A Profile of Older Americans: 2011. [online] Available from: www.aoa.gov/Aging_Statistics/Profile/2011/docs/2011profile.pdf. [Accessed December, 2013].
23. Cleland JG, Swedberg K, Follath F, et al. The Euro Heart Failure Survey programme—a survey on the quality of care among patients with heart failure in Europe. Part 1: patient characteristics and diagnosis. Eur Heart J. 2003;24(5):442-63.
24. Levy D, Larson MG, Vasan RS, et al. The progression from hypertension to congestive heart failure. JAMA. 1996;275(20):1557-62.
25. Chobanian AV, Bakris GI, Black HR, et al. The Seventh Report of the Joint National Committee on Prevention, Detection, Evaluation and Treatment of High Blood Pressure: the JNC 7 report. JAMA. 2003;289(19):2560-72.
26. Ginghina C, Botezatu CD, Servan M, et al. A personalized medicine target: heart failure in women. J Med Life. 2011;4(3):280-6.
27. Stromberg A, Martensson J. Gender differences in patients with heart failure. Cur J Cardiovasc Nurs. 2003;2(1):7-18.
28. Regitz-Zagrosek V, Brokat S, Tschope C. Role of gender in heart failure with normal left ventricular ejection fraction. Prog Cardiovasc Dis. 2007;49(4):241-51.
29. Fisher M, Baessler A, Schukert H. Renin angiotensin system and gender differences in the cardiovascular system. Cardiovasc Res. 2002;53(3): 672-7.
30. Mejhert M, Holmgren J, Wandell P, et al. Diagnostic tests, treatment and follow-up in heart failure patients—is there a gender bias in the coherence to guidelines? Cur J Heart Fail. 1999;1(4):407-10.

31. Senni M, Rodenheffer RJ, Tribouilloy CM, et al. Use of echocardiography in the management of congestive heart failure in the community. J Am Coll Cardiol. 1999;33(1):164-70.
32. Topol E, Traill T, Fortunin N. Hypertensive hypertrophy cardiomyopathy of the elderly. N Engl J Med. 1985;312(2):277-83.
33. Wong, DT, Clark RA, Dondon BK, et al. Beware of quiet little old ladies: demographic features, pharmacotherapy, readmissions and survival in a 10-year cohort of patients with heart failure and preserved systolic function. Med J Aust. 2010;192(1):9-13.
34. Nieminen MS, Harjola VP, Hochadel M, et al. Gender related differences in patients presenting with acute heart failure. Results from the Euro Heart Failure Survey II. Eur J Heart Fail. 2008;10(2):140-8.
35. Galvao M, Kalman J, Demarco T, et al. Gender differences in in-hospital management and outcomes in patients with decompensated heart failure; analysis from the Acute Decompensated Heart Failure National Registry (ADHERE). J Card Fail. 2006;12(2):100-7.
36. Lee WY, Capra AM, Jensvold NG, et al. Gender and risk of adverse outcomes in heart failure. Am J Cardiol. 2004;94(9):1147-52.
37. Gustafsson F, Torp-Pedersen C, Burchardt H, et al. Female sex is associated with a better long-term survival in patients hospitalized with congestive heart failure. Eur Heart J. 2004;25(2):129-35.
38. O'Meara E, Clayton T, McEntegart MB, et al. Sex differences in clinical characteristics and prognosis in a broad spectrum of patients with heart failure: results of the Candesartan in Heart failure: Assessment of Reduction in Mortality and morbidity (CHARM) program. Circulation. 2007;115(24):3111-20.
39. Fairweather D, Cooper LT JR, Blauwet LA. Sex and gender differences in myocarditis and dilated cardiomyopathy. Curr Probl Cardiol. 2013;38(1): 7-26.
40. Iribarren C, Kater AJ, Go AS, et al. Glycemic control and heart failure among adult patients with diabetes. Circulation. 2001;103(22):2668-73.
41. Bibbins-Domingo K, Lin F, Vittinghoff E, et al. Predictors of heart failure among women with coronary disease. Circulation. 2004;110(11):1424-30.
42. Kannel WB, Hjortland M, Castelli WP. Role of diabetes in congestive heart failure: the Framingham study. Am J Cardiol. 1974;34(1):29-34.
43. Galderisi M, Anderson KM, Wilson PW, et al. Echocardiographic evidence for the existence of a distinct diabetic cardiomyopathy (the Framingham Heart Study). Am J Cardiol. 1991;68(1):85-9.
44. Meisinger C, Thorand B, Schneider A, et al. Sex differences in risk factors for incident type 2 diabetes mellitus: the MONICA Augsburg cohort study. Ach Intern Med. 2002;162(1):82-9.
45. Tanko LB, Bagger YZ, Alexandersen P, et al. Peripheral adiposity exhibits an independent dominant antiatherogenic effect in elderly women. Circulation. 2003;107(12):1626-31.
46. Kenchaiah S, Evans JC, Levy D, et al. Obesity and the risk of heart failure. N Engl J Med. 2002;347(5):305-13.
47. He J, Ogden L, Bazzaon L, et al. Risk factors for congestive heart failure in US men and women; NHANES I epidemiologic follow-up study. Arch Intern Med. 2001;161(7):996-1002.
48. Ghali JK, Krause-Steinrauf HJ, Adams KR, et al. Gender differences in advanced heart failure: insights from the BEST study. J Am Coll Cardiol. 2003;42(12):2128-34.
49. Hsich E, Chadalavada S, Krishnaswarmy G, et al. Long-term prognostic value of peak oxygen consumption in women versus men with heart failure and severely impaired left ventricular systolic function. Am J Cardiol. 2007;100(2):291-5.
50. Wilkins JT, Ning H, Berry J, et al. Lifetime risk and years lived free of total cardiovascular disease. JAMA. 2012;308(17):1795-801.
51. Lloyd-Jones DM, Larson MG, Beiser A, et al. Life-time risk of developing coronary heart disease. Lancet. 1999;353(9147):89-92.
52. Jessup M, Piña IL. Is it important to examine gender differences in the epidemiology and outcome of severe heart failure? J Thorac Cardiovasc Surg. 2004;127(5):1247-52.
53. Johnstone D, Limacher M, Roussear M, et al. Clinical Characteristics of patients in studies of left ventricular dysfunction (SOLVD). Am J Cardiol. 1992;70(9):894-900.
54. Mehta PA, Cowie MR. Gender and heart failure: a population perspective. Heart. 2006;92(Suppl 3):iii14-18.
55. Azevedo A, Bettencourt P, Pimenta J, et al. Clinical syndrome suggestive of heart failure is frequently attributable to non-cardiac disorders—population-based study. Eur J Heart Fail. 2007;9(4):391-6.
56. Seo Y, Yates B, Dizona P, et al. (2013). Predictors of cognitive/affective and somatic depression in heart failure patients. [online] Available from: cnr.sagepub.com/content/early/2013/01/28/1054773812473476. abstract. [Accessed December, 2013].
57. Angermann CE, Gelbrich B, Stork S, et al. Somatic correlates of comorbid major depression in patients with systolic heart failure. Int J Cardiol. 2011;147(1):66-73.
58. Sullivan M, Levy WC, Russo JE, et al. Depression and health status in patients with advanced heart failure: A prospective Study in Tertiary Care. J Card Fail. 2004;10(5):390-6.
59. Maisel AS, Bhalla V, Braunwald E. Cardiac biomarkers: a contemporary status report. Nat Clin Pract Cardiovasc Med. 2006;3(1):24-34.
60. Maisel AS, Krishnaswamy P, Nowak RM, et al. Rapid measurement of B-type natriuretic peptide in the emergency diagnosis of heart failure. N Engl J Med. 2002;347(3):161-7.
61. Bettencourt P, Azevedo A, Pimenta J, et al. N-terminal-pro-brain natriuretic peptide predicts outcome after hospital discharge in heart failure patients. Circulation. 2004;110(15):2168-74.
62. Maisel A, Hollander JE, Guss D, et al. Primary results of the Rapid Emergency Department Heart Failure Outpatient Trial (REDHOT). A multicenter study of B-type natriuretic peptide levels, emergency department decision making, and outcomes in patients presenting with shortness of breath. J Am Coll Cardiol. 2004;44(6):1328-33.
63. Weber M, Hamm C. Role of B-type natriuretic peptide (BNP) and NT-proBNP in clinical routine. Heart. 2006;92(6):843-9.
64. McDonagh TA, Holmer S, Raymond I, et al. NT-proBNP and the diagnosis of heart failure: a pooled analysis of three European epidemiological studies. Eur J Heart Fail. 2004;6(3):269-73.
65. Raymond I, Groenning BA, Hildebrandt PR, et al. The inuence of age, sex and other variables on the plasma level of N-terminal pro brain natriuretic peptide in a large sample of the general population. Heart. 2003;89(7):745-51.
66. Christ M, Laule-Kilian K, Hochholzer W, et al. Gender-specific risk stratification with B-type natriuretic peptide levels in patients with acute dyspnea. J Am Coll Cardiol. 2006;48(9):1808-12.
67. Redfield MM, Rodeheffer RJ, Jacobsen SJ, et al. Plasma brain natriuretic peptide concentration: impact of age and gender. JACC. 2002;40(5): 976-82.
68. Wang TJ, Larson MG, Levy D, et al. Impact of age and sex on plasma natriuretic peptide levels in healthy adults. Am J Card. 2002;90(3):254-8.
69. Velagaleti RS, Gona P, Larson MG, et al. Multimarker approaches for the prediction of heart failure incidence in the community. Circulation. 2010;122(17):1700-6.
70. Perna ER, Macin SM, Cimbaro, et al. Minor myocardial damage detected by troponin T is a powerful predictor of long-term prognosis in patients with acute decompensated heart failure. Int J Cardiol. 2005;99(2): 253-61.
71. Horwich TB, Patel J, MacLellan WR, et al. Cardiac troponin I is associated with impaired hemodynamic, progressive left ventricular dysfunction,

and increased mortality rates in advanced heart failure. Circulation. 2003;108(7):833-8.

72. deFilippi CR, de Lemos JA, Christenson RH, et al. Association of serial measures of cardiac troponin t using a sensitive assay with incident heart failure and cardiovascular mortality in older adults. JAMA. 2010; 304(22):2494-502.
73. Whitley H, Lindsey W. Sex-based differences in drug activity. Am Fam Physician. 2009;80(11):1254-8.
74. Shekelle PG, Rich MW, Morton SC, et al. Efficacy of angiotensin-converting enzyme inhibitors and beta-blockers in the management of left ventricular systolic dysfunction according to race, gender and diabetic status. JACC. 2003;41(9):1529-38.
75. Rathore SS, Wang Y, Krumholz HM. Sex-based differences in the effect of digoxin for the treatment of heart failure. N Eng J Med. 2002;347(18): 1403-11.
76. Kirkwood FA, Patterson JH, Gattis WA, et al. Relationship of serum digoxin concentration to mortality and morbidity in women in the digitalis investigation group trial: a retrospective analysis. J Am Coll Cardiol. 2005;46(3):496-504.
77. Jiménez-Navarro MF, Ramirez-Marrero MA, Anguita-Sánchez M, et al. Influence of gender on long-term prognosis of patients with chronic heart failure seen in heart failure clinics. Clin Cardiol. 2010;33(3):E13-8.
78. Piña IL, Kokkinos P, Kao A, et al. Baseline differences in the HF-ACTION trial by sex. Am Heart J. 2009;158(4 Suppl):S16-23.
79. Hernandez AF, Fonarow GC, Liang L, et al. Sex and racial differences in the use of implantable cardioverter-defibrillators among patients hospitalized with heart failure. JAMA. 2007;298(13):1525-32.
80. Arshad A, Moss, AJ, Foster E, et al. Cardiac resynchronization therapy is more effective in women than in men: the MADIT-CRT (Multicenter Automatic Defibrillator Implantation Trial with Cardiac Resynchronization Therapy) trial. J Am Coll Cardiol. 2011;57(7):813-20.
81. Aaronson KD, Schwartz JS, Goin JE, et al. Sex differences in patient acceptance of cardiac transplant candidacy. Circulation. 1995;91(11): 2753-61.
82. Regitz-Zagrosek V. Sex and gender differences in cardiovascular disease. In: Oertelt-Prigoione S, Regitz-Zagrosek V (Eds). Sex and Gender Aspects in Clinical Medicine. New York, USA: Springer-Verlag London Limited; 2012. pp. 32-7.

Chapter 38

Chronic Heart Failure in Geriatric Patients

José Tallaj, Kanan Patel, Ali Ahmed

ABSTRACT

Heart failure (HF) disproportionately affects older adults, due to a multitude of reasons including age-related changes in the cardiovascular system and the cumulative effect of multiple risk factors that is more likely to lead to the development of HF with preserved ejection fraction (HFpEF). Unlike other cardiovascular conditions, such as acute myocardial infarction that can present atypically or even be asymptomatic in older adults, clinical presentation of HF in older adults is rather similar regardless of age, except that older adults tend to attribute their HF symptoms to aging and respond by restricting physical activity thus delaying the presentation and diagnosis. Comorbidities and polypharmacy complicate the assessment and management of HF in older adults and the process may be simplified by the mnemonic DEFEAT (Diagnosis, Etiology, Fluid volume, Ejection fraction, And Treatment). Because HF is a clinical syndrome without a definite diagnostic test or procedure, a clinical diagnosis needs to be established based on the presence of constellation of symptoms and signs and underlying etiological risk factors need to be identified. It is often difficult to establish a direct causal role of multiple risk factors present in older HF patients. For optimal symptom management, euvolemia needs to be achieved by salt and fluid restriction and judicious use of diuretics. The latter is guided by fluid volume status assessed by jugular venous pressure using both internal and external jugular veins. Left ventricular ejection fraction (EF) needs to be determined using echocardiogram to identify HF with reduced EF who may benefit from evidence-based therapy with neurohormonal blockade and selective use of device and surgical therapies. Palliative care should be considered early and older adults with terminal HF should be referred for hospice care.

INTRODUCTION

Heart failure (HF) is a clinical syndrome that disproportionately affects older adults and is the leading cause for hospital admission and readmission for medicare beneficiaries in the United States. Like other geriatric syndromes, HF in older adults is often caused by multiple etiologic factors involving multiple pathogenetic pathways that lead to a common set of symptoms (Fig. 1).[1] These multiple etiologic factors often exist as multiple comorbidities in older adults with HF, which affect their management and prognosis. In the United States, about 10% of Medicare beneficiaries have six or more chronic conditions, a quarter of whom are readmitted within 30 days of hospital discharge.[2] HF is the only chronic condition with a similar readmission rate which in part is explained by the very high comorbidity in HF. Nearly half of all HF patients have five or more morbidities.[2] The diagnosis and management of HF in older adults can be confusing, but can be simplified by the use of the mnemonic Diagnosis, Etiology, Fluid volume, Ejection fraction, And Treatment (DEFEAT)-HF (Table 1).[3-6]

DIAGNOSIS

Because HF is a clinical syndrome, nearly all newly-diagnosed HF patients have one or more symptoms and signs of HF. Unlike other cardiovascular conditions, such as acute myocardial infarction that can present atypically or even be asymptomatic in older adults, HF symptoms

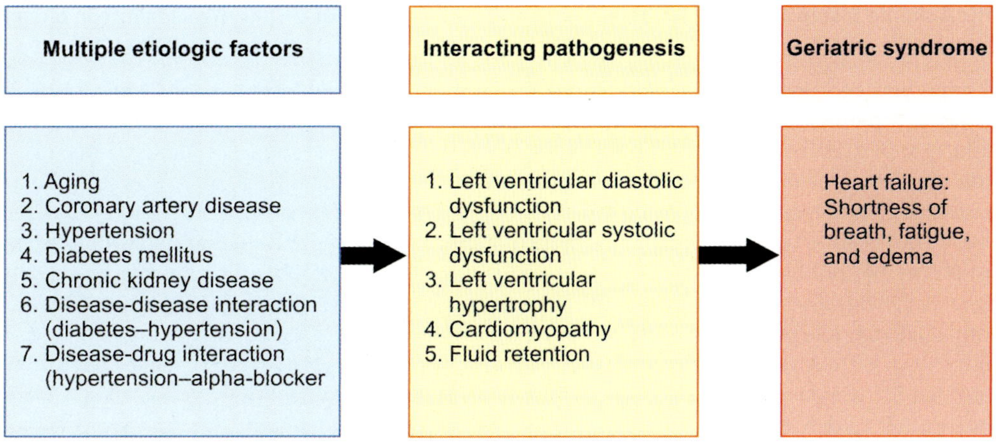

Fig. 1 Geriatric syndrome model of heart failure in older adults[1]

in older adults are generally similar regardless of age. Dyspnea on exertion (DOE) and fatigue are the most common symptoms of HF and nearly always present in all newly diagnosed HF patients. DOE is more common after abrupt activities, such as walking fast to pick up the phone from the other end of the room. Older adults often learn to avoid DOE by avoiding strenuous activities or by restricting physical activities that cause DOE. When an 85-year-old has DOE on walking four blocks that he/she could previously walk without DOE, he/she is more likely to attribute that to aging and it is not perceived as abnormal. These patients may even report no DOE when asked unless specifically asked about recent activity limitation. In some cases, older adults may continue to restrict activities until they have DOE on minimal exertion, such as walking around the house and in extreme cases, when they have dyspnea at rest. This may result in delayed diagnosis. Fatigue, on the other hand, results at the end of one's physiological exercise tolerance and often cannot be avoided. For example, a 75 year old with HF may get DOE on walking one block at a fast pace, but can walk up to four blocks at his/her own pace. They may not have DOE after that but they will report fatigue if they tried to walk longer without some rest. So, fatigue is probably more non-specific than DOE and when present without DOE, it is unlikely to be due to HF. Fatigue could also result from low cardiac output and indicates a more advanced disease. The other common HF symptom, swelling of the dependent parts of body, which is leg for the vast majority of ambulatory older adults, is also rather nonspecific. Bilateral leg swelling due to venous insufficiency is not uncommon in old age. When the onset of leg swelling is older than that of DOE, it is not very helpful in making a constellation of symptoms that would be suggestive of HF. However, when DOE and leg swelling are of similar duration, suspicion for HF should be higher.

Two other variants of dyspnea are also reported by patients with HF, orthopnea, and paroxysmal nocturnal dyspnea (PND). HF patients learn to use more pillows to avoid orthopnea. Some may even use blocks to raise the head of their beds and some may use hospital beds or sleep on a couch. Thus, a pillow count may not always inform about the presence of orthopnea. Patients are less likely to experience PND if they sleep on multiple pillows or sleep on a couch. Both orthopnea and PND are considered more specific HF symptoms and are major Framingham criteria for the diagnosis of HF which suggest that their presence would confirm a diagnosis of HF.[7] However, an analysis of 5,771 community-dwelling older adults in the Cardiovascular Health Study (CHS) suggested that only 388 (7%) reported both orthopnea and PND, and of these only 20% (76/388) had centrally-adjudicated HF.[8] When lower extremity edema was included, still only about 33% of older adults with all three symptoms of orthopnea, PND and lower extremity edema had centrally-adjudicate HF in the CHS. Thus, older adults with two very specific symptoms of HF and an important associated symptom may not have HF and other evidence must be sought before a diagnosis of HF may be made. It is also important to remember that the diagnosis of HF may be an ongoing process when early symptoms may not be associated with signs such as an elevation of JVP which may appear later in the course.

TABLE 1: DEFEAT-HF: A simple 5-step approach for assessment and management of chronic heart failure in older adults[4]

D	Diagnosis	There is no single test or procedure to establish a diagnosis of HF which needs to be done based on a constellation of symptoms and signs. Dyspnea and fatigue on exertion, often with simultaneous lower extremity edema are the earliest symptoms of HF in ambulatory older adults. Dyspnea is often precipitated by an abrupt activity, such as rushing to pick up the phone ringing on the other end of the room. Fatigue, on the other hand, sets in at the upper limit of exercise tolerance during activities performed at patients' own pace, such as walking on a level ground in a controlled environment, such as inside a mall. Orthopnea and paroxysmal nocturnal dyspnea (PND), when present, are helpful, but need to be interpreted in the context of other symptoms and signs as many older adults with both these symptoms may not have HF. The most useful sign of new-onset clinical HF is the fluid volume retention estimated by elevated JVP. Because nearly all incident HF patients are expected to have clinical HF, most will have elevated JVP and a normal JVP may rule out clinical HF during initial presentation in older adults without known HF. However, older adults with known HF receiving diuretics may have normal JVP, and some without diuretics may have normal JVP. Therefore, a normal JVP should not be used to rule out HF in a patient with known HF who was initially diagnosed elsewhere. Unlike other cardiovascular conditions, such as acute myocardial infarction, the clinical presentation of HF is rarely atypical in older adults although it may be delayed as older adults may attribute their HF symptoms to aging and avoid symptoms by restricting physical activity
E	Etiology	HF is a clinical syndrome and not a disease, and as such like fever, a diagnosis of HF is incomplete without an assessment of an underlying cause. In older adults with HF, these causes are often multiple and many HF risk factors, such as hypertension (HTN), coronary artery disease, diabetes, and atrial fibrillation are highly prevalent. Although it is often difficult to establish direct causal association, these should be identified for secondary prevention. When no known risk factors can be identified or a known risk factor such as an ongoing myocardial ischemia is active in an older adult with actively deteriorating HF, cardiology referral should be considered
F	Fluid volume	HF symptoms are most optimally controlled when patients are euvolemic and achieving euvolemia is an important clinical goal. In addition to salt and fluid restriction, diuretics are most frequently essential. Judicious use of diuretics needs to be guided by JVP estimated by a careful evaluation of internal or external jugular venous pulsation in the neck. JVP should be routinely assessed during all visits as it is the most important physical examination in HF and an elevated JVP is the most reliable sign of fluid volume retention. A determination of "no fluid retention" is not enough in patients with known HF as it is important to avoid hypovolemia due to overdiuresis. Therefore, JVP needs to be estimated in centimeters (cm) of water, which is "vertical" distance from the RA to the top of the jugular pulsation. Proper estimation of JVP is a multistep process that begins with positioning the patient so that the top of the jugular pulsation is visible in the middle of the neck, which could be supine when the JVP is low or sitting when the JVP is high. Then, the "vertical" distance from the SA to the top of the venous pulsation needs to be measured in cm. When the JVP is low, the top of the jugular pulsation may be at a lower level than the SA, and this number could be negative. The distance needs to be added to the distance between RA and SA. The RA-to-SA distance varies with body position and is 5 cm in supine position, 8 cm at 30°, and 10 cm at 45° or higher degrees of inclines
E	Ejection fraction (EF)	Left ventricular (LV) EF is the single most important test after a clinical diagnosis of HF has been made, and should be estimated using an echocardiogram. This information is necessary to categorize HF patients into those with reduced EF (HFrEF) and preserved EF (HFpEF). This classification has both prognostic and therapeutic significances: patients with HFrEF generally have poorer prognosis but that can be improved by use of disease-modifying neurohormonal antagonists
A	And	
T	Therapy	Guideline-recommended evidence-based HF therapy is restricted to HFrEF as there is no evidence of their benefit in HFpEF. Although nearly all randomized controlled trials (RCTs) are based on younger patients and older trial eligible patients often are prognostically better than real-world older patients, extrapolation of this evidence to older HFrEF patients, specifically those 65–79 years, are generally accepted. However, most RCTs systematically excluded older HF patients 80 years of age or older, and these drugs need to be used with caution in octogenarian patients with HFrEF. Because HF symptoms are similar for both HFrEF and HFpEF, therapy to relieve symptoms is generally similar for both types of HF

DEFEAT-HF, Diagnosis, Etiology, Fluid volume, Ejection fraction, And Treatment of Heart Failure; HF, heart failure; JVP, jugular venous pressure; SA, sternal angle; RA, right atrium

Heart failure patients may present with several clinical signs, including an elevation of jugular venous pressure (JVP), a positive hepatojugular reflux (HJR), a third heart sound (S3), pulmonary rales, ascites and edema of legs, or other dependent parts. All these signs are useful markers of right heart pressure, but only an elevated JVP is the best marker of an elevated pulmonary capillary wedge pressure (≥18 mmHg) with over 80% sensitivity, specificity and positive predictive values.[9] In fact, according to the American College of Cardiology (ACC) and American Heart Association (AHA) guideline for chronic HF, an elevated JVP is the most reliable sign of volume overload.[10] Because by definition, all new HF patients have clinical HF, they would have some degree of fluid volume retention. Confirmation of a normal JVP may be used to rule out an initial diagnosis of new HF in a patient who is not receiving diuretics. Similarly, an elevated JVP in the presence of other HF symptoms may be sufficient for an initial clinical diagnosis of HF. When internal jugular vein (IJV) cannot be viewed, which is not uncommon in chronic HF, one can estimate JVP from EJV. The IJV lies deep behind the sternocleidomastoid muscle for most of its course in the neck and its low pressure (10 cm of water = 7.4 mmHg) may not be transmitted to the surface of the neck, and may even be confounded by the adjacent high-pressure carotid pulsation and may be underestimated by experienced clinicians. Underestimation of JVP, presumably based on IJV, is well documented in literature. In two major randomized controlled trials (RCTs) of HF that enrolled nearly 10,000 patients and were examined by cardiologists, less than 15% of patients were reported to have JVP elevation.[11,12] This rate was similar in a group of older adults who presented at the emergency department with dyspnea,[13] and was slightly better (about 33%) in HF patients who were hospitalized for acutely decompensation.[14] Therefore, EJV needs to be used when IJV pulsation is not clearly visible and readable.[15]

Although the art of JVP estimation can be easily learned and mastered through practice, clinicians not comfortable with JVP estimation (a long-term handicap for HF care) may use serum B-type natriuretic peptide (BNP) and N-terminal pro-BNP (NT-proBNP) to help make a clinical diagnosis of HF. Although these neurohormones are secreted by the failing ventricle in HF, they may be elevated in other conditions and should not be used alone.[16] A normal level of BNP or NT-proBNP may be more helpful in ruling out HF than making a diagnosis with elevated levels. In one study of 1,586 younger (mean age, 64 years) patients with acute dyspnea who were examined by two independent cardiologists, 47% were diagnosed with HF but only 22% were reported to have JVP elevation.[17] In that study, 89% and 96% of those with BNP values less than 100 and less than 50 pg/mL respectively did not have HF.[17] Thus, although BNP was reported to be more accurate than physical signs in identifying HF, this was likely due to the fact that JVP elevation was missed in over half of the HF patients with acute dyspnea.[17] Older patients are also known to have higher circulating levels of natriuretic peptides,[18,19] and there are no standard cutoffs for these neurohormones for older adults,[16,20] it is strongly recommended that clinicians taking care of HF patients learn how to properly estimate JVP. Pulmonary rales are not a reliable sign of fluid retention in chronic HF as they are often absent as the fluid accumulated in the alveoli is rapidly cleared by the lymphatic system. However, when fluid buildup is rapid, pulmonary edema may develop.

All newly diagnosed HF patients have symptoms of HF and evidence of fluid volume retention, especially an elevated JVP, during the initial presentation. When patients with known HF who are already on diuretics are being seen for the first time as a new patient, it is important to confirm the diagnosis. Generally speaking, when HF patients are on diuretics and give a history of prior hospital admission due to acute decompensated HF, a diagnosis of HF is likely correct. However, if those patients give no history of DOE, orthopnea, PND, or leg swelling in the past, especially prior to the reported HF hospitalization, the diagnosis should be suspected. An older adult with signs and symptoms of HF who has reduced LV EF is more likely to have HF than if the EF is preserved, especially if the initial diagnosis was made in an ambulatory setting. However, EF should not be used to make an initial diagnosis of HF in older adults. Over half of all HF in older adults is HF due to preserved EF (HFpEF).[21] When data on a prior EF is available or an echocardiogram is done for another reason, it needs to be wisely incorporated in the diagnosis process. A low EF or severe impairment of diastolic filling by echocardiogram may help the initial diagnosis process, especially when a clinical diagnosis is not conclusive. However, a clinical diagnosis of HF should be made without using information on EF as clinical presentation of older adults with HFpEF and HFrEF is very similar.[14]

The terms acute HF and chronic HF are not synonymous with the terms newly-diagnosed HF and known HF. Because older adults often attribute their HF symptoms to aging and avoid symptoms by limiting physical activity, the process may continue until they have dyspnea at rest. Although these patients may present with New York Heart Association (NYHA) class IV symptoms, they did not develop them acutely, and can often be treated as an outpatient. On the other hand, an older adult with known HF may acutely decompensate after non-adherence with diet or medications, or from complications, such as severely uncontrolled blood pressure (BP) or acute myocardial ischemia. Therefore, HF symptoms may develop acutely or over time regardless of whether HF is new or known.

ETIOLOGY

A diagnosis of HF is incomplete without a determination of the underlying causes as a diagnosis of fever is incomplete without a determination of the underlying causes. Although HF in older adults is often described as due to hypertension (HTN), more often it has multiple etiological factors. As such, determining underlying causes may not always be easy. However, it is important for secondary prevention. As such when HF risk factors, such as HTN, coronary artery disease, diabetes, atrial fibrillation, obesity, and smoking are present as comorbidities, they should be identified and properly managed as appropriate. Although the extent to which each of these may be responsible for the development of HF cannot often be determined, it is also not clear to what extent it ought to be pursued. One of the reasons for the determination of potential etiological factors is to prevent continued insult that caused the HF in the first place. While that might be easy for some risk factors, it might be more complicated for others. For example, smoking is a risk factor for HF and also associated with poor outcomes.[22,23] Therefore, recommending smoking cessation to patients with HF who are smokers is rather straightforward even if smoking was not directly responsible for the development of HF. While diabetes is a risk factor for HF,[24] it cannot often be determined if it played a role in the development of HF. The comorbidity of diabetes may be of recent onset and thus may not have enough time to play a causal role, or it may have been a pre-existing condition but played no role (not everyone with diabetes develops HF). Although the presence of diabetes as a comorbidity maybe associated with poor outcomes,[25] there is no evidence that a more aggressive treatment of diabetes would improve outcomes. In contrast, HTN is also a risk factor for HF.[26] Yet, in patients with HF, low BP is often associated with poor outcomes.[27-29] Similarly, while obesity is a risk factor for HF,[30] once patients develop HF, obesity appears to provide paradoxical benefit.[31] It is recommended that reversible causes like myocardial ischemia be ruled out, especially when the EF is reduced. Another important etiology unique to the older HF population is amyloidosis, especially the senile type.[32] Cardiac amyloidosis should be suspected in patients with severe LV hypertrophy by echocardiogram with borderline EF, low voltage, and conduction abnormalities on the electrocardiogram or an accentuated response to digoxin.

FLUID VOLUME ASSESSMENT

Fluid volume assessment is the most important part of both initial and ongoing evaluations of older HF patients.[33] While pathophysiology of acute decompensation in HF is complex and some HF patients may decompensate due to redistribution of fluid rather than fluid overload,[34,35] the decompensation in the vast majority of HF patients is associated with fluid volume retention.[14] During initial evaluation of HF when prior data on weight are unavailable, it is often difficult to determine to what extent a weight gain was due to fluid retention. However, a weight gain or loss during a short period of time in a patient with chronic HF is usually due to fluid retention or response to diuretics. An elevated JVP is the most important physical sign of fluid volume overload and must be carefully estimated in all patients with HF. Proper estimation of JVP requires understanding three myths that surround it. First, the rule of IJV alone is likely to limit JVP estimation. Second, the rule of 45° is likely to preclude estimation of JVP when it is low or severely elevated without a plethoric EJV. The latter is important in the evaluation of chronic HF patients receiving diuretics. Finally, the rule of 5 cm is likely to underestimate true JVP. As mentioned earlier, anatomically IJV lies deep under the sternocleidomastoid muscle and in close proximity of the carotid artery, which often makes it difficult to estimate JVP from IJV. Therefore, clinicians should learn how to use EJV and understand its limitations. If no venous pulsation is visible in the neck at a 45° incline, then the JVP is not likely elevated and this is probably enough to rule out new-onset HF. However, this may be problematic when someone is on a high dose of diuretic and may be overdiuresed or hypovolemic and has low JVP. This could only be appreciated at a lower incline when the jugular pulsation would be visible in the neck. Similarly, in patients with severely elevated JVP, the pulsations might not be appreciated unless the patient is sitting at 90° or even standing at times.

The JVP is the vertical distance between the right atrium (RA) and the top of the jugular pulsation and is an estimate of the central venous or right atrial pressure that can only

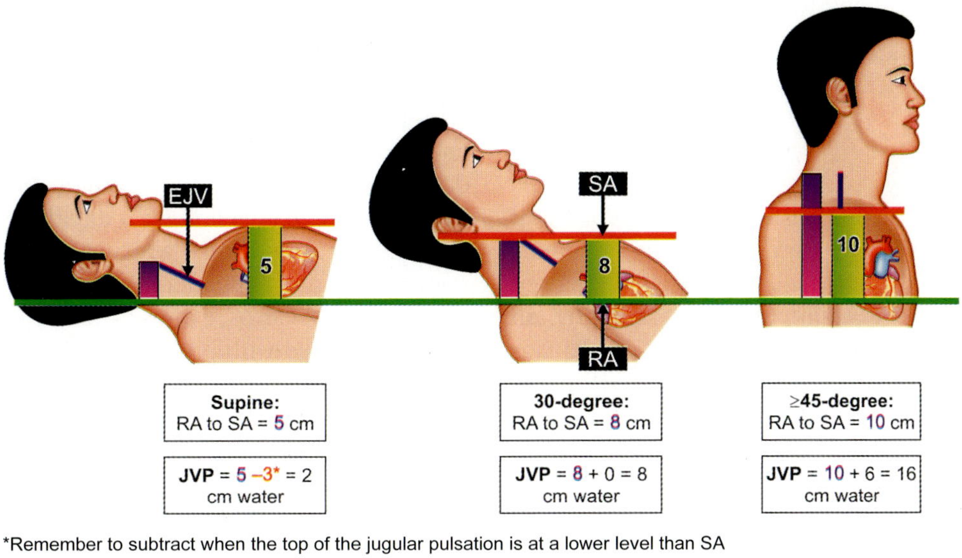

Fig. 2 Estimation of jugular venous pressure (JVP) in centimeters (cm) of water using external jugular vein (EJV). The vertical red-blue bar represents JVP and the vertical green bar represents the distances from right atrium (RA) to sternal angle (SA) in cm, which varies by body position

be accurately measured invasively. The JVP is estimated using two sets of numbers. First, one needs to estimate the vertical distance between the sternal angle (SA) and the top of the jugular pulsation, and then to that add (or subtract) the position-specific RA-to-SA distance. The first step in the estimation of JVP is the estimation of the distance from the SA to the top of the jugular pulsation. For this, one needs to position the patient so that the top of the jugular pulsation is visible in the middle of the neck. Generally speaking, if the JVP is low as it would be in a dry overdiuresed patient, it would only be visible while the patient is in a supine or near supine position (Fig. 2; left panel). In a euvolemic patient, it would be visible at inclines between 30° and 50° (Fig. 2; middle panel) and in patients with fluid volume overload, the patient may even needs to be seated (Fig. 2; right panel) to bring the top of the jugular pulsation in the middle of the neck. Once this distance has been estimated, then this needs to be added (or, subtracted if the SA to the top of the jugular pulsation distance is negative) to the RA-to-SA distance which varies according to the body position (Table 1 and Fig. 2).[36] The EJV is superficial and their contours can be seen like the veins on the back of one's hand. The EJV pulsation is almost always seen moving upward from the base of the neck. However, the IJV is deep and its pulsation is transmitted to the surface, at time can be confused with a nearly carotid pulsation. However, unlike the carotid pulsation, the jugular pulsation has double undulation (versus the single upward stroke of carotid pulsation), cannot be palpated, may be attenuate or disappear when gentle pressure is applied at the base of the neck, and responds to both gravity (body positions) and abdominal pressure (HJR). Flush HJR is common but to be considered positive, the top of the jugular pulsation needs to rise by 2–3 cm and remains elevated for about 10 seconds while a firm sustained pressure is being applied to the abdomen. When JVP is elevated, a positive HJR provides little additional information to assess fluid volume status. However, when JVP is normal, a positive HJR may suggest evidence of early fluid retention or mild residual fluid overload. Many of these patients are stable and have no bothersome dyspnea, and thus may be clinically insignificant. In one study, a positive HJR was both sensitive (100%) and specific (85%) for right atrial pressure greater than 9 mmHg.[37] Thus, for most practical purposed, HJR is often more helpful in identifying jugular pulsation and examining if the EJV is patent. One needs to remember that being a superficial vein, the EJV may look distended due to internal obstructions (thrombosis or sclerosis of valves) or external pressure (contraction of the overlying platysma muscle). Therefore, a distended EJV without visible pulsation may not be used to estimate JVP. Rarely, a distended EJV may not show pulsation but may disappear at a higher incline. This response to gravity may be used to get an estimate of JVP when there is no visible jugular pulsation. Clinicians skilled at using both IJV and EJV may estimate JVP or make an assessment of fluid volume status in nearly all patients.

EJECTION FRACTION

Aging is associated with diastolic dysfunction and the prevalence of HFpEF is very high in older adults, accounting for over half of the new cases of HF diagnosed annually. EF should be estimated, preferably by an echocardiogram, after a clinical diagnosis of HF has been made so that HF can be classified into HFrEF or HFpEF that has prognostic and therapeutic importance. Generally, older adults with HFrEF have poorer outcomes than those with HFpEF, who in turn have poorer outcomes compared to older adults without HF.[38,39]

TREATMENT

In general, treatment of HF needs to be guided by EF to ensure that those with HFrEF receive potentially life-prolonging therapies with neurohormonal inhibitors, namely, angiotensin-converting enzyme (ACE) inhibitors or angiotensin receptor blockers (ARBs), evidence-based beta-blockers, namely carvedilol, long-acting metoprolol succinate, and bisoprolol and aldosterone antagonists. In developing nations where estimation of EF may not always be possible, an option is to treat all HF patients as HFrEF and use neurohormonal antagonists whenever possible, especially, where indications for other comorbidities exist. For example, instead of treating coexisting HTN with a thiazide, use an ACE inhibitor or an ARB. Most of the older HF patients have HFpEF and there is no evidence that neurohormonal blockade improves outcomes in these patients. Further, patients with HFrEF receiving the full complement of neurohormonal blocking drugs may still have symptoms and be hospitalized. Therefore, HF therapy can be simplified by categorizing it into two broader groups: symptom relieving therapy and life-prolonging therapy. Because HF symptoms are similar in both HFpEF and HFrEF, symptom relieving therapy in HF is similar in both classes of HF and is primarily based on JVP-guided judicial use of diuretics.

Diuretics

Clinicians need to be familiar with the common diuretics, namely, furosemide, torsemide, and bumetanide. Furosemide 40 mg generally is equivalent to torsemide 10 mg or bumetanide 1 mg. Older adults may prefer a single morning dose to avoid overactive bladder symptoms.[40] However, some patients prefer to take it twice a day or a smaller afternoon dose, which may alleviate symptoms associated with fluid redistribution that occurs at night. Also, when patients are taking a rather large dose of diuretic, such as furosemide 480 mg daily, it may be preferable to give it twice a day to avoid hypotension. Diuretic use is associated with electrolyte imbalances and neurohormonal activation, both associated with poor outcomes.[41-44] Chronic diuretic use has also been shown to be associated with poor outcomes.[45,46] Therefore, only the lowest dose of diuretics needed to maintain euvolemia should be used and patients should be encouraged to adhere to a salt and fluid restricted diet to obviate the need for higher doses of diuretics. Older HF patients often cannot estimate salt contents of their diet. As such, general instructions, such as completely avoiding table salt and minimizing prepackaged and restaurant foods can be helpful. Patients should be advised to restrict their liquid intake to less than two L in 24 hours.

Neurohormonal activation and hypokalemia associated with torsemide use may be milder[47-49] and may be considered when potassium supplement is needed to maintain normokalemia. Serum potassium should be monitored to keep between 4 mEq/L and 5 mEq/L.[41,50,51] However, when potassium supplements are needed to maintain normokalemia in HFrEF patients, spironolactone or eplerenone may be preferable.[52-54] Combination diuretic therapy, such as a loop diuretic (furosemide 80 mg daily) and a thiazide-like diuretic (metolazone 2.5 mg daily) should be avoided whenever possible as they are more likely to cause electrolyte imbalance, necessitating closer monitoring of serum electrolytes and add to polypharmacy burden for older patients.

Renin-angiotensin System Blockade

An ACE inhibitor or an ARB should be considered for all older HFrEF patients without contraindication or intolerance. There is no need to use these drugs in the high doses used in RCTs. Most RCTs in HFrEF rather systematically excluded octogenarians,[55] and RCTs of ACE inhibitors were no exception. For example, in the Studies of Left Ventricular Dysfunction (SOLVD)-Treatment trial, the largest RCTs of ACE inhibitors in HFrEF, only eight patients were 80 years of age and none were more than or equal to 81 years of age.[56] Therefore, the evidence for the use of these drugs in octogenarians with HFrEF is weak at best. This disparity between efficacy (based on RCTs) and clinical effectiveness (in real-world patients) was demonstrated recently in a report that demonstrate that in a rigorously conducted observational study, aldosterone antagonists had no association with outcomes in real-world older HFrEF patients.[57,58] However, because mode of death changes with disease progression and more patients die from pump failure than sudden death,[59-61] and because ACE inhibitors reduce mortality primarily by reducing death due to pump failure, it may play a larger role in older patients with HFrEF.[56] Despite the overwhelming evidence of the beneficial effects of aldosterone antagonists in HFrEF,[52-54] their indication in older HFrEF may be limited by high prevalence of renal insufficiency and the risk of hyperkalemia, and lack of clinical effectiveness in real-world older HFrEF patients.[58]

Beta-blockers

Beta-blockers should be considered for older HFrEF patients without contraindications. The dose of the ACE inhibitor may be reduced to allow initiation of a beta-blocker and to avoid drop of systolic BP below 120 mmHg.[27-29] The beta-1 selective blocker, long-acting metoprolol succinate may be preferred in older HFrEF patients with normal or low-normal BP, while carvedilol, a non-selective beta-blocker with antihypertensive effect, may be preferred in those with high BP.[62]

Digoxin

Digoxin in low doses (0.125 mg/day or lower) should be considered for all older HFrEF patients who are symptomatic despite therapy with neurohormonal blockade.[63,64] Although low-dose digoxin leading to low (0.5–0.9 ng/mL) serum digoxin concentrations has been shown to be associated with lower mortality, it should not be prescribed before trying an ACE inhibitor (or, an ARB), a beta-blocker or when possible, an aldosterone antagonist. The Digoxin Investigation Group (DIG) trial, the largest RCT of digoxin in HFrEF, also excluded octogenarians, as only 5% of the participants were more than or equal to 80 years of age. Therefore, like all other HF drugs, digoxin should be used with extra caution in octogenarians with HFrEF.

Device-based Therapies

Like older adults in general, older HFrEF patients are heterogeneous by nature and any decision for device-based therapy for older HFrEF patients need to be individualized based on comorbidities and functional status. HFrEF is often associated with loss of synchronized intraventricular conduction and a wide (>120 ms) QRS complex on electrocardiogram. Cardiac resynchronization therapy (CRT) has been shown to improve outcomes in HFrEF patients with wide QRS complex.[65,66] Although this benefit was in older subgroup of patients, very few included octogenarians. Thus, CRT should be used with caution in octogenarians with HFrEF. Implantable cardioverter defibrillators (ICDs) may help reduce the risk of sudden cardiac death in HFrEF and may be of benefit when combined with CRT.[67,68] However, device-based therapy may play a lesser role in older HFrEF as the mode of death changes with disease progression from predominantly sudden death to pump failure death.[59-61]

MANAGEMENT OF HFPEF

There is little RCT evidence of benefit of therapy with ACE inhibitors or ARBs or beta-blockers reduce all-cause mortality in diastolic HF.[69-71] Digoxin has no effect on mortality, tends to reduce hospitalization due to HF, but this benefit appears to be cancelled by higher risk for hospitalization due to unstable angina.[72] In non-RCT studies, the associations of ARBs with outcomes appear to be similar to those observed in RCTs,[73] but ACE inhibitors appear to have a very modest association with outcomes.[74] Beta-blockers also do not seem to have any association with outcomes in HFpEF.[75,76] The effect of aldosterone antagonist awaits Treatment of Preserved Cardiac Function Heart Failure with an Aldosterone Antagonist (TOPCAT) trial. However, findings from non-RCT studies suggest no association with outcomes.[77] Because clinical presentation of HFrEF and HFpEF is similar, the general principle of diuretic use in HFpEF is very similar to that in HFrEF. The current standard therapy for HFpEF is largely anecdotal and directed to relieving congestion, control of BP, and tachycardia if present.

PALLIATIVE CARE

Because HFpEF is more common in older adults and because nearly half of older HFrEF patients are octogenarians, the primary goal of therapy is palliation and relief of symptoms. As such, palliative care can play a larger role in these patients. Older HFrEF patients with progressive disease may enter into a refractory end-stage despite the use of disease-modifying evidence-based therapy and may also benefit from palliative and hospice care. Medicare policy requires a life-expectancy of less than 6 months for hospice eligibility which may be difficult to predict in terminal HF as unlike terminal cancer, end-stage HF may follow an unpredictable course. Despite the fact that pump-failure death is more common than sudden death in advanced HF, both sudden death and acute decompensation are common occurrences. Therefore, a clinically useful rule of thumb is to ask if one would be surprised if a terminal HF patient died within 6 months. If the answer is no then the patient may be a potential candidate for hospice referral.

CONCLUSION

Most of the HF patients are older adults and HF is the leading cause of hospitalization among older adults. HF is a clinical diagnosis and can be difficult. However, the assessment and management of HF in older adults can be structured using the mnemonic DEFEAT: Diagnosis (clinical, and must not be ruled out based on normal LVEF), Etiology (often multifactorial, though preceded by HTN in the vast majority of the cases), Fluid volume (needs to be estimated by JVP using IJV or EJV to help achieve euvolemia), EF (necessary to categorize HF into HFrEF or HFpEF, important prognosis and treatment considerations), And Treatment (broadly categorized into life-prolonging evidence-based therapy for HFrEF and palliative or symptom-relieving therapy for all patients, especially for end-stage HF).

REFERENCES

1. Inouye SK, Studenski S, Tinetti ME, et al. Geriatric syndromes: clinical, research, and policy implications of a core geriatric concept. J Am Geriatr Soc. 2007;55(5):780-91.
2. The Centers for Medicare and Medicaid Services. (2011). Chronic Conditions among Medicare Beneficiaries, Chart Book. (online) Available from: www.cms.gov/Research-Statistics-Data-and-Systems/Statistics-Trends-and-Reports/Chronic-Conditions/Downloads/2011Chartbook.pdf. [Accessed December, 2013].
3. Ahmed A. Clinical manifestations, diagnostic assessment, and etiology of heart failure in older adults. Clin Geriatr Med. 2007;23(1):11-30.
4. Ahmed A. DEFEAT heart failure: clinical manifestations, diagnostic assessment, and etiology of geriatric heart failure. Heart Fail Clin. 2007; 3(4):389-402.
5. Ahmed A, Jones L, Hays CI. DEFEAT heart failure: assessment and management of heart failure in nursing homes made easy. J Am Med Dir Assoc. 2008;9(6):383-9.
6. Ahmed A. Chronic heart failure in older adults. Med Clin North Am. 2011;95(3):439-61.
7. Senni M, Tribouilloy CM, Rodeheffer RJ, et al. Congestive heart failure in the community: a study of all incident cases in Olmsted County, Minnesota, in 1991. Circulation. 1998;98(21):2282-9.
8. Ekundayo OJ, Howard VJ, Safford MM, et al. Value of orthopnea, paroxysmal nocturnal dyspnea, and medications in prospective population studies of incident heart failure. Am J Cardiol. 2009;104(2):259-64.
9. Butman SM, Ewy GA, Standen JR, et al. Bedside cardiovascular examination in patients with severe chronic heart failure: importance of rest or inducible jugular venous distension. J Am Coll Cardiol. 1993;22(4): 968-74.
10. Hunt SA, Abraham WT, Chin MH, et al. ACC/AHA 2005 Guideline Update for the Diagnosis and Management of Chronic Heart Failure in the Adult: a report of the American College of Cardiology/American Heart Association Task Force on Practice Guidelines (Writing Committee to Update the 2001 Guidelines for the Evaluation and Management of Heart Failure): developed in collaboration with the American College of Chest Physicians and the International Society for Heart and Lung Transplantation: endorsed by the Heart Rhythm Society. Circulation. 2005;112(12):e154-235.
11. Drazner MH, Rame JE, Stevenson LW, et al. Prognostic importance of elevated jugular venous pressure and a third heart sound in patients with heart failure. N Engl J Med. 2001;345(8):574-81.
12. Curtis JP, Selter JG, Wang Y, et al. The obesity paradox: body mass index and outcomes in patients with heart failure. Arch Intern Med. 2005;165(1):55-61.
13. Mueller C, Scholer A, Laule-Kilian K, et al. Use of B-type natriuretic peptide in the evaluation and management of acute dyspnea. N Engl J Med. 2004;350(7):647-54.
14. Fonarow GC, Stough WG, Abraham WT, et al. Characteristics, treatments, and outcomes of patients with preserved systolic function hospitalized for heart failure: a report from the OPTIMIZE-HF Registry. J Am Coll Cardiol. 2007;50(8):768-77.
15. Vinayak AG, Levitt J, Gehlbach B, et al. Usefulness of the external jugular vein examination in detecting abnormal central venous pressure in critically ill patients. Arch Intern Med. 2006;166(19):2132-7.
16. Dickstein K, Cohen-Solal A, Filippatos G, et al. ESC Guidelines for the diagnosis and treatment of acute and chronic heart failure 2008: the Task Force for the Diagnosis and Treatment of Acute and Chronic Heart Failure 2008 of the European Society of Cardiology. Developed in collaboration with the Heart Failure Association of the ESC (HFA) and endorsed by the European Society of Intensive Care Medicine (ESICM). Eur Heart J. 2008;29(19):2388-442.
17. Maisel AS, Krishnaswamy P, Nowak RM, et al. Rapid measurement of B-type natriuretic peptide in the emergency diagnosis of heart failure. N Engl J Med. 2002;347(3):161-7.
18. Blonde-Cynober F, Morineau G, Estrugo B, et al. Diagnostic and prognostic value of brain natriuretic peptide (BNP) concentrations in very elderly heart disease patients: specific geriatric cut-off and impacts of age, gender, renal dysfunction, and nutritional status. Arch Gerontol Geriatr. 2011;52(1):106-10.
19. Kim HN, Januzzi JL Jr. Natriuretic peptide testing in heart failure. Circulation. 2011;123(18):2015-9.
20. Nieminen MS, Bohm M, Cowie MR, et al. Executive summary of the guidelines on the diagnosis and treatment of acute heart failure: the Task Force on Acute Heart Failure of the European Society of Cardiology. Eur Heart J. 2005;26(4):384-416.
21. Kitzman DW, Gardin JM, Gottdiener JS, et al. Importance of heart failure with preserved systolic function in patients > or = 65 years of age. CHS Research Group. Cardiovascular Health Study. Am J Cardiol. 2001;87(4):413-9.
22. Gopal DM, Kalogeropoulos AP, Georgiopoulou VV, et al. Cigarette smoking exposure and heart failure risk in older adults: the Health, Aging, and Body Composition Study. Am Heart J. 2012;164(2):236-42.

23. Suskin N, Sheth T, Negassa A, et al. Relationship of current and past smoking to mortality and morbidity in patients with left ventricular dysfunction. J Am Coll Cardiol. 2001;37(6):1677-82.
24. Roy B, Pawar PP, Desai RV, et al. A propensity-matched study of the association of diabetes mellitus with incident heart failure and mortality among community-dwelling older adults. Am J Cardiol. 2011; 108(12):1747-53.
25. Deedwania PC, Ahmed MI, Feller MA, et al. Impact of diabetes mellitus on outcomes in patients with acute myocardial infarction and systolic heart failure. Eur J Heart Fail. 2011;13(5):551-9.
26. Ekundayo OJ, Allman RM, Sanders PW, et al. Isolated systolic hypertension and incident heart failure in older adults: a propensity-matched study. Hypertension. 2009;53(3):458-65.
27. Gheorghiade M, Abraham WT, Albert NM, et al. Systolic blood pressure at admission, clinical characteristics, and outcomes in patients hospitalized with acute heart failure. JAMA. 2006;296(18):2217-26.
28. Desai RV, Banach M, Ahmed MI, et al. Impact of baseline systolic blood pressure on long-term outcomes in patients with advanced chronic systolic heart failure (insights from the BEST trial). Am J Cardiol. 2010;106(2): 221-7.
29. Banach M, Bhatia V, Feller MA, et al. Relation of baseline systolic blood pressure and long-term outcomes in ambulatory patients with chronic mild to moderate heart failure. Am J Cardiol. 2011;107(8):1208-14.
30. Kenchaiah S, Evans JC, Levy D, et al. Obesity and the risk of heart failure. N Engl J Med. 2002;347(5):305-13.
31. Horwich TB, Fonarow GC, Hamilton MA, et al. The relationship between obesity and mortality in patients with heart failure. J Am. Coll Cardiol. 2001;38(3):789-95.
32. Kapoor P, Thenappan T, Singh E, et al. Cardiac amyloidosis: a practical approach to diagnosis and management. Am J Med. 2011;124(11):1006-15.
33. Applefeld MM. (1990). The Jugular Venous Pressure and Pulse Contour. [online] Available from: www.ncbi.nlm.nih.gov/pubmed/21250143. [Accessed December, 2013].
34. Cotter G, Felker GM, Adams KF, et al. The pathophysiology of acute heart failure—is it all about fluid accumulation? Am Heart J. 2008;155(1):9-18.
35. Metra M, Dei Cas L, Bristow MR. The pathophysiology of acute heart failure—it is a lot about fluid accumulation. Am Heart J. 2008;155(1):1-5.
36. Seth R, Magner P, Matzinger F, et al. How far is the sternal angle from the mid-right atrium? J Gen Intern Med. 2002;17(11):852-6.
37. Sochowski RA, Dubbin JD, Naqvi SZ. Clinical and hemodynamic assessment of the hepatojugular reflux. Am J Cardiol. 1990;66(12):1002-6.
38. Ahmed A. Association of diastolic dysfunction and outcomes in ambulatory older adults with chronic heart failure. J Gerontol A Biol Sci Med Sci. 2005;60(10):1339-44.
39. Gottdiener JS, McClelland RL, Marshall R, et al. Outcome of congestive heart failure in elderly persons: influence of left ventricular systolic function. The Cardiovascular Health Study. Ann Intern Med. 2002;137(8):631-9.
40. Ekundayo OJ, Markland A, Lefante C, et al. Association of diuretic use and overactive bladder syndrome in older adults: a propensity score analysis. Arch Gerontol Geriatr. 2009;49(1):64-8.
41. Alper AB, Campbell RC, Anker SD, et al. A propensity-matched study of low serum potassium and mortality in older adults with chronic heart failure. Int J Cardiol. 2009;137(1):1-8.
42. Ahmed A, Zannad F, Love TE, et al. A propensity-matched study of the association of low serum potassium levels and mortality in chronic heart failure. Eur Heart J. 2007;28(11):1334-43.
43. Bowling CB, Pitt B, Ahmed MI, et al. Hypokalemia and outcomes in patients with chronic heart failure and chronic kidney disease: findings from propensity-matched studies. Circ Heart Fail. 2010;3(2):253-60.
44. Francis GS, Benedict C, Johnstone DE, et al. Comparison of neuroendocrine activation in patients with left ventricular dysfunction with and without congestive heart failure. A substudy of the Studies of Left Ventricular Dysfunction (SOLVD). Circulation. 1990;82(5):1724-9.
45. Ahmed A, Husain A, Love TE, et al. Heart failure, chronic diuretic use, and increase in mortality and hospitalization: an observational study using propensity score methods. Eur Heart J. 2006;27(12):1431-9.
46. Ahmed A, Young JB, Love TE, et al. A propensity-matched study of the effects of chronic diuretic therapy on mortality and hospitalization in older adults with heart failure. Int J Cardiol. 2008;125(2):246-53.
47. Lopez B, Querejeta R, Gonzalez A, et al. Effects of loop diuretics on myocardial fibrosis and collagen type I turnover in chronic heart failure. J Am Coll Cardiol. 2004;43(11):2028-35.
48. Cosin J, Diez J, TORIC investigators. Torasemide in chronic heart failure: results of the TORIC study. Eur J Heart Fail. 2002;4(4):507-13.
49. Murray MD, Deer MM, Ferguson JA, et al. Open-label randomized trial of torsemide compared with furosemide therapy for patients with heart failure. Am J Med. 2001;111(7):513-20.
50. Ahmed MI, Ekundayo OJ, Mujib M, et al. Mild hyperkalemia and outcomes in chronic heart failure: a propensity matched study. Int J Cardiol. 2010;144(3):383-8.
51. Ekundayo OJ, Adamopoulos C, Ahmed MI, et al. Oral potassium supplement use and outcomes in chronic heart failure: a propensity-matched study. Int J Cardiol. 2010;141(2):167-74.
52. Pitt B, Zannad F, Remme WJ, et al. The effect of spironolactone on morbidity and mortality in patients with severe heart failure. Randomized Aldactone Evaluation Study Investigators. N Engl J Med. 1999;341(10):709-17.
53. Pitt B, Remme W, Zannad F, et al. Eplerenone, a selective aldosterone blocker, in patients with left ventricular dysfunction after myocardial infarction. N Engl J Med. 2003;348(14):1309-21.
54. Zannad F, McMurray JJ, Krum H, et al. Eplerenone in patients with systolic heart failure and mild symptoms. N Engl J Med. 2011;364(1):11-21.
55. Masoudi FA, Havranek EP, Wolfe P, et al. Most hospitalized older persons do not meet the enrollment criteria for clinical trials in heart failure. Am Heart J. 2003;146(2):250-57.
56. Effect of enalapril on survival in patients with reduced left ventricular ejection fractions and congestive heart failure. The SOLVD Investigators. N Engl J Med. 1991;325(5):293-302.
57. Curtis LH, Mi X, Qualls LG, et al. Design and rationale of a retrospective clinical effectiveness study of aldosterone antagonist therapy in patients with heart failure. Am Heart J. 2012;163(6):946-53.
58. Hernandez AF, Mi X, Hammill BG, et al. Associations between aldosterone antagonist therapy and risks of mortality and readmission among patients with heart failure and reduced ejection fraction. JAMA. 2012;308(20):2097-107.
59. Zile MR, Gaasch WH, Anand IS, et al. Mode of death in patients with heart failure and a preserved ejection fraction: results from the Irbesartan in Heart Failure With Preserved Ejection Fraction Study (I-Preserve) trial. Circulation. 2010;121(12):1393-405.
60. Carson P, Anand I, O'Connor C, et al. Mode of death in advanced heart failure: the Comparison of Medical, Pacing, and Defibrillation Therapies in Heart Failure (COMPANION) trial. J Am Coll Cardiol. 2005;46(12):2329-34.
61. Mehta PA, Dubrey SW, McIntyre HF, et al. Mode of death in patients with newly diagnosed heart failure in the general population. Eur J Heart Fail. 2008;10(11):1108-16.
62. Ahmed A, Dell'Italia LJ. Use of beta-blockers in older adults with chronic heart failure. Am J Med Sci. 2004;328(2):100-11.
63. Ahmed A. Digoxin and reduction in mortality and hospitalization in geriatric heart failure: importance of low doses and low serum concentrations. J Gerontol A Biol Sci Med Sci. 2007;62(3):323-9.

64. Ahmed A, Pitt B, Rahimtoola SH, et al. Effects of digoxin at low serum concentrations on mortality and hospitalization in heart failure: a propensity-matched study of the DIG trial. Int J Cardiol. 2008;123(2):138-46.
65. Cleland JG, Daubert JC, Erdmann E, et al. The effect of cardiac resynchronization on morbidity and mortality in heart failure. N Engl J Med. 2005;352(15):1539-49.
66. Abraham WT, Fisher WG, Smith AL, et al. Cardiac resynchronization in chronic heart failure. N Engl J Med. 2002;346(24):1845-53.
67. Tang AS, Wells GA, Talajic M, et al. Cardiac-resynchronization therapy for mild-to-moderate heart failure. N Engl J Med. 2010;363(25):2385-95.
68. Bristow MR, Saxon LA, Boehmer J, et al. Cardiac-resynchronization therapy with or without an implantable defibrillator in advanced chronic heart failure. N Engl J Med. 2004;350(21):2140-50.
69. Massie BM, Carson PE, McMurray JJ, et al. Irbesartan in patients with heart failure and preserved ejection fraction. N Engl J Med. 2008;359(23): 2456-67.
70. Cleland JG, Tendera M, Adamus J, et al. The perindopril in elderly people with chronic heart failure (PEP-CHF) study. Eur Heart J. 2006;27(19):2338-45.
71. Yusuf S, Pfeffer MA, Swedberg K, et al. Effects of candesartan in patients with chronic heart failure and preserved left-ventricular ejection fraction: the CHARM-Preserved Trial. Lancet. 2003;362(9386):777-81.
72. Ahmed A, Rich MW, Fleg JL, et al. Effects of digoxin on morbidity and mortality in diastolic heart failure: the ancillary digitalis investigation group trial. Circulation. 2006;114(5):397-403.
73. Patel K, Fonarow GC, Kitzman DW, et al. Angiotensin receptor blockers and outcomes in real-world older patients with heart failure and preserved ejection fraction: a propensity-matched inception cohort clinical effectiveness study. Eur J Heart Fail. 2012;14(10):1179-88.
74. Mujib M, Patel K, Fonarow GC, et al. Angiotensin-converting enzyme inhibitors and outcomes in heart failure and preserved ejection fraction. Am J Med. 2013;126(5):401-10.
75. Flather MD, Shibata MC, Coats AJ, et al. Randomized trial to determine the effect of nebivolol on mortality and cardiovascular hospital admission in elderly patients with heart failure (SENIORS). Eur Heart J. 2005;26(3): 215-25.
76. Hernandez AF, Hammill BG, O'Connor CM, et al. Clinical effectiveness of beta-blockers in heart failure: findings from the OPTIMIZE-HF (Organized Program to Initiate Lifesaving Treatment in Hospitalized Patients with Heart Failure) Registry. J Am Coll Cardiol. 2009;53(2):184-92.
77. Patel K, Fonarow GC, Kitzman DW, et al. Aldosterone Antagonists and Outcomes in Real-World Older Patients With Heart Failure and Preserved Ejection Fraction. JACC Heart Fail. 2013;1(1):40-47.

Chapter 39

How to Diagnose and Treat Anemia in Patients with Heart Failure

Ewa A Jankowska, Piotr Ponikowski

ABSTRACT

Anemia is a common comorbidity in patients with heart failure (HF). The pathophysiology of anemia in HF is complex, multifactorial and has not been comprehensively established. Among several pathologies associated with anemia, iron deficiency, diminished erythropoietin (EPO) production and EPO resistance, are of a particular importance. The development of anemia in the course of HF interferes with the pathophysiology of HF syndrome, accelerates the progression of heart disease and worsens prognosis, all of which justifies that anemia could be a therapeutic target in patients with HF. In the chapter, we provide an algorithm which patients with HF should be screened for anaemia and when, recommend several tests to identify the major most likely cause of anemia, and associated treatment strategies.

INTRODUCTION

Recent European Society of Cardiology (ESC) guidelines on the management of heart failure (HF) emphasize the need to identify concomitant diseases in patients with HF.[1] And what is the most important, the optimal therapy of comorbidities is considered as a crucial element of the treatment plan of these patients.[1]

PREVALENCE

Anemia is a common comorbidity in patients with HF. Its prevalence ranges from approximately 10% to 55%, as the consequence of the differences in either the severity of heart disease in studied populations of HF patients or the applied definition of anemia.[2-5] Subjects with the following risk factors are characterized by the particularly high prevalence of anemia: older age, female gender, low socioeconomic status, advanced HF, cachexia, high circulating natriuretic peptides, impaired renal function, therapy with antiplatelet, and/or anticoagulant drugs, history of ulcerative disease.[2-5]

PATHOPHYSIOLOGY

The pathophysiology of anemia in HF is complex and has not been comprehensively established.[2,3,6-8] Taken into consideration the fact that patients with HF are relatively older, there are pathophysiological similarities regarding the anemia in elderly subjects and the anemia in patients with HF.[9,10]

In general, the origin of anemia is multifactorial. The following pathologies are considered as factors contributing to the development of anemia in the course of HF: (1) hemodilution; (2) gastrointestinal blood loss due to impaired integrity of intestinal mucosa and/or antiplatelet/anticoagulant treatment; (3) vitamin B_{12} and folic acid deficiencies; (4) iron deficiency (ID); (5) augmented inflammatory processes, potentially associated with diminished erythropoietin (EPO) production, EPO resistance, and also probably functional ID; (6) chronic kidney disease (CKD) (accompanied by pronounced inflammation and metabolic abnormalities); (7) insulin resistance and/or diabetes mellitus; (8) drugs being an element of standard therapy of HF, such as angiotensin-converting enzyme inhibitor (ACEI) and/or angiotensin receptor blocker (ARB) therapy; and (9) other drugs directly interfering with erythropoiesis and/or iron metabolism.[2,3,6-8,11,12]

In most cases, anemia occurring in patients with HF represents an anemia of chronic disease (ACD) or/and an iron deficiency anemia (IDA).[2,3,6-8] There are premises that the augmented inflammation demonstrated in patients with HF also negatively affects the function of erythropoietic system. Proinflammatory mediators [interleukin 6 (IL-6)] diminish the EPO production by the kidneys, induce the EPO resistance within both hematopoietic and extra-hematopoietic tissues, and reduce iron availability for cells metabolizing iron, including erythroid cells.[13,14] According to Opasich et al., 36% anemic patients with systolic HF have ID, whereas 64% of them have ACD.[15] In the analysis of the data from national and healthcare insurance systems performed by Ezekowitz et al., anemia was seen in 17% of patients hospitalized due to HF, and ID was demonstrated in 21% of anemia cases.[16] Nanas et al. revealed the presence of depleted iron stores in bone marrow in 73% of anemic patients with decompensated HF in New York Heart Association (NYHA) class IV.[17] Importantly, approximately 30% non-anemic patients with systolic HF have ID,[18] which implies the iron supplementation regardless of the presence of anemia itself.

The origin of depleted iron stores in the course of HF remains unknown.[6,19] Among the most likely causes of ID seen in HF there are: (1) poor nutrition without sufficient iron supply; (2) reduced gastrointestinal absorption; (3) gastrointestinal blood loss; (4) excessive menstrual bleedings; (5) medications favoring bleeding; and (6) other drug interactions.[6,19,20] So far, the role of inflammatory stimuli (IL-6) inducing the liver synthesis of hepcidin in the development of functional ID has not been confirmed in patients with HF,[21] which on the contrary is a characteristic feature of ID seen in patients with CKD. Hepcidin orchestrates the systemic iron metabolism, and when released from hepatocytes into the circulation, blocks the intestinal iron absorption, traps iron in the reticuloendothelial cells, and as a consequence results in a blockade of iron influx to iron metabolizing cells, resulting in the so-called functional ID.[20,22,23] Iron deficient patients with systolic HF demonstrate low (not high) circulating hepcidin and IL-6.[21]

CLINICAL AND PROGNOSTIC CONSEQUENCES

The development of anemia in the course of HF interferes with the pathophysiology of HF syndrome, and may accelerate the progression of heart disease.[2-4,24] Therefore, anemia is related with augmented HF symptoms, impaired exercise capacity (expressed as reduced 6-minute walking distance and diminished peak oxygen consumption), poor quality of life, advanced depressive symptoms,[4,25] as well as increased hospitalization rates and high cardiovascular and total mortality.[4,24,26,27] Anemia is associated with poor outcome also in patients with acute HF.[28] Importantly, the reduction of hemoglobin level in the course of HF is a strong risk factor of high morbidity and mortality in these patients.[26,27] All these facts justify that anemia should be an obligatory therapeutic target in patients with HF.

WHICH PATIENTS WITH HEART FAILURE SHOULD BE SCREENED FOR ANEMIA AND WHEN?

According to the ESC guidelines, all patients with HF should be screened for the presence of anemia.[1] It seems reasonable to assess hemoglobin level: (1) during the baseline assessment when the diagnosis of HF is established; (2) during any clinical deterioration; and (3) at least once per year during routine outpatient visits, even when the patient remains stable (Flowchart 1). It is worthy to remember that in elderly subjects (particularly with cardiovascular disease), angina, and/or dyspnea are commonly the first symptoms of anemia. Subjects with the aforementioned risk factors for the development of anemia should be more frequently screened (Flowchart 1).

HOW TO DIAGNOSE ANEMIA IN ADULTS WITH HEART FAILURE?

The diagnosis of anemia is straightforward. According to the World Health Organization, anemia is diagnosed when hemoglobin is less than 13 g/dL in men and less than 12 g/dL in postmenopausal women. However, there is no unified treatment of anemia in patients with HF. The therapeutic decisions regarding the anemia treatment depend on: (1) the clinical status (stability) of the patient, and the acuteness of the diagnosis of anemia;

Which patients with HF should be screened for anemia and when?

All patients with HF should be screened for the presence of anemia

- At baseline assessment
- During any deterioration of clinical condition
- At least once per year during routine outpatient visits

! In elderly subjects (particularly with cardiovascular disease), angina and/or dyspnea are commonly the first symptoms of anemia

! Subjects with the following risk factors are particularly fragile to develop anemia, and follow-up hemoglobin assessments should be performed more frequently in these subgroups: older age, female gender, low socioeconomic status, advanced HF, cachexia, high circulating natriuretic peptides, reduced GFR, therapy with antiplatelet and/or anticoagulant drugs, history of ulcerative disease

How to diagnose anemia in adults with HF?

Anemia is diagnosed when hemoglobin level is <13 g/dL in men and <12 g/dL in women (a WHO definition).

Question	Yes	No
Unstable clinical condition: Clinical signs and/or symptoms of hypovolemia and/or hypoperfusion (dizziness, hypotension, anuria, dyspnea, angina)?	Administer IV fluids, including colloids	→ next
Severe anemia (hemoglobin level <8 g/dL and hematocrit <25%)?	Perform erythrocyte mass transfusion	→ next
Certain/likely acute/subacute external/internal bleeding?	Urgent consultation with a gastroenterologist and/or a surgeon (work out the source of bleeding, consider invasive/ surgical treatment of the bleeding, consider cessation of antiplatelet, and anticoagulant drugs)	→ next

Has the patient experienced any of the following common conditions which may accompany HF?

Question	Yes	No
Chronic kidney disease (preceding the occurrence of HF), particularly in advanced stages, when treated with dialysis or after kidney transplantation?	Most commonly – anemia of chronic disease with concomitant functional iron deficiency Consult the patient with a nephrologist (in some cases, SC erythropoietin-stimulating agents and/or IV iron supplementation can be applied)	→ next
Certain/likely diagnosis of neoplasm?	Most commonly – anemia of chronic disease with concomitant functional iron deficiency Consult the patient with an oncologist (in most cases, anemia is not corrected, but in rare cases IV iron supplementation could be carefully considered)	→ next
Middle-aged premenopausal women with intense menses?	Most commonly – iron deficiency anemia due to menstrual blood loss Consult the patient with a gynecologist (consider additional gynecological and hormone tests, consider hormone therapy with PO/IV iron supplementation	→ next
Drugs toxic for bone marrow and causing anemia (hydroxyurea, AZT)?	Consult the patient with a specialist who administered the drug (consider the cessation of this drug and theadministration of alterative drugs)	→ next

Contd..

Contd..

The diagnostic tests to be performed in patients with HF and anemia

- Complete blood count with platelet count and automated differentiation including RBC indies (MCV, MCH, MCHC) and RDW
- Blood smear
- Reticulocytes
- Bilirubin, LDH
- Creatinine and eGFR
- Serum vitamin B_{12} serum FA
- TSH, fT3, fT4
- Serum ferritin, tsat = a ration of serum iron and TIBC
- hsCRP
- History of excessive alcohol use
- Screening for asymptomatic bleeding/suspicion of neoplasm: Chest X-ray, ultrasound imaging of abdomen; in certain clinical cases, consider gynecological consultation, gastroscopy, colonoscopy

! At the moment, the numerous biomarkers (sTfR, hepcidin, EPO, EPO receptor, and hemojuvelin) are used for research purpose in anemic patients with HF, however, still their value for clinical practice has not been established

! Classification of anemia according to MCV may be useful; however in HF, this parameter has low specificity and sensitivity, and its value can be only supportive

Microcytic anemia (MCV <80 fL) is typical for: iron deficiency, anemia of chromic disease (autoimmue diseases, infections, chronic kindney disease), myelofibrosis, and thalassemia

Normocytic anemia (MCV ≥80 fL and ≤100 fL) is typical for: anemia of chromic disease, also seen in iron deficiency, B_{12} deficiency and FA deficiency

Macrocytic anemia (MCV ≥100 fL) is typical for: B_{12} deficiency and FA deficiency, hemolysis, excessive alcohol use, liver failure, myelodysplastic syndrome

Abnormality	Recommendation
Positive screening tests for bleeding or neoplasms	Consult the patients with respective specialists, and treat the pathologies specifically, and reassess hematological status afterwards
Excessive alcohol use	Cessation of alcohol drinking, and reassess hematological status afterwards
Abnormal thyroid function	Consult the patient with an endocrinologist, treat thyroid pathology, and reassess hematological status afterwards
Reduced serum B_{12} or reduced serum FA	Supplement with depleted B_{12} (IM) or FA (PO)
Abnormal blood smear + clinical and laboratory features of inflammation	Confirm and treat inflammation (pneumonia, endocarditis)
Abnormal blood smear	Consult the patient with a hematologist (primary hematological disease is very likely)
High bilirubin, high LDH, high reticulocytes indicating hemolysis	Consult the patient with a hematologist (primary hematological disease or secondary cause of hemolysis is very likely)
Serum ferritin < 100 μg/L, or serum ferritin 100–299 μg/L with Tsat, indicating iron deficiency	Supplement iron (preferably IV)
Unclear cases	Consider the consultation with a hematologist (additional test may be needed: bone marrow biopsy, blood smear, hemoglobin electrophoresis, genetic tests, etc.)

! Recommendations to use IV iron in anemic patients with HF and iron deficiency are based on the entrance criteria and the results of FAIR-HF study.

! Currently, there is no indication for ESA administration in anemic patients with HF (RED-HF study).

HF, heart failure; GFR, glomerular filtration rate; WHO, World Health Organization; IV, intravenous; SC, subcutaneously; AZT, zidovudine; RBC, red blood cell; MCV, mean corpuscular volume; MCH, mean corpuscular hemoglobin; MCHC, mean corpuscular hemoglobin concentration; RDW, red cell distribution width; LDH, lactate dehydrogenase; eGFR, estimated glomerular filtration rate; TSH, thyroid-stimulating hormone; fT3, free triiodothyronine; fT4, free thyroxine; Tsat, transferrin saturation; TIBC, total iron-binding capacity; hsCRP, high-sensitivity C-reactive protein; sTfR, soluble transferrin receptor; EPO, erythropoietin; IM, intramuscular; ESA, erythropoiesis-stimulating agents; FAIR-HF, Ferinject Assessment in Patients with Iron Deficiency and Chronic Heart Failure trial; RED-HF, Reduction Event with Darbepoetin alfa in Heart Failure study

Flowchart 1 Which patients with heart failure should be screened for anemia and when?

(2) the presence/absence of several clinical conditions, which when present imply the implementation of other algorithms; and (3) the identification of the major (primary) cause of anemia based on additional diagnostic tests (Flowchart 1).

Therefore, the first step in the algorithm is *the confirmation/exclusion of acute/subacute bleeding*, which is accompanied by clinical features of hypovolemia/hypoperfusion, rather severe anemia and sometimes during physical examination and/or in additional tests the source of bleeding can be identified. In such a situation, the following actions need to be taken urgently: a surgical/invasive attempt to cease the bleeding, a discontinuation of antiplatelet and/or anticoagulant drugs, a fluid administration, a transfusion of erythrocyte mass (Flowchart 1).

The second step in the algorithm is *the identification of some relatively common clinical conditions* (primary CKD, cancer, intense menstrual bleedings, and drugs affecting erythropoiesis), which when present imply the implementation of other algorithms (Flowchart 1). It should be emphasized that there are several differences in the pathophysiology of anemia (and ID) between patients with CKD (due to primary kidney disease) and patients with HF.[21] These facts have serious therapeutic implications. In some cases of CKD, EPO or erythropoiesis-stimulating agents (ESA) therapy with or without iron supplementation can be administered by nephrologists, whereas the EPO/ESA therapy is not currently recommended in patients with HF (see further paragraphs).

The third step is associated with *the identification of the major (primary) cause of anemia based on additional diagnostic tests*. There is a list of standard assessments which are available for clinical practice, which are sufficient to work out the major cause of anemia in approximately 90% of cases (Flowchart 1). It should be emphasized that when diagnosing the cause of anemia in patients with HF (who in most cases are elderly subjects), the exclusion of thyroid dysfunction and cancer is obligatory, as these conditions are relatively common in elderly anemic patients with HF with subtle (if any) symptomatology. Currently, the numerous biomarkers [soluble transferrin receptor (sTfR), hepcidin, EPO, and EPO receptor] are used for research purposes in anemic and non-anemic patients with HF, however, still their value for clinical practice has not been established.

Based on the list of diagnostic tests, the several therapeutic pathways can be followed as described in the algorithm (Flowchart 1). It should be emphasized that all unclear cases, particularly when accompanied by severe abnormalities in other tests, should be consulted with a hematologist.

It is worthy to note that contrary to the treatment of anemia in patients with HF, there is no evidence to recommend the EPO/ESA therapy in anemic patients with HF. Indeed, few mainly uncontrolled small studies demonstrated some beneficial effects of the EPO/ESA therapy in patients with HF: the lessening of HF symptoms, the improvement in exercise capacity and quality of life, the reduction in circulating natriuretic peptides, the reduction in daily diuretic dose, and the improvement in systolic and diastolic function of left ventricle.[2,3,29,30] Unfortunately, the results of Reduction Event with Darbepoetin alfa in Heart Failure (RED-HF) study did not confirm the previous promising effects of the EPO/ESA therapy in anemic patients with HF.[31] The RED-HF study was a multicenter placebo-controlled double-blind study, where 2,278 patients with systolic HF and mild-to-moderate anemia (hemoglobin level between 9 g/dL and 12 g/dL) were treated with darbapoietin alpha (to increase hemoglobin level up to 13 g/dL) versus placebo.[31] There were no significant between-group differences in the rates of either the primary end-point (a composite of all-cause death or HF hospitalization) or any of the secondary endpoints. Fatal and nonfatal strokes as well as cancer-related adverse events had the similar occurrence in both studied groups, whereas thromboembolic events were reported more frequently in the group treated with darbapoietin alfa as compared to the group receiving placebo.[31] The futility of EPO/ESA therapy is suggested to be the consequence of EPO resistance, which is associated with concomitant inflammation and/or ID.[2,3,29,30] Therefore, currently the EPO/ESA therapy is not recommended in anemic patients with HF.

In recent years, ID has emerged as a potential therapeutic target in both anemic and non-anemic patients with HF.[6,19] Absolute ID (i.e., defined as insufficient iron stores) is assessed using circulating ferritin, which is secreted from iron-storing cells. In a general population, serum ferritin less than 30 μg/L indicates the presence of absolute ID.[32-34] In patients with inflammatory chronic diseases (such as HF) higher cut-offs of serum ferritin (<100 μg/L) are used, because inflammatory stimuli increase ferritin secretion, irrespectively of iron status. Reduced transferrin saturation (Tsat) (<20%) reflects insufficient iron available for metabolizing cells. Even when serum ferritin is between 100 μg/L and 299 μg/L (i.e., when iron stores are normal/slightly increased), Tsat less than 20% allows to identify patients with functional ID.[32-34] Therefore, in patients with HF, ID is suggested to be diagnosed when serum ferritin is less than 100 μg/L, or when serum ferritin is between 100 μg/L and 299 μg/L with Tsat less than 20%.[6,35] Patients with systolic HF with ID defined as described above demonstrate reduced peak oxygen consumption and increased ventilatory response to exercise[36] and the increased risk death and heart transplantation during the 3-year follow-up, irrespectively of hemoglobin and other clinical prognosticators.[18]

The recommendation for supplementing IV iron in patients with ID defined as described above in patients with systolic HF has resulted from the Ferinject assessment in patients with IRon deficiency and chronic Heart Failure (FAIR-HF) study.[35] It was the greatest randomized double-blind placebo-controlled multicenter trial, where a 24-week IV ferric carboxymaltose therapy (or placebo) was administered to 459 iron-deficient patients with systolic HF (both anemics and non-anemics), and iron supplementation reduced NYHA class and improved patient global assessment.[35] All these beneficial effects were seen in several clinical subgroups (including those with/without anemia, those with/without impaired renal function), without an increased risk of any side-effects.[35,37] There was also a trend toward a reduced rate of the first cardiovascular hospitalization in those treated with IV iron.[35] Further analyses provided evidence that IV iron supplementation also improves quality of life[38] and is cost-effective.[39] Undoubtedly, further large and longer-running trials are needed to prove the effects of IV iron supplementation on morbidity and mortality in iron-deficient patients with HF, both with and without anemia.

Therefore, anemic patients with ID defined as in the FAIR-HF trial can be considered for the IV iron supplementation. The dose is established using the Ganzoni equation. The monitoring of efficacy and safety of such a therapy should be based on the assessments of hemoglobin, ferritin, Tsat, as well as other indices of erythropoiesis [mean corpuscular volume, content of hemoglobin in reticulocytes may be useful here]. There is no evidence if PO iron supplementation is effective and safe in patients with HF. Due to enteropathy commonly seen in patients with HF, particularly in those with recent episodes of decompensations, the intestine iron absorption is difficult to be predicted, and gastrointestine side-effects may occur.

REFERENCES

1. McMurray JJ, Adamopoulos S, Anker SD, et al. ESC Guidelines for the diagnosis and treatment of acute and chronic heart failure 2012: The Task Force for the Diagnosis and Treatment of Acute and Chronic Heart Failure 2012 of the European Society of Cardiology. Developed in collaboration with the Heart Failure Association (HFA) of the ESC. Eur Heart J. 2012;33(14):1787-847.
2. Silverberg DS, Wexler D, Iaina A, et al. The role of correction of anemia in patients with congestive heart failure: a short review. Eur J Heart Fail. 2008;10(9):819-23.
3. Von Haehling S, Jankowska EA, Ponikowski P, et al. Anemia in heart failure: an overview of current concepts. Future Cardiol. 2011;7(1):119-29.
4. Tang YD, Katz SD. The prevalence of anemia in chronic heart failure and its impact on the clinical outcomes. Heart Fail Rev. 2008;13(4):387-92.
5. Tang WH, Yeo PS. Epidemiology of anemia in heart failure. Heart Fail Clin. 2010;6(3):271-8.
6. Jankowska EA, von Haehling S, Anker SD, et al. Iron deficiency and heart failure: diagnostic dilemmas and therapeutic perspectives. Eur Heart J. 2013;34(11):816-29.
7. Anand IS. Heart failure and anemia: mechanisms and pathophysiology. Heart Fail Rev. 2008;13(4):379-86.
8. Anand IS. Pathophysiology of anemia in heart failure. Heart Fail Clin. 2010;6(3):279-88.
9. Röhrig G, Doehner W, Schaefer RM, et al. [Anemia and iron deficiency in the elderly. Prevalence, diagnostics and new therapeutic options]. Z Gerontol Geriatr. 2012;45(3):191-6.
10. Berliner N. Anemia in the elderly. Trans Am Clin Climatol Assoc. 2013;124:230-7.
11. Ishani A, Weinhandl E, Zhao Z, et al. Angiotensin-converting enzyme inhibitors as a risk factor for the development of anemia, and the impact of incident anemia on mortality in patients with left ventricular dysfunction. J Am Coll Cardiol. 2005;45(3):391-9.
12. Van der Meer P, Lipsic E, Westenbrink BD, et al. Levels of hematopoiesis inhibitor N-acetyl-seryl-aspartyl-lysyl-proline partially explain the occurrence of anemia in heart failure. Circulation. 2005;112(12):1743-7.
13. van der Putten K, Braam B, Jie KE, et al. Mechanisms of Disease: erythropoietin resistance in patients with both heart and kidney failure. Nat Clin Pract Nephrol. 2008;4(1):47-57.
14. Weiss G. Iron metabolism in the anemia of chronic disease. Biochim Biophys Acta. 2009;1790(7):682-93.
15. Opasich C, Cazzola M, Scelsi L, et al. Blunted erythropoietin production and defective iron supply for erythropoiesis as major causes of anaemia in patients with chronic heart failure. Eur Heart J. 2005;26(21):2232-7.
16. Ezekowitz JA, McAlister FA, Armstrong PW. Anemia is common in heart failure and is associated with poor outcomes: insights from a cohort of 12,065 patients with new-onset heart failure. Circulation. 2003;107(2):223-5.
17. Nanas JN, Matsouka C, Karageorgopoulos D, et al. Etiology of anemia in patients with advanced heart failure. J Am Coll Cardiol. 2006;48(12): 2485-9.
18. Jankowska EA, Rozentryt P, Witkowska A, et al. Iron deficiency: an ominous sign in patients with systolic chronic heart failure. Eur Heart J. 2010;31:1872-80.
19. van Veldhuisen DJ, Anker SD, Ponikowski P, et al. Anemia and iron deficiency in heart failure: mechanisms and therapeutic approaches. Nat Rev Cardiol. 2011;8(9):485-93.
20. Hentze MW, Muckenthaler MU, Galy B, et al. Two to tango: regulation of Mammalian iron metabolism. Cell. 2010;142(1):24-38.

21. Jankowska EA, Malyszko J, Ardehali H, et al. Iron status in patients with chronic heart failure. Eur Heart J. 2013;34:827-34.
22. Nemeth E, Ganz T. The role of hepcidin in iron metabolism. Acta Haematol. 2009;122(2-3):78-86.
23. Kemna EH, Tjalsma H, Willems HL, et al. Hepcidin: from discovery to differential diagnosis. Haematologica. 2008;93:90-7.
24. Salisbury AC, Kosiborod M. Outcomes associated with anemia in patients with heart failure. Heart Fail Clin. 2010;6(3):359-72.
25. Ingle L, Rigby AS, Nabb S, et al. Clinical determinants of poor six-minute walk test performance in patients with left ventricular systolic dysfunction and no major structural heart disease. Eur J Heart Fail. 2006;8(3):321-5.
26. Anand IS, Kuskowski MA, Rector TS, et al. Anemia and change in hemoglobin over time related to mortality and morbidity in patients with chronic heart failure: results from Val-HeFT. Circulation. 2005;112(8):1121-7.
27. Tang WH, Tong W, Jain A, et al. Evaluation and long-term prognosis of new-onset, transient, and persistent anemia in ambulatory patients with chronic heart failure. J Am Coll Cardiol. 2008;51:569-76.
28. von Haehling S, Schefold JC, Hodoscek LM, et al. Anaemia is an independent predictor of death in patients hospitalized for acute heart failure. Clin Res Cardiol. 2010;99(2):107-13.
29. Agarwal AK, Singh AK. Therapy with erythropoiesis-stimulating agents and renal and nonrenal outcomes. Heart Fail Clin. 2010;6(3):323-32.
30. Lawler PR, Filion KB, Eisenberg MJ. Correcting anemia in heart failure: the efficacy and safety of erythropoiesis-stimulating agents. J Card Fail. 2010;16:649-58.
31. Swedberg K, Young JB, Anand IS, et al. Treatment of anemia with darbepoetin alfa in systolic heart failure. N Engl J Med. 2013;368:1210-9.
32. Wish JB. Assessing iron status: beyond serum ferritin and transferrin saturation. Clin J Am Soc Nephrol. 2006;1(Suppl 1):S4-8.
33. Goodnough LT, Nemeth E, Ganz T. Detection, evaluation, and management of iron-restricted erythropoiesis. Blood. 2010;116(23):4754-61.
34. Pasricha SR, Flecknoe-Brown SC, Allen KJ, et al. Diagnosis and management of iron deficiency anaemia: a clinical update. Med J Aust. 2010;193(9):525-32.
35. Anker SD, Colet JC, Filippatos G, et al. Ferric carboxymaltose in patients with heart failure and iron deficiency. N Engl J Med. 2009;361:2436-4.
36. Jankowska EA, Rozentryt P, Witkowska A, et al. Iron deficiency predicts impaired exercise capacity in patients with systolic chronic heart failure. J Card Fail. 2011;17:899-906.
37. Filippatos G, Farmakis D, Colet JC, et al. Intravenous ferric carboxymaltose in iron-deficient chronic heart failure patients with and without anaemia: a subanalysis of the FAIR-HF trial. Eur J Heart Fail. 2013;15(11):1267-76.
38. Comin-Colet J, Lainscak M, Dickstein K, et al. The effect of intravenous ferric carboxymaltose on health-related quality of life in patients with chronic heart failure and iron deficiency: a subanalysis of the FAIR-HF study. Eur Heart J. 2013;34(1):30-8.
39. Gutzwiller FS, Schwenkglenks M, Blank PR, et al. Health economic assessment of ferric carboxymaltose in patients with iron deficiency and chronic heart failure based on the FAIR-HF trial: an analysis for the UK. Eur J Heart Fail. 2012;14:782-90.

Chapter 40

Diabetes Management in Heart Failure

Rajiv Choudhary, Alan S Maisel

ABSTRACT

Heart disease is the number one cause of death in patients with diabetes. The risk of mortality is significantly elevated in the presence of comorbid conditions such as uncontrolled hypertension, obesity, dyslipidemia, smoking and physical inactivity. Managing diabetics with heart failure (HF) can be challenging in itself due to the complex nature of the disease. Poorly controlled diabetes leads to several pathophysiological changes, leading to HF. Moreover, poorly controlled blood sugar can affect other vital organs such as the kidneys resulting in renal failure. Controlling elevated blood sugars can lead to favorable outcomes by preventing the progression of the disease process. Glycemic control in diabetic patients with HF has become increasingly important but the "one size fits all" paradigm does not work in this case. Depending on patient background, medications must be titrated to avoid unnecessary side-effects and prevent conditions of hypoglycemia. Moreover, several factors must be considered when prescribing medications such as patient health literacy level, medication compliance, cost and medication availability. This chapter briefly highlights the underlying pathophysiological changes occurring in diabetic patients with HF along with review of current treatment strategies.

INTRODUCTION

Heart failure (HF) is one of the potentially serious comorbidities seen in diabetes. With a rapid increase in the number of individuals diagnosed with diabetes, one can safely assume a steady rise in the comorbid conditions associated with diabetes. Conducted more than 2 decades ago, the Framingham study delineated the associated risks in patients with HF.[1,2] The study revealed that HF was found to be twice as common in male diabetics and almost five times more common in female diabetics.[2] Interestingly the association was even stronger in individuals aged 65 years or less resulting in higher risk (fourfold) of HF in male diabetics compared to double the risk (eightfold) in female diabetics. The presence of other risk factors such as hypertension, cardiac conditions, dyslipidemia and cigarette smoking significantly increased the mortality.[2]

The Candesartan in Heart failure—Assessment of Reduction in Mortality and morbidity (CHARM) programme[3] randomized 7,599 participants with New York Heart Association (NYHA) classes II–IV HF and not on angiotensin-receptor blocker (ARB) to any of the three ongoing parallel concurrent trials based on ejection fraction (EF) and treatment with angiotensin-converting enzyme inhibitor (ACEI). The prevalence of diabetics in all three arms was around 28.5%. Diabetes was found to be significantly associated with an increased risk of cardiovascular (CV) death and readmissions due to worsening HF. When compared to the low EF group, those with preserved EF almost doubled their risk of CV death or HF hospitalizations [hazard ratio (HR) = 2.0 vs HR = 1.60; $p < 0.0001$ for both groups]. Diabetes was found to be an independent predictor of risk across all groups of EF, with greater risk in the preserved EF group. The stronger interaction between diabetes and preserved EF was explained by the time at risk for HF hospitalizations. Due to a high rate of mortality in the low EF group they were more likely to have lesser time at risk for HF hospitalizations when compared to the preserved EF group.

In an attempt to identify the risk and prognostic predictors of HF hospitalizations in survivors of acute myocardial infarction (MI), a secondary analysis of the multicenter international randomized VALsartan In Acute myocardial iNfarcTion (VALIANT) trial[4] identified diabetes as one of the most important predictors of HF hospitalization. The study demonstrated that among stable post-acute MI survivors, risk of developing HF and subsequent HF-related hospitalization was highest in the first 6 months with diabetes being one of the strong predictors of HF in long-term survivors.

Several population databases and clinical trials have alluded to the increasing risk of HF among diabetics with an approximate overall prevalence of diabetes to be around 25% in HF patients.[5] Among other factors, the effect of diabetes in ischemic heart disease has been partially explained by the presence of chronic atherosclerosis leading to ventricular remodeling and subsequent HF. A retrospective analysis of the Studies of Left Ventricular Dysfunction (SOLVD) trial[6] demonstrated a risk ratio (RR) of 2.16 for HF hospitalizations in diabetics. Moreover, in asymptomatic patients with ischemic cardiomyopathy, the risk of developing HF symptoms was markedly elevated in diabetics. This said, Cubbon et al.,[5] demonstrated that diabetes remained an adverse prognostic indicator of HF independent of underlying etiology of HF (ischemic or non-ischemic).

PATHOPHYSIOLOGY OF HEART FAILURE IN DIABETES

Patients with diabetes fall into two categories: type 1 diabetics wherein the pancreatic beta cells are unable to produce insulin due to destruction or deficiency; and type 2 diabetics wherein insulin insensitivity is increased. Type 2 diabetics are more likely to be undiagnosed for longer periods of time, suggesting a possibility of advanced stage cardiac disease present at the time of symptom onset.[7] With an estimated exponential rise in diabetes, understanding the underlying pathophysiological mechanism to better target therapy is imperative. Although a detailed explanation delving into the pathophysiology is beyond the scope of this chapter, an attempt to highlight the salient molecular and structural changes will be made.

Oxidative Stress

Oxidative stress results from the overproduction of reactive oxygen species (ROS) leading to cellular degradation, apoptosis and modification of the extracellular matrix. The detrimental effects of oxidative stress have been implicated in development of cardiac hypertrophy and progression to cardiomyocyte fibrosis leading to HF.[8-10] ROS are byproducts of cellular metabolism and are chemically unstable. Metabolic processes, which utilize oxygen as the electron acceptor, result in the release of ROS, such as nicotinamide adenine dinucleotide phosphate (NADPH) oxidase enzymes, nitric oxide synthase, and the mitochondrial chain electron transport. Experimental research demonstrates a direct correlation between upregulation of NADPH oxidase enzymes and myocyte hypertrophy by upregulation of profibrotic genes.[11-13] The adverse effect of ROS on the vasodilatory effect of NOS results in endothelial dysfunction, affecting ventricular relaxation of the ventricle. The mitochondrial production of ROS is mediated via activation of nuclear factor-kappa B (NF-κB), which triggers the inflammatory cascade leading to deoxyribonucleic acid (DNA) protein damage and cellular apoptosis.[12,13]

Extracellular Matrix Remodeling

Advanced glycation end-products (AGE) refer to a series of chemical rearrangements of glycated proteins to form complex compounds with crosslinking.[14,15] In diabetics, hyperglycemia results in elevated glucose levels unable to undergo reduction resulting in elevated NADPH levels. This causes a breakdown of the electron transport chain and activation of the poly-ADP (adenosine diphosphate)-ribose polymerase (PARP) enzyme, which is a compensatory response to the mitochondrial ROS production.[14,15] The PARP enzyme then induces ADP-ribosylation of glyceraldehyde-3-phosphate dehydrogenase (GAPDH) resulting in its inactivation and accumulation of glycated metabolites. This accumulation of AGE has shown to promote cardiac fibrosis and arterial stiffness. Furthermore, oxidative stress also induces expression of AGE and receptors for AGE, which result in alteration of cardiac contractility by activating NF-κB.[16] AGE levels in the serum have been shown to positively correlate with ventricular isometric relaxation time, arterial stiffness and carotid intimal thickness in diabetics.[17,18]

Impaired Excitation Contraction Coupling

Myocardial contractility is principally regulated by calcium. Diabetes impairs calcium cycling in myocytes by specifically affecting the sarcoplasmic/endoplasmic reticulum Ca^{2+} -ATPase (SERCA2).[19,20] The myocardial contractile elements function by an influx of intracellular calcium, which then bind the myofilaments resulting in cardiac contractility. SERCA2 is responsible for the movement of calcium out of the cytosol into the lumen in order to facilitate relaxation.[21,22] In diabetics, impaired SERCA2 functionality results in improper calcium handling and increased intracellular calcium levels which result in impaired cardiac relaxation. Furthermore, formation of AGE and ROS also depresses SERCA2 and further worsen myocardial relaxation and contractility.[22]

Endothelial Dysfunction

In diabetics, the myocardial vascular integrity is altered by a series of processes. Activation of inflammatory cytokines along with oxidative stress and impaired NOS vasodilatory effects, endothelial dysfunction adversely affects coronary and capillary blood flow resulting in micro- and macroangiopathy.[19,21] With the presence of receptors for AGE in the endothelial wall, inhibition of nitric oxide (NO) production by AGE and ROS, increased expression of cell adhesion molecules results in hardening of coronary vasculature and fibrosis. The cumulative effect is cardiac dysfunction due to repeated vasoconstriction and reperfusion injuries. Moreover, in diabetic patients, the suppression of vascular endothelial growth factor (VEGF) results in interstitial fibrosis, reduced capillary density and apoptosis of endothelial cells.[19-21]

ROLE OF GLYCEMIC CONTROL

Controlling elevated blood sugars is not only important to prevent the deleterious effects of hyperglycemia, but also to suppress free fatty acid production, which has shown to suppress cardiac contractility.[23,24] Elevated free fatty acid levels have been shown to disrupt plasma membrane functionality and increase cardiac workload by increasing intracellular calcium.[25,26] Iribarren et al.[27] assessed predominantly type 2 diabetic patients from the Kaiser Permanente Diabetes Registry to evaluate the association of glycated hemoglobin (HBA_{1c}) levels and incident HF. The results revealed that after adjusting for age and sex, every 1% rise in HBA_{1c} was associated with 12% increased risk of HF. Relative to patients with HBA_{1c} of less than 7% those with HBA_{1c} of greater than 10% were at 1.56 higher risk of HF.

Dungan et al.[28] assessed 748 patients with congestive HF to investigate the association between inpatient glycemic control and readmission rates. Results revealed that readmitted patients had a HBA_{1c} level of about 8.3% compared to 7.5% in those that were not readmitted. The study demonstrated 2% higher odds for readmission for every 1% increase in HBA_{1c} levels. Finally, the study concluded that elevated mean glucose and HBA_{1c} levels were associated with higher risk of HF readmission in the intermediate period of 30–90 days, but not in short-term period of 30 days or less. The Heart and Soul study[29] evaluated the association between diabetes and HBA_{1c} levels with incident HF in 839 individuals with stable coronary artery disease without a history of HF. The study demonstrated a 36% increased risk of HF hospitalization with every 1% rise in HBA_{1c} levels. Furthermore, participants with diabetes were at an increased risk of HF (HR = 2.17) compared to those without. HBA_{1c} levels of greater than 6.5% was associated with an increased risk of developing HF.

Although maintaining glucose control is crucial in preventing the development and readmission due to HF, strict regimens attempting to achieve an HBA_{1c} of 6% or less should be avoided, especially in the elderly (age > 65 years) due to higher incidence of hypoglycemia and increased risk of mortality.[30] In both the Action in Diabetes and Vascular Disease: Preterax and Diamicron MR Controlled Evaluation (ADVANCE) and Action to Control Cardiovascular Risk in Diabetes (ACCORD) clinical trials,[31,32] no benefit was shown with strict glucose control (HbA_{1c} 6.5% vs 6%, respectively). Moreover, patients with type 2 diabetes in the ACCORD trial with HBA_{1c} control of 6% or lower were found to be at a higher risk of complications such as hypoglycemia. Conversely, in the UK Prospective Diabetes Study (UKPDS) 10-year follow-up of newly diagnosed type 2 diabetes treated with intensive therapy, risk reduction in microvascular disease and MI was observed. Results were most significant in the metformin treatment arm of the study achieving a 27% risk reduction in death due to any cause and 30% for diabetes-related death.[33]

Thus, adequate glucose control measured by HBA_{1c} levels should be tailored to suit the patient's clinical and demographic profile in order to achieve maximum treatment benefit. In elderly and nursing home patients, stricter regimens must be avoided, whereas in the general population, depending on the CV risk profile, treatment should be titrated to achieve HBA_{1c} levels less than 6.5–7%.

ANTIDIABETIC AGENTS

Metformin

Considered as the first-line drug of choice in managing type 2 diabetics, metformin has been used extensively since 1957 following its documented use in lowering blood sugar in humans.[34] Belonging to the biguanide class of antidiabetic drugs, metformin prevents hyperglycemia via variety of mechanisms. Metformin prevents rise in blood glucose by inhibiting hepatic gluconeogenesis.[34] Furthermore, metformin increases insulin sensitivity by promoting peripheral glucose uptake, decreased gastrointestinal absorption and decreasing circulating levels of nonesterified free fatty acids. Metformin has also been shown to activate adenosine monophosphate-activated protein kinase (AMPK), the enzyme responsible for insulin signaling and regulating cellular energy.[35] Its use in HF has been controversial due to its primary side-effect of lactic acidosis, which leads to it being contraindicated in such patients. In a retrospective analysis of diabetic patients aged more than 65 years and with HF, use of metformin was associated with a significant reduction in 1-year mortality risk [HR = 0.87, 95% confidence interval (CI) = 0.78–0.97]. Moreover, those patients on metformin treatment were also found to have a low risk of readmission due to HF compared to those treated with thiazolidinediones (HR = 0.92 vs 1.06).[36]

Similarly, Eurich et al.[37] conducted a meta-analysis of randomized controlled trials in order to evaluate the association between use of antidiabetic medications and death and/or readmission. Results demonstrated a reduction in all-cause mortality and identified metformin as the only antidiabetic agent among insulin, sulfonylureas and thiazolidinediones not associated with harm in HF patients.

Shah et al.[38] demonstrated that in 401 patients with diabetes and advanced HF, of the 25% treated with metformin, 1-year survival was 91% compared to 76% in the nonmetformin treatment group. With several such clinical trials demonstrating a minimal risk in its use in HF patients, the Food and Drug Administration lifted the contradiction in 2006 and replaced it with a warning.

Finally although there have been experimental studies that have demonstrated a "cardioprotective effect" of metformin use by slowing HF progression, improving left ventricular ejection fraction (LVEF) and diastolic function, its exact role in preventing HF progression remains uncertain and more research is warranted in better understanding that effect.

Sulfonylureas

The other antidiabetic agent widely used in treating hyperglycemia is sulfonylurea. They act by binding adenosine triphosphate (ATP)-dependent potassium (K^+) channels located on the cell membrane of pancreatic beta cells.[39] Resultant effect is change in membrane potential due to increased intracellular K^+, which in turn leads to cell depolarization and opening of voltage-gated Ca^{2+} channels and release of insulin due to increased intracellular calcium.[39] To investigate the association between oral antidiabetic agents and congestive HF, risk of MI and all-cause mortality, a retrospective cohort analysis of UK general practice database revealed an increased risk of mortality in those using second- and first-generation sulfonylureas compared to metformin monotherapy.[40] The detrimental effect of sulfonylureas in patients with HF may be linked to the increased calcium influx into cells as a result of hyperpolarization by blocking ATP-dependent K^+ channels. In cardiac myocytes, under normal physiological conditions, the voltage-gated calcium channels remain closed and the calcium influx is avoided to prevent ischemic injury.[40] The inhibitory effect on the myocyte K^+ channels of sulfonylureas and influx of calcium can lead to impaired myocardial contractility and relaxation. Furthermore, sulfonylureas are notorious for causing hypoglycemic episodes and must be used with caution in the elderly or in patients with poor health literacy.

Thiazolidinediones

Thiazolidinediones refer to a class of drugs, which exert an insulin-sensitizing effect by activating peroxisome proliferator-activated receptor gamma (PPAR-γ).[41,42] Activation of the receptors along with formation of heterodimer results in upregulation of specific genes, which reduce insulin resistance, inhibit VEGF-induced angiogenesis, and increase appetite by lowering circulating leptin levels. Moreover they have a beneficial effect on the lipid profile by increasing high-density lipoprotein and decreasing triglycerides.[41,42] Thiazolidinediones have also demonstrated a positive effect on the vascular endothelium and myocardium possibly due to its suppressive effect on circulating free fatty acids and inflammatory cytokines. Their use in HF patients is highly controversial, especially in advance systolic HF due to the increased risk of developing fluid retention.[41-43]

A randomized double-blinded multicenter trial assessing the association between pioglitazone use and HF in type 2 diabetics demonstrated a high incidence of HF hospitalization with pioglitazone use.[42] Participants consisted of systolic dysfunction and NYHA classes II/ III HF. In the pioglitazone treatment arm, incidence of HF was 13% compared to the glyburide treatment arm, although there was no increase in CV mortality or worsening cardiac function on echocardiography. The PROspective pioglitAzone Clinical Trial In macrovascular Events (PROACTIVE) study[44] similarly showed a significant increase in HF with pioglitazone use whereas mortality and CV events were unaffected.

The underlying pathophysiological mechanisms of thiazolidinediones-causing fluid retention are multifactorial and can be partly explained by their synergistic effect with insulin-causing arterial vasodilation and subsequent renal sodium reabsorption thereby increasing extracellular fluid volume, resulting in pedal edema.[40] Moreover, changes in vascular endothelial permeability along with VEGF-induced effects via PPAR-γ activation also play a role.[40] Although no effect on myocardium has been demonstrated.

Clinical trials have also demonstrated a beneficial effect of using thiazolidinediones by improving cardiac function and improving risk of mortality. In a recently concluded double-blinded randomized controlled trial investigating the effects of pioglitazone on myocardial function, revealed an improvement in cardiac function in patients taking pioglitazone.[43] In the absence of cardiac ischemia and uncomplicated type 2 diabetes, when compared to metformin use, only pioglitazone use increased left ventricular (LV)-end-diastolic volume and compliance without concurrent changes in N-terminal prohormone brain natriuretic peptide (NT-proBNP) and early transmitral-to-early diastolic annular velocity ratio (E/Ea).[43] The use of other thiazolidinediones such as rosiglitazone has demonstrated an increased risk of MI.

The retrospective analysis by Masoudi et al.[36] of older patients (age > 65 years) on antidiabetic medications for diabetes and a discharge diagnosis of HF revealed treatment with thiazolidinediones was associated with a significant lower risk of death (HR = 0.87, 95% CI = 0.80–0.94) even after adjusting for covariates. Moreover the combined use of metformin and thiazolidinediones achieved an even more lower risk of death (HR = 0.76, 95% CI = 0.58–0.99).

Insulin

Clinical studies evaluating insulin use in diabetics with HF have provided equivocal results. Studies have shown an increased risk of HF with insulin use.[45,46] Several factors have been cited as possible causes relating insulin use to risk of mortality in diabetic patients with HF. The Outcome Reduction With Initial Glargine Intervention (ORIGIN) trial[47] demonstrated that in patients receiving basal insulin compared to standard care, neither an increase nor a decrease in CV outcomes was observed. In patients receiving insulin glargine, 4.9% had HF hospitalization compared to 5.5% in the standard care group. Also, the study by Eurich et al.[37] in assessing the benefits and harms of antidiabetic medications revealed no increase in mortality as mentioned in the metformin section.

Glucagon-like Peptide-1 Analogs

Glucagon-like peptide-1 (GLP-1) analogs belong to the class of drugs known as "incretin mimetics". Incretin hormones refer to a class of gut hormones namely GLP-1 and gastric inhibitory polypeptide (GIP), which inhibit glucagon release and increase insulin secretion from the pancreatic beta cells.[39,48] Similarly, GLP-1 analogs are secreted by the gut and regulate postprandial insulin release resulting in enhanced insulin sensitivity. Moreover, they delay gastric emptying thus slowing the rate of nutrient absorption and allowing for a more effective insulin secretion and response. The CV effects of GLP-1 analogs are promoting weight loss indirectly by affecting early satiety, promoting insulin sensitivity and thus improving glycemic control.[39] Given the relatively new nature of these drugs, more research investigating their properties and characteristics in diabetics with HF are needed.

Dipeptidyl Peptidase-4 Inhibitors

Dipeptidyl peptidase-4 (DPP-4) is a class of novel drugs, which act by increasing incretin hormone levels by inhibiting the enzyme DPP-4.[39,49] Also referred to as gliptins, DPP-4 inhibitors can be orally administered and exert their effect by inhibiting the degradation of GLP-1 and GIP. Due to the new nature of these drugs, clinical trials are lacking in respect to characterizing their effects on diabetics with HF. Although promising in nature, robust clinical evidence regarding their use is warranted.

CONCLUSION

With diabetic cases on the rise, effective treatment strategies are needed to avoid exacerbating underlying heart disease. With the documented risk of HF in diabetics, therapy should be tailored to fit the individual clinical profile. The "one size fits all" paradigm must be avoided and treatment should be titrated based on their CV risk in short term and long term. Improving CV-related mortality and HF readmission rate are essential in lowering the health and economic burden of the disease. With clinical trials demonstrating a measurable risk with use of oral antidiabetic drugs, treatment regimens employing a more stricter glycemic control approach must be avoided, especially in the older population. Pathophysiological effects of hyperglycemia are apparent, leading to molecular and structural changes in the heart and resulting in systolic and diastolic dysfunction. These changes have now been shown to occur at a more initial stage in asymptomatic prediabetics. Thus, with the longer time to presentation and diagnosis in type 2 diabetics, more care should be taken to monitor these patients and screen them for development of HF to appropriately tailor therapy. More clinical trials and translational studies investigating the effect of antidiabetic agents in HF patients with diabetes may allow a better understanding of the risks involved and possibly establish newer treatment guidelines in the future.

REFERENCES

1. Kannel WB, McGee DL. Diabetes and cardiovascular disease: the Framingham study. Circulation. 1979;59(1):8-13.
2. Kannel WB. Hazards, risks, and threats of heart disease from the early stages to symptomatic coronary heart disease and cardiac failure. Cardiovasc Drugs Ther. 1997;11(Suppl 1):199-212.
3. MacDonald MR, Petrie MC, Varyani F, et al. Impact of diabetes on outcomes in patients with low and preserved ejection fraction heart failure: an analysis of the Candesartan in Heart failure: Assessment of Reduction in Mortality and morbidity (CHARM) programme. Euro Heart J. 2008;29(11):1377-85.
4. Lewis EF, Velazquez EJ, Solomon SD, et al. Predictors of the first heart failure hospitalization in patients who are stable survivors of myocardial infarction complicated by pulmonary congestion and/or left ventricular dysfunction: a VALIANT study. Euro Heart J. 2008;29(6):748-56.
5. Cubbon RM, Adams B, Rajwani A, et al. Diabetes mellitus is associated with adverse prognosis in chronic heart failure of ischemic and non-ischemic aetiology. Diab Vasc Dis Res. 2013;10(4):330-6.
6. Vermes E, Ducharme A, Bourassa MG, et al. Enalapril reduces the incidence of diabetes in patients with chronic heart failure: insight from the Studies Of Left Ventricular Dysfunction (SOLVD). Circulation. 2003;107(9):1291-6.
7. Tribouilloy C, Rusinaru D, Mahjoub H, et al. Prognostic impact of diabetes mellitus in patients with heart failure and preserved ejection fraction: a prospective five-year study. Heart. 2008;94(11):1450-5.
8. Devereux RB, Roman MJ, Paranicas M, et al. Impact of diabetes on cardiac structure and function: the strong heart study. Circulation. 2000;101(19):2271-6.
9. Nichols GA, Hillier TA, Erbey JR, et al. Congestive heart failure in type 2 diabetes: prevalence, incidence and risk factors. Diabetes Care. 2001;24(9):1614-9.
10. Berry C, Brosnan MJ, Fennell J, et al. Oxidative stress and vascular damage in hypertension. Curr Opin Nephrol Hypertens. 2001;10(2):247-55.
11. Van Heerebreek L, Meischl C, Stooker W, et al. NADPH oxidase(s): new source(s) of reactive oxygen species in the vascular system? J Clin Pathol. 2002;55(8):561-8.
12. Griendling KK. Novel NAD(P)H oxidases in the cardiovascular system. Heart. 2004;90(5):491-3.
13. Ritchie RH, Quinn JM, Cao AH, et al. The antioxidant tempol inhibits cardiac hypertrophy in the insulin-resistant GLUT4-deficient mouse in vivo. J Mol Cell Cardiol. 2007;42(6):1119-28.
14. Aragno M, Mastrocola R, Medana C, et al. Oxidative stress-dependent impairment of cardiac-specific transcription factors in experimental diabetes. Endocrinology. 2006;147(12):5967-74.
15. Verzijl N, DeGroot J, Thorpe SR, et al. Effect of collagen turnover on the accumulation of advanced glycation end products. J Biol Chem. 2000;275(50):39027-31.
16. Berg TJ, Snorgaard O, Faber J, et al. Serum levels of advanced glycation end products are associated with left ventricular diastolic function in patients with type 1 diabetes. Diabetes Care. 1999;22(7):1186-90.
17. Yoshida N, Okumura K, Aso Y. High serum pentosidine concentrations are associated with increased arterial stiffness and thickness in patients with type 2 diabetes. Metabolism. 2005;54(3):345-50.
18. Lapolla A, Piarulli F, Sartore G, et al. Advanced glycation end products and antioxidant status in type 2 diabetic patients with and without peripheral artery disease. Diabetes care. 2007;30(3):670-6.
19. Chavali V, Tyagi SC, Mishra PK. Predictors and prevention of diabetic cardiomyopathy. Diabetes Metab Syndr Obes. 2013;6:151-60.
20. Asghar O, Al-Sunni A, Khavandi K, et al. Diabetic cardiomyopathy. Clin Sci (Lond). 2009;116(10):741-60.
21. Matheus AS, Tannus LR, Cobas RA, et al. Impact of diabetes on cardiovascular disease: an update. Int J Hypertens. 2013;2013:653789.
22. Miki T, Yuda S, Kouzu H, et al. Diabetic cardiomyopathy: pathophysiology and clinical features. Heart Fail Rev. 2013;18(2):149-66.
23. Malmberg K. Prospective randomized study of intensive insulin treatment on long term survival after acute myocardial infarction in patients with diabetes mellitus. DIGAMI (Diabetes Mellitus, Insulin Glucose Infusion in Acute Myocardial Infarction) Study Group. BMJ. 1997;314(7093):1512-5.
24. Malmberg K, Ryden L, Hamsten A, et al. Effects of insulin treatment on cause-specific one-year mortality and morbidity in diabetic patients with acute myocardial infarction. DIGAMI Study Group. Diabetes Insulin-Glucose in Acute Myocardial Infarction. Eur Heart J. 1996;17(9):1337-44.
25. Oliver MF, Opie LH. Effects of glucose and fatty acids on myocardial ischemia and arrhythmias. Lancet. 1994;343(8890):155-8.
26. Mjos OD. Effects of free fatty acids on myocardial function and oxygen consumption in intact dogs. J Clin Invest. 1971;50(7):1386-9.
27. Iribarren C, Karter AJ, Go AS, et al. Glycemic control and heart failure among adult patients with diabetes. Circulation. 2001;103(22):2668-73.
28. Dungan KM, Osei K, Nagaraja HN, et al. Relationship between glycemic control and readmission rates in patients hospitalized with congestive heart failure during the implementation of hospital-wide initiatives. Endocr Pract. 2010;16(6):945-51.
29. van Melle JP, Bot M, de Jonge P, et al. Diabetes, glycemic control, and new-onset heart failure in patients with stable coronary artery disease: data from the heart and soul study. Diabetes Care. 2010;33(9):2084-9.

30. Eshaghian S, Horwich TB, Fonarow GC. An unexpected inverse relationship between HbA1c levels and mortality in patients with diabetes and advanced systolic heart failure. Am Heart J. 2006;151(1):377-84.
31. ADVANCE Collaborative Group, Patel A, MacMahon S, et al. Intensive blood glucose control and vascular outcomes in patients with type 2 diabetes. N Engl J Med. 2008;358(24):2560-72.
32. Action to Control Cardiovascular Risk in Diabetes Study Group, Gerstein HC, Miller ME, et al. Effects of intensive glucose lowering in type 2 diabetes. N Engl J Med. 2008;358(24):2545-59.
33. Holman RR, Paul SK, Bethel MA, et al. 10-year follow-up of intensive glucose control in type 2 diabetes. N Engl J Med. 2008;359(15):1577-89.
34. Rojas LB, Gomes MB. Metformin: an old but still the best treatment for type 2 diabetes. Diabetol Metab Syndr. 2013;5(1):6.
35. Yin M, van der Horst IC, van Melle JP, et al. Metformin improves cardiac function in a nondiabetic rat model of post-MI heart failure. Am J Physiol Heart Circ Physiol. 2011;301(2):H459-68.
36. Masoudi FA, Inzucchi SE, Wang Y, et al. Thiazolidinediones, metformin, and outcomes in older patients with diabetes and heart failure: an observational study. Circulation. 2005;111(5):583-90.
37. Eurich DT, McAlister FA, Blackburn DF, et al. Benefits and harms of antidiabetic agents in patients with diabetes and heart failure: systematic review. BMJ. 2007;335(7618):497.
38. Shah DD, Fonarow GC, Horwich TB. Metformin therapy and outcomes in patients with advanced systolic heart failure and diabetes. J Card Fail. 2010;16(3):200-6.
39. Fisman EZ, Tenenbaum A. A cardiologic approach to non-insulin antidiabetic pharmacotherapy in patients with heart disease. Cardiovasc Diabetol. 2009;8:38.
40. Tzoulaki I, Molokhia M, Curcin V, et al. Risk of cardiovascular disease and all cause mortality among patients with type 2 diabetes prescribed oral antidiabetes drugs: retrospective cohort study using UK general practice research database. BMJ. 2009;339:b4731.
41. Nesto RW, Bell D, Bonow RO, et al. Thiazolidinediones use, fluid retention, and congestive heart failure: a consensus statement from the American Heart Association and American Diabetes Association. October 7, 2003. Circulation. 2003;108(23):2941-8.
42. van der Meer RW, Rijzewijk LJ, de Jong HW, et al. Pioglitazone improves cardiac function and alters myocardial substrate metabolism without affecting cardiac triglyceride accumulation and high-energy phosphate metabolism in patients with well-controlled type 2 diabetes mellitus. Circulation. 2009;119(15):2069-77.
43. Delea TE, Edelsberg JS, Hagiwara M, et al. Use of thiazolidinediones and risk of heart failure in people with type 2 diabetes: a retrospective cohort study. Diabetes Care. 2003;26(11):2983-9.
44. Wilcox R, Kupfer S, Erdmann E, et al. Effects of pioglitazone on major adverse cardiovascular events in high-risk patients with type 2 diabetes: results from PROspective pioglitAzone Clinical Trial In macro Vascular Events (PROactive 10). Am Heart J. 2008;155(4):712-7.
45. Currie CJ, Johnson JA. The safety profile of exogenous insulin in people with type 2 diabetes: justification for concern. Diabetes Obes Metab. 2012;14(1):1-4.
46. Melbin LG, Malmberg K, Norhamar A, et al. Prognostic implications of glucose-lowering treatment in patients with acute myocardial infarction and diabetes: experience from an extended follow-up of the Diabetes Mellitus Insulin-Glucose Infusion in Acute Myocardial Infarction (DIGAMI) 2 Study. Diabetologia. 2011;54:1308-17.
47. ORIGIN Trial Investigators, Gerstein HC, Bosch J, et al. Basal insulin and cardiovascular and other outcomes in dysglycemia. N Engl J Med. 2012;367(4):319-28.
48. Bell DS. Heart failure: the frequent, forgotten, and often fatal complication of diabetes. Diabetes Care. 2003;26(8):2433-41.
49. Tschöpe D, Hanefeld M, Meier JJ, et al. The role of co-morbidity in the selection of antidiabetic pharmacotherapy in type-2 diabetes. Cardiovasc Diabetol. 2013;12:62.

Chapter 41

Heart Failure in Europe

John GF Cleland, Pierpaolo Pellicori, Benjamin Dicken, Ahmad Shoaib, Sunaina Parsons, Riet Dierckx

ABSTRACT

Any discussion of the epidemiology of heart failure (HF) in Europe, as elsewhere, is fraught with uncertainty due to the lack of robust criteria for its definition. This is further complicated by reporting incidence and prevalence only in certain age groups rather than the whole population. Most cases are diagnosed during a hospital admission, only a minority of patients is managed by cardiologists in most countries and many cases probably go undiagnosed. Depending on the definition applied, between 5% and 10% of all emergency hospital admission are caused or complicated by HF. More than 2% of the entire population of Western Europe is taking loop diuretics for no obvious reason other than HF but less than half are labelled as such. In general, it appears that the prevalence of HF is similar across European countries. Poverty is associated with higher age-adjusted incidence rates for heart failure. However, because the development of HF is strongly associated with older age and because wealth is a major determinant of longevity, socioeconomic conditions have little or no impact on prevalence rates. Indeed, anything that increases longevity may increase the overall incidence and prevalence of HF. The management of HF by expert centers across European countries appears fairly uniform but great disparity in care may exist amongst the majority of patients who do not receive specialist care. About half of patients hospitalized with new onset or decompensated chronic HF will die within 1 year but this is strongly age-related, ranging from about 25% in those aged less than 75 years to greater than 60% in those aged greater than 85 years. For patients with chronic stable HF receiving expert care, the annual mortality is 5–10%.

INTRODUCTION

Europe is a large, ethnically, culturally, linguistically, and geographically diverse continent extending from the Ural Mountains and the Caspian Sea in the East to Iceland, Ireland and Spain in the West, and from the Arctic Ocean in the North to the Mediterranean Sea in the South. The European Society of Cardiology (ESC) extends the geography even further to the Pacific Ocean, Middle East, Persian Gulf, and the North African Coast covering a total population of about 1.5 billion people with great variations in affluence. It would be remarkable if the epidemiology of heart failure (HF) and clinical practice was similar across this region. However, in many respects, it is the similarities rather than the differences that are surprising, at least in the published evidence.

When considering the information presented in this chapter, it is important to realize that data are usually recorded only in healthcare systems that have either administrative or professional incentives to gather and report information. This creates bias toward more affluent systems and healthcare funded by the state or large insurance organizations. Professionally, those with a special interest in cardiology are more likely to collect relevant information and this will introduce bias toward younger patients with fewer comorbidities. A universally accepted definition of HF remains elusive and it is not clear that attempting to create a single definition would serve a useful purpose. A more useful approach is to consider how certain the diagnosis is. Almost everyone would agree that a patient with a left ventricular ejection fraction (EF) of 30% and persistent exertional breathlessness with an N-terminal B-type natriuretic peptide (NT-proBNP) of 1,200 ng/L despite 80 mg of furosemide per day had HF. However, the vast majority of patients treated with loop diuretics do not fulfill more than one of these criteria and yet get hospitalized for worsening peripheral edema and breathlessness and have a poor prognosis, consistent with a malign underlying disease, such as HF. Finally, clinical practice guidelines for HF have really only taken hold over the last 15 years stimulated by the advent of diagnostic testing with natriuretic peptides and treatments including beta-blockers (BB), aldosterone antagonists, implantable cardiac-defibrillators (ICD), and cardiac resynchronization therapy (CRT). Prior to this time, the treatment of HF relied only on digoxin, diuretics, and angiotensin-converting-enzyme inhibitors (ACEIs). Data gathered before the turn of the century may be out of date.

Heart failure is not only heterogeneous in its etiology and clinical presentation, but also in how it is defined. Patient characteristics will vary considerably depending on the method of case-ascertainment and the person making that judgment. Key epidemiological studies are reported that provide information on incidence and prevalence (Table 1). However, most reports describe the characteristics, treatment, and outcome in cohorts of patients. For the purposes of this chapter, HF has been grouped into three settings: (1) primary care; (2) outpatient clinic; and (3) hospital admissions.

EPIDEMIOLOGICAL STUDIES OF INCIDENCE AND PREVALENCE (TABLE 1)

Great care is required in interpreting such data on incidence and prevalence. Pay particular attention to the denominator and the case-definition for HF. Many epidemiological studies exclude younger people and sometimes also have an upper age limit. Overall, the data are consistent with a population annual incidence of about 0.3% or 3,000 new cases per million population per year or 180,000 in a United Kingdom (UK) sized population (63 million) or about 1 million per year in the United States of America (USA) population (316 million). The best estimate of the prevalence of symptomatic HF in the overall population may be similar to the proportion of patients taking a loop diuretic in the community, which is 2.4%.[13,14] This would translate into 1.5 million people in the UK and 7.6 million in the USA. Some patients will have HF but be treated either with thiazide diuretics or none at all. A substantial proportion of patients taking loop diuretics will have no other evidence of cardiac dysfunction. Perhaps only half of patients who are subsequently confirmed to have HF will have overt left ventricular systolic dysfunction (LVSD); others will have valve disease, atrial fibrillation (AF) and little or no reduction in left ventricular EF.[13]

HEART FAILURE IN PRIMARY CARE (TABLES 2 AND 3)

Information on this aspect of HF is dominated by the IMprovement PROgram in eValuation and managEMENT of Heart Failure (IMPROVEMENT-HF) survey that enrolled 11,062 patients in primary care.[15] Key differences of note were that women constituted a far higher proportion of primary care doctors and that patients were younger in Central and Eastern Europe. These factors may have influenced, respectively, therapy and comorbidity. Only about 50% of patients had LVSD but 60% were treated with ACEIs, with little regional variation, suggesting a high uptake of these agents in appropriate patients. The study was conducted only shortly after publication of the landmark studies and guidelines supporting the benefits of BB and mineralocorticoid antagonists, which accounts for their relatively low use. The most striking difference in clinical practice was preference for thiazide rather than loop diuretics in some countries. Patients included in surveys from primary care tended to be older, were more often women and presumably more often had HF with normal ejection fraction (HFnEF) and a substantially better prognosis, despite apparently poorer treatment. This may reflect the inaccuracy of diagnosis in primary care and the need for improved diagnostic testing.

OUTPATIENTS WITH HEART FAILURE (TABLE 4)

There are many small audits of local clinical practice but these are often from tertiary care centers associated with transplant programs. For the purposes of this report, we have focused on larger studies. These studies show that outpatients attending cardiology clinics are generally younger patients with LVSD and although they have high rates of comorbidity, they probably have less than most patients with HF.[21-23]

HOSPITAL ADMISSIONS WITH HEART FAILURE (TABLES 5–8)

The first EuroHeart Failure Survey (EHFS) provides epidemiological data that allows patient characteristics to be compared across a broad range of European

TABLE 1: Studies of the Prevalence and Incidence of heart failure (pay close attention to age-range studied)

Study and countries	*Collection period*	*Population*	*Age range surveyed*	*Number surveyed*	*Number with HF*	*Follow-up*	*Prevalence*	*Age and sex of patients with HF*	*Comments*
Prevalence									
England ECHOES Taylor et al. 2011[1]	1995–1999	Primary care registers	>45 years	6,162	449	NA	7.3%	64 years (mean) W: 50%	
England GPRD Hawkins et al. 2012[2]	Continuous 1999–2007	UK GPRD	>25 years	~2 million	13,330		2000: 1.08% 2007: 0.83%	1999 W: 56% >75 years 69% 2007 W: 51% >75 years 68%	
England Newcastle 85+ study Yousaf et al. 2012[3]	17 months 2006–2007	>84 years	87–89 years	376	51.6%	NA	LVSD: 32% (Mod/Sev 9%) LVDD: 88% (Mod/Sev 25%)	88 years W: 62%	
England E-ECHOES Gill et al. 2011[4]	2006–2009	Ethnic minorities	>45 years	5,354	59 (1.1%)	NA	EF <40%: 1.1%, HFnEF: 1.0% AF: 1.0%	South Asian M: 49% 59 years (mean) Afro-Caribbean M: 45% 63 years (mean)	Study of ethnic minority groups in England
Spain Cadiz study Gomez-Soto et al. 2011[5]	2000–2007	Community aged >13 years	>14 years	267,231	4,793		2000: 0.9% 2007: 2.1%	2000 W: 53% 67 years (mean) 2007 W: 53% 72 years (mean)	In 2007, risk-adjusted 30-day, 1-year and 4-year mortality was 12.1%, 28.8%, and 61.4%
Spain Madrid Prevalence Study Carmona et al. 2011[6]	2007	Community health records	All ages	198,670	1,377	NA	6.9%, out of these Cardiac arrhythmia 45.3%	78 years (mean) W: 52%	High rate of comorbidity with average of 5.2 ± 2.1 chronic diseases

Contd...

Contd...

Study and countries	*Collection period*	*Population*	*Age range surveyed*	*Number surveyed*	*Number with HF*	*Follow-up*	*Prevalence*	*Age and sex of patients with HF*	*Comments*
Sweden Stockholm Zarrinkoub et al. 2103[7]	2006 and 2010	Health register	All ages	2.1 million	88,038		2.2%	W: 51%	0.32% pa
Portugal EPICA Ceia et al. 2002[8]	1998	Primary care visits	>25 years	Estimated	551		4.4% HFrEF: 1.3%		
Portugal EPIPorto cohort study Severo et al. 2012[9]	2006–2008	Community	≥45 years	1,115	7.1%	7 years (mean)	7.1% LVSD: 3.5% LVDD: 14.5% NYHA >2 13.1% BNP >100 6.3%	57 years (mean) W: 61%	<5% had LVSD and HF LA Dil: 17% Valve Dis: 2.8%
Hull Administrative Data (unpublished)	2011	GP prescription of loop diuretic	Whole population				2.4% (3.1% of those aged >20 years)		
Incidence							**Incidence**	Age and sex at onset of HF	
The Netherlands PREVEND Brouwers et al. 2013[10]	1997–1998	Age 28-75 years ~60% selected by MAU	28–75 years	8,592	374	12 years	HF: 0.37% pa[#] HFrEF: 0.24% pa HFnEF: 0.13% pa	62 years (mean) W: 36%	
England GPRD Hawkins et al. 2012[2]	Continuous 1999–2007	Primary care Registers	Numerator: patients >25 years Denominator: unclear	~2 million	13,330	Continuous	2000: 0.2% pa 2007: 0.06% pa	1999 W: 56% >75 years 69% 2007 W: 51% >75 years 68%	1 year mortality unchanged between 1999 and 2007 = 5.2%
Sweden The Malmo preventative project Tasevska-Dinevska et al. 2009[11]	1974–1992	Community		33,342 (46 ± 7 years) W: 33%	W: 120 (1.1%) M: 644 (2.9%)	FU for average 21.7 ± 4.3 years	W: 1.1% (0.06% pa) M: 2.9% (0.12% pa)		Among HF patients, 55% of deaths amongst women and 41% amongst men was for non CV causes. Overall, 8% of deaths were due to HF

Contd...

Contd...

Study and countries	*Collection period*	*Population*	*Age range surveyed*	*Number surveyed*	*Number with HF*	*Follow-up*	*Prevalence*	*Age and sex of patients with HF*	*Comments*
Sweden Stockholm Zarrinkoub et al. 2103[7]	2006 and 2010	Health register		2.1 million	88,038		HF: 4.2% (0.38% pa)	W: 51%	
Spain Cadiz study Gomez-Soto et al. 2011[5]	2000–7	Community aged >13 years		267,231	4,793	8 years	2000: 0.30% pa 2007: 0.39% pa	2000 W: 53% 67 years (mean) 2007 W: 53% 72 years (mean)	
England UK GPRD De Giuli et al. 2005[9]	1991–1994	Regional GPRD	Patients aged >45 years	696,884	6,478		1.0% definite and 2.0% possible heart failure. New prescriptions for loop diuretics but not diagnosed as heart failure 0.9%	Definite HF W: 55% 77 years (mean)	65% of patients with definite heart failure died within 3 years

[#]This is likely to be a gross overestimate of overall population incidence since people aged <28 years were excluded and ~60% were selected because they had MAU

HF, heart failure; NA, not available; pa, per annum; ECHOES, Ethnic-Echocardiographic Heart of England Screening Study; GPRD, General Practice Research Database; E-ECHOES, Ethnic-ECHOES; UK, United Kingdom; LVSD, left ventricular systolic dysfunction; LVDD, left ventricular end-diastolic dimensions; EF, ejection fraction; HFnEF, heart failure with normal ejection fraction; AF, atrial fibrillation; HFrEF, heart failure with reduced ejection fraction; NYHA, New York Heart Association; LA, left atrial; BNP, brain natriuretic peptide; GP, general practice; MAU, microalbuminuria; CV, cardiovascular; FU, follow-up; PREVEND, Prevention of Renal and Vascular End Stage Disease

TABLE 2: Studies showing characteristics and treatment of patients with heart failure in primary care

Countries and name of the study	*Duration of collection and years of study*	*Number of GPs*	*Number of patients with HF (N)*	*Mean age*	*Women (%)*	*Key clinical characteristics*	*Treatment*	*Comments*
ECHOES Taylor et al. (2012)[1]	GP register (1995-1999)	16 GPs	449 HFnEF 230 LVSD 219	HFnEF 76 years LVSD 71 years	52% 31%	HFnEF: DM 11%, MI 20%, HTN 44% LVSD: DM 20%, MI 55%, HTN 41%	HFnEF: Diuretics 81%, ACEI 37%, ARB 2%, BB 7% LVSD: Diuretics 76%, ACEI 59%, ARB 2%, BB 11%	10-year mortality HF: 73% ALVSD: 62% No HF/no LVSD: 24%
15 ESC Countries IMPROVEMENT-HF Cleland et al. (2002)[15]	GP register (1999-2000)	1,363 GPs	11,062	70 years 54% ≥70 years	45%	IHD: 57% DCM: 6% HTN: 48% DM: 18% AF: 22% Valve disease: 15% COPD: 24% ECHO done: 82% (of which 51% LVSD)	ACEI: 60% BB: 34% Combined: 20%	41% had been hospitalized in previous year, including 27% for HF
Portugal EPICA Ceia et al. (2002),[8] (2004)[16]	6 months (1998)	365 GPs	551 (age <25 years excluded)	65 years	62%	IHD: 29% HTN: 66% DM: 11% AF: 13% Valve disease: 26% COPD: 20% LVSD: 43%	Diuretic: 78% ACEI: 58% BB: 7%	
Austria AUSTRIA Fruhwald et al. (2004)[17,*]	4 months (2004)	96 centers	1,880	71 years	50%	IHD: 47% HTN: 37%	Diuretic: 78% Digoxin: 36% ACEI: 78% BB: 50% ARA: 16%	
Spain GALICAP Otero-Raviña et al. (2009)[18]	6.5 months (2006)	149 GPs	1,195	76 years	52.1%	IHD: 32% HTN: 82% DM: 31% AF: 49% Valve disease 35% COPD: 28% GFR <60 mL/min: 63% BMI >30: 37% ECHO done: 67% HFnEF: 61% of echoes	Diuretic: 82% ACEI: 48% ARB: 29% ARB/ACE: 74% BB: 27% Spironolactone: 16%	Overall mortality 7.9% with median follow-up 6.5 months (80% CV) All-cause hospitalization 29% CV hospitalization 19.7% (ECHO only done in 67% of cases)

Contd...

Contd...

Countries and name of the study	*Duration of collection and years of study*	*Number of GPs*	*Number of patients with HF (N)*	*Mean age*	*Women (%)*	*Key clinical characteristics*	*Treatment*	*Comments*
Spain INCA de Rivas et al. (2008)[19]	Primary care group only (2006), cross-sectional	415 GPs	1,412	72.2 years	48.5%	HTN: 80% DM: 37% Anemia: 15% DCM: 14% IHD: 27% Mean EF: 50% HFnEF: 68%	Diuretics: 83.7% ACE: 47% ARB: 46% ACE/ARB: 88% BB: 35% MRA: 20%	Outcome: Health-related quality of life
England UK GPRD Hawkins et al. (2012)[20]	Continuous (1999-2007)	Regional GPRD	13,330 (age <25 years excluded)	>75 years 1999 (69%) 2007 (68%)	1999 (56%) 2007 (51%)		1999/2007 ACEI: 46%/64% BB: 12%/41% ARA: 3%/20%	One year mortality 5.2% in both 1999 and 2007

*A minority of patients were recruited from cardiology outpatient clinics

GP, general practice; HF, heart failure; ECHOES, Ethnic-Echocardiographic Heart of England Screening Study; HFnEF, heart failure with normal ejection fraction; LVSD, left ventricular systolic dysfunction; MI, myocardial infarction; HTN, hypertension; DM, diabetes mellitus; ACEI, angiotensin converting enzyme inhibitor; ARB, angiotensin II receptor blockers; BB, beta-blockers; ALVSD, asymptomatic left ventricular systolic dysfunction; EPICA, Elderly Patients Followed by Italian Centers for Anticoagulation; IHD, ischemic heart disease; AF, atrial fibrillation; COPD, chronic obstructive pulmonary disease; ESC, European Society of Cardiology; IMPROVEMENT-HF, IMprovement PROgram in eValuation and managEMENT of Heart Failure Study; GALICAP, Galician study of heart failure in primary care; AUSTRIA, Austrian survey of treating heart failure; GFR, glomerular filtration rate; BMI, body mass index; CV, cardiovascular; DCM, dilated cardiomyopathy; EF, ejection fraction; MRA, magnetic resonance angiography; ARA, adenine-regulating agent

countries.[15] Administrative and national audit data from England and Wales also provides a very large body of data.[36] The Efficacy of Vasopressin Antagonism in Heart Failure Outcome Study with Tolvaptan (EVEREST) and ProBNP Outpatient Tailored Chronic Heart Failure Therapy (PROTECT) clinical trials provide regional data for patients with acute HF participating in clinical trials.[40,41] These data sets should be seen as complimentary, and help extrapolate information from a strictly cardiology perspective to a much broader view of the HF "universe".

The EHFS-I asked investigators to report all deaths and discharges with HF or those discharged on a loop diuretic over the previous 6 weeks from cardiology and general internal medicine wards.[15] More than 10,000 patients were enrolled over this period from 115 hospitals. In some countries, such as the UK and Sweden, it appears that there was rather little selection bias but in some countries, such as Germany and Georgia, investigators appeared to focus mainly on cardiology wards. The most remarkable difference observed was in the age of patients. Patients were up to a decade older in Western compared to Eastern Europe. This fits with the concept that higher cardiovascular (CV) risk, due to smoking and poorer control of hypertension (HTN) and hyperlipidemia, leads to earlier onset of ischemic heart disease (IHD) and, therefore, of HF. Control of CV risk factors will delay the onset of HF and reduce the age-adjusted incidence of HF but ultimately, as longevity increases, the overall rate of HF is similar or higher. The etiology of HF may also shift from predominantly LVSD due to IHD to HFnEF due to HTN and arteriosclerosis. Data from the EVEREST and PROTECT clinical trials are consistent with this hypothesis.

Hospital administrative data from England and Wales show a 60% increase in deaths and discharges due to HF between 2005 and 2012. This may reflect a greater awareness of HF as well as a true increase in activity. Of note, only 18% of patients came under the care of a cardiologist. One-year mortality in both the audit and administrative data is strongly age-related ranging from an inpatient mortality of 5% for those aged less than 65 years to 18% in those aged greater than 84 years and a 1-year mortality amongst those surviving to discharge of 19% and 56%, respectively. The duration of hospital admission is also strongly age-related, ranging from 5 days in those aged less than 65 years to 10 days in those aged greater than 84 years. Although data from other Western European countries may appear different, this more likely reflects differences in the way the data are collected rather than true differences. The National Audit

TABLE 3: IMprovement PROgram in eValuation and managEMENT of Heart Failure (IMPROVEMENT-HF) survey conducted in 1999/2000 amongst primary care physicians. Treatment patterns are likely to have changed dramatically in the intervening years[15]

Parameters	Belgium	Czech or Slovak	France	Germany	Hungary	Italy	Nether-lands	Poland	Russia	Spain	Sweden	Swiss	Turkey	UK
PCP who were women	10%	73%	6%	31%	47%	12%	13%	52%	89%	36%	39%	8%	33%	23%
Number of patients (N)	621	849	1,227	873	861	778	769	681	900	705	663	660	876	599
Age (mean) (years)	73	68	73	72	66	71	72	66	65	70	76	72	64	72
Age ≥70 years	66%	50%	63%	62%	40%	58%	61%	42%	36%	56%	77%	65%	32%	58%
Women	49%	40%	40%	53%	45%	42%	40%	45%	53%	40%	44%	40%	52%	41%
Moderate/severe symptoms	48%	47%	42%	42%	40%	36%	50%	36%	44%	30%	25%	36%	57%	35%
Ankle swelling	62%	49%	54%	60%	63%	59%	42%	60%	73%	40%	40%	51%	67%	39%
IHD	58%	83%	48%	54%	77%	67%	52%	65%	74%	38%	48%	46%	48%	50%
Current SBP (mmHg)	134	139	137	140	141	137	139	144	152	136	142	136	146	138
AF	23%	21%	26%	21%	23%	19%	24%	16%	29%	31%	23%	18%	6%	22%
DM	20%	26%	16%	23%	28%	18%	17%	20%	14%	19%	12%	15%	11%	12%
COPD	31%	26%	21%	21%	24%	24%	22%	21%	32%	20%	16%	24%	32%	24%
ECHO	91%	88%	96%	83%	85%	87%	84%	69%	81%	78%	68%	82%	63%	95%
LVSD	70%	60%	62%	58%	58%	65%	38%	45%	50%	40%	34%	55%	20%	34%
Valve disease	26%	17%	15%	14%	12%	14%	19%	13%	14%	19%	9%	16%	6%	11%
Loop diuretics	53%	39%	58%	42%	54%	58%	59%	38%	52%	48%	74%	46%	28%	67%
Thiazide diuretics	10%	22%	9%	32%	20%	15%	10%	17%	33%	14%	4%	23%	30%	9%
ACEI/ARB	66%	63%	58%	61%	76%	70%	52%	65%	68%	51%	48%	52%	53%	60%
BB	38%	43%	34%	36%	56%	26%	38%	34%	35%	19%	49%	31%	10%	26%
MRA	17%	8%	15%	5%	10%	15%	14%	20%	14%	9%	10%	10%	9%	8%
Hospital admission for any reason in previous year	49%	48%	40%	40%	55%	43%	44%	44%	49%	36%	40%	34%	13%	47%
Prior admission for HF reported at any time	40%	29%	31%	20%	35%	24%	15%	20%	30%	25%	21%	20%	38%	31%

PCP, primary care physician; IHD, ischemic heart disease; SBP, systolic blood pressure; AF, atrial fibrillation; DM, diabetes mellitus; COPD, chronic obstructive pulmonary disease; LVSD, left ventricular systolic dysfunction; ACEI, angiotensin-converting enzyme inhibitor; ARB, angiotensin II receptor blockers; BB, beta-blockers; MRA, magnetic resonance angiography

TABLE 4: Studies showing characteristics and treatment of patients with heart failure attending hospital outpatient clinics

Countries and name of the study	Duration of collection and years of study	Number of centers	Number of patients	Age	Proportion that were women	Key clinical characteristics	Treatment	Comments
Spain INCA de Rivas et al. (2008)[19]	Cardiology patients only	93 Cardiologist and 415 PCP	2,161	71 years	44%	IHD: 31% HTN: 76% Valve: 19% DM: 35% Anemia (Hb <12 g/L): 15% ECHO done: 100% HFnEF: 62% had LVEF >40%	Diuretics: 85% Digoxin: 33% ACEI or ARB: 89% BB: 44 ARA: 25% Treatment compliance: 93%	Quality of life is significantly impaired in HF patients
12 European Countries EuroHeart Failure Observatory Maggioni et al. (2013),[21] (2010)[22]	One day per week for 8 months	136 centers	3,226	67 years (46% >70 years), but mean 63–68 years across regions Patients were older in South and North Europe	30%	IHD: 40% (40–43%) HTN: 58% DM: 29% (16–33%) AF: 39% (37–48%) eGFR <30: 5% ECHO done: around 80% HFnEF: 30% of patients had LVEF >45%	Diuretics: 83% Digoxin: 21% ACEI: 65% ARB: 27% Combined: 89% BB: 87% ARA: 44% Nitrate: 16% ICD: 5–18% CRT-P: 0.3–2.4 % CRT-D: 2–12%	1-year FU; all- cause mortality 7.2% (range 5–9%) HF hospitalized: 13% (range 12–17%) Major regional differences in 1-year mortality across regions Differences in characteristics and treatment of the patients could explain these findings
Italy IN-CHF Registry Tavazzi et al. (2013)[23]	24 months 2007-09 (minimum FU 1 year)	61	3,755	69 years 56% >70 years	24%	IHD: 46% HTN: 43% DM: 30% AF: 30% COPD: 21% CKD: 21% ECHO done: 57% HFnEF: 40% had LVEF > 40%	ACEI/ARB: 90% BB: 79% ARA: 38%	Mortality at 1 year: 6%, of which 65% were CV Age, higher heart rate Advanced NYHA class, anemia, large QRS, high creatinine level, and severe MR were independently associated with a worse outcome
Italy IN-CHF Registry Pulignano et al. (2002)[24]	33 months 1995-98	133	3,327	63 years 31% >70 years	Age <70 years 21% Age >70 years 35%	Age <70 years or >70 years IHD: 38%/50% DCM: 38%/17% HTN: 9%/9%	Age <70 years or >70 years Diuretic: 85%/90%	Age <70 years or >70 years Death: 14%/22% Readmission: 25%/24%

Contd...

Contd...

Countries and name of the study	*Duration of collection and years of study*	*Number of centers*	*Number of patients*	*Age*	*Proportion that were women*	*Key clinical characteristics*	*Treatment*	*Comments*
						Valve: 11%/19% AF: 19%/31% NYHA > II: 28%/40% ECHO done: 67%/61% HFnEF: 23%/ 33%	Digoxin: ACEI: 85%/75% BB: 13%/7% ARA: NR Nitrate	Readmission rate in older patients reduced by higher mortality
France Allaert et al. (2008)[25]	Prior to 2007	500	1,941	68 years 56% > 70 years	25%	IHD: 41% DCM: 34% HTN: 10% (49%*) Valve: 9% DM: 21% AF: 37% COPD: 11% CKD: 10% ECHO done: 91% HFnEF: 33% had LVEF >45%	Diuretics: 86% Digoxin: 30% ACEI: 76% ARB: 13% BB: 58% Nitrate: 20%	By 1 year: 37% hospitalized Non-CV: 13%; MLOS 8 days CV 24%; MLOS 13 days HF: 15%; MLOS 16 days Mortality 10% (78% CV)
Poland Patients with HF >64 years Rywik et al. (2004)[26] Rywik et al. (2000)[27]	6 months (1998)	417 physicians GPs 19% GIM: 68% Card: 7% Other: 6%	10,579	74 years 37% >75 years	63%	Gender M/F IHD: 87%/80% DCM: 8%/6% HTN: 64%/77% Valve: 7%/8% AF:19% Peripheral edema: 54%/64%	Diuretics: 55% Digoxin: 31% ACEI: 68% BB: 22% Nitrate: 62% CaB: 29%	The sickest patients were more likely to receive ACEI, digoxin, long-acting nitrates, and diuretics High number (29%) patients prescribed CaB
Norway Hole et al. (2010)[28] Brandsaeter et al. (2011)[29]	2000-06	24	3,632	71 years	30%	IHD: 57% DCM: 14% HTN: 9% Valve: 6% DM: 19% AF: 23% COPD: 18% CKD: around 50% $\geq$ mild CKD ECHO done: 100% HFnEF: 9% had LVEF > 50%	Diuretics: 87% ACEI: 73% ARB: 14% BB: 83% ARA:26% Statin: 50% Aspirin: 41% Warfarin: 48%	Mortality ranged from 8% to 11% at 12 months and 14% to 22% at 24 months Age and MLHF score were the most important predictors of mortality

Contd...

Contd...

Countries and name of the study	Duration of collection and years of study	Number of centers	Number of patients	Age	Proportion that were women	Key clinical characteristics	Treatment	Comments
Spain EPISERVE González-Juanatey et al. (2008)[30]	5 months (2005)	507 physicians Primary care 36% Cardiologist 34% GIM: 30%	2,249	72 years	45%	IHD: 39% DCM: 6% HTN: 30% Valve: 8% DM: 38% AF: 46% COPD: 24% CKD: 7% ECHO done: 61% HFnEF: 57% had LVEF >40%	Diuretics: 98% Digoxin:35% ACEI: 57% ARB: 47% BB: 54% ARA: 29% CaB: 21%	Only 20% of patients received the treatment recommended by guidelines, and those treated by cardiologist received a more appropriate treatment
France, Germany, Spain Salvador et al. (2004)[31]	Spain: 466 France: 271 Germany: 461 1-day data (26/04/2001)	465 cardiologists	1,252	68 years	38%	IHD: 35% DCM: 27% HTN: 71% Valve: 15% DM: 29% AF: 36% Hypercholesterol-emia: 26% Smoking: 29% ECHO done: 60%	Diuretics: 80% Digoxin: 32–52% ACEI: 72% ARB: 13–16% BB: 48% ARA: 23–34%	In Spain HTN is a common, etiology of HF. Use of BB low
MAHLER Komajda et al. (2005)[32]	6 month FU Nov 2001 till Apr 2002	150 cardiologists from 6 countries (France, Germany, Italy, Netherlands, Spain, UK)	1,410	69 years	31%	IHD: 68% HTN: 55% Valve: 7% DM: 23% ECHO done: >80%, but lower in UK	Diuretics: 79% Digoxin: 41% ACEI: 69% ARB: 18% BB: 53% ARA: 28% Nitrate: 32% Aspirin or clopidogrel: 36% Statin: 34% Warfarin: 35%	4% died during FU 17% of patients were hospitalized for a CV reason during follow-up (9% for worsening HF) Adherence of physicians to treatment guidelines are associated with decreased rates of HF and CV hospitalization

Contd...

Contd...

Countries and name of the study	Duration of collection and years of study	Number of centers	Number of patients	Age	Proportion that were women	Key clinical characteristics	Treatment	Comments
Netherlands Oudejans et al. (2012)[33]	2003-07 (minimum FU 3 years)	2 centers	93	83 years	63%	IHD: 27% HTN: 42% DM: 27% AF: 39% COPD: 27% Cancer: 16% NT-proBNP: 2.295 (791–5.543) pg/mL ECHO done: 100% HFnEF: 47% had LVEF >45%	Diuretics: 41% Digoxin: 24% ACEI or ARB: 38% BB: 28% ARA:11 %	The majority of geriatric outpatients with newly diagnosed HF die within 3 years after establishing the diagnosis due to different comorbidities
England Hull life laboratory (2010)[34]	10 years	Single clinic	2,271	72 years	25%	IHD: 67% HTN: 34% Valve: NR DM: 20% AF: 29% COPD: 10% Serum creatinine 120 µmol/L ECHO done: 100% HFnEF: LVSD only reported	At 1-year follow-up Loop diuretics: 82% Digoxin: 17% ACEI or ARB: 87% BB: 81% ARA: 35% Nitrate: NR	
England, Germany, Italy Poland, Russia SICA-HF (2013)[35]	3 years	12 partners across Europe and Russia	1,170	65 years (median 52–72 years across centers)	23%	IHD: 58% HTN: 63% (45–80%) DM: 35% (21–41%) AF: 20% (4–28%) NT-proBNP: 740 (292–1901) ng/L ECHO done: 100% HFnEF: 30% (LVEF > 50% ranges 0–39% across centers)	Treatment not reported	Large differences exist between characteristics of patients recruited in different centers

IN-CHF, Italian Network on Congestive Heart Failure; IHD, ischemic heart disease; DCM, dilated cardiomyopathy; HTN, hypertension; AF, atrial fibrillation; NYHA, New York Heart Association; ECHO, echocardiography; HFnEF, heart failure with normal ejection fraction; ACEI, angiotensin-converting enzyme inhibitor; BB, beta-blockers; ARA, adenine-regulating agent; NR, not recommended; DM, diabetes mellitus; AF, atrial fibrillation; COPD, chronic obstructive pulmonary disease; CKD, chronic kidney disease; LVEF, left ventricular ejection fraction; ARB, angiotensin II receptor blockers; MR, mitral regurgitation; CV, cardiovascular; GP, general practice; GIM, General Internal Medicine; CaB, cellulose acetate butyrate; MLHF, Minnesota Living with Heart Failure Questionnaire; MLOS, median length of stay; NT-proBNP, N-terminal pro-brain natriuretic peptide; FU, follow-up; HF, heart failure; Hb, hemoglobin; INCA, Inspiratory Muscle Training in Patients with Chronic Heart Failure; SICA-HF, Studies Investigating Co-morbidities Aggravating Heart Failure; eGFR, estimated glomerular filtration rate; ICD, implantable cardioverter-defibrillator; CRT-P, cardiac resynchronization therapy pacemaker; CRT-D, cardiac resynchronization therapy defibrillator

TABLE 5: Studies showing characteristics and treatment of patients with heart failure (HF) admitted to hospital for worsening symptoms

Countries and name of the study	*Duration of collection and years of study*	*Number of centers*	*Number of patients*	*Age*	*Proportion that were women*	*Key clinical characteristics*	*Treatment at discharge*	*Comments*
EuroHeart Observatory[21,22]		136 centers from 12 European countries	1,892	70 years	37%	IHD: 51% HTN: 62% Valve: DM: 35% AF: 44% COPD: 19% EF ≥45%	Diuretics: ~ 90% ACEI/ARB ~ 78% BB: 80% MRA ~ 55% Digoxin ~ 30%	By 1-year mortality 17% Readmission 44% HF readmission 25%
IN-CHF Tavazzi et al. (2013)[23]	2 years 2007-09	61 Italian hospitals	1,855	72 years	40%	IHD: 51% HTN: 62% Valve: NR DM: 35% AF: 44% COPD: 19% Mean LVEF: 38% Median NT-proBNP (ng/L): 5168 (2,518–11,583)	Diuretics: 96% ACEI/ARB: 78% BB: 65% MRA: 55% Digoxin: 24%	By 1-year mortality 24% Readmission 31% CV readmission 24% HF readmission 16%
England and Wales National Audit[36]	2008-12	142 hospitals		78 years	45%	IHD: 42% DCM: NR HTN: 58% Valve: NR DM: 40% AF: 38% COPD: 30% EF ≥45%	Diuretics: Loop: 89% Thiazide: 4% ACEI: 72% ACEI/ARB: 84% BB: 78% MRA: 45% Digoxin: 23%	Age <75 years or >75 years Inpatient mortality Postdischarge mortality 1 year 3 years
UK Administrative Data (unpublished)	2006-12	145 Trusts (may be more than one hospital per Trust)	2.1 million admissions	Median 82 years for women and 76 years for men	47%	NA	NA	1-year mortality <65 years ~18% 65–74 years ~30% 75–84 years ~40% >85 years ~55%
EHFS-I[37]	6 weeks per hospital 2000-01	115 hospitals from 24 European countries	10,701	71 years	47%	IHD: 68% HTN: 53% Aortic valve disease: 10% MR: 29% DM: 27% AF: 23% COPD: 32% EF ≥45%: 42%	Diuretics: 87% ACEI: 62% ARB: 5% BB: 37% MRA: 21% Digoxin: 36%	12-week follow-up Mortality 14% (7% during index hospital) Readmissions 24% (about one-third due to HF)
EHFS-II[38,39]	11 months 2004-05	133 centers in 30 European countries	3,580	70 years	39%	IHD: 54% HTN: 63% Valve: 27% DM: 33% AF: 39% COPD: 19% EF ≥45%	Diuretics: 90% ACEI, ARB, BB, MRA, Digoxin	Hospital deaths: 7% 1-year mortality 21%

EHFS, EuroHeart Failure Survey; IHD, ischemic heart disease; HTN, hypertension; MR, mitral regurgitation; DM, diabetes mellitus; AF, atrial fibrillation; COPD, chronic obstructive pulmonary disease; EF, ejection fraction; LVEF, left ventricular ejection fraction; NT-proBNP, N-terminal pro-brain natriuretic peptide; DCM, dilated cardiomyopathy; NR, not recommended; ACEI, angiotensin-converting enzyme inhibitor; BB, beta-blockers; ARB, angiotensin II receptor blockers; MRA, magnetic resonance angiography; CV, cardiovascular; HF, heart failure; NA, not available; IN-CHF, Italian Network on Congestive Heart Failure

TABLE 6: EuroHeart Failure Survey-I (EHFS-I) of hospital admissions—conducted over 6 weeks (during 2000-01) screening 46,788 deaths and discharges from 115 hospitals in 24 European Society of Cardiology (ESC) countries. Of those screened, 11,327 had evidence of heart failure. Highlighted cells helps illustrate patterns of care. Treatment patterns are likely to have changed in the intervening years[37]

Parameters	UK and Eire	Scandinavia	Austria/ Germany/ Swiss	Belgium/ France/ Netherlands	Czech/ Slovak/ Slovenia/ Hungary	Poland/ Lithuania	Russia	Israel	Italy	Georgia	Greece	Portugal/ Spain
Number of patients (N)	1,953	1,318	1,208	459	1,525	1,162	370	584	545	187	410	980
Age (years)	74	75	68	71	70	68	65	75	70	65	68	72
Women (%)	51	55	42	54	45	51	44	43	43	49	32	49
IHD	65	63	71	53	55	72	77	76	57	57	55	37
Chronic AF	22	22	22	23	23	21	23	28	21	24	24	30
Any AF	42	42	40	55	48	43	43	42	31	38	41	48
DM	20	24	33	20	38	22	16	36	23	14	32	35
COPD	37	25	21	28	39	33	24	23	35	24	20	52
Managed by cardiology	25	38	61	78	46	52	52	13	52	87	69	30
ECHO done	58	59	86	93	80	64	59	47	73	81	80	60
Moderate/Severe LVSD	34	37	58	57	54	48	56	25	45	30	65	37
Therapy												
Loop diuretics	93	95	81	88	80	80	81	93	87	86	91	90
ACEI/ARB	52 + 3	47 + 6	70 + 8	66 + 6	71 + 3	71 + 2	85 + 2	49 + 7	60 + 4	59 + 1	72 + 8	54 + 4
BB	24	69	56	29	39	47	65	39	21	20	28	10
MRA	14	19	21	16	32	30	28	10	15	21	21	22
Outcome												
Length of stay (days)	12	11	11	13	11	14	19	7	11	7	8	11
Mortality; inpatient	9%	6%	7%	7%	8%	8%	2%	4%	4%	5%	7%	9%
Mortality; 12 week	15%	16%	11%	15%	14%	11%	4%	10%	12%	22%	12%	17%
Readmission by 12 week for/with HF	10%	14%	12%	8%	14%	7%	1%	11%	7%	3%	8%	13%
Readmission by	32%	47%	37%	28%	29%	12%	3%	28%	21%	5%	17%	26%

IHD, ischemic heart disease; AF, atrial fibrillation; DM, diabetes mellitus; COPD, chronic obstructive pulmonary disease; LVSD, left ventricular systolic dysfunction; ACEI, angiotensin-converting enzyme inhibitor; ARB, angiotensin II receptor blockers; BB, beta-blockers; MRA, magnetic resonance angiography; HF, heart failure

TABLE 7: Efficacy of Vasopressin Antagonism in Heart Failure: Outcome Study with Tolvaptan (EVEREST): a trial of hospital admissions with heart failure in which patients were randomized to tolvaptan, an anti-diuretic hormone antagonist, or placebo[40]

	North America	*South America*	*Western Europe*	*Eastern Europe*
Number of patients (N)	1,251	699	564	1,619
Patients/site	7	20	8	20
Age (years)	68	62	69	65
Women	25%	25%	21%	27%
IHD	77%	40%	64%	72%
Prior MI	56%	30%	49%	56%
AF	16%	24%	30%	36%
DM	52%	30%	42%	31%
Severe COPD	18%	6%	11%	5%
LVEF	25%	26%	27%	31%
Serum creatinine	133	124	133	106
BNP	1,031 (470–2,100)	694 (296–1,405)	720 (366–1,467)	533 (222–1,225)
Drugs at discharge				
Loop diuretics	93%	96%	98%	91%
Digoxin	49%	56%	37%	46%
ACEI/ARB	77%	90%	87%	91%
BB	82%	63%	72%	76%
MRA	43%	75%	48%	67%
ICD	34%	3%	13%	5%
ICD or pacemaker	48%	13%	28%	11%
1-year mortality	30%	27%	27%	21%
HR after adjusting for risk*	NA	0.91 (0.76–1.08)	0.97 (0.81–1.16)	0.63 (0.54–0.73)
CV death or HF hospitalization	53%	42%	47%	35%
HR after adjusting for risk*	NA	1.11 (0.94–1.32)	1.10 (0.93–1.28)	0.84 (0.73–0.97)

*Compared to North America

IHD, ischemic heart disease; MI, myocardial infarction; AF, atrial fibrillation; DM, diabetes mellitus; COPD, chronic obstructive pulmonary disease; LVEF, left ventricular ejection fraction; BNP, B-type natriuretic peptide; ACEI, angiotensin-converting enzyme inhibitor; ARB, angiotensin II receptor blockers; BB, beta-blockers; MRA, magnetic resonance angiography; ICD, implantable cardioverter-defibrillator, HF, heart failure; HR, hazard ratio; CV, cardiovascular

TABLE 8: PROTECT a trial of hospital admissions with heart failure in which patients were randomized to rolofylline, an adenosine antagonist, or placebo[41]

	Western Europe (N = 388)	*Russia (N = 283)*	*Eastern Europe (N = 676)*	*Israel (N = 318)*	*Argentina (N = 55)*	*North America (N = 313)*
Age (years)	75 (66–82)	69 (60–76)	71 (61–77)	76 (70–81)	72 (62–78)	67 (57–77)
Men (%)	70	58	68	62	39	74
Caucasian (%)	98	100	100	100	100	71
IHD	60	86	67	82	53	63

Contd...

Contd...

	Western Europe (N = 388)	*Russia (N = 283)*	*Eastern Europe (N = 676)*	*Israel (N = 318)*	*Argentina (N = 55)*	*North America (N = 313)*
Medical history						
Myocardial infarction	44	60	47	62	35	41
Diabetes mellitus	49	29	43	54	44	53
Asthma or COPD	21	25	14	16	15	30
AF/flutter	61	59	56	47	50	49
Biventricular pacing	13	0	6	12	0	24
AICD	21	0	9	15	2	44
LVEF (%)	30 (25–40)	34 (26–42)	30 (25–40)	30 (23–43)	30 (25–35.5)	25 (20–35)
Hospitalization for HF (prior year)	46	48	51	41	51	59
Physical examination						
BMI (kg/m^2)	27 (24–31)	29 (25–34)	27 (24–31)	28 (25–32)	27 (24–30)	29 (25–35)
Systolic blood pressure (mmHg)	120	130	125	128	120	114
Pulse (beats/min)	76 (68–87)	88 (76–99)	80 (70–92)	72 (66–81)	79.5 (70–91)	76 (67–87)
Respiratory rate (breath/min)	20 (18–24)	24 (22–26)	20 (17–22)	22 (20–24)	21 (19–23)	20 (18–22)
Severe orthopnea (breathlessness at rest)	39	42	47	42	45	47
Marked edema	60	86	67	65	80	64
eGFR (mL/min/1.73 m^2)	41	54	48	42	41	43
Hemoglobin (g/dL)	12.3	13.5	13.1	11.8	12.9	11.7
Medications at discharge						
ACEI/ARB	78	95	86	80	87	71
BB	79	78	88	85	87	88
MRA	49	80	75	41	66	41
Digoxin	28	52	37	13	26	32
Length of stay (LOS) (including in-hospital deaths)	10 (7–15)	15 (14–20)	8 (7–13)	5 (4–7)	4 (4–6)	5 (4–8.5)
Death or CV/renal rehospitalization (1–60 days)	117 (30.2)	34 (12.0)	171 (25.3)	117 (36.8)	9 (16.4)	112 (35.8)
	1.0	0.39 (0.23–0.64)	0.78 (0.58–1.04)	1.10 (0.80–1.52)	0.54 (0.26–1.11)	0.91 (0.66–1.26)
Death or rehospitalization (1–60 days)	143 (36.9)	39 (13.8)	184 (27.2)	139 (43.7)	11 (20.0)	136 (43.5)
Death to 60 days	39 (10.1)	23 (8.1)	67 (9.9)	23 (7.2)	1 (1.8)	22 (7.0)
	1.0#	0.97 (0.45–2.09)	1.24 (0.74–2.09)	0.40 (0.19–0.81)	0.23 (0.03–1.72)	0.42 (0.22–0.83)
Re-hospitalization to 60 days	116 (29.9)	18 (6.4)	131 (19.4)	128 (40.3)	10 (18.2)	123 (39.3)
Death through day 180	79 (20.4)	34 (12.0)	125 (18.5)	50 (15.7)	7 (12.7)	63 (20.1)
	1.0#	0.80 (0.46–1.41)	1.23 (0.85–1.78)	0.59 (0.37–0.94)	0.62 (0.24–1.57)	0.75 (0.49–1.16)

#Hazard ratio compared to Western Europe

PROTECT, Placebo-Controlled Randomized Study of the Selective Adenosine A1 Receptor Antagonist Rolofylline for Patients Hospitalized with Acute Decompensated Heart Failure and Volume Overload to Assess Treatment Effect on Congestion and Renal Function; IHD, ischemic heart disease; COPD, chronic obstructive pulmonary disease; AF, atrial fibrillation; AICD, automatic implanted cardioverter defibrillator; LVEF, left ventricular ejection fraction; HF, heart failure; BMI, body mass index eGFR, estimated glomerular filtration rate; ACEI, angiotensin-converting enzyme inhibitor; ARB, angiotensin II receptor blockers; BB, beta-blockers; MRA, magnetic resonance angiography; CV, cardiovascular data from England and Wales showed that even within one country the age at which HF develops is highly dependent on socioeconomic status.[36] A similar gradient between affluence and overall life expectancy can be observed. Thus, long-lived populations will develop HF at an older age but it seems almost an inescapable truth that the lifetime risk of developing HF is about one in five, or maybe higher. Good management can procrastinate but not prevent HF.

HOW THE SYSTEM LOOKS AFTER HEART FAILURE: VIGNETTES FROM AROUND EUROPE

Belgium

(*Riet Dierckx*)

In Belgium, healthcare is managed through private and public systems. The level of reimbursement for examinations, hospitalizations, and treatment is determined by the National Institute for Health and Disability Insurance (NIHDI). Doctors may or may not work in accordance with the NIHDI regulations. If they choose to accept these regulations, they must respect a predetermined tariff for examinations and consultations. In return, they are entitled to some benefits, especially in case of incapacity or retirement.

Patients are legally required to have health insurance in Belgium. Most, but not all, healthcare expenses are covered by health insurance companies. Patients can buy extra insurance to reduce their contribution to healthcare costs, or to avoid supplementary costs when treated by doctors outside of the NIHDI scheme.

Patients with HF are managed by general practitioners (GPs), office-based cardiologists, and/or HF clinics. Asymptomatic LVSD is usually diagnosed by coincidence during hospital admissions for other reasons. Symptomatic LVSD is most often suspected by the general physician (GP).[42] In order to confirm the diagnosis, laboratory examinations, X-rays, and echocardiograms (ECHO) are widely available in surgeries or hospitals. A national survey among sentinel primary care practices reported that GP's perform an electrocardiogram (ECG) in 64% of patients with suspected HF. Additional blood tests, chest X-ray, and ECHO are requested in respectively 57%, 50%, and 53% of patients.[43] Although NT-proBNP is well known as a diagnostic and prognostic biomarker, its use is limited in primary care (9% of suspected HF cases), probably due to lack of reimbursement.

Treatment for HF can be initiated by the GP, or after referral, by the cardiologist. When symptoms or signs of HF are worsening, the GP will usually refer the patient to secondary care.

Organization of follow-up after hospital discharge differs significantly among cardiology and noncardiology wards. Only 12.7% of patients with HF admitted to an elderly medicine ward are scheduled for an outpatient cardiology clinic but 82.6% of those admitted to a cardiology ward.[44] In large volume hospitals, HF management is usually organized through a multidisciplinary hospital-based HF clinic, involving HF nurses, cardiologists, social workers, a rehabilitation team, psychologists, and dieticians.

Nurses in Belgium are not allowed to prescribe medication or organize patient clinics. Although the HF nurse plays a central role in the multidisciplinary HF clinic, there is no system of home visits by HF nurses. Only a minority of hospitals have engaged in telehealth, which usually comprises remote monitoring of pacemaker or ICD data. An important barrier for widespread adoption of telehealth technologies in Belgium is the lack of reimbursement.

France

(*Thibaud Damy*)

In France, the French Social Security System was created in 1945 by De Gaulle in order to make it possible for everyone to support themselves and their family in decent conditions.[45] It is based on the principle of solidarity which guarantees financial protection against life's contingencies for everyone. It covers health insurance, compensation for occupational injuries and illnesses, pensions, and family benefits.[46]

Most healthcare expenses (76%) are covered by the healthcare system.[47,48] All residents are automatically enrolled with an insurance fund based on their occupational status. Workers and their families are in the general scheme that accounts for about three quarters of the total expenditure incurred by the basic social security schemes. Ninety percent of the population takes out supplementary private health insurance. Unemployed people's health expenses are covered by a special care system and doctors are obliged to apply the lowest predetermined tariff. In 2011, total net expenditure was €320 billion for the general scheme and about €442.2 billion for all schemes combined. The French Social Security System is financed by contributions from employers and employees, a general social welfare contribution (CSG), and various other contributions and taxes. Patients are free to take on extra health insurance to avoid supplementary costs when they are treated by doctors who are authorized to raise additional charges (sector 2, see below).

In France, healthcare is managed through private and public systems. The private sector includes "private" office-based surgery and hospitals. Three types of private hospitals exist with different levels of commitment to the public healthcare system. Public hospitals comprise local, regional, and University hospitals. About 52% of doctors are GPs and 48% are specialists with at least 4 years training. Most specialist doctors work in private office-based clinics. In 2001, of 196,000 doctors in France, 36% worked only as employees and 56% privately or with mixed activity. In contrast with other countries, there is no "gatekeeper" regulating access by patients to specialist care.

The level of reimbursement for examinations, hospitalizations, and treatment is determined by the "Caisse Primaire d'Ássurance Maladie" (CPAM).[46] Most doctors work in accordance with the regulations (not mandatory). There are two sectors of activity: 1 and 2. In sector 1, doctors must respect a predetermined tariff for examinations and consultations. In return, they are entitled to some benefits, especially in case of incapacity or retirement. Only specialists can apply to sector 2, which allows them to do a "dépassement d'honoraires" which means that they can add honorariums to the predetermined tariff (sector 1). The added honorarium is not yet limited but it might change.

Heart failure patients are managed by GPs, office-based cardiologists, and/or mainly public HF clinics. In order to confirm the diagnosis, patients are usually referred to an office-based cardiologist (private) who can do an ECG and ECHO. In the PRINCEPS (Prise en charge des Insuffisants Cardiaques: Enquête chez les Patients Symptomatiques) study,[49] GPs reported that 81% of their patients had confirmation of their diagnosis by a cardiologist. ECHOs are widely available in clinics but this examination is only performed by cardiologists in France. Asymptomatic LVSD is usually diagnosed by coincidence during hospital admissions for other reasons. Additional blood tests (NT-proBNP, troponin) are also available and reimbursed in private laboratories.

Symptomatic treatment for HF can be initiated by the GP or after referral by the office-based cardiologist. Organization of follow-up after hospital discharge differs significantly among cardiology and noncardiology wards. Few elderly patients with HF are scheduled for an outpatient cardiology clinic. In large volume hospitals, HF management is usually organized through a multidisciplinary[50] hospital-based HF clinic, involving nurses, cardiologists, social workers, a rehabilitation team, psychologists, and dieticians. Educational HF programs have obtained reimbursement since last year. Nurses specialized in HF are rare compared to the UK system and are not allowed to prescribe medication or organize patient clinics. There is no system of home visits by HF nurses. Only a minority of hospitals have engaged in telehealth, which usually comprises remote monitoring of pacemaker or ICD data. An important barrier for widespread adoption of telehealth technologies in France is the lack of reimbursement.

Germany

(Lutz Frankenstein)

In 2011, about 11.3% of the gross domestic product of Germany was spent on healthcare (approximately €300 billion or €4,000 per capita).[51] The public health care system contributed about €170 billion and the rest was covered by private healthcare insurance or direct payment by patients.

Germans are legally required to have health insurance and a compulsory client of one of the more than 200 public insurance companies. The social security contributions are split 50/50 between employers and employees. Once the gross income exceeds a certain limit, one can opt out and become a client of a private health insurance company. In addition, anyone can take out additional insurance to obtain access to extra benefits offered by private insurers. In order to receive payment from public insurers, doctors must be panel accredited.

The hospital sector is regulated via the G-DRG (Diagnosis Related Groups in Germany) reimbursement scheme. This scheme is mandatory for settlement with private and public insurers alike. In 2010, 2,065 hospitals with 502,716 beds and 826,732 employees treated 18,024,447 cases with an average length of stay (LOS) of 8 days.[51]

In 2011, 373,575 patients were hospitalized for cardiac decompensation.[52] Of these, 15,921 patients were categorized as the DRGs F62A (complex HF) with a median LOS of 14 days, 81,136 patients as F62B with a median LOS of 12 days, and 211,844 patients with a median LOS of 8 days. There are many hurdles to overcome in the transition between inpatient and outpatient care, leading the German government to name HF as one of nine specific diseases that require an interdisciplinary approach due to the complexity of management [Section 116b German Social Code Book V (116b SGB V)].

Most patients with HF are managed by GPs.[53] In general, awareness of HF in the German population is low[54] and despite its high socioeconomic impact,[55] treatment is often still suboptimal.[53] Treatment for HF is usually initiated by the GP and only a minority of patients will be referred to a cardiologist.[56] When symptoms or signs of HF are worsening, the GP will usually refer the patient to secondary care, mostly in-hospital or specialist outpatient HF clinics like the comprehensive cardiomyopathy center at the University Hospital, Heidelberg.

As in Belgium and in contrast to the UK system, nurses in Germany are not allowed to prescribe medication or organize patient clinics. Similarly, only a minority of hospitals have engaged in telehealth, which usually comprises remote monitoring of pacemaker or ICD data. An important barrier for widespread adoption of telehealth technologies in Germany is the lack of reimbursement.

Greece
(*Stamatia Prapa*)

In Greece, the healthcare system differs significantly from the British National Health Service (NHS) as care in the community is provided mostly by cardiologists rather than GPs. Hospital care is free to all acutely ill patients with no additional charges for elective investigations upon discharge.

Patients presenting with acute decompensated HF are treated in either district general hospitals or specialized tertiary centers, depending on the locality. Standard investigations in the emergency room include chest X-ray, ECHO and blood tests (biochemical profile, full blood count, and inflammatory markers). Natriuretic peptides are rarely measured in an acute setting, and are usually ordered by treating physicians at a later stage. Following initial treatment, patients with acute HF are transferred to the cardiology ward for further investigations and management. Patients with inherited cardiomyopathies or requiring advanced treatments, such as left ventricular assist devices or transplantation are referred to tertiary care center with most cases treated at the Onassis Cardiac Surgery Centre in Athens.

Upon discharge, patients are followed-up by local cardiologists with no additional charges. Similarly, a patient presenting with stable symptoms for the first time, can visit the local practice of a cardiologist for initial investigations and subsequent management at a community level. As a result of specialist-based community care, most patients with HF have regular ECHO. An exception to this rule is patients requiring more intensive treatment and follow-up who continue to be followed-up by highly specialized centers following initial referral.

Italy
(*Pierpaolo Pellicori*)

In Italy, the healthcare system provides free hospital care for all acutely ill patients. After discharge, these patients have to pay a small prescription charge (ticket) for medications, specific outpatients investigations like ECHO and/or specialist visits unless the patient has exemptions.

Data published in 2007 from *Ministero della Salute*[57] indicates that HF might affect around 3 million people in the country (around 5% of the total population) and that this disease is the leading cause of acute admissions (around 190,000 in 2003) with a great impact on national economic resources, consuming around 2% of the total healthcare budget.

Most patients with acute decompensation are treated in district general hospitals or tertiary centers. Recent results from an Italian Registry,[58] show that in-patients with acute HF often undergo ECHO (91%), probably because Italian cardiologists do ECHO themselves, but measurement of natriuretic peptides is not very common (30% of patients) in the emergency room. Use of inotropic agents including dobutamine, dopamine, or levosimendan is common whilst ultrafiltration and/or noninvasive ventilation are rarely used.

Patients with HF are usually managed primarily by GPs that have no specific training in HF management after discharge from hospitals.[59,60] In 2004, only a minority of outpatients with HF had an ECG or ECHO during the same year. To improve the management of outpatients with HF, in 2006 the Italian Association of Hospital Cardiologists (ANMCO) promoted a multidisciplinary Consensus Conference to create a network to improve HF management in the community.[61] Regional variations exist, depending on geography, local priorities, skills and resources.[62]

The main caregivers are family members who follow instructions given by doctors. Only more severe cases are mainly under specialist care.[63] Better communication between hospital cardiologists and GPs is a pressing need.[63,64]

Poland
(*Pawel Rubis*)

After the fall of Communism, the healthcare system has been constantly undergoing reforms since 1998. The health system is financed partly from contributions from employees and employers (for those in work) and directly from the Ministry of Health. Public healthcare is organized in two sectors: primary care that provides community-based services and a secondary, hospital-based sector. Primary care physicians (PCPs) (GP, family doctor) provide ambulatory care for all residents, including patients with HF. In most stable patients, GPs decide on management and referrals to specialists. Specialist outpatient clinics are usually located on hospital premises or non-hospital trusts that encompass several specialisms (polyclinics: cardiology, lung specialists, endocrinology, minor surgery, etc.). The next tier of healthcare is hospitals. District hospitals offer basic noninvasive services and provide initial care for the great majority of patients with acute decompensated HF. Regional hospitals offer both noninvasive and invasive diagnostic and therapeutic services, including expert pharmacological management and invasive diagnostics and treatments including devices. There are six or seven tertiary centers in Poland that provide cardiac surgery, usually including heart transplantation, expert management of pulmonary HTN, and genetic testing. Generally, only patients on heart transplant (HTX) lists, surgical patients [coronary artery bypass graft (CABG), valve surgery], or cardiomyopathy for extensive diagnostic work-up are accepted.

Heart failure does not constitute a separate specialty. Patients are diagnosed by general cardiologists, either after referral to a cardiology clinic or after first-ever decompensation in district hospitals. When an ischemic cause is suspected, the patient is usually further referred for coronary angiography. After hospital discharge, the patient is referred back to the GP with instructions on further management. The GP is responsible for continuation of pharmacotherapy. In most cases, the GP lacks in-depth knowledge on HF and cannot interpret specialist tests including ECG or natriuretic peptides. Many GPs try to discharge HF patients to permanent specialist care and although it is discouraged they often succeed. This may not be good for patients because they may have to travel long distances and wait for hours to be seen and then often only by a cardiology trainee. If stable, the patient is usually annually (or biannually) seen by general cardiologist in the outpatient clinic.

The system is similar for most medical conditions and that for HF management is not unusual. There is no national HF program and quality of care varies depending on the skill, attitude, and interest of the GP and cardiologist. There are few or no HF-specialist nurses, no physical/social rehabilitation, and no telemonitoring. The cost of typical HF drugs is not high but patients usually have to pay themselves with rather small reimbursement. This raises the question of medical compliance, which is probably not very high.

In outpatient's clinics and even district hospitals, access to ECHO and natriuretic peptides is relatively good. Invasive cardiology is well financed and so patients are easily accepted for invasive studies and percutaneous coronary interventions (PCIs) and revascularization procedures (particularly PCIs) may be overused. Device therapy is not so well distributed and still underused, particularly CRT. The other problem is that patients often have to wait for 6 or more months for ICD implantation for primary sudden cardiac death (SCD) prevention.

The private medical sector is rapidly evolving but is mainly restricted to outpatient clinics as there are few private hospitals in Poland. There is no special incentive for private care to manage patients with HF.

United Kingdom
(*John GF Cleland*)

In the UK, more than 95% of patients with HF are managed by the NHS which employs healthcare personnel to deliver care both in the community and hospitals. Only a small number of patients are managed predominantly by private healthcare. The UK NHS provides free hospital care for all patients and makes only a small prescription charge (about €10) for medicines for people who are working (a small proportion of those with HF). HF is usually recognised when it has provoked symptoms severe enough to require hospitalization and, therefore, the diagnosis is usually made during hospitalization. Most patients (80%) admitted with HF are managed by physicians with an internal medicine specialty other than cardiology.

After discharge, patients are referred back to a primary care physician (PCP), who usually has no specialist HF training. Some patients may also be given a hospital outpatient appointment with a general physician or cardiologist. Hospital physicians are currently strongly discouraged from following up patients with HF regularly, although some do. Unlike for other malignant disease, such as cancer, the NHS encourages follow-up to be done by PCPs. Education and training of specialist HF nurses, an initiative of the British Heart Foundation, has transformed management for many patients. Specialist nurses may be considered in two broad groups although with some crossover. One group focuses on care in the community, either visiting patients at home or running follow-up clinics in primary care. These typically have 50–100 patients under their care at any time. Patients will usually be discharged from their care after treatment optimization and a period of stability. Another growing group is hospital nurse specialists who identify patients on the wards, ensure accurate diagnosis, and an effective care-plan and will offer hospital clinic follow-ups, although not usually home visits or community clinics. Many patients are treated with loop diuretics in the community (about 3% of adults) but only a minority are investigated for HF. PCPs increasingly have access to natriuretic peptides for diagnosis (although probably still not the majority), and are encouraged to ensure ECHOs are done, usually by referral to an ECHO service or to a cardiologists (there is great regional variation in practice). The UK is a leader in implementing telehealth for the management of HF but still only a minority of patients are managed in this way, often only to optimise medication and stabilize the patients in the months after an episode of decompensation.

REFERENCES

1. Taylor CJ, Roalfe AK, Iles R, et al. Ten-year prognosis of heart failure in the community: follow-up data from the Echocardiographic Heart of England Screening (ECHOES) study. Eur J Heart Fail. 2012;14(2):176-84.
2. Hawkins NM, Petrie MC, MacDonald MR, et al. Selecting patients for cardiac resynchronisation theraoy: electrical or mechanical dyssynchrony? Eur Heart J. 2006;27(11):1270-81.
3. Yousaf F, Collerton J, Kingston A, et al. Prevalence of left ventricular dysfunction in a UK community sample of very old people: the Newcastle 85+ study. Heart. 2012;98(19):1418-23.
4. Gill PS, Calvert M, Davis R, et al. Prevalence of heart failure and atrial fibrillation in minority ethnic subjects: the Ethnic-Echocardiographic Heart of England Screening Study (E-ECHOES). PLoS One. 2011;6(11):e26710.
5. Gomez-Soto FM, Andrey JL, Garcia-Egido AA, et al. Incidence and mortality of heart failure: a community-based study. Int J Cardiol. 2011;151(1):40-5.
6. Carmona M, Garcia-Olmos LM, Alberquilla A, et al. Heart failure in the family practice: a study of the prevalence and co-morbidity. Fam Pract. 2011;28(2):128-33.
7. Zarrinkoub R, Wettermark B, Wändell P, et al. The epidemiology of heart failure, based on data for 2.1 million inhabitants in Sweden. Eur J Heart Fail. 2013;15(9):995-1002.
8. Ceia F, Fonseca C, Mota T, et al. Prevalence of chronic heart failure in Southwestern Europe: the EPICA study. Eur J Heart Fail. 2002;4(4):531-9.
9. Severo M, Gaio AR, Lourenco P, et al. Diagnostic value of patterns of symptoms and signs of heart failure: application of latent class analysis with concomitant variables in a cross-sectional study. BMJ Open. 2012;2(6). pii: e001510.
10. Brouwers FP, de Boer RA, van der Harst P, et al. Incidence and epidemiology of new onset heart failure with preserved vs. reduced ejection fraction in a community-based cohort: 11-year follow-up of PREVEND. Eur Heart J. 2013;34(19):1424-31.
11. Tasevska-Dinevska G, Kennedy LM, Nilsson PM, et al. Gender aspects on heart failure incidence and mortality in a middle-aged, urban, community-based population sample: the Malmo preventive project. Eur J Epidemiol. 2009;24(5):249-57.
12. de Giuli F, Khaw KT, Cowie MR, et al. Incidence and outcome of persons with a clinical diagnosis of heart failure in a general practice population of 696,884 in the United Kingdom. Eur J Heart Fail. 2005;7(3):295-302.
13. Cleland JG, Khand A, Clark A. The heart failure epidemic: exactly how big is it? Eur Heart J. 2001;22(8):623-6.
14. Clarke KW, Gray D, Hampton JR. How common is heart failure? Evidence from PACT (prescribing analysis and cost) data in Nottingham. J Public Health Med. 1995;17(4):459-64.
15. Cleland JG, Cohen-Solal A, Aguilar JC, et al. Management of heart failure in primary care (the IMPROVEMENT of Heart Failure Programme): an international survey. Lancet. 2002;360(9346):1631-9.
16. Ceia F, Fonseca C, Mota T, et al. Aetiology, comorbidity and drug therapy of chronic heart failure in the real world: the EPICA substudy. Eur J Heart Fail. 2004;6(6):801-6.
17. Fruhwald FM, Rehak P, Maier R, et al. Austrian survey of treating heart failure—AUSTRIA. Eur J Heart Fail. 2004;6(7):947-52.
18. Otero-Ravina F, Grigorian-Shamagian L, Fransi-Galiana L, et al. Morbidity and mortality among heart failure patients in Galicia, N.W. Spain: the GALICAP study. Int J Cardiol.2009;136(1):56-63.
19. de Rivas B, Permanyer-Miralda G, Brotons C, et al. Health-related quality of life in unselected outpatients with heart failure across Spain in two different health care levels. Magnitude and determinants of impairment: the INCA study. Qual Life Res. 2008;17(10):1229-38.
20. Hawkins NM, Scholes S, Bajekal M, et al. Community care in England: reducing socioeconomic inequalities in heart failure. Circulation. 2012;126(9):1050-7.
21. Maggioni AP, Dahlström U, Filippatos G, et al. EURObservational Research Programme: regional differences and 1-year follow-up results of the Heart Failure Pilot Survey (ESC-HF Pilot). Eur J Heart Fail. 2013;15(7):808-17.
22. Maggioni AP, Dahlström U, Filippatos G, et al. EURObservational Research Programme: The Heart Failure Pilot Survey (ESC-HF Pilot). Eur J Heart Fail. 2010;12(10):1076-84.
23. Tavazzi L, Senni M, Metra M, et al. Multicenter prospective observational study on acute and chronic heart failure: one-year follow-up results of IN-HF (Italian Network on Heart Failure) outcome registry. Circ Heart Fail. 2013;6(3):473-81.
24. Pulignano G, Del Sindaco D, Tavazzi L, et al. Clinical features and outcomes of elderly outpatients with heart failure followed up in hospital cardiology units: data from a large nationwide cardiology database (IN-CHF Registry). Am Heart J. 2002;143(1):45-55.
25. Allaert FA, Mosnier M. Analysis of ambulatory heart failure management and its incidence on one-year survival. Ann Cardiol Angeiol (Paris). 2008;57(1):22-8.
26. Rywik TM, Rywik SL, Korewicki J, et al. A survey of outpatient management of elderly heart failure patients in Poland-treatment patterns. Int J Cardiol. 2004;95(2-3):177-84.
27. Rywik SL, Wàgrowska H, Broda G, et al. Heart failure in patients seeking medical help at outpatients clinics. Part I. General characteristics. Eur J Heart Fail. 2000;2(4):413-21.
28. Hole T, Grundtvig M, Gullestad L, et al. Improved quality of life in Norwegian heart failure patients after follow-up in outpatient heart failure

clinics: results from the Norwegian Heart Failure Registry. Eur J Heart Fail. 2010;12(11):1247-52.
29. Brandsaeter B, Atar D, Agewall S. Gender differences among Norwegian patients with heart failure. Int J Cardiol. 2011;146(3):354-8.
30. Gonzalez-Juanatey JR, Alegria Ezquerra E, Bertomeu Martinez V, et al. [Heart failure in outpatients: comorbidities and management by different specialists. The EPISERVE Study]. Rev Esp Cardiol. 2008;61(6):611-9.
31. Salvador MJ, Sebaoun A, Sonntag F, et al. [European study of ambulatory management of heart failure by cardiologists]. Rev Esp Cardiol. 2004;57(12):1170-8.
32. Komajda M, Lapuerta P, Hermans N, et al. Adherence to guidelines is a predictor of outcome in chronic heart failure: the MAHLER survey. Eur Heart J. 2005;26(16):1653-9.
33. Oudejans I, Mosterd A, Zuithoff NP, et al. Comorbidity drives mortality in newly diagnosed heart failure: a study among geriatric outpatients. J Card Fail. 2012;18(1):47-52.
34. Futter JE, Cleland JG, Clark AL. Body mass indices and outcome in patients with chronic heart failure. Eur J Heart Fail. 2011;13(2):207-13.
35. Pellicori P, von Haehling S, Jankowska EA, et al. Regional differences in characteristics of patients enrolled in an epidemiological study of heart failure: SICA-HF. Heart Fail. 2013:1226.
36. Cleland JG, McDonagh T, Rigby AS, et al. The national heart failure audit for England and Wales 2008-2009. Heart. 2011;97(11):876-86.
37. Cleland JG, Swedberg K, Follath F, et al. The EuroHeart Failure survey programme—a survey on the quality of care among patients with heart failure in Europe. Part 1: patient characteristics and diagnosis. Eur Heart J. 2003;24(5):442-63.
38. Nieminen MS, Brutsaert D, Dickstein K, et al. EuroHeart Failure Survey II (EHFS II): a survey on hospitalized acute heart failure patients: description of population. Eur Heart J. 2006;27(22):2725-36.
39. Harjola VP, Foilath F, Nieminen MS, et al. Characteristics, outcomes, and predictors of mortality at 3 months and 1 year in patients hospitalized for acute heart failure. Eur J Heart Fail. 2010;12(3):239-48.
40. Blair JE, Zannad F, Konstam MA, et al. Continental differences in clinical characteristics, management, and outcomes in patients hospitalized with worsening heart failure results from the EVEREST (Efficacy of Vasopressin Antagonism in Heart Failure: Outcome Study with Tolvaptan) program. J Am Coll Cardiol. 2008;52(20):1640-8.
41. Fiuzat M, Massie BM, Chiswell K, et al. International differences in acute heart failure (AHF) patients: insight from the PROTECT trial. J Card Fail. 2011;17(8):S59-60.
42. Cosyns B, Claeys M. Management of heart failure in Belgium. Eur J Heart Fail. 2001;3(4):509-12.
43. Devroey D, Van Casteren V. The incidence and first-year mortality of heart failure in Belgium: a 2-year nationwide prospective registration. Int J Clin Pract. 2010;64(3):330-5.
44. De Geest S, Scheurweghs L, Reynders I, et al. Differences in psychosocial and behavioral profiles between heart failure patients admitted to cardiology and geriatric wards. Eur J Heart Fail. 2003;5(4):557-67
45. Direction de la Sécurité sociale. (2012). Les chiffres clés de la Sécurité sociale. [online] Available from: www.securite-sociale.fr/IMG/pdf/2013_chiffres_cles.pdf. [Accessed January, 2014].
46. l'Assurance Maladie. Caisse Primaire d'Ássurance Maladie. [online] Available from: www.ameli.fr. [Accessed January, 2014].
47. World Health Organization. (Year). Article. [online] Available from: www.who.int/health_financing/le_financt_du_sys_de_sante_en_france_dp_f_05_1.pdf. [Accessed January, 2014].
48. Rodwin VG. The health care system under French national health insurance: lessons for health reform in the United States. Am J Public Health. 2003;93(1):31-7.
49. Jondeau G, Allaert FA, Leurs I. [Management of heart failure by French general practitioners in 2003]. Arch Mal Coeur Vaiss. 2004;97(9):833-9.
50. Selke B, Brunot A, Lebrun T. [Economic repercussions of cardiac insufficiency in France]. Arch Mal Coeur Vaiss. 2003;96(3):191-6.
51. Statistisches Bundesamt. (2013). Öffentliches Finanzierungsdefizit im 1.-3. Quartal 2013 auf 28,7 Milliarden Euro gestiegen. [online] Available from: www.destatis.de/DE/Startseite.html. [Accessed January, 2014].
52. German Social Code Book V. Data following publication from Section 17b Abs 8 Hospital Financing Act KHG.
53. Rauch B, Dietz R, Cline C, et al. Für die SHAPE-Studiengruppe. Diagnostik und Therapie der chronischen Herzinsuffizienz durch niedergelassene Allgemeinärzte in Deutschland im Vergleich zu Frankreich und England. Z Kardiol. 2004;93(Suppl 3):447.
54. Remme W, Cline C, Cohen Solal A, et al. A Pan-European general public heart failure awareness and perception survey. Circulation. 2003;108(Suppl 4):693.
55. Remme W, McMurray J, Rauch B, et al. SHAPE (Study of Heart Failure Awareness and Perception in Europe): a pan-european general public survey on awareness and perception of the clinical, social and Economic Importance of Heart Failure. Eur Heart J. 2003;24(Suppl):178.
56. Hobbs FD, Jones MI, Allan TF, et al. European survey of primary care physician perceptions on heart failure diagnosis and management (Euro-HF). Eur Heart J. 2000;21(22):1877-87.
57. Ministero Della Salute. (2007). Regioni e Province autonome - Progetti. [online] Available from: www.salute.gov.it/portale/temi/p2_6.jsp?lingua=italiano&id=1095&area=Ricerca%20sanitaria&menu=finalizzata. [Accessed January, 2014].
58. Oliva F, Mortara A, Cacciatore G, et al. Acute heart failure patient profiles, management and in-hospital outcome: results of the Italian Registry on Heart Failure Outcome. Eur J Heart Fail. 2012;14(11):1208-17.
59. Filippi A, Sessa E, Pecchioli S, et al. Homecare for patients with heart failure in Italy. Ital Heart J. 2005;6(7):573-7.
60. Cancian M, Battaggia A, Celebrano M, et al. The care for chronic heart failure by general practitioners. Results from a clinical audit in Italy. Eur J Gen Pract. 2013;19(1):3-10.
61. Consensus conference on the management of heart failure. G Ital Cardiol (Rome). 2006;7(6):383-432.
62. Mangano A. An analysis of the regional differences in health care utilization in Italy. Health Place. 2010;16(2):301-8.
63. De Maria R, Misuraca G, Milli M, et al. Role of outpatient heart failure clinics and primary care physicians in the tailored follow-up of heart failure patients. G Ital Cardiol (Rome). 2010;11(5 Suppl 2):38S-44S.
64. Tavazzi L, Senni M, Metra M, et al. Multicenter prospective observational study on acute and chronic heart failure: one-year follow-up results of IN-HF (Italian Network on Heart Failure) outcome registry. Circ Heart Fail. 2013;6(3):473-81.

Chapter 42

Heart Failure in Southeast Asia

Raymond CC Wong, Carolyn SP Lam

ABSTRACT

Southeast Asia is witnessing a rising tide of cardiovascular risk factors, in particular, diabetes mellitus and hypertension. With increasing affluence and aging societies, heart failure (HF) is expected to reach epidemic proportions in Southeast Asia. Thus far, limited data in clinical HF patients from the region indicate that symptomatic decompensation occurs at a younger age, and is associated with a unique metabolic profile of high prevalence of diabetes mellitus despite relative lack of obesity, compared to Western cohorts. Interethnic differences in HF probably exist within the populations, which need to be accounted for in the management of these socioculturally diverse societies. Endothelial dysfunction leading to micro- and macrovascular dysfunction in HF presents particularly attractive therapeutic targets in Southeast Asian patients with stage C HF. There remain large gaps in knowledge pertaining to the prevalence of HF with preserved ejection fraction, ethnicity specific pathophysiologic mechanisms, prognosis and clinical outcomes, the role of device therapy, barriers to expensive recommended therapies, and cost-effectiveness of treatment strategies. Ongoing studies will hopefully address some of these issues in future.

INTRODUCTION

Southeast Asia refers to the geographic subregion of Asia south of China, east of India, west of New Guinea and north of Australia. It consists of a collection of varied island fragments unique in their history and sociocultural heterogeneity, and home to a rapidly growing population of almost 600 million people, most of whom are younger than 65 years and in the most productive years of their lives. Recent globalization and development have combined to create a potent force for convergence in terms of accessibility, communication, commerce, and culture within the region. Along with this convergence, there has been rapid epidemiological transition in the region, characterized by a reduction in deaths from communicable diseases, an increase in average life expectancy and an epidemic rise in chronic noncommunicable diseases such as heart disease.[1]

Heart failure, is the final common pathway of a myriad of heart diseases. Contemporary international HF guidelines emphasize that HF is a progressive disease syndrome with four stages (A–D)[2] beginning with cardiovascular risk factors alone in stage A, leading to structural cardiovascular abnormalities without symptoms in stage B and progressing to symptomatic manifestations of HF in stage C followed by terminal disease in stage D. Accordingly, we will review HF in Southeast Asia following these stages, with an emphasis on region specific characteristics and their practical implications at each stage.

STAGE A HEART FAILURE (CARDIOVASCULAR RISK FACTORS)

The 2004 World Health Organization estimated prevalence of cardiovascular risk factors for HF in Southeast Asia, compared to Europe and the Americas, is summarized in table 1. Most notably, the prevalence of diabetes mellitus was strikingly high in Southeast Asia (17%)—1.7 times that in the Americas and more than 1.4

TABLE 1: Prevalence of cardiovascular risk factors in Southeast Asia (WHO estimates for 2004)

Risk factor	*Prevalence measure*	*Southeast Asia*	*The Americas*	*Europe*
High blood pressure	Mean systolic pressure (mmHg)	125.3	125.6	133.7
	Systolic 142 mmHg or more (%)	19	21	36
High cholesterol	Mean serum cholesterol (mmol/L)	5.1	5.3	5.5
	Cholesterol level 6 mmol/L or more	21	28	34
High blood glucose	Mean fasting plasma glucose (mmol/L)	5.6	5.4	5.4
	Diabetic (FPG >7 mmol/L) (%)	17	10	12
Overweight and obesity	Mean BMI (kg/m^2)	22.1	27.9	26.9
	Overweight and obese (BMI >25) (%)	22	70	65
	Obese (BMI >30) (%)	2	33	24
Low fruit and vegetable intake	Mean fruit and vegetable intake (g/day)	239	244	376
	Less than five serves per day	80	69	56
Physical inactivity	Inactive (%)	16	22	20
	Insufficiently active (%)	38	38	43
	Moderately active (%)	17	19	18
	Highly active (%)	28	21	20
Tobacco use	Current smokers (%)	21	24	33
	Smoking impact ratio (%)	12	25	36

WHO, World Health Organization; FPG, fasting plasma glucose; BMI, body mass index

Source: Global health risks: mortality and burden of disease attributable to selected major risks. Geneva, World Health Organization 2009. Available at www.who.int/evidence/bod

times that in Europe—despite a much lower mean body mass index (~22 kg/m^2 in Southeast Asians compared to ~27 kg/m^2 in the Americas and Europe) and 12- to 17-fold lower prevalence of obesity (body mass index >30 kg/m^2) in Southeast Asians. Accordingly, the attributable deaths and disability-adjusted life years (DALYs) for high blood sugar in Southeast Asia exceeded that in the Western countries (Table 2).

A more recent estimation in 2010 illustrates the epidemiologic transition with increasing affluence in Southeast Asian countries (Fig. 1). When countries were arranged according to gross national income, a clear pattern was observed for diabetes prevalence, which was highest in the more affluent countries of Brunei, Malaysia, and Singapore (10.2–12.6%) and lowest in the less affluent nations of Myanmar, Cambodia, Laos, Vietnam, and Indonesia (3.2–5.6%). Mean levels of blood pressure were highest in Indonesia (a middle-income country) while total cholesterol levels were highest in Vietnam (a low-income country).

Practical point: Given the epidemiologic transition and rising tide of cardiovascular risk factors in Southeast Asia, it is paramount to employ effective community surveillance for early risk factors such as diabetes mellitus. Preventive measures to control these risk factors, before the development of adverse cardiovascular changes, could potentially avert progression of stage A to stage B HF. This may be realized by public health bodies working in partnership with charitable bodies to focus on public education and community health screening.

STAGE B HEART FAILURE (PRECLINICAL STRUCTURAL HEART DISEASE)

Published data from our Echocardiography Core Lab[3] show that reference values for left ventricular mass (LVM) among healthy Southeast Asians are consistently smaller than that in Western cohorts, even after correcting for body surface area (BSA). The 95th percentile of LVM (n = 198) in healthy, normotensive men and women were 189 g (106 g/m^2) and 148 g (96 g/m^2), respectively. These values are consistently smaller than published values from the West.[4] Age ($r = 0.27$, $p < 0.001$), gender ($r = 0.30$, $p < 0.001$), and systolic blood pressure ($r = 0.25$, $p = 0.003$) were important univariate predictors of LVM. These data highlight the potential for underdiagnosis

TABLE 2: Attributable deaths (000s) and DALYs (000s) by risk factor (WHO estimates for 2004)

Cause	*Southeast Asia*		*The Americas*		*Europe*	
Population (000)	1,671,904		879,899		883,705	
	Deaths	DALYs	Deaths	DALYs	Deaths	DALYs
High blood pressure						
Hypertensive heart disease	108.5	1,029.0	116.6	746.6	154.6	935.6
Ischemic heart disease	749.2	7,297.9	399.5	2,514.9	1,244.9	8,780.1
High cholesterol						
Ischemic heart disease	702.1	8,936.8	316.7	3,018.6	871.7	7,845.1
High blood glucose						
Diabetes mellitus	280.2	4,891.9	261.7	4,131.6	155.5	2,660.6
Ischemic heart disease	545.7	6,076.1	180.7	1,363.2	219.2	2,003.3
Overweight and obesity						
Diabetes mellitus	63.8	1,197.8	155.5	2,821.9	33.9	690.5
Hypertensive heart disease	29.9	369.1	73.1	635.9	32.5	277.6
Ischemic heart disease	187.3	2,601.9	242.5	2,498.8	305.1	3,462.3

WHO, World Health Organization; DALYs, deaths and disability-adjusted life years

Source: Global health risks: mortality and burden of disease attributable to selected major risks. Geneva, World Health Organization 2009. Available at www.who.int/evidence/bod

of left ventricular hypertrophy in Asian adults using cutoffs derived from Western populations, with resultant underrecognition of the transition from stage A and stage B of HF.

Practical point: To accurately identify stage B HF, clinicians must recognize that LVM index cutoffs for the diagnosis of left ventricular hypertrophy may need to be lowered in Asians.

STAGE C HEART FAILURE (SYMPTOMATIC HEART FAILURE)

In sharp contrast to the wealth of information regarding HF in Western populations, data in Asian patients are scarce, and even more limited in the subpopulation of Southeast Asia.

Incidence and Prevalence of Symptomatic Heart Failure in Southeast Asia

While data are available regarding Asian ethnic groups in Western countries, such as the United Kingdom[5,6] and Canada,[7] there are few published data from Southeast Asian countries. In this section, we focus on available data from Singapore (Table 3), a Southeast Asian country with a unique multiethnic population of 5.31 million (as of 2012). The ethnic composition of Singapore includes Southeast Asian ethnic Chinese (74.2%), Malay (13.3%), Indian (9.2%), and others (3.3%);[8] thus being highly representative of the mix of ethnicities found in urban Southeast Asia.

In Singapore, HF is the most common cardiac cause of hospitalization, accounting for 17% of all cardiac admissions. This translates to about 5,000 admissions a year. Ng and Niti[9] showed the unambiguous rising trend of incident HF admissions amongst those aged more than 65 years from 1991 to 1998, where the final 3 years showed an acute rise in rates (Fig. 2). Admission rates per 10,000 population rose from 85.4 (1991) to 110.3 (1998). The absolute change was +38.4% in the overall HF admissions, affecting both genders and all ethnic groups. Yet, the mortality directly caused by HF syndromes remained stable between 11.4% and 14.9%.

More contemporary trends are available from our single center registry (unpublished, personal communication) indicating growing rates of hospitalization between 1980s and 1990s through to the 21st century, from 225 unique admissions annually in 1998 to 980 in the year 2010. The most plausible explanation for this rising trend is a combination of changing population demographics where older age groups now account for 9.9% of the 5.31 million population compared to 6% of the

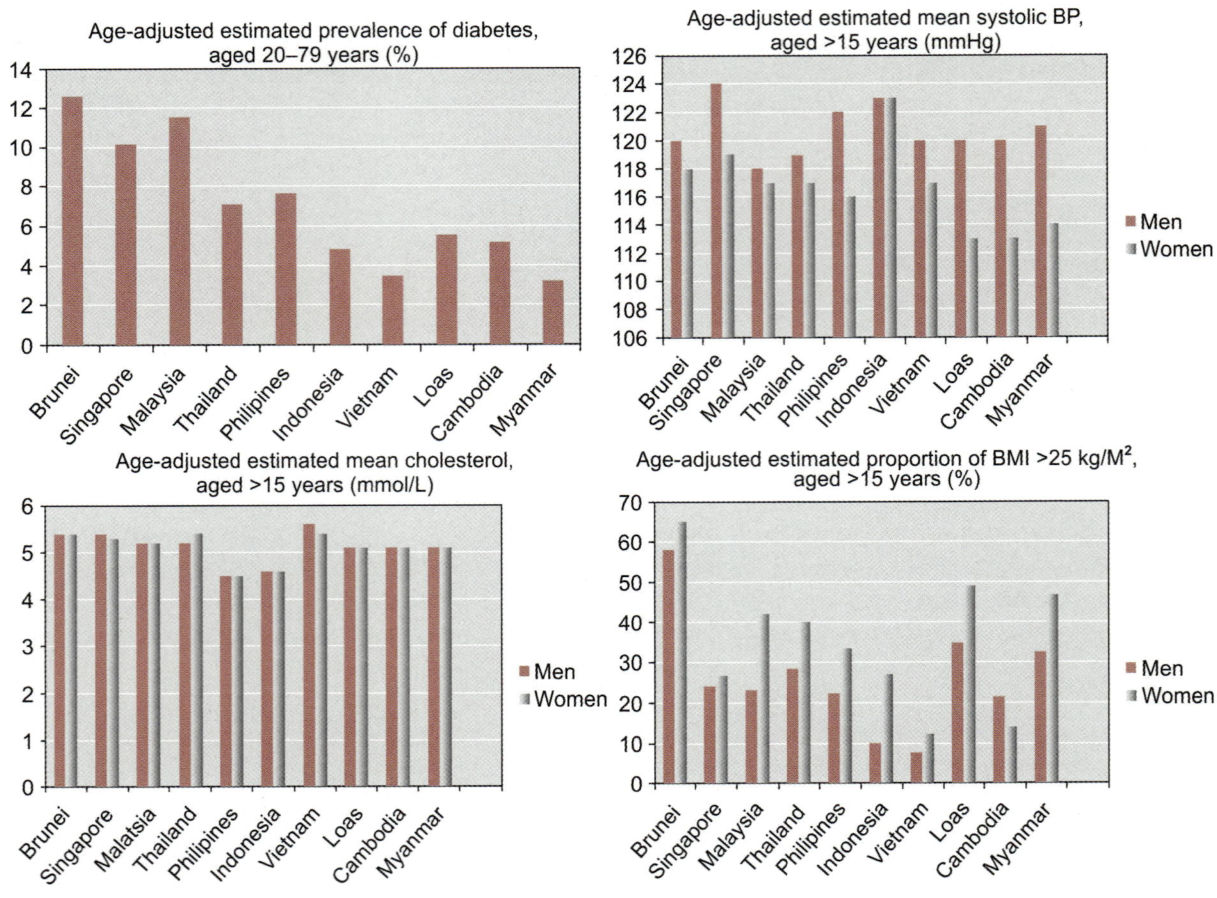

BP, blood pressure; BMI, body mass index

Fig. 1 Distribution of cardiovascular risk factors in Southeast Asian countries ranked by gross national income[1]

3.05 million in 1990, as well as the changing landscape of cardiovascular therapy, wherein effective management of acute myocardial infarctions reduced short-term mortality but was followed by adverse cardiac remodeling. Furthermore, our data indicate that HF in Southeast Asians is a recurrent and progressive disease, constituting the top contributor to 30-day rehospitalization, alongside chronic obstructive pulmonary disease in 2009 (18.5% vs 13% respectively). Nationwide, the corresponding figures were 14.9% and 22.3% respectively.

Practical point: The older age group is most vulnerable to HF in Southeast Asians. With increasing affluence and aging societies, HF is expected to reach epidemic proportions in Southeast Asia. Early recognition of the public health burden of HF and proper resource allocation to manage this growing population are important for Southeast Asian nations in epidemiologic transition.

Unique Characteristics of Southeast Asian Patients with Symptomatic Heart Failure

There is a paucity of direct comparisons between Southeast Asian and Western patients with HF in the existing literature. In the Acute Decompensated Heart Failure Registry (ADHERE) International-Asia Pacific study,[10] Asia Pacific patients hospitalized for acute decompensated HF were found to be younger, but with more patients exhibiting severe clinical symptoms and signs and higher rates of mechanical ventilation, compared with similar registries in the United States and Europe.[11-13] This was attributed to differences in the underlying risk factor profile and socioeconomic factors related to epidemiologic transition of emerging economies. In-hospital mortality was higher for patients enrolled in ADHERE-Asia Pacific compared

TABLE 3: Published studies based on heart failure cohorts in Southeast Asia

Author	Year	Cohort	Study design	Sample size	Age	Male (%)	Ethnicity (%)	Risk factors (%)	Mortality	Drugs (%)	Comments
Leong et al.	2007	Hospital-based	Observational prospective	173	68.7	51.4	C 52; M 33.5; I 10.4	DM 50.3; HTN 67.6; CAD 46.8; AF 16.5	20.8% in one year	ACEI/ ARB 75.1; BB 41.6	35.8% of cohort had LVEF ≤45%
Seow et al.	2007	Hospital-based	Retrospective	225	68.5	56.4	C 60; M 24; I 14.7	DM 52.1; HTN 53.5; CAD 83.1	67.5% in 5 years	ACEI 79.1; BB 6.2	All had LVEF ≤40%. More deaths in females than males (75.3% vs 62.7%)
Lee et al.	2007	Hospital-based	Retrospective	668	66	67.4	C 72; M 17.1; I 10.9	DM 48.5; HTN 72.6; CAD 68.5	C 14.3%; M 27%; I 18.6% in 24 months	ACEI/ ARB 86.5; BB 66.6	17% had LVEF >40%. Indians had more deaths
Omar et al.	2007	Program-based	Retrospective	154	65	54	C 56; M 26; I 17	DM 62; HTN 79; CAD 63	None in 6 months	ACEI/ ARB 96; BB 70	High usage of guideline-based drugs

C, Chinese; M, Malay; I, Indian; DM, diabetes mellitus; HTN, hypertension; CAD, coronary artery disease; AF, atrial fibrillation; ACEI, angiotensin-converting enzyme inhibitor; ARB, angiotensin receptor blocker; BB, beta-blocker; LVEF, left ventricular ejection fraction

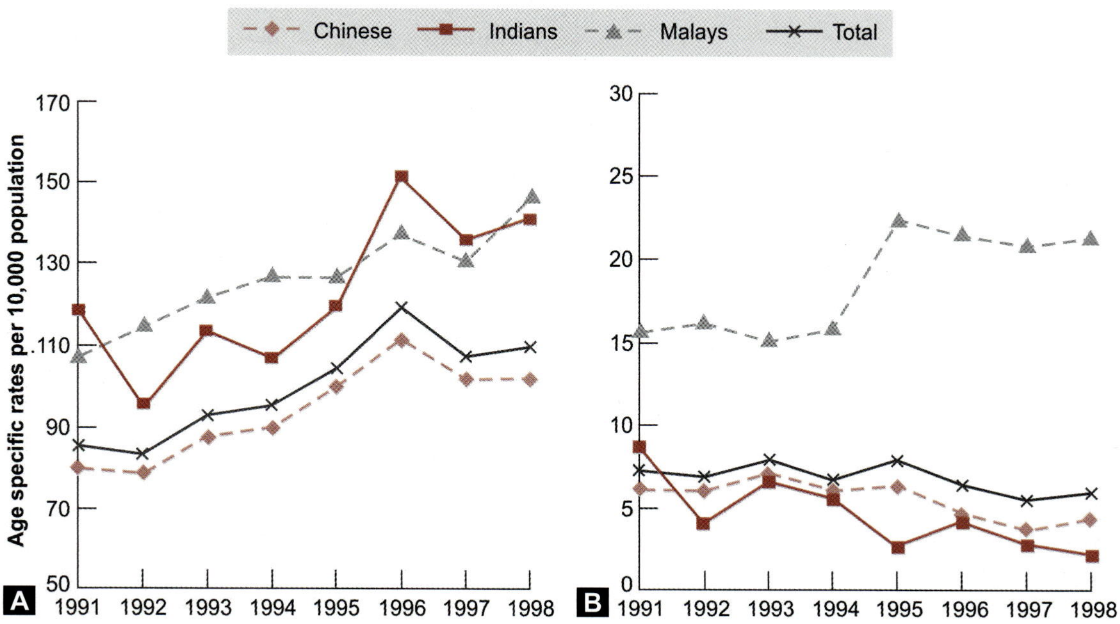

Fig. 2 Trends in hospital admissions and mortality from congestive heart failure (age standardized) in elderly people (≥65 years) by ethnicity, Singapore, 1991 to 1998[9]

with the US-based ADHERE.[13] Robust comparisons of echocardiographic and electrocardiographic data between Asian and Western patients were not available in this prior study, largely due to missing data.

Specifically among Southeast Asian patients with HF, published data from the region show a mean age of 65–68.7 years, diabetes mellitus in 48.5–62%, hypertension in 53.5–79%, and coronary artery disease in 46.8–83.1% (Table 3). Ongoing efforts to address the need for direct comparisons between Asian and Western patients include parallel multicenter studies in Singapore [Singapore Heart Failure Outcomes and Phenotypes (SHOP) Study] and New Zealand [Outcome in Patients with Heart Failure with Preserved Left Ventricular Ejection Fraction (PEOPLE) Study].[14] Preliminary results in 911 patients with HF recruited from nine centers across Singapore (n = 618; majority Chinese descent, SG-Asian group) and New Zealand (n = 293; majority European descent, NZ group) show that, compared to the NZ group, SG Asians were almost a decade younger on average (69 ± 13 years vs 60 ± 11 years), and had strikingly higher prevalence of diabetes (32% vs 55%) and hypertension (58% vs 69%) despite having smaller body mass index (30 ± 7 kg/m^2 vs 26 ± 5 kg/m^2) (all $p < 0.05$).

Practical point: Heart failure tends to occur at a younger age in Southeast Asians and is associated with a unique metabolic profile of high prevalence of diabetes mellitus despite relative lack of obesity compared to Western cohorts.

Ethnic Differences among Southeast Asian Patients with Symptomatic Heart Failure

Ng and Niti[9] examined HF admissions between 1991 and 1998 across all ethnic groups in Singapore (n = 15,774; Chinese 37.9%, Malay 47.4%, and Indians 30%). However, only Indians showed higher mortality rate of +54.3%, whereas reverse trends were seen in Chinese (-36.3%) and Malay (-70.3%). Indian ethnicity independently gave a rate ratio of 3.48 [2.38–5.08, 95% confidence interval (CI)].

In another single hospital-based observational study, Lee et al.[15] aimed to assess the impact of race on clinical outcome in the multiracial Singapore HF population (n = 668). The mean age was 66 ± 12 years, left ventricular ejection fraction (LVEF) 29 ± 13%, and ethnic mix were 72% Chinese, 17% Malays, and 11% Indians. After mean follow-up of 24 months, composite end-point of all-cause mortality or HF readmission occurred in 198 patients, with ethnic composition being 64.1% Chinese (underrepresented), 21% Malays, and 14.9% Indians (both overrepresented) compared to total recruited cohort. A trend towards a higher all-cause mortality rate was seen in Malays. Diabetes mellitus, peripheral vascular disease and hyperlipidemia were more prevalent in Indians compared to Malays or Chinese (all $p < 0.05$) suggesting the impact of comorbid conditions on outcome. Similar findings were reported by Leong et al.[16] where Chinese and Malay ethnicity were univariate predictors of lower 1-year mortality [odds ratio (OR) 0.229, 95% CI 0.058–0.907 and OR 0.194, 95% CI 0.044–0.854, respectively]. However, Seow et al.[17] had conflicting results against other authors when they did observe ethnic differences in mortality rates.

Practical point: Ethnic specific risk factors are evident from small studies performed in multiethnic Southeast Asian cohorts. To what extent these differences represent actual ethnicity specific pathophysiologic pathways, versus sociocultural/lifestyle differences, is unclear. Further research is warranted and the optimal management of Southeast Asian patients with HF should account for these ethnic differences.

Heart Failure with Preserved Ejection Fraction

A wealth of epidemiologic data from Western countries has shown that HFpEF accounts for almost 50% of the HF population in Western cohorts. In contrast, very little is known regarding the prevalence and outcome of patients with HFpEF from Southeast Asian populations. In Singapore, Lee et al.[15] reported 17% prevalence of HFpEF (out of 668 HF patients) in a study; while Leong et al.[16] observed 35.8% in another public hospital cohort (n = 173). The high prevalence of hypertension—the leading risk factor for HFpEF—as well as the rapidly aging societies in Southeast Asia, portends a large increase in the prevalence of HFpEF in this region. Clearly much more work is needed to define the relative prevalence, characteristics, and outcomes of patients with HFpEF compared with those with HF and reduced LVEF (HFrEF) as well as to look for any interethnic differences. These are, indeed, the aims of the ongoing nationwide HF surveillance study (SHOP study) in Singapore.[14]

To understand HFpEF versus HFrEF in our Southeast Asian cohort of SHOP, we measured circulating levels of growth differentiation factor 15 (GDF15), ST2, high-sensitivity troponin T (hsTnT), and N-terminal pro-brain natriuretic peptide (NT-proBNP) in 51 patients with HFrEF, 50 patients with HFpEF, and 50 community-based controls. Among these biomarkers, GDF15 distinguished HFpEF from controls with the largest area under curve (0.936; $p < 0.001$); NT-proBNP and hsTnT levels were higher in HFrEF than in HFpEF; and the ratio of NT-proBNP: GDF15 best distinguished between HFpEF and HFrEF. These data suggest a prominent role for myocardial injury (hsTnT) with increased wall stress (NT-proBNP) in HFrEF and systemic inflammation (GDF15) in HFpEF among Southeast Asian patients.[18] Additionally, we found an optimal NT-proBNP cutoff value of 288 pg/mL for the diagnosis of HFpEF, similar to the European Society of Cardiology recommendation of more than 220 pg/mL.[19]

Practical point: Aging populations in Southeast Asia are likely to see a rise in HFpEF prevalence. Further work is urgently needed to understand this complex syndrome in Southeast Asians.

Pathophysiology of Heart Failure

As discussed above, diabetes mellitus and hypertension are predominant risk factors in Southeast Asian patients with symptomatic HF. Both risk factors are known to induce microvascular and macrovascular dysfunction, leading to end-organ damage. Recent data have highlighted the central role of endothelial dysfunction in mediating these adverse effects of cardiovascular risk factors on micro- and macrovasculature.[20-22] Endothelial dysfunction is clinically assessed as a deficient vasodilatory response to various stimuli, indicating impaired endothelium mediated nitric oxide (NO) bioavailability. In the presence of diabetes mellitus and hypertension, redox imbalances induce oxidative stress that causes endothelial dysfunction. Lack of NO bioavailability to vascular media cells and cardiomyocytes in contact with the dysfunctional endothelial cells results in reduced activation of intracellular soluble guanylyl cyclase (sGC) and impairment of cyclic guanosine monophosphate-protein kinase G (cGMP-PKG) dependent mechanisms. Indeed, the NO-cGMP-PKG pathway is critical for cardiovascular homeostasis and structural remodeling. Impairment of this pathway leads to vascular stiffening, ventricular systolic and diastolic dysfunction, adverse cardiac remodeling and ventricular-vascular fibrosis—all hallmarks of HF regardless of ejection fraction.[23,24]

Specifically in the Asian context, Murphy et al.[25] showed in their sample of healthy young men from the United Kingdom (UK) that healthy South Asians had worse parameters of endothelial function compared with healthy whites. In patients with HF and reduced ejection fraction, Shantsila et al.[26] further showed that South Asian ethnicity was associated with more severe endothelial dysfunction compared to White and African Caribbean ethnicities in their UK cohort, even after adjustment for age, presence of hypertension and diabetes mellitus, blood pressure, and glucose levels. More recently, Akiyama et al.[27] demonstrated the prognostic significance of endothelial dysfunction in a sample of Japanese patients with HFpEF, suggesting a primary pathophysiologic role of endothelial dysfunction in the progression of HFpEF. Our own data in Singapore confirm the high prevalence of endothelial dysfunction in HF regardless of EF: endothelial dysfunction, defined as a reactive hyperemia peripheral arterial tonometry index less than 1.67 was present in 38% of HF patients versus 16% of controls ($p < 0.001$), a difference which persisted after adjustment for age, sex, body size, cardiovascular risk factors and medications ($p = 0.002$).[28]

Practical point: The prominent role of endothelial dysfunction in Southeast Asian patients with HF suggests that endothelial dysfunction may be an important therapeutic target in these patients. This opens the door to several therapeutic options that deserve further study in Southeast Asian patients with HF: NO donors, such as isosorbide dinitrate + hydralazine combinations, statins, cGMP stimulators or activators, and phosphodiesterase-5 inhibitors.

Management of Symptomatic Heart Failure: Adherence to Guideline-based Medications

The ADHERE-AP reported suboptimal usage of angiotensin-converting enzyme inhibitor (ACEI) and angiotensin receptor blocker (ARB) as well as beta-blocker in the Asia-Pacific countries on discharge, at 63.5% and 41%, respectively. In patients with moderate/severe left ventricular systolic dysfunction, ACEI/ARB usage increased to 72%, but beta-blocker use remained under 50%. Local publications suggested a higher usage of these guideline-based medications (Table 3); nonetheless only Lee et al. observed a "protective" effect of beta-blocker in their HF cohort.[15] An important gap in knowledge is with regards to the dosages of these drugs in Southeast Asian populations where the smaller body sizes may impact the maximum tolerated doses or prescription habits of doctors.

Management of Symptomatic Heart Failure: Role of Implantable Devices

There is very little published data relating to the use of implantable devices in Southeast Asian patients with

HF, specifically cardiac resynchronization therapy-pacemakers and defibrillators (CRT-P or CRT-D). Single center unpublished data showed a rising trend of implantation of both CRT-P and CRT-D from 2008 (24 cases) to 2012 (52 cases). Several important questions remained unanswered and represent important barriers to the widespread application of device therapy in Southeast Asian nations: firstly, the cost-effectiveness of device therapy within the Southeast Asian populations has not been established; secondly, the health economic impact of such devices on aging Southeast Asian communities is unknown, and thirdly the rates of key clinical events (such as, sudden cardiac death) in the baseline Southeast Asian HF population are still unclear.

Limited outcome data in Asian HF populations describe the following: In Singapore, Leong et al.[16] reported 54.3% of 1-year cardiovascular death or readmissions and 20.8% on 1-year mortality. Seow et al.[17] reported 67.5% mortality in a cohort of HFrEF in 5 years (mean survival 2.7 years) of which 69.7% were attributable to cardiovascular causes. A disproportionally smaller composite end-points of death and readmissions were reported by Lee et al.[15] (29.6% in mean follow-up of 24 months). In a Japanese cohort, when second Multicenter Automatic Defibrillator Implantation Trial (MADIT-II) criteria were applied to a Japanese cohort, 12 patients who were eligible but did not undergo implantable cardioverter-defibrillator (ICD) implantation showed significantly lower risk of sudden cardiac death and even better overall survival than the historical Western MADIT-II population.[29] In contrast, when applied to a Chinese cohort, those satisfying the MADIT-II criteria were found to be at similar risk of sudden cardiac death compared to the original Western MADIT-II population.[30] Both prior Asian studies have been criticized for their small sample sizes, possible selection bias, and retrospective nature. However, they clearly demonstrate the ambiguity regarding the risk of sudden cardiac death among Asian patients, an issue that may be depriving Asian patients of potentially lifesaving therapy, and one that needs to be urgently addressed so that patients, doctors and policymakers can make informed healthcare decisions.

The Asian Sudden Cardiac Death in Heart Failure (ASIAN-HF) Registry (ClinicalTrials.gov Identifier: NCT01633398) is an ongoing study designed to determine mortality and morbidity in Asian patients under clinical management for HF. Specifically, the incidence of, and risk factors for, sudden cardiac death will be characterized, as well as the sociocultural factors influencing therapeutic choices in these patients. ASIAN-HF is a prospective observational multinational Asian registry of 5,000 patients with symptomatic HF (Stage C) and left ventricular systolic dysfunction (ejection fraction <40%) involving 40 centers across 10 Asian regions (Korea, Thailand, Indonesia, Philippines, India, Japan, Malaysia, Hong Kong, China, and Singapore). Patients will be followed over 3 years for outcomes of death or hospitalization.

Practical point: The ASIAN-HF Registry aims to advance fundamental understanding of the burden and predictors of death and hospitalization among Asian patients with stage C HF. The knowledge gained will be important for guiding resource allocation and planning preventive strategies to address the unmet and growing clinical needs of patients with cardiovascular disease in Asia.

Management of Symptomatic Heart Failure: Role of Chronic Disease Management Program

A multidisciplinary chronic disease management program (CDMP) in chronic HF has been shown to improve clinical outcome measures in Southeast Asian patients with Stage C HF.[31] Of the 154 patients (54% male, mean age 65 years) with a primary diagnosis of HF, New York Heart Association (NYHA) class III/IV and LVEF less than 40% enrolled in HF-specific CDMP, improvement in the quality of life and activity status ($p < 0.001$) was observed at 6 months. Proportions of patients in NYHA class I/II rose from 48% to 97%. six-minute walk test (6MWT) increased significantly from mean 273 m to 316 m ($p < 0.001$). ACE inhibitors/ARB were maintained in 97% of the patients and there was an increase of beta-blockers use ($p = 0.001$). Quality of life assessed by Minnesota Living with Heart Failure Questionnaire (MLHFQ) dropped significantly from mean 43 to mean 24 points. HF admissions were reduced by 68% ($P < 0.001$). The primary drivers for the effectiveness of HF-specific CDMP are behavioral and lifestyle modifications, ease of access of expert intervention from multiple disciplines making up the program and interpersonal connection made via telephonic interviews with the HF coordinators, who in turn bring into proximity physicians' input beyond regular clinic visits. Above all, CDMP mandates active patient and caregiver participations in the disease monitoring and therapeutic processes, and empowers them to make many basic decisions from day to day. Omar et al. did not, however, study the effectiveness of CDMP based on ethnicity nor gender.

Practical point: HF specific CDMPs hold promise as an effective tool for management of Southeast Asian patients with stage C HF. While additional funding is required to initiate and sustain such a program, the long term payoffs in terms of reduction in HF admissions and mortality may lead eventually to cost saving for the patients and reduced economic burden of public healthcare. CDMP also provides a platform for effective dialogue between healthcare workers from different disciplines, a crucial step in reducing misinformation and service gaps that commonly exist in all large healthcare organizations. Above all, CDMP databases are convenient yet critical administrative audit tools for healthcare authorities who frequently make use of the data to apportion health budget and lead quality improvement initiatives.

STAGE D HEART FAILURE (ADVANCED HEART FAILURE)

Data are very limited regarding the management of end-stage HF in Southeast Asian nations. We summarize available data from our experience in Singapore and highlight areas for further development.

Role of Heart Transplantation and Ventricular Assist Devices

Heart transplant program started in Singapore in 1990. It was aimed at offering definitive treatment for intractable or end-stage HF patients. Sivathasan reviewed the database of 40 consecutive heart transplantations performed in Singapore from July 1990 through December 2007.[32] The mean age of recipients was 45 years (range 14–64 years). Ischemic cardiomyopathy (52.5%) and dilated cardiomyopathy (42.5%) were the major indications. From 1990 to 2007, the average donor age increased from 28.3 years to 38.1 years. The 30-day mortality was 10% and half-life was 10 years. Cardiac allograft vasculopathy and sepsis caused 41.7% of mortality each. 11.7% of the mortality was due to cerebrovascular accident. The overall outcome was comparable to 2008 registry data of the International Society for Heart and Lung Transplantation (ISHLT). Figure 3 illustrates donor availability and selection statistics between 2001 and 2007. Ventricular assist device (VAD) program started in 2001 and had over the years seen the change of preferred VADs from HeartMate vented electric (VE) left ventricular assist system (LVAS) (Thoratec Corp.) to HeartMate II (Thoratec Corp.) and HeartWare ventricular assist device (HVAD) (HeartWare International, Inc.). With few donor

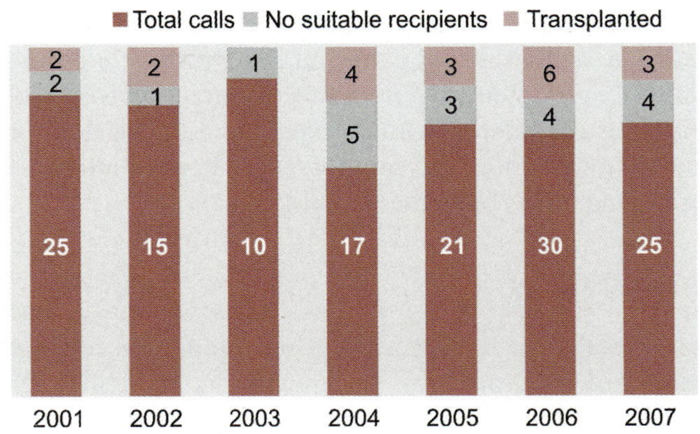

Fig. 3 Annual statistics of donors for heart transplant, year 2001–2007[32]

hearts available locally for transplantation, the move towards longer duration on bridge to transplant (BTT) as well as destination therapy (DT) using VAD becomes a reality. Both HeartMate II and HVAD are small built continuous pumps particularly suited to be implanted in Asians who have smaller BSA, some as small as 1.2 m^2. Comfort aside, smaller devices are associated with less pump pocket related infections. Presently, six to eight VADs are implanted annually in Singapore.

Role of Advanced Care Planning and Home-based Palliative Disease Management

The Advance Care Planning Program (ACP) is a structured process of assisting local stage D HF patients to reflect on their health condition and make rational choices about future treatment preferences in the event they are rendered incapable of making end-of-life decisions. Presently, the ACP is a nationwide, government funded program incorporated into respective HF CDMP in Singapore. In our institution, dedicated counseling sessions and in-depth interviews are conducted by care specialists with patients and care givers covering issues such as disease acceptance, symptom palliation, and care designation. In Singapore, an integrated, healthcare authority-funded home-based palliative care program exists to rightsite the delivery of palliative care right in patients' homes. Our unpublished audit data showed that this strategy effectively reduced HF readmissions of stage D HF (mean time to death 5.5 months) where mean all-cause and HF hospitalizations were 3.6 and 2.0 per patient before enrolment, but improved to 1.0 and 0.6, respectively, after ACP. Two-thirds experienced fewer HF hospitalizations after recruitment into the home-based program.

Practical point: End stage HF is an expensive disease to manage. Heart transplantation and VAD programs require upfront investments of enormous resources. These needs must be considered within the unique socioeconomic and cultural contexts of Southeast Asia where nations are at varying stages of epidemiologic transition.

CONCLUSION

Southeast Asia is witnessing an epidemic of non-communicable diseases along with its epidemiologic transition. The rising tide of cardiovascular risk factors, especially diabetes mellitus and hypertension indicates that there is a rapidly growing population with stage A HF in Southeast Asia. These patients should be targeted for surveillance and preventive measures. In assessing patients for structural cardiac changes (i.e., stage B HF) ethnicity specific cutoffs should be used. Limited data in stage C HF patients from Southeast Asia indicate that symptomatic decompensation occurs at a younger age (almost a decade younger) and is associated with a unique metabolic profile of high prevalence of diabetes mellitus despite relative lack of obesity compared to Western cohorts. Important interethnic differences may exist within Southeast Asian populations which deserve further study and need to be accounted for in the management of these patients. Endothelial dysfunction leading to micro- and macrovascular dysfunction in HF represents a particularly attractive therapeutic target in Southeast Asian patients with stage C HF. There are large gaps in knowledge pertaining to the prevalence of HFpEF, ethnicity-specific pathophysiologic mechanisms, clinical outcomes, the role of device therapy, barriers to recommended therapies, and cost-effectiveness of treatment strategies. Ongoing studies (SHOP, PEOPLE, and ASIAN-HF) will hopefully address some of these issues in future. Such knowledge will be important for guiding resource allocation and planning preventive strategies to address the unmet and growing clinical needs of patients with HF in Southeast Asia.

REFERENCES

1. Dans A, Ng N, Varghese C, et al. The rise of chronic non-communicable diseases in southeast Asia: time for action. Lancet. 2011;377(9766):680-9.
2. Hunt SA, Baker DW, Chin MH, et al. ACC/AHA Guidelines for the Evaluation and Management of Chronic Heart Failure in the Adult: Executive Summary A Report of the American College of Cardiology/American Heart Association Task Force on Practice Guidelines (Committee to Revise the 1995 Guidelines for the Evaluation and Management of Heart Failure): Developed in Collaboration With the International Society for Heart and Lung Transplantation; Endorsed by the Heart Failure Society of America. Circulation. 2001;104(24):2996-3007.
3. Wong RC, Yip JW, Gupta A, et al. Echocardiographic left ventricular mass in a multiethnic Southeast Asian population: proposed new gender and age-specific norms. Echocardiography. 2008;25(8):805-11.
4. Shub C, Klein AL, Zachariah PK, et al. Determination of left ventricular mass by echocardiography in a normal population: effect of age and sex in addition to body size. Mayo Clin Proc. 1994;69(3):205-11.
5. Lip G, Zarifis J, Beevers DG. Acute admissions with heart failure to a district general hospital serving a multiracial population. Int J Clin Pract. 1997;51(4):223-7.
6. Lip GY, Khan H, Bhatnagar A, et al. Ethnic differences in patient perceptions of heart failure and treatment: the West Birmingham heart failure project. Heart. 2004;90(9):1016-9.
7. Singh N, Gupta M. Clinical characteristics of South Asian patients hospitalized with heart failure. Ethn Dis. 2005;15(4):615-9.
8. Singapore Department of Statistics. (2013). [online] Available from: www.singstats.gov.sg. [Accessed December, 2013].
9. Ng TP, Niti M. Trends and ethnic differences in hospital admissions and mortality for congestive heart failure in the elderly in Singapore, 1991 to 1998. Heart. 2003;89(8):865-70.
10. Atherton JJ, Hayward CS, Wan Ahmad WA, et al. Patient characteristics from a regional multicenter database of acute decompensated heart failure in Asia Pacific (ADHERE International-Asia Pacific). J Card Fail. 2012;18(1):82-8.
11. Cleland JG, Swedberg K, Follath F, et al. The EuroHeart Failure survey programme—a survey on the quality of care among patients with heart failure in Europe. Part 1: patient characteristics and diagnosis. Eur Heart J. 2003;24(5):442-63.
12. Owan TE, Hodge DO, Herges RM, et al. Trends in prevalence and outcome of heart failure with preserved ejection fraction. N Engl J Med. 2006;355(3):251-9.
13. Yancy CW, Lopatin M, Stevenson LW, et al. Clinical presentation, management, and in-hospital outcomes of patients admitted with acute decompensated heart failure with preserved systolic function: a report from the Acute Decompensated Heart Failure National Registry (ADHERE) Database. J Am Coll Cardiol. 2006;47(1):76-84.
14. Santhanakrishnan R, Ng TP, Cameron VA, et al. The Singapore Heart Failure Outcomes and Phenotypes (SHOP) study and Prospective Evaluation of Outcome in Patients with Heart Failure with Preserved Left Ventricular Ejection Fraction (PEOPLE) study: rationale and design. J Card Fail. 2013;19(3):156-62.
15. Lee R, Chan SP, Chan YH, et al. Impact of race on morbidity and mortality in patients with congestive heart failure: a study of the multiracial population in Singapore. Int J Cardiol. 2009;134(3):422-5.
16. Leong KT, Goh PP, Chang BC, et al. Heart failure cohort in Singapore with defined criteria: clinical characteristics and prognosis in a multi-ethnic hospital-based cohort in Singapore. Singapore Med J. 2007;48(5):408-14.
17. Seow SC, Chai P, Lee YP, et al. Heart failure mortality in Southeast Asian patients with left ventricular systolic dysfunction. J Card Fail. 2007; 13(6):476-81.
18. Santhanakrishnan R, Chong JP, Ng TP, et al. Growth differentiation factor 15, ST2, high-sensitivity troponin T, and N-terminal pro brain natriuretic peptide in heart failure with preserved vs. reduced ejection fraction. Eur J Heart Fail. 2012;14(12):1338-47.
19. Paulus WJ, Tschope C, Sanderson JE, et al. How to diagnose diastolic heart failure: a consensus statement on the diagnosis of heart failure with normal left ventricular ejection fraction by the Heart Failure and Echocardiography Associations of the European Society of Cardiology. Eur Heart J. 2007;28(20):2539-50.
20. Taddei S, Ghiadoni L, Virdis A, et al. Mechanisms of endothelial dysfunction: clinical significance and preventive non-pharmacological therapeutic strategies. Curr Pharm Des. 2003;9(29):2385-402.

21. Brutsaert DL. Cardiac endothelial-myocardial signaling: its role in cardiac growth, contractile performance, and rhythmicity. Physiol Rev. 2003;83(1):59-115.
22. Lam CS, Brutsaert DL. Endothelial dysfunction: a pathophysiologic factor in heart failure with preserved ejection fraction. J Am Coll Cardiol. 2012;60(18):1787-9.
23. Ferrari R, Bachetti T, Agnoletti L, et al. Endothelial function and dysfunction in heart failure. Eur Heart J. 1998;19 Suppl G:G41-7.
24. Borlaug BA, Olson TP, Lam CS, et al. Global cardiovascular reserve dysfunction in heart failure with preserved ejection fraction. J Am Coll Cardiol. 2010;56(11):845-54.
25. Murphy C, Kanaganayagam GS, Jiang B, et al. Vascular dysfunction and reduced circulating endothelial progenitor cells in young healthy UK South Asian men. Arterioscler Thromb Vasc Biol. 2007;27(4):936-42.
26. Shantsila E, Wrigley B, Shantsila A, et al. Ethnic differences in macrovascular and microvascular function in systolic heart failure. Circ Heart Fail. 2011;4(6):754-62.
27. Akiyama E, Sugiyama S, Matsuzawa Y, et al. Incremental prognostic significance of peripheral endothelial dysfunction in patients with heart failure with normal left ventricular ejection fraction. J Am Coll Cardiol. 2012;60(18):1778-86.
28. Shir Lynn L, Rajalakshmi S, Carolyn SP L. Endothelial Dysfunction Is Associated With The Cardiorenal Syndrome In Asian Patients With Heart Failure. Abstract, Asian-Pacific Society of Cardiology Congress 2013.
29. Tanno K, Miyoshi F, Watanabe N, et al. Are the MADIT II criteria for ICD implantation appropriate for Japanese patients? Circ J. 2005;69(1):19-22.
30. Siu CW, Pong V, Ho HH, et al. Are MADIT II criteria for implantable cardioverter defibrillator implantation appropriate for Chinese patients? J Cardiovasc Electrophysiol. 2010;21(3):231-5.
31. Omar AR, Suppiah N, Chai P, et al. Efficacy of community-based multidisciplinary disease management of chronic heart failure. Singapore Med J. 2007;48(6):528-31.
32. Sivathasan C. Heart transplantation in Singapore. Ann Acad Med Singapore. 2009;38(4):309-14.

Chapter 43

Heart Failure in India

Ajay Bahl, Inder S Anand

ABSTRACT

The profile of heart failure (HF) patients in India has changed over the past few decades and this evolution is likely to continue in the coming years. Straddling several ages of the epidemiological transition, India is burdened with degenerative diseases like coronary artery disease, hypertension, and diabetes mellitus while infections and rheumatic heart disease continue to remain a major public health problem. Occurrence of coronary artery disease and diabetes mellitus at a younger age is largely attributable to lifestyle and dietary changes. Prevention of these risk factors is needed to reduce the burden of HF. Unique genetic factors like a deletion in MYBPC3 add to the heart failure burden. Based on the limited data, we can infer that Indians do not show any differences in the responses to standard HF medications as compared to the Western population. Optimising use of drugs and devices as per the guidelines can improve outcomes. As the Indian population ages, the prevalence of HF will continue to increase and diastolic HF is likely encountered much more frequently in clinical practice.

INTRODUCTION

Cardiovascular diseases are the commonest cause of mortality and morbidity in adults and the elderly in India[1,2] and heart failure, is the final common pathway of most of these diseases. Despite being a major clinical problem, there is a dearth of reliable data on prevalence, incidence, and current etiological factors associated with the development of HF, and use of evidence based therapies in the Indian subcontinent. The limited data available is derived from the small epidemiological studies on risk factors associated with HF.

However, there are several aspects of the etiology and management of HF that are uniquely different in Indian population and need to be highlighted. Although ischemic heart disease and hypertension have now become the commonest causes of HF in India, rheumatic heart disease and cardiomyopathies are still highly prevalent. In addition, certain uncommon conditions like endomyocardial fibrosis and Takayasu arteritis also cause HF and are more often seen in India as compared to the West. Moreover, some genetic factors like a specific polymorphism in MYBPC3 is a condition restricted almost exclusively to people of South Asian descent.

SCOPE OF THE PROBLEM

India is a large and diverse country, and therefore, geographical variations in cardiovascular diseases are expected to be seen in different states. In addition, the causes of HF have significantly changed over time. Etiology of HF in India was first studied by Rustom Jal Vakil in 1949.[3] He reported on 1,281 patients based on his hospital clinical practice in Bombay (now, Mumbai). HF was common even at that time and accounted for 4.8% of all patients admitted to the medical wards. Hypertension and coronary artery disease accounted for 31.3% of patients, rheumatic heart disease was seen in 29.3%, and syphilis accounted for 11.7% of the remaining.[3] Compared to that, the scenario is now markedly different; syphilitic heart disease has virtually disappeared, rheumatic heart disease continues to be common, but the burden of degenerative diseases like coronary artery disease, hypertension, and diabetes mellitus have strikingly increased, and are the commonest causes of HF today.[4] This reflects the major epidemiological transition that is currently occurring in India and which needs to be understood to gain an insight into the problem of HF facing the country today.

EPIDEMIOLOGICAL TRANSITION AND ITS IMPLICATIONS

Cardiovascular diseases have evolved variably in different regions of the world in the last century. The concept of epidemiologic transition helps us understand these changes.[5,6] Accordingly, epidemiological transition stages cardiovascular diseases from the age of pestilence and famine, seen in primitive societies, to the age of delayed degenerative diseases seen in developed countries today.[6] India has undergone rapid industrialization, urbanization with marked social and economic changes over the past 60 years. Transition from a rural agriculture based society to a more urban service based and industrial society has been comparatively recent and uneven. Major social and economic disparities continue to be present within towns and cities as well as between different parts of the country. While India has rapidly moved to the stage of degenerative and man-made diseases, infectious disease epidemics and malnutrition commonly seen in the past have not been fully controlled. As a result, poorer social groups may still be in the age of pestilence and famine and receding pandemics. The same issues of uneven development also apply to the problem of HF in India resulting in a double burden. Like other major public health problems, HF also straddles several different stages in the epidemiological transition. While the incidence of degenerative diseases like coronary artery disease, hypertension, and diabetes mellitus have markedly increased and are the major causes of HF today, infectious conditions like rheumatic heart disease and tuberculous pericarditis still remain widely prevalent and are important causes of HF.[4]

RISK FACTORS

While robust data on HF in India is lacking, reasonable epidemiological data on the prevalence of important risk factors and underlying conditions leading to HF like coronary artery disease, hypertension, diabetes mellitus, and rheumatic heart disease is available from both urban and rural areas. Analysis of these underlying conditions can help us understand the scope of the problem and management issues in India.

Coronary Artery Disease

Coronary artery disease as a cause of left ventricular systolic dysfunction is a common cause of HF in Indians.[1,2] Cross-sectional studies have shown that the prevalence of coronary artery disease has increased over the last 3–4 decades in both urban and rural India. In urban areas, the reported prevalence of coronary artery disease in adults is 7–9.6% while in rural areas it is 1.7–3.5%.[7-11] Scope of the problem is huge considering the 17.5 % of the world's population resides in India (1.22 billion). Thirty million people were estimated to have coronary artery disease in India, in 2000.[4] If we consider that approximately 2% of coronary artery disease patients are likely to develop symptomatic HF each year,[12] around 600,000 new cases of symptomatic HF would be expected to occur due to coronary artery disease alone.

It is well-established that South Asians are at a higher risk of coronary artery disease and get the disease at younger age.[13-15] In the absence of reliable epidemiological data, the increased risk was to a large extent attributable to nonconventional risk factors.[16-17] However, the *interheart* study dispelled the myth of nonconventional risk factors in South Asian population. In this large case control study of 15,152 cases of the first acute myocardial infarction, 2171 of whom were of South Asian descent, the population attributable risk due to the nine conventional risk factors (abnormal lipids, smoking, hypertension, diabetes, abdominal obesity, psychosocial factors, consumption of fruits, vegetables and alcohol, and regular physical activity) was 92%.[18] This was similar to that seen in all other ethnic groups in that study. The first myocardial infarction, however, occurred at a younger age in South Asians. The median age for the first myocardial infarction was 52 years for South Asians as compared to 62 years in Europeans. Also young individuals less than 40 years of age formed 11·7% of the South Asian cohort as compared to only 3.8% among Europeans. We can, therefore, conclude that the Indian patients have their first myocardial infarction at a younger age and that the conventional risk factors are largely responsible for the risk. Two of these risk factors, i.e., elevated apolipoprotein B100/apolipoprotein AI ratio (43.8% vs 31.8%) and history of diabetes (9.5% vs 7.2%) were more common in South Asians as compared to individuals from other countries.[19] It is, therefore, important to target the conventional coronary risk factors in order to cut the risk of HF due to coronary artery disease in the population. The important modifiable risk factors that should be targeted include tobacco use, obesity, hyperlipidemia, hypertension, diabetes mellitus, low consumption of fruits and vegetables, and sedentary lifestyles.[20,21] In addition, increasing access to cardiovascular healthcare in rural areas and to the poorer sections of society could improve outcomes after myocardial infarction and reduce the burden of HF.

Hypertension

The prevalence of hypertension has increased in both rural and urban areas. In epidemiological studies, prevalence of hypertension in adults in urban areas is 30–47% in men and 33–48% in women.[7,22-24] In rural areas, the prevalence is 3–24% in men and 5.8–17% in women.[25,26] As in the West, the prevalence of hypertension in India shows an increase with age with the highest prevalence in the seventh decade.[27] With an adult population of over 600 million, the burden of hypertension is enormous and is probably the most common risk factor for development of HF. Since, it is potentially treatable, effective anti-hypertensive therapy is probably the most important effective public health measure in preventing HF.

Diabetes Mellitus

India has the dubious distinction of having the largest number of diabetics in the world and these numbers are projected to increase markedly in future. From 31.7 million in 2000, the number of diabetics are expected to reach 79.4 million by 2030.[28] This high prevalence of diabetes is attributable to the "Indian phenotype" which includes insulin resistance, higher waist circumference despite a lower body mass index and higher high sensitive C-reactive protein levels. Rapid epidemiological transition to an urban society resulting in decreased physical activity and dietary changes is largely responsible for the increasing prevalence of metabolic syndrome. These factors are also responsible for onset of diabetes at a younger age in Indians.[29,30] In addition, India is also facing a problem of obesity especially in urban areas with 6.8% Indians being obese.[31]

Increasing burden of the major risk factors; hypertension, diabetes mellitus, and obesity is largely attributable to lifestyle changes associated with increased urbanization. These risk factors are more prevalent in urban as compared to rural areas although a significant increase is also seen in rural areas. Lifestyle and dietary changes for primary prevention and adequate treatment of these risk factors is urgently needed to control the increasing burden of HF.

Rheumatic Heart Disease

Rheumatic heart disease continues to be a common cause of HF in India. Prevalence of rheumatic heart disease in school children varies from 1–5.4/1,000.[32-36] According to the 2001 census, children in the age group 7–14 years numbered almost 200 million. This would mean an estimated 0.2–1.8 million cases of rheumatic heart disease in this age group alone. Rheumatic HF contributes significantly to the burden of HF since these patients require frequently hospitalizations. Of the 12 million estimated cases of rheumatic heart disease worldwide in 1994, 3 million required hospitalizations.[37]

Some surveys from India have indicated a decline of rheumatic heart disease in school. These surveys have reported prevalence of 0.5–0.68/1,000.[38-40] These surveys cannot be extrapolated to the entire country since other studies have not shown a decline.[41,42] The incidence of rheumatic fever in school children is 0.17–0.7/1,000 per year.[32,34,35] Such a high incidence of rheumatic fever will continue to add to the burden of rheumatic heart disease and HF. We can, therefore, conclude that there may be a decline in the prevalence in some parts of the country; however, rheumatic fever and rheumatic heart disease are still a major public health problem. Rheumatic heart disease occurs at a younger age in India. Juvenile rheumatic heart disease has several special characteristics. The disease is more severe and rapidly progressive. Mitral stenosis, severe pulmonary artery hypertension, organic tricuspid valve disease, and HF are more common. Juvenile disease presents some unique management problems. Small mitral annular size is a concern while inserting prosthetic valves in children. As a result, smaller size prosthesis is often used in children resulting in higher gradients across the valve. Another important issue is the development of HF during pregnancy in patients with rheumatic heart diseases. Mitral stenosis is the commonest condition presenting during pregnancy and is responsible 71% of valvular lesions.[43] Many of these patient require a balloon mitral valvotomy during pregnancy to prevent and relieve HF.

As in Western countries, improvement of living conditions is likely to reduce the prevalence of rheumatic heart disease ultimately. Early treatment of streptococcal sore throat, penicillin prophylaxis, and availability of affordable valvular surgery to all patients will reduce the burden of HF due to rheumatic heart disease.

Endomyocardial Fibrosis

Endomyocardial fibrosis is reported in only certain parts of India and passes through three phases. An acute phase of myocarditis that presents as a febrile illness, sometimes associated with HF. This acute phase is rarely recognized. In the subacute phase, thrombi form on the damaged endocardium. The chronic phase is characterized by endocardial fibrosis, affecting mainly the apices and the inflow tract of the either or both ventricles resulting in restrictive cardiomyopathy. Common complications include atrioventricular valve regurgitation, atrial fibrillation, and thromboembolism.

Endomyocardial fibrosis is possibly the only cause of HF that has witnessed a definite decline over the past 3 decades.[44,45] This disease was most commonly found in the South Indian coastal state of Kerela, but sporadic cases were reported across India. Even at its peak, endomyocardial fibrosis was not as prevalent as other causes of HF with only 295 cases being registered in a large institute in Kerela over a 16 year period from 1975–1991.[46] It was, however, more common in young and accounted for 2.5% of cardiac admissions below the age of 40 years in the state of Kerala during late 1970s and 1980s.[44] The reasons for the decline in the incidence of endomyocardial fibrosis in Kerala are not clear. During the last 30 years, Kerala has seen a rapid epidemiological transition. Nutritional deficiency disorders have declined. In fact, the problem Kerala now faces is problem of overnutrition. Kerala has the highest prevalence of diabetes mellitus in India. There have been marked improvements in health parameters, economic standards, and literacy. Cassava and plantain are no longer the staple diet. Filariasis, worm infestations, and eosinophilia have also declined. Although, the etiology of endomyocardial fibrosis is not known, all these factors have been implicated in its causation. This epidemiological transition correlates temporally with the decline in the prevalence of endomyocardial fibrosis and is possibly responsible for this decline.

Takayasu Arteritis

Takayasu arteritis is an uncommon cause of HF that may be potentially treatable. HF in Takayasu arteritis is multifactorial. Possible causes of HF include hypertension, stenosis of the aorta, left main coronary artery stenosis, pulmonary artery stenosis, or myocardial involvement in the form of inflammatory myocarditis.[47-49] Hypertension is often refractory and requires high doses of multiple drugs. In patients with aortic stenosis, balloon dilatation or stenting of the lesion results in improvement of left ventricular ejection fraction and relieve HF.[50] Aortic lesions are hard and often result in long segment stenosis. Thus, balloon dilatation of the aorta often requires higher pressures and may have significant residual gradients. Also, patients with long segment stenosis may have restenosis rates as high as 30%.[50]

Heart Failure with Systolic Versus Preserved Left Ventricular Dysfunction

Prevalence of HF with preserved ejection fraction (HFpEF) in India is not known. Physicians in India are far more likely to encounter HF with reduced ejection fraction. The situation may be different from the Western countries where HFpEF or diastolic HF is responsible for almost half the cases of HF. There may be several reasons for these differences. The most important is the age profile of Indian patients. India patients are usually young and as per the 2001 census, individuals more than 60 years of age constitute only 7.5% of the population. HFpEF is predominantly a disease of the elderly. The younger Indian patients are more likely to have systolic HF, particularly because of a higher incidence of coronary artery disease and myocardial infarction, conditions that cause systolic HF. Regurgitant rheumatic valvular lesions and dilated cardiomyopathy also contribute to the burden of systolic HF. It is possible that the physicians in India are missing patients with HFpEF because ejection fraction is not routinely measured in all patients with HF. This situation is likely to change as the Indian population ages and the physicians become aware of the condition. Indians have a high prevalence of hypertension and diabetes. Both these are important risk factors for diastolic HF. As the elderly population increases in number, the incidence of diastolic HF is also likely to increase progressively in future.

Genetic Factors

Unique genetic factors may contribute to HF in the Indian population. The best studied among these is a 25-bp (base pair) deletion in intron 32 of MYBPC3. This particular polymorphism is found exclusively in the Indian subcontinent and in the South East Asian region and is not found in the African and Caucasian population.[51,52] Studies suggest that this deletion arose around 33,000 years ago from a common ancestor and spread throughout the Indian subcontinent . This deletion is seen in around 3–8% of the Indian population and is found in all parts of India except the North East.[51,52] It causes loss of the regular splicing branch point in the intron 32 and results in skipping of exon 33. This results in a change in the amino acid sequence of MYBPC3 that disrupts the cardiomyocyte structure.[52,53] This deletion is associated with dilated, hypertrophic, and restrictive various cardiomyopathies, and is over-represented in patients with cardiomyopathies as compared to controls with an odd's ratio of around 7. The phenotype is characterized by delayed onset of symptoms and is influenced by other risk factors of HF. Presence of this deletion may also aggravate HF due to other etiologies. Patients with coronary artery disease who carry this deletion have a lower ejection fraction.[54] Thus, this deletion increases susceptibility to left ventricular dysfunction. Thus, this common deletion, almost exclusive to the Indian subcontinent contributes significantly to HF. There is an urgent need to assess whether the presence of this mutation affects response to therapy, disease progression, and HF outcomes.

Like other populations, inherited cardiomyopathies also make a significant contribution to the burden of HF in India. No epidemiological data is available on the prevalence of these disorders. Several mutations found in Indians have also been found in other populations.[55,56] In addition, novel mutations, not described in other populations have also been found to cause cardiomyopathies in Indians.[56-58] The clinical implications of these novel mutations needs further study.

MANAGEMENT

Several ethnic differences have been reported in the responsiveness to HF medications. Thus it cannot be assumed that treatments shown to work for Caucasians will be equally efficacious for patients from other ethnic groups.[59-61] Indian patients have constituted only a very tiny proportion of patients in clinical trials on HF, although this situation is rapidly changing. No large HF clinical trials on the standard of care drugs and devices have been carried out exclusively in Indian patients. Data on Indian patients can thus only be derived from the subgroup analyses of some multinational trials. There are 19 drug trials on HF registered with the clinical trials registry, India, or with www.clinicaltrials.gov, which have Indian sites. Most of these trials are studying newer investigational drugs. EMPHASIS-HF was the only trial that assessed the effect of epleronone, a standard of care drug, in Indian patients.[62] Even in this trial, data on Indian patients was not reported separately. Indian patients has been clubbed together with Asians and Africans patients in the subgroup analysis, which showed that effect of eplerenone in this subgroup was no different from that in the entire population.[62] Therefore, in view of the sparse data, it is difficult to make any firm conclusions about the responsiveness of Indians to standard HF medications. The clinical impression is that Indian subpopulations do not show any differences in the responses to standard HF medications and these drugs work just as well in Indian patients.[62] Realiable data on the usage of drugs in Indians with HF is not available. Affordability and accessibility to medical care are the most important factors that may limit the optimal use of drug therapy. Analysis of the coronary artery database suggests that significant proportion of patients do not receive medications as per the guidelines.[63,64] In addition, dosage of beta blockers and angiotensin-converting-enzyme (ACE) inhibitors prescribed may be lower than recommended. However, analysis of the MUSIC (multicentre ultrasound study in coronaries) trial, a devise based study conducted in India, showed that used of angiotensin converting enzyme inhibitor (ACEI)/angiotensin receptor blocker (ARB) and betablockers in Indian patients with moderate severe HF is similar to that reported in the Western patients, at least in the setting of a clinical trial. [65] There is a wide variation in the quality of care. Hospitals attached to medical colleges are more likely to adhere to guidelines.[66] Increasing adherence to guidelines is a simple measure that is likely to improve outcomes.

Implantable cardioverter-defibrillators and cardiac resynchronization devices have a very low usage in India.[67,68] In 2008, only 700 implantable cardioverter-defibrillators and 600 cardiac resynchronization devices were implanted in India.[68] This would imply a cardioverter-defibrillator implant rate of less than 1/million when compared as compared to an implant rate of 300/million population in the United States.[68] Though the number of implants are increasing each year, vast majority of patients who would benefit from these implants still do not receive them. The main factor limiting the use of these implants is the high cost, however, this is not the only factor. Even if we assume that 10% of Indians have access to these devices, an implant rate of around 10–20/million population would be expected. This implies that increasing access to tertiary healthcare and physician education can optimize device use even within existing resources. In view of high costs, explanted implantable cardioverter-defibrillators have been successfully reused in India.[69] Explanted devices with remaining battery life are frequently reused after resterilization without an increased risk for complications. These devices have functioned normally and delivered appropriate life-saving therapies.[69]

REFERENCES

1. Joshi R, Cardona M, Iyengar S, et al. Chronic diseases now a leading cause of death in rural India—mortality data from the Andhra Pradesh Rural Health Initiative. Int J Epidemiol. 2006;35:1522-9.
2. Indian Council of Medical Research (2009), Study on causes of death by verbal autopsy in India. [online]. Available from: www.icmr.nic.in/final/causes_death/causes_death.htm. [Accessed December, 2012].
3. Vakil RJ. A statistical study of 1281 cases of congestive cardiac failure or myocardial insufficiency in India. Indian Physician. 1949;8:281-9.
4. Huffman MD, Prabhakaran D. Heart failure: epidemiology and prevention in India. Natl Med J India. 2010;23:283-8.
5. Omran AR. The epidemiologic transition: a theory of the epidemiology of population change. 1971. Milbank Q. 2005;83:731-57.
6. Yusuf S, Ounpuu S, Anand S. The global epidemic of atherosclerotic cardiovascular disease. Med Princ Pract. 2002;11 Suppl 2:3-8.
7. Gupta R, Gupta VP, Sarna M, et al. Prevalence of coronary heart disease and risk factors in an urban Indian population: Jaipur Heart Watch-2. Indian Heart J. 2002;54:59-66.
8. Chadha SL, Radhakrishnan S, Ramachandran K, et al. Epidemiological study of coronary heart disease in urban population of Delhi. Indian J Med Res. 1990;92:424-30.
9. Kumar R, Singh MC, Singh MC, et al. Urbanization and coronary heart disease: a study of urban-rural differences in northern India. Indian Heart J. 2006;58:126-30.
10. Wander GS, Khurana SB, Gulati R, et al. Epidemiology of coronary heart disease in a rural Punjab population—prevalence and correlation with various risk factors. Indian Heart J 1994;46:319-23. J Clin Epidemiol. 1997;50:203-9.
11. Gupta R, Prakash H, Gupta VP, et al. Prevalence and determinants of coronary heart disease in a rural population of India. J Clin Epidemiol. 1997;50(2):203-9.
12. Yusuf S, Sleight P, Pogue J, et al. Effects of an angiotensin-converting-enzyme inhibitor, ramipril, on cardiovascular events in high-risk patients. The Heart Outcomes Prevention Evaluation Study Investigators. N Engl J Med. 2000 20;342:145-53.
13. Balarajan R. Ethnic differences in mortality from ischaemic heart disease and cerebrovascular disease in England and Wales. BMJ. 1991;302:560-4.
14. Enas EA, Yusuf S, Mehta JL. Prevalence of coronary artery disease in Asian Indians. Am J Cardiol. 1992;70:945-9.
15. Enas EA, Garg A, Davidson MA, et al. Coronary heart disease and its risk factors in first-generation immigrant Asian Indians to the United States of America. Indian Heart J. 1996;48:343-53.
16. Enas EA. Hypertriglyceridemia and elevated lipoprotein(a) are major risk factors for coronary events in middle-aged men. Am J Cardiol. 1996;78:859-60.
17. Puri A, Gupta OK, Dwivedi RN, et al. Homocysteine and lipid levels in young patients with coronary artery disease. J Assoc Physicians India. 2003;51:681-5.
18. Yusuf S, Hawken S, Ounpuu S, et al. Effect of potentially modifiable risk factors associated with myocardial infarction in 52 countries (the INTERHEART study): case-control study. Lancet. 2004;364:937-52.
19. Joshi P, Islam S, Pais P, et al. Risk factors for early myocardial infarction in South Asians compared with individuals in other countries. JAMA. 2007;297:286-94.
20. Prabhakaran D, Singh K. Premature coronary heart disease risk factors & reducing the CHD burden in India. Indian J Med Res. 2011;134:8-9.
21. Ajay VS, Prabhakaran D. Coronary heart disease in Indians: implications of the INTERHEART study. Indian J Med Res. 2010;132:561-6.
22. Gupta R, Guptha S, Gupta VP, et al. Prevalence and determinants of hypertension in the urban population of Jaipur in western India. J Hypertens. 1995;13:1193-200.
23. Gupta PC, Gupta R, Pednekar MS. Hypertension prevalence and blood pressure trends in 88,653 subjects in Mumbai, India. J Hum Hypertens. 2004;18:907-10.
24. Joseph A, Kutty VR, Soman CR. High risk for coronary heart disease in Thiruvananthapuram city: a study of serum lipids and other risk factors. Indian Heart J. 2000;52:29-35.
25. Gupta R, Sharma AK. Prevalence of hypertension and subtypes in an Indian rural population: clinical and electrocardiographic correlates. J Hum Hypertens. 1994;8:823-9.
26. Malhotra P, Kumari S, Kumar R, et al. Prevalence and determinants of hypertension in an un-industrialised rural population of North India. J Hum Hypertens. 1999;13:467-72.
27. Yadav S, Boddula R, Genitta G, et al. Prevalence & risk factors of pre-hypertension & hypertension in an affluent north Indian population. Indian J Med Res. 2008;128:712-20.
28. Wild S, Roglic G, Green A, et al. Global prevalence of diabetes: estimates for the year 2000 and projections for 2030. Diabetes Care. 2004;27:1047-53.
29. Ramachandran A, Snehalatha C, Kapur A, et al. High prevalence of diabetes and impaired glucose tolerance in India: National Urban Diabetes Survey. Diabetologia. 2001;44:1094-101.
30. Mohan V, Deepa M, Deepa R, et al. Secular trends in the prevalence of diabetes and impaired glucose tolerance in urban South India—the Chennai Urban Rural Epidemiology Study (CURES-17). Diabetologia. 2006;49:1175-8.
31. Reddy KS, Prabhakaran D, Shah P, et al. Differences in body mass index and waist: hip ratios in North Indian rural and urban populations. Obes Rev. 2002:197-202.
32. Grover A, Dhawan A, Iyengar SD, et al. Epidemiology of rheumatic fever and rheumatic heart disease in a rural community in northern India. Bull World Health Organ. 1993;71:59-66.
33. Padmavati S. Present status of rheumatic fever and rheumatic heart disease in India. Indian Heart J. 1995;47:395-8.
34. Avasthi G, Singh D, Singh C, Aggarwal SP, Bidwai PS, Avasthi R. "Prevalence survey of rheumatic fever (RF) and rheumatic heart disease (Rhd) in urban & rural school children in Ludhiana". Indian Heart J 1987;39:26-8.
35. Patel DC, Patel NI, Patel JD, et al. Rheumatic fever and rheumatic heart disease in school children of Anand. J Assoc Physicians India. 1986;34:837-9.
36. Indian Council of Medical Research. Community control of rheumatic fever and rheumatic heart disease. Report of ICMR task force study. New Delhi: Indian Council of Medical Research; 1994.
37. World Health Organization. Rheumatic fever and rheumatic heart disease: Report of a WHO expert consultation. World Health Organ Tech Rep Ser. 2004;923:1-122.
38. Jose VJ, Gomathi M. Declining prevalence of rheumatic heart disease in rural schoolchildren in India: 2001-2002. Indian Heart J 2003;55:158-60.
39. Misra M, Mittal M, Singh R, et al. Prevalence of rheumatic heart disease in school-going children of Eastern Uttar Pradesh. Indian Heart J. 2007;59:42-3.
40. Periwal KL, Gupta BK, Panwar RB, et al. Prevalence of rheumatic heart disease in school children in Bikaner: an echocardiographic study. J Assoc Physicians India. 2006;54:279-82.

41. Mishra TK, Routray SN, Behera M, et al. Has the prevalence of rheumatic fever/rheumatic heart disease really changed? A hospital-based study. Indian Heart J. 2003;55:152-7.
42. Deshpande J, Vaideeswar P, Amonkar G, et al. Rheumatic heart disease in the past decade: an autopsy analysis. Indian Heart J. 2002;54:676-80.
43. Guleria R, Vasisht K, Dhall GI, et al. Pregnancy with heart disease. Experience at Postgraduate Institute of Medical Education and Research, Chandigarh. J Assoc Physicians India 1990;38:902-6.
44. Vijayaraghavan G, Sivasankaran S. Tropical endomyocardial fibrosis in India: A vanishing disease! Indian J Med Res. 2012;136:729-38.
45. Sivasankaran S. Restrictive cardiomyopathy in India: the story of a vanishing mystery. Heart.. 2009;95:9-14.
46. Valiathan MS, Somers K, Kartha CC. Endomyocardial fibrosis. Delhi: Oxford University Press; 1993.
47. Talwar KK, Kumar K, Chopra P, et al. Cardiac involvement in nonspecific aortoarteritis (Takayasu's arteritis). Am Heart J. 1991;122:1666-70.
48. Panja M, Kar AK, Dutta AL, et al. Cardiac involvement in non-specific aorto-arteritis. Int J Cardiol. 1992;34:289-95.
49. Sharma BK, Jain S, Radotra BD. An autopsy study of Takayasu arteritis in India. Int J Cardiol. 1998;66 Suppl 1:S85-90; discussion S91.
50. Tyagi S, Khan AA, Kaul UA, et al. Percutaneous transluminal angioplasty for stenosis of the aorta due to aortic arteritis in children. Pediatr Cardiol. 1999;20:404-10.
51. Simonson TS, Zhang Y, Huff CD, et al. Limited distribution of a cardiomyopathy-associated variant in India. Ann Hum Genet. 2010;74: 184-8.
52. Dhandapany PS, Sadayappan S, Xue Y, et al. A common MYBPC3 (cardiac myosin binding protein C) variant associated with cardiomyopathies in South Asia. Nat Genet. 2009;41:187-91.
53. Waldmüller S, Sakthivel S, Saadi AV, et al. Novel deletions in MYH7 and MYBPC3 identified in Indian families with familial hypertrophic cardiomyopathy. J Mol Cell Cardiol. 2003;35:623-36.
54. Srivastava A, Garg N, Mittal T, et al. Association of 25 bp deletion in MYBPC3 gene with left ventricle dysfunction in coronary artery disease patients. PLoS One. 2011;6:e24123.
55. Rai TS, Ahmad S, Ahluwalia TS, et al. Genetic and clinical profile of Indian patients of idiopathic restrictive cardiomyopathy with and without hypertrophy. Mol Cell Biochem. 2009;331:187-92.
56. Rai TS, Ahmad S, Bahl A, et al. Genotype phenotype correlations of cardiac beta-myosin heavy chain mutations in Indian patients with hypertrophic and dilated cardiomyopathy. Mol Cell Biochem. 2009;321:189-96.
57. Boda U, Vadapalli S, Calambur N, et al. Novel mutations in beta-myosin heavy chain, actin and troponin-I genes associated with dilated cardiomyopathy in Indian population. J Genet. 2009;88:373-7.
58. Pamuru PR, Maithili DV, Mohiuddin K, et al. Novel mutations in arrhythmogenic right ventricular cardiomyopathy from Indian population. Indian J Hum Genet. 2011;17:70-6.
59. Carson P, Ziesche S, Johnson G, et al. Racial differences in response to therapy for heart failure: analysis of the vasodilator-heart failure trials. Vasodilator-Heart Failure Trial Study Group. J Card Fail. 1999;5: 178-87.
60. Exner DV, Dries DL, Domanski MJ, et al. Lesser response to angiotensin-converting-enzyme inhibitor therapy in black as compared with white patients with left ventricular dysfunction. N Engl J Med.. 2001; 344:1351-7.
61. Domanski MJ, Krause-Steinrauf H, Massie BM, et al. A comparative analysis of the results from 4 trials of beta-blocker therapy for heart failure: BEST, CIBIS-II, MERIT-HF, and COPERNICUS. J Card Fail. 2003;9:354-63.
62. Zannad F, McMurray JJ, Krum H, et al. Eplerenone in patients with systolic heart failure and mild symptoms. N Engl J Med. 2011;364:11-21.
63. Mendis S, Abegunde D, Yusuf S, et al. WHO study on Prevention of recurrences of myocardial infarction and stroke (WHO-premise). Bull World Health Organ. 2005;83:820-9.
64. Karthikeyan G, Xavier D, Prabhakaran D, et al. Perspectives on the management of coronary artery disease in India. Heart. 2007;93:1334-8.
65. Anand IS, Tang WH, Greenberg BH, et al. Design and performance of a multisensor heart failure monitoring algorithm: results from the multisensor monitoring in congestive heart failure (MUSIC) study. J Card Fail. 2012;18(4):289-95.
66. George E, Hunsberger S, Savitha D, et al. Treatment of acute myocardial infarction: does the type of hospital make a difference? PPAMI Study Group. Indian Heart J. 1999;51:161-6.
67. Sethi KK, Dhall A. Optimal utilization of defibrillators and CRT in India—awareness, guidelines and financing—the cardiologist's viewpoint. Indian Heart J. 2011;63:347-50.
68. Mehra R, Dasgupta S, Radhakrishnan R. Optimal use of defibrillators and CRT in India—awareness, guidelines and finances: the industry view point. Indian Heart J. 2011;63:351-5.
69. Pavri BB, Lokhandwala Y, Kulkarni GV, et al. Reuse of explanted, resterilized implantable cardioverter-defibrillators: a cohort study. Ann Intern Med. 2012;157:542-8.

Chapter 44

Heart Failure in India: Clinical Perspective

Hardeep K Grewal, Manish Bansal, Ravi R Kasliwal

ABSTRACT

Heart failure (HF) is rapidly growing into an enormous health problem in India. Ironically, while the prevalence of atherosclerotic vascular disease continues to rise in India, the infectious diseases, such as rheumatic heart disease (RHD) and cardiac tuberculosis also remain widely prevalent. These etiological differences, coupled with the socioeconomic characteristics, account for the differences observed in the clinical presentation, overall diagnostic work-up and management of HF in Indian patients.

INTRODUCTION

India is currently facing the epidemic of cardiovascular diseases (CVD), with more than half of the world's heart disease population already living in India. Greater genetic propensity and rapid economic growth with resultant lifestyle changes have been attributed as the causes of rapid increase in the burden of CVD in India. At the same time, nonuniform economic growth and poor health care infrastructure have ensured that the pretransition diseases, such as RHD also remain equally prevalent. The combination of these factors is resulting in an exponential increase in the incidence and prevalence of HF which has rapidly grown into one of the biggest health challenges of our time.

While clinical presentation, diagnostic work-up, and management of HF in Indian patients is largely similar to that in the western countries, there are several distinct aspects of HF in India related primarily to the underlying etiology and the socioeconomic environment prevalent in India (Table 1). This chapter highlights how these differences impact day-to-day management of HF in Indian patients.

EPIDEMIOLOGY OF HEART FAILURE IN INDIA

As discussed above, India is experiencing the dual burden of lifestyle-related disorders, such as hypertension, diabetes, obesity, and CVD as well as pretransition diseases, such as RHD, chronic constrictive pericarditis (CCP), anemia, etc., which together are the major determinants of HF burden in India. Based on the disease-specific estimates of prevalence and incidence rates of HF, it is estimated that the prevalence of HF in India due to coronary artery disease (CAD), hypertension, obesity, diabetes, and RHD ranges from 1.3 million to 4.6 million, with an annual incidence of 0.5–1.8 million.[1] The prevalence of HF is uniformly high, irrespective of the gender and rural-urban distribution. More importantly, while HF in Western populations is predominantly a disease of elderly, it tends to occur at a much younger age in Indian patients. Both, a high prevalence of diseases like RHD and CCP, as well as earlier occurrence of CVD in Indians are responsible for younger age-onset of HF in India. It is estimated that out of total CVD deaths in India, approximately 52% occur below the age of 70 years in comparison to only 23% in the developed nations.[2]

TABLE 1: Salient differences in the characteristics of heart failure patients in India as compared to the developed countries

Characteristic	Differences
Major etiologies	CAD and RHD are the most common causes, unlike the developed countries where RHD is uncommon. CCP, EMF, anemia, other nutritional deficiencies, etc. are also common
Age of onset	Onset at younger age is common in India
Presenting symptoms	Atrial fibrillation is more common. Previous history suggestive of acute rheumatic fever is also common. Constitutional symptoms of tuberculosis will be present in patients with CCP
Examination findings	Evidence of nutritional deficiencies and atrial fibrillation are common. Valvular involvement is common and the clinical findings vary accordingly. Peripheral signs of acute rheumatic fever and infective endocarditis can also be seen
Diagnostic work-up	Detailed diagnostic work-up often not possible due to financial constraints. However, evidence of valvular and pericardial diseases needs to be actively looked for in younger patients
Prognosis and management	HF in India is often due to treatable causes such as RHD, CCP, etc. and hence these patients have better prognosis if managed appropriately. However, affordability and availability of advanced treatment modalities is an issue. In addition, certain ethnic variations exist in the drug management of HF

CAD, coronary artery disease; RHD, rheumatic heart disease; CCP, chronic constrictive pericarditis; EMF, endomyocardial fibrosis; HF, heart failure

COMMON CAUSES OF HEART FAILURE IN INDIA

A host of clinical conditions can result in development of HF. Among them, the most common encountered in Indian patients are:

- Coronary artery disease
- Valvular heart disease (RHD being the most common etiology)
- CCP (the most often tubercular)
- Cardiomyopathies, including dilated cardiomyopathy, endomyocardial fibrosis (EMF), etc.
- Myocarditis
- Diastolic HF as in diabetes, hypertension, and chronic kidney disease
- Nutritional deficiencies like anemia, beriberi, etc.

Coronary artery disease is currently the leading cause of death and also the leading cause of HF in India. It is estimated that roughly 120,000–690,000 Indians could develop symptomatic HF due to CAD every year.[3,4] Hypertension, diabetes, and obesity are estimated to further contribute upto almost 1.2 million HF patients every year.

However, unlike the Western countries, acute rheumatic fever, chronic RHD, CCP, and EMF contribute to a sizeable portion of HF in India, and are particularly common in young individuals. The prevalence rates for RHD remain high in India, reaching 1.0–5.4 cases per 1,000 school children in one study.[5] RHD is the most common cause of valvular heart disease in India and a major source of morbidity and mortality. Approximately 98,000 people died from RHD in India in 2004, which would add to the total estimated HF prevalence given above.[6] CCP is yet another common cause of HF in India and is most often caused by tuberculosis.[7-9] In contrast, the etiology of CCP in the Western world has undergone a significant change over the years, with tuberculosis reported in only 0–1% of cases in some recent series.[10,11] The leading identifiable causes of CCP in developed countries include postcardiac surgery, radiation therapy, and viral pericarditis, all of which are relatively less important causes of CCP in Indian patients.

CLINICAL PRESENTATION

The aforementioned etiological differences as well as socioeconomic circumstances result in several distinct differences in the clinical presentation of HF in India, which need to be recognized.

The patients usually present late in the course of illness because of lack of awareness and limited healthcare facilities. There is often history of irregular treatment under the guidance of local medical practitioners who may not be adequately trained and skilled to manage such patients. As a result, by the time patient presents to an appropriate healthcare facility, the disease is already fairly advanced and is, therefore, associated with much worse clinical outcomes.

A thorough and intelligent clinical examination is critical to optimum management of HF patients. It will not only establish the diagnosis of HF, but also provide information that may have significant prognostic and therapeutic implications. Importance of detailed history and physical examination is even greater in developing countries like India where diagnostic tests are not readily available and affordability is always an issue.

The clinical features of HF in most etiologies are generally common. Depending on the nature and the severity of HF, the patients can present with symptoms, such as dyspnea, orthopnea, paroxysmal nocturnal dyspnea, easy fatigability, leg edema, and generalized body swelling. The common physical findings are tachycardia, tachypnea, raised jugular venous pulse, hepatomegaly, loud pulmonary component of second heart sound, audible left or right third heart sound, and basal crepitations. However, in addition to these, there may be certain clues in the history and clinical examination that can hint toward the underlying etiology (Flowchart 1).

Acute rheumatic fever can present with HF if there is carditis and valvulitis. Patients are usually young with history of pharyngitis for 2–4 weeks. There may be chest discomfort due to pericardial involvement. The discomfort is usually pleuritic in nature and a pericardial rub can often be heard on auscultation. In addition, cardiac examination may reveal new or changing murmurs. Because mitral regurgitation is the most common lesion in acute rheumatic fever, systolic murmur is the most commonly heard murmur. Isolated aortic regurgitation and hemodynamically significant stenotic lesions are unusual. In addition to the features of HF, patients often have noncardiac symptoms also. Joint pains and swelling involving predominantly knees, elbows, ankles, and wrist joints may be seen and are usually migratory in nature.

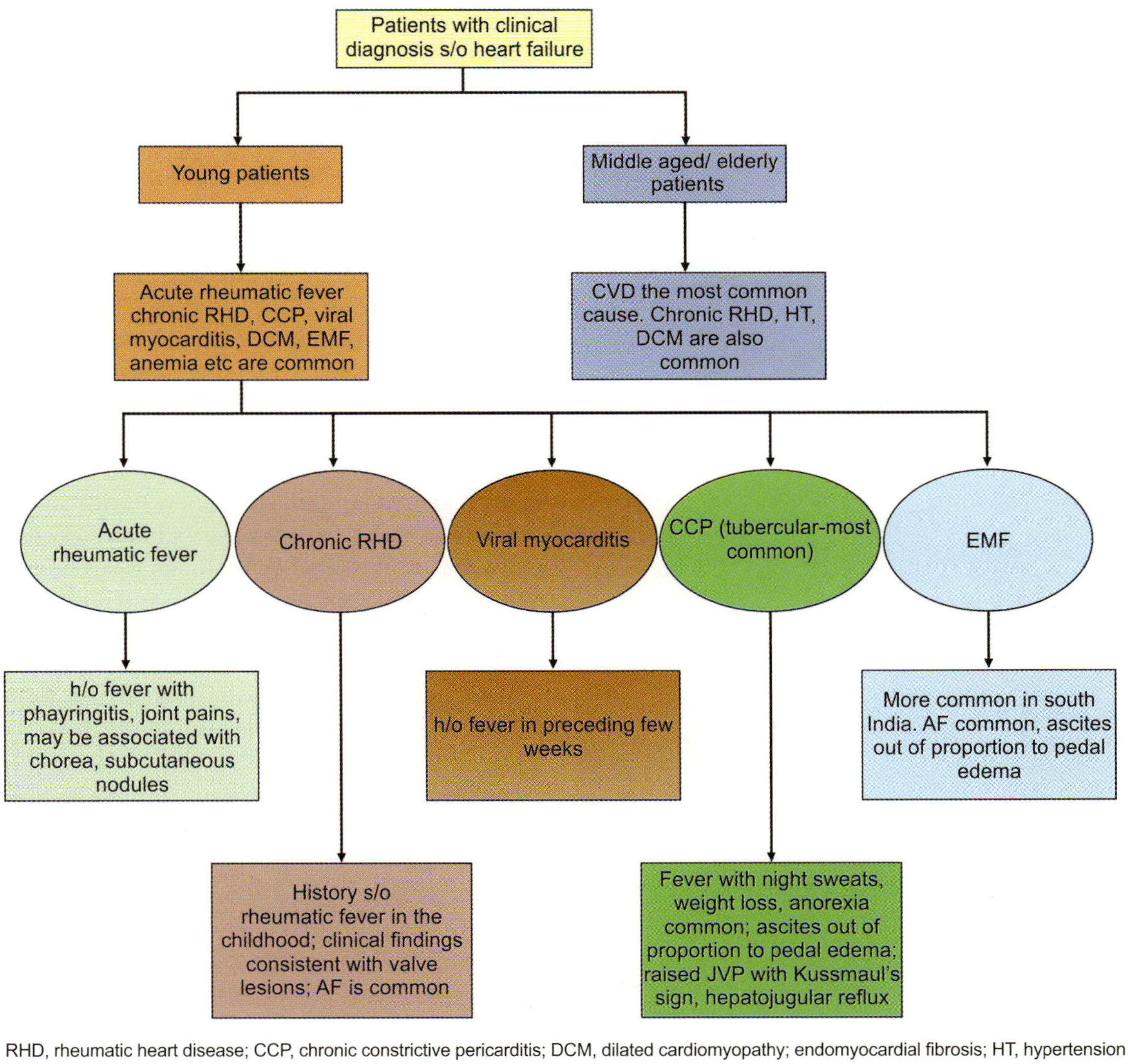

Flowchart 1 Salient clinical features helpful in suggesting the underlying etiology of heart failure in Indian patients

Subcutaneous nodules and erythema marginatum are also relatively more common in patients with carditis. Subcutaneous nodules are painless, firm collections of collagen fibers over bones or tendons, and commonly appear on the back of the wrist, the outside elbow, and the front of the knees (Fig. 1). Erythema marginatum is characterized by erythematous, macular, non-pruritic, non-indurated rash with pale centers and rounded or serpiginous margins, which blanches completely on pressing (Fig. 2). These lesions are commonly seen in bathing-suit distribution, occurring mainly on the trunk and proximal extremities but not on the face or below elbows and knees. In patients with dark complexion, these lesions can be easily missed as they are not that prominent. Sydenham's chorea or chorea minor (also referred to as Saint Vitus' dance) is a late manifestation of acute rheumatic fever, occurring upto 6 months after the acute infection, but may occasionally be the presenting symptom of rheumatic fever. It is characterized by rapid, uncoordinated jerking movements affecting primarily the face, feet, and hands; is reported to occur in 20–30% of patients with acute rheumatic fever, and is more common in females.

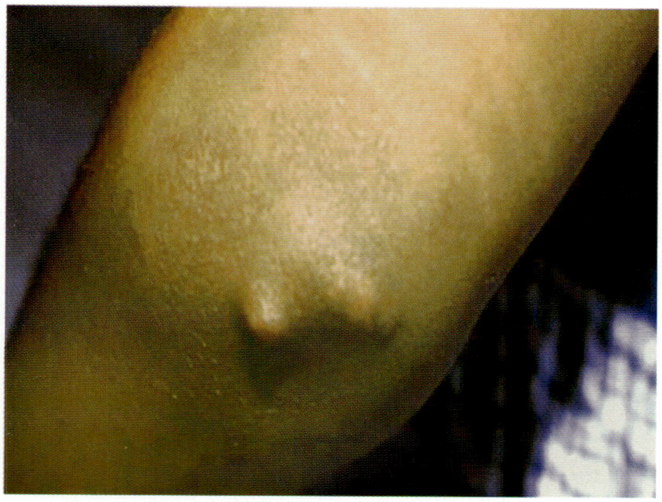

Fig. 1 Subcutaneous nodules seen in acute rheumatic fever

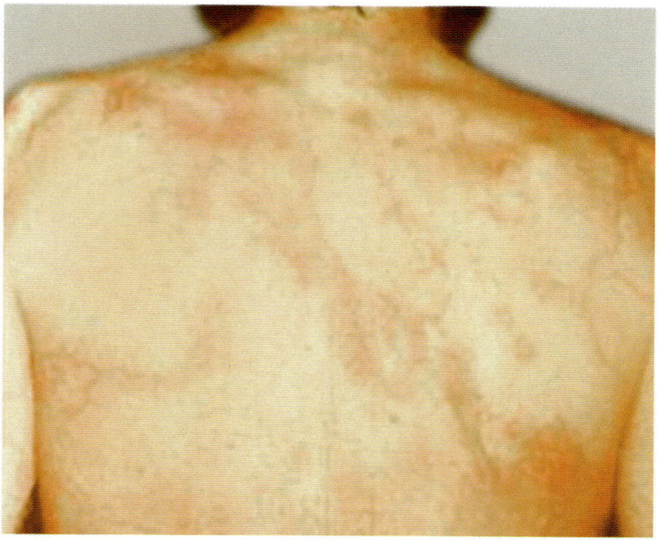

Fig. 2 Erythema marginatum of acute rheumatic fever

Chronic RHD is the most common form of valvular heart disease seen in India. Approximately 25% of all patients with RHD have isolated mitral stenosis and 40% have both mitral stenosis and mitral regurgitation.[12] Nearly 40% of the patients with mitral stenosis also have associated valvular involvement with aortic valve involvement in 35% and tricuspid valve involvement seen in 6% of patients. Pulmonary valve is rarely involved. In contrast, aortic valve involvement is invariably associated with mitral valve involvement. Two-thirds of all the patients with rheumatic mitral stenosis are females,[13] whereas mitral regurgitation is more common in males. The patients can present at any age, with the most common age of presentation being third to fifth decades. However, severe mitral stenosis can develop even in children as young as 6–12 years. This entity, which is known as juvenile mitral stenosis, was first described in India and is particularly common in this subcontinent.

The most common symptom in RHD is dyspnea and usually the first episode of dyspnea is precipitated by fever, anemia, exercise, pregnancy, or atrial fibrillation. Atrial fibrillation is common in patients with mitral stenosis and the prevalence increases with age. General physical examination may also reveal malar rash (brownish tint or flush), seen on face, cheeks, ears, and nose. It is observed in patients with chronic mitral stenosis, and is caused by veno-capillary metastasis due to persistently low cardiac output. The cardiovascular (CV) examination will reveal findings commensurate with the type and severity of valvular involvement. Of note, presence of audible opening snap is an important finding in patients with mitral stenosis and indicates a pliable valve which is likely to be suitable for balloon mitral valvotomy.

The patients with valve diseases can present with infective endocarditis also, which often leads to acute worsening and precipitates HF. There are several important clinical features of infective endocarditis including anemia, petechiae, clubbing, janeway lesions, Osler's nodes, etc., many of which may not be commonly seen. Janeway lesions—one of the minor criteria of Duke's criteria for diagnosis of infective endocarditis—are small erythematous or hemorrhagic, painless, non-tender macular lesions on the palms and soles, and develop as a consequence of septic embolization (Fig. 3). Osler's nodes too are among the minor criteria for diagnosis of infective endocarditis but are tender subcutaneous nodules seen on the pads of fingers or toes and palms or soles (Fig. 4). Both of these lesions are seen in roughly 6–10% of the patients.

Chronic constrictive pericarditis, unlike other causes of HF, has several unique clinical features. In CCP, ascites occur earlier than peripheral edema and is out of proportion to edema. Exertional dyspnea and orthopnea are other common symptoms of CCP but acute-onset chest pain typical of pericarditis is unusual. In India, as tuberculosis is still the most common underlying etiology and, therefore, the patients often present with constitutional symptoms also, such as fever, night sweats, malaise, loss of appetite and weight loss.

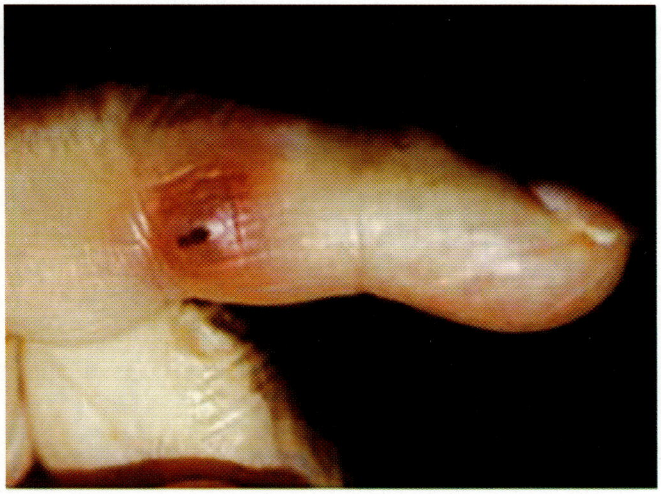

Fig. 3 Janeway lesions seen in infective endocarditis

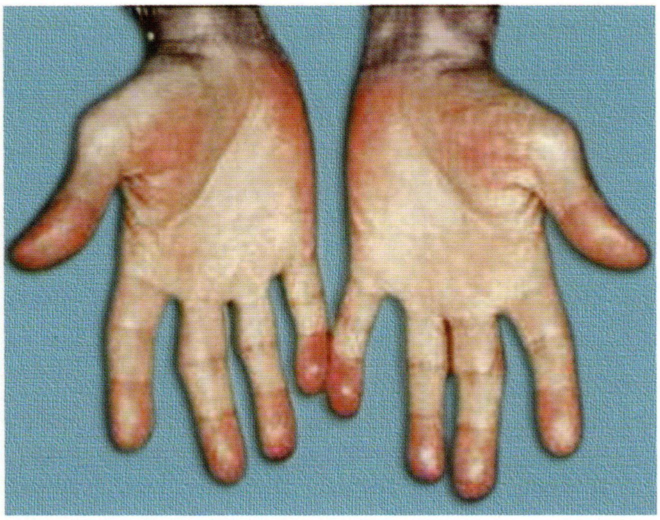

Fig. 4 Osler's nodes seen in infective endocarditis

Endomyocardial fibrosis was a common medical problem in South India but the incidence has now decreased. The early part of the disease is rarely clinically recognized in India and most patients come to clinical attention in the chronic burnt-out phase. The triad of elevated jugular venous pulse, ascites, and hepatomegaly forms the hallmark of right ventricular EMF, which can also present with cyanosis and clubbing because of stretch opening of foramen ovale. Similar to CCP, ascites in EMF is also out of proportion to pedal edema. In contrast, mild cardiomegaly, loud left ventricular third heart sound, short systolic murmur and severe pulmonary hypertension are the classical features of left ventricular EMF.

In high output HF, patients are likely to have warm rather than cold peripheries. Anemia is one of the common causes of high output cardiac failure. Another common condition causing high output cardiac failure is beriberi (wet beriberi with CV involvement) disease caused by thiamine deficiency. A more rapid form of wet beriberi is termed as acute fulminant CV beriberi, or Shoshin's beriberi. In this condition, edema may not be present. Instead, cyanosis of the hands and feet, tachycardia, distended neck veins, restlessness, and anxiety occur.

INVESTIGATIONS

In a developing country like India where cost is an important factor, the most cost-effective diagnostic modality would be a complete history and physical examination. Nevertheless, investigations are invariably required to not only confirm the diagnosis, but also to characterize the nature and severity of the disease which is essential for planning appropriate treatment strategy.

Electrocardiogram (ECG) should be performed in all patients suspected of having HF. Though abnormal findings on ECG are not specific for a diagnosis of HF, a normal ECG is rarely seen in patients with HF. More importantly, in Indian scenario, presence of atrial fibrillation or evidence of left atrial enlargement and/or right ventricular hypertrophy in a young patient presenting with HF will strongly suggest the possibility of rheumatic mitral stenosis. In patients with acute rheumatic carditis, ECG may reveal prolonged PR interval.

Chest X-ray is another cost-effective, diagnostic modality in the initial evaluation of HF. Besides features of pulmonary edema, certain findings can point toward specific etiology. In mitral stenosis, there is left atrial enlargement which causes straightening of left heart border and "double density" in the midportion of the cardiac silhouette on the frontal view. The cardiac size is usually normal. In tubercular constrictive pericarditis, pericardial calcification is an uncommon but important radiological finding. In addition, pleural effusion is common in these patients and is often bilateral. Chest X-ray may also reveal evidence of concurrent pulmonary tuberculosis.

Biochemical markers, particularly natriuretic peptides, may be quite helpful in establishing the diagnosis of HF when there is dilemma between cardiac or non-cardiac causes of dyspnea. However, because of the cost constraints, in Indian setting, biochemical markers are often not utilized for this purpose.

Echocardiography remains the most important diagnostic modality in patients with HF, and provides comprehensive information about cardiac structure, function and intracardiac hemodynamics. Such information is extremely useful in guiding therapeutic strategy, as well as monitoring response to treatment in these patients. For these reasons, coupled with the noninvasive nature and safety, echocardiography is today the cornerstone of diagnostic work-up of any patient presenting with suspected cardiac illness. Unfortunately, echocardiography is not performed in many patients with HF in rural India because of lack of availability as well as affordability.

MANAGEMENT

Heart failure is a progressive disorder, extending through the stages of initially asymptomatic to very symptomatic, severe HF in the late stages. Accordingly, the management of HF also has several components, depending on the disease stage, ranging from lifestyle modification to use of drugs, and lastly to devices and surgery. The American College of Cardiology/American Heart Association has described four stages of HF and the physicians in India can use the same paradigm for guiding management of HF in their own practice. Special emphasis needs to be given on early recognition of HF patients because if the patients are identified during the initial stages and treatment is instituted, that will effectively reduce the morbidity and mortality arising from HF. This is particularly important in developing countries like India where healthcare facilities are limited and advanced therapies required at advanced stages of disease are either not available at many places or not feasible because of financial constraints.

Once a patient has been identified to have HF, then the treatment is instituted as per the stage of HF in which patient has presented. The basic principles that need to be followed include:

- It is important to identify the underlying etiology which has led to the development of HF. As discussed above, RHD and CCP are common and treatable causes of HF in India and should not be missed. It is common to come across patients of HF who are receiving treatment from local practitioners for temporary relief of symptoms without being evaluated thoroughly
- In addition, it is equally important to recognize clinical conditions which can either lead to HF or precipitate HF of other etiologies:
    - Nutritional deficiencies like anemia and beriberi are common in India which can be easily corrected. Similarly, hormonal disorders like thyroid disorders can also lead to HF and need to be recognized
    - Identify risk factors like hypertension, diabetes, dyslipidemia, and treat appropriately
    - Identify rhythm disturbances like atrial fibrillation. As discussed, atrial fibrillation is usually seen in elderly patients but in India, even younger patients who have underlying rheumatic mitral valve disease can develop atrial fibrillation. Control of heart rate, reversion to sinus rhythm if required, and anticoagulation are very helpful in improving symptomatic status and preventing thromboembolic complications in these patients
- *Pharmacotherapy*: Till 1980s, HF management consisted predominantly of bed rest, digoxin and diuretics. But now with the availability of better cardioprotective medicines like beta-blockers, angiotensin-converting enzyme (ACE) inhibitors, angiotensin-receptor blockers (ARBs), and aldosterone antagonists, there has been substantial reduction in morbidity and mortality from HF. Unfortunately, their use in India, especially in rural populations, is significantly limited with most of the patients still being treated with drugs aimed at symptomatic relief only, such as diuretics. Drugs like beta-blockers and ACE inhibitors with effect on mortality and long-term survival are not routinely taken by most patients. Lack of awareness among treating physicians, cost considerations, and false beliefs among patients are

the major reasons responsible for the under use of these potentially lifesaving drugs in India. In a study it was found that Indians were less compliant to HF drugs[14] and almost two-thirds of Indo-Asians felt that God or fate controlled their health rather than the treating doctors.[15] Besides these general principles underlying pharmacological management of HF, there are important points related to each of the individual classes of drugs that need to be considered:

- *Diuretics*: Diuretics relieve symptoms and signs of pulmonary and systemic venous congestion in patients with HF. Though torsemide is more potent than furosemide and side effects are also less with torsemide, furosemide is cheaper than torsemide. Therefore, compliance is likely to be better with furosemide, which may be a preferable option.
- *ACE inhibitors and ARBs*: ACE inhibitors should be prescribed to all patients with symptomatic HF and left ventricular ejection fraction (LVEF) less than 40%, if there is no contraindication. The available data do not suggest superiority of any particular ACE inhibitor. Hence, a cheaper ACE inhibitor, such as enalapril should be used to enhance compliance. Those who are not able to tolerate ACE inhibitors, should be prescribed ARBs and once again, a cost-effective agent should be used
- *Beta-blockers*: Similar to ACE inhibitors, beta-blockers should also be used in all patients with HF and LVEF less than 40% if there is no contraindication. The treatment with beta-blockers is usually initiated when patients are stable and are in compensated phase. When there is worsening HF, the dose needs to be reduced or the medicine may have to be temporarily discontinued. However, the patients with severe mitral stenosis often develop HF because of either sinus tachycardia or atrial fibrillation with fast ventricular rate. These patients improve with beta-blockers even when given during the decompensated phase
- *Aldosterone antagonists*: Unless contraindicated or not tolerated, the addition of a low dose of an aldosterone antagonist should be considered in all patients with an LVEF less than 35% and severe symptomatic HF
- *Digoxin*: Although digoxin was earlier one of the most commonly used medicines for HF, its role in the present day practice is limited primarily to management of atrial fibrillation in HF patients. The metabolism of digoxin, especially its inactivation by anaerobic gut flora, has been an area of interest and has been shown to have ethnic variations. Studies in normal healthy volunteers from Southern India and the United States have revealed that only 1.0% of Indians (urbans > rural villagers) are metabolizers in comparison to 14% of Americans. Since the patients in whom digoxin is actively metabolized by gut flora require higher dose of the medicine, these findings suggest that Indian patients may be better managed with lower doses of digoxin as compared to their western counterparts
- *Devices and surgical procedures*: Surgical correction of valvular lesions and myocardial revascularization can result in significant reduction in morbidity and mortality from HF and should be performed whenever indicated

  Cardiac resynchronization therapy (CRT) is recommended to all patients with HF who have LVEF less than 35% and wide QRS (>120 ms) on ECG and who remain symptomatic despite optimal medical therapy. However, despite careful patient selection, nearly one-third of all the patients undergoing CRT fail to show any benefit with the therapy. Since this is an expensive form of therapy, any nonresponse has major financial implications, particularly in countries like India. In this context, echocardiographic assessment of dyssynchrony, though not recommended by the guidelines, may prove to be helpful in improving patient selection and in reducing nonresponse to CRT
- *Ventricular assist devices, artificial hearts, and heart transplants*: Although in end-stage HF, ventricular assist devices and heart transplant are the only viable treatment options, they are prohibitively expensive and out of the realms for majority of HF patients in India. Not only the procedure cost is very high, subsequent immunosuppressive therapy is also very expensive and cannot be easily afforded by most of the Indian patients. In addition, the availability of donor hearts is also very limited, both because of a general lack of awareness as well as the reluctance toward organ donation due to social and cultural reasons. Approximately 60% of world's population is in Asia but accounts for only 4% of heart transplantations performed, whereas only 5% of world's population is in North America and accounts for 71% of heart transplantations performed[16]

- *Nonpharmacological measures*: Nonpharmacological measures play an important role in the management of HF and are especially relevant for Indian patients. Careful attention needs to be paid to fluid restriction, reduced sodium intake, weight monitoring, smoking cessation, etc. Regular, moderate daily physical activity is equally important for all patients with HF. However, in comparison to the Western countries, the adoption of comprehensive cardiac rehabilitation program is still limited in India.

PREVENTION

Given the chronic nature of HF, significant morbidity, high mortality rate, and the enormous economic burden associated with HF, its prevention remains the most cost-effective and the most desirable option. Most of the strategies for prevention of HF in India are same as anywhere else in the world and include:

- *Reduction in alcohol consumption*: Excessive alcohol intake causes cardiomyopathy, and is an important cause of beriberi which can also lead to HF. Alcohol consumption has been steadily increasing in developing countries like India, as compared to the developed countries where it has been on a decline since the 1980s
- *Smoking cessation*: Smoking is a major risk factor for CVD, and is also responsible for numerous other health hazards including a wide range of malignancies. Socioeconomic milieu strongly influences smoking habits in the community. For example, despite financial constraints, smoking is more common among underprivileged sections because of the lack of knowledge about its harmful health effects. The World Health Survey (WHS) conducted by the World Health Organization (WHO) has found that 46.7% of the poor men smoke in India as against 21.8% of the rich men. Furthermore, consumptions of *bidis*, an indigenous, leaf-rolled cigarette is the dominant form of smoking in India. Nearly 4.52 trillion cigarettes and 40.3 trillion *bidis* have been produced between 1910 and 2010 and are estimated to have caused nearly 100 million premature deaths in adult men of more than or equal to 35 years of age. Of these, more than three-fourths were likely to be caused by *bidis* alone. While increasing health awareness among general population is important for reducing smoking in the society, tobacco taxation can also be of great help. Taxation has been shown to reduce tobacco consumption in high-income countries and the reduction is likely to be much higher in India due to higher price sensitivity of tobacco consumers in India[17]
- *Prevention of CVD*: Given the role of CVD in causation of HF, prevention of CVD through aggressive lifestyle measures including smoking cessation, increased physical activity, dietary changes as well as appropriate pharmacological treatment of CV risk factors, as and when needed, is extremely important for reducing the burden of HF. In addition, even in patients with established CVD, timely detection and treatment of the disease helps minimize myocardial damage and prevents progression to the stage of HF
- *Prevention of RHD*: RHD remains the most common cause of valvular heart disease in India. Improvements in public hygiene through improvement in socioeconomic status and proper treatment of sore throat during childhood are measures that can be very effective in prevention of RHD. In addition, penicillin prophylaxis for secondary prevention reduces progression of valvular damage and delays development of symptomatic HF. The vaccines against rheumatic fever are currently under development, and will take some time before they become available for regular use
- *Tuberculosis prevention*: Although there has been a decline in the incidence and prevalence of tuberculosis in India, the disease still remains widely prevalent. Vaccination against tuberculosis is a standard practice at birth in India but it has only modest efficacy in preventing tubercular infection. Aggressive management of all active cases of tuberculosis is required to prevent transmission to and development of disease in others. At the same time, antitubercular treatment will also reduce morbidity and mortality associated with tubercular pericarditis. In fact, it has been estimated that the advent of antitubercular drugs for treatment of pericardial tuberculosis has been associated with a decline in estimated case fatality rate from nearly 100% to as low as 8%.[18]

CONCLUSION

Heart failure is a widely prevalent health problem in India and a major cause of morbidity and mortality. Unlike the Western populations, in India, both CVD as well as pretransition diseases, such as RHD and CCP are responsible for causing HF and the problem is further compounded by nutritional deficiencies which too are quite common in India. Accordingly, HF in India is characterized by relatively younger age of onset, greater prevalence of valvular involvement, and higher incidence of atrial fibrillation. These differences have important diagnostic, prognostic and therapeutic implications that need to be considered while managing HF patients in India.

REFERENCES

1. Huffman MD, Prabhakaran D. Heart failure: epidemiology and prevention in India. Natl Med J India 2010;23:283-8.
2. Gupta R. Recent trends in coronary heart disease epidemiology in India. Indian Heart J. 2008;60:B4-18.
3. Yusuf S, Sleight P, Pogue J, Bosch J, Davies R, Dagenais G. Effects of an angiotensin-converting-enzyme inhibitor, ramipril, on cardiovascular events in high-risk patients. The Heart Outcomes Prevention Evaluation Study Investigators. N EnglJ Med. 2000;342:145-53.
4. Fox KM; European trial on reduction of cardiac events with perindopril in stable coronary artery disease investigators. Efficacy of perindopril in reduction of cardiovascular events among patients with stable coronary artery disease: Randomised, double-blind, placebo-controlled, multicentre trial (the EUROPA study). Lancet. 2003;362:782-8.
5. Thakur JS, Negi PC, Ahluwalia SK, Vaidya NK. Epidemiological survey of rheumatic heart disease among school children in the Shimla hills of northern India: Prevalence and risk factors. J Epidemiol Community Health. 1996;50:62-7.
6. World Health Organization. Global burden of disease—2004 update. Geneva: Switzerland; 2004.
7. Bashi VV, John S, Ravikumar E, Jairaj PS, Shyamsunder K, Krishnaswami S. Early and late results of pericardiectomy in 118 cases of constrictive pericarditis. Thorax. 1988;43:637-41.
8. Pedreira Perez M, Virgos Lamela A, Crespo Mancebo FJ, Cervantes JL, Fernandez de la Reguera G, Barragan Garcia R. [40 years' experience in the surgical treatment of constrictive pericarditis]. Arch Inst Cardiol Mex. 1987;57:363-73
9. Arsan S, Mercan S, Sarigul A, Atasoy S, Demircin M, Dogan R, et al. Long-term experience with pericardiectomy: analysis of 105 consecutive patients. Thorac Cardiovasc Surg. 1994;42:340-4.
10. Ling LH, Oh JK, Schaff HV, Danielson GK, Mahoney DW, Seward JB, et al. Constrictive pericarditis in the modern era: evolving clinical spectrum and impact on outcome after pericardiectomy. Circulation. 1999;100:1380-6.
11. Oh KY, Shimizu M, Edwards WD, Tazelaar HD, Danielson GK. Surgical pathology of the parietal pericardium: a study of 344 cases (1993–1999). Cardiovasc Pathol. 2001;10:157-68.
12. Otto CM, Bonow RO. Valvular heart disease. In: Libby P, Bonow RO, Mann DL, Zipes DP, editors. Braunwald's heart disease: A textbook of cardiovascular medicine, 8th ed. Saunders, Philadelphia: 2008. p. 1625-712.
13. Bonow RO, Carabello BA, Chatterjee K, de Leon AC, Jr., Faxon DP, Freed MD, et al. ACC/AHA 2006 guidelines for the management of patients with valvular heart disease: a report of the American College of Cardiology/ American Heart Association Task Force on Practice Guidelines (writing Committee to Revise the 1998 guidelines for the management of patients with valvular heart disease) developed in collaboration with the Society of Cardiovascular Anesthesiologists endorsed by the Society for Cardiovascular Angiography and Interventions and the Society of Thoracic Surgeons. J Am Coll Cardiol. 2006;48:e1-148.
14. Joshi PP, Mohanan CJ, Sengupta SP, Salkar RG. Factors precipitating congestive heart failure – role of patient non-compliance. J Assoc Physicians India. 1999;47:294-5.
15. Lip GY, Khan H, Bhatnagar A, et al. Ethnic differences in patient perceptions of heart failure and treatment: the West Birmingham heart failure project. Heart. 2004;90:1016-9.
16. Sivathasan C. Heart transplantation in Singapore. Ann Acad Med Singapore. 2009;38:309-14.
17. Chaloupka FJ, Hu TW, Warner KE, Jacobs R, Yurekli A. The taxation of tobacco products. In: Jha P, Chaloupka F, editors. Tobacco control in developing countries. Oxford: Oxford University Press; 2000. p. 877-83.
18. Ntsekhe M, Wiysonge C, Volmink JA, Commerford PJ, Mayosi BM. Adjuvant corticosteroids for tuberculous pericarditis: Promising, but not proven. QJM. 2003;96:593-9.

Chapter 45

Heart Failure in China

Yuhui Zhang, Jian Zhang

ABSTRACT

Heart failure (HF) has become a serious medical burden in China because of the increase of aging population and patients with high risk of cardiovascular disease. The China HF registry was started to collect data on the epidemiology and medical therapy of HF. The highlights of treatment to HF patients in China are as follows: Intravenous β-blocker in ischemic heart disease with acute HF in China. The therapy of recombinant human neuregulin-1, traditional Chinese medicine, cardiac resynchronisation therapy and implantable cardioverter-defibrillator, and ultrafiltration for patients with HF in China. The surgical management of HF includes coronary artery bypass surgery in combination with cell transplantation or "hybrid" strategy, a left ventricular (LV) assist device named FW-II axial flow pump and heart transplantation In China. The Chinese guidelines for diagnosis and therapy of HF (2014) has been published on February, 2014. In the future, further HF research and clinical study should be done to obtain more evidence of diagnosis and therapy for Chinese HF patients.

INTRODUCTION

Heart failure (HF) has became a serious medical burden in China for several reasons: the increased aging population, numerous poorly controlled hypertensive and diabetic patients, and more patients are at risk for developing HF after surviving through acute coronary syndrome with the popularization of interventional therapy. HF research and clinical study were developed rapidly in recent years in China. Here, we give a brief description from several aspects.

EPIDEMIOLOGY AND REGISTERY STUDY OF HEART FAILURE IN CHINA

Epidemiology Study of Heart Failure in China

It is a little regretful that there is no new robust data on the epidemiology of HF in China in recent years. A new epidemic study is ongoing. The main cause of HF in China is similar to that in Western countries, the percentages of coronary heart disease, hypertension, rheumatic valvular disease, and DCM are 55.7%, 13.9%, 8.9%, and 7.5%, respectively.[1] An echocardiography study showed that the age and sex adjusted prevalence of HCM was about 80 per 100,000 adults, while DCM was 19 per 100,000 adults in China [2,3]

Registery Study of Heart Failure in China

In 2012, as the national 12.5 project [National Science and Technology Support Program (2011BAI11B00)], the China HF registry study was carried on under the leader of HF center of Fuwai Hospital. This is a comprehensive, large-scale, prospective, and multicenter study in China, it would be developed into a long-term, permanent national data platform of HF. The aims of the study are as follows:

- To set up the national database platform for patients with HF; to learn the demographics, risk factors,

etiology, comorbidities, clinical diagnosis, therapy status, prognosis, and cost of acute and chronic HF in different levels of hospitals in different provinces of China
- To evaluate the gap between the evidence-based guideline-recommended medicine and the real status of clinical diagnosis and therapy in China, ensure the appropriate use of evidence-based medicine
- To set up and generalize the standard process and algorithms for HF diagnosis and therapy which is suitable to the actual situation in China
- To set up biological specimen banks in order to screen the biomarkers and other risk factors which can provide the effect of early-warning, risk stratification and prognosis evaluation, and set up the risk scoring system for Chinese patients with HF
- To explore the genetic mechanism for Chinese patients with HF.

At the first 5 years' stage, about 70 hospitals (level 2-3) in nearly all provinces of China have been recruited.

THE HIGHLIGHTS OF TREATMENT TO PATIENTS WITH HEART FAILURE IN CHINA

Intravenous β-blocker in Ischemic Heart Disease with Acute Heart Failure

Doctors in HF care unit of Fuwai Hospital accumulated clinical experience of using intravenous β-blocker in ischemic heart disease patients with acute HF as early as 2003. At that time, this was not recommended by the guideline until 2005. A retrospectively study of 16 ischemic heart disease patients with acute HF received routine management and could not get recovery. Every patients demonstrated pulmonary edema on X-ray, the average blood pressure (BP) increased by 10 mmHg and the average heart rate (HR) increased by 10 beat per minute during the acute HF exacerbation. The intravenous BB was infused and the dosage was adjusted according to the BP and HR, all of the patients improved their clinical symptoms and signs within a few hours, 62.5% of patients showed decreased rales, and disappearance of pulmonary congestion on X-ray later, and 87.5% of patients had improved electrocardiogram for their ischemic condition. The mechanism is that BB can break the vicious cycle of ischemic, sympathetic activation, ischemia, and HF. Until now, the usage of intravenous BB in ischemic heart disease patients with acute HF attack is also an symbol of the combination of individualization and standardization therapy in acute HF.[4,5]

Recombinant Human Neuregulin-1: The New Drug for Heart Failure

Neuregulin-1 plays important roles in maintaining adult heart structural and functional integrity. Recombinant human neuregulin-1 (rhNRG-1), which contains 61 amino acid residues and covers the epidermal growth factor-like domain (the domain necessary for ErbB2/ ErbB4 activation).[6] Since 2004, series of clinical trials were carried out [the China Food and Drug Authority (CFDA) study number 2004L02304, 2005L04180, and 2010L00444] in China. Phase I and IIA trials in China confirmed the safety of rhNRG-1 in both healthy individuals and congestive heart failure (CHF) patients. Phase II trial was both started in China and Australia in 2006. The phase II clinical trial showed rhNRG-1 improved the cardiac function of chronic HF patients by increasing the left ventricular ejection fraction (LVEF) and the capability of anti-remodeling by decreasing end-systolic volume and end-diastolic volume (EDV), EDV levels continued to decrease at day 90 (-20.79 ± 17.03% and -14.03 ± 13.17%, respectively), accompanied by a sustained increase in LVEF%.[7] Another phase II clinical trial enrolled a total of 195 patients showed 0.6 μg/kg dosage level can increase LVEF%, decrease N-terminal brain natriuretic peptide (NT-proBNP) at 30, 90 days, and decrease the rate of readmission 30-day. In 2010, phase III trial which takes the one year's all-cause death as the main endpoint is being carried on in China.

Traditional Chinese Medicine

The traditional Chinese medicine (TCM) has its advantages in treating chronic HF, a lot of research and clinical trials of TCM are done in recent years. Animal experiments showed that the some of the TCM can restrain renin-angiotensin-aldosterone system (RAAS), inhibit the development of cardiac hypertrophy, remodeling, improve hemodynamics of dog HF model obviously, increase urine volume, and decrease the whole heart quality index and BNP levels obviously.[8-10]

A study on Qili Qiangxin capsules was published on 2013 [Efficacy and Safety of Qili Qiangxin Capsules for Chronic Heart Failure: A Multicenter, Randomized, Double-Blind, Parallel-group, Placebo-Controlled Trial (ChiCTR-TRC-11001478)], 512 patients with LVEF ≤40% and New York Heart Associarion (NYHA) II-III were randomized into Qili Qiangxin and placebo group on the basis of accepted standardized treatment. At the 12-week follow-up, Qili Qiangxin capsule group demonstrated a significantly greater reduction of NT-proBNP level and NT-proBNP levels of at least 30% than the placebo group ($p < 0.002$ and $p < 0.001$, respectively). Treatment with Qili Qiangxin capsules also demonstrated superior performance in comparison to the placebo with respect to New York Heart Association functional classification, LVEF, 6-min walking distance, and quality of life.[11]

Cardiac Resynchronization and Implantable Cardioverter-defibrillator Therapy in China

The first use of cardioverter-defibrillator therapy (CRT) in China was in 1999 and the first use of CRT-defibrillator (CRTD) was in 2002. The implanting number for CRT, CRTD, and implantable cardioverter-defibrillator (ICD) increased gradually in recent years, the number of CRT is 1,573, 1,876, 2,210, and 2,198 from 2010, 2011, 2012, and 2013, respectively. However, only 4.3% patients who have indication for CRT accepted the therapy, this ratio is much lower than the level in developed countries. Among all patients who have accepted CRT, the mean age was about 62.37, 71.76% were men, 75.3% patients (LVEF ≤35%), 40.0% patients (QRS ≥150 ms), 53.9% patients (QRS = 120–150 ms), 66.74% patients (left bundle branch block), and 55.65% and 27.03% patients were NYHA III and IV, respectively. There may be many reasons for this, such as a shortage of doctors who have mastered pacing technology, electrophysiology knowledge and some interventional technology, all of the CRT, CRTD, and ICD are relatively expensive to most HF patients and not covered by medical insurance now.

The most causes of death for HF are deterioration of cardiac failure and/or sudden cardiac death (SCD), and the latter is mostly caused by the malignant ventricular arrhythmia (ventricular tachycardia and ventricular fibrillation). Recently, the Chinese national "10.5" key project announced the survey of SCD in China. Approximately more than 500,000 people suffer from SCD every year in China. HF is one of the most important factor of SCD.[12] The percentage of CRTD in the total number of CRT is about 56% in 2013.

Ultrafiltration Therapy in Heart Failure in China

A new ultrafiltration device which is made by a Chinese Medical company finished it's phase II multicenter clinical trial in China since December 2009 to April 2011, this ultrafiltration device has the function same as the Aquadex^{TM} System which is the production of The CHF Solution Company. This trial included 60 cases of congestive HF (NYHA classification IV) with liquid retention, the dose of oral furosemide is ≥80 mg/day (or other equivalent diuretics), the average LVEF was 41.45 ± 15.16%. The main results were as follows: the average amount of removed fluid is 4297 ± 2152 mL, the efficacy rate of ultrafiltration dehydration is 100%. Twenty four-hour weight loss is from 72.7 ± 15.38 kg to 68.4 ± 15.12 kg and 24-hour dyspnea relief is from 6.6 ± 5.72 to 13.4 ± 2.62. No hypotension events happened during ultrafiltration. Now, the CFDA had approved the clinical application of this ultrafiltration device.

Surgical Management of Heart Failure: The Experiences in China

We discuss the surgical management of patients with HF in the setting of coronary artery disease (CAD) with a reduced ejection fraction (EF), which focus on the experiences and researches in China.

Coronary Artery Bypass Grafting Combines with Cell Transplantation or "Hybrid" Strategy

- A single-center prospective observational study involves 239 ischemic heart failure (IHF) patients with EF <35% who undergo isolated coronary artery bypass surgery (CABG) in Fuwai Hospital, the results show that the operative mortality is 2.9% and 5-year survival rate is 89.3% at a 62.3-month mean follow-up interval, which is comparable to counterpart studies in the world[13]
- *Coronary artery bypass grafting combined with cell transplantation:* Isolated CABG cannot reverse pathological ventricular remodeling as a result of substantial cardiomyocyte loss secondary to massive myocardial infarction (MI). Professor Hu and colleagues carried out the first prospective randomized controlled clinical trials on CABG combined with cell transplantation of autologous bone marrow mononuclear cells (BMNCs) for treatment of IHF with old MI [Stem Cell Therapy to Improve Myocardial Function in Patients Undergoing Coronary Artery Bypass Grafting (NCT00395811)]. From November 2006 to June 2009, they recruited 65 consecutive advanced CAD patients with old MI and LVEF <35%, 31 patients randomized to receive concurrent cell transplantation via bypass graft. After 6-month follow-upresults showed that CABG plus cell transplantation had a better effect on the structural and functional changes of LV before and after surgery

as well as 6-minute walking distance in comparison with isolated CABG. In conclusion, CABG plus cell transplantation provides an alternative treatment option for advanced CAD patients with severe LV dysfunction[14]

- *Coronary artery bypass grafting combines with "hybrid" strategy:* Professor Hu and colleagues pioneer a study hypothesis of "hybrid" strategy which combines atrial appendage tissue with Greater momentum cover plus CABG to improve cardiac function and inhibit LV remodeling, They firstly carry out the Phase I clinical study [CABG Combined Pedicled Omentum Wrapped Autologous Atrial Tissue Patch Cardiomyoplasty for Ischemic Cardiomyopathy (NCT00972114)] to validate the safety of aforementioned "hybrid" surgical techniques on 11 patients. Phase II treatment trial including 60 cases is underway currently.

Left Ventricular Assisted Device in China

In China, the left ventricular assist device (LVAD) is totally imported now and the high cost limits its widespread application. To impel the clinical use of domestic LVAD in Chinese advanced HF patients, a fully implantable FW-II axial flow pump has been developed in Fuwai Hospital. This LVAD can deliver 5 L/min for pressure of 100 mmHg over 8,000 rpm. A series of *in vitro* and *in vivo* studies have shown that the blood pump can be used to assist left ventricular circulation for a short time with a satisfactory biocompatibility and reliable. Further clinical trials are ongoing in Fuwai Hospital.[15]

Heart Transplantation in China

In China, first case of human heart transplantation was performed in Shanghai in 1978, it was also the first case of orthotopic heart transplant in Asia, considerable progress has been made recently. In 2010, Fuwai Hospital was committed to establish the national cardiac transplantation network registry system. According to the data collected, a total of 1,139 cases of cardiac transplantation were performed in 31 centers from 1995 to 2013 in China. In Fuwai Hospital, a total of 414 cases of cardiac transplantation were performed between 2004 and 2013, and the annual number of cardiac transplantation has been up to 45 to 65 Since 2010. The average early survival rate within 30-day is 92.2%, the overall survival rate at 1-, 3-, 5-, and 7-year after transplantation was 94.7%, 91.6%, 88.0%, and 82.6%, respectively, which showed a better outcome than that of the International Registry for Heart and Lung Transplantation (ISHLT) statistics, namely, 84.9%, 78.0%, 72.2%, and 66.8% at 1-, 3-, 5-, and 7-year after transplantation, respectively. In China, patients with cardiomyopathy accounted for 80.9% of recipients, among them, about 70% is dilated cardiomyopathy, whereas coronary artery disease only accounted for 10.8%, which is different from that in ISHLT statistics result. The mean age of Chinese recipients was 43.6 years, about 9 years younger than that of patients of ISHLT.

THE CHINESE GUIDELINES FOR THE DIAGNOSIS AND TREATMENT OF ACUTE AND CHRONIC HEART FAILURE 2014

This guideline includes three main parts: the clinical evaluation of HF, the therapy of HF, and the holistic management of HF.[16] There are six parts in the therapy of HF: the chronic HF with reduced LVEF (HF-REF), HF with preserved LVEF (HF-PEF), the acute HF, the right HF, the end-stage and refractory HF, and the comorbidity and the cause of HF. Flowcharts 1–3 demonstrate the treatment of symptomatic chronic HF and acute HF.

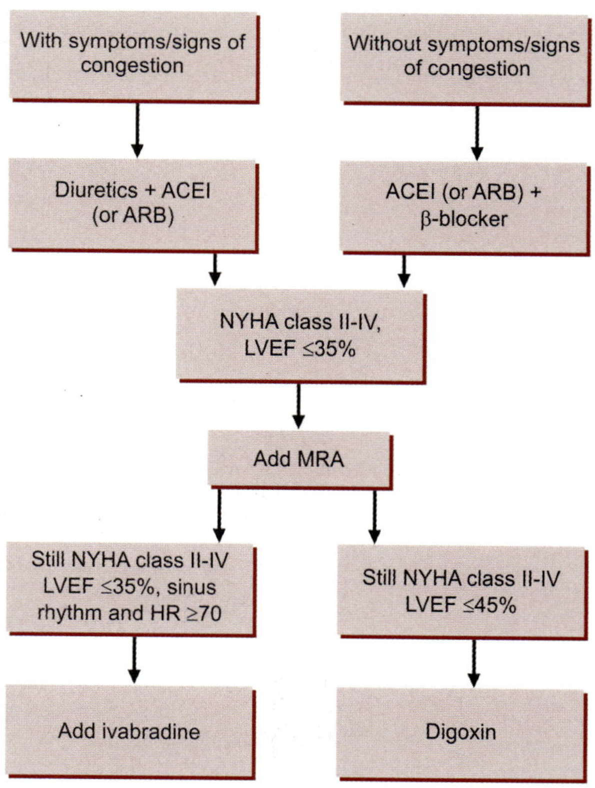

ACEI, angiotensin converting enzyme inhibitor; ARB, angiotensin receptor blocker; NYHA, New York Heart Association; LVEF, left ventricular ejection fraction; MRA, magnetic resonance angiography; HR, heart rate

Flowchart 1 Algorithm for medication treatment of chronic symptomatic heart failure (New York Heart Association II-IV)

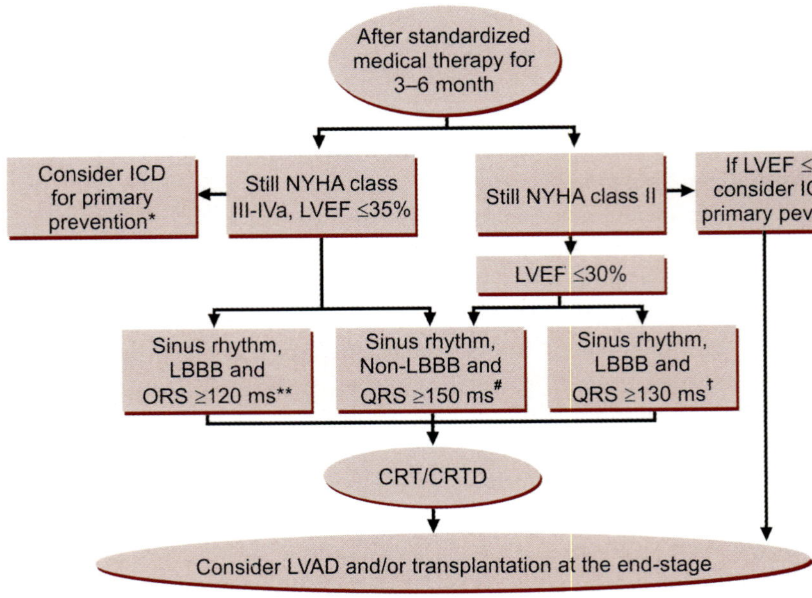

*It is not indicated for NYHA class IV; for ischemic HF, it is only indicated for patients at least 40 days after AMI with a class I, level A recommendation; for non-ischemic HF, it is a class I, level B recommendation

**When QRS ≥150 ms, recommendation is class I, level A; when 120 ≤QRS <150 ms, recommendation is class IIa, level B

#For NYHA class II, recommendation is class IIb, level B; for NYHA class III or IVa, recommendation is class IIa, level A

†When QRS ≥150 ms, recommendation is class I, level A; when 130 ≤QRS <150 ms, recommendation is class IIa, level B

ICD, implantable cardioverter-defibrillator; New York Heart Association; LVEF, left ventricular ejection fraction; LBBB, Left bundle branch block; CRT, cardioverter-defibrillator therapy; CRTD, defibrillator; LVAD, left ventricular assist device

Flowchart 2 Algorithm for non-medication treatment of chronic symptomatic heart failure (New York Heart Association II-IV)

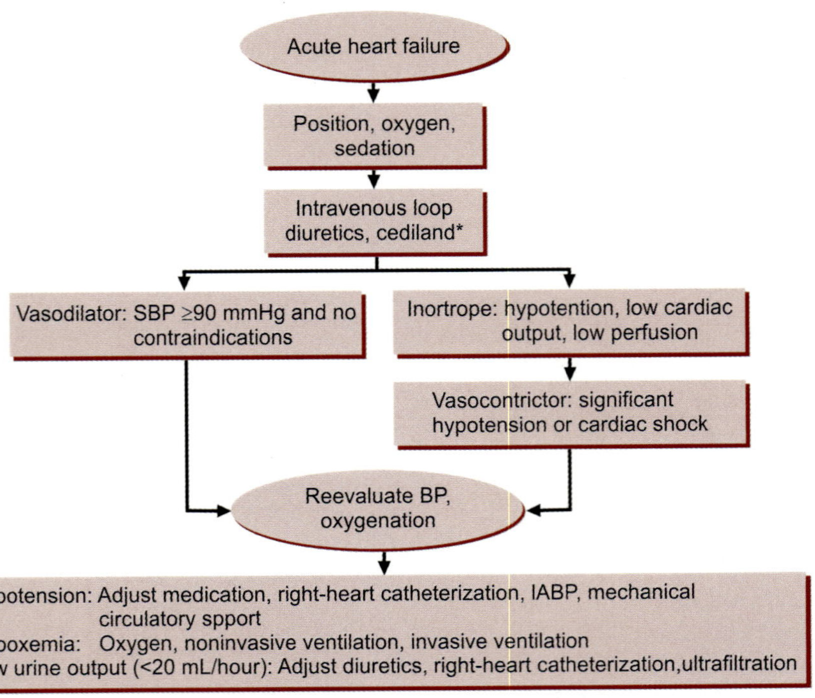

*Indicated for patients with atrial fibrillation accompanied by fast ventricular rates or severe systolic dysfunction

BP, blood pressure; IABP, intra-aortic balloon pump

Flowchart 3 Algorithm for non-medication treatment of chronic symptomatic heart failure (New York Heart Association II-IV)

REFERENCES

1. Shanghai Investigation Group of Heart Failure. The evolving trends in the epidemiologic factors and treatment of hospitalized patients with congestive heart failure in Shanghai during the years of 1980, 1990 and 2000. Chin J Cardiol. 2002;30:24-6.
2. Jiang H, Ge J. Epidemiology and clinical management of cardiomyopathies and heart failure in China. Heart. 2009;95(21):1727-31.
3. Zou Y, Song L, Wang Z, et al. Prevalence of idiopathic hypertrophic cardiomyopathy in China: a population-based echocardiographic analysis of 8080 adults. Am J Med. 2004;116(1):14-8.
4. Li J, Dou KF, Kang LM, et al. Summary of intravenous a-blocker infusion for ischemic heart disease patients with acute heart failure attack. Chinese. Circulation J. 2010;25(6):449-52.
5. Zhang J, Dou KF, Yang YJ, et al. Intravenous beta-blocker infusion for ischemic heart disease patients with acute heart failure. Chinese Circulation J. 2006;21(3):175-7.
6. Xu Y, Li X, Liu X, et al. Neuregulin-1/ErbB signaling and chronic heart failure. Adv Pharmacol. 2010;59:31-51.
7. Gao R, Zhang J, Cheng L, et al. A Phase II, randomized, double-blind, multicenter, based on standard therapy, placebo-controlled study of the efficacy and safety of recombinant human neuregulin-1 in patients with chronic heart failure. J Am Coll Cardiol. 2010;55(18):1907-14.
8. Yunzeng Zou, Li Lin, Yong Ye, et al. Qiliqiangxin inhibits the development of cardiac hypertrophy, remodeling, and dysfunction during 4 weeks of pressure overload in mice. J Cardiovasc Pharmacol. 2002;59(3):268-80.
9. Liu W, Chen J, Xu T, et al. Qiliqiangxin improves cardiac function in spontaneously hypertensive rats through the inhibition of cardiac chymase. Am J Hypertens. 2012;25(2):250-60.
10. Xiao H, Song Y, Li Y, et al. Qiliqiangxin regulates the balance between tumor necrosis factor-alpha and interleukin-10 and improves cardiac function in rats with myocardial infarction. Cell Immunol. 2009;260(1):515.
11. Li X, Zhang J, Huang J, et al. A multicenter, randomized, double-blind, parallel-group, placebo-controlled study of the effects of qili qiangxin capsules in patients with chronic heart failure. J Am Coll Cardiol. 2013; 17:1065-72.
12. Zhang S. Sudden cardiac death in China. Pacing Clin Electrophysiol. 2009;32(9):1159-62.
13. Y Li, Z Zheng, S Hu, et al. The Chinese coronary artery bypass grafting registry study: analysis of the national multicentre database of 9248 patients. Heart. 2009;95(14):1140-4.
14. Hu S, Liu S, Zheng Z, et al. Isolated coronary artery bypass graft combined with bone marrow mononuclear cells delivered through a graft vessel for patients with previous myocardial infarction and chronic heart failure: a single-center, randomized, double-blind, placebo-controlled clinical trial. J Am Coll Cardiol. 2011;57(24):2409-15.
15. Zhang Y, Hu SS, Zhou JY, et al. Design and performance testing of an axial-flow ventricular assist device developed at the Fuwai Hospital in Beijing. Int J Artif Organs. 2008;31(11):983-7.
16. Chinese society of cardiology, Editing committee of Chinese Journal of Cardiology. China Guidelines for the diagnosis and treatment of heart failure. Chinese J Cardiol. 2014;42(2):98-122.

Chapter 46

Heart Failure from the US Veterans Health Administration Perspective: A Patient-centered Approach to Care

Robert L Jesse

ABSTRACT

The strategic imperative for the Veterans Health Administration is to provide proactive, personalized, and patient-driven care. The premise that any patient with a given diagnosis will absolutely benefit from guideline-driven care is inherently flawed. The management of patients with chronic heart failure (CHF) is an excellent example of why care must be individualized. This chapter lays out the step-wise approach to optimizing care for the patient with CHF through a personalized and proactive approach that engages patients in their care. The principles to this approach are straightforward: know the unique disease that each patient has; manage that disease to the unique needs of each patient; and chronic disease management is not an event, it is an ongoing relationship between providers, patients, and their support systems. We believe that these are the crucial constructs that must be embraced to support the transformation toward patient-centered care, and from there to patient-driven care. This approach (proactive, personalized, and patient-driven care enabled through connected health), will result in optimal outcomes for patients with heart failure (HF) whatever the etiology.

INTRODUCTION

We in healthcare will continue to think of heart failure (HF) as a singular entity, at great peril. First and foremost, HF is not one disease, but is in fact an encompassing term that covers a number of clinical manifestations and underlying etiologies. Even among those patients with impaired ejection fractions, there are wide variations in etiology, presentation, and response to therapies. For this reason alone, I can think of no more compelling a reason to always take a patient-centered approach; in this context, patient-centered means both personalized and proactive care that ensures optimal treatment for each and every individual. Toward that end, in the Veterans Health Administration (VHA), we are focusing the mission of our quality and delivery systems toward, "Quality for an 'n' of one, insight to an 'n' of 6 million".

The cost of managing cardiovascular disease in the United States accounts for approximately 43 cents of every medicare dollar spent. The proportion of that attributable to HF is increasing through the sheer weight of demographics and the improved survival in patients with ischemic heart disease. So, the fundamental question is whether we can substantively reduce the cost of managing patients with HF, without compromising the quality of care or outcomes. A comparison of HF trends from 1993 versus 2006 noted a trade-off between a reduced length of stay (LOS) of 8.6–6.4 days against a higher 30-day readmission rate of 17.3–20.1%.[1] There was also a decrease in the proportion of patients being discharged to home versus those discharged to skilled nursing facilities, including hospice. Data from VHA, by Kaboli et al., questions this trade-off between LOS and readmission.[2] And, more recent studies have questioned whether readmission necessarily reflects the quality of care.[3]

Rather than engage in debate over the implications of readmission on patients with HF hospitalizations, understanding the reasons why patients get readmitted might be more instructive toward improving care. These

Box 1: Why patients get readmitted

- Disease specific factors
- Patient dependent conditions
- Clinician associated decisions
- Systems related issues

can be parsed into several unique categories (Box 1), each of which can be further attributed to either medical-related or social-related influences, but regardless of the contributing factors involved, a little over one-third of the readmissions following HF discharges are for the same issue as the index admission.[4]

Because this is so clearly multifactorial, it is by its very nature complex. Let us just take patient-specific factors as an example. How do we evaluate the impact of a given patient's habits and behaviors, which are often not visible to those in the healthcare system? How do we measure and account for adherence, not just with the medications but with diet and exercise prescriptions? How does this impact sleep, or better yet, what is the impact of sleep on outcomes? What are the social determinants of health that have the most impact on a given HF patient's outcome, and can these contribute to both personalized and predictive assessments that can be leveraged to improve outcomes? Can culture and language inherently be impediments to care, and if so, how do we ensure equity across these boundaries? What is the contribution related to verbal understanding where comprehension is not necessarily limited to a lack of competence with the English language, i.e., how do we ensure that the "Language of Medicine" is understood? The issue of health literacy is very much a critical factor contributing to patient behavior and outcomes, and this is not to imply that it is just the patient that is lacking in this regard—it may well be us.

We believe that improvement in outcomes for patients with HF can be managed through a few key principles that are predicated on a foundation of personalized, proactive, and patient-driven care.

RULE 1: KNOW THE DISEASE

First, are we dealing with a chronic disease, an acute disease, or an acute manifestation of a chronic disease? This is an essential distinction necessary for optimal outcomes, yet fragmentation in healthcare can be problematic in this regard. For instance, a patient with chronic HF managed primarily in the outpatient setting who is admitted acutely to a hospital may well be managed by providers with little insight into either the remote or recent history. So, as a fundamental construct for effective management across multiple domains, there must be continuity of health information. In principle, an individual patient's aggregated health information is the basis for continuity of care. And only when we have that we can actually answer the opening question.

Understanding the nature of a patient's HF is also crucial for initiating applicable clinical practice guidelines. All too often the guidelines that may be applicable to a studied population may not be beneficial to a unique patient. Think, "Guidelines are us", but the "n of 1" is always "me". Regardless there remains great pressure, from internal and external influences, to conform with guidelines as these are considered the bellwether of quality for both individual practitioners and health systems. Process measures used as quality indicators run the risk of actually promoting worse outcomes when used to drive systems on performance alone: I believe that there is an operational correlate to the Frank-Starling curve (Fig. 1).

The individualization of evidence-based treatments to optimize outcomes and minimize adverse events is the overarching goal of the personalized medicine movement.[5] However, the term should not refer solely to the genomic construct but to the entirety of data available to individualize treatment. Toward that end, the level of precision we are pursuing will eventually be achieved through biomarkers. That includes proteomics, metabolomics, and all the other "omics"; functional and imaging data; social determinants and patient-preference data; all integrated into an individualized plan. Since VHA delivers both healthcare and important social resources needed to engender health and well-being, as a system, VHA has incredible insight and capability in these areas.

Many see the answer in "big data" analytics. It is clear that there is great potential in this. In addition, there is now the emergence of individuals willing to contribute their data obtained outside of the typical healthcare stream through the proliferation of personal-monitoring devices. Regardless of the type of patient worn-devices, these will most certainly contribute to our understanding of both population- and individual-based HF management. The acquisition of this level of data is easy. What to do with it, how to validate it, where to store it, what analytic engines can contribute by using it, and defining a user experience around it, is not so easy. Further, patient data acquired within the healthcare system comes with situational awareness, but the situational metadata for that acquired

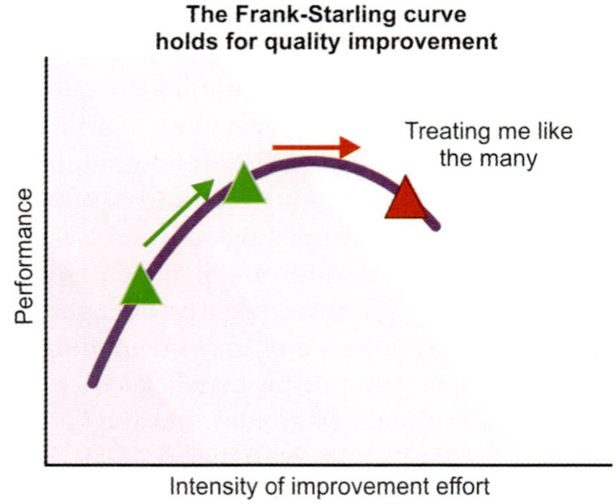

Fig. 1 The Frank-Starling curve for myocardial performance defines the relationship between sarcomere length and force generation (or end-diastolic pressure and stroke volume). It essentially describes the optimal preload state for the heart that supports optimal contractile force generation (or cardiac output), but at some point there results a diminishing return. The correlate in quality improvement is the relationship between the intensity of effort put into improvement and the resulting change in performance. Just as for the heart, there is a point of diminishing return where performance can actually begin to degrade in the face of an increased intensity of efforts to improve. Reasons include, among others, the application of guideline driven treatments to inappropriate individuals. A goal of personalized medicine is to concentrate a given intervention on those who will most likely benefit, sparing side effects and cost from those who will not. The pressure to treat all HF individuals according to a guideline (treating me like the many) in order to meet a performance measure, without considering the specific appropriateness for that unique individual, can result in harm.

outside of the system is itself of unique value and could be considered the informing "small data" that is often overlooked.

RULE 2: MAKE IT ABOUT THE PATIENT

Why is this even an issue? Historically we had been taught (and had taught others) that it is the physician who is responsible for "continuity of care". That only works when *one* physician is "in charge", and given the fragmentation of the delivery system there is risk to that construct breaking down. There is growing distinction between primary care clinicians, the hospitalists, and specialty care, which is particularly evident between inpatient and outpatient environments. However, it is clear that patient engagement leading to increased self-management, with the care team in a supporting role, is a preferred scenario, particularly for those with chronic diseases including HF.

Much of the attention directed toward HF readmissions centers is on the handoffs between these elements as patients move from one environment to another. In that regard, in VHA we prefer to eschew the concept of "admission" and "discharge", but rather to operate on the simple notion that, "...we help care for patients in the environment most appropriate for their needs at the time". It has been our belief that physicians/clinicians are not the axis of continuity, but rather that role belongs to the aggregate of individual's health information: in VHA the single and robust electronic medical record (VistA) for each Veteran provides the coherent health information to serve as the hub for continuity of care.

There are also issues between physicians, nurses, and other elements of the delivery system, but the ability to coordinate care across all of these is the intent of VHA's patient aligned care teams, similar to the Medical Home initiatives. The obvious advantage in VHA is the coherence brought by VistA, which is agnostic to the clinician or location of care such that all health information is available to all in an integrated record.

For patients with HF there is a growing appreciation of the importance of patient-reported outcomes (I briefly mentioned the concept of small data earlier) and the ability to include health-status and functional capability are both valuable and complex. Several instruments have been published (Box 2) and are increasingly being utilized in practice. The real challenge is to incorporate this data into the management strategies and protocols as a means of individualizing therapy, which can truly make it about the patient.

Box 2: Patient-reported health status patient outcomes in the era of small data

- Minnesota Living with Heart Failure
  - Physical, emotional
- Kansas City Cardiomyopathy Questionnaire
  - Physical limitation, symptoms, self-efficacy, quality of life, social
- Chronic Heart Failure Questionnaire
  - Dyspnea, fatigue, emotional
- Quality of Life Questionnaire for Severe heart failure
  - Psychosocial, physical, symptoms, life dissatisfaction

RULE 3: HEALTHCARE MUST CHANGE FROM BEING ENCOUNTER-BASED TO BEING RELATIONSHIP-BASED

When Rule 1 and Rule 2 have been implemented, there will follow a fundamental change in the dynamic of healthcare, which presently remains a transaction-based industry. The change must be away from a system based on volume of encounters toward one based on sustained relationships that is driven by the patient who is in charge of their health. "Connected Health" defines the relationship between patient and healthcare systems/providers, and is enabled through a myriad of technological solutions. Toward that end, VHA has invested heavily over the past 10 years in deploying connected health strategies, including infrastructure, capacity, and capability to bridge that gap and provide enhanced and seamless continuity to improve the management of HF and other conditions. However, this must never be about the technology itself, which is only an enabling function, and is rapidly evolving. What is clear is that self-management can be greatly enhanced through connecting patients to a supportive delivery system, and that insight from patient generated data can be leveraged to improve outcomes.

Connected health must encompass all modalities available to engage patients and provide care. This includes secure messaging, mobile apps, home telehealth, teleconsultation, biosensors, self-monitoring, etc. The ability to deliver care away from the bricks and mortar anchors of the health system through connected health technologies permits a greater level of patient engagement and the "management of me" as the foundation of personalized patient-driven care. It is about the ability to manage that relationship across time and distance in both synchronous and asynchronous domains. But most importantly, it is never about the device, it is about the relationship it enables.

Veterans Health Administration's historical investment has been for the management of HF with home-based devices that capture vital signs and weight. It also includes teleconsultation to support primary care providers and to improve inherent capability to manage HF patients when cardiologists may not be readily accessible. We are now deploying tablet-based applications, for both patients, caregivers, and clinicians, having a broad array of capabilities. It is anticipated that the smart phone/tablet will become the primary instrument for patient engagement in connected health, and that "applications" will emerge that improve both care and communication.

CONCLUSION

The effective management of HF requires personalized, proactive, and patient-driven healthcare. This is the model being deployed in VHA today, including primary and specialty care venues, there are three unifying goals: (1) decrease unnecessary hospitalizations, tests, and treatments for patients with HF. The overall aim is to increase the efficiency of VA HF care; (2) increase the use of life-improving therapy; and (3) increase the use of therapy that prolongs life. This includes the need to increase the capability of caregivers and patients to optimize self-care, maximize home care, and to improve palliative care.

An extensive resource of VHA's programs to improve HF care can be obtained from the CHF-QUERI website (Congestive Heart Failure Quality Enhancing Research Initiative). This includes publications, presentations, tool kits, fact sheets, implementation guides, quality improvement products, and links for patients, caregiver, researchers, etc.[6]

As noted, in the VHA model, we care for patients in the environment that is most suitable for their needs at the time. Patients with HF, especially those HF patients with more advanced and complex disease will move across boundaries frequently. So, to summarize, the VHA approach to patients with HF:

- Personalized, means that there is a complete understanding of each patient's unique disease, and that we address all the factors that impact on the course of the disease including both medical and social determinants. Proactive, means that if we understand the disease we can anticipate problems; big data and small data will be leveraged to optimize outcomes. That is rule 1 - *Know the disease*
- Personalized, means that patients are empowered and educated about their disease, especially including issues that impact on the outcomes patient perceive as important to them. When proactive, patients are engaged in the management of their health issues; education and understanding are crucial if patients are to be able to make informed decisions. That is Rule 2 - *Make it about the patient*
- Personalized, means that patients have a defined relationship with their healthcare providers in a system that is open, collaborative, consistent and constant,

unconstrained by time and distance. Proactive, means that communication and information between patients and providers flows both synchronously and asynchronously, moving information and decisions more closely time. That is Rule 3 - *Relationship based.*

When the above all occur, then healthcare can transition from system-centric, or even patient-centered, to patient-driven. Better information leads to better decisions and to better health. In VHA, we believe that this state will result in the most optimal outcomes for patient with HF, whatever the etiology or presentation.

ACKNOWLEDGMENT

I would like to acknowledge the seminal work of Dr Ralph Snyderman toward defining the importance of personalized, proactive patient driven care,[7] and to thank him for the many thoughtful conversations and insight he has shared with us as we have worked to adopt these concepts in VHA.

REFERENCES

1. Bueno H, Ross JS, Wang Y, et al. Trends in length of stay and short-term outcomes among Medicare patients hospitalized for heart failure, 1993-2006. JAMA. 2010;303(21):2141-7.
2. Kaboli PJ, Go JT, Hockenberry J, et al. Associations between reduced hospital length of stay and 30-day readmission rate and mortality: 14-year experience in 129 Veterans Affairs hospitals. Ann Intern Med. 2012;157(12):837-45.
3. Krumholz HM, Lin Z, Keenan PS, et al. Relationship between hospital readmission and mortality rates for patients hospitalized with acute myocardial infarction heart failure, or pneumonia. JAMA. 2013;309(6): 587-93.
4. Dharmarajan K, Hsieh AF, Lin Z, et al. Diagnoses and timing of 30-day readmissions after hospitalization for heart failure, acute myocardial infarction, or pneumonia. JAMA. 2013;309(4):355-63.
5. President's Council of Advisors on Science and Technology. (2008). Priorities for Personalized Medicine. [online] Available from: www.whitehouse.gov/files/documents/ostp/PCAST/pcast_report_v2.pdf. [Accessed December, 2013].
6. Alto P. (2013). Chronic Heart Failure (CHF) Quality Enhancement Research Initiative. [online] Available from: www.queri.research.va.gov/chf/. [Accessed December, 2013].
7. Snyderman R, Dinan M. Improving health by taking it personally. JAMA. 2010;303(4):363-4.

Chapter 47

Heart Failure in the Nursing Home Setting

Corrine Y Jurgens, Mary A Dolansky, Harleah G Buck

ABSTRACT

Management of residents with heart failure (HF) in long-term care facilities such as nursing homes pose unique challenges for delivery of quality care. Residents are complex in terms of older age, frailty, comorbid illness, polypharmacy, and atypical HF symptom profiles. Detecting changes in status is difficult as residents with limitations in function or cognition may not experience typical exertional symptoms of HF or be able to report changes in health status. Therefore, a comprehensive and systematic approach is recommended for ongoing interdisciplinary education and strategies for monitoring quality of care.

INTRODUCTION

Nursing home residents diagnosed with heart failure (HF) pose several unique challenges for health care providers. Challenges include accurate diagnosis in the context of comorbid illness, cognitive dysfunction, and an atypical HF symptom profile associated with an older population.[1,2] Many nursing home residents can be characterized as a vulnerable population being among the oldest-old with multiple comorbid illnesses.[3] Comorbidity complicates accurate attribution of symptoms to HF or less threatening illnesses because of overlapping symptom profiles. Other management challenges associated with nursing home care include lack of routine monitoring of HF status and reliance on direct care personnel to report changes in condition to licensed providers.[4] These challenges are formidable as currently, approximately 1.5 million Americans reside in nursing homes. Of those, almost 20% have a diagnosis of HF.[5]

For patients both with and without a known diagnosis of HF at the time of admission, detecting a change in HF status is particularly difficult. Early symptoms of impending decompensation of HF such as fatigue or activity intolerance are nonspecific and easily missed. Cognitive dysfunction is common, further limiting nursing home residents' ability to report symptoms. Importantly, symptoms of HF may be atypical in older adults based on sedentary lifestyles and compensatory changes in the pulmonary vasculature. As a result, hallmark symptoms of HF such as exertional dyspnea, orthopnea and nocturnal dyspnea may not be evident.[2,6,7] Atypical HF signs also may include loss of appetite and lower body mass index.[7] In adults older than 80 years of age, common symptoms of HF that would be unusual in younger patients include changes in mental status such as confusion, somnolence, irritability and fatigue.[1,2,8] Accordingly, acute changes in mental status should prompt an evaluation of cardiac status in residents with a history or risk factors for HF.

Comorbid illness is common among residents of nursing homes. The most frequently occurring comorbid illnesses in addition to HF are hypertension, dementia, depression, diabetes mellitus, chronic obstructive lung disease, stroke and arthritis.[3,5,9] Many of these diagnoses require ongoing pharmacotherapy. As a result, polypharmacy is common. When combined with management of HF congruent with national guidelines,[10-12] pharmacological management becomes a balancing act in a population with decreasing metabolic reserves. Pharmacotherapy of HF for the older, frail nursing home residents is largely empirical as most studies were conducted with younger and healthier populations. Quality of life over longevity is preferred by some patients with HF.[13] Accordingly, guideline therapy must be individualized to maximize quality of life, minimize symptom burden, and avoid both negative side-effects and drug-to-drug interactions. Cardiac medications outlined in the Beers criteria as potentially inappropriate in older adults include several antiarrhythmic drugs and higher doses of spironolactone and digoxin, to name a few. The full list can be found at website (onlinelibrary.wiley.com/doi/10.1111/j.1532-5415.2012.03923.x/pdf). Consideration of the resident's and family goals, functional and cognitive status is paramount when determining the plan of care including medications.

Finally, monitoring the status of residents with HF is challenging as it is not typically part of routine care in many nursing home facilities.[4] Lack of regular tracking of HF indices is problematic as symptoms can escalate insidiously over days to weeks resulting in the need for hospitalization. Health care providers also rely on direct caregivers for detection of a change in status necessitating ongoing education and monitoring of quality indicators. To "do it right" and achieve quality outcomes for nursing home residents with HF, an appreciation of age-related differences in presentation and management within the context of a nursing home health delivery system is important.

HEART FAILURE DISEASE MANAGEMENT IN THE NURSING HOME SETTING

Management of HF in long-term care is complex and frequently ignored.[14] Successful HF management requires coordination of care among interdisciplinary professional personnel, physicians, nurse practitioners, nursing assistants, residents and family members. As HF is a chronic and progressive illness, management typically entails periodic transitions in delivery of care. Changes in HF status that nursing home personnel must address include awareness of movement from a stable HF status to unstable, potentially requiring skilled transfer to and from the hospital, to end of life, including eventual crucial conversations related to palliative and hospice care. However, minimizing unnecessary transitions to acute care facilities is generally preferred as hospitalization is associated with increased risk of iatrogenic complications and increased healthcare costs.[15] With careful planning and training, particularly of licensed nursing home personnel, acute clinical events can potentially be managed in the nursing home setting. Several tools and resources designed to guide nursing home personnel on avoidable hospitalizations are available at website (interact2.net).[15]

Content of Heart Failure Disease Management in Nursing Homes

Heart failure disease management education is an important component supporting delivery of quality of care by nursing home personnel.[4] The content of HF disease management education must be consistent with national evidenced-based guidelines for HF[11,12] as well as those specific to long-term care systems.[16,17] Table 1 summarizes the essential components of the HF disease management content.

Heart failure residents must be identified so that all staff understand, who the residents with HF are, to ensure implementation of vigilant monitoring and treatment of acute decompensation as appropriate (Flowchart 1).[11,12] Residents with devices such as implantable cardioverter-defibrillators (ICD) and pacemakers should be clearly identified in the event the device deactivation is necessary.[18] The cardiologist managing the device and schedule of follow-up care should be documented in the medical record. In the event of inappropriate ICD shocks or emergent need to disable the device, ICDs can be deactivated by placing a donut magnet over the device.[19] Accordingly, access to a magnet with accompanying policies for use are needed in nursing home facilities. Systems for identification may include heart stickers, arm bands, or a special code next to their name.

The next essential content component is to have a HF assessment protocol in place so personnel, residents and family understand the critical importance of accurate daily weights, reporting of signs and symptoms, low sodium diet, and medications. This step can be facilitated using pocket cards, posters, and notations in the medical record.[16] The pocket card with the acronym *A NEW LEAF* can be used as a screening tool designed for direct caregivers for detection of changes in HF status (Box 1).[16]

The last content component is a mechanism to report the status of the resident from shift-to-shift and a summary tracking sheet used to report the HF trajectory of each resident. Clearly, direct caregivers will come to know and recognize subtle differences in

TABLE 1: Essential elements of heart failure disease management in nursing homes

Content components	
Identification of HF and devices	• Armband, sticker, reminder in chart, family awareness
Assessment: • Daily for high risk • Weekly for low risk	• Weights: Must be GRAPHED • Signs and symptoms (use pocket card/posters of symptoms and NYHA classification) • Vital signs
Report of status shift-to-shift for high-risk residents	• Keep a log of all the HF patients and current status for RN to review daily
Tracking HF	• A mechanism that summarizes the HF status of each resident (Fig. 1) • Continual assessment of the residents change in status and need to be moved to palliative/hospice care
Organizational implementation components	
Staff education	• Orientation • Continual reminders include: Basic physiology of HF, treatment, skill of accurate weights, signs and symptoms of worsening condition • Review of implantable devices and emergent deactivation of cardioverter defibrillator with donut magnet • National Heart Failure Training Program (N-HeFT™); website (www.nheft.org)
Family and resident education	• Information on HF monitoring, treatment, disease process and palliative/hospice services, website (www.hfsa.org/heart_failure_education_modules.asp)
Implementation plan	• Creating a climate for change, engage and enable the whole organization, implement and sustain change
Monitoring plan	• Monitoring adherence to protocols developed by leadership
Transition to hospital plan	• Standardization of communication both written and verbal between nursing and providers at both institutions
Transition to palliative care/hospice plan	• Partnering with local hospices and developing joint management plans

HF, heart failure; NYHA, New York Heart Association; RN, Registered nurse

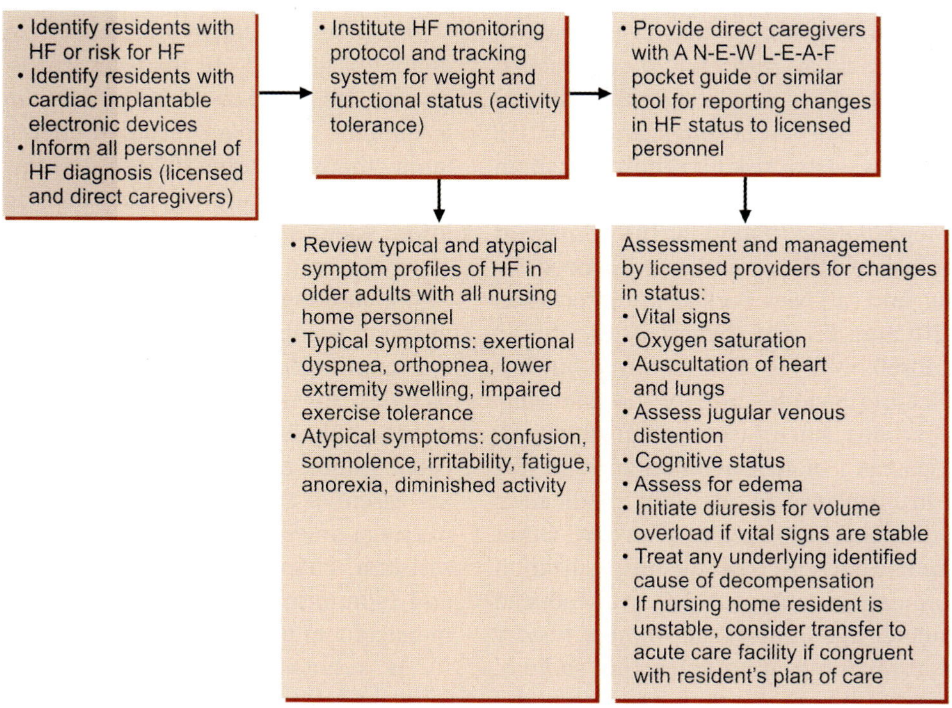

HF, heart failure

Flowchart 1 Algorithm for heart failure assessment and management in nursing homes

Box 1: A N-E-W L-E-A-F: a heart failure screening tool for direct caregivers[16]

A: Acute agitation/anxiety
N: Nighttime shortness of breath or increase in nighttime urination
E: Edema in lower extremities
W: Weight gain (2–4 pounds per week)
L: Lightheadedness
E: Extreme shortness of breath lying down
A: Abdominal symptoms (nausea, pain, decreased appetite, distention)
F: Fatigue

residents under their care. It is critically important to appreciate and act on their reports of residents' changes in cognition or functional status. Figure 1 displays the essential elements of a HF disease management tracking sheet. Knowledge of the condition and treatments over time is a key strategy for the successful management of residents diagnosed with HF. The tracking sheet provides the "forest" view to monitor the dynamic trajectory of HF care. Examination of HF status over time, comparing functional status and symptoms with activity from day to day, and reporting changes to licensed nursing home personnel and medical staff is essential for averting hospitalization.

The Minimum Data Set mandated by the Centers of Medicare and Medicaid Services is a comprehensive assessment used in nursing homes that is impractical for identifying residents at risk for a HF-related hospitalization. Accordingly, a simple algorithm (Fig. 1) for identifying those at risk for hospitalization for HF management is as follows. High risk for rehospitalization is defined as any of the following: (i) hospitalized during the last 6 months for HF exacerbation, or (ii) primary or a secondary diagnosis of HF that indicated a need for vigilant monitoring, and (iii) New York Heart Association (NYHA) classes III and IV, (iv) hypertension [blood pressure (BP) >150/90 mmHg]. The category for low risk for rehospitalization includes both of the following: (a) more than 6 months since last hospitalization for HF or (b) NYHA classes I or II. Documentation of risk is recommended to be placed in the daily medication administration record and in the resident's chart. Other risk factors reported to increase risk for hospitalization within 6 months among patients with HF with reduced ejection fraction include age greater than 70 years, history of diabetes, stroke, arrhythmia, abnormal serum sodium, blood urea nitrogen (BUN) greater than 43 mg/dL, and absence of beta-blocker therapy.[20,21]

Organizational Level Components Required for Heart Failure Disease Management

Organizational components are essential for a HF disease management program in nursing homes.[22] Table 1 displays organizational components of a disease management program to consider. Education must occur during orientation and quarterly as continual reminders to the staff. The education should include basic physiology of HF, treatment, skill of accurate weights, and signs and symptoms of worsening condition. Organizationally, a plan for implementation needs to be developed and disseminated.[23] The principles consist of three distinct phases: (i) creating a climate for change, (ii) engaging and enabling the whole organization, and (iii) implementing and sustaining change. Tools, such as HF pocket cards and weight booklets can be provided to staff as reminders to enhance daily integration.

Implementing a HF disease management program presents challenges less likely to be encountered in acute care settings.[17,22] The absence of a standard weight protocol for residents results in errors in daily weights (variation of blankets, shoes, different scales and wheelchairs). Therefore, a weight protocol to specify how to obtain accurate weights and a visual graphic of what 3 pounds of water is equal to needs to be posted to ensure consistency and awareness of the severity of the problem.

Balancing dietary preferences in the context of quality of life and HF management is often an issue in nursing homes. Lowering the sodium content in food is difficult as not all facilities offer low sodium diets, family members bring in high sodium content food, and residents potentially decrease their food intake with a lower sodium diet. Furthermore, resident weight loss can be a confounding condition for patients with HF. Although weight loss related to treatment of volume overload is appropriate for patients with HF, weight gain is often considered a sign of quality care in long-term care facilities. For residents without a diagnosis of HF, weight loss is a marker of inadequate nutrition. Interdisciplinary collaboration and HF dietary education for all personnel are essential components in the management of HF in nursing homes. A physician/nurse practitioner/physician assistant champion, weekly interdisciplinary rounds, and monitoring the implementation of the HF disease management program are keys to success.[22]

As rehospitalizations are a major concern and frequent,[4,21,24,25] a transitional care plan needs to be established. Having an institutional policy on

Heart Failure Disease Management in Nursing Homes

HF protocol initiated date_____________

Protocol type (circle any one):

- High risk
- Low risk

Date(s) of change in status_______________

- High risk (one of the following):
  - Hospitalized in last 6 months for HF
  - Primary or ACTIVE secondary diagnosis of HF
  - NYHA class III or IV
  - Hypertensive BP >150/90 mmHg
- Low risk (both must be present):
  - More than 6 months since last HF hospitalization
  - NYHA class I or II

Echocardiogram Report in Chart (Circle Any One) Yes No

- If NO, echocardiogram-ordered date ordered________
- Diet: No added sodium (NAS)_________date ordered_________
- Baseline weight__________________
- NYHA classification (circle one) I, II, III, IV
- Blood pressure__________ Pulse__________
- Weight Graph initiated________date

Heart Failure Medications (List Name, Dose and Frequency)

- ACE inhibitor__________________________
  - If no ACE inhibitor, ARB___________
  - If on neither state why – if known ___________
- Beta blocker__________________________
- Diuretic ______________________________

List of ACE inhibitors	benazepril, captopril, enalapril, fosinopril, lisinopril, perindopril, quinapril, ramipril, trandolapril, zestril
List of angiotensin II receptor blockers (ARB)	Candesartan (Atacand), eprosartan, irbesartan, losartan (Cozaar), telmisartan, valsartan (Diovan)
Potential reasons for why no ACE or ARB	History of adverse reaction (angioedema or cough), creatinine >2.5, hypotension, hyperkalemia, other
List of beta-blockers	Bisoprolol, metoprolol (Toprol, Lopressor), carvedilol (Coreg), atenolol (Tenormin)
List of diuretics	Furosemide (Lasix), bumetanide (Bumex), torsemide (Demadex)

Education Materials Given

- ______Resident (signs to report)
- ______Family (bringing in food)
- ______2 gm Na diet

Heart Failure Etiology

____Ischemic

____Non-ischemic

____Other

Heart failure type

______HF preserved ejection fraction

______HF reduced ejection fraction

______% left ventricular ejection fraction

Implanted Devices

- Implantable cardiac device_____________
- Resident activation/deactivation preference___________
- Physician managing device________________________; Follow-up appointment____________

Health Service Use

- Rehospitalization history ____
- Emergency room history____
- Palliative care consults____
- Hospice ____

HF, heart failure; NYHA, New York Heart Association; BP, blood pressure; ACE, angiotensin converting enzyme; Na, sodium

Fig. 1 Heart failure disease management tracking sheet

communication between the nursing home and the hospital or emergency department is essential for continuity of care. Similarly, a plan for transitioning HF residents to palliative care and hospice needs to be articulated so all members of the team (nurses, physicians, resident, family) can be involved in the decision making.

TRANSITION TO END-OF-LIFE CARE

Though the focus of care in a nursing home is aimed at quality of life, it is prudent to thoughtfully assist residents and families to plan for end of life. However, the trajectory for end of life among patients with HF is unpredictable and may span 1–2 years making the decision to initiate palliative care difficult.[26] For HF patients with significant cardiac dysfunction, current national HF guidelines recommend end-of-life care, such as hospice, as an option for stage D heart failure.[12,27] Specifically, recommendations are that clinicians conduct careful discussions of prognosis, goals of care and options available for end of life when all conventional strategies used in evidence based HF care have been implemented and no further therapies are deemed appropriate.[27] Options include continuing HF therapies from earlier stages that stabilize the patient, provide symptom relief or improve quality of life.[12] Aggressive procedures that do not potentiate recovery or increase quality of life are not deemed appropriate in the last months of life.[28] The setting of care, such as found in nursing homes, provides contextual issues but principles remain the same. Every resident with HF should receive optimal, guideline directed care.[29] The National Consensus Project for Quality Palliative Care[30] addresses contextual issues related to delivery of end-of-life care. Patient safety and privacy, open and flexible visiting hours, family support, and access to both palliative care teams and other professionals are criteria of quality end-of-life care in nonhome settings.

Challenges for Clinical Management in End of Life

While the setting of care provides unique challenges, common quandaries for managing any HF patient remain. Specifically, issue of prognosis, symptom management, and ethical issues are similar across settings. Prognostic factors in HF for a median survival of equal to or less than 6 months in those with three or more factors include increased age, poor left ventricular ejection fraction, elevated serum B-type natriuretic peptide, elevated cardiac troponin I, or C-reactive protein, multiple hospitalizations and/or critical events, decreased functional status, malnutrition, systolic hypotension and renal, vascular, or other comorbid diseases.[31] Retrospectively, admission hypotension, age, serum creatinine, anemia, comorbidities, left ventricular ejection fraction less than 40%, hyponatremia, cachexia, and depression have all been found to predict early postdischarge mortality.[32-34] Definitive prospective data is lacking. What is known is that HF patients managed by HF specialists are more likely to die of metabolic irregularity and subsequent coma or sudden death rather than by poor disease management evidenced by volume overload or severe dyspnea.[35,36]

Recommendations for HF management at end of life in the nursing home setting include aggressive symptom management, patient and family discussions, decision making, education, psychosocial and spiritual care, and possible interventions.[28,29,37] Palliation of symptoms becomes a primary focus in end-of-life care and regular assessment, ideally by resident rating is preferred.[30] The most common symptoms are dyspnea, pain, depression, fatigue, and edema.[29,38-40] These symptoms are related to HF or to comorbidities or common geriatric syndromes. Unfortunately, no rigorous evidence exists to address the best management of dyspnea, pain, or depression for end of life with HF.[39] Evidence from earlier in the HF trajectory and expert clinician opinion support the continued use of diuretics[41,42] and introduction of oxygen[37] for dyspnea and edema, opioids for moderate to severe pain[28] and dyspnea,[37] selective serotonin reuptake inhibitors and emotional or spiritual support for depression,[37,43] stimulants[37] and the exploration of secondary causes for fatigue, including anemia, depression, and sleep disordered breathing.[28,43] All treatments ordered earlier in HF including ICD devices should be reevaluated in light of the goals of care. Only essential pharmacological agents should be used. Therapies that are burdensome or not symptom focused may need to be discontinued or titrated down. Therapies that manage neurohormonal or sympathetic disorders should be continued as long as the patient tolerates them.[37] Open and caring discussions between clinicians and residents/families are a key element of quality palliative care.[30] Psychosocial and spiritual support are part of best practice palliative care.[30] Consultative services can be used by nursing home personnel without current resources to provide this interprofessional level of care.

Hospice as an Earlier Option

Many of the clinical management challenges discussed earlier can be addressed by earlier referral to hospice. Hospice has been shown to reduce hospitalizations and improve pain management in nursing homes.[44] However, the lack of recognition of HF as a terminal diagnosis, the unpredictable disease trajectory of HF, and a lack of coordination and communication are often cited as barriers to earlier referral.[29,44,45] New models of care, specifically palliative care consultative services, or nursing home based teams, or nursing home/hospice partner relationships are infusing the principles of palliative care into nursing homes.[45]

HEART FAILURE MANAGEMENT AND QUALITY OF CARE IN THE NURSING HOME SETTING

Providing quality care for nursing home residents diagnosed with HF requires systematic initiation and maintenance of processes to ensure accurate assessment of HF status. Education of nursing home personnel at all professional and support levels is critical in creating an environment attuned to assessment of residents who may have diminished capacity to report changes in their health. In the event of escalating HF symptoms, early detection may avert hospitalization with treatment in the nursing home setting. To maximize improvement of HF disease management in nursing homes, quality must be systematically tracked and evaluated. Monitoring quality indicators via chart audits, feedback of results to personnel, clinical decision support, and reminder systems for use of HF medications and tests have been shown to be effective.[11,46,47]

CONCLUSION

Heart failure, prevalent among nursing home residents, requires recognizing subtle changes in status to support early intervention of volume overload. In addition to maintaining pharmacological therapies to control symptoms, routine monitoring similar to tracking blood glucose levels for diabetes is paramount. Vigilant monitoring includes carefully tracking weight and activity tolerance from day to day. Worsening HF can occur insidiously over several weeks. Therefore, all staff interacting with residents should be trained to observe and report changes in symptom burden. To "do it right", a comprehensive systems approach in conjunction with interdisciplinary HF management and palliative care strategies will support quality of care for residents in nursing homes.

REFERENCES

1. Rich MW. Heart failure in older adults. Med Clin North Am. 2006;90(5):863-85.
2. Tresch DD. Clinical manifestations, diagnostic assessment, and etiology of heart failure in elderly patients. Clin Geriatr Med. 2000;16(3):445-56.
3. Kasper HJ, O'Malley M, Kaiser Commission on Medicaid and the Uninsured. (2007) Changes in characteristics, needs, and payments for elderly nursing home residents: 1999 to 2004. Washington, DC: Kaiser Family Foundation. [online] Available from kff.org/medicaid/report/changes-in-characteristics-needs-and-payment-for/. [Accessed December, 2013].
4. Boxer RS, Dolansky MA, Frantz MA, et al. The Bridge Project: improving heart failure care in skilled nursing facilities. J Am Med Dir Assoc. 2012;13(1):83.e1-7.
5. Moore KL, Boscardin WJ, Steinman MA, et al. Age and sex variation in prevalence of chronic medical conditions in older residents of U.S. nursing homes. J Am Geriatr Soc. 2012;60(4):756-64.
6. Ahmed A, Allman RM, Aronow WS, et al. Diagnosis of heart failure in older adults: predictive value of dyspnea at rest. Arch Gerontol Geriatr. 2004;38(3):297-307.
7. Oudejans I, Mosterd A, Bloemen JA, et al. Clinical evaluation of geriatric outpatients with suspected heart failure: value of symptoms, signs, and additional tests. Eur J Heart Fail. 2011;13(5):518-27.
8. Rich MW, Kitzman DW. Heart failure in octogenarians: A fundamentally different disease. Am J Geriatr Cardiol. 2000;9(Suppl):97-104.
9. Daamen MA, Schols JM, Jaarsma T, et al. Prevalence of heart failure in nursing homes: a systematic literature review. Scand J Caring Sci. 2010;24(1):202-8.
10. American Geriatrics Society updated Beers Criteria for potentially inappropriate medication use in older adults. J Am Geriatr Soc. 2012;60(4):616-31.
11. Hunt SA, Abraham WT, Chin MH, et al. 2009 Focused update incorporated into the ACC/AHA 2005 Guidelines for the Diagnosis and Management of Heart Failure in Adults: A Report of the American College of Cardiology Foundation/American Heart Association Task Force on Practice Guidelines Developed in Collaboration with the International Society for Heart and Lung Transplantation. J Am Coll Cardiol. 2009;53(15):e1-90.
12. Heart Failure Society of America, Lindenfeld J, Albert NM, et al. HFSA 2010 Comprehensive Heart Failure Practice Guideline. J Card Fail. 2010;16(6):e1-194.
13. Stanek EJ, Oates MB, McGhan WF, et al. Preferences for treatment outcomes in patients with heart failure: symptoms versus survival. J Card Fail. 2000;6(3):225-32.
14. Dolansky MA, Zullo MD, Hassanein S, et al. Cardiac rehabilitation in skilled nursing facilities: a missed opportunity. Heart Lung. 2012;41(2):115-24.
15. Ouslander JG, Lamb G, Tappen R, et al. Interventions to reduce hospitalizations from nursing homes: evaluation of the INTERACT II collaborative quality improvement project. J Am Geriatr Soc. 2011;59(4):745-53.
16. Harrington CC. Assessing heart failure in long-term care facilities. J Gerontol Nurs. 2008;34(2):9-14.
17. Martinen M, Freundl M. Managing congestive heart failure in long-term care: development of an interdisciplinary protocol. J Gerontol Nurs. 2004;30(12):5-12.
18. Goldstein N, Carlson M, Livote E, et al. Brief communication: Management of implantable cardioverter-defibrillators in hospice: A nationwide survey. Annals Int Med. 2010;152(5):296-9.

19. Lampert R, Hayes DL, Annas GJ, et al. HRS Expert Consensus Statement on the Management of Cardiovascular Implantable Electronic Devices (CIEDs) in patients nearing end of life or requesting withdrawal of therapy. Heart Rhythm. 2010;7(7):1008-26.
20. Allen LA, Gheorghiade M, Reid KJ, et al. Identifying patients hospitalized with heart failure at risk for unfavorable future quality of life. Circ Cardiovasc Qual Outcomes. 2011;4(4):389-98.
21. Allen LA, Hernandez AF, Peterson ED, et al. Discharge to a skilled nursing facility and subsequent clinical outcomes among older patients hospitalized for heart failure. Circ Heart Fail. 2011;4(3):293-300.
22. Dolansky MA, Hitch JA, Piña IL, et al. Implementation of a heart failure management program in skilled nursing facilities: lessons learned. Clin Nurs Res. 2013;22(4):432-47.
23. Stoller JK. Implementing change in respiratory care. Respir Care. 2010; 55(6):749-57.
24. Chen J, Ross JS, Carlson MD, et al. Skilled nursing facility referral and hospital readmission rates after heart failure or myocardial infarction. Am J Med. 2012;125(1):100.e1-9.
25. Mor V, Intrator O, Feng Z, et al. The revolving door of rehospitalization from skilled nursing facilities. Health Aff (Millwood). 2010;29(1):57-64.
26. Sullivan MD, O'Meara ES. Heart failure at the end of life: symptoms, function, and medical care in the Cardiovascular Health Study. Am J Geriatr Cardiol. 2006;15(4):217-25.
27. Jessup M, Abraham WT, Casey DE, et al. 2009 focused update: ACCF/AHA Guidelines for the Diagnosis and Management of Heart Failure in Adults: a report of the American College of Cardiology Foundation/American Heart Association Task Force on Practice Guidelines: developed in collaboration with the International Society for Heart and Lung Transplantation. Circulation. 2009;119(14):1977-2016.
28. Adler ED, Goldfinger JZ, Kalman J, et al. Palliative care in the treatment of advanced heart failure. Circulation. 2009;120(25):2597-606.
29. Goodlin SJ, Hauptman PJ, Arnold R, et al. Consensus statement: Palliative and supportive care in advanced heart failure. J Card Fail. 2004;10(3): 200-9.
30. National Consensus Project for Quality Palliative Care. (2009). Clinical Practice Guidelines for Quality Palliative Care, 2nd edition. [online] Available from www.nationalconsensusproject.org/guideline.pdf. [Accessed February, 2014].
31. Salpeter SR, Luo EJ, Malter DS, et al. Systematic review of noncancer presentations with a median survival of 6 months or less. Am J Med. 2012;125(5):512.e1-6.
32. O'Connor CM, Abraham WT, Albert NM, et al. Predictors of mortality after discharge in patients hospitalized with heart failure: an analysis from the Organized Program to Initiate Lifesaving Treatment in Hospitalized Patients with Heart Failure (OPTIMIZE-HF). Am Heart J. 2008;156(4):662-73.
33. Coventry PA, Grande GE, Richards DA, et al. Prediction of appropriate timing of palliative care for older adults with non-malignant life-threatening disease: a systematic review. Age Ageing. 2005;34(3):218-27.
34. Lee DS, Austin PC, Rouleau JL, et al. Predicting mortality among patients hospitalized for heart failure: derivation and validation of a clinical model. JAMA. 2003;290(19):2581-7.
35. Teuteberg JJ, Lewis EF, Nohria A, et al. Characteristics of patients who die with heart failure and a low ejection fraction in the new millennium. J Card Fail. 2006;12(1):47-53.
36. Derfler MC, Jacob M, Wolf RE, et al. Mode of death from congestive heart failure: implications for clinical management. Am J Geriatr Cardiol. 2004;13(6):299-304.
37. Goodlin SJ. Palliative care in congestive heart failure. J Am Coll Cardiol. 2009;54(5):386-96.
38. Goodlin SJ. Palliative care for end-stage heart failure. Curr Heart Fail Rep. 2005;2(3):155-60.
39. Lorenz KA, Lynn J, Dy SM, et al. Evidence for improving palliative care at the end of life: a systematic review. Ann Intern Med. 2008;148(2): 147-59.
40. Abraham A, Kutner JS, Beaty B. Suffering at the end of life in the setting of low physical symptom distress. J Palliat Med. 2006;9(3):658-65.
41. Faris R, Flather MD, Purcell H, et al. Diuretics for heart failure. Cochrane Database Syst Rev. 2006;(1):CD003838.
42. Cheng JW, Nayar M. A review of heart failure management in the elderly population. Am J Geriatr Pharmacother. 2009;7(5):233-49.
43. Goodlin SJ. End-of-life care in heart failure. Curr Cardiol Rep. 2009;11(3):184-91.
44. Stevenson DG, Bramson JS. Hospice care in the nursing home setting: a review of the literature. J Pain Symptom Manage. 2009;38(3):440-51.
45. Carlson MD, Lim B, Meier DE. Strategies and innovative models for delivering palliative care in nursing homes. J Am Med Dir Assoc. 2011;12(2):91-8.
46. Fonarow GC, Abraham WT, Albert NM, et al. Influence of a performance-improvement initiative on quality of care for patients hospitalized with heart failure: results of the Organized Program to Initiate Lifesaving Treatment in Hospitalized Patients With Heart Failure (OPTIMIZE-HF). Arch Intern Med. 2007;167(14):1493-502.
47. Fonarow GC, Albert NM, Curtis AB, et al. Improving evidence-based care for heart failure in outpatient cardiology practices: primary results of the Registry to Improve the Use of Evidence-Based Heart Failure Therapies in the Outpatient Setting (IMPROVE HF). Circulation. 2010;122(6):585-96.

Chapter 48

Heart Failure from the Nursing Perspective

Nancy M Albert

ABSTRACT

Heart failure management is complex. Nurses who apply management approaches directed by medical or licensed independent nurse care providers must consider patient and family needs and issues surrounding multiple foci of care, complexity of care, desire and ability to adhere to the plan of care, and knowledge about treatments and responsibilities in self care. Further, nurse variability in knowledge about heart failure assessment and management and in available resources and support structures, systems and processes, may affect nursing management of heart failure and ultimately, patient outcomes. This chapter will discuss global differences in nursing training and background and the three primary groups of clinically based nurses. Nursing perspectives in managing adults with chronic heart failure will be discussed throughout the continuum of care. Changes in hospital reimbursement for heart failure care have prompted administrators to call upon nurses to lead change in managing patients during care transitions, especially from hospital to the next site of care. The emergence of new or redefined roles may create opportunities that strengthen nursing coordination, collaboration, and teamwork with other healthcare professions.

INTRODUCTION

Nurses are holistic in their approach to patient management. Holistic management refers to caring for the whole person. In heart failure (HF) management, holistic nursing involves consideration for the interconnectedness of the mind, body, emotion, environment, relationships, and social, cultural, economic and spiritual being. The following discussion are global themes that nurses understand (or must quickly learn and master) about heart failure management in order to be an effective and responsive healthcare provider, no matter the setting or circumstances of care delivery. Although the themes may seem fairly basic and maybe even intuitive to expert HF clinicians, nurses providing or overseeing direct patient care face intermittent and ongoing barriers and issues when managing HF:

- HF pathophysiology is complex, involves multiple etiologies and foci, and may be asymptomatic or symptomatic
- Comorbidities that mask or mimic HF signs and symptoms are prevalent and must be managed effectively
- Hospitalization, rehospitalization, and mortality rates are high
- Fluid overload may be an important precipitant to or objective marker of acute decompensation
- Optimal medical management includes core vasodilator [angiotensin-converting enzyme inhibitors (ACEIs), angiotensin receptor blockers (ARBs), and hydralazine/nitrate (H/N) combination], beta blocker, and aldosterone antagonist therapies delivered at target doses; as well as cardiac device therapies, when warranted[1,2]
- Processes involving reconciliation of pharmacologic therapies and facilitation of patient adherence to core HF pharmacologic therapies must be routinely implemented at transitions of care and routine nurse patient encounters

- Application of disease management or team approaches in assessing, planning and evaluating care is critical to meeting patient management goals, promoting patient safety, facilitating family/caregiver support and decreasing mortality[3,4]
- Individualized, face-to-face processes that promote or enhance patient adherence to nonpharmacologic, guideline recommended self-care expectations (such as activity and exercise, diet, fluid management and monitoring of signs and symptoms of worsening condition) are time intensive to clinicians, patients and families/caregivers, but development and implementation are critical to supporting patients' need to control HF and manage health[5,6]
- Patient education about HF requires delivery of information about what HF means (including the cause if known and that it is chronic, even when asymptomatic), its timeline, consequences and how to monitor and control it. Education must be individualized to patient's learning styles and include assessment of patient understanding of education taught[7,8]
- Patients generally have multiple care providers. Systems and processes of open, ongoing patient provider communication and collaboration can assure consistent, high quality healthcare delivery and optimal responsiveness to changing patient needs
- Physician and administrative leadership, support, and commitment to adherence of contemporary, guideline recommended HF management is critical to nurses' ability to plan and deliver evidence based, best practice nursing care and create innovative systems and processes that advance quality of care[9]
- Excellence in delivery of family centered HF care requires continual nurse education and understanding about new and changing evidence related to HF care. Nurse education should include assessment, diagnostic measures and risk stratification tools, management therapeutics, cardiac and mechanical circulatory devices, surgical approaches and advanced care strategies.

This chapter will describe and discuss what HF management really looks like from a nursing perspective. First, global differences in nursing training and background will provide context for differences in the delivery of nursing care to manage HF. There are three primary groups of clinically based nurses. Although each group has similarities, it is the unique perspective each group brings that enhances the management of HF. The second focus is on nursing perspectives in managing adults previously diagnosed with HF. Content will span the continuum of patient stability from being asymptomatic, to maintaining symptoms at a stable clinical status, to overcoming episodes of acute decompensation, and to encouraging palliation at end-of-life.

NURSE TRAINING AND ROLE

Nurses caring for patients with HF have varies by basic training that generally spans a range from receiving a 2-year community college associate nursing degree, 3-year diploma certificate, or a 4-year bachelor degree. Regardless of differences in basic education that affects how nurses view patient management responsibilities, hospital and ambulatory-based clinical nurses make patient care decisions aimed at bolstering heart function and clinical outcomes. Nurses make practice-centered decisions that optimize patient quality and safety and promote evolution in clinical care. Moreover, nurses aim to overcome complexities in care planning. They foster interdisciplinary collaboration to enhance culturally sensitive and economically and emotionally responsive care to patients who are generally elderly and have multiple comorbidities.

Beyond basic training, nurses on the other end of the spectrum are advanced practice nurses (APNs) with graduate degrees, who are trained as clinical nurse specialists or nurse practitioners. APNs understand the importance of and have necessary training and skills in translating research and other best practice evidence into clinical practice. APNs also carry out patient advocacy roles that include measuring patient outcomes (at the patient, local practitioner, system and national levels), and participating actively on teams aimed at transforming health care systems to ensure quality and safety. As an example, APNs may be on HF transition of care or performance measures work groups aimed at creating or adapting local agendas based on national governmental policies and healthcare reform.

Regardless of nurse training, nursing roles can influence clinical nursing management of HF.[10] Nurse clinicians provide routine care based on physician leadership and administrator goals and level of support and specific care under the direction of a physician or licensed independent provider. APNs with a clinical practitioner focus prescribe medications, order consultative services (cardiac rehabilitation, pulmonary care, or hospice services) and make decisions about the need for hospitalization or long-term care in addition to basic care services. Alternately, APNs may have a clinical focus that is population-based. Nurses with a population-based focus have responsibilities in assuring quality care and best practices for a population of patients, rather than individual patients (for a cardiovascular service line or HF service team). They create and ensure opportunities for optimal evidence based clinical practices, efficient care delivery processes among team members, clinical nursing research, and use creativity and innovation to improve practices in an evolving healthcare system. Population-based APNs address issues and overcome barriers on a global level and may have responsibilities in a hospital, ambulatory setting, skilled nursing facility, or in multiple settings across the continuum of care.

Variation in highest nurse training, environment of clinical care and nurse roles affects how individual patients and patient populations are managed. Perceived importance of role expectations, such as patient family centered care planning and education delivery, can affect care quality and capability of achieving outcomes consistent with nursing excellence. Moreover, policies and procedures, resources (human, supplies, equipment), interdisciplinary support systems, time to carry out roles, administrative guidance, leadership oversight, and attention to quality monitoring are all facilitating and constricting forces in patient management. Table 1 provides general nursing management capabilities based on training as a nurse clinician working in a general cardiac or HF environment of care versus an advanced care, HF specialty or critical care area, and for APNs, based on a clinical practitioner or population based focus. Table 1 is not inclusive, many nursing team members have eclectic roles not discussed; for example, education specialists, case managers, transition coaches, and unit or department managers or coordinators. When nurses with expertise in eclectic HF roles are part of the healthcare team, management goals are strengthened. In addition, non-nurse interdisciplinary providers may be called upon to enhance patient and family centered care, especially when nurse retention or other factors limit nurses' ability to carry out patient care expectations. For example, pharmacists, dieticians and exercise physiologists can provide individualized medication, diet and exercise instructions, respectively, to hospitalized patients before discharge.

Healthcare providers, especially physician leaders, need to understand the scope and capabilities of nurses based on training and roles. For example, developing a home care program in HF that includes extensive patient education and nurse assessment for fluid status may be beyond the knowledge level of home care nurse clinicians who serve multiple populations and lack intensive patient care experiences or formal training in managing patients with HF. Nurses may have completed continuing education classes on reviewing food labels for sodium content, and the importance of exercise; however, lack of confidence or comfort in teaching specific details about low sodium diet and exercise may become a barrier to delivering expected patient education content.[11-14] Failure to deliver HF education with enough breadth and depth, may affect 6-month clinical outcomes, especially rehospitalization.[5,6,15] Nurses untrained in advanced assessment of fluid status beyond identifying rales, lower extremity edema and ascites may not recognize new or worsening fluid overload manifested as a new S3 heart sound, murmur, or jugular venous distension or elevated pulsation. Failure to identify early worsening of status could impair patient quality of life and precipitate rehospitalization. The literature includes many examples of heterogeneous results of hospital, home care service, community, cardiac rehabilitation, telemonitoring, and mixed site disease management programs,[3,4,16-18] that may have been dependent on clinical nurse delivery of services that were beyond the nurses' level of training or expertise. Ultimately, a strong match between nurse strengths and role demands will increase success of disease management programs and lead to desired outcomes.

MANAGING ADULTS WITH HEART FAILURE

Asymptomatic Heart Failure

In this section, it is assumed that physicians have already confirmed presence of HF, diagnosed HF etiology, and staged the syndrome's severity as stage C. Nurses have multiple roles in managing patients currently in asymptomatic status or New York Heart Association (NYHA) functional class (FC) I. Heart failure is chronic and progressive; thus, an asymptomatic condition may be perceived as a stable state. However, thorough subjective and objective assessments can help determine if the asymptomatic state is due to a truly stable state or a purposeful change in patient behaviors designed to eliminate symptoms. For example, patients who become dyspneic when walking to the mailbox or carrying groceries into the house may forgo these behaviors, then report not having symptoms when questioned. Nurses must be diligent in questioning patients and using objective markers to verify findings; for example, brain natriuretic peptide (BNP) less than 100 pg/mL or

TABLE 1: General nursing capabilities based on training and role in managing heart failure

General nurse capabilities in accurately managing patients with heart failure (examples in parentheses are not inclusive)	*Nonadvanced practice nurse clinicians*		*Advanced practice nurses*	
	Ambulatory or hospital, general care settings	*Critical or advanced heart failure specialty care*	*Clinical practitioner focus*	*Population focus*
Provide gross objective assessment of excessive intravascular and interstitial volume overload (edema, lung crackles, dyspnea)	+	+	+	+
Provide gross objective assessment of excessive intravascular volume depletion (orthostatic symptoms from excessive diuretic use, diarrhea, fever, sweating)	+	+	+	+
Provide fine objective assessment of fluid status (S3, JVD-P, new/ worsening murmur, paroxysmal nocturamal dyspnea, sleep apnea; hepatojugular reflex; serum laboratory changes)	–	~	+	+
Provide fine objective assessment of left ventricular dysfunction (laterally displaced point of maximal impulse; pulsus alternans; chest pain or palpitations in left lateral position; echocardiogram findings—left ventricular end-diastolic pressure or volume)	–	-/~	~/+	+
Understand hemodynamics beyond high or low blood pressure, oxygen saturation or respirations; and tachy- or bradycardiac heart rate	–	+	+	+
Understand physical examination findings that differentiate systolic from diastolic dysfunction (S3, S4, peripheral edema, JVD-P and cardiomegaly) and those that are similar (rales)	~	~	+	+
Provide subjective assessment of new or worsening status, assuming appropriate time is allotted	~	~	+	+
Provide assessment of patients' current knowledge of heart failure and barriers to readiness to change; assuming appropriate time is allotted	–/~	+	+	+
Deliver in depth patient education on core heart failure medications; assuming appropriate time is allotted	–/~/+	~/+	~/+	~/+
Deliver in depth patient education on self-care expectations related to diet, fluid management and signs and symptoms of worsening heart failure; assuming appropriate time is allotted	–/~/+	+	~/+	~/+
Assess and provide patient education about factors that increase risk for worsening condition (obesity, smoking, alcohol or substance abuse)	+	+	+	+
Determine a patients'"dry" weight (weight without excess fluid) and assess for optimization of weight	–	-/~	~/+	~/+
Determine current New York Heart Association-functional status and stage of heart failure	–/~/+	~/+	+	+
Determine atrial fibrillation contribution to current subjective/objective health status	~/+	+	+	+
Use serum laboratory changes plus current medications and subjective/ objective health status to determine dilutional hyponatremia, worsening renal or liver function, and myocardial instability requiring emergency care, hospitalization or readiness for hospice or palliative care	–	~/+	~/+	~/+
Use echocardiogram, subjective/objective health status and other measures to determine need for surgical care approaches (coronary artery bypass surgery, or valvular procedures)	–	-/~/+	+	+

Contd...

Contd...

General nurse capabilities in accurately managing patients with heart failure (examples in parentheses are not inclusive)	*Nonadvanced practice nurse clinicians*		*Advanced practice nurses*	
	Ambulatory or hospital, general care settings	*Critical or advanced heart failure specialty care*	*Clinical practitioner focus*	*Population focus*
Assess psychosocial, cultural and economic care needs and patient preferences, assuming appropriate time is allotted	+	+	+	+
Assess cognitive, psychological, literacy, health literacy and preferred method of learning, assuming appropriate time is allotted	+	+	+	+
Assess use of prescription (thiazolidinediones, dronedarone) and over-the-counter substances (nonsteroidal anti-inflammatory drugs, ephedrine, effervescent antacids) that should be avoided or are contraindicated	–/~	~	+	+
Assess readiness for a cardiac device (cardiac resynchronization or implantable cardioverter defibrillator) based on QRS width, presence of Q waves and/or left bundle branch block	–	-/~	+	~/+
Screen patients for advanced therapies or need for change in setting (home to hospital; hospital floor to critical care)	~/+	+	+	+
Assess patients for non heart failure conditions that could worsen heart failure or require use of therapies that could cause progressive worsening of condition (anemia, thyroid disease, chronic lung diseases, peripheral vascular diseases, sleep disorders, gout, cardiac dysrhythmias, hypertension, hypotension, degenerative joint disease)	~	+	+	+
Evaluate effectiveness of current medication therapies and need for up- or down-titration	~	+	+	+
Evaluate effectiveness of current nonpharmacological therapies and need for revision or consultation of other healthcare personnel	~	+	+	+
Participate in developing, implementing and routinely assessing the effectiveness of unit based quality or process improvement activities	–/~/+	–/~/+	+	+
Participate in gap analysis of issues with healthcare provider performance	–	–	~/+	~/+
Participate in gap analysis of issues with clinical care delivery and/or outcomes of clinical care (rehospitalization, mortality, quality of life)	–	–	~/+	~/+
Request internal or external interdisciplinary care consultation to advance clinical therapies	~/+	~/+	+	+
Communicate with physician and other non-nurse healthcare providers to advance clinical therapies	+	+	+	+
Communicate with physician and other non-nurse healthcare providers to minimize gaps in care and promote evidence-based practices	–/~	–/~	+	~/+
Review heart failure literature for highest strength and quality of research evidence on clinical and non clinical management topics important to managing patients clinically	–/~	–/~	+	+
Translate best practice, research-based evidence in clinical setting	–/~	–/~	+	+

+, yes; –, no; ~ yes, with formal training and/or practical application experiences.

JVD-P, jugular venous distension-pressure elevation

N-terminal pro-brain natriuretic peptide (NT-proBNP) less than 400 pg/mL; stable blood pressure and slow heart rate (HR) (<80 beats per minute at rest when on optimal core HF therapies). A systematic plan of assessing 6 minute walk test distance will facilitate reliability in testing and accuracy of results when changes in meters walked are observed from visit to visit.

Nurses must understand that asymptomatic HF should not prompt lackadaisical HF treatment. Patients on the right core HF therapies, but not on ideal doses based on multicenter evidence from large randomized controlled trials, need to have therapies optimized. When patients are in asymptomatic HF, they should be encouraged to routinely complete aerobic exercises and maintain a low sodium diet when dining outside the home. Nurses must remember to educate patients about normal short term effects of exercise; such as dyspnea, diaphoresis and elevated HR, so that patients do not perceive a need to stop exercising when they experience normal effects. Education about subtle signs and symptoms of excess intravascular sodium and fluid could create greater awareness of the effects of a high sodium meal on subsequent physical functioning.

For APNs who treat patients independently, it is important to obtain yearly assessments of serum laboratory results for anemia, thyroid function, hypercholesterolemia, diabetes, and other medical conditions. An electrocardiogram is needed to assess heart rhythm, findings consistent of previous ST elevated myocardial infarction, and determine QRS width. An echocardiogram may be needed to assure stable myocardial function (Box 1).

Box 1: Nurse management of asymptomatic heart failure

- Assure delivery of tailored heart failure medication therapies
- Assess adherence to prescribed heart failure medication therapies
- Aerobic activity and exercise training, cardiac rehabilitation, and assessment of adherence to activity counseling
- Moderate sodium restriction (3,000 mg sodium per day) and assessment of adherence to dietary counseling
- Optimization of weight if under or overweight
- Daily weight monitoring, understanding of dry weight, assessment of adherence to daily weight counseling, and self-care measures to control weight when changes occur
- Smoking and alcohol cessation counseling
- Counseling of individualized patient factors to attenuate risk of onset of symptoms
- Assure minimum of yearly to biyearly ambulatory follow-up
- Assess laboratory, electrocardiogram, echocardiogram findings at follow-up
- Consult with electrophysiologist (cardiac devices), pulmonologist (sleep disordered breathing), endocrinologist (diabetes, thyroid disease, or other endocrine abnormalities), or other services, as needed
- Family counseling to promote self-care monitoring and management

Patients with Symptomatic Heart Failure and Stable Status

Stable symptomatic status may reflect NYHA-FC II or III status. Disease management is an important means of preventing acute decompensation, promoting continued stable status and facilitating improved cardiac function. Nurses are the lead care providers in disease management programs and are responsible for directing and delivering care (APNs) or carrying out nursing actions based on healthcare provider orders (nurse clinicians). The scope of disease management services is wide, and may involve all aspects of the plan of care (assessment, planning interventions, implementing interventions, and evaluating interventions and outcomes); or may be focused on HF counseling and education; or monitoring for worsening status through telemonitoring or other means. Management principles discussed in asymptomatic patients apply here (Box 1); however, there are common pitfalls in treating stable HF that can lead to worsening of status and warrant discussion (Box 2).

There is an assumption that nurses understand medication management in HF: not just the right drug, dose, timing and frequency of administration; but also, pathophysiologic effects in HF, expected versus adverse events, and monitoring needs at initiation or uptitration. However, research on nurse understanding of medications commonly used in HF was highest for aspirin, warfarin and diuretics and low for drug therapies of most importance in keeping HF stabilized (ACEI, ARB, and aldosterone antagonists).[19] Nurse understanding of HF medications requires regular updates through continuing education. Better nurse understanding of medication therapies may facilitate greater depth and breadth of information delivered to patients during medication counseling. Further, nurses will be better able to advocate for patients.

Congestive Heart Failure Patients with Acute Decompensation

As previously mentioned, HF is a complex condition. In the acute care setting, nurses are always part of a team

Box 2: Common pitfalls nurses must consider in maintaining patient stability

- Recognize the presence of noncardiac related comorbidities since a noncardiac, nonheart failure condition (such as chronic obstructive pulmonary disease, asthma, bronchitis, pneumonia, and hypoventilation from sleep disordered breathing) may be the cause of current symptoms, even if stable
- Assure that patients understand that heart failure is chronic, not episodic, and that stable status requires ongoing adherence to drug therapies and nonpharmacologic self-care expectations
- Assure correction of reversible causes of heart failure and/or conditions that could worsen silently and affect heart failure outcomes. Correction may involve counseling (alcohol and/or substance abuse) or treatment of myocardial ischemia, hypertension, hyperlipidemia, atrial fibrillation, or diabetes
- Failure to recognize and make changes in pharmacologic therapies as needed (nonexhaustive list):
    - Inappropriate decrease in ACEI, ARB, or hydralazine/nitrate (H/N) combination due to transient asymptomatic hypotension or lightheadedness
    - Inappropriate decrease in ACEI or ARB due to a transient, mild increase in creatinine or blood urea nitrogen (especially when associated with aggressive diuretic therapy)
    - Inappropriate decrease in beta-blocker therapy for asymptomatic bradycardia when heart rate is 50 beats per minute or higher (and not receiving amiodarone)
    - Failure to use evidence based beta-blocker therapies (carvedilol, metoprolol succinate, or bisoprolol)
    - Ineffective diuretic therapy prescription or excessive diuresis requiring a decrease in diuretic therapy
    - Failure to use aldosterone antagonist therapy in patients with symptomatic heart failure and left ventricular systolic dysfunction, who meet criteria
    - Failure to decrease digoxin dose in patients with renal insufficiency
    - Failure to decrease digoxin dose in patients receiving amiodarone therapy
    - Failure to add nitrate therapy (preload reduction) to improve dyspnea and signs of fluid overload when diuretic therapy (in addition to other core heart failure therapies) does not resolve the problem
    - Inappropriate use of the combination of ACEI, ARB or renin inhibitor and aldosterone antagonist therapies
    - Failure to use anticoagulant therapy in concomitant atrial fibrillation (when not contraindicated)
    - Failure to reassess timing of medication doses when hypotension or lightheadedness occurs
        - Switch twice daily beta blocker from breakfast and dinner to breakfast and bedtime and once daily vasodilator therapy (ACEI or ARB) to dinner time
        - Administering aldosterone antagonist or vasodilator therapy before the loop diuretic morning dose (for example, 30 minutes), to enhance the effectiveness of the loop diuretic
    - Failure to consider and control polypharmacy, when appropriate
    - Failure to promote delivery of medications during hospitalization on a schedule that mimics the patients preferred home schedule
- Failure to provide individualized self-care education and assure patient understanding
    - Focusing on "what" to do; rather than on "how" to do it based on current lifestyle and limiting (social, cultural, and economic) factors
    - Failure to provide the full scope of education needed to apply principles in everyday life; i.e. discusses low sodium diet but fails to discuss how to prevent relapse when depressed, socializing with friends/family or at a restaurant; provides fluid restriction (when warranted) but does not provide instructions on how to overcome thirst
    - Failure to assure that patients understand the rationale for self-care instructions and notification of healthcare providers when changes occur; especially related to weight monitoring and monitoring of signs of worsening condition, since patients may not feel different (no new or worsening symptoms) with an increase in weight or edema

ACEI, angiotensin-converting enzyme inhibitor; ARB, angiotensin receptor blocker

of healthcare providers. Nurses need to understand that pulmonary congestion may be substantial, even when patients do not have rales or jugular venous distension. Team management is important since patients may have liver congestion, impaired mental acuity, sleep disordered breathing, anxiety, atrial and ventricular dysrhythmias, renal insufficiency, polypharmacy, and other factors that affect decompensation severity and treatment options. Nurses are key participants in general management aimed at improving signs and symptoms of hypervolemia (very common) and low cardiac output (less common); as well as dealing with comorbid medical diagnoses

Box 3: Transition care nursing roles*

- Focused assessments to identify early signs of problems and changes in health status (in hospital)
- Identifies the primary caregiver postdischarge
- Creates an evidence based care plan
- Utilizes shared decision making
- Implements strategies to prevent onset of symptoms or minimize symptom effects†
- Collaborates with patients' physicians regarding adjustments in medications and other therapies (in postdischarge setting or among multiple ambulatory providers)
- Shares discharge and hospital information with post hospital care providers:
  - Outstanding patient care issues
  - Tests and serum laboratory findings that were completed after discharge
  - Appointments and follow-up plans
- Communicates with patients and families early after discharge (generally within 72 hours) to:
  - Assure understanding of daily self-care expectations and promotes self-care maintenance and management
  - Assess clinical status and risk for readmission
  - Complete medication reconciliation with prehospital medications
  - Assure medication prescriptions were filled and available
  - Alleviate barriers that interfere with maintaining early postdischarge care expectations and follow-up appointment
  - Schedule follow-up, as needed
- Provides heart failure education to patients and caregivers and coordinates education delivery by other disciplines; uses teach back or other system to assess patient understanding
- Acts as single source contact for patients 24/7 to minimize patient, provider, systems and process issues affecting heart failure care
- Facilitates access to community resources

*All roles are not carried out in each transition care initiative

†Carried out by advanced practice nurses (APNs) with prescriptive privileges

and attending to holistic patient needs. Further, long-standing Joint Commission and Centers of Medicare and Medicaid performance measures; most notably, HF patient education and smoking cessation counseling, have shaped discharge planning priorities of nurses caring for patients with acutely decompensated HF.

More recently, potential penalties associated with the Affordable Care Act have led to an increased focus on implementing care transitions aimed at decreasing 30-day rehospitalization. When acute care APNs are clinical practitioner-focused, they may be called upon to determine treatment priorities or they may be transition leaders in initiatives aimed at improving communication and collaboration during the transition from the acute care setting (emergency department or hospital) to the next setting of care (independent home care; skilled home health services, assisted living; skilled nursing facility or acute rehabilitation). Moreover, new nurse positions with multiple titles, including transition coach, patient navigator and care coordinator, are responsible for ensuring transitions initiatives are completed. Nurses are often the single link between patients, families, multiple healthcare providers, and systems/services. Box 3 provides common nursing responsibilities completed during the transition period. Of note, the transition period timeline may vary by program type but is usually initiated during the index hospitalization, before discharge. The transition period generally lasts from as little as 72 hours postdischarge (after one follow-up telephone contact) and may continue up to 3 months postdischarge (to coordinate patient services using an individualized, holistic social service, care coordination approach).[20-22] In some programs, the nurse coach or coordinator collaborates directly with the patients' primary care provider, but not all programs include this expectation. Patients who are rehospitalized (for any reason) early after discharge (during the transition period) should receive follow-up from the same transitions coach or care coordinator whenever possible, to enhance consistency of care and create greater awareness of gaps and barriers that must be overcome to promote optimal clinical outcomes.

Palliation and End-of-life Care

In the United States, palliative and end-of-life care are often ordered very late in the patients' life cycle, even if the transition to advanced HF was previously determined. Palliation or hospice care services should be offered to patients with serious, ongoing signs and symptoms of HF (stage D, NYHA-FC IV) and poor quality of life, to relieve suffering and meet holistic needs. Prognostic models are available for hospitalized and ambulatory patients, but there is still a need for reliable estimates of risk of death. Nurses are often team members involved in patient and family discussions that involve learning patient preferences and emotional readiness, discussing current and potential therapies or treatments available, and discussing expectations related to implantable cardioverter defibrillator operation.

Advanced HF resulting in palliation or hospice care is discussed more fully in chapter 51. From a nursing perspective, patient-clinician communication is a key component in decision making, preventing misperceptions and creating ease as patients and families make a transition toward end of life. Open-ended questions that help determine what patients know and what they want to know will help clear up unanswered questions. Nurses are often uncomfortable with end-of-life discussions and feel uncertain about their ability to meet patients' needs, especially when time allotment to initiate and complete a complex conversation is inadequate. Nurses may benefit from educational workshops that teach techniques related to improving empathetic communication, understanding family dynamics, resolving conflicts related to culture, religion, and language differences, and exploring patients' hidden and transparent emotions. Workshops that provide opportunities for nurses to demonstrate tools learned in role play may enhance practical application of skills. It may be helpful to have an algorithm available to use as a resource; especially if end-of-life situations are uncommon.[23]

In conclusion, from the nursing perspective, HF involves team management, as nurses are never managing patients' lives in isolation; no matter if they are nurse clinicians or APNs. Nursing roles in HF management must be tailored to nurses training, knowledge and capabilities. When role expectations and nurse capabilities are aligned, patients receive safe, quality care and have the best opportunity for optimal clinical outcomes. Nurses who care for patients with HF understand that there are many challenges associated with managing a chronic, complex condition. Further, nurses appreciate receiving continuing education to enhance current skill sets and perform new skills that increase their capability of meeting patients' needs and using evidence based practices.

REFERENCES

1. Hunt SA, Abraham WT, Chin MH, et al. ACC/AHA 2005 Guideline Update for the Diagnosis and Management of Chronic Heart Failure in the Adult: a report of the American College of Cardiology/American Heart Association Task Force on Practice Guidelines (Writing Committee to Update the 2001 Guidelines for the Evaluation and Management of Heart Failure): developed in collaboration with the American College of Chest Physicians and the International Society for Heart and Lung Transplantation: endorsed by the Heart Rhythm Society. Circulation. 2005;112(12):e154-235.
2. Heart Failure Society of America, Lindenfeld J, Albert NM, et al. HFSA 2010 Comprehensive Heart Failure Practice Guideline. J Card Fail. 2010;16(6):e1-194.
3. Drewes HW, Steuten LM, Lemmens LC, et al. The effectiveness of chronic care management for heart failure: meta-regression analyses to explain the heterogeneity in outcomes. Health Serv Res. 2012;47(5):1926-59.
4. Savard LA, Thompson DR, Clark AM. A meta-review of evidence on heart failure disease management programs: the challenges of describing and synthesizing evidence on complex interventions. Trials. 2011;12:194.
5. Kozak AT, Rucker-Whitaker C, Basu S, et al. Elements of nonpharmacologic interventions that prevent progression of heart failure: a meta-analysis. Congest Heart Fail. 2007;13(5):280-7.
6. Koelling TM, Johnson ML, Cody RJ, et al. Discharge education improves clinical outcomes in patients with chronic heart failure. Circulation. 2005;111(2):179-85.
7. Kommuri NV, Johnson ML, Koelling TM. Relationship between improvements in heart failure patient disease specific knowledge and clinical events as part of a randomized controlled trial. Patient Educ Couns. 2012;86(2):233-8.
8. Fredericks S, Beanlands H, Spalding K, et al. Effects of the characteristics of teaching on the outcomes of heart failure patient education interventions: a systematic review. Eur J Cardiovasc Nurs. 2010;9(1):30-7.
9. Naylor MD. Advancing high value transitional care: the central role of nursing and its leadership. Nurs Adm Q. 2012;36(2):115-26.
10. Bettger JP, Sochalski JA, Foust JB, et al. Measuring nursing care time and tasks in long-term services and supports: one size does not fit all. J Nurs Res. 2012;20(3):159-68.
11. Prasun MA, Casida J, Howie-Esquivel J, et al. Practice patterns of heart failure nurses. Heart Lung. 2012;41(3):218-25.
12. Albert NM, Collier S, Sumodi V, et al. Nurses's knowledge of heart failure education principles. Heart Lung. 2002;31(2):102-12.
13. Washburn SC, Hornberger CA, Klutman A, et al. Nurses' knowledge of heart failure education topics as reported in a small midwestern community hospital. J Cardiovasc Nurs. 2005;20(3):215-20.
14. Willette EW, Surrells D, Davis LL, et al. Nurses' knowledge of heart failure self-management. Prog Cardiovasc Nurs. 2007;22(4):190-5.
15. Krumholz HM, Amatruda J, Smith GL, et al. Randomized trial of an education and support intervention to prevent readmission of patients with heart failure. J Am Coll Cardiol. 2002;39(1):83-9.
16. Lambrinou E, Kalogirou F, Lamnisos D, et al. Effectiveness of heart failure management programmes with nurse-led discharge planning in reducing re-admissions: a systematic review and meta-analysis. Int J Nurs Stud. 2012;49(5):610-24.

17. Giamouzis G, Mastrogiannis D, Koutrakis K, et al. Telemonitoring in chronic heart failure: a systematic review. Cardiol Res Pract. 2012;2012:410-820.
18. Gurné O, Conraads V, Missault L, et al. A critical review on telemonitoring in heart failure. Acta Cardiol. 2012;67(4):439-44.
19. Albert NM, Aspinwall L, Liu X, et al. Heart failure hospital nurses need help (health education and logical planning) to educate patients. Heart Lung. 2011;40(4):363.
20. Stamp KD, Machado MA, Allen NA. Transitional Care Programs Improve Outcomes for Heart Failure Patients: An Integrative Review. J Cardiovasc Nurs. 2014;29(2):140-54.
21. Stauffer BD, Fullerton C, Fleming N, et al. Effectiveness and cost of a transitional care program for heart failure: a prospective study with concurrent controls. Arch Intern Med. 2011;171(14):1238-43.
22. Naylor MD, Aiken LH, Kurtzman ET, et al. The care span: The importance of transitional care in achieving health reform. Health Aff (Millwood). 2011;30(4):746-54.
23. Allen LA, Stevenson LW, Grady KL, et al. Decision making in advanced heart failure: a scientific statement from the American Heart Association. Circulation. 2012;125(15):1928-52.

Chapter 49

Developing Heart Failure Service in a Developing Nation: Borneo Malaysia Perspective

Houng-Bang Liew, Siow-Yen Liau, Jia Hoong Chi

ABSTRACT

Heart failure (HF) is an emerging major cardiovascular morbidity even in developing nation like Malaysia. This chapter highlights the "start-up" of HF program within a tertiary referral centre, in the Borneon state of Sabah, East Malaysia; whereby the philosophy of patient-centred care and organizational transformation are key to implementation of evidence-based HF management from admission, to discharge and beyond. Under the circumstances of limitation in human and material resources, the "delivery" system, is as important, as the drugs and devices, to provide quality care for these patients.

INTRODUCTION

Sabah is one of the 13 states of Malaysia, a tropical country located in Southeast Asia. Malaysia is divided by South China Sea into two parts, at the west is Peninsular Malaysia, and at the east are Sabah and Sarawak states on Borneo, the third largest island in the world. Sabah is at the north of Borneo with a population of 3.1 million. The capital is Kota Kinabalu city with a population of approximately 750,000. This chapter aims to showcase the planning and implementation of heart failure (HF) management program at a newly established tertiary heart center in a developing nation and to highlight the successful implementation of evidence-based care for HF patients through organisational commitment, smart partnertship, and multidisciplinary teamwork.

The Sabah Heart Center is established within the main city hospital, Queen Elizabeth Hospital II, a 455-bedded public hospital. This is developed by Ministry of Health as the regional referral center to provide tertiary cardiology and cardiothoracic surgery service (Table 1). At present this is the only center providing interventional cardiology service in the state. The center has three resident cardiologists, two cardiothoracic surgeons, a team of medical officers, and allied health workers. The scope of services includes outpatient and inpatient: eight-bedded coronary care unit (CCU), 24-bedded ward, and one cathlab. In 2012, the center received 6,921 cardiac outpatients, 2,113 inpatients of which 399 patients were admitted in CCU. A total of 1,090 diagnostic catheterization, 374 percutaneous coronary intervention (PCI), and 63 pacemaker implantations were performed in 2012.

Amongst these patients, an estimate of 30% of admissions is HF-related. A clinical audit of HF patients at discharge found that majority of patients were warm

TABLE 1: Ministry of Health, Malaysia, Health Facts 2012

	MYR	USD
Total MOH budget	16,870,767,600	5,407,823,330
MOH operating budget	14,998,120,400	4,807,557,506
MOH development budget	1,872,647,200	600,265,824
Per capita income	30,856	9,890.71
Total expenditure on health	33,691	10,799.45

MYR, Malaysian Ringgit; USD, US dollar; MOH, Ministry of Health
(Based on currency exchange on 17 Mar 2013: 1.00 MYR = 0.320544 USD)

(81%) and dry (78%) with mean systemic blood pressure of 132/75 mmHg. However, there is underdosing of HF medications at discharge and only a minority (21%) were given a 2-week review appointment.

Heart failure management is amongst the key missions identified for the 5-year plan. This includes improvement in care of acute decompensated heart failure (ADHF), early postdischarge care, optimal medical therapy, device implant in appropriate patients, cardiac rehabilitation program, and eventually palliative care.

HEART FAILURE EPIDEMIOLOGY: MALAYSIA PERSPECTIVE

Heart failure is a major challenge of our time, even in the developing world. Prevalence of HF is estimated at 3–20 per 1,000 population. For age more than 65-year-old, it could be as high as 100 per 1,000 population, accounting for about 10% of all medical admissions in Malaysia with an inpatient mortality rate of 11%. About 45% of HF patients are admitted at least once within 12 months for acute decompensation (reference: Malaysian Clinical Practice Guideline for Heart failure, 2007). Our National Cardiovascular Database (NCVD) maintains acute coronary syndrome (ACS) registry, which revealed 7% of ACS patients have preexisting HF at presentation. A national clinical practice guideline (CPG) for HF was produced in 2007 in recognition of the increasing burden of this chronic disease.

In the north Borneon state of Sabah, we face a "dual challenge" as we reach the crossroad from third world status to developed nation: ischemic heart disease, attributed by rising prevalence of noncommunicable diseases (NCD), like diabetes mellitus, hypertension, dyslipidemia, and obesity at the same time, we are still plagued by rheumatic heart disease (RHD), which comprised of 15% of our outpatients.

As a consequence, our HF management program needs to deal with the complexities of underlying diseases and the consequent HF that has both acute and chronic dimensions.

The goal of such program is to achieve "right patient, right place, right time, right level of care" and last but not least, within the finite resources of a developing nation. The clinical objectives include reduction in mortality and morbidity of multiple readmissions, and improvement in quality of life, and lastly, good end-of-life care.

Our philosophy is to develop patient centered care, i.e., "walk with the patient, as we designed the program" with a strong emphasis of implementing evidence-based medicine, especially the optimal use of pharmacotherapy. This is achieved by training of staff, incorporation of clinical pathway, and ready reference of drug titration algorithms at point of care.

While we establish HF management program, we must also address the root causes in our state, in order to curb the rise, whenever we can. For practical purpose, our HF patients are broadly classified into ischemic versus nonischemic cardiomyopathy. This simplistic dichotomy serves to focus our strategy to reperfuse coronaries, an important reversible cause of HF. Keeping in mind; the nonischemic represents a heterogeneous group of etiology for HF.

In Sabah, valvular heart disease, notably RHD, remains the second commonest cause of HF admissions. Aside RHD, other causes include chronic hypertensive, chronic renal failure, thyroid disease, peripartum cardiomyopathy, tachycardia-induced cardiomyopathy, thalassemia, alcohol-related, and presumably post-myocarditis and idiopathic dilated cardiomyopathy, after no discernable causes are found.

"HOW WE DO IT?" HEART FAILURE: ACUTE CARE

Hospital admissions are indicated for acute disabling dyspnea in HF patients. Level of care depends on acuity of illness. For those with hemodynamic instability, ischemia, arrhythmia, and respiratory failure, they should ideally be admitted to CCU and high dependency unit (HDU). For those who are relatively stable, be admitted to cardiac rehabilitation ward (CRW). In reality, the overwhelming number of patients presenting to hospital often outnumber the CCU, HDU, CRW capacity, and many patients are admitted to general medical wards. There are ongoing efforts to implement our management protocols to these HF patients. Currently, priorities are given to newly diagnosed HF patients to expedite investigations for reversible causes, notably ischemic heart disease.

At this point, this includes patients who have known history of chronic HF and clarified etiology, but presented with ADHF. It is important to investigate for contributing factors in order to target treatment strategy and long-term prevention of readmissions. Common factors include:

- Noncompliance to dietary restriction of salt, fluid intake, weight monitoring
- Noncompliance to medications
- Myocardial ischemia/infarct

- Arrhythmia, e.g., new onset atrial fibrillation with loss of "atrial kick" can be critical in severe systolic ventricular dysfunction
- Valvular dysfunction
- Any other pathophysiology stress that overwhelm the balance of cardiac output and demand, e.g., infection, bleeding, sepsis, anemia, and dehydration
- Exacerbation of other comorbidities, e.g., hypoxia in chronic obstructive pulmonary disease, renal failure, and thyrotoxicosis.

One of the key success factors in disease management of acute decompensated HF is intensive decongestion. The triage of patients based on Stevenson HF Class, "wet/dry" for evidence of congestion and "cool/warm" for perfusion provides early bedside stratification of in hospital mortality risk and also guide the usage of diuretics and intravenous inotropic agents.

In order to implement evidence-based practice, the following are introduced as standard operational procedures (SOP) for all HF admissions:

1. Heart failure admission checklist
    - To standardize the clinical evaluation of HF by ward staff: clinical triage, investigations, and early implementation of nondrug interventions, e.g., education, low salt diet, fluid intake restriction
    - Early recognition and reminder of both short-term and mid-term treatment modalities, beyond drugs, devices, interventions, and surgery (Appendix)
2. Pharmacologic treatment algorithms (Flowcharts 1 to 3)
    - Beyond the use of diuretics and inotropes, we emphasize on early initiation of pharmacotherapy that targets the pathophysiology of HF, i.e., renin-angiotensin aldosterone system and sympathetic hyperactivation. Based on hemodynamic status, and degree of congestion versus perfusion, patients are started on beta-blocker, angiotensin-converting enzyme inhibitor (ACEI), spironolactone, often in combination. However, we advocate early achievement of maximal or most tolerable "target dose" of these drugs during their hospitalization. For the relatively stable patients, "start low, but not too slow" to uptitrate doses on one to two daily basis instead of two-weekly basis
3. Heart failure patient daily review chart (Table 2)
    - To closely monitor during intensive phase of decongestion, with or without inotropic support
    - The emphasis on daily weight change as compared to urine output *per se*, to evaluate response to diuretic and need to escalate dose, either in oral or intravenous bolus as well as infusion regime, to target 0.5–1 kg of weight loss per day
4. Heart failure patient discharge planning (Box 1)
    - To assess readiness for discharge in order to prevent premature discharge of patients and hence unscheduled rehospitalization for another decompensation

HEART FAILURE "DAYCARE" AFTER DISCHARGE

Upon discharge, majority of patients are still vulnerable to further decompensation. Up to a quarter of patients may be rehospitalized within 1 month of discharge. We piloted the HF "daycare" for early review of HF patients post discharge, which was run on a weekly basis at our outpatient unit within the center.

Patients who were discharged were given scheduled appointments to review at 2-weekly interval, i.e., week-2, -4, -6, -8, and so forth.

The objective of this "daycare" service is to reduce early relapse by providing continuity of patient education initiated from index hospitalization on issues of diet, fluid intake, dry weight maintenance, medication compliance, smoking cessation, and the opportunity to uptitrate the anti-HF pharmacotherapy.

Resident medical officers of the department, assisted by pharmacists, run this "daycare" program. The junior doctors go through a training session of "how-to" disease management for HF, followed by "hands-on" patient management, under direct supervision of cardiologists in the preparatory phase and continual supervision by proxy through case discussions in the implementation phase.

A "HF outpatient care bundle" is conceptualized and developed as a framework for clinical management strategies: beyond disease management with emphasis on patient-centered, value-based care. The concept is based on four-step systematic approach of focused history, targeted examination, need assessment, and personalized care plan (Table 3).

This is provided at consultation rooms for quick reference at point of care with HF patients during their visits. The HF drugs algorithms are provided at consultation rooms for continuity of titration after discharge. The aim is to maintain patients at euvolemic state, i.e., dry and warm.

A recent review of our 1st-year experience was presented at the 2013 Asia Pacific Society of Cardiology Congress (APCC). We noted amongst the HF patients

Patients with heart failure and systolic dysfunction
Asymptomatic, mild, moderate, or severe symptoms

Patient exclusion criteria

ACEIs: ACEI allergy, angioedema, intolerable cough, moderate or severe aortic/mitral stenosis, shock, symptomatic hypotension, hyperkalemia (K^+ > 5.5 mmol/L), bilateral renal artery stenosis, pregnancy

ARBs: Hypersensitivity to ARBs, moderate or severe aortic/mitral stenosis, shock, symptomatic hypotension, hyperkalemia (K^+ >5.5 mmol/L), bilateral renal artery stenosis, pregnancy

Start ACEI or ARB (with a diuretic if volume overload present)

Dosage initiation and titration

Rapid uptitration to the target dose is recommended except when limited by borderline BP and/or renal function

	ACEIs				ARBs#		
	Captopril	**Enalapril**	**Perindopril**	**Ramipril**	**Valsartan**	**Losartan**	**Candesartan**
Initial dose	6.25 mg TDS	2.5 mg BD	2 mg OD	2.5 mg OD	40 mg BD	25 mg OD	4 mg OD
Titration steps (typically double dose at each step	12.5 mg TDS	5 mg BD	4 mg OD	5 mg OD	80 mg BD	50 mg OD	8 mg OD
	25 mg TDS	10 mg BD	*6 mg OD	*7.5 mg OD	*120 mg BD	*75 mg OD	16 mg OD
Traget dose	50 mg TDS	20 mg BD	8 mg OD	10 mg OD	160 mg BD	100 mg OD	32 mg OD

Outpatient monitoring
- Heart failure symptoms
- Serum K^+
- Serum Cr/renal function
- BP
- Concomitant drug interactions
- Volume status/diuretic dose

Serum Cr may increase after addition of ACEI. If the increase plateaus or returns to baseline, maintain dose titration. If serum Cr con-tinues to increase (>30%), down titrate the dose till SrCr stabilized. To with hold the drugs and to dis-cuss with doctor if SrCr continues to increase.

Serum K^+ increases an average of 0.3 mmol/L on ACEI therapy. Adjust potassium supplementation, aldosterone antagonist and potassium-containing salt substitutes as clinically indicated.

Note: Careful consideration of patient characteristics and choice of drug is warranted.

#ARBs are most frequently used in place of ACEIs when side effects limit ACEI use (intolerable cough may occur in as many as 20% of patients receiving ACEIs)

*Suggested dose when a slower dose titration is preferred for patients' condition.

ACEI, Angiotensin-converting enzyme inhibitor(s); ARB, Angiotensin receptor blocker; BP, Blood pressure; TDS, three times a day; OD, once a day

Flowchart 1 Angiotensin-converting enzyme inhibitor/angiotensin receptor blocker treatment algorithm[1-4]

who were in NYHA II-IV (77%) at index admission, were able to stabilize in NYHA I (83%) (Fig. 1).

The usage of medications at admission compared to follow-up at "daycare" for beta-blockers, ACEI/ARB, and spironolactone were 43% versus 97%, 37% versus 73%, and 23% versus 57%, respectively (Fig. 2).

Heart failure daycare program also reduces hospital readmissions to 10% over 1 year (Fig. 3).

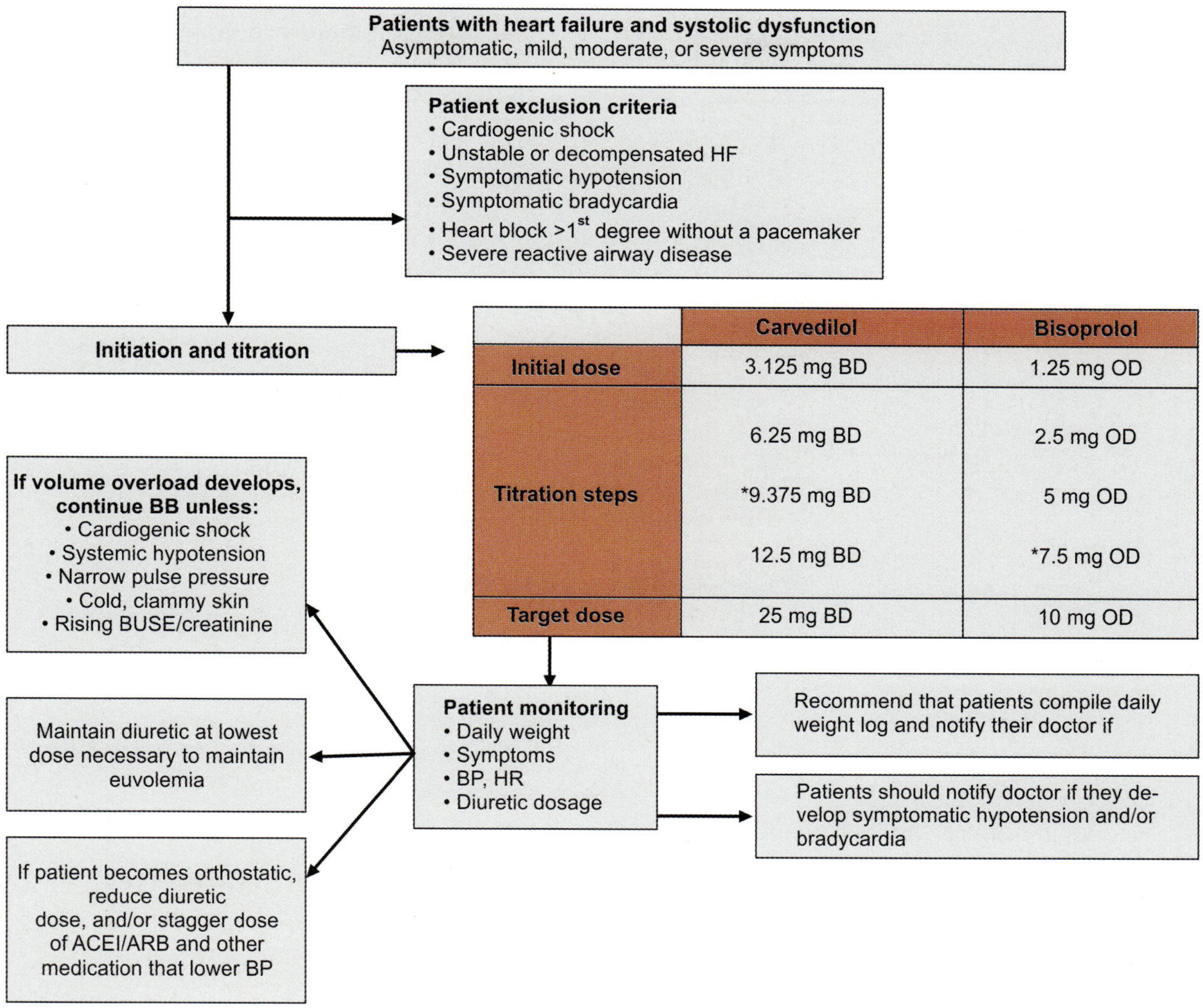

Note:

- ACC/AHA 2005 guidelines recommend using only those B-blockers proven to be effective in heart failure (carvedilol, sustained –release metoprolol succinate and bisoprolol) at the doses studied in large clinical trials. If patient is currently on a B-blocker other than listed, consider switching.
- B-blocker titration steps are generally at 2-week intervals. BP and HR should be carefully monitored. If SBP <80 mmHg or HR is <55 bpm, assess the dose and recheck patient carefully for signs of hypoperfusion. Recheck status as needed.
- Patients who cannot achieve target dose of the B-blocker should be maintained on the highest tolerated dose.

HF, heart failure; ACEI, angiotensin-converting enzyme inhibitor; ARB, angiotensin receptor blocker; BP, blood pressure; SBP, systolic blood pressure; HR, heart rate; BB, beta-blockers; BUSE, blood urea and serum electrolyte

Flowchart 2 Beta-blocker treatment algorithm[1,5-7]

HEART FAILURE CLINIC

Once the patients are stabilized in the early postdischarge phase, they are "step-down" to the "heart failure clinic" which is established with a vision to anchor the cardiac rehabilitation program, whereby a multidisciplinary team including nurses, pharmacists, physiotherapists, and occupational therapists will collaborate to provide optimal care to these patients.

Aside cardiac rehabilitation, the clinic shall also coordinate the appropriate use of cardiac rhythm management devices like cardiac resynchronization therapy and implantable cardioverter defibrillator.

Beyond the hospital setting, this HF clinic has also established "shared care" with family medicine physicians who are based in primary healthcare centers. These patients may then be reviewed at longer intervals, i.e., 3–6 monthly at the tertiary HF clinic, while maintaining

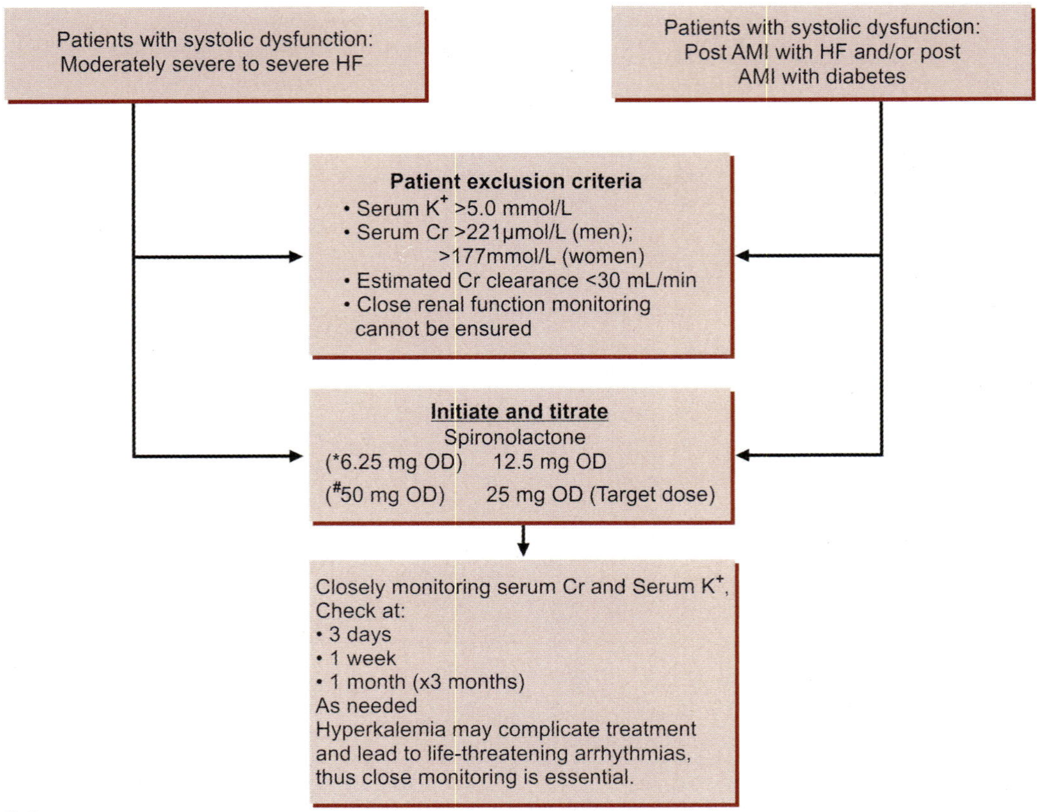

Note:

*Start at 6.25 mg OD in patients at high risk for hyperkalemia

#Maximum daily dose of 50 mg is used when existing dieresis is inadequate to relieve the congestion.

- Impaired renal function is a risk factor for hyperkalaemia during treatment with spironolactone. The risk of hyperkalemia increases progressively when serum Cr >142 mmol/L
- Hyperkalemia risk is increased with concomitant use of higher dose of ACEIs or ARBs.
- NSAIDs and COX-2 inhibitors should be avoided.
- Potassium supplements should be discontinued or reduced.
- Dehydration, by diarrhea or other causes, should be addressed emergently.

AMI, acute myocardial infarction; HF, heart failure; OD, once a day; NSAID, nonsteroidal anti-inflammatory drug; COX-2 cyclooxygenase-2; ACEI, angiotensin converting enzyme inhibitor; ARB, angiotensin receptor blockers; Cr, creatine

Flowchart 3 Spironolactone treatment algorithm[1,8,9]

TABLE 2: Heart failure patient daily review chart

	Day: *Date:*	*Day:* *Date:*	*Day:* *Date:*	*Day:* *Date:*	*Day:* *Date:*	*Day:* *Date:*
Perfusion (warm/cool)						
If SBP <100: check standing BP						
Body weight						
Fluid status (volume overload/over-diuresis)						
Estimated "dry weight"						
(Target 1–2 kg/day weight loss)						
Diet : low salt (<2,000 mg Na)/normal						
Fluid restriction: 5,00 mL/1,000 mL/ 1,500 mL/other (please specify)						
I-O chart (According to diuretic regime)	8 hourly/ 12 hourly/ 24 hourly	8 hourly/ 12 hourly/ 24 hourly	8 hourly/ 12 hourly/ 24 hourly	8 hourly/ 12 hourly/ 24 hourly	8 hourly/ 12 hourly/ 24 hourly	8 hourly/ 12 hourly/ 24 hourly

Contd...

Contd...

	Day: Date:	Day: Date:	Day: Date:	Day: Date:	Day: Date:	Day: Date:
If applicable: frusemide IV dose						
Inotropes IV dose: • Dobutamine • Dopamine • Noradrenaline • Milrinone						

*Inform doctor immediately if find out any of the following:

HR <60 bpm/>120 bpm;SBP <80 mmHg/>150 mmHg; O_2 Saturation <90%; Temp >38oC; K_+ <3.0 mmol/L/>5.0 mmol/L

HF, heart failure; BP, blood pressure; SBP, systolic blood pressure; IV, intravenous; HR, heart rate; I-O chart, input-output chart

TABLE 3: Systemic approach (care bundle) to outpatient management for chronic heart failure

S.O.A.P	Aspects	Focus information	Knowledge and analysis
Focused Hx	Past Hx, Rx Hx	Causes of CHF: Hx of CAD, MI, valvular heart disease, congenital heart disease, arrhythmia, hpt, DM Hx of precipitating condition, e.g., anemia, thyroid problem CVD risk factors: smoking	Status @last visit/ review Med compliance, side effects of Rx
	Present symptom review	Activity level/ employment/ exercise/sport Systemic review: other organ functions, comorbidities?	NYHA for HF
Targeted Ex	Evidence, extent, severity of disease	HR (?AF), BP control, perfusion (warm vs cool), weight, severity of heart failure	
	Relevant Lx findings	Echo, ECG, CXR, coronary anatomy CVD screening (lipid, glucose), RFT, INR, Hb, TFT	Echo report INR target achieved?
Assessment	Disease status (stability, progression, response)	Compare to last review: status quo, better or worse?	Room for improvement? Step-up/ step-down Rx?
	Needs: priority, outstanding issues	Influence clinical outcomes? If yes, prioritize Potential life-threatening, disabling? If yes, urgent	
	Patient profile: functional level, knowledge, expectation	Are symptoms limiting/affecting lifestyle of patients? Assess knowledge and comprehension of disease; psychosocial status, personal and carer adjustment, expectation	ADL, QOL?
	Prognosis, complication risk	Assessment of risk of MACE, SCD	
Plan	Expected clinical outcomes measures	Reduce morbidity and mortality, reduce hospitalization, improve QOL	Individualize according to disease stage, comorbidities, patient expectation
	Short- vs long-term goals (symptom-control, definitive, rehab, palliative)	Consider Rx options that may impact on agreed goals; Conservative vs drugs/device/intervention/surgery, etc.	Education and counseling
	Disease-specific vs patient-focused plan	Apt application of EBM (CPG/ consensus); Individualized Rx plan according to patient profile	Discuss feasible treatment options
	Review and monitoring schedule	Review schedule according to anticipation of Rx end-point, timeframe of clinical response; Share-care arrangement	Aim to achieve optimal benefit, minimize/ monitor risk

SOAP, subjective, objective, assessment, plan; Mx, management; Hx, history (of); Rx, prescription drug; Ex, examination; Lx, laboratory; CHF, congestive heart failure; CAD, coronary artery disease; MI, myocardial infarction; DM, diabetes mellitus; CVD, cardiovascular disease; NYHA, New York Heart Association; HF, heart failure; HR, heart rate; BP, blood pressure; ECG, electrocardiogram; CXR, chest X-ray; AF, atrial fibrillation; RFT, renal function test; INR, international normalized ratio; Hb, hemoglobin; TFT, thyroid function tests; ADL, activities of daily living; QOL, quality of life; MACE, major adverse cardiac events; SCD, sudden cardiac death; EBM, evidence-based medicine; CPG, clinical practice guidelines

Box 1: Heart failure patient discharge planning

- Symptoms improved? Ask patient the following:
  - Self care/previous level of functional status
  - Ready returning to home environment
  - Return to work
- Fluid status:
  - Achieved target "dry weight"
  - Pulmonary edema or pleural effusion resolved/improved
  - Peripheral edema resolved/improved
- Vital signs stable:
  - SBP >90 mmHg (adequate perfusion)
  - No symptomatic orthostatic hypotension/BP drop >10 mmHg
- Not require O_2 therapy >2 days (Except for patient on long term O_2 therapy at home)
- Not on IV infusion drug including inotropes
- Tolerating discharge medical regimens >24 hours
- Patient and/or family are counseled regarding:
  - Dietary change especially salt restriction
  - Fluid management
  - Daily weight monitoring
  - Medication education
  - Ambulate and level of activity
  - Patient education pamphlet
- Review plan :____________________
- Daycare plan:____________________
- Action plan: Return to ward or clinic when warning signs noticed:-
  - Body weight increased >2 kg/week
  - Breathlessness
  - Peripheral edema/abdominal distension

HF, heart failure; BP, blood pressure; SBP, systolic blood pressure; IV, intravenous

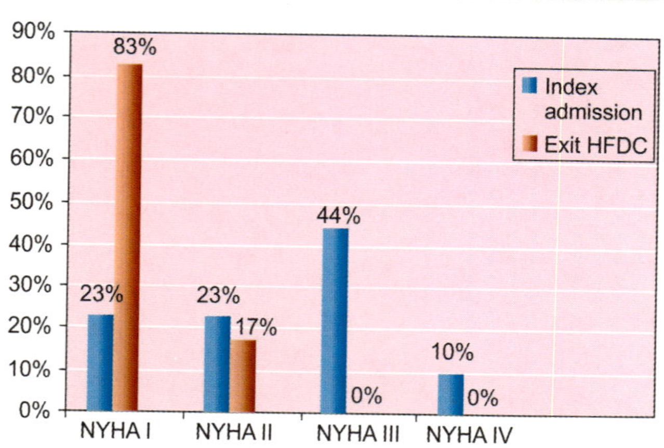

HFDC, heart failure daycare; NYHA, New York Heart Association

Fig. 1 Heart failure daycare improves New York Heart Association

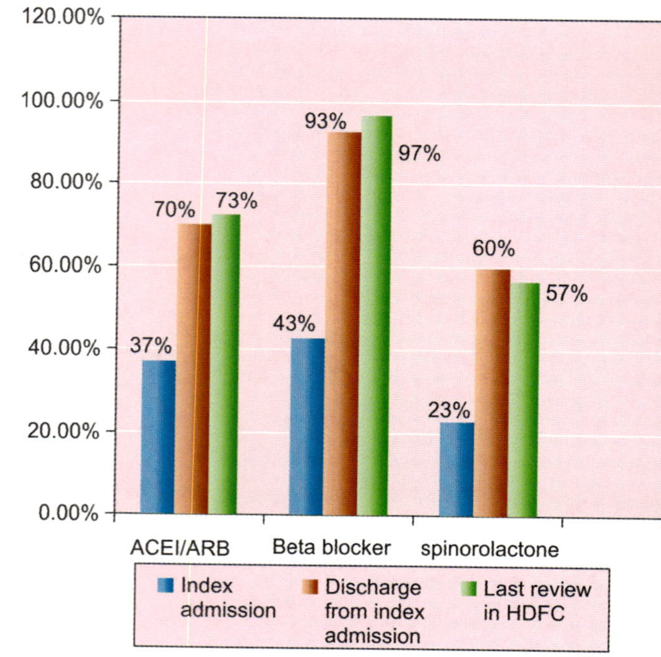

HFDC, heart failure daycare; ACEI, angiotensin-converting enzyme inhibitor; ARB, angiotensin receptor blocker

Fig. 2 Heart failure daycare improves use of heart failure medications

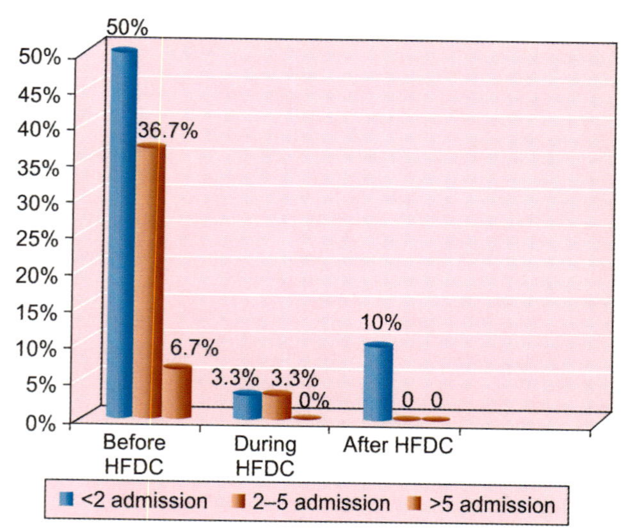

HFDC, heart failure daycare

Fig. 3 Heart failure daycare reduces hospital readmissions

monthly visits to the family medicine specialist. It is hoped that in the future, HF clinic can be established *in situ* within primary healthcare centers.

An ongoing HF registry has also recently been established in order to collect information which may assist in quality and outcome measures in order to improve management of HF.

REFERENCES

1. Hunt SA, Abraham WT, Chin MH, et al. ACC/AHA 2005 guideline update for the diagnosis and management of chronic heart failure in the adult—summary article: a report of the American College of Cardiology/American Heart Association Task Force on Practice Guidelines (Writing Committee to update the 2001 Guidelines for the Evaluation and Management of Heart Failure. Circulation. 2005;112:1825-52.
2. Garg R, Yusuf S. Overview of randomized trials of angiotensin-converting enzyme inhibitors on mortality and morbidity in patients with heart failure. Collaborative Group on Ace Inhibitor Trials. JAMA. 1995;273:1450-6.
3. Young JB, Dunlap ME, Pfeffer MA, et al. Mortality and morbidity reduction with candesartan in patients with chronic heart failure and left ventricular systolic dysfunction: results of the CHARM low-left ventricular ejection fraction trials. Circulation. 2004;110:2618-26.
4. Pfeffer MA, McMurray J, Velazquez EJ, et al. Valsartan, captopril or both in myocardial infarction complicated by heart failure, left ventricular dysfunction or both. NEJM. 2003;349:1893-906.
5. Packer M, Coats AJ, Fowler MB, et al. Effect of carvedilol on survival in severe chronic heart failure. NEJM. 2001;344:1651-8.
6. Hjalmarson A, Goldstein S, Fagerberg B, et al. The MERIT-HF Study Group. Effects of controlled-release metoprolol on total mortality, hospitalizations, and well-being in patients with heart failure (MERIT-HF). JAMA. 2000;283: 1295-302.
7. CIBIS II Investigators and Committees. The Cardiac Insufficiency Bisoprolol Study II (CIBIS-II): a randomised trial. Lancet. 1999;353:9-13.
8. Swedberg K, Cleland J, Dargie H, et al. Guidelines for the diagnosis and treatment of chronic heart failure: executive summary (update 2005): The Task Force for the Diagnosis and Treatment of Chronic Heart Failure of the European Society of Cardiology. Eur Heart J. 2005;26:1115-40.
9. Pitt B, Zannad F, Remme WJ, et al. The effect of spironolactone on morbidity and mortality in patients with severe heart failure. Randomized Aldactone Evaluation Study Investigators. NEJM. 1999;341:709-17.

5

SECTION

Advanced Heart Failure

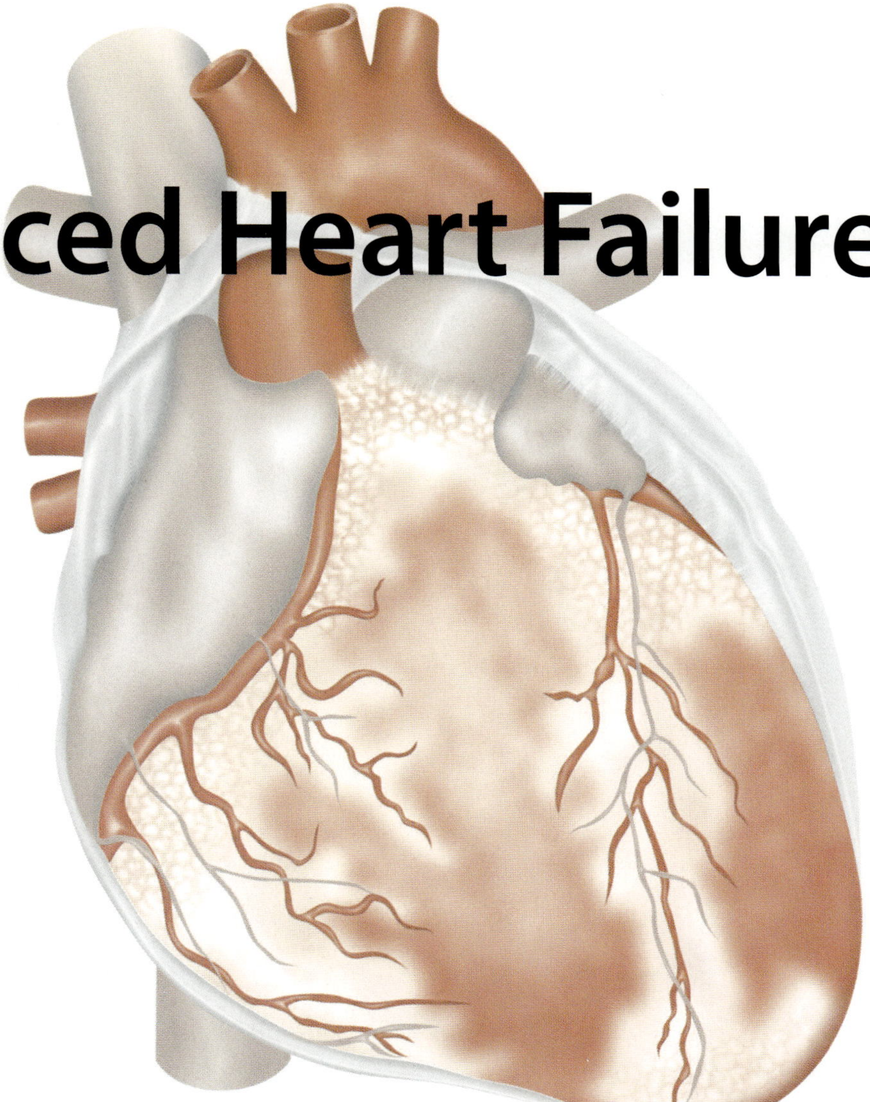

Chapter 50

Approach to the End-stage Heart Failure Patient

Joyce W Wald, Mariell Jessup

ABSTRACT

The patient with end-stage heart failure (ESHF) is identified as one who has refractory heart failure (HF) symptoms despite attempts at optimal medical therapy. These patients may also be categorized as advanced HF. A thorough evaluation for maximal medical and device therapy is warranted and only if intolerant, should the patient be deemed refractory to therapy.

If it is determined that the patient has received appropriate medical and/or device therapy, clinicians should then monitor diligently for signs or symptoms of decline. These include worsening exercise tolerance, arrhythmias, intolerance to disease modifying HF medications, escalating diuretic need, echocardiographic signs of continued remodeling, and recurrent hospitalizations. The identification, evaluation, and management of such patients are reviewed in this chapter.

INTRODUCTION

The end-stage heart failure (ESHF) patient must first be identified, and only then can the approach to care proceed. This requires the practice of both the art of medicine, as well as the science of inquiry—the essence of clinical skill. In general, the definition of ESHF is a constellation of heart failure's (HF) signs and symptoms that have persisted despite optimal medical and device therapy (OMDT). For the purpose of this chapter, we will focus only on the patient with chronic, low left ventricular (LV) ejection fraction, or heart failure with reduced ejection fraction (HFrEF), primarily because the therapy for these patients has been so well defined. The patient with acute, cardiogenic shock is a different phenotype and is covered in other sections of this book. The American College of Cardiology (ACC)/American Heart Association's (AHA) HF-staging system has classified these patients as stage D, or refractory HF; others prefer the term "advanced HF". In this review, these terms will be used interchangeably. These patients may be encountered in either the outpatient or in the hospitalized setting and each requires a unique, but complementary approach.

OPTIMAL MEDICAL AND DEVICE THERAPY

The OMDT has been reviewed in detail in other chapters of this book and can also be found in either the European Society of Cardiology's (ESC) or ACC/AHA HF guidelines; the evidence-based approach to patients with HFrEF will not be reviewed here. Thus, patients with refractory HF symptoms have either failed to respond to optimal therapy, have not received optimal therapy, have an underlying pathophysiologic process that is causing progressive myocardial dysfunction despite optimal therapy, and/or finally, have been noncompliant with their prescribed regimen. The definition of advanced HF is precisely outlined by the ESC's statement with the same name, as shown in Box 1. Note in particular that there are multiple components to the criteria that must be fulfilled before the patient has been declared as advanced.[1]

Box 1: Definition of advanced chronic heart failure

- Severe symptoms of heart failure with dyspnea and/or fatigue at rest or with minimal exertion (New York Heart Association functional class III or IV)
- Episodes of fluid retention (pulmonary and/or systemic congestion, peripheral edema) and/or of reduced cardiac output at rest (peripheral hypoperfusion)
- Objective evidence of severe cardiac dysfunction, shown by at least one of the following:
  - A low left ventricular ejection fraction (<30%)
  - A severe abnormality of cardiac function on Doppler-echocardiography with a pseudonormal or restrictive mitral-inflow pattern
  - High left ventricular filling pressures (mean pulmonary capillary wedge pressure >16 mmHg, and/or mean right atrial pressure >12 mmHg by pulmonary artery catheterization)
  - High brain natriuretic peptide or N-terminal prohormone of brain natriuretic peptide plasma levels, in the absence of noncardiac causes
- Severe impairment of functional capacity shown by one of the following:
  - Inability to exercise
  - Six-minute walk test distance <300 m or less in females and/or patients aged >75 years
  - Peak oxygen consumption <12–14 mL/kg/min
- History of >1 heart failure hospitalization in the past 6 months
- Presence of all the previous features despite "attempts to optimize" therapy including diuretics, inhibitors of the renin–angiotensin–aldosterone system, and beta blockers, unless these are poorly tolerated or contraindicated, and cardiac resynchronization therapy, when indicated

Source: Adapted from Metra M, Ponikowski P, Dickstein K, et al. Advanced chronic heart failure: A position statement from the Study Group on Advanced Heart Failure of the Heart Failure Association of the European Society of Cardiology. *Eur J Heart Fail*. 2007;9(6-7):684-94, *with permission*

The first step, then, in the approach to the advanced HF patient is to review very carefully their past medical history. Important historical information to elicit is shown in Table 1. The goal of this meticulous review is to determine for how long the patient has had the benefit of optimal medical therapy, or alternatively, why the patient has not been prescribed optimal medical treatment. Has the patient been able to achieve goal doses of angiotensin-converting-enzyme inhibitors (ACEI) or angiotensin-receptor blockers (ARBs), and if not, why not? An ominous note in the patient's history is their inability to tolerate ACEI or ARBs because of renal dysfunction. The inability to tolerate these important drugs reflects a poor prognosis and implicates important renal dysfunction as well. A similar question may be asked about beta-blockers. These two classes of drugs are not only life prolonging, but have been shown to improve symptoms and favorably reverse adverse ventricular remodeling in the patient with HFrEF. Mineralocorticoid antagonists (MRAs) such as spironolactone or eplerenone may often improve symptoms and facilitate optimal volume control, in addition to enhancing survival—have they been tried? Most importantly, one must get a sense of the patient's typical volume status. Do they frequently have edema, or orthopnea? Are they drinking excessive liquids during the day or using excessive salt? Not infrequently, the clues to improving a patient's symptoms will be revealed during this fact finding, and increased diuretics are all that is needed.

A special note should be emphasized about the patient with a device, either an implantable cardioverter-defibrillator (ICD) or cardiac resynchronization therapy (CRT) or both. It is important to learn the detailed history about the reasons and setting for which the device(s) were implanted. Is the patient using the ICD more often for right ventricular pacing? Has the CRT been optimized? Have arrhythmias interfered with the mandatory pacing in the patient with CRT? A particularly concerning patient is one who has been stable and suddenly converts to atrial fibrillation (AF) or who has received multiple ICD shocks for ventricular arrhythmias. These clinical scenarios are often the prelude to a rapid and progressive deterioration in the course of the patient with HFrEF.

After a thorough discussion about evidence-based therapy with the patient, potential additional pathophysiologic processes must be excluded. Some of the important diseases that can impact the course of HFrEF (as well as incite the myocardial dysfunction) include ongoing ischemia from coronary artery disease, uncontrolled hypertension and poorly managed arrhythmias, especially AF with a rapid ventricular response. These conditions are reviewed elsewhere in this book; successful management may also result in marked functional improvement of individual patients, and enhance myocardial recovery and clinical stabilization of the HF syndrome. Next, the physical examination may often reveal the severity of the HF process. Is there pronounced LV enlargement or a very loud S3 gallop? Are the neck veins markedly distended or is there obvious right ventricular distension? Other important clues during the physical examination that suggest that the patient has far advanced HFrEF are listed in Table 2. Finally, a careful review of the echocardiogram will often be the source of important confirmatory evidence that

TABLE 1: Important historical information in the assessment of advanced heart failure

Historical information	*Clinical implications*
Duration of HF symptoms	Longer duration suggests more advanced disease
Multiple hospitalizations for HF	Progressive disease, poorly controlled
Need for inotropic therapy during hospitalization	Progressive disease, poorly controlled
Less than optimal medical and device therapy	Potential to improve with evidence-based therapy
Recent need to reduce evidence-based therapy due to hypotension or renal function	Progressive HF syndrome
New-onset AF	Progressive cardiac dysfunction
Recent or multiple defibrillator shocks	Poor prognostic sign
Presence of new cardiac ischemia or angina	Possibility to address symptoms with revascularization
Weight loss or poor appetite	Marked right HF or cardiac cachexia
Progressive renal insufficiency	Worsening cardiac function leading to cardiorenal syndrome
Poorly controlled AF	Potential to improve cardiac function with better rate control
Cardiac resynchronization therapy implanted without clinical improvement	May imply significant myocardial fibrosis
Patient cannot relate details of regimen	Possible medical noncompliance
Patient misses appointments frequently	Possible medical noncompliance
Presence of negative inotropic drugs (verapamil, nifedipine, diltiazem)	Potential to improve clinical syndrome with elimination
Presence of drugs that increase salt retention (steroids, thiazolidinediones, NSAIDs)	Potential to improve clinical syndrome with elimination

AF, atrial fibrillation; HF, heart failure; NSAIDs, nonsteroidal anti-inflammatory drugs

TABLE 2: Signs and symptoms of advanced heart failure

Symptoms	*Signs*
Frequent paroxysmal nocturnal dyspnea	Resting tachycardia
Severe orthopnea	Hypotension
Poor appetite	Resting tachypnea
Weight loss with edema	Cachectic appearance
Frequent palpitations	Anasarca, ascites
Frequent dizziness	Somnolence
Nocturnal angina	Right ventricular lift
Abdominal bloating	Marked neck vein distension, loud S3 gallop

the patient has advanced disease. Ominous findings on the echocardiogram include marked LV dilatation, especially if the resultant LV shape is more spherical than the normal ellipsoid shape of the LV. Severe functional mitral or tricuspid regurgitation, or severe pulmonary hypertension are likewise poor prognostic signs.

It must be acknowledged that compliance with a HF regimen is not always easy. Following a strict, low-salt diet and taking many pills several times a day is challenging for the best of patients. Nevertheless, some patients have what appears to be refractory HF because they are importantly noncompliant with their lifestyle and/or medications. Excessive alcohol and illegal street drugs make adherence to a regimen difficult and may contribute to the decreased myocardial contractility in these patients. Gentle questioning may reveal that a patient has not been able to afford their prescriptions, or that an inability to read the written word has resulted in a failure to follow written instructions. We often suspect noncompliance in the patient who is admitted frequently to the hospital with marked volume overload, only to respond quickly to a single dose of intravenous diuretics. Other important steps are to question the patient's family members or the nurses on the hospital units; they often will corroborate a patient's nonadherence.

OUTPATIENT

In the patient who has achieved maximal medical and device therapy, or has been proven to be intolerant to target doses, or has achieved a reasonable regimen but remains symptomatic with shortness of breath, edema, or fatigue, the next step is to acertain that the symptoms are indeed related to the HF syndrome. Two tests are important to utilize in this setting: (i) the cardiopulmonary stress test and (ii) the right heart catheterization to assess cardiac filling pressures, cardiac output (CO), and systemic and pulmonary vascular resistances.

Much has been written about the cardiopulmonary stress test, and there are some aspects of the testing that remain in debate. In experienced laboratories, however, the maximal exercise test with oxygen utilization has the ability to objectively measure exercise capacity, the contributory component of pulmonary abnormalities (in part, related to the resting ventilatory measurements done at baseline), the heart rate and blood pressure response to exercise, accordingly the stroke volume response to exercise and the maximal or peak oxygen update during exercise. In the patient with HF and no other obvious disease abnormalities, peak oxygen uptake is equal to the peak CO times the peak arteriovenous oxygen difference; assuming that the patient can extract oxygen maximally (eliminating metabolic diseases and pulmonary disease that interferes with oxygenation) then peak oxygen uptake is equivalent to peak CO. Multiple studies have shown, beginning with the description by Mancini et al.[2] that a measurement of maximal oxygen uptake (VO_2max) is a useful way to triage patients requiring advanced therapies. Indeed, measurement of functional capacity is a key component of describing the patient with advanced HF, as noted by the ESC's important scientific statement (Table 1). In general, a VO_2max less than 12–14 mL/kg/min is worrying for the patient with HFrEF who is on optimal medical therapy.

The maximal oxygen uptake exercise test is probably best followed by a right heart catheterization to objectively assess hemodynamic performance. A number of studies have shown that a CO alone or an assessment of filling pressures alone is not adequate to predict the full hemodynamic profile of a patient.[3] Moreover, a full hemodynamic assessment will often give clues to further understanding of management difficulties or options. For example, the patient with very low right-sided pressures may explain why vasodilator therapy escalation was associated with hypotension. The patient with severe, chronic, biventricular failure and a very low systemic vascular resistance may have cirrhosis from chronic hepatic congestion. The patient with severe, secondary pulmonary arterial hypertension may benefit from specific therapy aimed at pulmonary vasodilatation. Finally, the resting CO, as with the surrogate of VO_2max,

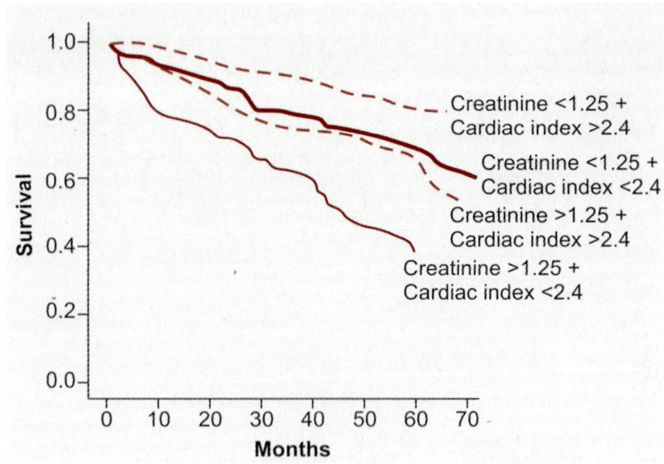

Fig. 1 Kaplan–Meier curves of survival by medians of serum creatinine (mg/dL) and cardiac index (L/min/m^2). Log rank for all curves ($p < 0.0001$)

Source: Adapted from Mullens W, Abrahams Z, Skouri HN, et al. Prognostic evaluation of ambulatory patients with advanced heart failure. *Am J Cardiol*. 2008;101(9):1297-302, *with permission*

is an important gauge of prognosis. In addition, coupling measurement of CO with other important prognostic information, such as renal function, is very useful to help stage the risk profile of a patient with severe HF, as shown in Figure 1.[3]

IN-HOSPITAL PATIENT

There are two types of patients with severe HF and HFrEF encountered in the hospital: (i) the patient with new-onset HF and (ii) the patient with chronic HF who has progressed despite apparent treatment. As reviewed elsewhere in this book, the management of the patient with new-onset HF is to attempt to institute evidence-based therapy in gradually increasing doses. Most clinicians find it useful to assess patients with acute HF using an algorithm suggested by Nohria et al.[4] (Fig. 2). Based on a physical examination, the clinician should determine if the patient is volume overloaded or *wet*, or euvolemic-*dry*. Second, the examining clinician should assess whether the patient is *warm*, e.g., well-perfused, or *cold*-suggesting the shock syndrome. The management tasks are defined by this initial assessment: patients who are volume overloaded need diuresis; patients with physical findings suggesting low CO or low blood pressure need hemodynamic support-typically with inotropic agents, such as dopamine, dobutamine, or milrinone.

The routine use of intravenous inotropic agents or right heart catheterization has not been shown to be beneficial to outcomes when used in all decompensated HF patients. Indeed, there are almost no studies showing the therapeutic efficacy of either strategy. It is only after a failure to begin the approach of standard HF therapy for HFrEF, either because of hemodynamic instability, hypotension, or arrhythmias that hemodynamic evaluation is necessary. Invasive hemodynamic monitoring is a tool to be utilized in a selected group of patients. The indications for invasive hemodynamic assessment include obvious fluid overload in the setting of worsening renal function despite diuresis, signs of end-organ hypoperfusion, such as decreased mental status, hepatic insufficiency, renal insufficiency, and/or cool extremities or hypotension. This can be summarized by the simple dictate as follows: when the patient is not clinically improving with the initial treatment, or the exact clinical scenario is not clear, a right heart catheterization can be done with little risk and may help further define next steps.

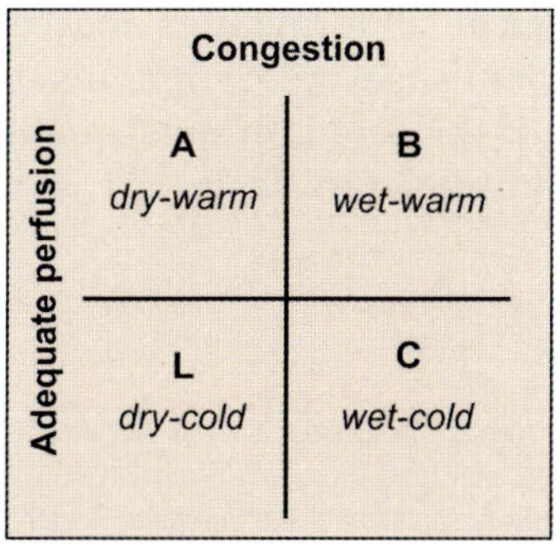

Fig. 2 Schematic for assessment of clinical profiles; congestion was assessed by the presence of orthopnea, jugular venous distention, rales, hepatojugular reflux, ascites, peripheral edema, leftward radiation of the pulmonic heart sound, or a square-wave blood pressure response to the Valsalva maneuver. Compromised perfusion was assessed by the presence of a narrow proportional pulse pressure, pulsus alternans, symptomatic hypotension (without orthostasis), cool extremities, and/or impaired mentation

Source: Adapted from Nohria A, Tsang SW, Fang JC, et al. Clinical assessment identifies hemodynamic profiles that predict outcomes in patients admitted with heart failure. *J Am Coll Cardiol*. 2003;41(10):1797-804, *with permission*

In the patient with new-onset HF, the initiation of inotropic therapy is hopefully a supportive measure, or bridge, to the slow titration of evidence-based medications. In the chronic patient who has failed medical and device therapy, as outlined above, the initiation of inotropic therapy is an ominous prognostic event, and should be accompanied by an immediate determination about the patient's candidacy for advanced therapies such as mechanical circulatory assist devices or heart transplantation. For patients who are obviously not suited

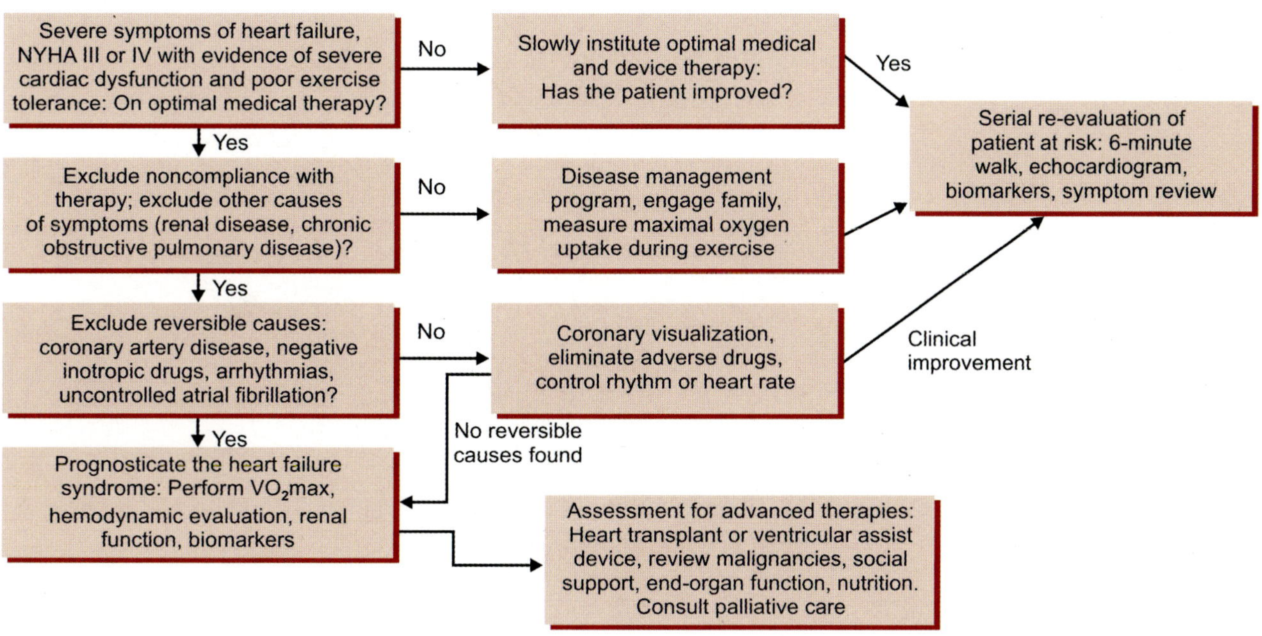

NYHA, New York Heart Association functional class; VO_2max, maximal oxygen uptake exercise test

Flowchart 1 An approach to the patient with refractory heart failure symptoms for such advanced therapies, consideration of a consult for palliative care or hospice should be undertaken. If not done already, end-of-life preferences should be elicited by a gentle discussion with the patient and family.

ADVANCED THERAPIES FOR HEART FAILURE WITH REDUCED EJECTION FRACTION

Appropriate candidates for heart transplantation or mechanical circulatory support devices known more commonly as left ventricular-assist devices (LVADs) have been well described in a number of guidelines and reviews. Social support and compliance with a medical regimen are key essentials to both therapies. The absence of irreversible pulmonary arterial hypertension is likewise a barrier to the successful implementation of either. Significant right HF with dilatation, especially in the setting of normal pulmonary pressures, suggests that LVAD alone may not be possible for the patient with right ventricular insufficiency. These decisions are shown in Flowchart 1.

CONCLUSION

The approach to the patient with suspected refractory or advanced HF is similar to most other issues in cardiovascular medicine. Much depends on the cataloguing of historical events leading to the acute clinical syndrome, the length of the illness and the details of the treatment strategies utilized. An accurate representation of the signs and symptoms of the patient with severe HF is mandatory. An assessment of the pathophysiological abnormalities that determines an individual patient's severe symptoms is logical and straight forward. The details of subsequent management and triage to advanced therapies are as varied as each patient.

REFERENCES

1. Metra M, Ponikowski P, Dickstein K, et al. Advanced chronic heart failure: A position statement from the Study Group on Advanced Heart Failure of the Heart Failure Association of the European Society of Cardiology. Eur J Heart Fail. 2007;9(6-7):684-94.
2. Mancini D, Katz S, Donchez L, et al. Coupling of hemodynamic measurements with oxygen consumption during exercise does not improve risk stratification in patients with heart failure. Circulation. 1996;94(10):2492-6.
3. Mullens W, Abrahams Z, Skouri HN, et al. Prognostic evaluation of ambulatory patients with advanced heart failure. Am J Cardiol. 2008; 101(9):1297-302.
4. Nohria A, Tsang SW, Fang JC, et al. Clinical assessment identifies hemodynamic profiles that predict outcomes in patients admitted with heart failure. J Am Coll Cardiol. 2003;41(10):1797-804.

Chapter 51

Left Ventricular Assist Device Versus Transplantation: How to Decide

Patrick McCann, Eric Adler

ABSTRACT

Advanced heart failure (HF) is a dynamic disease process that requires the synthesis of complex data points including, but not limited to, volume status, comorbidities, exacerbating factors and prognosis. Treatment of stage D HF is essentially limited to three options: (i) mechanical circulatory support (MCS); (ii) heart transplantation; and (iii) hospice. Historically heart transplantation provided the only option for patients with stage D HF refractory to medical therapy. With significantly limited donor heart availability, patients experienced extended waiting periods with extremely reduced functional capacity and many die (approximately 10%) while waiting. However, recent advances in technology and outcomes with ventricular assist devices (VADs) have markedly changed the approach to advanced HF management. VADs are mechanical circulatory devices that are surgically implanted to support either the left (LVAD), right (RVAD), or both (BIVAD) ventricle(s) and improve blood flow generated by the failing heart. As only a minority of patients with advanced HF ultimately undergo cardiac transplantation, VADs have revolutionized care for these patients.

This chapter provides an overview of the indications for LVAD and transplant with a focus on how to choose the appropriate therapy for appropriate patient.

INTRODUCTION

Despite great efforts, end-stage heart failure (HF) remains a leading cause of morbidity and mortality worldwide. Estimates suggest that end-stage HF [American Heart Association (AHA)/American College of Cardiology (ACC) stage D HF] accounts for 5–10% of the total HF population and is associated with a mortality of roughly 50% annually.[1-4] Advanced HF is a dynamic disease process that requires the synthesis of complex data points including, but not limited to, volume status, comorbidities, exacerbating factors and prognosis. Treatment of stage D HF is essentially limited to three options: (i) mechanical circulatory support (MCS); (ii) heart transplantation; and (iii) hospice. Historically, heart transplantation provided the only option for patients with stage D HF refractory to medical therapy. With significantly limited donor heart availability, patients experience extended waiting periods with extremely reduced functional capacity and many die (approximately 10%) while waiting.[5] However, recent advances in technology and outcomes with ventricular assist devices (VADs) have markedly changed the approach to advanced HF management. This chapter provides an overview of the indications for advanced therapies with a focus on VAD and transplant.

INDICATIONS FOR MECHANICAL CIRCULATORY SUPPORT

The indications for VAD use have evolved over time with experience and duration of use. Originally, VADs were used to support patients that could not be weaned from cardiopulmonary bypass after cardiotomy. This type of support was initially designed for use for hours to a few days. Rapid development of technology provided pumps that could supply support for months. As the technology continued to evolve the indications for MCS expanded.

Short-term circulatory support devices for left ventricular (LVAD) or right ventricular (RVAD) support are indicated for refractory cardiogenic shock. Examples include acute severe myocarditis and cardiac arrest during interventional cardiac procedures. The decision between an LVAD or RVAD or both primarily depends on RV function and pulmonary artery resistance.

Longer-term circulatory support devices are typically indicated for patients with advanced HF [New York Heart Association (NYHA) IV] who continue to worsen despite optimal medical and/or resynchronization therapy. Three groups exist that benefit from long-term devices. The first group consists of patients with severe HF who remain hemodynamically unstable despite maximal pharmacologic support and meet criteria for cardiac transplantation. These patients undergo LVAD implantation as a "bridge to transplant" (BTT). The second group encompasses patients with NYHA Class IV advanced HF who are not transplant candidates. These patients have a surgically implanted LVAD for "destination therapy" (DT). The last group of patients usually present with cardiogenic shock in circumstances where candidacy for cardiac transplantation cannot be determined. These patients receive MCS as a "bridge to decision" (BTD). Occasionally, patients are implanted with the expectation that their cardiac function will recover , aka a "bridge to recovery" (BTR).

Bridge to Transplant

Currently, the most common indication for MCS is BTT in patients who deteriorate and develop refractory HF while awaiting heart transplant.[6] Historically, 20–30% of patients who had a VAD implanted as a BTT did not survive to transplantation regardless of the device used or year of implantation owing to the severity of HF and complications associated with the device.[7] However, this mortality has been reduced significantly with the use of newer generation continuous flow devices.[8,9] Recent changes to prioritize use of donors for 1A patients by the United Network for Organ Sharing (UNOS) guidelines for organ sharing have also had a significant impact on the use of LVADs. This change in approach to transplantation and the reduction in mortality with newer generation VADs have contributed to a rapid increase in the use of LVADs.

Other than MCS, the only other option for unstable patients awaiting heart transplant is intravenous continuous inotropes. Data from several studies have shown the outcome with VADs is significantly better than therapy with intravenous inotropes.[10] Furthermore, the Investigation of Nontransplant-Eligible Patients Who are Inotrope Dependent (INTrEPID) trial that declined LVAD implantation showed a 20% survival at 1 year.[11] The success of LVADs compared to the low survival rates of intravenous inotropes has nearly eliminated inotrope therapy as a long-term option for advanced HF. In patients with shorter expected waiting times for heart transplant being treated with inotropes, delay in VAD transplant should be approached with extreme caution.

Destination Therapy

In contrast to patients that are transplant eligible, DT is reserved for patients who are deemed ineligible for heart transplant. The development of DT is partially attributable to an aging population and limited donor availability.[12] Two prospective trials[6,13] have examined the outcome of MCS in patients that are not eligible for transplant. The first study was the Randomized Evaluation of Mechanical Assistance for the Treatment of Congestive Heart Failure (REMATCH) trial which compared the outcome of first-generation LVADs versus medical therapy in patients that were not eligible for transplant.[13] The primary endpoint was death from any cause. The trial showed an absolute risk reduction of 27% at 1 year. However, the authors noted significant morbidity and mortality with the LVAD resulting in a 2-year survival rate of 23%.

More recently the outcomes with MCS in DT patients were examined comparing the first generation pulsatile XVE device versus the second generation continuous flow HeartMate II device.[6] The primary endpoint was a composite of survival at 2 years, free of disabling stroke or reoperation to replace the device. The survival estimate at 2 years in the continuous flow device was 55% compared to 24% with the pulsatile flow device. However, the risk of death from index hospitalization was 56% regardless of device, similar to results noted in the REMATCH trial. These data emphasize the importance of candidate selection in determining the outcomes with MCS.

Bridge to Decision

Mechanical circulatory support must be initiated in an appropriate and timely fashion to achieve the best outcomes. It is not uncommon for patients to present with cardiogenic shock, multisystem organ failure and uncertain neurologic status. Such patients present a unique situation where implantation of durable MCS may be associated with poor outcomes and is not cost-effective. These clinical circumstances may require nondurable MCS support as a BTD to provide support until the clinical situation allows for the implantation of a permanent device. A multidisciplinary approach and excellent communication between local hospitals and specialized MCS centers can make this an effective strategy.[14]

It is important for medical teams to consider which patients will benefit from nondurable MCS and what modality of MCS device should be used. The ongoing evolution of these devices presents a challenging landscape to navigate when evaluating the appropriateness of a device for a particular patient. The current recommendation is to use the device that is familiar to the team and can best serve the needs of the patient.[15] Quick and appropriate intervention with MCS can provide stabilization which may ultimately improve survival.

INDICATIONS FOR TRANSPLANT

Cardiac transplantation remains the treatment of choice for patients with end-stage HF who are symptomatic despite optimal medical therapy. Unfortunately, this therapy is not available to the majority of people who need it secondary to a shortage of available donors. In the past 2 decades approximately 2,200 heart transplants have been performed annually. As a result, screening for transplant, which will be reviewed later in this chapter, involves an extensive evaluation to identify factors that may increase perioperative risk or decrease long-term survival.

Multiple indications for heart transplant exist and are outlined by Mancini and Lietz in selection of cardiac transplantation candidates.[16] The following circumstances are indicated for cardiac transplant: cardiogenic shock requiring continuous intravenous inotrope therapy or MCS with an intra-aortic balloon pump device or MCS; persistent NYHA class IV congestive HF symptoms refractory to maximal medical therapy [left ventricular ejection fraction (LVEF) <20%; peak VO2 <12 mL/kg/min]; intractable or severe angina symptoms in patients with coronary artery disease not amenable to percutaneous or surgical revascularization; intractable life-threatening arrhythmias unresponsive to medical therapy, catheter ablation and/or implantation of intracardiac defibrillator.

PATIENT SELECTION FOR ADVANCED THERAPIES

The approach to implementing advanced therapies for HF is determined by the trajectory of HF progression, etiology of the HF and overall clinical status. Appropriate patient selection is essential for achieving excellent clinical outcomes. This principle extends to all therapies including MCS and heart transplant. Before evaluation for any therapy can proceed, a candid discussion between the HF team and the patient regarding prognosis and postoperative care/responsibilities is paramount as caregiver burden after advanced therapies is high. In addition to a review of advanced therapies, the benefits and risks of therapies, resuscitation and deactivation of devices should be explained to the patient and the patient's family.

Whether patients receive MCS or cardiac transplant is determined by a variety of medical factors which will be reviewed below. Psychosocial factors including barriers to care, informed consent, end-of-life care and patient preferences should all be discussed prior to MCS or transplant. Consent should be discussed with both the patient and the patient's family. Both parties should be made aware of all the risks and benefits, including lifestyle changes that are required for both MCS and heart transplant. Furthermore, end of life discussions, including palliative care, availability of hospice and device deactivation need to be reviewed. Lastly, patient preferences must be identified before proceeding with evaluation for MCS or transplant. This may take time as patients consider their diagnosis, prognosis and treatment options. Occasionally, an ethics consult may be helpful in decision-making for the patients and their families. Patients may also benefit from meeting others that have undergone LVADs and/or cardiac transplantation so they can ask them questions about their lifestyle post-surgery.

As previously noted, medical factors play a significant role in screening patients for MCS or transplant. Univariate and multivariate analyses have examined the data to develop predictors of survival in HF. These analyses have also tried to compare predictors for subgroups of HF including systolic versus diastolic, acute versus chronic and outpatient versus inpatient with HF and will be reviewed below.

Risk Stratification for Outpatients with Heart Failure

Two multivariable risk stratifications for outpatients with HF are available for individual patient risk stratification:

the Heart Failure Survival Score (HFSS)[12] and the Seattle Heart Failure Model (SHFM).[17] The HFSS was the first prospectively validated multivariable risk stratification to predict survival in patients with HF.[18] Ambulatory patients with medium and high risk were considered for cardiac transplant referral. However, the HFSS was developed in an era that preceded the use of beta-blockers, aldosterone antagonists, defibrillators and resynchronization therapy. Butler and colleagues[19] examined the HFSS on an improved background of HF therapies including beta-blockers and aldosterone antagonists and concluded patients receiving a beta-blocker who are at medium risk may have transplant deferred with close monitoring as survival rates were similar between those groups.

The SHFM was also prospectively validated to predict survival in outpatients with HF based on severity of disease. The model was developed by Levy and coworkers[20] to predict 1-year, 2-year and 3-year survival in patients with HF. The model is predictive of mortality in HF and may be used to identify at-risk patients.[21] However, it may overestimate survival when used to stratify patients with advanced HF. The SHFM has been investigated in a sample of patients presenting to an advanced HF clinic for transplant evaluation.[22] The validation study using patients considered for MCS or heart transplant found the model to underestimate the mortality in patients with the greatest observed mortality. The hope is that use of SHFM in future trials will provide further validation.

Risk Stratification for Inpatients with Heart Failure

Similarly, many factors influence mortality risk in the inpatient setting. Again multiple data parameters have been analyzed to determine risk stratification in patients who are hospitalized for decompensated HF. The Acute Decompensated Heart Failure National Registry (ADHERE) provides a predictive model for hospitalized patients based on three readily available variables at HF admission: systolic blood pressure less than 115 mmHg, blood urea nitrogen more than or equal to 43 mg/dL and serum creatinine more than or equal to 2.75 mg/dL.[23] In this analysis, a 10-fold increase in mortality was observed between the low-risk group and high-risk group. Additionally, HF mortality was noted to increase significantly after each HF admission[24] and is directly related to the duration and frequency of HF admissions.[25] Patients with progressive symptoms, multiple admissions for HF and who are intolerant to conventional medical therapy should be considered for MCS and/or transplant.

Comorbidities

Often patients with advanced HF exhibit multiple comorbidities. Screening these patients for MCS or transplant involves an evaluation of significant comorbidities that can increase the short-term peri-operative risk or effect long-term survival. Considerable overlap exists between contraindications for MCS and heart transplant. Absolute indications for both therapies include medical nonadherence, severe psychosocial limitations, terminal illness (life expectancy of <2 years), active systemic infection, severe chronic obstructive pulmonary disease (COPD), irreversible neurologic, hepatic or renal dysfunction. Relative contraindications shared by both therapies include poor functional status, previous substance abuse within 6 months, impaired cognitive function and morbid obesity. These lists are not all inclusive and a specific therapy must be tailored to the needs of the individual.

Age

Age remains one of the most controversial aspects of patient selection for cardiac transplant. Today, 50% of transplanted patients are between 50 years and 64 years of age.[12] Currently, 65 years is considered the upper limit for age. A large registry database analysis indicates decreased long-term survival in older patients.[26,27] Patients more than 65 years of age have lower rates of rejection, likely secondary to physiologic changes which occur with aging. This immune senescence is linked to a decrease in the body's ability to defend against carcinogens and foreign pathogens. Unsurprisingly, older age is associated with a greater morbidity and mortality from infectious diseases and malignancy.

With the advent of DT, MCS for patients more than 80 years of age has now become a relative contraindication. The approval of MCS for DT has provided additional options for advanced HF in elderly patients. As previously mentioned, survival data from the REMATCH trial[13] and the HeartMate II DT trial[6] supports the use of DT. Patients experience significant improvement in quality of life in addition to the survival benefits. In the HeartMate II DT trial patients had NYHA class I or II symptoms at 24 months and a doubling of the mean distance on the 6-minute walk test.[6] Moreover, patients selected for DT may have significant improvement of heart transplantation contraindications and ultimately be selected for transplantation.[11]

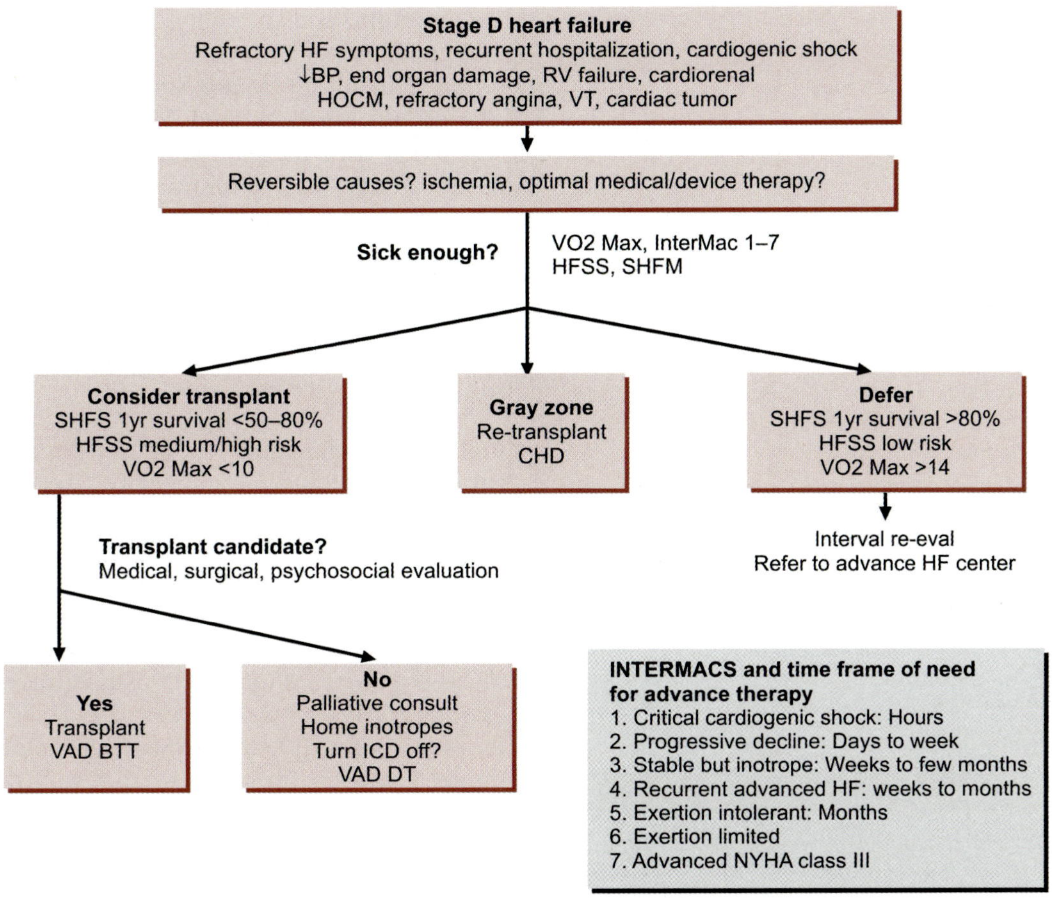

HF, heart failure; BP, blood pressure; RV, right ventricle; HOCM, hypertrophic obstructive cardiomyopathy; VT, ventricular tachycardia; HFSS, Heart Failure Survival Score; SHFM, Seattle Heart Failure Model; CHD, coronary heart disease; VAD, ventricular assist device; BTT, bridge to transplant; ICD, implantable cardioverter-defibrillator; DT, destination therapy

Flowchart 1 Sample treatment algorithm for Stage D heart failure

PATIENT EVALUATION

Clinicians are responsible for determining which HF patients should be referred for MCS or transplant. The selection process is dynamic and dependent on multiple variables. Specific selection criteria for cardiac transplantation have been established and endorsed by the International Society for Lung and Heart Transplantation (ISHLT) and the ACC/AHA/Heart Failure Society of America (HFSA) and updated by Mehra et al.[12] However, until recently, no guidelines had been approved for MCS. These new guidelines have been endorsed by the ISHLT and include a section on candidate selection. These guidelines help aid clinicians in determining the most appropriate therapy for their patients (Flowchart 1).

Mechanical Circulatory Support

The leading causes of mortality and morbidity with VAD use have remained unchanged since their initial use. These include sepsis, bleeding, renal failure, right HF, multiorgan failure and stroke.[9] Many of these complications may be recognized prior to VAD implantation. The recognition of significant risk factors prior to MCS may help prevent adverse outcomes. General indications and contraindications for LVAD are summarized in Boxes 1 and 2.

Renal Function

Renal dysfunction presents a consistent challenge with the use of LVADs. It is often one of the greatest risk factors

Box 1: Indications for left ventricular assist device implantation

- NYHA class IV symptoms
- Life expectancy <2 years*
- Not a candidate for heart transplantation*
- Failure to respond to optimal medical therapy for at least 60 of the last 90 days*
- Left ventricular ejection fraction ≤25%*
- Refractory cardiogenic shock or cardiac failure
- Peak oxygen consumption ≤12 mL/kg/min with cardiac limitation
- Continued need for intravenous inotropic therapy limited by symptomatic hypotension, decreasing kidney function, or worsening pulmonary congestion*
- Recurrent, refractory symptomatic sustained ventricular tachycardia or ventricular fibrillation
- Body surface area >1.5 m^2*°

*Requirements necessary for "destination therapy" (Centers for Medicare and Medicaid Services)

°Smaller devices may be used in smaller patients

NYHA, New York Heart Association

Box 2: Contraindications

- Potentially reversible cause of heart failure
- High surgical risk for successful implantation
- Recent or evolving stroke
- Neurological deficits impairing the ability to manage device
- Coexisting terminal condition (e.g., metastatic cancer, cirrhosis)
- Abdominal aortic aneurysm ≥5 cm
- Biventricular failure in patients older than 65 years
- Active or chronic infection
- Fixed pulmonary hypertension or portal hypertension
- Severe pulmonary dysfunction
- Impending kidney or liver failure
- Inability to tolerate anticoagulation, e.g., active bleeding
- Significant underlying psychiatric illness or lack of social support that impair ability to maintain and operate VAD

Relative contraindications

- Age >65 years, unless minimal or no other clinical risk factors
- Chronic kidney disease with serum creatinine level >3.0 mg/dL
- Severe chronic malnutrition (BMI <21 kg/m^2 in males and <19 kg/m^2 in females)
- Morbid obesity (BMI >40 kg/m^2)
- Mechanical ventilation
- Severe mitral stenosis or moderate to severe aortic insufficiency, or uncorrectable mitral regurgitation

VAD, Ventricular assist device; BMI, Body mass index

for morbidity and mortality. Several measures of renal function have been proposed to define this risk including serum creatinine greater than 2.5 mg/dL, estimated glomerular filtration rate less than 0.5 mL/kg/min and blood urea nitrogen greater than 40 mg/dL. All of these variables are continuous with increased risk with progressive abnormality of the variable. It is often difficult to assess the reversibility of renal dysfunction.[28] Generally, patients who are on long-term dialysis support are considered high-risk candidates for MCS as DT.

Right Ventricular Function

Right ventricular failure is one of the most important causes of mortality or morbidity after LVAD therapy. RV failure contributes to bleeding, renal failure and prolonged hospitalization which may lead to other adverse events. RV failure occurring after implantation of MCS may be anticipated preoperatively. It is estimated to occur in 20–30% of patients undergoing MCS. RV failure after LVAD usually results from pre-existing RV failure. Matthews et al. developed a model for prediction of RV failure after LVAD implantation. The model has been shown to predict survival with RVAD support.[29]

Hemodynamics

Hemodynamic assessment with a Swan Ganz catheter is essential to the evaluation of patient who may be a candidate for MCS. Data from invasive hemodynamics is lacking in showing an individual parameter as a predictor of adverse outcomes. Both Fick and thermodilution should be used to determine cardiac output. Patients with pulmonary artery pressures less than 25–30 mmHg and poor RV function on echocardiogram are at higher risk of RV failure.

Pulmonary Function

Patients with severe obstructive or restrictive pulmonary disease are at risk of prolonged time in the intensive care unit (ICU) and mechanical ventilation following LVAD implantation. Severe cardiac dysfunction may preclude accurate assessment of pulmonary function or give falsely low values if pulmonary congestion is present at the time of the test.[30] When the forced vital capacity, forced expiratory volume at 1 second and carbon monoxide diffusing capacity all are less than 50% predicted, exclusion from LVAD should be considered. Patients should also be screened for obstructive sleep apnea if screening tests are suggestive.

Hepatic Function

Hepatic dysfunction has long been shown to be associated with poor outcomes after LVAD implantation.[31] The most common biomarker of hepatic dysfunction is hyperbilirubinemia, which may be the result of "cardiac congestion". Patients should be screened for other causes of abnormal liver function tests including hepatitis, alcohol abuse and infiltrative diseases. Cirrhosis is a poor predictor of outcome. Many centers screen patient with evidence of hepatic dysfunction with ultrasound and/or liver biopsy.

Hematologic Function

Thrombocytopenia and anemia are two hematologic markers associated with poor outcomes for MCS candidates. These problems should be thoroughly assessed and attempts to correct the underlying cause should be made prior to device implantation. Preoperative platelet counts less than 149,000/μL have been shown to have higher risk of death before discharge. Lietz and colleagues showed that the cause of death before discharge was directly linked to preoperative laboratory abnormalities and the closest correlation was abnormal coagulation values and death caused by bleeding.[9]

Additional risk factors exist that should be evaluated prior to MCS implantation which include gastrointestinal bleeding, peripheral vascular disease, infection, nutrition, neurologic, psychiatric and malignancy. Many investigators have examined composite risk factors associated with early mortality in the use of VADs. The largest series was reported by Lietz and colleagues. Lietz et al. developed a weighted risk score based on a multivariate analysis of data obtained in the REMATCH study. The scores were analyzed and shown to have a strong predictive accuracy. The score was not derived to exclude patients but rather identify patients at high risk who may need more intensive therapy prior to MCS. Currently, there are no prospective data confirming preoperative optimization can reduce a patient's risk of adverse events.

Cardiac Arrhythmia

Ventricular arrhythmia is common in patients with stage D HF. Furthermore, malignant ventricular arrhythmias may be a primary indication for advanced therapies. Patients with LVADs may tolerate arrhythmias for a short period of time, but ultimately are at risk for RV failure. Hence, transplant is generally a preferable option for these patients. If they are too unstable to wait for transplant, MCS with biventricular support or a total artificial heart may be indicated.

CONCLUSION

Surgical therapy for stage D HF has undergone a radical transformation as a result of the rapid development and evolution of MCS. Selection of appropriate therapeutics has become a complicated multifactorial decision that is influenced by the etiology of the HF, the severity of disease and patient preferences. A multidisciplinary systematic approach is clearly required to maximize the likelihood of a good outcome in this highly morbid patient population. A summary of our approach to patient selection in MCS is summarized in Flowchart 1.

REFERENCES

1. Stevenson LW, Pagani FD, Young JB, et al. INTERMACS profiles of advanced heart failure: the current picture. J Heart Lung Transplant. 2009;28(6):535-41.
2. Lloyd-Jones D, Adams RJ, Brown TM, et al. Heart disease and stroke statistics-2010 update: a report from the American Heart Association. Circulation. 2010;121:e46-215.
3. Redfield MM. Heart failure—an epidemic of uncertain proportions. N Engl J Med. 2002;347(18):1442-4.
4. Miller LW, Missov ED. Epidemiology of heart failure. Cardiol Clin. 2001;19(4):547-55.
5. Mulligan MS, Shearon TH, Weill D, et al. Heart and lung transplantation in the United States, 1997-2006. Am J Transplant. 2008;8(4 Pt 2):977-87.
6. Slaughter MS, Rogers JG, Milano CA, et al. Advanced heart failure treated with continuous-flow left ventricular assist device. N Engl J Med. 2009;361(23):2241-51.
7. Deng MC, Edwards LB, Hertz MI, et al. Mechanical circulatory support device database of the International Society for Heart and Lung Transplantation: third annual report—2005. J Heart Lung Transplant. 2005;24(9):1182-7.
8. Miller LW, Pagani FD, Russell SD, et al. Use of a continuous-flow device in patients awaiting heart transplantation. N Engl J Med. 2007;357(9):885-96.
9. Lietz K, Long JW, Kfoury AG, et al. Outcomes of left ventricular assist device implantation as destination therapy in the post-REMATCH era: implications for patient selection. Circulation. 2007;116(5):497-505.
10. Stevenson LW, Miller LW, Desvigne-Nickens P, et al. Left ventricular assist device as destination for patients undergoing intravenous inotropic therapy: a subset analysis from REMATCH (Randomized Evaluation of Mechanical Assistance in Treatment of Chronic Heart Failure). Circulation. 2004;110(8):975-81.
11. Rogers JG, Butler J, Lansman SL, et al. Chronic mechanical circulatory support for inotrope-dependent heart failure patients who are not transplant candidates: results of the INTrEPID Trial. J Am Coll Cardiol. 2007;50(8):741-7.

12. Mehra MR, Kobashigawa J, Starling R, et al. Listing criteria for heart transplantation: International Society for Heart and Lung Transplantation guidelines for the care of cardiac transplant candidates—2006. J Heart Lung Transplant. 2006;25(9):1024-42.
13. Rose EA, Gelijns AC, Moskowitz AJ, et al. Long-term use of a left ventricular assist device for end-stage heart failure. N Engl J Med. 2001;345(20):1435-43.
14. Haft JW, Pagani FD, Romano MA, et al. Short- and long-term survival of patients transferred to a tertiary care center on temporary extracorporeal circulatory support. Ann Thorac Surg. 2009;88(3):711-7.
15. Peura JL, Colvin-Adams M, Francis GS, et al. Recommendations for the use of mechanical circulatory support: device strategies and patient selection: a scientific statement from the American Heart Association. Circulation. 2012;126(22):2648-67.
16. Mancini D, Lietz K. Selection of cardiac transplantation candidates in 2010. Circulation. 2010;122(2):173-83.
17. Teuteberg JJ, Lewis EF, Nohria A, et al. Characteristics of patients who die with heart failure and a low ejection fraction in the new millennium. J Card Fail. 2006;12(1):47-53.
18. Aaronson KD, Schwartz JS, Chen TM, et al. Development and prospective validation of a clinical index to predict survival in ambulatory patients referred for cardiac transplant evaluation. Circulation. 1997;95(12):2660-7.
19. Butler J, Khadim G, Paul KM, et al. Selection of patients for heart transplantation in the current era of heart failure therapy. J Am Coll Cardiol. 2004;43(5):787-93.
20. Levy WC, Mozaffarian D, Linker DT, et al. The Seattle Heart Failure Model: prediction of survival in heart failure. Circulation. 2006;113(11):1424-33.
21. Levy WC, Mozaffarian D, Linker DT, et al. Can the Seattle heart failure model be used to risk-stratify heart failure patients for potential left ventricular assist device therapy? J Heart Lung Transplant. 2009;28(3):231-6.
22. Kalogeropoulos AP, Georgiopoulou VV, Giamouzis G, et al. Utility of the Seattle Heart Failure Model in patients with advance heart failure. J Am Coll Cardiol. 2009;53(4):334-42.
23. Fonarow GC, Adams KF Jr, Abraham WT, et al. Risk stratification for in-hospital mortality in acutely decompensated heart failure: classification and regression tree analysis. JAMA. 2005;293(5):572-80.
24. Setoguchi S, Stevenson LW, Schneeweiss S. Repeated hospitalizations predict mortality in the community population with heart failure. Am Heart J. 2007;154(2):260-6.
25. Solomon SD, Dobson J, Pocock S, et al. Influence of nonfatal hospitalization for heart failure on subsequent mortality in patients with chronic heart failure. Circulation. 2007;116(13):1482-7.
26. Morgan JA, John R, Mancini DM, et al. Should heart transplantation be considered as a treatment option for patients aged 70 years and older? J Thorac Cardiovasc Surg. 2004;127(6):1817-9.
27. Morgan JA, John R, Weinberg AD, et al. Long-term results of cardiac transplantation in patients 65 years of age and older: a comparative analysis. Ann Thorac Surg. 2003;76(6):1982-7.
28. Smith GL, Vaccarino V, Kosiborod M, et al. Worsening renal function: what is a clinically meaningful change in creatinine during hospitalization with heart failure. J Card Fail. 2003;9(1):13-25.
29. Matthews JC, Koelling TM, Pagani FD, et al. The right ventricular failure risk score a pre-operative tool for assessing the risk of right ventricular failure in left ventricular assist device candidates. J Am Coll Cardiol. 2008;51(22):2163-72.
30. Aaronson KD, Patel H, Pagani FD. Patient selection for left ventricular assist device therapy. Ann Thorac Surg. 2003;75(6 Suppl):S29-35.
31. Reinhartz O, Farrar DJ, Hershon JH et al. Importance of preoperative liver function as a predictor of survival in patients supported with Thoratec ventricular assist devices as a bridge to transplantation. J Thorac Cardiovasc Surg. 1998;116(4):633-40.

Chapter 52

Approach to Left Ventricular Assist Devices and Follow-up in Advanced Congestive Heart Failure

Anthony Choi, Keshav R Nayak, Brian E Jaski

ABSTRACT

Patients afflicted with advanced heart failure (HF) derive improved functional capacity, quality of life and survival when they receive critical mechanical circulatory support with implanted flow left ventricular assist devices (LVADs). The pioneering development of smaller, more durable continuous flow devices has dramatically improved treatment of advanced HF making it standard therapy for patients as a bridge-to-transplant or destination therapy (DT). Major determinants of successful LVAD therapy include patient selection, optimization of right heart function, followed by proper timing of device implantation. In this chapter, we outline a general approach to LVAD support, patient selection and preoperative work-up, postoperative management, as well as troubleshooting and monitoring stable device function.

INTRODUCTION

Heart failure (HF) is a circulatory state where demands of tissue perfusion may exceed an impaired cardiac output. A cascade of maladaptive processes including activation of neurohormonal mediators, myocyte hypertrophy, and changes to vascular endothelial function may result in progressive worsening of heart failure. The original Framingham Heart Study cohort and their offspring demonstrated a staggering 70–80% mortality rate over a span of 8 years amongst patients with heart failure diagnosed at less than 65 years of age.[1] In patients with progressive HF who are deemed unsuitable for cardiac transplantation, mechanical assistance with a left ventricular assist devices (LVAD) may provide critical hemodynamic support and improve survival. LVADs, by virtue of replacing or augmenting left ventricular (LV) function, were designed to improve cardiac output, coronary perfusion, and perhaps reverse the maladaptive metabolic and hemodynamic consequences of terminal heart failure.[2] In fact, recent studies of second-generation LVADs have shown promising results of improved functional capacity, quality of life, and survival.

Mechanical circulatory systems had their putative start during development of blood pumps to allow temporary cessation of cardiac function during open heart surgery. Although, the first cardiopulmonary bypass was developed in 1953, it would not be until the establishment of a Total Artificial Heart Program by the National Heart, Lung and Blood Institute (NHLBI) that contracts were awarded to support the technical development of an implanted heart or heart assist device.[3] To accomplish this, biocompatible materials that could withstand the stresses of several thousand cycles, as well as a drive system, and a flow system that would not result in thrombus required laborious investigative development. Early attempts at mechanical support utilized volume displacement to create pulsatile flow LVADs (HeartMate XVE and Novacor). These first-generation devices were typically larger in profile with a volume of 450 mL and a weight of 1,250 g. Unfortunately the pulsatile LVADs were hampered by routine valve or bearing failure limiting device durability. Despite these design flaws, the landmark Randomized Evaluation of Mechanical Assistance for the Treatment of Congestive Heart Failure (REMATCH) trial studying the first-generation LVADs versus medical therapy showed a significantly improved 2-year survival with mechanical-assist therapy (23% vs 8%).[4] However, long-term therapy with the pulsatile LVAD was impossible due to poor device durability, bulky size of the pump, and driveline predisposing to bleeding, infection, and higher incidence of adverse events. This led to the development of second-generation devices that employed newer rotary-pump technology which extended the duration of mechanical circulatory support (MCS). These continuous flow LVADs (also known as axial flow or centrifugal pumps) are as small as 45 mL of displacement and weigh as little as 145 g, more durable, and are both preload and afterload-dependent. These continuous flow LVADs have all but replaced the pulsatile flow LVADs and have demonstrated improved hemodynamic profiles, increased functional capacity and quality of life, as well as survival benefit in recent studies[5] (Fig. 1). Successful MCS in advanced heart failure is crucially dependent

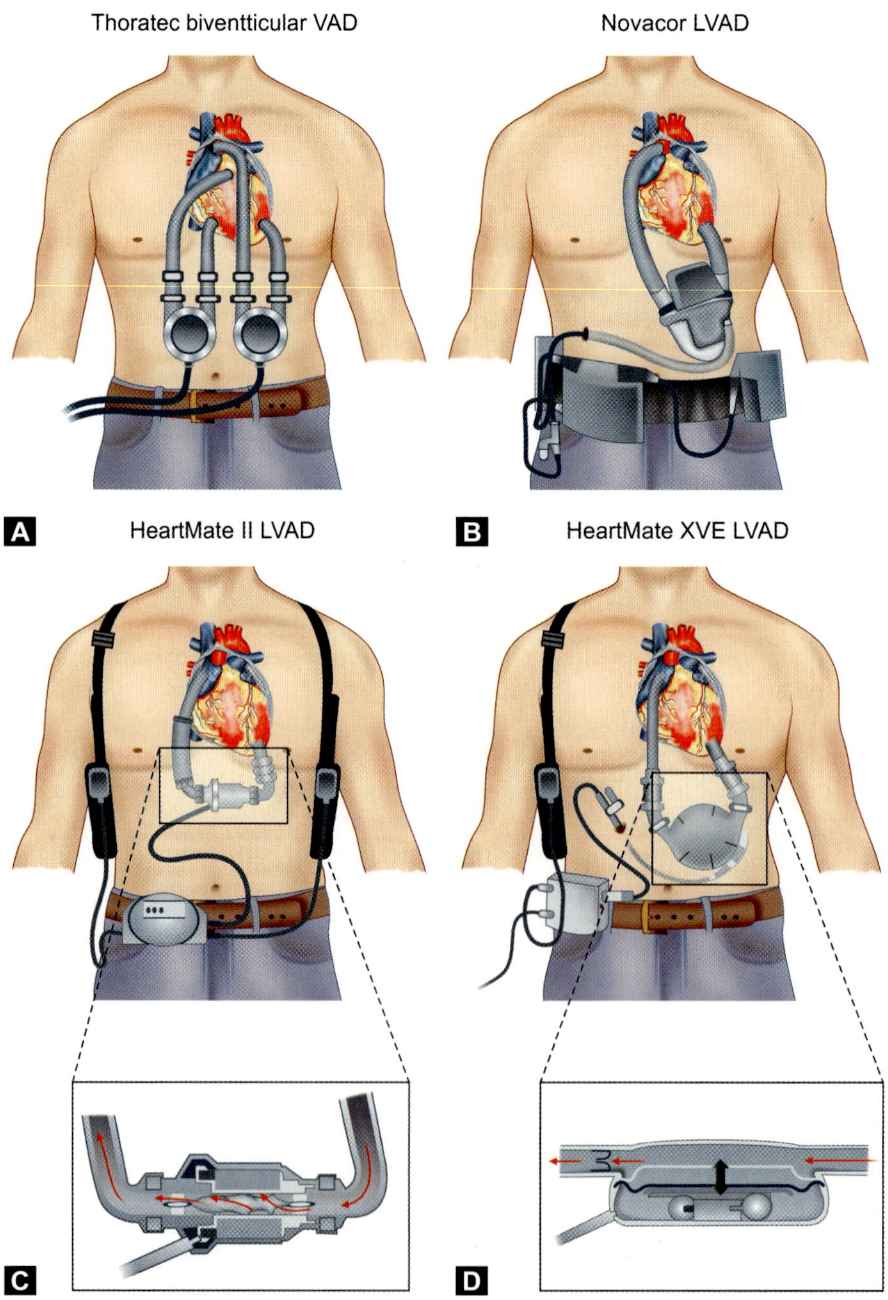

Fig. 1 Schematic representation of left ventricular assist devices (LVADs) in use. **A,** Thoratec bi-ventricular assist device (VAD); **B,** Novacor LVAD; **C,** HeartMate II LVAD; **D,** HeartMate XVE LVAD[6]

on proper patient selection, preoperative optimization of the neurohormonal axis, and right heart function, culminating in the proper timing of LVAD implantation. The following sections will review these critical steps for successful LVAD support in advanced heart failure with a focus on the more commonly used continuous flow LVAD.

PATIENT SELECTION AND PREOPERATIVE OPTIMIZATION

Currently, Food and Drug Administration (FDA) approval for LVADs exists for bridge-to-transplant therapy or bridge-to-destination therapy (DT). Patients selected for bridge-to-transplant therapy receive MCS awaiting a transplant and DT patients are those who are not initially offered transplant. However, evidence in patients who have had long-term mechanical support suggests improvement of structural and functional maladaptive processes seen in heart failure (i.e., regression of cellular hypertrophy and improvement in neurohormonal derangements). This has dramatically broadened the use of mechanical assist devices to include bridges to candidacy, recovery, and decision therapies, respectively (Flowchart 1).

The selection process of patients who are suitable for LVAD implantation should be carried out in a careful, methodical and multidisciplinary manner. Assessments should take into consideration medical appropriateness, ability of the patient to successfully undergo surgery and the patient's access to dependable home support with adequate family/caregiver involvement. Additionally, implantation should not be considered for patients with comorbidities that would preclude a good outcome despite MCS. Lastly, psychosocial concerns, such as poor family/caregiver involvement, unresolved psychological/psychiatric issues, and compliance issues should be carefully weighed before consideration of MCS[7] (Flowchart 2).

The Interagency Registry for Mechanically Assisted Circulatory Support (INTERMACS) registry follows all FDA approved long-term MCS systems in the United States. They have defined patient profiles to assist in timing for initiation MCS[8] (Table 1).

Risk models can predict patient risk category and survival to discharge during the patient selection process. Data from the HeartMate XVE LAD DT Registry allows estimation of 1-year mortality derived from a cumulative weighted risk score[9] (tables 2 and 3). A newer risk score, the HeartMate II risk score (HMRS), has been proposed to predict outcomes in the new era of continuous flow LVADs.[10] The HMRS will require further validation for use in the highest risk LVAD patients.

Proper patient selection together with preoperative optimization impacts timing and success of LVAD implantation. The general work-up for patients to

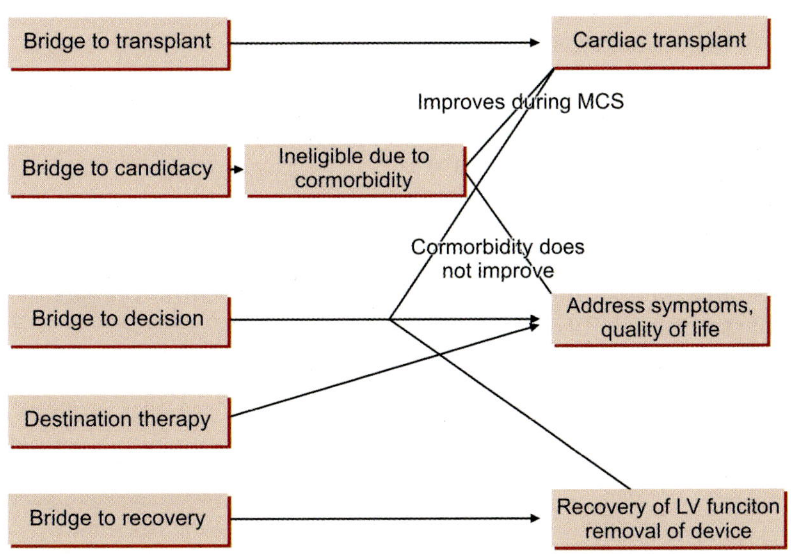

MCS, mechanical circulatory support; LV, left ventricular

Flowchart 1 Nomenclature of indication of mechanical circulatory support

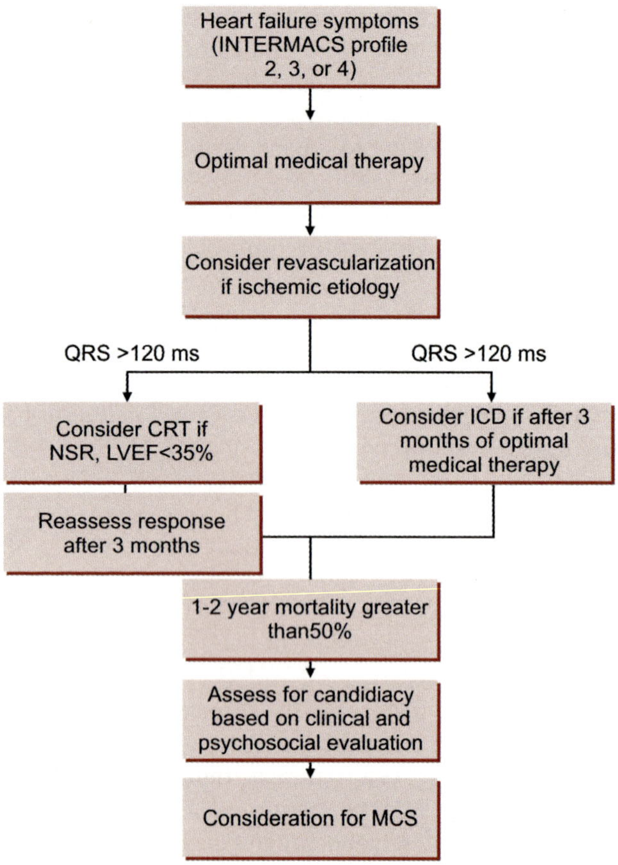

INTERMACS, Interagency Registry for Mechanically Assisted Circulatory Support; CRT, cardiac resynchronization therapy; NSR, normal sinus rhythm; LVEF, left ventricular ejection fraction; ICD, implantable cardioverter-defibrillator; MCS, mechanical circulatory support

Flowchart 2 Clinical pathway for mechanical circulatory support

undergo LVAD implantation, as well as preoperative metabolic goals are shown in Table 4. Ideally, right ventricular (RV) function should be optimized by addressing pulmonary hypertension and circulatory volume status in the preoperative period. Intraoperative hypoxia or pulmonary insult can result in RV dysfunction. In addition, preoperative assessment of cardiac valvular testing, bleeding risk and nutrition can help reduce intraoperative and postoperative complications.

Right Ventricular Function

Right ventricular function is essential to determine while considering candidacy for an LVAD as RV failure is a significant cause of morbidity and death in patients receiving an LVAD. RV stroke work index (RVSI) is a well-

TABLE 1: Interagency Registry for Mechanically Assisted Circulatory Support (INTERMACS) patient profiles and timing of left ventricular assist device support

Profile no	*Description*	*Time to LVAD*
1	Crashing and burning: Critical cardiogenic shock	Within hours
2	Progressive decline: Inotrope dependence with continuing deterioration	Within a few days
3	Stable but inotrope-dependent	Within a few weeks
4	Recurrent advanced heart failure: With recurrent rather than refractory decompensation	Within weeks to months
5	Exertion intolerant: Comfortable at rest, but exercise intolerant	Variable
6	Exertion limited: Patient who is able to do some mild activity, but fatigue within a few minutes	Variable
7	Advanced NYHA II: Reasonably stable, able to tolerate reasonable level of comfortable activity; decompensation history that is not recent	Not a candidate

LVAD, left ventricular assist device; NYHA, New York Heart Association

TABLE 2: Risk factors for 90-day mortality and the weighted scores

Risk factors	*Score*
Platelet count <148 × 10^3/μL	7
Serum albumin <3.3 g/dL	5
INR >1.1	4
Vasodilator therapy	4
Mean PAPs <25 mmHg	3
Aspartate aminotransferase >45 U/mL	2
Hematocrit <34%	2
Blood urea nitrogen >51 mg/dL	2
No intravenous inotropes	2

INR, international normalized ratio; PAPs, pulmonary artery pressures

TABLE 3: Risk category and survival to hospital discharge

Score	*Risk category*	*1-year survival (%)*
0–8	Low risk	81
9–16	Medium risk	62
17–19	High risk	28
>20	Very high risk	11

TABLE 4: Preoperative assessment for patients undergoing left ventricular assist devices

Laboratory tests	*Studies*	*Other*
• CBC with differential and platelet count • Complete chemistry panel • Uric acid • Thyroid profile • Lactate dehydrogenase • PT/PTT, INR • Plasma renin activity • Pregnancy test in women • Iron, transferrin, ferritin • HbA1c • HIT antibody if clinically suspected. Should be followed by a serotonin release assay if HIT antibodies are positive • Urinalysis, culture, and sensitivity	• Chest X-ray (AP and lateral) • Carotid Doppler if history of CAD or >5 years old • Chest/abdominal CT if prior surgery • ABI if history of claudication or diabetes • Abdominal ultrasound for AAA if >60 years old or if PAD • EGD or colonoscopy in the last 2 years • Echocardiography • Right heart catheterization	• Dental evaluation with Panorex image

CBC, complete blood count; PT, prothrombin time; PTT, partial thromboplastin time; INR, international normalized ratio; HbA1c, glycated hemoglobin; HIT, heparin-induced thrombocytopenia; AP, anteroposterior; CAD, coronary artery disease; CT, computed tomography; ABI, ankle-brachial index; AAA, abdominal aortic aneurysm; PAD, peripheral artery disease; EGD, esophagogastroduodenoscopy

defined predictor of RV dysfunction and can be computed by:

$$\text{RVSI} = \frac{\text{SV (mean-PAP) CVP}}{\text{BSA}}$$

where SV stands for stroke volume; PAP, pulmonary artery pressure; CVP, central venous pressure; and BSA, body surface area.

A RVSI value of less than 300 mmHg × mL/m^2 connotes preserved RV function. Additional hemodynamic and valvular indices, such as central venous pressure (CVP) less than 15 mmHg, mild-to-moderate tricuspid regurgitation, pulmonary vascular resistance less than 4 Woods units, transpulmonary gradient less than 15 mmHg, absence of RV dilation, and absence of preoperative ventilatory support are desirable prior to LVAD implantation.[7]

Valvular Disease

Aortic valve: Insufficiency of the aortic valve in the setting of LVAD support can create a circular shunt from the aortic outflow cannula to left ventricle to LVAD, to outflow tract again. Aortic insufficiency can be underestimated in patients with high LV filling pressures, and may worsen with reduction of pressures in the presence of an LVAD. Furthermore, aortic insufficiency is likely to progress. Aortic insufficiency can be addressed by valve replacement, oversewing the aortic valve (not desirable in bridge to possible recovery patients as this renders the patient dependent on the LV conduit to aortic outflow cannula), or aortic patch. Preexisting mechanical prosthesis in the aortic position must be replaced with a bioprosthetic valve to attenuate risk of thrombotic events. Aortic stenosis does not require correction as this has an insignificant effect on LVAD performance.

Mitral valve: As LVADs are preload-dependent, significant mitral valve disease can impair LV filling. Furthermore, elevated left atrial pressures can result in pulmonary hypertension and subsequent RV dysfunction. Valve repair or, if needed, a bioprosthetic valve replacement should be considered.

Tricuspid valve: Right heart function should be evaluated as part of the selection process for patients with LVAD. Severe tricuspid insufficiency should be corrected to preserve RV function. Mild-to-moderate insufficiency may improve with reduction of RV afterload.

Patent Foramen Ovale

Preoperative and intraoperative echocardiography can aid in the detection of a persistent patent foramen ovale (PFO). All PFOs should be closed at the time of LVAD implant to prevent right-to-left shunting which can induce hypoxemia and worsen RV function in the postoperative period. It is advisable for implanting surgeons to visually inspect the interatrial septum for PFOs due to false-negative bubble studies.

Bleeding

Bleeding is a leading cause of adverse events. Bleeding can result in hemodynamic shifts resulting in right heart failure, whereas hematoma formation can result in infection, and severe anemia can result in a requirement for additional transfusions. Reoperation due to bleeding carries increased morbidity and mortality in patients. If possible, antiplatelet and anticoagulant medication should be stopped 3–7 days prior to surgery and the international normalized ratio (INR) should be normalized prior to surgery. If necessary, enoxaparin can be used upto 24 hours prior to surgery.

Nutrition

Poor nutritional status is common in patients with advanced heart failure. Patients with malnutrition are at risk for infection, poor wound healing, and specific clinical markers may predict increased mortality (Table 5).[11] Cachexia, per se, is associated with increased perioperative mortality.[12] Increased risk has been demonstrated in patients with prealbumin levels less than 15 mg/dL 2 weeks after implant.[13] If feasible the prealbumin level should be optimized to greater than 15 mg/dL and should be checked every 2 weeks.

Summary

- Preoperative selection of patients should include consideration of the following:
  - Surgical risk
  - Dependable home support
  - Adherence to medication and therapeutic regimen
- Preoperative optimization of comorbid conditions should include:
  - Nutritional status
  - Optimize right heart function
  - Appropriately timing anticoagulation and correcting coagulopathy

TABLE 5: Markers of nutritional deficiency

Body mass index	*<20 kg/m^2*
Albumin	<3.2 g/dL
Prealbumin	<15 mg/dL
Total cholesterol	<130 mg/dL
Lymphocyte count	<100 × 10 μL

- Patients with valvular disease:
  - Mechanical aortic valve should be replaced with a bioprosthetic valve
  - Aortic insufficiency, mitral regurgitation, mitral stenosis, and tricuspid regurgitation should be addressed during the time of surgery
- Anatomic shunting should be evaluated for and corrected if necessary prior to procedure
- Preoperative prealbumin level should be >15 mg/dL prior to implant surgery.

POSTOPERATIVE MANAGEMENT

Blood Pressure

In patients with axial flow devices, there is frequently little pulse pressure and Korotkoff sounds are diminished. Routine blood pressure measurements should be obtained by Doppler for uniformity. The desired goal mean arterial pressure is between 70 mmHg and 90 mmHg. Blood pressure should be addressed as hypertension and increased afterload is associated with device cannula valve deterioration. Furthermore, continuous flow devices rely on LV to aortic pressure gradient for flow and thus a decrease in this gradient by increase in afterload can result in a low flow states. In approximately 50% of patients, blood pressure can be estimated by automatic blood pressure cuff.[14]

Right Ventricular Function

Right ventricular dysfunction is a key predictor of morbidity and mortality in patients with LVADs, particularly in the postoperative period. Furthermore, early postoperative changes can result in considerable volume shifts affecting RV function. Loading of LV pressures can also profoundly affect RV geometry and function resulting from leftward septal shift. Reduction of RV preload can translate to LV preload reduction, thus affecting preload seen by the device. As these changes are seen early in the postoperative course, RV evaluation by echocardiography with a range of LVAD speeds (ramp study) is recommended.

Anticoagulation

Continuous flow LVADs require chronic oral anti-coagulation with warfarin. Patients in the immediate postoperative period should not be given anticoagulation unless there is another indication (known atrial or

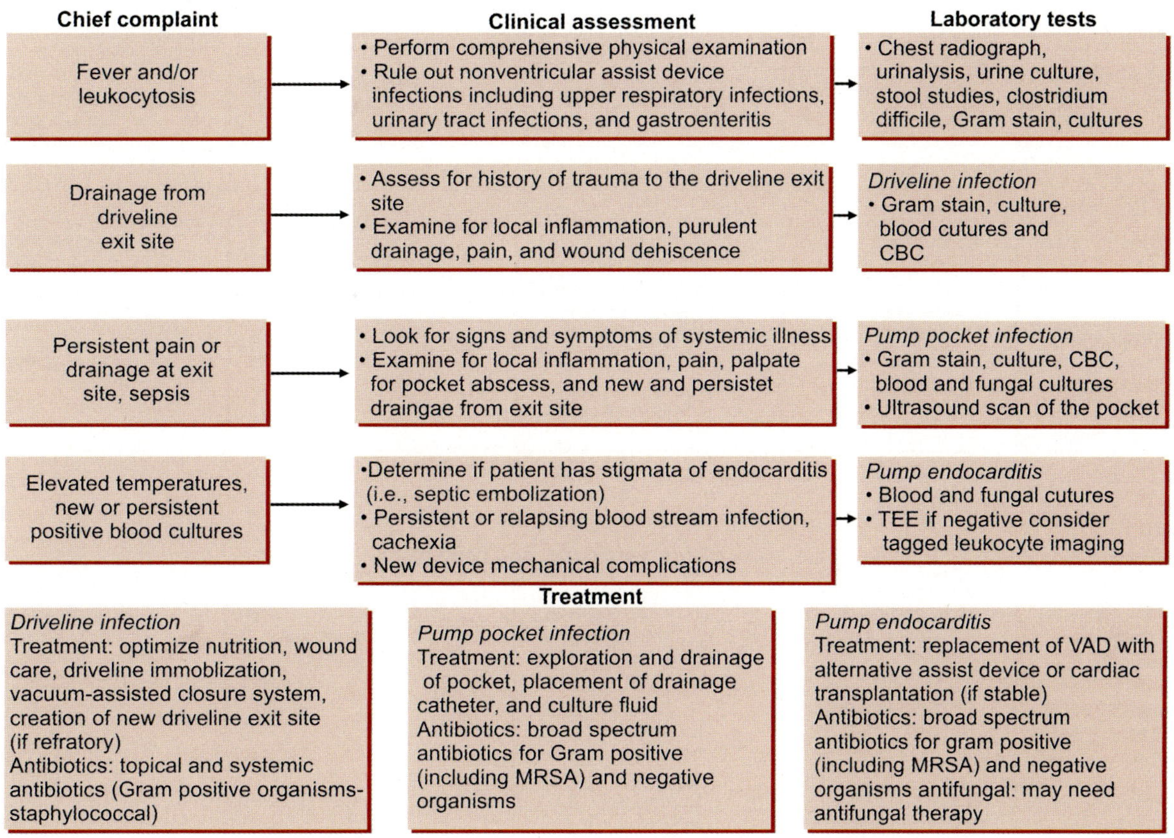

CBC, complete blood count; TEE, transesophageal echocardiography; VAD, ventricular assist device; MRSA, methicillin-resistant Staphylococcus aureus

Flowchart 3 Approach to patient with suspected left ventricular assist device (LVAD) infection[6]

ventricular thrombus). Warfarin should be initiated when chest tubes have been removed and there is less concern for post operative bleeding. Target INR for HeartMate II is 1.8–2.4, for the HeartWare the goal is 2–3, and the pulsatile HeartMate XVE does not require anticoagulation. A low dose aspirin should be given daily.

Infection

Infection is a frequent cause of readmission at any time after implant, and is the cause of 10–26% of readmissions.[15] LVAD infection is associated with a 30% reduced survival when compared to patients who did not have infections of the LVAD.[16] The entire LVAD system is susceptible to infection and thus a patient presenting with fever or leukocytosis should have a thorough physical examination as well as targeted laboratory and imaging studies.[6] Three categories of LVAD infection are: (1) driveline infection, (2) pump pocket infection, and (3) pump endocarditis (Flowchart 3).

Summary

- Mean arterial pressure should be targeted to 70–90 mmHg
- Early echocardiography is recommended to guide management of RV function
- Anticoagulation goals are as follows:
  - HeartMate II: 1.8-2.4
  - HeartWare: 2-3
  - HeartMate XVE (pulsatile): no warfarin required
- Patients with fever or leukocytosis should be scrutinized with high suspicion for system infection or pump endocarditis.

TROUBLESHOOTING AND MONITORING STABLE DEVICE FUNCTION

Proper LVAD function can be monitored by parameters provided by the LVAD to include pump speed, power, pulsatility index, and estimated flow. These parameters

Problem				
Inflow onstruction (without contact with LVAD rotor)	Outflow obstruction (without cobtact with LVAD rotor)	Suction event	Percutaneous lead or motor failure	Thrombus in pump in contact with LVAD rotor
LVAD Response				
Decreased pump power Decreased pulsatility index Decreased flow Suction events	Decreased pump power Decreased pulsatility index Decreased flow Suction events	Pump speed decreases below set speed to low speed limit and ramps back up to set speed Decreased pump flow	Pump vibrates, Not maintaining set pump speed PI > 10	High power and estimated flow Decreased PI Sound of pump changes
Workup **In all patients evaluate for volume status, heart failure symptoms, and hemolysis**				
Chest X-ray, echocardiography. (observed for septal shift) Ramped speed study for LV size change Diastolic arterial blood pressure change with speed change	Chest X-ray, echocardiography (assess for graft kink) rampeed speed study for LV size change Diastolic arterial blood pressure with speed change	Chest X-ray, echocardiography. (inflow position, LV size, septal position) Evaluate RV function Screen for arrythmia	Arterial blood pressure decreases with increased pulse pressure	Echocardiography and angiography to confirm lack of pump inflow
Management				
Ensure that patient is hydrated Consider reducing pump speed to relieve septal or free wall obstruction against inlet Optimize right heart function Consider throacotomy to adjust pump position or to relieve tamponade	Consider throacotomy to relive outflow obstruction	Ensure adequate hydration	Contact manufacturer to see if lead repair is feasible May need to replace system	Consider thrombolytic therapy IV heparin may prevent progression of thrombus Consider pump replacement

LVAD, left ventricular assist device; PI, pulsatile index; LV, left ventricular; RV, right ventricular; IV, intravenous

Flowchart 4 Troubleshooting of the continuous flow left ventricular assist device

along with surveillance echocardiography provide excellent indicators of device function. Physicians caring for LVAD patients should be familiar with the following LVAD conditions and their acute management (Flowchart 4).

Left ventricular suction event: Suction and associated flow events are most commonly a result of low LV filling pressures or LV free wall excursion into the LV inflow cannula. This can occur if the pump speed is higher than the volume available to the LVAD. This may be due to dehydration or less commonly if the pump speed is set too high. In patients with a suction event, echocardiography and chest X-ray is indicated to evaluate for inflow cannula position and LV size. Evaluation for arrhythmia should be considered as both a cause and effect of suction events. RV dysfunction can also impair preload to the inflow cannula. Treatment can include hydration or adjustment of pump speed.[5]

Ventricular arrhythmias: Patients with cardiomyopathy and especially ischemic cardiomyopathy are susceptible to ventricular tachycardia (VT) or ventricular fibrillation (VF). VT/VF is a marker for increased mortality risk.[17] VT/VF as a result of a suction event should be considered. Most patients have implantable cardioverter-defibrillator (ICDs) to allow antitachycardia pacing and some require VT radiofrequency ablation.

Pump thrombus: Thrombus in the pump can affect speed, power, flow and pulsatile index (PI). Etiologies include an embolic capture of thrombus into the device or growth of thrombus from prior deposits.[18] In patients who are hemodynamically stable, heparin drip or thrombolysis may resolve the clinical syndrome. If the device function is significantly affected by the presence of thrombus, LVAD replacement should be considered.[5]

Summary

- LVAD function assessments should include pump speed, power, PI, and estimated flow
- Ventricular arrhythmia in patients with LVAD should include consideration of a suction event of the LV free wall or septum
- New onset hemolysis during LVAD support should lead to assessment for pump thrombosis.

CONCLUSION

Improvement in clinical and surgical expertise in LVAD has improved the quality of life in well selected patients. New continuous flow devices have largely replaced pulsatile flow devices as they are smaller, lighter, and confer improvement in survival and quality of life when compared to pulsatile flow devices. Congestive heart failure patients have enjoyed expanding indications for mechanical assist devices to include bridge-to-recovery or bridge-to-DT. Careful selection of patients is essential in identifying patients who may benefit the most from LVAD therapy. The presence of valvular disease, anatomic shunting, nutritional status, and psychosocial factors has measurable impact on survival and should be optimized prior to implantation. As indications and number of patients with LVADs expand, these patients will increasingly seek medical attention outside of advanced heart failure centers. Physicians involved in primary care, general cardiologists and acute caregivers will benefit from familiarization with indications and patient selection for LVAD therapy as well as the evaluation of the patient with an LVAD, goals for anticoagulation therapy, and have a high suspicion for common LVAD complications.

REFERENCES

1. Rosamond W, Flegal K, Furie K, et al. Heart disease and stroke statistics—2008 update: a report from the American Heart Association Statistics Committee and Stroke Statistics Subcommittee. Circulation. 2008;117(4):e25-146.
2. Frazier OH. Ventricular assistance: a perspective on the future. Heart Fail. 1994;10(6):259-64.
3. Poirier V. The LVAD: a case study. Bridge. 1997;27:14-20.
4. Rose EA, Gelijns AC, Moskowitz AJ, et al. Long-term use of a left ventricular assist device for end-stage heart failure. New Engl J Med. 2001;345(20):1435-43.
5. Slaughter MS, Rogers JG, Milano CA, et al. Advanced heart failure treated with continuous-flow left ventricular assist device. New Engl J Med. 2009;361(23):2241-51.
6. Wilson SR, Givertz MM, Stewart GC, et al. Ventricular assist devices the challenges of outpatient management. J Am Coll Cardiol. 2009; 54(18):1647-59.
7. Slaughter MS, Pagani FD, Rogers JG, et al. Clinical management of continuous-flow left ventricular assist devices in advanced heart failure. J Heart Lung Transplant. 2010;29(4 Suppl):S1-39.
8. Kirklin JK, Naftel DC, Kormos RL, et al. Second INTERMACS annual report: More than 1,000 primary left ventricular assist device implants. J Heart Lung Transplant. 2010;29(1):1-10.
9. Lietz K, Long JW, Kfoury AG, et al. Outcomes of left ventricular assist device implantation as destination therapy in the post-REMATCH era: implications for patient selection. Circulation. 2007;116(5):497-505.
10. Cowger J, Sundareswaran K, Rogers JG, et al. Predicting survival in patients receiving continuous flow left ventricular assist devices: the HeartMate II risk score. J Am Coll Cardiol. 2013;61(3):313-21.
11. Holdy K, Dembitsky W, Eaton LL, et al. nutrition assessment and management of left ventricular assist device patients. J Heart Lung Transplant. 2005;24(10):1690-6.
12. Mano A, Fujita K, Uenomachi K, et al. Body mass index is a useful predictor of prognosis after left ventricular assist system implantation. J Heart Lung Transplant. 2009;28(5):428-33.
13. Lockard KL, DeGore L, Schwarm P, et al. Lack of improvement in pre-albumin at two weeks predicts a poor outcome after mechanical circulatory support. J Heart Lung Transplant. 2009;28(2):S66.

14. Bennett MK, Roberts CA, Dordunoo D, et al. Ideal methodology to assess systemic blood pressure in patients with continuous-flow left ventricular assist devices. J Heart Lung Transplant. 2010;29(5): 593-4.
15. Hasin T, Marmor Y, Kremers W, et al. Readmissions after implantation of axial flow left ventricular assist device. J Am Coll Cardiol. 2013;61(2): 153-63.
16. Simon D, Fischer S, Grossman A, et al. Left ventricular assist device-related infection: treatment and outcome. Clin Infect Dis. 2005;40(8):1108-15.
17. Bedi M, Kormos R, Winowich S, et al. Ventricular arrhythmias during left ventricular assist device support. Am J Cardiol. 2007;99(8):1151-3.
18. Goldstein DJ, John R, Salerno C, et al. Algorithm for the diagnosis and management of suspected pump thrombus. J Heart Lung transplant. 2013;32(7):667-70.

Chapter 53

How to Approach Palliative and End-of-life Care

Tiny Jaarsma, Anna Strömberg

ABSTRACT

Along the heart failure (HF) disease trajectory, the condition of the patient with HF often changes and symptoms may progress over time. HF is equivalent to malignant disease in terms of symptom burden and mortality and therefore patients are in need of care that prepares them to live optimally with their disease and plan and discuss the importance of the disease in the phases of their life. Communication with the patients and patient-centered decision making are integral to optimal HF management and should also include discussions around preferences of palliation and end-of-life care. In this chapter, we will provide practical pointers with regard to palliative care and communication with HF patients related to end-of-life decisions in the HF trajectory. Important issues in communication include a comprehensive assessment of understanding and needs, planning for the future, including advance directives, discussing the potential need for device withdrawal and symptom management. These issues need to be discussed within the broader context of multidisciplinary HF management, include patients and their caregivers and have a place in the whole HF trajectory.

INTRODUCTION

Professional consensus papers advise provision of palliative or supportive care concurrent with efforts to prolong life in heart failure (HF) and at the end of life.[1-4] However, in daily practice far from all HF patients receive adequate palliative care. This is due to several barriers such as the unpredictable nature of the HF condition, the attitude of health care providers that a palliative care approach is of less importance in HF or due to organizational issues such as less priority or lack of time. Communication with the patient and his/her family and patient-centered decision making are integral to optimal HF management and should also include discussions around preferences of palliation and end-of-life care. In this chapter we will provide basic background and practical pointers with regard to palliative care and on communication with patients related to end-of-life decisions in the HF trajectory.

PALLIATIVE AND END-OF-LIFE CARE IN HEART FAILURE

Definitions

Palliative care is defined by the World Health Organization (WHO)[5] as care that improves the quality of life of patients and families who face life-threatening illness, by providing pain and symptom relief, and psychosocial support from diagnosis to the end of life. Palliative care focuses on relief of pain and other distressing symptoms, affirms life, and regards dying as a normal process. Palliative care intends neither to hasten nor postpone death and offers a support system to help patients live as actively as possible until they die. This holistic approach also addresses emotional and spiritual aspects of patient care and supports the family and informal caregivers during the illness and into bereavement.[5] *Supportive care* is a description of care that is often used as a synonym for palliative care and is described as care focusing on alleviating symptoms, complications and side-effects of HF interventions, including supporting patients and families to cope with the disease and the effects of treatment. The term "end-of-life care" is variously used either signifying terminal care of dying patients and/or also interchangeably as "palliative care". End-of-life care may begin as soon as an irreversible progressive illness is diagnosed.

Terminal care often refers to the care during the last days or weeks of the patient's life.

Hospice care is often used to describe service models and is inconsistently used for mobile outpatient hospice teams, inpatient hospices, and also describing a financial model in some countries.[5]

The Need for Palliative and End-of-life Care During the Illness Trajectory

Heart failure is a progressive disease with an often unpredictable course (Fig. 1). HF often changes and progresses in different phases along a trajectory. The phases can be referred to as crisis, chronic and terminal. The crisis phase refers both to the period between the prediagnostic phase when symptoms start occurring to the initial period after the diagnosis when the patient starts adapting to the disease and periods of deterioration. The chronic phase is defined as the period between the initiation of treatment and the transition to the terminal stage of the illness. Crisis can occur during the chronic phase and the terminal phase is, as stated before, sometimes difficult to define. Each phase is associated with different demands.[6] As depicted in Figure 1, HF patients often have several exacerbations during their disease trajectory, which mostly are accompanied by rehospitalizations or extra visits to a health care professional.[4] These rehospitalizations are responsible for high costs in health care and have major negative impact on the quality of life of patients and their families.

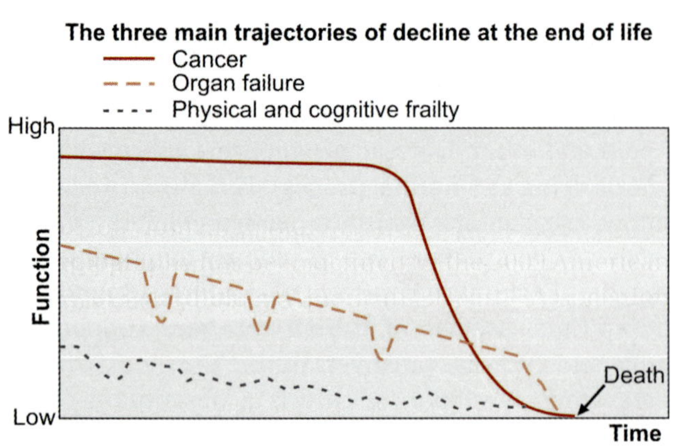

Fig. 1 Trajectories of decline

Health care professionals seem to be more used to handling the cancer trajectory where patients have a clear breakpoint where palliative and end-of-life care is needed and are less skilled to have an ongoing assessment of needs. Although it is generally recognized that HF is a serious condition and equivalent to malignant disease in terms of symptom burden and mortality, only a limited number of HF patients receive care that prepares them to live optimally with their disease and plan and discuss the importance of the disease in the phases of their life.[1,4] Such poor communication with the patient might be due to a lack of awareness or skills of current health care professionals.

Communication on Palliative and End-of-life Care

The lack of clear terminology and the unpredictability of the course of HF may hinder the provision of palliative care to patients with HF. However, in accordance with the WHO definition, a palliative care approach is applicable earlier in the course of HF in parallel with treatment options directed at improving cardiac function and prognosis.[1,4] In addition to the appropriateness of a palliative care approach for "typical" older HF patients, a palliative approach may also become relevant for relatively younger patients being considered for heart transplant of left ventricular assist device (LVAD) implantation.[4]

Open and clear communication is vital to ensure good quality of care at the end of life of the HF patients, their family and caregivers. Ineffective communications on prognosis and needs of patients can increase anxiety and uncertainty in patients affecting their outcomes. HF patients have a lot of thoughts about their future and their prognosis. Higher levels of anxiety/depression can be correlated to fear of death and patients might be afraid of pain, loss of independence and dignity.[7] Some patients are afraid that health care will not be able to support them and treat their symptoms and others are afraid to be a burden to their family.[8] The cardiology team does not always have enough clarity regarding what had been previously discussed with and disclosed to patients regarding prognosis in palliative care and different health care providers argue on who should be responsible for the communication.[8,9] It is quite common that every health care provider expects that someone else have addressed prognosis, preferences for life-supporting and palliative care.

Previous research in the cancer field has suggested that poor communication practices can affect cancer patients' psychological adjustment, quality of life, satisfaction and understanding of their condition.[10,11] From the perspective of the HF patients we know that they have little insight into the nature of their disease, or their prognosis and are rarely offered discussion on palliative care with their professional caregivers.[12,13] Patients also believe that doctors do not want to provide patients with too much knowledge.[14] Some patients also may have an ambivalent attitude toward gaining greater knowledge of their condition.[15]

General communication rules are applicable to all chronically ill patients, but there might be some more specific issues relevant to HF patients. Improving communication between the attending physician and the seriously ill patient and family has been defined by chronically ill patients and family members as a key factor related to quality of end-of-life care.[15,16]

Box 1: Principles of a "good death"[17]

- To know when death is coming, and to understand what can be expected
- To be able to retain control of what happens
- To be afforded dignity and privacy
- To have control over pain relief and other symptom control
- To have choice and control over where death occurs (at home or elsewhere)
- To have access to information and expertise of whatever kind is necessary
- To have access to any spiritual or emotional support required
- To have access to hospice care in any location, not only in hospital
- To have control over who is present and who shares the end
- To be able to issue advance directives which ensure wishes are respected
- To have time to say goodbye, and control over other aspects of timing
- To be able to leave when it is time to go, and not to have life prolonged pointlessly

A PRACTICAL APPROACH TO END-OF-LIFE CARE: WHAT, WHEN, HOW AND WHO

What to Discuss and Decide

In the approach to end-of-life care of patients with HF, both general principles and heart failures' specific issues need to be considered. General principles of a "good death" are presented in Box 1, and are important to consider during different stages in the HF trajectory.

Important issues in communication include a comprehensive assessment of understanding and needs, planning for the future, including advance directives, discussing the potential need for device withdrawal and symptom management. Discussions and decisions should be clearly documented, regularly reviewed and routinely communicated to all those involved in the patient's care.[18]

Comprehensive Assessment of Understanding and Needs

To adequately cope with HF, patients need to understand their prognosis and have a realistic view and expectations of their future. Previous research has shown that elderly patients with HF often think about death and some fear death in general. However, most patients stated that they only fear disability, helplessness, dependence, uncontrolled or unbearable symptoms of pain or shortness of breath, and not receiving adequate care.[7]

In the case of device therapy [cardiac resynchronization therapy (CRT), implantable cardioverter-defibrillator (ICD), LVAD], it is advocated that advance care planning and the potential needs such as device withdrawal are discussed in the preoperative phase (before implantation), in addition to informed consent.[19-21]

Family caregivers play an important role in supporting the patient and should also be involved in the palliative care plan.

Advance Directives

An open and clear discussion addressing expectations with regard to survival, consequences of the treatment for the patient and family and "what to do in case of..." needs to be included in the management of HF patients.[22] Advance directives refer to discussing preferences regarding the possible need for therapeutic interventions such as cardiopulmonary resuscitation or mechanical ventilation with patients, families and caregivers. Advance directives are recognized as important for the quality of end-of-life care in HF patients. However, many patients never have advance directives, and even among LVAD patients, where one might expect clear discussions, those patients who do have advance directives, the possible need for withdrawal of the LVAD support at the end of life is often not mentioned.[23] It is very important that advance directives are documented and preferences discussed repeatedly during the illness trajectory.

Discussing the Potential Need for Device Withdrawal

In the terminal phase of HF, ICD therapy may lead to an uncomfortable dying process with repeated shock during the last weeks or days of life.[24] Deactivation of the ICD allows death to occur naturally without painful shocks. Hence, deactivation may be perceived by patients, families and health care professionals as an act of euthanasia.[25,26] This underlines the delicate human and ethical aspects of this therapy that needs to be discussed, between health care providers and patients and their caregivers before implantation or battery replacements and at the end of life. The current guidelines in Europe and the United States[27,28] recommend that elective ICD deactivation should be communicated to the patient. Effective communication should be tailored to the patients' preferences and needs.[29] Unfortunately, health care professionals avoid discussing end-of-life management of the ICD or termination of LVAD therapy with their patients.[30,31] Patients on the other hand, may also be reluctant about having discussions when and how they would prefer to deactivate the ICD.[31-33] This may be due to lack of knowledge on the goal of LVAD and ICD treatment and the risk of complications in the terminal phase, but may also involve other psychological processes that need to be understood and respected.

With regard to LVAD support is important to realize that if LVAD support will no longer meet its goal (to prolong life and improve quality of life) or even cause serious complications, mechanical support is no longer indicated and can be considered to be withdrawn.[34] Preparing the patient, his family and caregivers (preparedness planning) for those moments in end-of-life care is important in order to reduce the distress and ethical dilemmas in both the patients' families and health care providers during this critical situation.[35]

In the professional literature, there has been a lot of discussion on how to place withdrawal of LVAD support within the legal and ethical perspectives.[20,23] Since LVAD support is not seen as a replacement therapy, withdrawing such a support is described as ethically and legally permissible and is considered different to assisted suicide or euthanasia. Since many LVAD supported patients also have an ICD, it is also appropriate to deactivate those functions (defibrillation, not pacing) as part of end-of-life care to avoid the risk of patients being shocked.[35] There may be a great variability in how patients and families from different cultures perceive the discussion to device withdrawal or other issues related to end of life.[36]

Symptom Management at the End of Life

Patients with HF often experience distressing symptoms that might be caused by HF or by comorbidities, the side effects of drugs or by the psychological and practical consequences of disease progression. They often stay untreated for one of three reasons:[3,18]

1. They are not identified or addressed by the health care team.
2. Patients do not mention them.
3. The symptoms are resistant to conventional treatment.

Symptom control in HF poses specific challenges. For example, palliation of dyspnea underscores the need to maintain patients on optimal active HF medication.[4] Since the majority of patients with end-stage HF have multiple medical conditions, strategies for optimal symptom management need to accommodate both cardiovascular and noncardiovascular conditions.

Treatment options should be discussed openly with patients and their families and their preferences taken into account when reviewing their medication and management.[18]

Some patients will want to continue all treatment that might extend their lives. Others find complex drugs regimens burdensome and want these simplified. Concrete guiding can be obtained from local palliative care guidelines or by consultation with local palliative care specialists.

When to Consider and Discuss Palliative Care

Since palliative care as defined by the WHO[5] is care focusing on symptom relief and spiritual and psychosocial support from diagnosis to the end of life, the palliative care communication and planning should start already when a patient is diagnosed with HF, often the main responsibility of patient care is in the primary care. Being admitted to hospital due to deteriorating HF is an indicator that the prognosis of the patient is poorer.[4] Palliative care then needs to be refocused including more education on monitoring and management of symptoms of deterioration, e.g., daily weighing and symptom control and flexible diuretic intake in case of congestion. Patients and their families often need psychosocial support from health care professionals to handle the physical and psychosocial aspects of the HF syndrome and HF self-

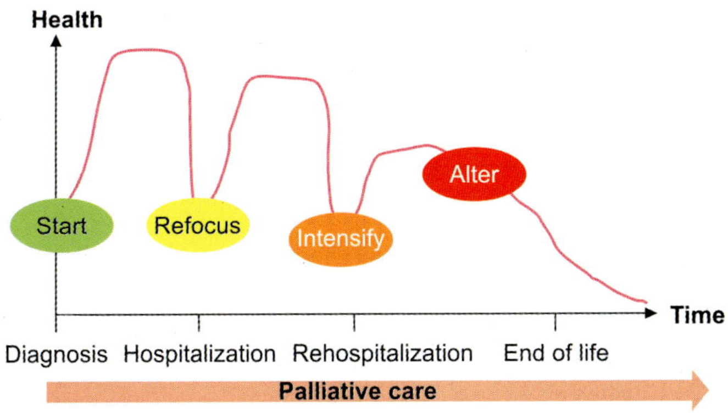

Fig. 2 Palliative care in the heart failure trajectory: room for improvement!

care. Patients suffering from repeated hospitalizations have a very poor prognosis. They often suffer from several handicapping symptoms, have a decreased quality of life and more depressive symptoms. At this stage of medical and device treatment, psychosocial support and educational initiatives need to be intensified. Somewhere after this stage the patients with HF enter the terminal phase. The care then needs to be intensified and home-based care is often the most convenient alternative for the patient and his/her family. However, home-based palliative care services are not always available for patients with HF. Palliative care in the HF trajectory is shown in Figure 2.

Preferences for treatment, deactivation of the ICD, termination of LVAD therapy, resuscitation might change over time during illness trajectory necessitating regular open discussions. Clinicians may be reluctant to discuss advance directives and resuscitation preferences, fearing that these interactions may be distressing for patients. However, as evident in the Surfactant, Positive Pressure, and Oxygenation Randomized Trial (SUPPORT) study, resuscitation preferences are inconstant and therefore discussion on end-of-life issues should be undertaken and frequently revisited.[4,37]

How to Discuss Palliative Care and End-of-life Issues

Good communication about the nature of disease is described as a primary need, identified by HF patients and their caregivers. They described the importance of an open, two-way dialogue about the patient's condition.[22] However, cognitive problems and fatigue might pose barriers to active communication.[38] Health care professionals need to:[18]

- Establish a process of open and interactive discussion with patients and caregivers
- Explain the nature of the condition and agree to a management plan
- Acknowledge and discuss the unpredictability inherent in the natural history of HF, including the possibility of sudden death
- Encourage a positive but realistic approach to treatment and care
- Promote patient and family/caregiver participation in decision making
- Discuss advanced care planning and foster achievable goals of care
- Discuss any personal, social or spiritual issues raised by patients and carers.

Practical key points for communication are presented in Box 2.

Box 2: Key points for communication[39]

- Encourage the patient to bring a caregiver (e.g., family member), if wished
- Ensure sufficient time and privacy, if possible
- Make sure you know the facts
- Make sure that all realize that the discussion is important
- Establish what the patient and caregiver already knows
- Be open and honest
- Maintain hope wherever possible
- Do not make the patient feel "given up"
- It is always possible to offer the patient something: symptom control, psychological support or practical help
- Explain further if the patient and caregiver wishes
- Listen to concerns
- Allow expression of emotion
- Involve the patient and caregiver in decision making
- Avoid premature or unrealistic reassurance
- Summarize the discussion
- Provide opportunity to rediscuss
- Provide a point of contact in case of questions

Who to Involve in Palliative Care and End-of-life Issues

In HF care, a team approach is increasingly advocated. Specifically in end-stage HF, several initiatives are under way to integrate palliative and HF teams; these initiatives include the use of models where HF specialist care have access to palliative care consultancy, where palliative

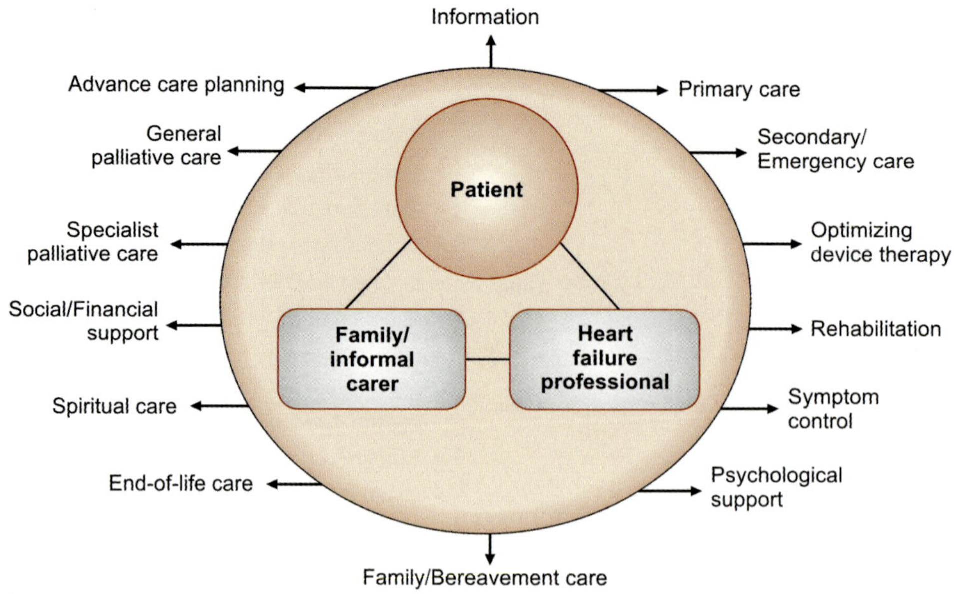

Fig. 3 Patient-centered heart failure care

Source: Adapted from Connolly M, Beattie J, Walker D, Dancy M. End of life care in heart failure. A framework for implementation. Heart Improvement Programme, NHS Improvement 2010, *with permission*

care services assume responsibility for the basic care of the patient and his/her family, or where HF specialists serve as consultants on specific treatment issues.[4,40,41] Members of multiprofessional palliative care teams can include consultants in palliative medicine, clinical nurse specialists, chaplains, social workers, pharmacists and appropriate allied health professionals (Fig. 3). Specialist palliative care teams may be available to advise colleagues in primary and secondary care as well as offering a specialist assessment or direct involvement in patient care, if appropriate. In all care settings, an awareness of when to seek advice or refer can be crucial in ensuring that the palliative care needs of patients and families are met appropriately.[18] Integrating HF and palliative care teams combines unique expertise from both cardiology and palliative care. Although healthcare systems and legal regulations differ from country to country, issues relating to end-of-life care for patients with advanced HF need to be highlighted.

CONCLUSION

Since palliative care focuses on symptom relief and spiritual and psychosocial support from diagnosis to the end of life, the palliative care communication and planning should start already early in the HF trajectory. Multidisciplinary HF management should include discussions around preferences of palliation and end-of-life care and good communication about the nature of the disease is described as a primary need by HF patients and their caregivers. This includes an assessment of understanding and needs, planning for the future, including advance directives, discussing the potential need for device withdrawal and symptom management. In the approach to end-of-life care of patients with HF, both general principles and heart failures' specific issues are important and should be discussed with patients and their caregivers. Discussions and decisions should be clearly documented, regularly reviewed and routinely communicated to all those involved in the patient's care.

REFERENCES

1. Goodlin SJ, Hauptman PJ, Arnold R, et al. Consensus statement: Palliative and supportive care in advanced heart failure. J Card Fail. 2004;10(3):200-9.
2. Allen LA, Stevenson LW, Grady KL, et al. Decision making in advanced heart failure: a scientific statement from the American Heart Association. Circulation. 2012;125(15):1928-52.
3. Metra M, Ponikowsky P, Dickstein K, et al. Advanced chronic heart failure: A position paper from the Study Group on Advanced Heart Failure Association of the European Society of Cardiology. Euro J Heart Fail. 2007;9(6-7):684-94.
4. Jaarsma T, Beattie JM, Ryder M, et al. Palliative care in heart failure: a position statement from the palliative care workshop of the Heart Failure Association of the European Society of Cardiology. Eur J Heart Fail. 2009;11(5):433-43.
5. World Health Organization. (2009). WHO Definition of Palliative Care. [online] Available from www.who.int/cancer/palliative/en/. [Accessed December, 2013].

6. Rolland JS. Chronic illness and the life cycle: a conceptual framework. Family Process. 1987;26(2):203-21.
7. Strömberg A, Jaarsma T. Thoughts about death and perceived health status in elderly patients with heart failure. Eur J Heart Fail. 2008;10(6):608-13.
8. Harding R, Selman L, Beynon T, et al. Meeting the communication and information needs of chronic heart failure patients. J Pain Symptom Manage. 2008;36(2):149-56.
9. Goodlin SJ, Quill TE, Arnold RM. Communication and decision-making about prognosis in heart failure care. J Card Fail. 2008;14(2):106-13.
10. Ong LM, Visser MR, Lammes FB, et al. Doctor-patient communication and cancer patients' quality of life and satisfaction. Patient Educ Couns. 2000;41(2):145-56.
11. Gysels M, Richardson A, Higginson IJ. Communication training for health professionals who care for patients with cancer: a systematic review of effectiveness. Support Care Cancer. 2004;12(10):692-700.
12. Murray SA, Sheikh A. Palliative care beyond cancer: Care for all at the end of life. BMJ. 2008;336(7650):958-9.
13. Horowitz CR, Rein SB, Leventhal H. A story of maladies, misconceptions and mishaps: effective management of heart failure. Soc Sci Med. 2004;58(3):631-43.
14. Willems DL, Hak A, Visser F, et al. Thoughts of patients with advanced heart failure on dying. Palliat Med. 2004;18(6):564-72.
15. Heyland DK, Dodek P, Rocker G, et al. What matters most in end-of-life care: perceptions of seriously ill patients and their family members. CMAJ. 2006;174(5):627-33.
16. Barclay S, Momen N, Case-Upton S, et al. End-of-life care conversations with heart failure patients: a systematic literature review and narrative synthesis. Br J Gen Pract. 2011;61(582):e49-62.
17. Henwood M. Debate of the Age Health and Care Study Group. The future of health and care of older people: the best is yet to come. London, United Kingdom: Age Concern England; 1999.
18. Scottish Partnership for Palliative Care. (2008). Living and dying with advanced heart failure: a palliative care approach. [online] Available from www.palliativecarescotland.org.uk/content/publications/HF-final-document.pdf. [Accessed December, 2013].
19. Brouwers C, Denollet J, de Jonge N, et al. Patient-reported outcomes in left ventricular assist device therapy: a systematic review and recommendations for clinical research and practice. Circ Heart Fail. 2011;4(6):714-23.
20. Brush S, Budge D, Alharethi R, et al. End-of-life decision making and implementation in recipients of a destination left ventricular assist device. J Heart Lung Transplant. 2010;29(12):1337-41.
21. Clark AM, Jaarsma T, Strachan P, et al. Effective communication and ethical consent in decisions related to ICDs. Nat Rev Cardiol. 2011;8(12): 694-705.
22. Low J, Pattenden J, Candy B, et al. Palliative care in advanced heart failure: an international review of the perspectives of recipients and health professionals on care provision. J Card Fail. 2011;17(3):231-52.
23. Mueller PS, Swetz KM, Freeman MR, et al. Ethical analysis of withdrawing ventricular assist device support. Mayo Clin Proc. 2010;85(9):791-7.
24. Goldstein NE, Lampert R, Bradley E, et al. Management of implantable cardioverter defibrillators in end-of-life care. Ann Intern Med. 2004; 141(11):835-8.
25. Goldstein NE, Mehta D, Teitelbaum E, et al. "It's like crossing a bridge" complexities preventing physicians from discussing deactivation of implantable defibrillators at the end of life. J Gen Intern Med. 2008; 23(Suppl 1):2-6.
26. Kramer DB, Kesselheim AS, Brock DW, et al. Ethical and legal views of physicians regarding deactivation of cardiac implantable electrical devices: a quantitative assessment. Heart Rhythm. 2010;7(11):1537-42.
27. Lampert R, Hayes DL, Annas GJ, et al. HRS Expert Consensus Statement on the Management of Cardiovascular Implantable Electronic Devices (CIEDs) in patients nearing end of life or requesting withdrawal of therapy. Heart Rhythm. 2010;7(7):1008-26.
28. Padeletti L, Arnar DO, Boncinelli L, et al. EHRA Expert Consensus Statement on the management of cardiovascular implantable electronic devices in patients nearing end of life or requesting withdrawal of therapy. Europace. 2010;12(10):1480-9.
29. Glanz K, Rimer B, Lewis F. Health Behaviour and Health Education - Theory, Research, and Practice, 4th edition. San Francisco, USA: Jossey-Bass; 2002.
30. Davidson PM. Difficult conversations and chronic heart failure: do you talk the talk or walk the walk? Curr Opin Support Palliat Care. 2007;1(4):274-8.
31. Sherazi S, Daubert JP, Block RC, et al. Physicians' preferences and attitudes about end-of-life care in patients with an implantable cardioverter-defibrillator. Mayo Clin Proc. 2008;83(10):1139-41.
32. Fluur C, Bolse K, Strömberg A, et al. Patients' experiences of the implantable cardioverter defibrillator (ICD); with a focus on battery replacement and end-of-life issues. Heart Lung. 2013;42(3):202-7.
33. Herman D, Stros P, Curila K, et al. Deactivation of implantable cardioverter-defibrillators: results of patient surveys. Europace. 2013;15(7):963-9.
34. MacIver J, Ross HJ. Withdrawal of ventricular assist device support. J Palliat Care. 2005;21(3):151-6.
35. Ben Gal T, Jaarsma T. Self-care and communication issues at the end of life of recipients of a left-ventricular assist device as destination therapy. Curr Opin Support Palliat Care. 2013;7(1):29-35.
36. Swetz KM, Freeman MR, AbouEzzeddine OF, et al. Palliative medicine consultation for preparedness planning in patients receiving left ventricular assist devices as destination therapy. Mayo Clin Proc. 2011;86(6):493-500.
37. Krumholz HM, Phillips RS, Hamel MB, et al. Resuscitation preferences among patients with severe congestive heart failure: results from the SUPPORT project. Study to Understand Prognoses and Preferences for Outcomes and Risks of Treatments. Circulation. 1998;98(7):648-55.
38. Barnes S, Gott M, Payne S, et al. Communication in heart failure: perspectives from older people and primary care professionals. Health Soc Care Community. 2006;14(6):482-90.
39. Lawrie I, Kite S. Communication in heart failure. In: Johnson M, Lehman R, Twycross R (Eds). Heart Failure and Palliative Care: A Team Approach, 1st edition. Oxford, UK: Radcliffe Publishing Limited; 2006.
40. Brännström M, Boman K. A new model for integrated heart failure and palliative advanced home care--rationale and design of a prospective randomized study. Eur J Cardiovasc Nurs. 2013;12(3):269-75.
41. Johnson MJ, Maccallum A, Butler J, et al. Heart failure specialist nurses' use of palliative care services: a comparison of surveys across England in 2005 and 2010. Eur J Cardiovasc Nurs. 2012;11(2):190-6.

Chapter 54

Percutaneous Mechanical Circulatory Support in Cardiogenic Shock

Scott Hopkins, Justin Cox, Keshav R Nayak

ABSTRACT

Percutaneous mechanical circulatory support may be necessary in the setting of severe refractory cardiogenic shock. This chapter gives a brief overview of devices available for rapid placement either at the bedside or in the cardiac catheterization laboratory. The devices described include: the intra-aortic balloon pump, percutaneous extracorporeal membrane oxygenator, the Impella and TandemHeart devices. These devices are used as a temporizing measure while the patient can be either urgently revascularized or undergo surgical implantation of a more durable device, or until recovery of their myocardial function. This chapter reviews the physiologic effects, indications, relevant literature, proper placement and proper use of the devices.

INTRODUCTION

In severe refractory cardiogenic shock, mechanical circulatory support may be necessary in the acute setting to augment cardiac output until the patient can be revascularized, a more durable device can be surgically implanted, or until recovery of myocardial function. This chapter briefly outlines devices and their applications in this setting.

DEVICES

Intra-aortic Balloon Counterpulsation

The intra-aortic balloon counterpulsation (IABP) device was pioneered at Grace Sinai Hospital in Detroit, USA, during the early 1960s by Dr Adrian Kantrowitz and his team. The device was developed for use in heart surgery by Dr David Bregman in 1976 at NewYork-Presbyterian Hospital in New York City. The first clinical implant was performed at Maimonides Medical Center, Brooklyn, New York in October, 1967.[1]

Intra-aortic balloon counterpulsation is an intravascular balloon which is placed in the descending aorta from a percutaneous vascular sheath in the femoral artery. The balloon is deflated during systole just prior to aortic valve opening and inflates during diastole. Diastolic inflation displaces blood volume and causes an increase in diastolic blood pressure and coronary artery perfusion pressure. Deflation of the balloon during systole decreased afterload and myocardial oxygen consumption (Fig. 1).[2]

Indications

- Cardiogenic shock
- Acute myocardial infarction (MI)
- High-risk percutaneous coronary intervention (PCI)
- Mechanical complications of acute MI
    - Acute mitral regurgitation
    - Ventricular septal defect
- Post coronary artery bypass graft
- Refractory angina
- Refractory polymorphic ventricular tachycardia.

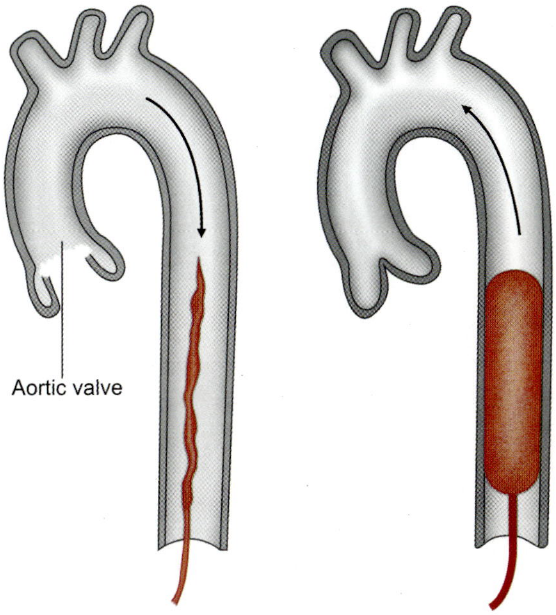

Fig. 1 Intra-aortic balloon pump

Contraindications

- Aortic dissection
- Aortic aneurysm
- Severe peripheral vascular disease
- Limb ischemia
- Coagulopathy (cannot receive heparin)
- > Mild aortic insufficiency
- Prosthetic aortic tree grafts
- Local sepsis
- Not effective in low cardiac index of less than 1.2 L/min/m^2 and tachyarrhythmias.

Effects

Increased: Diastolic blood pressure, cardiac output, myocardial blood flow
Decreased: Systolic blood pressure, pulmonary capillary wedge pressure (PCWP), myocardial oxygen demand.

Evidence and Recommendations

- Class I indication for use in cardiogenic shock complicating an MI or mechanical complications of an MI including acute severe mitral regurgitation and ventricular septal defect
- Class IIa indication for treatment of refractory angina in unstable angina/non-ST elevation myocardial infarction (UA/NSTEMI) despite intensive medical therapy
- Intra-aortic balloon support for myocardial infarction with cardiogenic shock (IABP-SHOCK) II trial (2012) showed no 30-day mortality benefit from IABP insertion for cardiogenic shock following MI when early revascularization was planned[3]
- Sjauw et al. (2009) systematic review found that only low quality observational studies support IABP use post-STEMI for thrombolysis, not for PCI. There was no support from randomized studies[4]
- Treat angina with Aggrastat and determine cost of therapy with an invasive or conservative strategy (TACTICS) trial (2005) was a smaller trial that showed no mortality benefit for IABP in addition to thrombolysis for STEMI, but there was a trend to improved Killip class in patients with severe heart failure/cardiogenic shock[5]
- The randomized IABP study group trial (1994) found that patients randomized to aortic counterpulsation following revascularization for MI had significantly less reocclusion rates of the infarct-related artery during follow-up (median 5 days) compared with control patients (8% vs 21%, $p < 0.03$).[6]

Insertion

- Percutaneous or surgical access into the femoral artery
- 0.03-inch J-guidewire inserted and advanced to the thoracic aorta
- 7–9.5 Fr balloon sheath is inserted
- Balloon is advanced over the guidewire till the proximal tip 1 cm distal to the left subclavian
- Intravenous heparin is started to maintain activated partial thromboplastin time (aPTT) at 50–70 seconds.

Tips

- Balloon can be inserted sheathless in patients with peripheral vascular disease reducing distal ischemia
- Use of a super-stiff wire can facilitate sheath placement in tortuous vessels.

Balloon Triggering and Timing

Triggering:
- Surface ECG—preferred mode triggered on R wave
- Arterial waveform
- Paced rhythm—triggered off pacer spikes
- Asynchronous timing mode—in the arresting patient or failure of other modes.

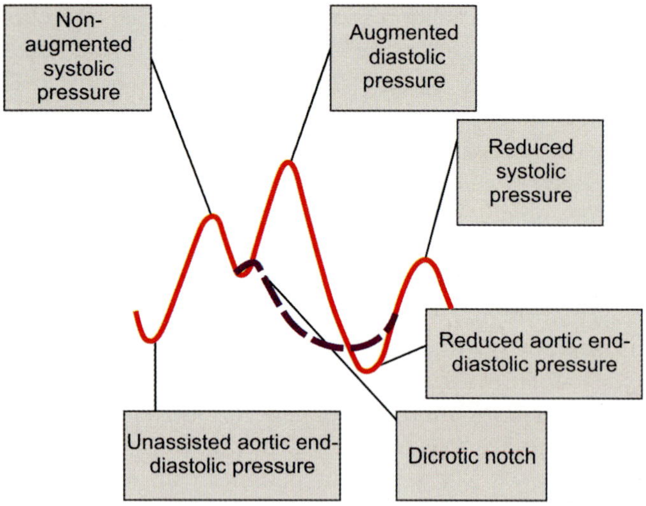

Fig. 2 Proper timing occurs when the balloon inflates on the downslope of the systolic pressure waveform and deflates before the onset of systole. Augmented diastolic pressure should be higher than systolic pressure while end-diastolic pressure is reduced from baseline[7]

Timing: Proper balloon timing has been shown in Figure 2.

Removal

- Change inflation to 1:2 then 1:3 over several hours
- Check aPTT to ensure less than 150 seconds
- Change settings to standby and disconnect gas line
- Pull balloon back until it is in the sheath (resistance felt) then remove sheath and balloon as one unit
- Allow puncture site to bleed back for 1–2 seconds
- Apply manual pressure until hemostasis achieved.

Complications

- Limb ischemia
- Bleeding
- Infection
- Balloon rupture
- Balloon entrapment
- Ischemia of intra-abdominal vessels
- Anemia and thrombocytopenia.

Percutaneous Extracorporeal Membrane Oxygenator

Percutaneous extracorporeal membrane oxygenator (ECMO), also called cardiopulmonary support (CPS) when set up in a venoarterial circuit, is a generic term for devices that provide oxygenation and continuous pumping for biventricular support. It consists of a venous cannula, an arterial cannula, a centrifugal pump and a membrane oxygenator. These devices may be favored for their ease of rapid, bedside placement and recent device miniaturization.[8] The downside of these devices is that they do not necessarily unload the left ventricle, especially at higher flow rates. This can cause an increase in myocardial work and myocardial oxygen demand. Worsening left ventricular (LV) function in this setting may require LV venting (Fig. 3).[9]

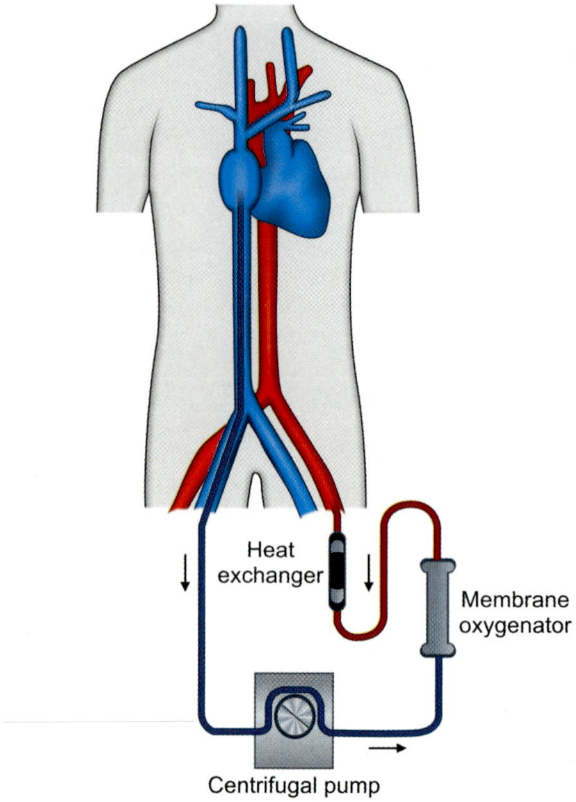

Fig. 3 Percutaneous extracorporeal membrane oxygenator

Indications

- Severe refractory cardiogenic shock
- Acute MI and cardiogenic shock
- Post cardiotomy cardiogenic shock.

Contraindications

- Coagulopathy

Effects

Increased: Mean arterial pressure (MAP), diastolic arterial pressure
Rate dependent: PCWP, LV end-diastolic pressure, myocardial oxygen demand, LV distention.[9]

Evidence and Recommendations

- Class I indication for use in cardiogenic shock complicating an MI
- Class IIb indication for elective insertion as an adjunct to PCI in carefully selected high-risk patients.[10]

Extracorporeal membrane oxygenator has been studied with favorable outcomes in post cardiotomy cardiogenic shock, fulminant myocarditis, as well as acute MI with severe cardiogenic shock. The latter study, a nonrandomized prospective study showed improved 30-day mortality in patients with profound cardiogenic shock after acute MI with the use of ECMO.[11-13]

It should be noted that insertion, monitoring, and removal are device specific.

Complications

- Thrombosis
- Bleeding
- Infection
- Access site complications
- Worsening LV function.

TandemHeart®

The TandemHeart® (CardiacAssist, Inc, Pittsburgh, PA) is a percutaneous ventricular assist device that can be quickly inserted in the catheterization laboratory. It uses a left atrial outflow cannula allowing for LV decompression. The device consists of a trans-septal cannula, femoral artery cannula, a centrifugal pump and a controller mechanism. The continuous pump allows up to 4 L/minute of augmented cardiac output (Fig. 4).[8]

Indications

- Severe refractory cardiogenic shock
- Acute MI and cardiogenic shock
- High risk PCI.

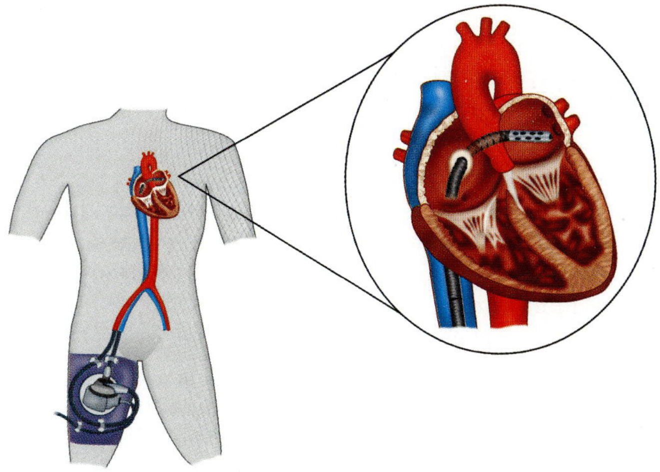

Fig. 4 TandemHeart® system and pump

Contraindications

- Biventricular failure
- Significant pulmonary dysfunction
- Coagulopathy.

Effects

Increased: Cardiac output, MAP, diastolic arterial pressure
Decreased: LV end-diastolic pressure, ejection fraction, PCWP, myocardial work and oxygen demand
Unaffected: Contractility.[9]

Evidence and Recommendations

- Class I indication for use in cardiogenic shock complicating an MI
- Class IIb indication for elective insertion as an adjunct to PCI in carefully selected high-risk patients.[10]

A retrospective study of 117 patients with severe refractory cardiogenic shock showed marked improvements in hemodynamics. The 30-day- and 6-month mortality rates were 40.2% and 45.3% respectively.[14]

Randomized trials comparing TandemHeart® to IABP in cardiogenic shock and with cardiogenic shock post MI both showed better hemodynamics and no difference in 30-day mortality. The latter study, however, had higher complication rates.[15,16]

Insertion

Requires insertion in a cardiac catheterization laboratory:
- Femoral vein access for trans-septal puncture
- After trans-septal puncture, heparin is started for activated clotting time (ACT) more than 300 seconds
- Over a stiff wire, the trans-septal sheath is exchanged for the TandemHeart® 14 Fr/21 Fr two-stage dilator
- The dilator is then exchanged for the 21 Fr trans-septal cannula into the left atrium
- The external end of the cannula is then sutured to the thigh
- Access of the femoral artery is then performed and a 17 Fr arterial cannula is placed in the femoral artery with the distal end advanced to above the aortic bifurcation
- The arterial cannula is then sutured to the thigh
- Once cannulae are in place, the pump, cannulae are de-aired and connected. The pump is then connected to the TandemHeart® controller.[17]

Monitoring

- Intensive care unit level monitoring including pulmonary artery catheter for cardiac output monitoring
- ACT: 180–220 seconds.[17]

Removal

- Wean flow rate by 50% for 1 hour (may be slower or faster). Do not reduce to less than 1 L/minute
- Turn off device if patient tolerates the wean
- Clamp outflow then the inflow cannulae
- Stop heparin
- Withdraw trans-septal cannula out of the left atrium
- Wait for acceptable ACT
- Remove both cannulae from the body
- Achieve hemostasis.[17]

Complications

- Thrombosis
- Limb ischemia
- Access site complications
- Tamponade
- Cannulae kinking
- Cannulae movement.

Impella®

Impella® is a form of axial flow pump which works on the principle of an Archimedes screw. The device is placed retrograde across the aortic valve into the left ventricle. A high-speed pump draws blood out of the left ventricle and ejects it into the ascending aorta. The Impella® 2.5 was approved by the Food and Drug Administration in 2008 (Fig. 5).

There are currently four devices available:
1. Impella® 2.5
2. Impella® CP
3. Impella® 5.0
4. Impella® LD.

Indications

- Cardiogenic shock
- Acute MI
- Off pump coronary artery bypass graft
- Support during high risk PCI
- Post PCI.

Contraindications

- Mechanical aortic valves
- Moderate to severe aortic stenosis or regurgitation
- Severe peripheral artery disease.

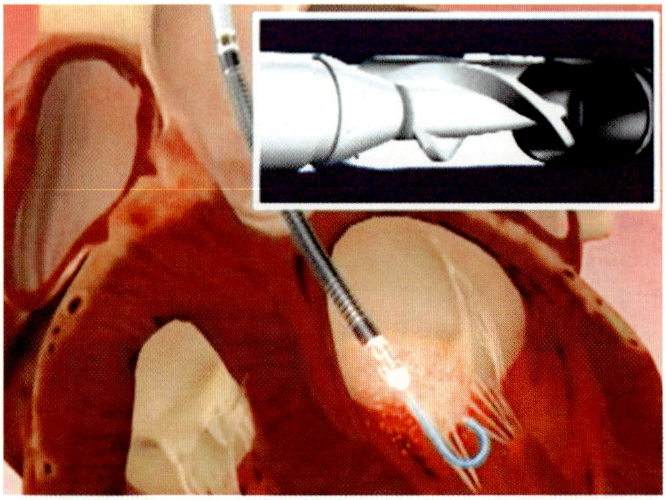

Fig. 5 Impella® showing a tiny screw-shaped propeller

Effects[18]

Increased: Cardiac output, myocardial blood flow, MAP
Decreased: PCWP, myocardial oxygen demand.

Evidence and Recommendations

- Class I indication for use in cardiogenic shock complicating an MI
- Class IIb indication for elective insertion as an adjunct to PCI in carefully selected high-risk patients.[10]

The Impella® LP2.5 versus IABP in cardiogenic shock (ISAR-Shock) trial (2008) randomized 25 patients with cardiogenic shock complicating an acute MI to IABP versus Impella® 2.5. The confidence interval (CI) after 30 minutes of support was significantly increased in patients with the Impella® LP2.5 compared with patients with IABP (Impella®: CI = 0.49 ± 0.46 L/minute/m^2; IABP: CI = 0.11 ± 0.31 L/minute/m^2; p = 0.02). Overall 30-day mortality was 46% in both groups (Fig. 6).[19]

The Prospective, Multicenter Randomized Controlled (PROTECT) II trial (2012) was designed to compare outcomes in over 600 symptomatic patients with complex three vessel or unprotected left main coronary artery disease and severely depressed LV function (LV ejection fraction ≤35%) who were to be randomly assigned to an Impella® (version 2.5) or an intra-aortic balloon pump. The trial was stopped for futility at 69% of planned enrollment. There was no significant difference in the primary end point of major adverse events at 30 days (35.1% vs 40.1% respectively) with a non-significant trend toward improvement at 90 days (Fig. 7).[20]

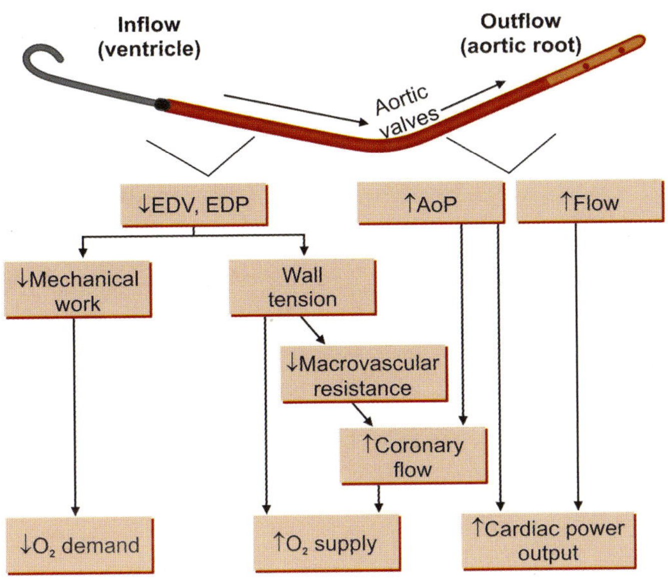

EDV, end-diastolic volume; EDP, end-diastolic pressure; AoP, aortic pressure

Fig. 6 Schematic of hemodynamic design principles of Impella®

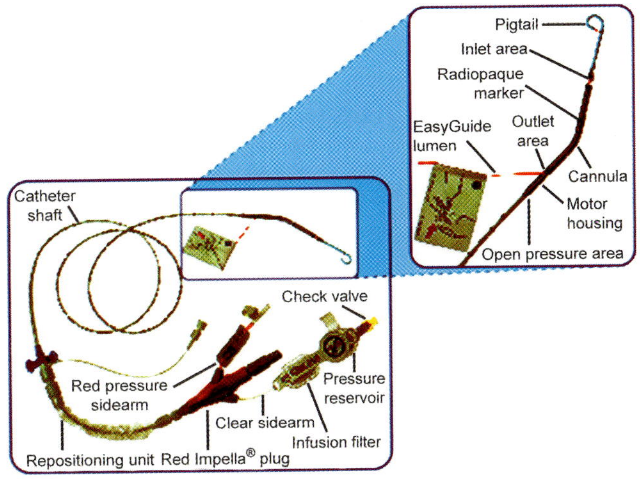

Fig. 7 Impella® 2.5 catheter

Insertion

Insertion technique varies significantly depending on the device chosen. For example, the Impella® 2.5 device can be inserted through a sheath, the Impella® 5.0 via femoral cut down, and the Impella® LD by direct insertion into the aorta. Please see ABIOMED specific instructions for each device.

Impella® 2.5

- Give heparin to maintain an ACT more than 250 seconds
- A 13-F peel away sheath is positioned in the femoral artery
- A 6-F coronary guiding catheter (JR-4, multipurpose, AL1) is placed in the left ventricle over a 0.035-inch guidewire
- A 0.018-inch guidewire is placed across the aortic valve into the left ventricle. Once the guidewire is across the aortic valve, the guiding catheter is removed
- The Impella® catheter is threaded onto the wire. With the device positioned in the ventricle, the wire is removed, and the performance level on the Impella® console is started at its minimum setting (just enough to counteract physiologic forces and stabilize the device position)

- Once positioned across the aortic valve, the console can be used to confirm that the device placement is proper and stable. At this point, the device performance is typically adjusted to a higher level.

Weaning and Removal

- Initiate weaning by decreasing catheter performance level in two-level steps over time as cardiac function allows (for example, P6 to P4 to P2). Do not decrease performance level to below P2 until just before removing the catheter from the ventricle
- When the performance level has been reduced to P2, maintain the patient on P2 support until the patient's hemodynamics remain stable before discontinuing circulatory support
- When the patient's hemodynamics remain stable, decrease the performance level to P1, pull the catheter into the aorta (approximately 30–40 cm), and stop the motor by decreasing the performance level to P0
- Remove the Impella® 2.5 catheter and insert an obturator into the sheath
- Disconnect the connector cable from the Impella® console
- Wait until ACT drops below 150 seconds
- When ACT is below 150 seconds, remove the introducer and apply manual compression for 40 minutes or per hospital protocol.

REFERENCES

1. Oberwalder P. Intra-aortic balloon pump (IABP) counterpulsation; theory and clinical applications. The Internet Journal of Thoracic and Cardiovascular Surgery. 1999;2(2).
2. Jaski BE. Basics of heart failure: a problem solving approach. Berlin: Kluwer Academic Pub;2000.
3. Thiele H, Zeymer U, Neumann F-J, et al. Intraaortic balloon support for myocardial infarction with cardiogenic shock. N Engl J Med. 2012;367(14): 1287-96.
4. Sjauw KD, Engström AE, Vis MM, et al. A systematic review and meta-analysis of intra-aortic balloon pump therapy in ST-elevation myocardial infarction: should we change the guidelines? European Heart Journal. 2009;30(4):459-68.
5. Ohman EM, Nanas J, Stomel RJ, et al. Thrombolysis and counterpulsation to improve survival in myocardial infarction complicated by hypotension and suspected cardiogenic shock or heart failure: results of the TACTICS trial. J Thromb Thrombolysis. 2005;19(1):33-9.
6. Ohman EM, George BS, White CJ, et al. Use of aortic counterpulsation to improve sustained coronary artery patency during acute myocardial infarction. Results of a randomized trial. The Randomized IABP Study Group. Circulation. 1994;90(2):792-9.
7. Griffin BP. Manual of Cardiovascular Medicine. Lippincott Williams & Wilkins; 2012.
8. Basra S, Loyalka P, Gregoric I, et al. Percutaneous assist devices for left ventricular shock. Interventional Cardiology Clinics. 2013;2(3):457-68.
9. Burkhoff D. Hemodynamic support science and evaluation of the assisted circulation with percutaneous assist devices. Intervent Cardiol Clin. 2013;2:407-16.
10. Levine G, Bates E, Blankenship J, et al. 2011 ACCF/AHA/SCAI guideline for percutaneous coronary intervention: a report of the American College of Cardiology Foundation/American Heart Association task force on practice guidelines and the Society for Cardiovascular Angiography and Intervention. Circulation. 2011;124(23):e574-651.
11. Asaumi Y, Yasuda S, Morii I, et al. Favourable clinical outcome in patients with cardiogenic shock due to fulminant myocarditis supported by percutatneous extracorporeal membrane oxygenation. Eur Heart J. 2005;26(20):2185-92.
12. Doll N, Kiaii B, Borger M, et al. Five-year results of 219 consecutive patients treated with extracorporeal membrane oxygenation for refractory postoperative cardiogenic shock. Ann Thorac Surg. 2004;77(1):151-7.
13. Sheu J, Tsai T, Lee F, et al. Early extracorporeal membrane oxygenator-assisted primary percutaneous coronary intervention improved 30-day clinical outcomes in patients with ST-segment elevation myocardial infarction complicated with profound cardiogenic shock. Crit Care Med. 2010;38(9):1810-7.
14. Kar B, Gregorie I, Basra S, et al. The percutaneous ventricular assist device in severe refractory cardiogenic shock. Journal of the American College of Cardiology. 2011;57(6):688-96.
15. Thiele H, Sick P, Boudriot E, et al. Randomized comparison of intra-aortic balloon support with a percutaneous left ventricular assist device in patients with revascularized acute myocardial infarction complicated by cardiogenic shock. Eur Heart J. 2005;26(13):1276-83.
16. Burkhoff D, Cohen H, Brunckhorst C, et al. A randomized multicenter clinical study to evaluate the safety and efficacy of the TandemHeart percutaneous ventricular assist device versus conventional therapy with intraaortic balloon pumping for treatment of cardiogenic shock. Am Heart J. 2006;152(3):469.e1-8.
17. Svitek R. The TandemHeart System: Device Description and Clinical Results. Mechanical Circulatory Support. McGraw-Hill Professional; 2011. pp. 154-9.
18. Weber DM, Raess DH, José PS, et al. Principles of Impella Cardiac Support. Principles of Hemodynamics. 2009;3-16.
19. Seyfarth M, Sibbing D, Bauer I, et al. A randomized clinical trial to evaluate the safety and efficacy of a percutaneous left ventricular assist device versus intra-aortic balloon pumping for treatment of cardiogenic shock caused by myocardial infarction. Journal of the American College of Cardiology. 2008;52(19):1584-8.
20. O'Neill WW, Kleiman NS, Moses J, et al. A prospective, randomized clinical trial of hemodynamic support with Impella 2.5 versus intra-aortic balloon pump in patients undergoing high-risk percutaneous coronary intervention: the PROTECT II study. Circulation. 2012;126(14):1717-27.

6

SECTION

Cardiomyopathies
Practical Recommendations to Diagnosis and Management

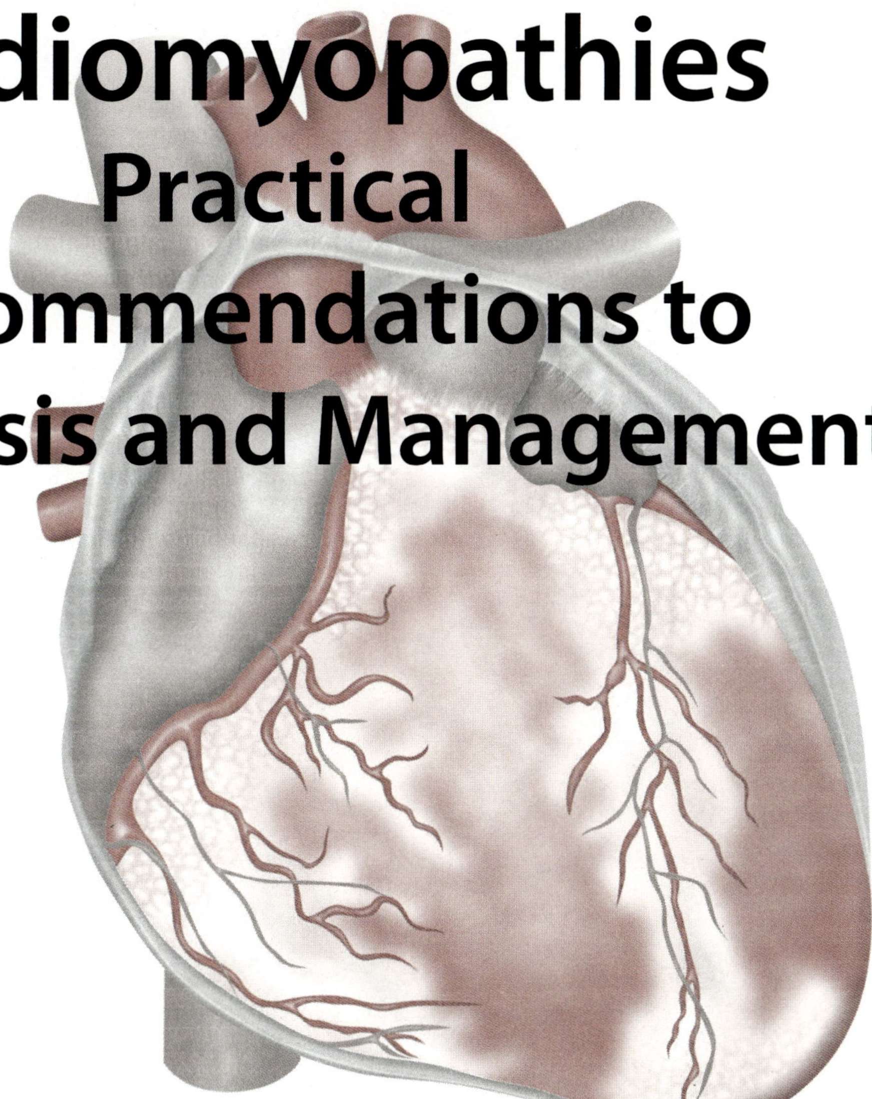

Chapter 55

New Onset Cardiomyopathy: Biopsy or MRI and Other Imaging Modalities

Khwaja S Alim, Matt M Kawahara

ABSTRACT

Cardiomyopathy is a disease of the heart causing cardiac muscle dysfunction. The main types of cardiomyopathies include dilated cardiomyopathy (DCM), hypertrophic cardiomyopathy (HCM), restrictive cardiomyopathy (RCM), and arrhythmogenic right-ventricular cardiomyopathy (ARVC). Ischemic cardiomyopathy is a major subtype of DCM.

The pathophysiology of each of these types of cardiomyopathies can be unique, and hence identification of the morphology, pathophysiology, and diagnosis of cardiomyopathies continues to be a challenge. For now, cardiac biopsy remains the gold standard for diagnosing different types of cardiomyopathies. Cardiac magnetic resonance (CMR) imaging is another very commonly used diagnostic tool which can differentiate different types of cardiomyopathies with great accuracy. This is a noninvasive test, hence offers a major advantage over the cardiac biopsy. Different types of infiltrative cardiomyopathies have distinct CMR images, e.g., cardiac amyloidosis causes qualitative global and subendocardial gadolinium enhancement of the myocardium. The subendocardial longitudinal relaxation time (T1) is shorter in amyloid patients when compared with the control group, and it indicates the increased myocardial amyloid load which causes increased left ventricular (LV) mass, wall thickness, interatrial septal thickness, and decline in diastolic function.

For a long time cardiac biopsy was the only definitive method of diagnosing different types of cardiomyopathies. Cardiac biopsy is an invasive procedure, and even in best of the hands, it is not risk free. Repeated cardiac biopsies can lead to scarring and fibrosis of the myocardium. CMR imaging is a noninvasive alternative to the cardiac biopsy.

INTRODUCTION

Cardiomyopathy is a disease of the heart causing cardiac muscle dysfunction. Degradation of myocardial performance, in regard to cardiomyopathies, occurs due to functional abnormalities of the heart; these abnormalities can be caused by mechanical or electrical dysfunction of the heart muscle which could lead to arrhythmias and heart failure.[1]

The main subtypes of cardiomyopathies include dilated cardiomyopathy (DCM), hypertrophic cardiomyopathy (HCM), restrictive cardiomyopathy (RCM) and arrhythmogenic right ventricular cardiomyopathy (ARVC). DCMs are characterized by increased left ventricle size. Additionally, increased left ventricular (LV) mass and normal or decreased LV wall thickness can be observed.[2] Ischemic cardiomyopathy is a major subtype of DCM. Unique to HCM is most often a thickening of the LV wall and a decrease in LV cavity size.[2,3] RCM is characterized by diastolic dysfunction of either or both ventricles and atrial dilation due to restrictive ventricular physiology.[2,3] ARVC is characterized by the replacement of cardiac myocytes by fibrofatty tissue.[3]

The pathophysiology of each of these types of cardiomyopathies can be unique and part of a generalized system of disorders. Thus, identification of the morphology, pathophysiology and diagnosis of cardiomyopathies continues to be a challenge in research and clinical settings. Identifying the type of cardiomyopathy is crucial for prognostication and the determination of treatment options. A commonly used diagnostic tool used to identify cardiac muscle dysfunction is cardiac magnetic resonance imaging (CMRI). CMRI offers a noninvasive method of observing myocardial tissues for morphological abnormalities.[4] Another method used to study or reveal potential cardiomyopathy is via endomyocardial biopsy (EMB). EMB is used to examine myocardial tissue physiology at a cellular level.[4]

Cardiac MRI and EMB each have unique advantages and disadvantages. The main issue is to discuss the utility of both techniques in the diagnosis of cardiomyopathy.

CARDIOMYOPATHY (TABLE 1)

Ischemic Cardiomyopathy

Ischemic cardiomyopathy is caused by a block in the coronary arterial circulation, which leads to myocardial infarction (MI). This is one of the most common causes of DCM.

Fortunately, with the advances made in the diagnostic modalities available at our disposal, early detection and optimal medical treatment can prevent this devastating condition in many patients.

Diagnostic Work Up

The fundamental approach to evaluate ischemic cardiomyopathy is the same as diagnosing any other medical condition which includes a detailed medical history, signs and symptoms, and family history.

Basic evaluation includes electrocardiogram (ECG) and two-dimensional echocardiogram (2D-ECHO), which can show wall motion abnormalities, reduced left ventricular ejection fraction (LVEF) as well as increase in the chamber size, more specifically increased left ventricular end-systolic volume (LVESV).

Other cardiac evaluations include stress tests like dobutamine stress ECHO and more invasive tests like cardiac angiogram. Newer approaches include nuclear studies like positron emission tomography (PET) scan single-photon emission computed tomography (SPECT) and CMRI. Cardiac biopsy is seldom used to diagnose ischemic cardiomyopathy.

After an ischemic event occurs, the ultimate goal is to limit the damage and to salvage the viable tissue. During a dobutamine stress ECHO, when a low dose of dobutamine is given and there is an improvement in the contractile function, followed by a deterioration of wall motion at a higher dose; it is called a biphasic response. This is the most specific sign of viability of the myocardium by dobutamine stress test.[5]

Cardiac MRI can also be used to determine the end-diastolic wall thickness; less than 5 mm thickness likely represents a nonviable transmural scar.[6,7] Additionally, the myocardial scar can be further analyzed by using delayed gadolinium contrast enhancing CMR. This technique requires delayed cardiac imaging at 5 minutes after the intravenous gadolinium contrast is administered. On delayed T1-weighted images, the scar has delayed uptake and delayed washout, hence has increased intensity. If the hyperenhanced area has less than 50% wall thickness, this is considered to be a viable tissue.[8] CMR has a superior spatial resolution; whereas 2D-ECHO has a superior temporal resolution.[9]

Nuclear studies include SPECT and PET scan. Both of these modalities have many protocols. SPECT and

TABLE 1: Classification of cardiomyopathies

Dilated cardiomyopathy (DCM)	*Hypertrophic cardiomyopathy (HCM)*	*Restrictive cardiomyopathy (RCM)*	*Arrhythmogenic right-ventricular cardiomyopathy (AVRC)*
• Ischemic • Alcoholic • Congestive • Diabetic • Familial dilated • Idiopathic • Peripartum • Primary	• Asymmetric septal • Familial hypertrophic • Hypertrophic nonobstructive • Hypertrophic obstructive • Idiopathic hypertrophic subaortic stenosis	• Idiopathic restrictive • Infiltrative	

Source: National Institutes of Health: National Heart, Lung, and Blood Institute (2013). Types of cardiomyopathy. [online] Available from www.nhlbi.nih.gov/health/health-topics/topics/cm/types.html. [Accessed December 2013].

PET perfusion tracers rely on both myocardial perfusion and cellular membrane integrity for the myocardial uptake and retention, but the assessment of myocardial glucose metabolism with PET contributes to its very high sensitivity for predicting regional contractile recovery after revascularization.[10]

Cardiac catheterization is a very commonly used minimally invasive procedure, which can be both diagnostic as well as therapeutic. Right-sided cardiac catheterization is commonly used to measure the intracardiac pressures. This information can be very important in diagnosing carcinogenic shock and then dynamically monitoring the response to therapy.

Left-sided cardiac catheterization is used to determine the coronary anatomy as well as to perform the ventriculogram which shows the global function of the left ventricle. Cardiac biopsy is very rarely performed in the setting of ischemic cardiomyopathy.

Nonischemic Cardiomyopathies

These cardiomyopathies are usually inherited conditions which are classified based on ventricular morphology and abnormal function. They are usually inherited as autosomal dominant conditions. They include HCM, DCM, ARVC, left ventricular noncompaction (LVNC) and RCM.[11]

Hypertrophic Cardiomyopathy

Hypertrophic cardiomyopathy is the most common inherited heart condition with an estimated prevalence of 1 in 500 in general population[12,13] and a leading cause of sudden cardiac death in young adults and competitive athletes in the United States.[14] HCM is primarily inherited in an autosomal dominant pattern, although reduced penetrance and clinical variability are not uncommon. Patients can remain completely asymptomatic, or present with an advanced heart failure followed by sudden cardiac death. HCM is usually diagnosed by using cardiac imaging techniques such as 2D-ECHO and CMRI. It usually presents as asymmetrical septal hypertrophy.[15]

Dilated Cardiomyopathy

Dilated cardiomyopathy is characterized by LV dilatation and LVEF less than 50% which can be seen on conventional 2D-ECHO. DCM can develop as a result of environmental exposures, including myocarditis and alcohol abuse or secondary to ischemic cardiomyopathy as mentioned above. Idiopathic DCM (IDCM) is a diagnosis of exclusion when other causes have been ruled out. In almost 50% of these patients, genetic etiology plays a role, with a high degree of locus heterogeneity; hence family history becomes very important.[16] It is most commonly inherited in an autosomal dominant pattern, although X-linked and autosomal recessive inheritances have also been described.

Idiopathic DCM is the most common indication for cardiac transplantation in the United States.[16] Most patients are diagnosed between 20 years and 50 years of age, although in some patients the symptoms can develop even in childhood.[17]

The pathophysiology causing IDCM includes high degree of locus heterogeneity, which affects the sarcomere, Z-disk, nuclear lamina proteins, intermediate filaments and the dystrophin-associated glycoprotein complex.[18] In contrast, HCM mainly affects the sarcomere. The histopathologic features of IDCM typically show myocyte hypertrophy and increased fibrosis.[19] In contrast to HCM, the myocite disarray is absent in IDCM, but ventricular remodeling and contractile dysfunction is typically progressive. This uncontrolled ventricular remodeling ultimately leads to arrhythmias, fatal end-stage heart failure and cardioembolic events (e.g., stroke). Hence, even patients with asymptomatic systolic dysfunction should be empirically started on appropriate cardioprotective medical therapy.[20]

Arrhythmogenic Right Ventricular Cardiomyopathy

Arrhythmogenic RV cardiomyopathy is a condition in which there is myocyte loss and fibrofatty infiltration of the myocardium which leads to an increased susceptibility to arrhythmias and sudden cardiac death. It accounts for a significant portion of sudden deaths in athletes and young adults.[21] It can affect both the ventricles,[22] although predominantly this is the disease of the right ventricle. ARVC is typically inherited in an autosomal dominant pattern with reduced penetrance. It affects men more frequently than women.[23] ARVC affects the desmosome, a multiprotein complex of proteins that are essential for cell-to-cell junctions, and links intermediate filaments of adjacent cells, as a result establishing a functional intercellular network. Desmosomes are especially prevalent in tissues like heart muscles and skin which are exposed to mechanical stress.

In these patients, 2D-ECHO shows dilatation of the right ventricle with reduced function with or without impairment of the left ventricle, regional right ventricular hypokinesis and localized RV aneurysms.

Cardiac MRI findings include fibrofatty infiltration, dilation and thinning of the right ventricle, regional RV hypokinesis, reduced RV function, trabecular disarray and RV aneurysms. But these CMR criteria have not yet been established to diagnose ARVC.

Left Ventricular Noncompaction

Left ventricular noncompaction is characterized by a heavily trabeculated or spongy appearance of the LV myocardium which is usually first seen on a routine 2D-ECHO. The left ventricle is typically affected, but in 50% of these patients the right ventricle may also be involved.[24,25] It is an X-linked condition characterized by early onset of cardiomyopathy (usually dilated). These patients may also develop other conditions like neutropenia, muscle weakness and growth retardation. These individuals may remain completely asymptomatic or may progressively develop poor cardiac function, ventricular hypertrophy and increased risk of thromboembolic events.[26]

Restrictive Cardiomyopathy

Restrictive cardiomyopathy is characterized by increased stiffness of the ventricular chambers, although ventricular wall thickness and systolic function is generally within normal limits. Most of these patients develop rapidly progressive fatal heart failure if they do not receive early aggressive treatment.[27] Idiopathic RCM is a rare condition, and develops due to variants in sarcomere protein genes.

Infiltrative cardiomyopathies: Infiltrative cardiomyopathies can cause wide spectrum of inherited and acquired conditions with varying clinical features, and most of these conditions fall under the subgroup of RCM.

AMYLOIDOSIS

Amyloidosis is a clinical disorder caused by extracellular deposition of insoluble abnormal fibrils which are derived from aggregation of normally soluble but misfolded protein.[28-30]

Systemic amyloidosis affects the viscera, blood vessel walls and connective tissues. It is usually a fatal condition. Amyloidosis can be further divided into systemic serum amyloid A protein (SAA) amyloidosis, previously known as secondary amyloidosis, systemic amyloid light-chain (SAL) amyloidosis formerly known as primary amyloidosis and the transthyretin-related cardiomyopathy which develops in senile systemic amyloidosis (SSA).

The SAA amyloidosis rarely affects the heart. SAL, on the other hand, is the most commonly diagnosed form of amyloidosis in the developed countries. The heart is affected in 90% of the SAL patients. SAL amyloidosis is associated with only slightly increased cardiac wall thickness, but has the highest frequency of hemodynamic derangement and low QRS voltage as seen on the ECG. Its clinical course is aggressive, with 50% of these patients progressively developing diastolic heart failure with right-sided heart failure and fatal arrhythmias.[29,30]

The SSA is associated with increased LV wall thickness but less frequent hemodynamic changes. Its clinical course is also less aggressive than the SAL amyloidosis, although the patients typically have more advanced age and greater morphological abnormalities. The aggressive nature of SAL amyloidosis is attributed to the direct toxic effects of the circulating free light chains that affect the myocardium whereas the SSA typically causes infiltrative cardiomyopathy which is less aggressive.

Echocardiography

Echocardiography can show several features that are suggestive of cardiac amyloidosis. The most common echocardiography feature is increased thickness of the LV wall, usually in the absence of hypertension. This is an infiltrative process and it is incorrectly referred to as "hypertrophy". It has very poor specificity since it occurs in other conditions like HCM, hypertensive heart disease and other infiltrative cardiac diseases. But the absence of high ECG voltage in the presence of increased LV mass is more specific for infiltrative process and amyloidisis is the most common condition with high sensitivity (72–79%) and specificity (91–100%).[31] When using the standard echocardiography (without tissue harmonics), granular or "sparkling" appearance has been reported in several studies. This can occur in other causes of left ventricular hypertrophy (LVH) and, although high specificity rates are quoted (71–81%), sensitivity tends to be low, with this pattern seen in 26–36% of cardiac amyloid cases.

Diastolic dysfunction typically develops in the early stages of the disease. LVEF does not get affected till later stages.

The progression of the disease not only correlates with severity of symptoms, but also parallels the decline in the diastolic function, with atrial enlargement and restrictive filling pattern (deceleration time < 150 ms) which is associated with 50% mortality at 1 year. Speckle tracking can show changes in the strain and strain rate which are more sensitive in detecting subtle changes in longitudinal contractions even in the early stages of the cardiac amyloidosis.[32] In the later stages, LVEF declines, RV dilatation as well as small to moderate size pericardial effusion may develop.

Cardiac Magnetic Resonance Imaging

Cardiac MRI using late gadolinium enhancement (LGE) has high spatial resolution and reproducibility, and hence can be used to diagnose various forms of cardiomyopathies.[33] Cardiac amyloidosis causes qualitative global and subendocardial gadolinium enhancement of the myocardium. The subendocardial longitudinal relaxation time (T1) is shorter in amyloid patients when compared with the control group and it indicates the increased myocardial amyloid load, which causes increase in LV mass, wall thickness, interatrial septal thickness and decline in diastolic function.

Cardiac MRI can also be used as a prognostic marker of the disease progression. In a study at a threshold value of 23 ms, the 2 minutes post-gadolinium intra-myocardial T1 difference between the subepicardium and subendocardium predicted mortality with 85% accuracy. The intramyocardial T1 gradient is a measure of the amount of amyloid deposit in the myocardium. The amount of subepicardial involvement is inversely proportional to the T1 and the intramyocardial T1 gradient is a better predictor of overall survival and diastolic dysfunction.[34]

Radiolabeled Serum Amyloid P Component Scintigraphy

Serum amyloid P (SAP) is a highly conserved, invariant plasma glycoprotein which belongs to the pentraxin family. SAP becomes specifically and highly concentrated in amyloid deposits of all types because of its calcium-dependent high affinity for all types of amyloid fibril.

Radiolabeled SAP can be used for the diagnosis, distribution and extent of amyloid deposits throughout the body. Serial scans can be used to monitor the progress and response to therapy. But unfortunately at this time this noninvasive technique is unable to image amyloid in the moving heart.

SARCOIDOSIS

Sarcoidosis is a systemic disorder of unknown etiology, which causes granulomatous infiltration of various organs, including the heart. The cardiac sarcoidosis is diagnosed in accordance to the Japanese Ministry of Health and Welfare (JMHW) guidelines which includes the use of ECG, CMR and histopathology.[35]

Echocardiography

Sarcoidosis of the heart produces nonspecific echocardiography abnormalities including the regional wall thinning and aneurysms, systolic and diastolic dysfunction, pulmonary hypertension and pericardial effusions.

Nuclear Imaging

In cardiac sarcoidosis, thallium-201 scintigraphy has a distinctive pattern of reverse redistribution in which a resting perfusion defect improves with stress imaging which is opposite to what happens in ischemic cardiomyopathy. However, in absence of cardiac symptoms these findings are nonspecific, hence are of limited value as a screening test.

Gallium-67 scintigraphy can also be used to diagnose cardiac sarcoidosis because it accumulates in the presence of active inflammation. Thus, the absence of uptake does not exclude cardiac sarcoidosis but it suggests lack of active disease. This can be used to predict response to corticosteroid therapy.[36]

Another technique called ^{18}F-fluoro-2-deoxyglucose PET (FDG-PET) shows a specificity of 90% and sensitivity of 85%[37] in diagnosis of cardiac sarcoidosis.

Cardiac Magnetic Resonance Imaging

In 73% of patients diagnosed with cardiac sarcoidosis, CMRI with LGE showed patchy involvement of the epicardium of the basal and lateral segments. In about half of these patients scintigraphy was normal, while patchy LGE was present, underlining the differences in spatial resolution. In other studies, subendocardial or transmural hyperenhancement has been also observed, which can also be seen in ischemic cardiomyopathy. Along with the changes seen on LEG, by using the functional and anatomical CMRI sequences, one can detect characteristic features of the cardiac sarcoidisis namely the septal thinning, LV/RV dilatation and systolic dysfunction and pericardial effusion. T2-weighted sequences can be used to identify the myocardial edema.[38] Other noncardiac features such as perihilar lymphadenopathy and pulmonary fibrosis can be seen on CMRI, which can further help to make the diagnosis.

ANDERSON–FABRY DISEASE

Fabry disease is an X-linked condition which has systemic and cardiac manifestations. It develops due to an enzyme deficiency of α-galactosidase, which results in the accumulation of glycosphingolipids in the lysosomes of various cells and organs. Heart is frequently involved and results in myocyte hypertrophy, vacuolation and regional fibrosis.[39-41]

Currently, the diagnostic criteria are based on genetic mapping, biochemical testing and EMB.

Myocardial imaging techniques are being explored as noninvasive ways of early screening and diagnosing these patients. Unlike many other forms of infiltrative cardiomyopathies, this condition is potentially reversible with treatment by enzyme replacement therapy,[42] and hence correct diagnosis is of utmost importance.

Echocardiography

The characteristic 2D-ECHO finding in Fabry disease is concentric LVH with preserved systolic function and without cavity dilatation. The main functional abnormality is diastolic dysfunction. The cardiac valves rarely develop dysfunctions, although they may be thickened. Aortic root dilatation quite often develops, and needs to be frequently monitored.

Tissue Doppler imaging can be used which shows reduction in both relaxation and contraction velocities. These changes develop even before the onset of LVH and other morphological changes.[43] Strain and strain rate imaging measures the regional myocardial function and contractility respectively and these are also reduced early in the disease process. With appropriate treatment these abnormalities can be reversed as the cardiac function improves.[42] Strain imaging has the advantage over tissue Doppler velocity in that it can detect regional heterogeneity in myocardial function. These changes are most pronounced in the inferolateral wall.

Cardiac Magnetic Resonance Imaging

Cardiac MRI with LGE technique has a unique distribution involving the basal inferolateral wall, sparing the endocardium. This pattern of distribution is seen in 50% of affected patients and it represents the area of myocardial fibrosis.[44] When enzyme replacement therapy is given, CMRI with LGE can be used to monitor the response to the therapy and patients without myocardial fibrosis have a significant reduction in LV mass, improvement in myocardial function and higher exercise capacity.[45]

Prolongation of myocardial T2 relaxation time has also been shown in studies of patients with genotype positive Fabry disease, probably related to the pronounced deposition of glycolipid in the myocardium, but this can occur in patients with LVH due to other conditions.[46]

CARDIAC SIDEROSIS

Cardiac siderosis develops due to intracellular iron deposition. This causes myocardial damage which ultimately leads to cardiac dysfunction.

Cardiac MRI T2-star (T2*) is a measure of myocardial relaxation and this is shortened when the excessive hemosiderin stored iron disturbs the magnetic microenvironment, causing decline in the myocardial T2*.[47] This decline in myocardial relaxation is associated with increasing risk of LV dysfunction.[48-50]

Hence, CMRI T2* plays an important role in diagnosing myocardial iron overload, and eliminate the need for heart biopsy.[50]

CONCLUSION

For a long time, cardiac biopsy was the only definitive method of diagnosing different types of cardiomyopathies. Cardiac biopsy is an invasive procedure, and even in best of the hands, it is not risk free. Repeated cardiac biopsies can lead to scarring and fibrosis of the myocardium.

Our colleagues in the "world of radiology" continued their relentless quest in refining the field, and today we are blessed with several different types of noninvasive imaging modalities which can be used for diagnosing cardiomyopathies including, echocardiography, speckle tracking, computed tomography (CT) scan, CMRI, SPECT, PET and hybrid techniques. Each of these techniques provides distinct properties and advantages, thus challenging the need for biopsy in every case of cardiomyopathy.

REFERENCES

1. Maron BJ, Towbin JA, Thiene G, et al. Contemporary definitions and classification of the cardiomyopathies: an American Heart Association Scientific Statement from the Council on Clinical Cardiology, Heart Failure and Transplantation Committee; Quality of Care and Outcomes Research and Functional Genomics and Translational Biology Interdisciplinary Working Groups; and Council on Epidemiology and Prevention. Circulation. 2006;113(14):1807-16.
2. Davies MJ. The cardiomyopathies: an overview. Heart. 2000;83(4):469-74.
3. Belloni E, De Cobelli F, Esposito A, et al. MRI of cardiomyopathy. AJR Am J Roentgenol. 2008;191(6):1702-10.
4. Dickerson JA, Raman SV, Baker PM, et al. Relationship of cardiac magnetic resonance imaging and myocardial biopsy in the evaluation of nonischemic cardiomyopathy. Congest Heart Fail. 2013;19(1):29-38.
5. Afridi I, Grayburn PA, Panza JA, et al. Myocardial viability during dobutamine echocardiography predicts survival in patients with coronary artery disease and severe left ventricular systolic dysfunction. J Am Coll Cardiol. 1998;32(4):921-6.
6. Baer FM, Voth E, Schneider CA, et al. Comparison of low-dose dobutamine-gradient-ECHO magnetic resonance imaging and positron emission tomography with [^{18}F]fluorodeoxyglucose in patients with chronic coronary artery disease. A functional and morphological approach to the detection of residual myocardial viability. Circulation. 1995;91:1006-15.
7. Cwajg JM, Cwajg E, Nagueh SF, et al. End-diastolic wall thickness as a predictor of recovery of function in myocardial hibernation: relation to rest-redistribution T1-201 tomography and dobutamine stress echocardiography. J Am Coll Cardiol. 2000;35(5):1152-61.
8. Kim RJ, Wu E, Rafael A, et al. The use of contrast-enhanced magnetic resonance imaging to identify reversible myocardial dysfunction. N Engl J Med. 2000;343(20):1445-53.
9. Go RT, O'Donnell JK, Underwood DA, et al. Comparison of gated cardiac MRI and 2D echocardiography of intracardiac neoplasms. AJR Am J Roentgenol. 1985;145(1):21-5.
10. Schinkel AF, Bax JJ, Poldermans D, et al. Hibernating myocardium: diagnosis and patient outcomes. Curr Probl Cardiol. 2007;32(7):375-410.
11. Callis TE, Jensen BC, Weck KE, et al. Evolving molecular diagnostics for familial cardiomyopathies: at the heart of it all. Expert Rev Mol Diagn. 2010;10(3):329-51.
12. Maron BJ, Gardin JM, Flack JM, et al. Prevalence of hypertrophic cardiomyopathy in a general population of young adults. Echocardiographic analysis of 4111 subjects in the CARDIA Study. Coronary Artery Risk Development in (Young) Adults. Circulation. 1995;92(4):785-9.
13. Zou Y, Song L, Wang Z, et al. Prevalence of idiopathic hypertrophic cardiomyopathy in China: a population-based echocardiographic analysis of 8080 adults. Am J Med. 2004;116(1):14-8.
14. Maron BJ, Casey SA, Hauser RG, et al. Clinical course of hypertrophic cardiomyopathy with survival to advanced age. J Am Coll Cardiol. 2003; 42(5):882-8.
15. Cirino AL, Ho C. (2011). Familial hypertrophic cardiomyopathy overview. [online] Available from www.ncbi.nlm.nih.gov/books/NBK1768/. [Accessed December, 2013].
16. Hershberger RE, Morales A. (2013). Dilated cardiomyopathy overview. [online] Available from www.ncbi.nlm.nih.gov/books/NBK1309/. [Accessed December, 2013].
17. Dec GW, Fuster V. Idiopathic dilated cardiomyopathy. N Engl J Med. 1994;331(23):1564-75.
18. Morita H, Seidman J, Seidman CE. Genetic causes of human heart failure. J Clin Invest. 2005;115(3):518-26.
19. Schönberger J, Seidman CE. Many roads lead to a broken heart: the genetics of dilated cardiomyopathy. Am J Hum Genet. 2001;69(2): 249-60.
20. Colucci WS, Kolias TJ, Adams KF, et al. Metoprolol reverses left ventricular remodeling in patients with asymptomatic systolic dysfunction: the REversal of VEntricular Remodeling with Toprol-XL (REVERT) trial. Circulation. 2007;116(1):49-56.
21. Corrado D, Basso C, Thiene G, et al. Spectrum of clinicopathologic manifestations of arrhythmogenic right ventricular cardiomyopathy/ dysplasia: a multicenter study. J Am Coll Cardiol. 1997;30(6):1512-20.
22. Sen-Chowdhry S, Syrris P, Prasad SK, et al. Left-dominant arrhythmogenic cardiomyopathy: an under-recognized clinical entity. J Am Coll Cardiol. 2008;52(25):2175-87.
23. Bauce B, Frigo G, Marcus FI, et al. Comparison of clinical features of arrhythmogenic right ventricular cardiomyopathy in men versus women. Am J Cardiol. 2008;102(9):1252-7.
24. Ritter M, Oechslin E, Sütsch G, et al. Isolated noncompaction of the myocardium in adults. Mayo Clin Proc. 1997;72(1):26-31.
25. Weiford BC, Subbarao VD, Mulhern KM. Noncompaction of the ventricular myocardium. Circulation. 2004;109:2965-71.
26. Pignatelli RH, McMahon CJ, Dreyer WJ, et al. Clinical characterization of left ventricular noncompaction in children: a relatively common form of cardiomyopathy. Circulation. 2003;108(21):2672-8.
27. Sen-Chowdhry S, Syrris P, McKenna WJ. Genetics of restrictive cardiomyopathy. Heart Fail Clin. 2010;6:179-86.
28. Merlini G, Westermark P. The systemic amyloidoses: clearer understanding of the molecular mechanisms offers hope for more effective therapies. J Intern Med. 2004;255:159-78.
29. Selkoe DJ. Folding proteins in fatal ways. Nature. 2003;426:900-4.
30. Rapezzi C, Merlini G, Quarta CC, et al. Systemic cardiac amyloidoses: disease profiles and clinical courses of the 3 main types. Circulation. 2009;120:1203-12.
31. Selvanayagam JB, Hawkins PN, Paul B, et al. Evaluation and management of the cardiac amyloidosis. J Am Coll Cardiol. 2007;50:2101-10.
32. Koyama J, Ray-Sequin PA, Falk RH. Longitudinal myocardial function assessed by tissue velocity, strain, and strain rate tissue Doppler echocardiography in patients with AL (primary) cardiac amyloidosis. Circulation. 2003;107:2446-52.
33. Maceira AM, Joshi J, Prasad SK, et al. Cardiovascular magnetic resonance in cardiac amyloidosis. Circulation. 2005;111:186-93.
34. Maceira AM, Prasad SK, Hawkins PN, et al. Cardiovascular magnetic resonance and prognosis in cardiac amyloidosis. J Cardiovasc Magn Reson. 2008;10:54.
35. Soejima K, Yada H. The work-up and management of patients with apparent or subclinical cardiac sarcoidosis: with emphasis on the associated heart rhythm abnormalities. J Cardiovasc Electrophysiol. 2009;20:578-83.
36. Ishimaru S, Tsujino I, Takei T, et al. Focal uptake on ^{18}F-fluoro-2-deoxyglucose positron emission tomography images indicates cardiac involvement of sarcoidosis. Eur Heart J. 2005;26:1538-43.
37. Langah R, Spicer K, Gebregziabher M, et al. Effectiveness of prolonged fasting ^{18}F-FDG PET-CT in the detection of cardiac sarcoidosis. J Nucl Cardiol. 2009;16:801-10.
38. Vignaux O, Dhote R, Duboc D, et al. Clinical significance of myocardial magnetic resonance abnormalities in patients with sarcoidosis: a 1-year follow-up study. Chest. 2002;122:1895-901.
39. Kampmann C, Baehner F, Whybra C, et al. Cardiac manifestations of Anderson-Fabry disease in heterozygous females. J Am Coll Cardiol. 2002;40:1668-74.

40. Chimenti C, Pieroni M, Morgante E, et al. Prevalence of Fabry disease in female patients with late-onset hypertrophic cardiomyopathy. Circulation. 2004;110:1047-53.
41. Funabashi N, Toyozaki T, Matsumoto Y, et al. Images in cardiovascular medicine. Myocardial fibrosis in Fabry disease demonstrated by multi-slice computed tomography: comparison with biopsy findings. Circulation. 2003;107:2519-20.
42. Weidemann F, Breunig F, Beer M, et al. Improvement of cardiac function during enzyme replacement therapy in patients with Fabry disease: a prospective strain rate imaging study. Circulation. 2003;108: 1299-301.
43. Pieroni M, Chimenti C, Ricci R, et al. Early detection of Fabry cardiomyopathy by tissue Doppler imaging. Circulation. 2003;107:1978-84.
44. Moon JC, Sachdev B, Elkington AG, et al. Gadolinium enhanced cardiovascular magnetic resonance in Anderson-Fabry disease. Evidence for a disease specific abnormality of the myocardial interstitium. Eur Heart J. 2003;24:2151-5.
45. Weidemann F, Niemann M, Breunig F, et al. Long-term effects of enzyme replacement therapy on Fabry cardiomyopathy: evidence for a better outcome with early treatment. Circulation. 2009;119:524-9.
46. Imbriaco M, Spinelli L, Cuocolo A, et al. MRI characterization of myocardial tissue in patients with Fabry's disease. AJR Am J Roentgenol. 2007;188(3):850-3.
47. Carpenter JP, Pennell DJ. Role of T2* magnetic resonance in monitoring iron chelation therapy. Acta Haematol. 2009;122(2-3):146-54.
48. Anderson LJ, Holden S, Davis B, et al. Cardiovascular T2-star (T2*) magnetic resonance for the early diagnosis of myocardial iron overload. Eur Heart J. 2001;22(23):2171-9.
49. Wood JC, Tyszka JM, Carson S, et al. Myocardial iron loading in transfusion-dependent thalassemia and sickle cell disease. Blood. 2004; 103(5):1934-6.
50. Sibley CT, Noureldin RA, Gai N, et al. T1 mapping in cardiomyopathy at cardiac MR: comparison with endomyocardial biopsy. Radiology. 2012;265(3):724-32.

Chapter 56

Hypertrophic Cardiomyopathy

Christian Prinz, Lothar Faber, Alan S Maisel

ABSTRACT

Hypertrophic cardiomyopathy (HCM) is the most common cardiac hereditary disease. Several hundred mutations in more than 30 genes, most of which encode sarcomeric structures, are associated with the phenotype of HCM. This condition can be thought of as a sarcomeric disease, with myocardial fiber disarray as its histological hallmark. A more common, obstructive type [hypertrophic obstructive cardiomyopathy (HOCM), 70%] and a less common, nonobstructive type can be distinguished. The symptoms of HCM include dyspnea, angina pectoris, palpitations, dizziness and occasionally syncope. Particularly in young and asymptomatic patients sudden cardiac death (SCD) is the most serious complication of HCM. Therefore, correct diagnosis, followed by risk stratification of patients with regard to the need for prophylactic implantation of an implantable cardioverter defibrillator (ICD), can be of life-saving importance. The pharmacotherapy of symptomatic hypertrophic nonobstructive cardiomyopathy (HNCM) consists of the treatment of heart failure with a normal ejection fraction (HFNEF). In HOCM, the patient's symptoms and the obstructive gradient are the guide to treatment with beta-blockers or verapamil. For patients with drug-resistant disease, surgical myectomy and percutaneous septal ablation are now standard treatments. A near-normal life expectancy and a highly satisfactory quality of life are now realistic treatment goals for patients with HCM.

INTRODUCTION

The prevalence of hypertrophic cardiomyopathy (HCM) is estimated to be one case per 500–1,000 in the overall population. The hallmark of this cardiomyopathy is an excessive thickening of the left ventricular myocardium, occasionally also of the right ventricular myocardium, without any other identifiable causes such as arterial hypertension or valve disease. It is possible to distinguish two phenotypes of HCM. Most commonly is the obstructive type [hypertrophic obstructive cardiomyopathy (HOCM), 70%] in which there is left ventricular outflow tract obstruction (LVOTO) and a less common the nonobstructive type [hypertrophic nonobstructive cardiomyopathy (HNCM)] is present. The extent and localization of the wall thickening is highly variable. Oftentimes the interventricular septum is involved. This also led to the alternative name, asymmetric septal hypertrophy. An American working group on cardiomyopathies suggested that HCM should be defined rather genetically than morphologically. However, for better clinical and practical use the European Society of Cardiology (ESC) Working Group on Myocardial and Pericardial Diseases recommends the morphological classification of the disease.[1-4]

CLINICALLY IMPORTANT PATHOPHYSIOLOGICAL PRINCIPLES

The left ventricular ejection fraction (LVEF) usually remains normal for several years in patients with HCM. However, due to myocardial fibrosis and hypertrophy almost all patients present some degree of diastolic dysfunction which is often already present at the time of diagnosis. Depending on the morphology of the left ventricle (LV), a dynamic obstruction with formation of

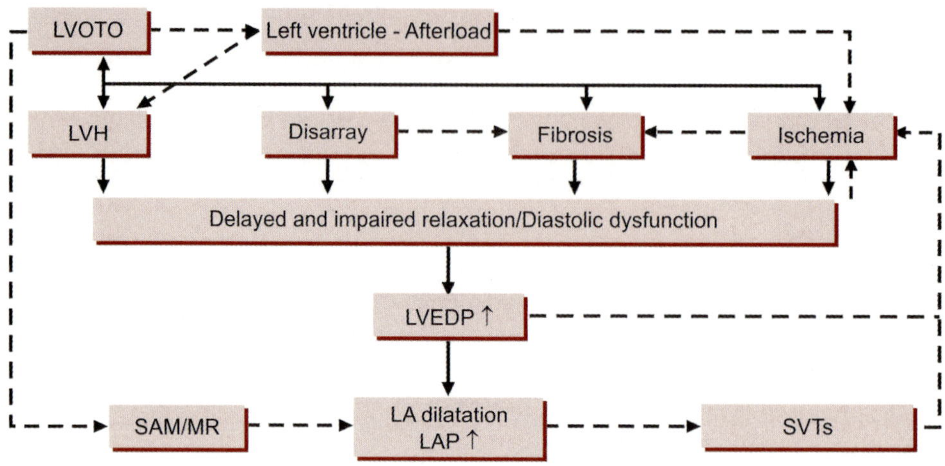

LVOTO, left ventricular outflow tract obstruction; LVH, left ventricular hypertrophy; LVEDP, left ventricular end-diastolic pressure; SAM, systolic anterior movement; MR, mitral regurgitation; LA(P), left atrial (pressure); SVTs, supraventricular tachycardias

Flowchart 1 The chart summarizes the underlying and clinically important pathophysiological principles causing diastolic dysfunction in hypertrophic cardiomyopathy

an intracavitary systolic pressure gradient may occur. We recommend in all patients to perform an exercise test since 50% of all HOCM patients only exhibit this LVOTO under provocation. Therefore, older references that indicate that HNCM is the most common form must be considered to be superseded. Due to high blood flow velocities in the narrowed left ventricular outflow during early systole Venturi forces create suction which draws the mitral valve leaflets toward the interventricular septum. This phenomenon is called systolic anterior motion (SAM phenomenon) of the mitral valve. Afterwards, the mitral valve leaflets are then dragged by the blood flow. This causes the valve to make contact with the interventricular septal wall (drag effect). All these conditions cause the mechanical outflow obstruction in HOCM. Furthermore, in most patients a mitral regurgitation due to the valve's deformation can be observed. An increased systolic left ventricular end-diastolic pressure (LVEDP) is an additional stimulus for the progression of the myocardial hypertrophy. Hypertrophy, microvascular ischemia, displacement fibrosis and an abnormal formation of the myocytes (so called "myocardial disarray") are contributors to ongoing diastolic dysfunction (Flowchart 1).

CLINICAL OBSERVATIONS AND SYMPTOMS

Patients may be completely asymptomatic or severely restricted by the disease. Classical findings in history or on clinical examination are dyspnea and angina pectoris under stress. Furthermore, dizziness, palpitations and occasionally syncope are common. The most devastating symptom remains sudden cardiac death (SCD), which is most common in young and previously asymptomatic patients. Death may be explained by malignant arrhythmias like ventricular fibrillation and occurs predominantly during or after strenuous physical exercise. HCM is the most common cause of sudden death in athletes. Identification of patients with HCM at high-risk of SCD has gained considerable clinical attention and routine management therefore includes repeated risk stratification.

DIAGNOSTIC ALGORITHMS

Physical Examination

The physician should first take a detailed clinical history of the patients pertaining to signs and symptoms and possible risk factors for SCD (see Flowchart 2). Furthermore, a detailed physical examination should be performed.

The nonobstructive form (HNCM) is typically silent on auscultation. Sometimes a fourth heart sound can be heard due to the increased atrial pressure. In HOCM a systolic murmur can usually be detected on auscultation due to the dynamic LVOTO which is often associated with at least mild-to-moderate mitral regurgitation. Due to the low risk of serious side effects we recommend to perform a Valsalva maneuver which may result in an increased degree of obstruction or an increase in the intensity of the auscultatory findings. Alternatively, short-acting preload reducers (acute nitrate therapy) can be given carefully to achieve the same effects. In all patients, the physician should be aware of the stigmata of systemic diseases occasionally associated with left ventricular hypertrophy such as Noonan's syndrome (facial dysmorphia) or Anderson-Fabry disease (typical maculopapular skin lesions) since these disorders may require specific therapeutic approaches.

Electrocardiography

Most HCM patients (75–95%) show unspecific electrocardiogram (ECG) changes, oftentimes in the form of left ventricular hypertrophy. A left anterior hemiblock or complete left bundle branch block can be found in up to 25% of all patients. Hypervoltage and giant negative T waves are typical signs for HNCM. Pseudoinfarct Q waves may be seen in HOCM. In patients with an apical form of HCM hyperacute negative T waves are characteristic findings. Peripheral low voltage may be seen in storage disorders like Fabry's disease or cardiac amyloidosis. Due to important therapeutic consequences, we recommend myocardial biopsy in such patients. However, a normal ECG does never exclude the presence of HCM but suggests a mild manifestation of the disease.

Echocardiographic Evaluation

Due to the absence of radiation and broad availability, echocardiography remains the perfect "working horse" for the management and follow-up of HCM patients. The morphological findings may range from isolated thickening of individual myocardial segments that deviate from the normal LV wall thickness (<12 mm) by only a few millimeters to diffuse and massive hypertrophy and wall thicknesses up to 60 mm. We recommend the performance of echocardiography in all patients with HCM (also using of axis views) since a maximal wall thickness of more than 30 mm is an established risk marker for SCD.

As already mentioned, the right ventricle is only rarely involved. In particular, attention must be paid to the presence of LVOTO causing SAM and mitral regurgitation. Doppler echocardiography can be used to quantify the severity of LVOTO and to calculate the pressure gradients. Furthermore, severity of mitral regurgitation can by assessed by Doppler echocardiography. Also by using echocardiography provocation is mandatory and can be induced pharmacologically or using the Valsalva maneuver or ergometric exercise. Postextrasystolic potentiation of outflow gradients (Brockenbrough sign) can be observed sometimes. On principle, an increase in the afterload (blood pressure increase) or negative inotropic substances can reduce the gradients. This may explain possible variabilities in assessing intraventricular pressure gradients at different times. As indirect but reliable sign an enlargement of the left atrium reflects ventricular relaxation disturbances. Furthermore, a flattening of the EF slope of the anterior mitral leaflet and a reduction or prolongation of the rapid filling phase all indicate diastolic ventricular dysfunction. Also on echocardiography attention must be paid to signs for cardiac storage disorders or myocardial hypertrophy due to secondary causes such as valve diseases.

Use of Other Imaging Modalities

In patients with insufficient acoustic window maximal wall thicknesses and determination of the left ventricular muscle mass can also be determined by using cardiac magnetic resonance (CMR) imaging or cardiac computed tomography (CT). Myocardial scars can be detected by using late gadolinium-enhanced cardiac magnetic resonance imaging (LGE-CMR). Early gadolinium enhancement imaging enables the detection of hypovascular regions such as dark, unenhanced intracardiac thrombi and microvascular obstruction (postmyocardial infarction). LGE imaging also detects accumulation of contrast in areas of myocardial fibrosis due to slower contrast kinetics and greater volume of distribution in the extracellular matrix. However, it must be mentioned that not all areas of LGE represent scar, particularly in HCM. The presence of fibrosis in LGE-CMR in cases of HCM may either be judged visually, or may be quantified as percentage of total LV mass using dedicated software. On principle, all quantification techniques rely on the fact that LGE makes the scar appear brighter. A signal intensity of two or more standard deviations above normal myocardium can be defined as fibrosis. However, it has been stated that two standard deviations as threshold will likely overestimate the amount of scar. The so-called full-width half-maximum technique, using half of the maximal signal intensity within the scar as the threshold, has been suggested to be the most reproducible method of fibrosis quantification. We believe that the cutoff point is somewhere between 5 and 6 standard deviations which correlates well with visual LGE assessments. Recent reports indicate that there may be a causal relationship between the extent of fibrosis and the risk of ventricular arrhythmias. A relationship has been described between disrupted microcirculation and subsequent scar formation with a tendency toward arrhythmia.

Use of Biomarkers

On principle, we recommend baseline assessment of brain natriuretic peptide (BNP) or N-terminal pro-brain natriuretic peptide (NT-proBNP) in HCM patients with clinical signs and symptoms of heart failure. BNP levels can be used for therapy guidance and to assess the success of medical therapy in decompensated patients.

Recent reports have also focused on the role of myocardial fibrosis in HCM. Different degrees of collagen turnover in patients with left ventricular hypertrophy with and without heart failure symptoms suggest that serum markers of collagen synthesis or turnover could be used as biomarkers for fibrosis (and perhaps for risk stratification). A marker of collagen type I degradation, serum carboxy-terminal telopeptide of collagen type I (CITP), was reduced in hypertensive patients, providing a plausible explanation for the increased collagen deposition and fibrosis. Using endomyocardial biopsies from hypertensive patients, a direct correlation was found between serum collagen I propeptide (PICP) as a marker of collagen synthesis and tissue collagen volume. In heart failure patients of different etiologies, high serum levels of cardiac fibrosis markers [collagen III propeptide (PIIINP) and PICP] were significantly associated with a poor outcome. Recently, galectin-3 has also been found to correlate with left ventricular mass and to predict heart failure incidents in large community samples. In HCM, extracellular matrix turnover also seems to be a determinant of cardiac remodeling. However, until now the role of biomarkers for the detection of myocardial fibrosis in HCM remains unclear. Probably in the future clinical management and risk stratification will be changed by integrating biomarkers for the detection of myocardial fibrosis in HCM.

Exercise Tests

We recommend determining the objective workload capacity in patients with HCM using spiroergometry because a subjective estimate of symptoms is often misleading due to prolonged restriction and adaptation. This method also provides information about blood pressure response at rest and under load (risk stratification) and provides information about therapeutic success.

Rhythm Diagnostics

Established risk stratification requires a 48-hour (ambulatory) Holter ECG recording to detect non-sustained ventricular tachycardia (nsVT). In the last years invasive electrophysiological examination has become less important. We only carry out this type of recording for specific instances (for example, suspicion of concomitant Wolff-Parkinson-White syndrome).

Invasive Diagnostics

In order to exclude or verify coexistent coronary sclerosis, to evaluate the vascular supply to the septum prior to planned septal ablation and to verify prognostically relevant myocardial bridging we recommend invasive diagnostics. As earlier mentioned, myocardial storage diseases (amyloidosis) should be excluded by myocardial biopsies. Due to noninvasive imaging invasive gradient determination is rarely necessary today (poor echo window). Elevated LVEDP is usually an expression of a lack of distensibility and a sign for diastolic dysfunction. With corresponding clinical staging [New York Heart Association (NYHA) III], invasive examination should be used as part of a step-by-step diagnostic approach.

Molecular Genetics

We recommend evaluating first-degree relatives for the presence of HCM. If genetic diagnostics are not possible, adolescents between 12 years and 18 years of age should be examined annually, and adults over 18 years of age every 5 years using echocardiography (see above).

THERAPEUTIC ALGORITHMS

Since HCM is a rare disease with a low prevalence, large randomized clinical trials are missing. Therefore, therapeutic recommendations are mostly based on observational studies or case series. Until now, results for symptomatic therapy using alcohol-induced myocardial ablation are only available from medium-term studies. Despite an updated American College of Cardiology Foundation (ACCF)/American Heart Association (AHA) guideline from 2011 for the diagnosis and treatment of HCM, the essentials of the recommendations developed in 2003 by an international expert committee are still valid. Physical endurance activity should be performed in the aerobic range (abstaining from high-performance sports, athletics or competitive sports). However, we recommend not a general prohibition on sports. Smoking should be avoided and alcohol should not be ingested since outflow tract obstruction can be aggravated by reduction of afterload and cause arrhythmias. The earlier indication for infective endocarditis prophylaxis with HOCM has since been qualified.

Risk Stratification

Treatment of high-risk HCM patients with implantable cardioverter defibrillator (ICD) has proven to prevent SCD. However, the correct identification of high-risk HCM patients remains a particular challenge (Flowchart 2).

Until now, five major risk factors have been identified. Each individual risk factor has a relatively low predictive value, but combining them increases their significance considerably. High-risk patients with more than or equal to two risk factors are considered to have an annual SCD rate of approximately 4%. The single risk factors are:

- There is a positive family history of premature SCD caused by HCM in about 25% of the affected families (<45 years of age)
- Documented nsVT is a sensitive marker for increased risk of suffering SCD. The absence of nsVT is also diagnostically useful because of the high negative predictive value
- Syncope at rest or during exercise is an important risk marker for all age groups
- An abnormal blood pressure response during exercise is defined as an increase in the systolic blood pressure of less than 20 mmHg from the baseline value. A progressive fall in blood pressure during exercise or a fall in the systolic value by 20 mmHg after an initial increase, particularly in younger patients (<40 years of age) is also assessed as being associated with risk

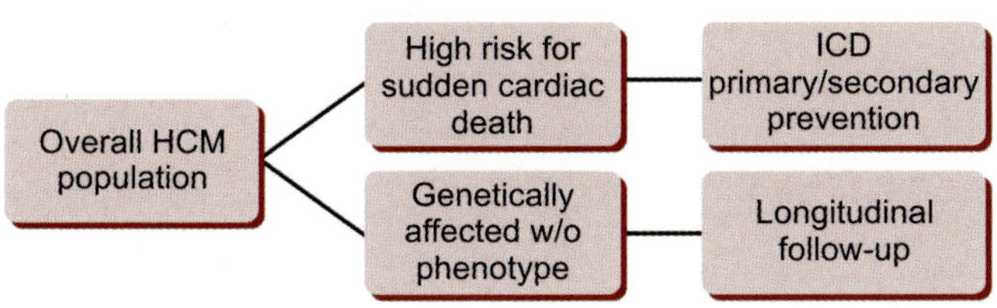

HCM, hypertrophic cardiomyopathy; ICD, implantable cardioverter defibrillator

Flowchart 2 The chart summarizes the importance of identifying hypertrophic cardiomyopathy patients at high risk for sudden cardiac death. Such patients should be treated by an implantable cardioverter defibrillator. All other patients should undergo longitudinal follow-up

- Extreme left ventricular hypertrophy with wall thicknesses more than 30 mm is also associated with risk. The highest rate of cases of SCD in adolescents was linked with pronounced hypertrophy.

Additional risk factors that may support implantation of an ICD and which were only studied in smaller patient collectives are listed in Table 1. More recent studies consider marked fibrosis (cardiac MRI) to be an additional risk factor. Table 1 demonstrates the algorithm used by us to identify at-risk HCM patients. Patients without any of the listed risk markers have a high probability of a good prognosis. We consider two first-degree risk markers to be an indication for primary prophylactic ICD implantation. An individual decision must be made for patients with one first-degree risk marker. Second-degree risk factors may provide additional support for decisions. A previously survived cardiac arrest or documentation of sustained ventricular tachycardia are clear indications for an ICD implantation.

Asymptomatic Patients

In asymptomatic patients, there is no clear indication for pharmacotherapy due to an absence of data. For pathophysiological considerations, we advise initiating pharmacotherapy using beta-blockers. The role of an upstream medical therapy to prevent myocardial fibrosis including statins, omega-3 polyunsaturated fatty acids or aldosterone receptor blockers remains unclear until now. However, risk evaluation should be performed precisely in this group of patients. We recommend strict control of any coexistent arterial hypertension (reduction of the myocardial growth stimulus) which is of particular importance.

Symptomatic Hypertrophic Nonobstructive Cardiomyopathy Patients

Beta-blockers or verapamil-type calcium antagonists should be used for rate control due to the ubiquitous presence of diastolic dysfunction in HCM (Flowchart 3). In patients with signs of congestion or concomitant hypertension, we recommend the use of diuretics and angiotensin-converting enzyme (ACE) inhibitors/ angiotensin (AT) receptor antagonists. It is important to perform a tight monitoring because we and others observed in individual cases induction of an outflow tract obstruction in patients who were initially recorded as having HNCM. Recent data postulate a reversal of fibrosis with favorable long-term effects

TABLE 1: The table gives an algorithm to identify at-risk hypertrophic cardiomyopathy patients for implantation with an implantable cardioverter defibrillator. If two first-degree risk factors are present, an implantable cardioverter defibrillator should be implanted. In case of one present risk factor, an individualized approach should be used. Presence or absence of second risk factors may be helpful for decision-making

Algorithm to identify at-risk HCM patients for implantation with an implantable cardioverter defibrillator	
First-degree risk factors	**Definition**
• Positive family history of SCD	Ad 1: Cases with SCD <45 years
• Recurrent syncope	Ad 2: ≥2 incidents
• Left ventricular hypertrophy	Ad 3: ≥30 mm at any side in the LV
• Abnormal blood pressure response during exercise	Ad 4: Increase <20 mmHg or fall >20 mmHg
• Nonsustained VT in Holter ECG	Ad 5: ≥3 consecutive QRS complexes with HR ≥120 BPM
Second-degree risk factors	**Definition**
• Atrial fibrillation/atrial flutter	Any form
• Left atrium dilatation	>45 mm (M-Mode echo)
• High LVOT gradient at rest	>80 mmHg (CW-Doppler)
• Evidence of myocardial ischemia during exercise	
• Early manifestation of HCM	<30 years of age
• Myocardial bridging near the LAD	In younger patients (<45 years)
• Marked fibrosis in cardiac MRI	Fibrosis ≥2 segments in 17-segment model of the LV

HCM, hypertrophic cardiomyopathy; SCD, sudden cardiac death; VT, ventricular tachycardia; ECG, electrocardiography; LVOT, left ventricular outflow tract; LAD, left anterior descending coronary artery; HR, heart rate; BPM; beats per minute; CW-Doppler, continuous wave Doppler; LV, left ventricle

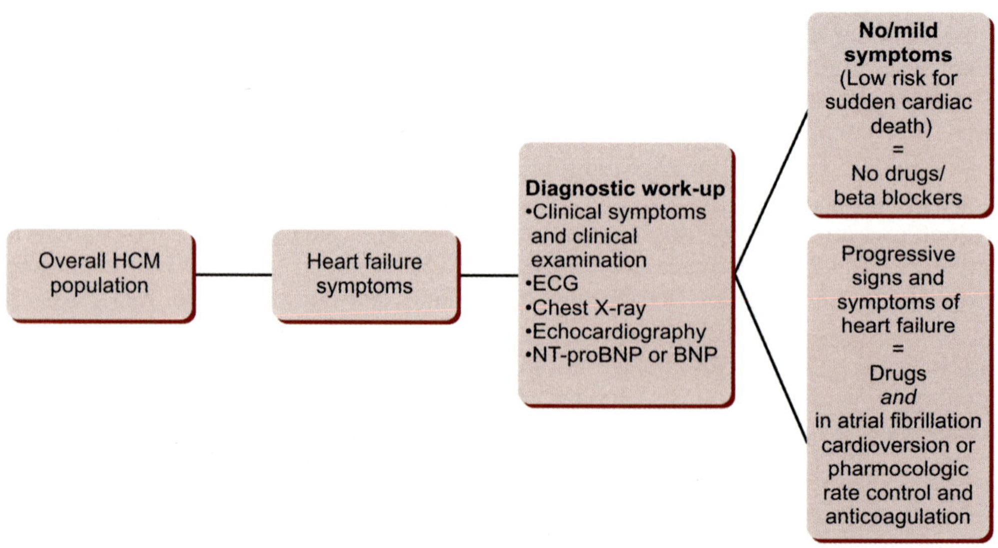

HCM, hypertrophic cardiomyopathy; NT-proBNP, N-terminal pro-brain natriuretic peptide; BNP, brain natriuretic peptide

Flowchart 3 An algorithm for the treatment of hypertrophic cardiomyopathy patients affected by heart failure symptoms. However, each patient needs an individualized therapeutic approach

with treatment using AT receptor antagonists, statins, or spironolactone. If atrial fibrillation occurs, patients develop oftentimes with loss of an active ventricular filling a considerable drop in output and are at higher risk of cardiac embolic events. We recommend the promptly use of anticoagulants. Despite amiodarone can prevent recurrence of atrial fibrillations, there is evidence that medical treatment with amiodarone does not reduce the risk of SCD. Due to structural heart disease different methods available for ablation of atrial fibrillation have less favorable outcomes in this cohort of patients.

CONCLUSION

Due to the complexity and low prevalence of the disease, patients with HCM require continuous monitoring in, or in collaboration with, specialized centers. Every patient, even asymptomatic patients, should undergo adequate risk stratification in terms of the risk of SCD, with subsequent ICD implantation if required. Symptomatic treatment of patients with HNCM corresponds to specific treatment of heart failure. For symptomatic HOCM septal ablation and septal myectomy are now comparable procedures. The choice of method depends on an individual approach. In addition to optimizing risk stratification, by also integrating additional procedures (MRI, CT, biomarkers) for example, longitudinal observation of patients who have received different treatments remains a priority.

REFERENCES

1. Maron BJ, McKenna WJ, Danielson GK, et al. American College of Cardiology/European Society of Cardiology Clinical Expert Consensus Document on Hypertrophic Cardiomyopathy. A report of the American College of Cardiology Foundation Task Force on Clinical Expert Consensus Documents and the European Society of Cardiology Committee for Practice Guidelines. Eur Heart J. 2003;24(21):1965-91.
2. Gersh BJ, Maron BJ, Bonow RO, et al. 2011 ACCF/AHA guideline for the diagnosis and treatment of hypertrophic cardiomyopathy: executive summary: a report of the American College of Cardiology Foundation/ American Heart Association Task Force on Practice Guidelines. Circulation. 2011;124(24):2761-96.
3. Prinz C, Farr M, Hering D, et al. The diagnosis and treatment of hypertrophic cardiomyopathy. Dtsch Arztebl Int. 2011;108(13):209-15.
4. Prinz C, Farr M, Laser KT, et al. Determining the role of fibrosis in hypertrophic cardiomyopathy. Expert Rev Cardiovasc Ther. 2013;11(4): 495-504.

Chapter 57

Takotsubo Cardiomyopathy

Andrew C Morley-Smith, Alexander R Lyon

ABSTRACT

Takotsubo cardiomyopathy (TTC) is a stress-associated reversible cause of ventricular dysfunction which remains an underdiagnosed, variably managed and incompletely understood cause of acute heart failure. In the last decade, the growth of urgent coronary angiography for acute coronary syndrome (ACS) has yielded a greater appreciation of its true incidence and a more unified approach to clinical management of this often challenging patient group. The growing identification of individuals with this syndrome has fuelled clinical, registry and laboratory research programs to better understand its epidemiology and underlying pathophysiology. This wealth of accumulating data is generating important implications for frontline clinicians. Here, we assimilate this understanding and take a practical approach, in turn covering initial diagnosis, approach to clinical investigation, in hospital management and follow-up protocols.

INTRODUCTION

Takotsubo cardiomyopathy (TTC) is an increasingly recognized, but still underdiagnosed cause of reversible acute cardiomyopathy. TTC was first described in Japan and named Takotsubo after the left ventricle's resemblance to the Japanese fisherman's octopus trap at ventriculography. Also known as stress cardiomyopathy, or "broken heart syndrome" in the context of bereavement, it is a clinical syndrome mimicking acute ST-elevation myocardial infarction (STEMI) but in the absence of causative obstructive coronary artery disease. Catecholamine surge is the etiological cornerstone in TTC with serum levels at presentation significantly elevated compared both to resting levels in the same patient and to levels in comparable patients with acute ischemic heart failure. As such TTC is usually triggered by an event causing sympathetic activity with catecholamine release that induces characteristic patterns of left ventricular (LV) wall motion abnormalities with systolic dysfunction. The "classic" pattern of marked apical hypokinesia with compensatory basal hyperkinesia is now recognized as one phenotypic subtype with basal and midventricular variants also recognized with increasing frequency. Whatever the form it takes, the changes typically resolve completely, at least macroscopically in a period of days to weeks depending on the severity of the acute abnormalities. We have focused here on practical management from the emergency room through to discharge from hospital.

EPIDEMIOLOGY

The incidence of TTC is almost certainly underestimated, but with increasing awareness and more widespread access to early coronary angiography it is now recognized more frequently. Several series in Asian and Western, predominantly Caucasian populations suggest around 1–2% of patients with suspected acute coronary syndrome (ACS) are eventually diagnosed with TTC.[1] Within the United Kingdom, this would equate to approximately 3,000 cases per annum. The distribution is strikingly skewed with postmenopausal women account for 70–90% of reported cases.[2] TTC is uncommon (<3% of cases) in those under 50 years. Unlike ACS and other atherosclerosis related conditions, presentation is more common in the summer months and lacks the early morning peak associated with plaque rupture events.

PATTERNS OF DISEASE

Despite common perception, the cardiac morphology associated with TTC is heterogeneous. The classic description is akin to "Takotsubo octopus pot", with the LV apex typically akinetic or markedly hypokinetic and accompanied by compensatory hypercontractility of the base. In a cardiac magnetic resonance (CMR) imaging series, this group constituted 82% of TTC presentations.[3] However, variant midventricular and basal forms are now recognized, comprising 17% and 1% respectively in the same CMR series and each with sparing of apical segments. Atypical morphologies are often associated with atypical clinical presentations such as younger patients, males and those with a comorbid trigger, though beyond this the significance of the variance in LV morphology is unclear. Those cases with biventricular involvement (34%) have a more severe disease, but otherwise there is no evidence to date that atypical TTC morphology carries an adverse prognosis.

CLINICAL PRESENTATION

Most patients with TTC present to the emergency department, often arriving by ambulance with suspected ACS heralded by acute chest pain (67.8%) and/or dyspnea (17.8%), and sometimes with ventricular arrhythmia or cardiogenic shock (1.5% and 4.2% respectively). Typically there is a history of recent emotional event (26.8%; e.g., bereavement, major argument, gambling losses), physical stress (37.8%; e.g., exhausting work, asthma attack, neuromuscular crisis), or a combination (e.g., suicide attempt), though in a significant minority no preceding stressor can be identified (34.3%).[1] Iatrogenic causes are also recognized, including various drugs, induction of general anesthetic, adrenaline administration and dobutamine stress echocardiography. From a medicolegal perspective, there is suspicion that physical restraint or electrical stunning (e.g., Taser weapons) might also trigger the condition.

On bedside assessment, particular suspicion could be brought by description of symptoms typical for ACS in the context of a precipitating stressful event, particularly in postmenopausal women. Clinically, patients show signs of sympathetic overdrive with profound sweatiness, hypertension and anxiety.

INVESTIGATIONS

The different modalities of investigation are targeted toward rapid and precise distinction of TTC from STEMI, and subsequent determination of severity.

Electrocardiogram

The electrocardiogram (ECG) is invariably abnormal in the ST and T-wave segments, normally prompting immediate cardiac catheterization.

The ECG in Takotsubo cardiomyopathy patients shows a series of typical changes.

Firstly, there is ST-segment elevation present in 80% of cases, which appears early in the presentation and is greatest in the precordial leads.[1] As the ST elevation resolves, a negative T-wave pattern develops, which deepens progressively over the first few days.[4] The changes are widespread, involving multiple coronary artery territories, and raising suspicion of myo- or pericarditis.

Secondly, there is transient QTc prolongation associated with the deep T-wave inversion which resolves to normal during the recovery phase. This is often very pronounced (>500 ms), which would rarely be seen in STEMI due to coronary occlusion, and increases the risk for malignant arrhythmias (in particular *torsades de pointes*). If present, management of arrhythmia risk becomes a management priority as this is an easily treatable complication (see below). The duration of T-wave abnormalities and QTc prolongation are highly variable. The QTc may normalize rapidly,[4] and this emphasizes the need for early imaging to identify the structural abnormalities before they resolve, in turn avoiding mistaken diagnosis of inherited long QT syndrome and unnecessary therapy such as defibrillator implantation.

Differences between the ECG patterns seen in TTC and STEMI have been proposed as a tool for early triage, with the presence of ST-segment depression in lead aVR alongside absence of ST-segment elevation in lead V_1 identifying TTC with 91% sensitivity and 96% specificity in one series of Asian patients, though this has not been replicated in Caucasian populations. In practice, this would not preclude the need for cardiac catheterization in the context of acute chest pain with new ST-segment elevation.

Cardiac Catheterization

Most TTC patients will proceed directly to the cardiac catheterization laboratory for urgent angiography to exclude STEMI. In TTC the epicardial coronary arteries are typically normal, though bystander atherosclerotic coronary artery disease can be present. This is incidental to the index presentation, and insufficient to cause the degree or pattern of LV dysfunction. In one cohort of Japanese patients with TTC, 10% had coronary artery disease judged incidental to the primary diagnosis of TTC.[5] Once causative coronary occlusion has been excluded, left ventriculography should be performed (unless contraindicated). In TTC, this will often be the diagnostic investigation (Figs 1 and 2), with patterns of wall motion abnormality as described above. After diagnostic cardiac catheterization, early access to high-quality cardiac imaging is essential, in particular echocardiography and, where available, CMR imaging.

Bystander coronary disease has been controversial in TTC, and "aborted myocardial infarction" has been proposed on the basis of the association. In this paradigm, coronary plaque rupture with thrombus formation then dissipation leaves an acute myocardial stunning that subsequently resolves. A case was initially made for patients with abnormal left anterior descending (LAD) artery anatomy, such that the acutely occluded vessel supplies an unusually large area of the LV anterior wall and apex (so called "wrap-around" LAD) accounting for the large distribution, and there were reports of acute plaque rupture in this context. However, a recent study using intravascular ultrasound has not corroborated these results,[6] and a retrospective analysis of coronary anatomy in a cohort of TTC patients showed no increased frequency of wrap-around LAD anatomy.[7] These studies are supported by a further prospective study,[8] largely dismissing aborted STEMI as a mechanism. We feel that there is little to support a macrovascular cause for TTC on current evidence.

Echocardiography

Echocardiography is readily available, aids diagnostic confirmation and provides early triage for complications. The most prominent feature is reduced LV systolic function, with or without accompanying right ventricle (RV) dysfunction. Depending on the disease variant there will be characteristic pattern of wall motion abnormality as discussed above (Fig. 3). The degree of dysfunction is variable, though some patients in the acute phase can have normal or near normal stroke volume with preserved cardiac output.[2] Diastolic dysfunction is often present, though in practice will not assist differentiation from STEMI. Left ventricular outflow tract obstruction (LVOTO) occurs in at least 25% of presentations, especially in patients with septal hypertrophy. Assessment for this is important in the presence of hypotension, as this has immediate implications for management as discussed further below. Contrast echocardiography may be helpful to exclude thrombosis in the akinetic LV apex.

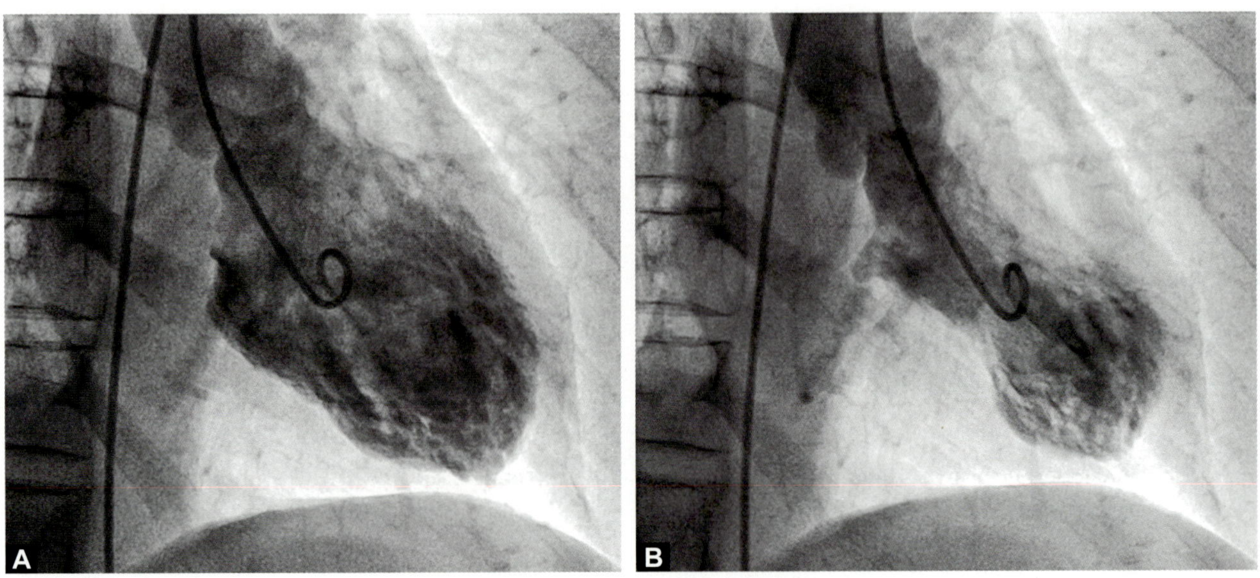

Fig. 1 Ventriculography of a classic apical pattern of Takotsubo cardiomyopathy: **A,** at end-diastole and **B,** end-systole, with akinesis of the mid-ventricle and compensatory hyperkinesias of apical and basal regions

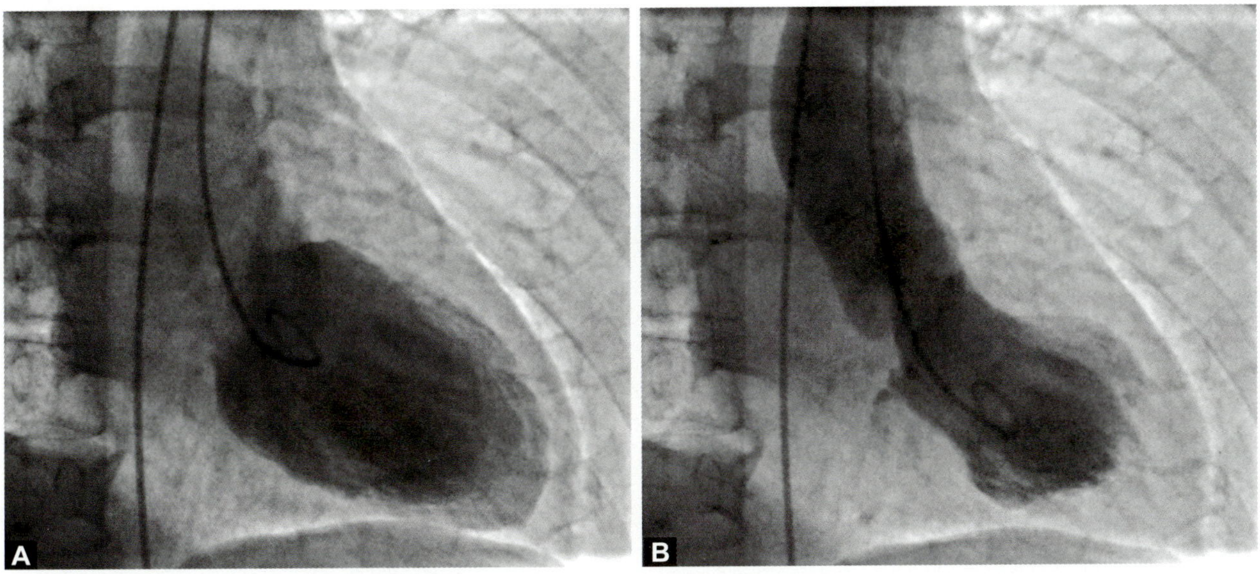

Fig. 2 Ventriculography of a midventricular variant of Takotsubo cardiomyopathy: **A,** at end-diastole and **B,** end-systole, with akinesia of the mid-ventricle and compensatory hyperkinesia of apical and basal regions

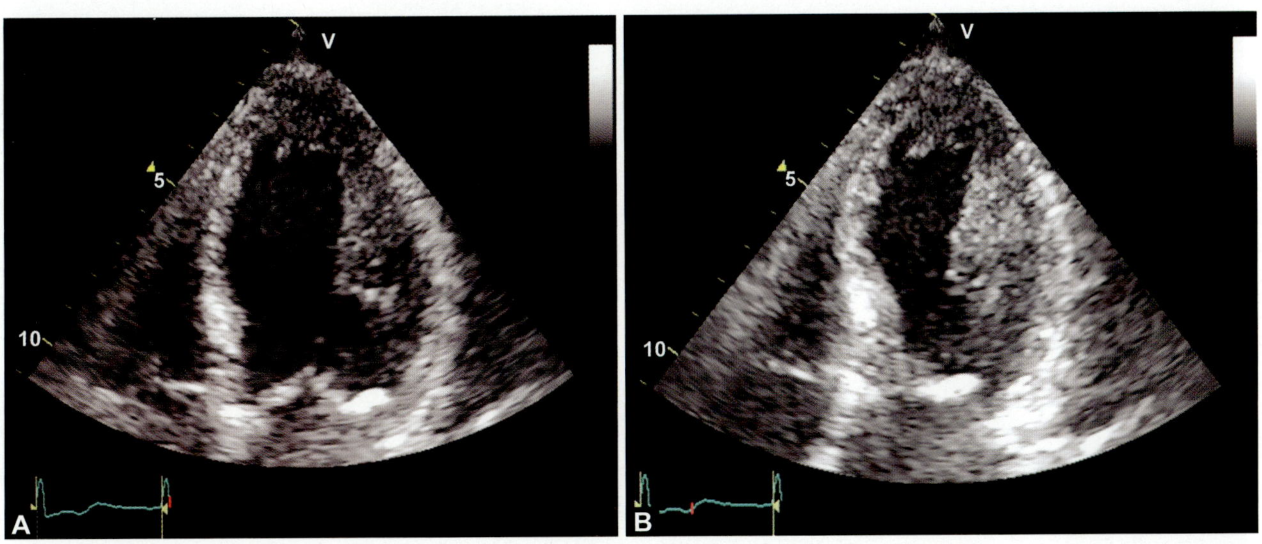

Fig. 3 Apical four chamber images at: **A,** end-diastole and **B,** end-systole, from a transthoracic echocardiogram in the classic apical pattern of Takotsubo cardiomyopathy, showing marked apical hypokinesia

Cardiovascular Magnetic Resonance

Acute cardiovascular magnetic resonance imaging is extremely helpful in TTC patients in confirming diagnosis, assessing for complications and establishing a baseline for follow-up comparison[3] (Fig. 4). In most cases all these abnormalities will have resolved at follow-up scanning at 2 months.

Baseline images will show LV dysfunction with a characteristic wall motion abnormality, and can be used alongside ventriculography and echocardiography to define precisely which disease pattern is present (Fig. 4). After infusion of the contrast agent gadolinium, the early phase scan will delineate any LV apical thrombus present. The delayed phase scan will demonstrate absence of the intense subendocardial to transmural

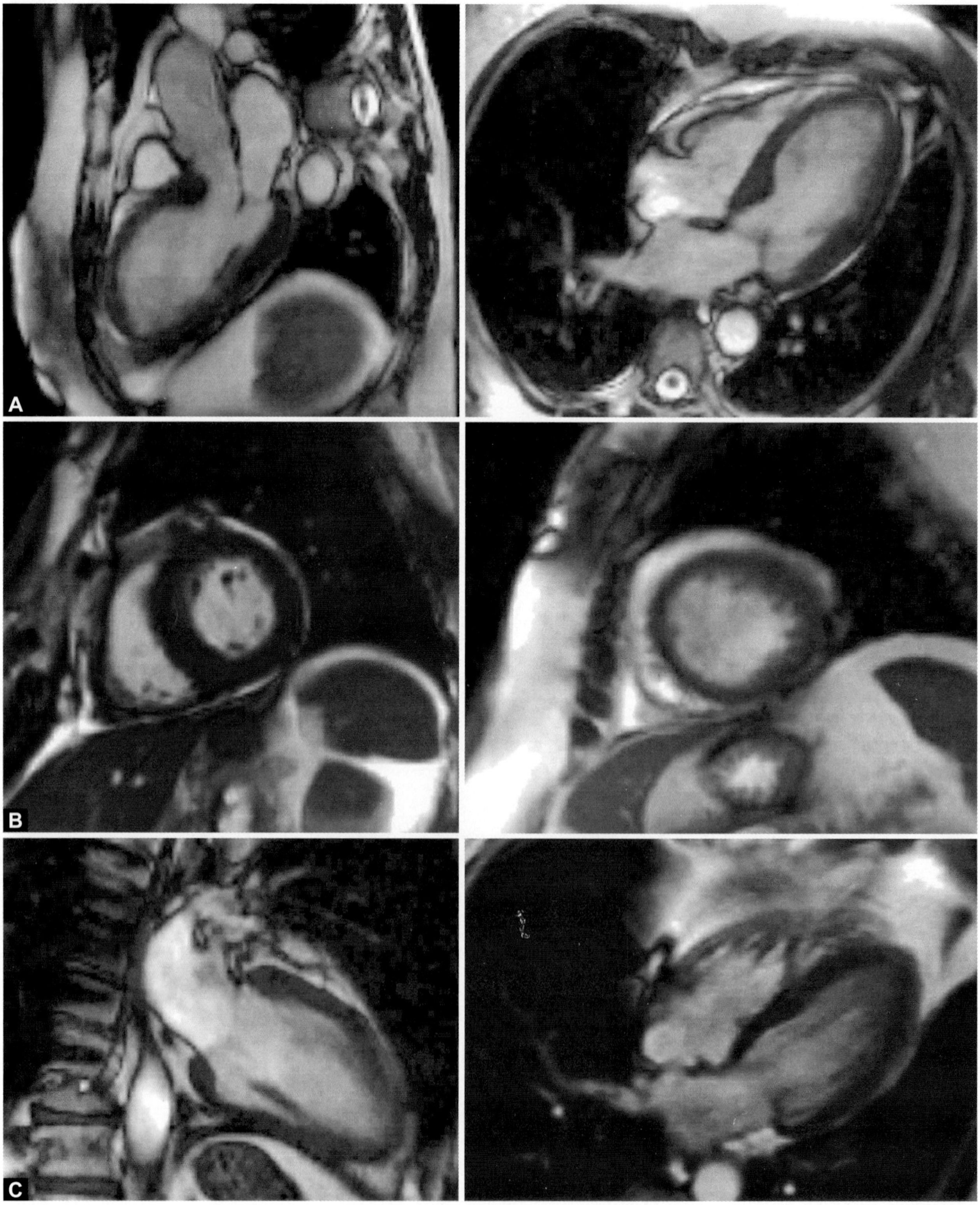

Contd...

Contd...

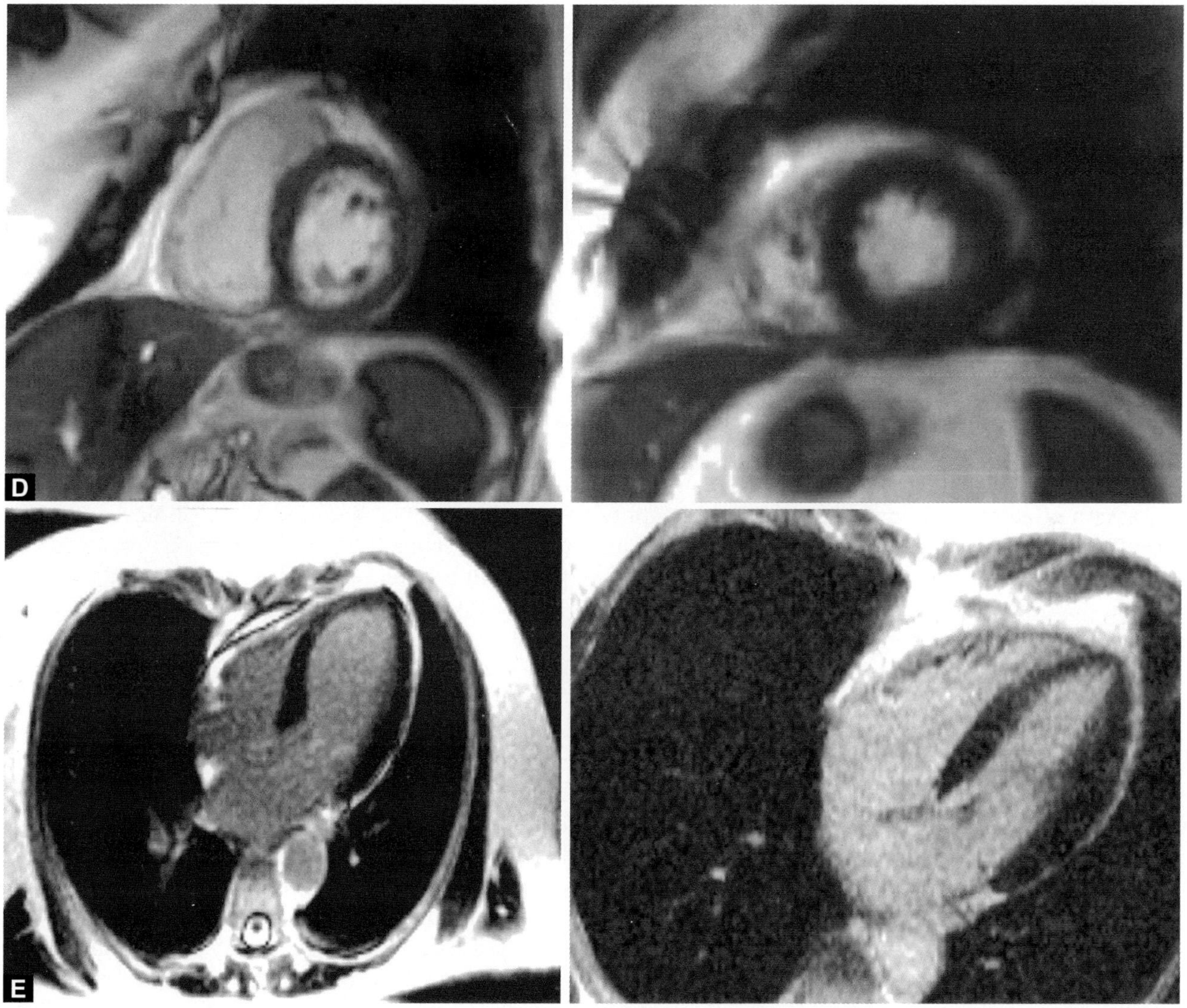

Fig. 4 Cardiac magnetic resonance imaging in Takotsubo cardiomyopathy with "typical" pattern in the acute phase and at 3 month follow-up. **A** and **B** show noncontrast images taken in the acute phase. In **A,** there is pronounced thickening of basal myocardium with akinesia at the apex; **B,** the typical Takotsubo pattern in short-axis views, with thickened, active myocardium in the basal slice contrasting with the thin, akinetic walls in the apical slice; **C** and **D** show comparable images acquired at 3-month follow-up, with resolution of the wall motion abnormality; and **E** shows slices acquired after infusion of gadolinium contrast, showing absence of late enhancement in the acute phase (left) and at 3-month follow-up (right)

pattern of late gadolinium enhancement (LGE) that is typical of myocardial infarction. Patchy LGE during the acute phase has been reported but is usually absent at follow-up,[9] though in a subgroup of patients a pattern of small, transmural LGE persists in the ventricular apex. In the absence of coronary atherosclerosis, and with the original hypokinesis during the acute phase involving a much wider volume of myocardium, this should not be considered a conventional myocardial infarction. This may reflect pressure-induced myocardial edema and necrosis due to the extremely high intraventricular pressures which can be generated during the acute stress, with the thin-walled apex most susceptible. Histological confirmation of myocardial changes reflecting this underlying cause for the LGE pattern is lacking, but it does not appear to be fibrosis. Finally, T2-weighted studies can show increased regional water content, probably due to myocardial inflammation, typically collocated with the areas of LV dysfunction, though this is less specific for TTC.

In those patients with suspected STEMI but normal coronaries, the ability of CMR to show virtual myocardial tissue characterization provides an excellent technique for further assessment and differentiation of TTC from other acute heart failure syndromes such as acute myocarditis.[10] In addition, its ability to reliably exclude myocardial infarction, through analysis of distribution of wall motion abnormalities as well as with LGE, has important implications for the individual patients and the health economy in removing the need for long-term secondary prevention of atherosclerosis. Its weakness is limited availability outside large centers, and a time lapse from presentation to scanning may allow abnormalities to resolve in some cases before being fully appreciated.

Biomarkers

Serum assays of cardiac troponins, myoglobin, creatine kinase-MB (CK-MB), natriuretic peptides [brain natriuretic peptide (BNP) and N-terminal pro-brain natriuretic peptide (NT-proBNP)] can, and usually are, all elevated in TTC, but none carries sufficient specificity for diagnostic purposes. In most cases, a patient with TTC will have a dramatically elevated BNP alongside a marginally elevated troponin, reverse to the biomarker profile typically observed in STEMI.[11] Ratios of different biomarkers at presentation could help differentiate TTC from STEMI, though this needs to be further validated. For prognostication, marked or persistent elevation in NT-proBNP or BNP levels carries worse prognosis and correlates with the extent of catecholamine release, and severity of LV dysfunction.[12]

ACUTE CARDIAC COMPLICATIONS

Takotsubo cardiomyopathy patients are a heterogeneous group, and as such there is a spectrum of disease severity in TTC. Mild cases may exhibit only a minimal degree of LV dysfunction and resolve quickly, whilst more severe cases presenting with cardiogenic shock make a more protracted recovery. In this latter group there are several factors contributing to the abrupt loss of cardiac output. The akinesia of the LV apex causes an acute LV systolic impairment, which results in marked reduction of ventricular ejection. With this, the hyperdynamic contraction in the base of the LV may cause acute LVOTO, usually associated with septal hypertrophy, systolic anterior motion of the mitral valve and acute mitral regurgitation that may exacerbate the hemodynamic instability and pulmonary congestion. These factors together can cause a severe acute pump failure and the clinical cardiogenic shock.

Other problems include complete atrioventricular block, which may require temporary pacing, but will usually resolve quickly in parallel to the functional recovery; cardiac rupture, usually fatal without urgent surgery, which is more common in older hypertensive females; and *torsades de pointes* or other ventricular tachyarrhythmias consequent to the QTc prolongation. Importantly, the apical wall motion abnormality predisposes to formation of thrombus within the LV cavity (2% of cases in one CMR study),[3] and systemic embolic events (3%)[2] can be encountered.

DIAGNOSTIC CRITERIA AND RISK PREDICTION

Diagnostic criteria based on expert consensus have been proposed by both the Mayo Clinic[13] and a Swedish group[14] (Table 1). In practice, a nuanced clinical judgment is often required. Some cases will be obviously TTC, with a clear stress precipitant, normal coronary arteries, marked apical hypokinesis on ventriculography and echocardiography, and no LGE on CMR.

But many are less clear and fall in a clinical "gray zone", perhaps giving a convincing history but with areas of coronary atherosclerosis ("Is this causative or bystander disease?"), a less convincing pattern or degree of hypokinesis ("Has the dysfunction already resolved, or is this an atypical pattern?") and patchy LGE on the acute phase CMR ("Does this represent an area of infarction, inflammation in myocarditis, or TTC?"). Clinical experience and multidisciplinary discussion are required in the acute phase to resolve the diagnostic dilemma and decide initial management. Follow-up at 6 weeks often resolves these unclear cases, as in more than 90% of TTC the dysfunction and patchy CMR LGE will have resolved by this time.

In those patients with a confirmed diagnosis of TTC, it is important to anticipate those patients at high risk of complications. Factors associated with worse outcome include older age, greater myocardial injury as indexed by greater release of cardiac troponin and lower ejection fraction (EF), and trigger by a stressful physical rather than emotional event. The Mayo Clinic validated a risk score based on these findings (omitting troponin due to variation in laboratory assays between centers). With one point allocated for each risk factor present (age >70 years, presence of physical stressor and EF <40%), acute heart failure occurred in 28%, 58% and 85% of patients with one, two and three points respectively.[15] Tools such as

TABLE 1: Modified Mayo Clinic (left) and Gothenburg (right) criteria for diagnosis of Takotsubo cardiomyopathy[13,14]

Modified Mayo Clinic criteria: all four required for diagnosis		Gothenburg criteria: all three required for diagnosis	
A	Transient hypokinesis, akinesis, or dyskinesis in the left ventricular mid-segments with or without apical involvement; regional wall motion abnormalities that extend beyond a single epicardial vascular distribution; and frequently, but not always, a stressful trigger	1	Transient hypokinesis, akinesis, or dyskinesis in the left ventricular segments and frequently, but not always, a stressful trigger (psychological or physical)
B	The absence of obstructive coronary disease or angiographic evidence of acute plaque rupture	2	The absence of other pathological conditions (e.g., ischemia, myocarditis, toxic damage, tachycardia, etc.) that may more credibly explain the regional dysfunction
C	New ECG abnormalities (ST-segment elevation and/or T-wave inversion) or modest elevation in cardiac troponin	3	No elevation or modest elevation in cardiac troponin (i.e., disparity between the troponin level and the amount of the dysfunctional myocardium present)
D	The absence of pheochromocytoma and myocarditis		

this may assist clinicians identify early those patients at higher risk.

MANAGEMENT

The central tenet of TTC is that ultimately the myocardial function will return to normal, and so the priority lies with aggressive supportive care to sustain life and minimize complications until full recovery is achieved. In mild cases, no treatment or a short course of medical therapy may be sufficient; in severe cases, consideration for mechanical support as a "bridge to recovery" may be necessary. The general principles and priorities of management are summarized in Flowchart 1.

Takotsubo cardiomyopathy is a recently recognized entity and so there is still little evidence on which to base management rationale. This discussion is based on available evidence, current consensus, and the viewpoint of the authors.

Diagnosis and Initial Management

In the initial phase, standard protocols for management of STEMI should be followed until this has been excluded with cardiac catheterization confirming no culprit coronary lesions (Flowchart 2). The importance of early diagnosis is underlined by potential for complications of STEMI therapy, particularly antiplatelet and anticoagulant therapy. Ventriculography at the time of coronary angiography is essential and often diagnostic in TTC, and an early complete echocardiogram will demonstrate the LV dysfunction and characteristic pattern of wall motion abnormality (Fig. 3). In some patients LV function may normalize within 2–3 hours which strengthens the need for the early assessment of LV function.

Patients should be admitted to an acute cardiac or medical unit with continuous cardiac ECG monitoring given the risk of acute arrhythmias, particularly in the setting of significantly prolonged QTc interval. We would advise monitoring continues until the QTc interval has returned to a level considered low risk for sudden cardiac death (e.g., QTc <500 ms). Noninvasive monitoring of hemodynamics parameters such as cardiac output, stroke volume, peripheral vascular resistance (PVR), for example with impedance electrocardiography, may be helpful in continuous assessment of patients' stability, and for evaluation of the hemodynamic consequences of pharmacological treatment. Contrast echocardiography and CMR in the early phase post gadolinium will exclude LV thrombus, and the late post gadolinium phase will provide further evidence to exclude myocardial infarction (Flowchart 1).

Once STEMI has been excluded, antiplatelet and anticholesterol drugs can be reviewed for discontinuation. Systemic anticoagulation should be initiated if LV thrombus is confirmed.

Mild Cases

Mild cases with rapid symptomatic improvement may require no therapy and early discharge. Patients with persistent symptoms and LV dysfunction often warrant conventional heart failure therapy with graded introduction of angiotensin-converting enzyme (ACE) inhibitors and beta-blockers licensed for heart failure. However, bear in mind that some TTC patients can have

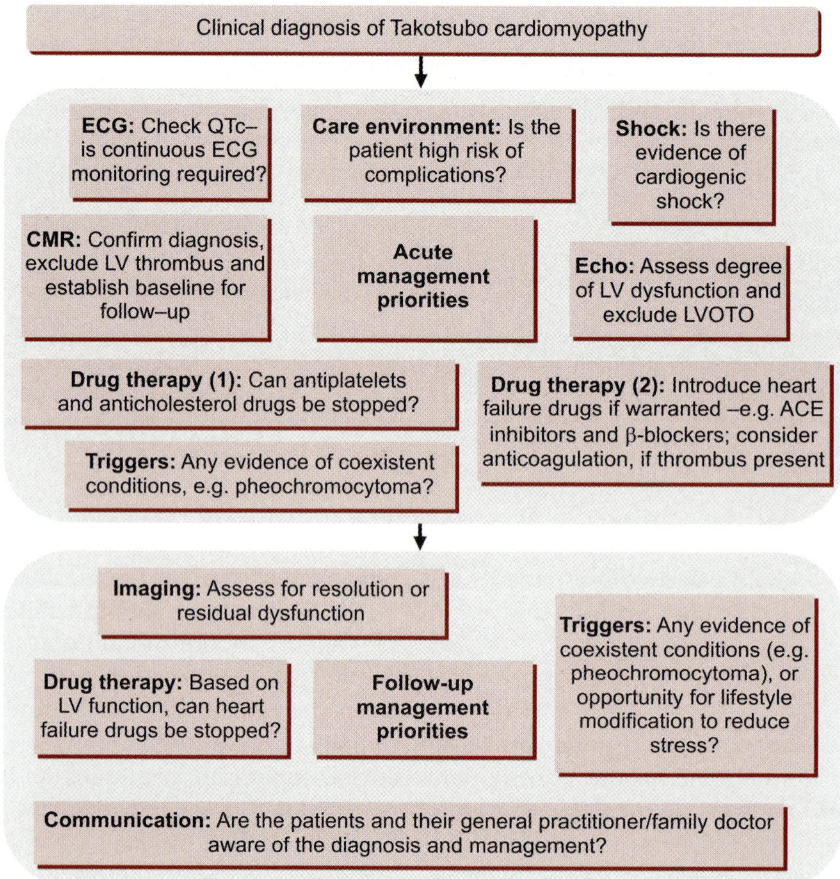

CMR, cardiac magnetic resonance imaging; LV, left ventricular; LVOTO, left ventricular outflow tract obstruction; ACE, angiotensin-converting enzyme

Flowchart 1 Management priorities in Takotsubo cardiomyopathy

altered peripheral sympathetic nerve activity associated with low PVR, which may warrant avoiding vasodilators such as ACE inhibitors. There is no clinical evidence for superiority of one specific drug over another, though studies in a novel animal model in our laboratory have suggested carvedilol may have a beneficial effect above other beta-blockers.[16] Beta-blockers may also reduce the risk of cardiac rupture.

Severe Cases with Cardiogenic Shock

Takotsubo cardiomyopathy with severe hemodynamic instability provides unique challenges (Flowchart 3). Urgent echocardiographic assessment is essential both to establish the degree of LV systolic impairment and crucially to define the presence or absence of dynamic LVOTO (which may have already been identified at cardiac catheterization by pull-back across the aortic valve). If LVOTO is identified, beta-blockers should be cautiously introduced to prolong diastolic filling time and increase in LV end-diastolic volume, reducing the LV outflow gradient and improving cardiac output, and electrical pacing of the right ventricular apex could be considered. In this situation, and in cases where the low cardiac output is associated with low PVR, afterload reduction with intravenous nitrates and ACE inhibitors can be detrimental and should be avoided (Flowchart 3).

Intra-aortic balloon counterpulsation (IABP) has hemodynamic benefit largely through afterload reduction in the systolic phase and improved coronary perfusion in the diastolic phase. Theoretically, it avoids complications of positive inotropy such as increased myocardial oxygen demand, though absolute benefit in patients with normal coronary arteries will be less than for those patients with cardiogenic shock in the context of myocardial infarction. Patient selection is critical if considering IABP, especially

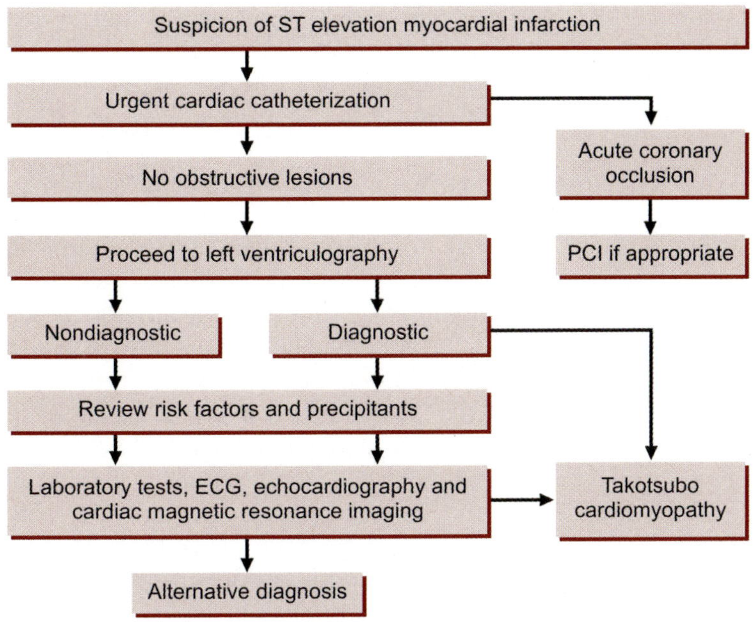

PCI, percutaneous coronary intervention

Flowchart 2 Diagnostic management algorithm for patients with suspected Takotsubo cardiomyopathy

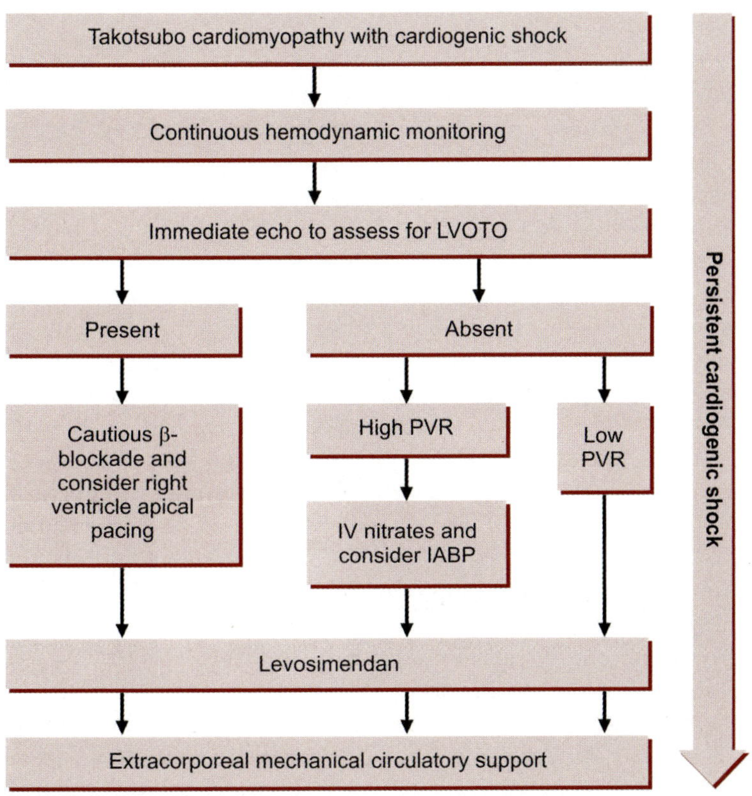

LVOTO, left ventricular outflow tract obstruction; PVR, peripheral vascular resistance; IABP, intra-aortic balloon counterpulsation

Flowchart 3 Management algorithm for patients with confirmed Takotsubo cardiomyopathy complicated by cardiogenic shock in light of recent neutral data from the Intra-aortic Balloon Support for Myocardial Infarction with Cardiogenic Shock (IABP-SHOCK) II trial, and given the theoretical risk (never described clinically in TTC) that IABP and afterload reduction could worsen dynamic LVOTO.

The decision to use sympathomimetic drugs for positive inotropy is challenging and counterintuitive in TTC. Given its etiology, further activation of catecholamine receptors or their downstream molecular pathways might worsen the LV dysfunction. In addition, dobutamine infusion may worsen dynamic LVOT obstruction, and many cases of dobutamine induced TTC have been described during stress protocols. In contrast, levosimendan is a positive inotrope that acts to sensitize cardiac myofilaments to calcium. Recent data shows levosimendan is safe to use in patients with TTC, and in our animal model it was shown to be effective rescue from cardiogenic shock.[16] Though further studies are necessary to define its role, levosimendan is our recommendation for inotropic drug therapy in TTC with cardiogenic shock. However, given its limited availability, medical practitioners may be forced to resort to alternatives (e.g., noradrenaline) as the only available inotrope until transfer to a tertiary center.

In patients with refractory cardiogenic shock and deteriorating multiorgan failure, there should be early referral for venoarterial extracorporeal membrane oxygenation (VA-ECMO) or for implantation of a left or biventricular assist device as a "bridge to recovery", given the ventricular function of these patients has an excellent chance of full recovery (Flowchart 3).

In the recovery phase, it is appropriate to introduce standard heart failure therapy as hemodynamics allow including ACE inhibitors, beta-blockers and potentially an aldosterone receptor antagonist.

Other Considerations

Takotsubo cardiomyopathy can be the herald for an underlying medical condition such as pheochromocytoma or intracranial pathologies, and consideration should be given to appropriate screening especially if the patient is young, male or has an atypical pattern of wall motion abnormality. Complete explanation of the diagnosis to the patient and appropriate communication with the primary care physician is essential. Patients must be aware that they have not suffered a "heart attack" and their primary care physician must be clear that—in the absence of comorbidities that would mandate it—there is no evidence to support long-term secondary prevention therapies started during an ACS protocol to target atherosclerosis.

PROGNOSIS AND OUTCOME

Takotsubo cardiomyopathy is an acute, reversible process and in the majority of cases the prognosis is excellent. LV systolic function on serial echocardiography improves over days to weeks, with one study showing resolution of mean EF from 20% to 60% by follow-up at mean of 21 days.[17] There are a proportion of patients who will have ongoing episodic chest pain (possibly up to 30%), and some will have a formal recurrence of TTC with varying frequency reported from 3.5% to 10%.[1]

However for a significant minority of patients the outcomes are less favorable. There is an in-hospital mortality of 0.5–1% and 30-day mortality of 5% associated with sudden cardiac death or cardiogenic shock and multiorgan failure.[2] Moreover, the potential of TTC to explain a cohort of stress-induced sudden cardiac death prior to hospitalization remains to be determined.

CONCLUSION

Takotsubo cardiomyopathy is a unique and intriguing syndrome that still frequently eludes diagnosis. Our understanding of TTC has increased exponentially over the past decade, with much greater clarity in approach to its diagnosis and best management. Ultimately, however, there remains only a partial awareness of TTC's true incidence in the emergency department, on the general medical take or in the catheter laboratory, and sparse clinical evidence for how to manage these patients. Coordinated epidemiological and pathophysiological studies will improve recognition, shed light on its mechanisms, and validate the theoretical and animal models that form the basis of our practice today. Our research group would be interested to review any confirmed or suspected cases of TTC, and be delighted to offer management advice regarding patients with this challenging condition.

KEY POINTS

- Takotsubo cardiomyopathy is an acute, reversible process most often seen in postmenopausal women and triggered by sudden catecholamine surge from an emotional or physical stress
- The presentation is suggestive of acute STEMI, but at cardiac catheterization the coronary arteries are

normal, and ventriculography shows a left ventricle resembling a Japanese octopus trap, the "takotsubo"

- There is a spectrum of disease from mild chest pain to refractory cardiogenic shock
- Management is aimed at supporting the hemodynamics until the abnormalities have resolved, employing mechanical circulatory support if necessary
- Acute complications are common, and in approximately 5–10% cases serious. However, prognosis is excellent in those surviving to discharge and the majority of patients make a complete recovery.

ACKNOWLEDGMENTS

Andrew C Morley-Smith is a British Heart Foundation Clinical Research Training fellow. Alexander R Lyon is a British Heart Foundation Intermediate Clinical Research fellow. Both authors are supported by the National Institute for Health Research Cardiovascular Biomedical Research Unit at the Royal Brompton Hospital.

REFERENCES

1. Gianni M, Dentali F, Grandi AM, et al. Apical ballooning syndrome or takotsubo cardiomyopathy: a systematic review. Eur Heart J. 2006;27(13):1523-9.
2. Schultz T, Shao Y, Redfors B, et al. Stress-induced cardiomyopathy in Sweden: evidence for different ethnic predisposition and altered cardio-circulatory status. Cardiology. 2012;122(3):180-6.
3. Eitel I, von Knobelsdorff-Brenkenhoff F, Bernhardt P, et al. Clinical characteristics and cardiovascular magnetic resonance findings in stress (takotsubo) cardiomyopathy. JAMA. 2011;306(3):277-86.
4. Kurisu S, Inoue I, Kawagoe T, et al. Time course of electrocardiographic changes in patients with tako-tsubo syndrome: comparison with acute myocardial infarction with minimal enzymatic release. Circ J. 2004;68(1):77-81.
5. Kurisu S, Inoue I, Kawagoe T, et al. Prevalence of incidental coronary artery disease in tako-tsubo cardiomyopathy. Coron Artery Dis. 2009;20(3):214-8.
6. Haghi D, Roehm S, Hamm K, et al. Takotsubo cardiomyopathy is not due to plaque rupture: an intravascular ultrasound study. Clin Cardiol. 2010;33(5):307-10.
7. Hoyt J, Lerman A, Lennon RJ, et al. Left anterior descending artery length and coronary atherosclerosis in apical ballooning syndrome (Takotsubo/stress induced cardiomyopathy). Int J Cardiol. 2010;145(1):112-5.
8. Delgado GA, Truesdell AG, Kirchner RM, et al. An angiographic and intravascular ultrasound study of the left anterior descending coronary artery in takotsubo cardiomyopathy. Am J Cardiol. 2011;108(6):888-91.
9. Naruse Y, Sato A, Kasahara K, et al. The clinical impact of late gadolinium enhancement in Takotsubo cardiomyopathy: serial analysis of cardiovascular magnetic resonance images. J Cardiovasc Magn Reson. 2012;13:67.
10. Monney PA, Sekhri N, Burchell T, et al. Acute myocarditis presenting as acute coronary syndrome: role of early cardiac magnetic resonance in its diagnosis. Heart. 2011;97(16):1312-8.
11. Madhavan M, Borlaug BA, Lerman A, et al. Stress hormone and circulating biomarker profile of apical ballooning syndrome (Takotsubo cardiomyopathy): insights into the clinical significance of B-type natriuetic peptide and troponin levels. Heart. 2009;95(17):1436-41.
12. Nguyen TH, Neil CJ, Sverdlov AL, et al. N-terminal pro-brain natriuretic protein levels in takotsubo cardiomyopathy. Am J Cardiol. 2011;108(9):1316-21.
13. Prasad A, Lerman A, Rihal CS. Apical ballooning syndrome (Tako-Tsubo or stress cardiomyopathy): a mimic of acute myocardial infarction. Am Heart J. 2008;155(3):408-17.
14. Omerovic E. How to think about stress-induced cardiomyopathy? –Think "out of the box"! Scand Cardiovasc J. 2011;45(2):67-71.
15. Madhavan M, Rihal CS, Lerman A, et al. Acute heart failure in apical ballooning syndrome (TakoTsubo/stress cardiomyopathy): clinical correlates and Mayo Clinic risk score. J Am Coll Cardiol. 2011;57(12):1400-1.
16. Paur H, Wright PT, Sikkel MB, et al. High levels of circulating epinephrine trigger apical cardiodepression in a â2-adrenergic receptor/Gi-dependent manner: a new model of Takotsubo cardiomyopathy. Circulation. 2012;126(6):697-706.
17. Wittstein IS, Thiemann DR, Lima JA, et al. Neurohumoral features of myocardial stunning due to sudden emotional stress. N Engl J Med. 2005;352(6):539-48.

Chapter 58

Myocarditis

Michel Noutsias

ABSTRACT

Acute myocarditis has a wide spectrum of clinical presentations. Moreover, the natural course of the disease can be highly diverse, spanning from spontaneous resolution to chronic dilated cardiomyopathy and death due to sudden cardiac death (SCD) or refractory heart failure. In addition to established clinical investigations (physical examination, blood sample analyses, echocardiography), cardiac magnetic resonance (CMR) imaging has gained substantial impact in the noninvasive diagnosis of myocarditis. The heart failure guidelines equally apply to clinically suspected myocarditis with reduced ejection fraction patients. The wearable cardioverter defibrillator is an acknowledged device, which prevents from SCD and from premature implantable cardioverter defibrillator implantation in light of the substantial potential of left ventricular ejection fraction improvement. Pericardial effusions in the context of myopericarditis respond to nonsteroidal anti-inflammatory drugs and/or colchicine. Contemporary endomyocardial biopsy (EMB) investigations, including the immunohistological detection of intramyocardial inflammation and the proof of viral genomes, are accredited as "diagnostic gold standard" for myocarditis. Recent research has identified the adverse prognostic impact of several clinical investigation parameters [New York Heart Association (NYHA) functional class III/IV, QRS 120 sec, sinus tachycardia, late gadolinium enhancement in CMR] and laboratory investigations (immunohistological proof of myocarditis in EMB, detectability of anticardiac antibodies). These parameters aid to segregate patient groups who need more close follow-up assessment. Several immunomodulatory studies have shown beneficial effects in selected patient groups. However, the results of multicenter investigations are needed to foster this evidence.

INTRODUCTION

From the clinicians' daily practice, myocarditis is often restricted to the clinical presentation of acute myocarditis (AMC). However, several developments have broadened the term of myocarditis to comprise both AMC and its chronic sequelae, namely dilated cardiomyopathy with inflammation (DCMi) as specific cardiomyopathy entity, being defined as cardiac dysfunction in association with myocarditis.[1] A meta-analysis calculated a transition rate of AMC to chronic dilated cardiomyopathy (DCM) of 21% within a follow-up time of 33 months.[2]

Several recent investigations on polymerase chain reaction (PCR) amplification of a given repertoire of viral genomes in endomyocardial biopsy (EMB) have suggested that the following of these viruses might be the leading causes of AMC and DCMi in the Western world: parvovirus B19 (B19V), human herpes-virus type 6 (HHV6), human herpes-virus type 7 (HHV7), Epstein-Barr virus (EBV), adenovirus (ADV), and enterovirus (EV). Of note, numerous other viruses, and infectious agents (bacteria, fungi, and protozoa), toxic agents, medications, physical conditions and systemic disorders affecting also the myocardium are known potential inducers of myocarditis (Table 1).

The three-phase model of coxsackie B virus (CBV)-induced murine myocarditis, which has been derived from experimental insights,[3,4] may be broadly valid also for the intricate processes involved in human virus-induced myocarditis. As summarized in figure 1, the initial viral infection induces the acute myocardial inflammation during AMC, which is pivotal for viral

TABLE 1: Infectious agents and toxic conditions associated with acute myocarditis, dilated cardiomyopathy with inflammation and dilated cardiomyopathy

Infectious agents	
Viruses	Adenovirus, arbovirus, arenavirus, coxsackievirus (especially coxsackie B virus), cytomegalovirus, dengue virus, echovirus, encephalomyocarditis, enteroviruses, Epstein-Barr virus, flavivirus, hepatitis A virus, hepatitis B virus, hepatitis C virus, herpes simplex virus, herpes zoster virus, human immunodeficiency virus, human herpes virus type 6 influenza virus, Junin virus, lymphocytic choriomeningitis virus, lyssavirus, measles virus, mumps virus, parvovirus B19, poliomyelitis virus, rabies virus, respiratory syncytial virus, rubella virus, rubeola virus, vaccinia virus, varicella-zoster virus, variola virus, yellow fever virus
Bacteria	*Actinomyces, Borrelia* species, *Brucella* species, *Chlamydia pneumoniae, Chlamydophila psittaci, Clostridium tetani, Corynebacterium diphtheriae, Coxiella burnetii, Francisella tularensis, Haemophilus influenzae, Legionella pneumophila, leptospira, Neisseria gonorrhoea, Meningococcus, Mycobacterium tuberculosis, Mycoplasma pneumoniae, Pneumococcus, Rickettsiae, Salmonella typhi, Serratia marcescens, Staphylococcus, Streptococcus pneumoniae, Streptococcus pyogenes, Treponema pallidum, Tropheryma whippelii, Vibrio cholerae*
Fungi	*Actinomyces* species, *Aspergillus, Blastomyces, Candida, Coccidioides, Cryptococcus, Histoplasma, mucormycosis, Nocardia, Sporothrix schenkii*
Protozoa	*Ascaris, Entamoeba histolytica*, echinococcosis, leishmaniasis, helminthic diseases, malaria, *Paragonimus westermani, Schistosoma* species, *Strongyloides stercoralis, Taenia solium, Trichinella spiralis, Toxoplasma gondii, trichinosis, Trypanosoma cruzi*, sleeping sickness/African trypanosomiasis, visceral larva migrans, *Wuchereria bancrofti*
Toxic conditions	
Animal toxic agents	Bee stings, wasp stings, scorpion bites, snake bites, spider bites
Medication	Acetazolamide, amitriptyline, aminophylline, amphotericin B, amphetamines, ampicillin, benzodiazepines, bumetanide, carbamazepine, catecholamines, cefaclor, cephalosporins, chemotherapeutics (especially anthracyclines), chloramphenicol, chlorthalidone, clozapine, colchicine, cocaine, cyclophosphamide, cyclosporine, dobutamine, ethanol, fluorouracil, furosemide, hemetine, hydralazine, hydrochlorothiazide, interleukin-2, isoniazid, lidocaine, lithium, metolazone, methyldopa, methysergide, nitroprusside, oxyphenbutazone, para-aminosalicylic acid, penicillin, phenindione, phenylbutazone, phenytoin, reserpine, spironolactone, sulfadiazine, sulfamethoxypyridine, sulfisoxazole, sulfonylureas, streptomycin, tetracycline, thiazides, triazolam, trastuzumab, tricyclic antidepressants
Physical conditions	Catecholamines, various cytokines (i.e., tumor necrosis factor, interleukin-2), electric shock, hyperpyrexia, radiation, sepsis
Toxic agents	Alcohol, arsenic, carbon monoxide, copper, diverse inhalants, iron, lead, lithium, phosphorus, tetanus toxoid
Cardiac involvement in systemic disorders	Celiac disease, Churg–Strauss syndrome, collagen-vascular diseases, inflammatory bowel disease, diabetes mellitus, hypereosinophilia, Kawasaki's disease, myasthenia gravis, polymyositis, sarcoidosis, scleroderma, systemic lupus erythematosus, thyrotoxicosis, Wegener's granulomatosis

The table is not deemed to present all known or suspected associations with acute myocarditis, dilated cardiomyopathy with inflammation, and dilated cardiomyopathy completely. In parts, the associations are based on case reports only, and a robust "proof of principle" causative relationship or pathogenic pathway is not established[4]

elimination, and which is not permanently detrimental to myocardial contractility. Following, some parallels being evident both for experimental murine and human AMC will be highlighted.

After acute viral infection, accompanied by viremia, with rise of antiviral IgM antibodies, a seroconversion to persisting antiviral IgG antibodies occurs. The evolution of the humoral antiviral immune response is paralleled by a substantial decrease of viral loads.[3,5,6] Myocardial expression of viral receptors [i.e., the coxsackie-adenovirus receptor (CAR)] may facilitate myocardial infection.[7,8] Depression of cardiac contractility is exerted among others by cytokines,[9] remodeling of the extracellular matrix,[10] and by myocytolysis carried out by cytotoxic T lymphocytes (CTL).[11,12] Cellular infiltration of the heart is orchestrated by cell adhesion molecules (CAM), which are induced by cytokines, and are expressed on endothelial cells and on leukocytes.[13-15] Malignant arrhythmias [sudden cardiac death (SCD); associated with strenuous exercise] and fulminant cardiac failure contribute to mortality during AMC.[16-19]

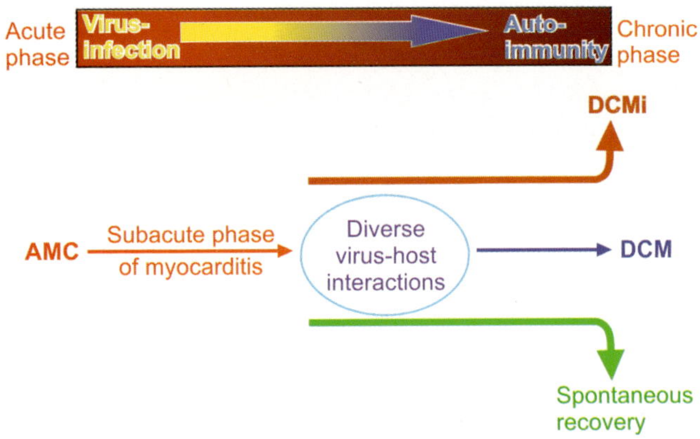

AMC, acute myocarditis; DCM, dilated cardiomyopathy; DCMi: dilated cardiomyopathy with inflammation

Fig. 1 Pathogenesis of virus-induced acute cardiomyopathy and its transition to either dilated cardiomyopathy with inflammation/dilated cardiomyopathy or to spontaneous resolution[4]

Immunosuppressive treatment irrespective of the dynamics of viral infection is rather detrimental at the early stage of AMC.[20,21]

During the subacute phase after AMC, highly complex interactions of the adaptive and the innate immune response, including direct cytopathic effects of the virus, virus-induced anticardiac immune responses, and the host's genetic susceptibility for the detrimental outcome of this intricate network, are decisively involved to guide the development to either spontaneous recovery, or to incomplete recovery and manifestation of DCM. The maladaptive general heart failure pathways gain importance in the chronic stage of the disease, and superimpose to the cardiodepressive effects of the detrimental immune regulation, and of relevant viral persistence. DCMi is characterized by low-level intramyocardial inflammation, accompanied by low-level persistence of viral loads in the absence of viremia.[3,14,22] In addition to cellular inflammation, anticardiac autoantibodies, which are possibly induced by molecular mimicry, are prevalent both in the chronic phase experimental murine myocarditis and human DCMi.[23-25] Although animal experiments provide important details on these intricate processes of immune and gene expression regulation,[26] these insights did not have substantial impact on the clinicians' practice and decisions, up-to-date. However, they are indispensable to explain the network which is responsible for the diverse outcomes after AMC, and especially the detrimental transition from AMC to DCMi. Overall, these insights convey the main message that after the initial cardiotropic viral infection during AMC, the resolution to the healed status after myocarditis is accompanied by an efficient immune mediated viral elimination, a decrement of the intramyocardial inflammation, and the noninitiation of anticardiac autoimmunity. In contrast, transition to DCMi is paralleled by the development of anticardiac autoimmunity, persistence of low-level intramyocardial inflammation, and possibly also viral persistence (Fig. 1).

EPIDEMIOLOGY

For human AMC, no detailed epidemiological survey is available, which is due to frequently insidious clinical presentations, and mainly due to inestimable subclinical courses. In a systematic investigation over 20 years carried out on 672,672 Finish young men at military service, an incidence of 0.17/1,000 man-year of AMC with acute myocardial infarction (AMI) presentation was reported, while the incidence for DCM like presentation accounted 0.02/1,000 man-years.[27] In another survey, the prevalence of DCM was calculated 29 per 10^6 persons/year, and the prevalence accounted 131 cases per 10^6 persons/year.[28] DCM is the leading indication for heart transplantation.[29] Myocarditis can be histologically confirmed in 10–20% of adult SCD cases at age less than 35 years.[19,30,31]

CLINICAL PRESENTATION

Acute myocarditis patients can present with a diverse spectrum of clinical scenarios: with an AMI-like situation, chest discomfort, arrhythmias, acute heart failure, palpitations, syncope or SCD (Fig. 2). AMC patients may report an antecedent (days to few weeks) flulike illness with respiratory or gastrointestinal tract infection before the onset of AMC symptoms. However, AMC may be missed frequently due to subclinical or virtually absent symptoms.[2,32-35] In AMC with preserved systolic function [myocarditis with preserved ejection fraction (MCPEF)], regional wall motion abnormalities, diastolic dysfunction, wall edema and pulmonary effusions (PEs) may be detected by echocardiography and by cardiac magnetic resonance (CMR) imaging. AMC can also present as new onset DCM. AMC with reduced left ventricular ejection fraction (LVEF) [myocarditis with reduced ejection fraction (MCREF)] is dominated by chronic and often progressive heart failure (CHF) symptoms (i.e., dyspnea on exertion or at rest, peripheral edema). Cardiomegaly, pulmonary congestion/edema and pleural effusions are frequently observed in chest X-ray.

Systolic and diastolic dysfunction, LV- or biventricular dilatation can be confirmed by echocardiography. LV-thrombi can cause thromboembolic complications. In the absence of troponin and/or creatine phosphokinase (CPK) elevations, a clear differentiation of MCREF and chronic DCM based on clinical investigations alone can be difficult or impossible. Further diagnostic procedures such as CMR and EMB, as well as the consideration of the further natural course of the disease under heart failure medication are needed to differentiate these distinct diseases.[4] The most severe presentation of MCREF is acute fulminant myocarditis (AFMC). By definition, inotropic support with high doses of catecholamines is required for this status.[18]

Both MCPEF and MCREF can present with various types of electrocardiography (ECG) abnormalities [right or left bundle branch block, ST-segment depression, Q-wave and T-wave inversions, atrioventricular (AV) block] and rhythm disturbances on Holter monitoring (sinus tachycardia/bradycardia, supra-/ventricular extrasystoles, atrial fibrillation/flutter and ventricular tachycardia/flutter/fibrillation). AMC is a frequent cause of SCD; up to 40% especially in the young, and is often associated with strenuous physical exertion.[17,19]

PROGNOSIS

Highly heterogeneous clinical courses have been observed after AMC, spanning from complete or partial healing, to indications for cardiac transplantation and lethal outcomes due to SCD and refractory end stage DCM (Fig. 2). Transition of AMC to DCM/DCMi has been reported in 20% of the patients.[2,36] This transition may be accompanied by recurrent myocarditis events.[37,38] After AMC, transplantation-free survival has been determined as 78% within a mean follow-up of 59 + 42 months.[15] This is not different compared with the survival of DCM patients.[39]

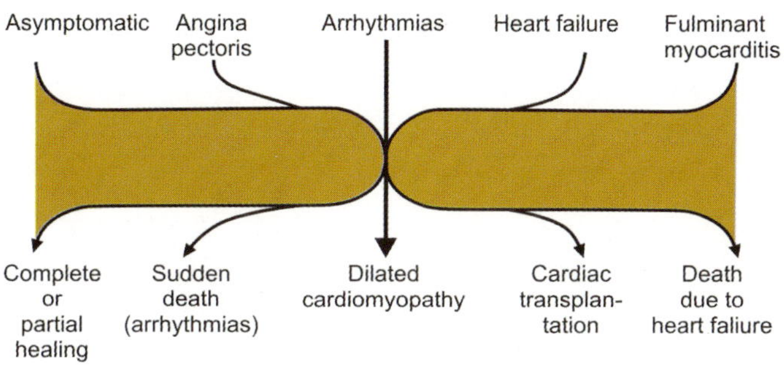

Fig. 2 Clinical presentation and outcomes of acute myocarditis[2]

The initial LVEF, LV end-diastolic pressure and left ventricular end-diastolic diameter (LVEDD) have no independent prognostic relevance in AMC,[15,18,40,41] which can be explained by the known highly variable natural courses of the disease.[2,4]

Recent research has elucidated the prognostic relevance of several clinical, CMR and EMB parameters for MCREF patients:

- The immunohistological proof of myocarditis/DCMi, which was present in 50% of the n = 181 consecutive MCREF patients, was one of the three independent prognostic parameters for adverse outcome (SCD, indication for heart transplantation and refractory end stage heart failure) [hazard ratio (HR): 3.46; 95% confidence interval (CI): 1.39–8.62; $p = 0.008$][15]
- New York Heart Association (NYHA) functional class III–IV at the initial clinical presentation was a further independent prognostic condition for adverse outcome in the above mentioned prospective investigation (HR: 3.20; 95% CI: 1.36–7.57; $p = 0.008$).[15] In a further prospective study, any New York Heart Association functional class greater than I proved as an independent predictor for incomplete recovery after myocarditis ($p = 0.03$)[41]
- The absence of beta blockers in CHF medication was the third independent prognostic condition for adverse outcome in the above mentioned study (HR: 0.43; 95% CI: 0.21–0.91; $p = 0.027$)[15]
- A prolonged QRS duration more than or equal to 120 msec proved as independent prognostic parameter for adverse outcome in a further analysis of this prospective study on n = 186 consecutive myocarditis patients (HR: 2.83; CI: 1.07–7.49; $p = 0.012$). A QTc prolongation more than or equal to 440 msec, an abnormal QRS axis, and premature ventricular beats, while showing significance in monovariate analysis, were not robust independent predictors in multivariate analysis.[42] The independent negative prognostic impact of QRS prolongation more than 110 msec was also confirmed in a further study on DCM patients[43]
- Reduced mean arterial blood pressure (MAP) less than 87 mmHg was independently associated with an adverse outcome in a prospective analysis on n = 175 myocarditis patients (HR: 2.58; 95% CI: 1.26–5.08; $p < 0.001$).[44] This was also true for the systolic arterial blood pressure less than 115 mmHg and for the diastolic arterial blood pressure less than 70 mmHg
- In a subgroup analysis (n = 62 patients without beta-blocker treatment, atrial fibrillation or pacemaker) of the before mentioned study, a high heart rate in

sinus rhythm more than 78/min was also associated with poor outcome (HR = 2.92, 95% CI = 1.02–8.29, p = 0.045)[44]

- Late gadolinium enhancement as detected by CMR proved as independent prognostic factor for adverse outcome in a study enclosing n = 184 DCM patients (HR: 3.4; 95% CI: 1.26–9). Late gadolinium enhancement (LGE) fraction of more than 4.4% of LV mass was determined as optimal discriminator for the composite end point (cardiac death, hospitalization due to decompensated heart failure, or appropriate implantable cardioverter defibrillator (ICD)-shock) by receiver operated characteristics-area under the curve (ROC-AUC). A stratification subanalysis revealed that the predictive relevance of LGE was confined to DCM patients with LVEF more than 30%. This subanalysis also identified those DCM patients with LVEF more than 30% without LGE did not experience higher rates of composite end point compared with the remaining subgroups.[45] The negative predictive role of CMR detected LGE has been also confirmed for patients with EMB confirmed myocarditis. In n = 203 consecutive patients, LGE was significantly associated with all-cause mortality (HR: 8.4) and with cardiac mortality (HR: 12.8), independent of clinical symptoms. Interestingly, no patient without LGE experienced SCD, and LGE was the best predictor for SCD (HR: 12.8; $p < 0.01$)[41]
- A further prospective study revealed the negative prognostic impact of inflammatory parameters for DCM patients with LVEF less than or equal to 45% and LVEDD more than 70 mm (41.7% vs 13.6%; HR: 1.14; p = 0.04)
- Acute fulminant myocarditis is defined by an AMC presentation with depressed LVEF requiring high doses of vasopressors (>5 µg of dopamine or dobutamine/kg/min, or indication for left ventricular assist device (LVAD) support, and more than or equal to two of the following clinical features: fever, distinct onset of symptoms of heart failure (fatigue, dyspnea on exertion or at rest, or edema that could be dated specifically to a one-to-two-day period), and a history consistent with the presence of a viral illness within the two weeks before hospitalization.[46] In a prospective study on n = 147 patients with EMB proven myocarditis (Dallas criteria), the 15 AFMC patients had an excellent long-term survival: while 93% of the AFMC patients were alive at 11 years follow-up time (HR for death or cardiac transplantation: 0.10; 95% CI: 0.01–0.88), only 45% of the remaining AMC patients were alive[18]

DIAGNOSIS

Endomyocardial Biopsy Technique

Endomyocardial biopsy can be obtained by venous or arterial percutaneous approach from the right ventricular (RV) septum or from the LV. Complications of EMBs obtainment are fairly rare in experienced centers, and serious periprocedural complications have been reported less than 0.5% in various studies.[15,47,48] LV-EMB may yield more diagnostic results compared to RV-EMB, however, the highest diagnostic yields were achieved by biventricular EMB procedures.[49] This investigation also contradicted previous reports, and did not confirm the notion of EMB obtainment guided by CMR/LGE.[49,50]

Histology of Endomyocardial Biopsy

By histological hematoxylin and eosin (HE) stainings, "active" (interstitial infiltrates with myocytolysis with/without fibrosis; Fig. 3) and borderline myocarditis (increased infiltrates with/without fibrosis) can be diagnosed according to the Dallas criteria.[51] However, myocarditis can be revealed only in a minority of the patients by histological assessment (5–20%).[14,52] Histological assessment of myocarditis is hampered by the substantial sampling error and interobserver-variability.[53-55] The Dallas criteria are neither relevant for prognostic assessment, nor the selection of patients

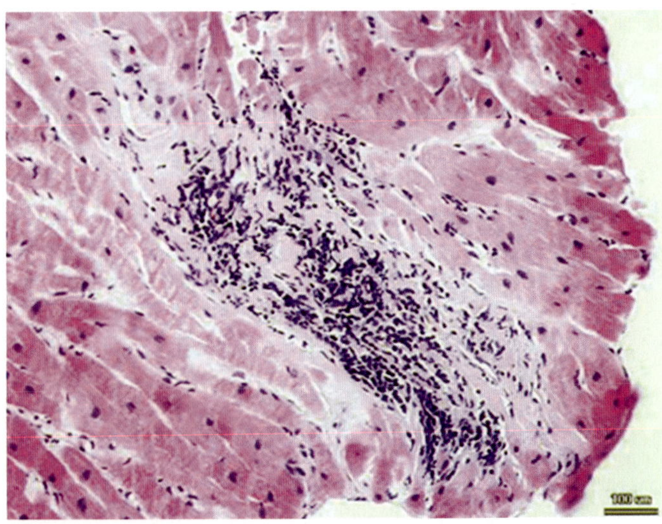

Fig. 3 Histological proof of myocarditis. Focal lymphomononuclear infiltrates with adjacent myocytolysis (active myocarditis; original magnification 200×)[58]

who benefit from immunosuppression.[15,39] However, histological EMB evaluation is essential for the diagnosis of further specific pathologies (i.e., giant cell myocarditis, myocardial storage diseases).[56-58]

Immunohistology of Endomyocardial Biopsy

By targeting specific epitopes with antibodies, immunohistology enables the specific detection and exact quantification of infiltrates and their detailed phenotypic characterization. Moreover, abundance of endothelial CAM expression has evolved to a further cornerstone of the immunohistological EMB assessment for myocarditis and DCMi.[14,15,59] The homogeneous CAM expression pattern likely reduces the sampling error.[14,60,61] Sarcolemmal expression of major histocompatibility complex (MHC) may be a suitable standalone criterion for the selection of DCM patients who benefit from immunosuppression.[60,62] Two immunohistological diagnostic concepts are available: more than 7.0 $CD3^+$/$CD2^+$ lymphocytes/mm^2 myocardial tissue area and concurrent abundance of several CAMs,[14,63] and furthermore more than 14.0 leukocytes/mm^2 with facultative CAMs abundance.[50,64-69] Intramyocardial inflammation can be detected in 50% of the AMC and DCM patients using these immunohistological concepts. Digital image analysis is a suitable standardization tool of the evaluation of immunohistological EMB stainings.[70] Representative findings of immunohistological EMB stainings are demonstrated in Figure 4.

The immunohistological proof of myocarditis has adverse prognostic impact in AMC patients.[15,44] More importantly, this diagnostic concept has proven suitable to select DCMi patients who will likely benefit from immunosuppression treatment.[60,67] These are the two major advantages of the immunohistological versus the histological proof of myocarditis in EMB.

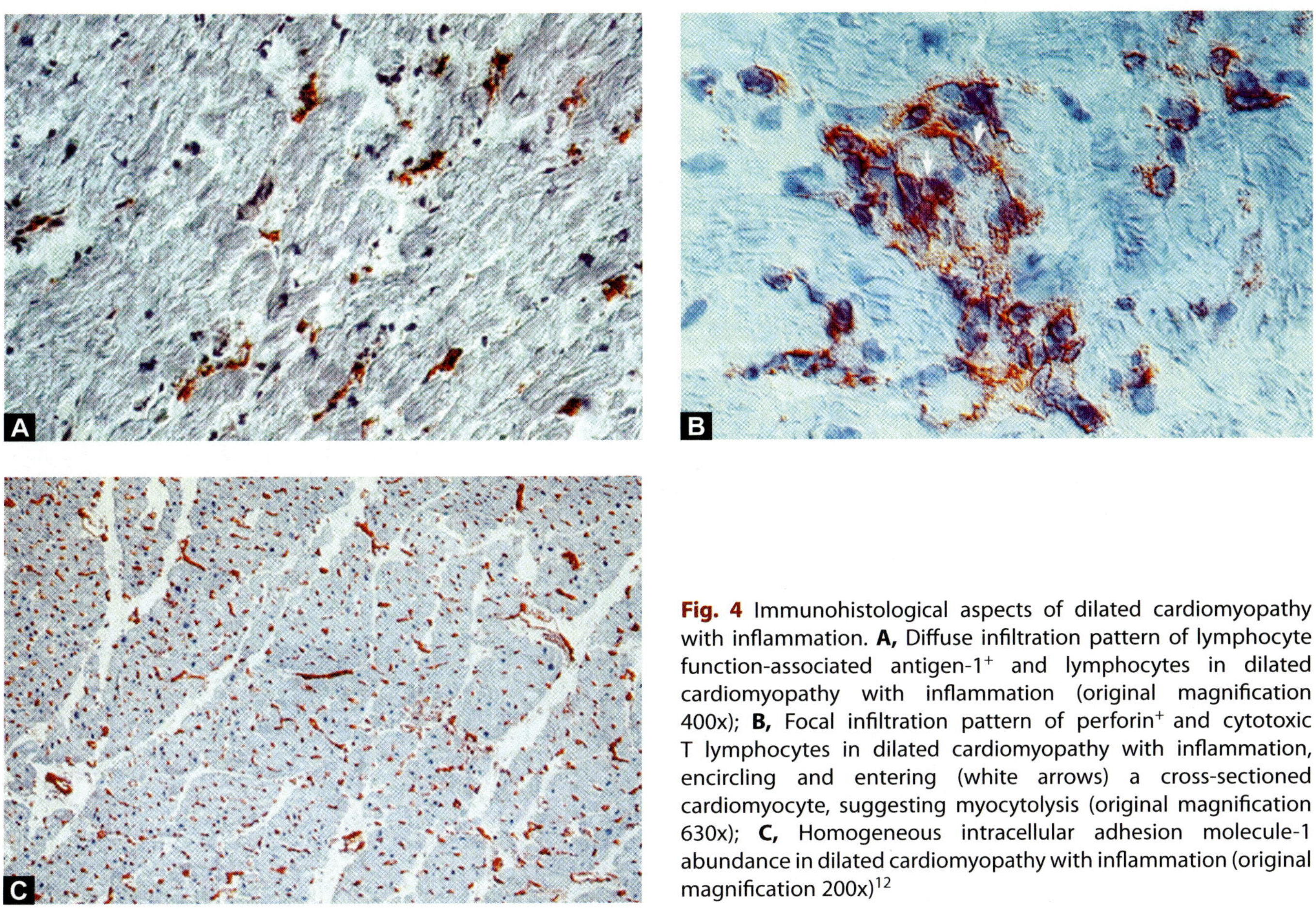

Fig. 4 Immunohistological aspects of dilated cardiomyopathy with inflammation. **A,** Diffuse infiltration pattern of lymphocyte function-associated antigen-1^+ and lymphocytes in dilated cardiomyopathy with inflammation (original magnification 400x); **B,** Focal infiltration pattern of $perforin^+$ and cytotoxic T lymphocytes in dilated cardiomyopathy with inflammation, encircling and entering (white arrows) a cross-sectioned cardiomyocyte, suggesting myocytolysis (original magnification 630x); **C,** Homogeneous intracellular adhesion molecule-1 abundance in dilated cardiomyopathy with inflammation (original magnification 200x)[12]

Virological Analyses of Endomyocardial Biopsy

The various infectious, toxic agents and further conditions, which have been etiologically associated with myocarditis are summarized in Table 1. It is assumed that the majority of AMC cases are induced by viral infections in the Western World in light of the often close preceding gastrointestinal or respiratory tract infections. PCR is the dominant technique of viral genome detection in EMB. The disease specificity of coxsackievirus/EV has been confirmed by meta-analysis.[71] EV/coxsackievirus B (CVB) infection has shown negative prognostic impact in one prospective investigation: In a cohort of 120 consecutive DCM patients, the 34% patients with PCR proven EV RNA in EMB were characterized by a statistically independent worse prognosis.[40] In a further prognostic study, EV replication was associated with adverse outcome after partial left ventriculotomy of DCM patients, which, however, does not reflect the natural course of the disease.[72] In a highly selected patient group, subjects with viral elimination over a follow-up period of 6 months demonstrated a significant improvement of LVEF, as opposed to further decrement observed in patients with EMB proven viral persistence.[73] EV persistence has been associated with significantly higher mortality compared to patients with EV elimination during the natural course of the disease.[74] However, the recent prospective studies failed to confirm any prognostic relevance of the detection of viral genomes by PCR at the initial presentation (including i.e. B19V, HHV6, ADV, EBV).[15,41,75] The lack of prognostic relevance of the detection of these viral genomes in EMB may be due to numerous factors, among others the negligence of viral loads especially for B19V,[76-78] and the lack of disease specificity of B19V genomes for AMC and DCM.[79,80] In fact, the "bioportfolio" role of lifelong persisting B19V genomes is well acknowledged for various tissues,[81] and is thus expectedly not different for myocardial tissues.[79,80] The clinical relevance of the mere B19V genome detection in EMB from AMC and DCM patients by PCR without proof of myocardial active infection is therefore controversial. The dynamics of dramatically decreasing B19V viral copies both in blood mononuclear cells and in EMB after acute B19V viremia and associated myocarditis can be witnessed, and a discernible type-1 anti-B19V-specific T-cell response is detectable in rare, exceptional cases.[76] The differentiation of the infection stage specific B19V antibody profiles as well as the classical seroconversion from IgM to IgG might prove helpful in this regard.[5,82,83] Nonetheless, in light of the multiple infectious agents which have been associated with myocarditis (Table 1), it appears possible that the majority of more disease specific viruses as compared to B19V, which account for the majority of viral genome detection with the "common PCR repertoire" used by several researchers in the past decade, may have been missed in these analyses and are therefore largely unknown.

Cardiac Magnetic Resonance Diagnosis of Myocarditis

Cardiac magnetic resonance has evolved to a well-acknowledged diagnostic tool for myocarditis.[50,84-86] The various diagnostic CMR parameters gave rise to the consensus "Lake Louise" criteria,[87] which require at least two of the following three parameters to be present:

1. At least one LGE focus with nonischemic regional distribution.
2. Early gadolinium enhancement ratio between myocardium and skeletal muscle in gadolinium-enhanced T1-weighted images.
3. Regional or global myocardial signal intensity increase in T2-weighted images.

The presence of LV dysfunction or PE provides additional, supportive evidence for myocarditis in the setting of CMR diagnosis. Further infrequent findings such as LV thrombus can be observed.[88]

Late gadolinium enhancement plays a major diagnostic role in CMR analyses. In AMC and DCM, the LGE pattern is typically subepicardial, has no association to ischemic regional distribution, and is often present in the lateral wall and midventricular within the septum.[89,90]

It is recommended to repeat CMR studies between 1 and 2 weeks after the initial CMR study in the case none of the criteria are present, but the onset of symptoms has been very recent and there is strong clinical evidence for myocardial inflammation.[87] The dynamics of inflammation and/or interstitial fibrosis can be evidenced by CMR (Fig. 5), as well as of LVEF and LV dilatation.[88,91,92] A high synergy between EMB diagnostics and LGE as assessed by CMR has been described.[68] However, viral genomes cannot be specifically detected by CMR.[86]

As described above in detail in the chapter "Prognosis", LGE as detected by CMR has proven as independent prognostic factor for adverse long-term prognosis in AMC and DCM patients, including all-cause mortality, cardiac mortality, and SCD.[41,45] The body of evidence supporting

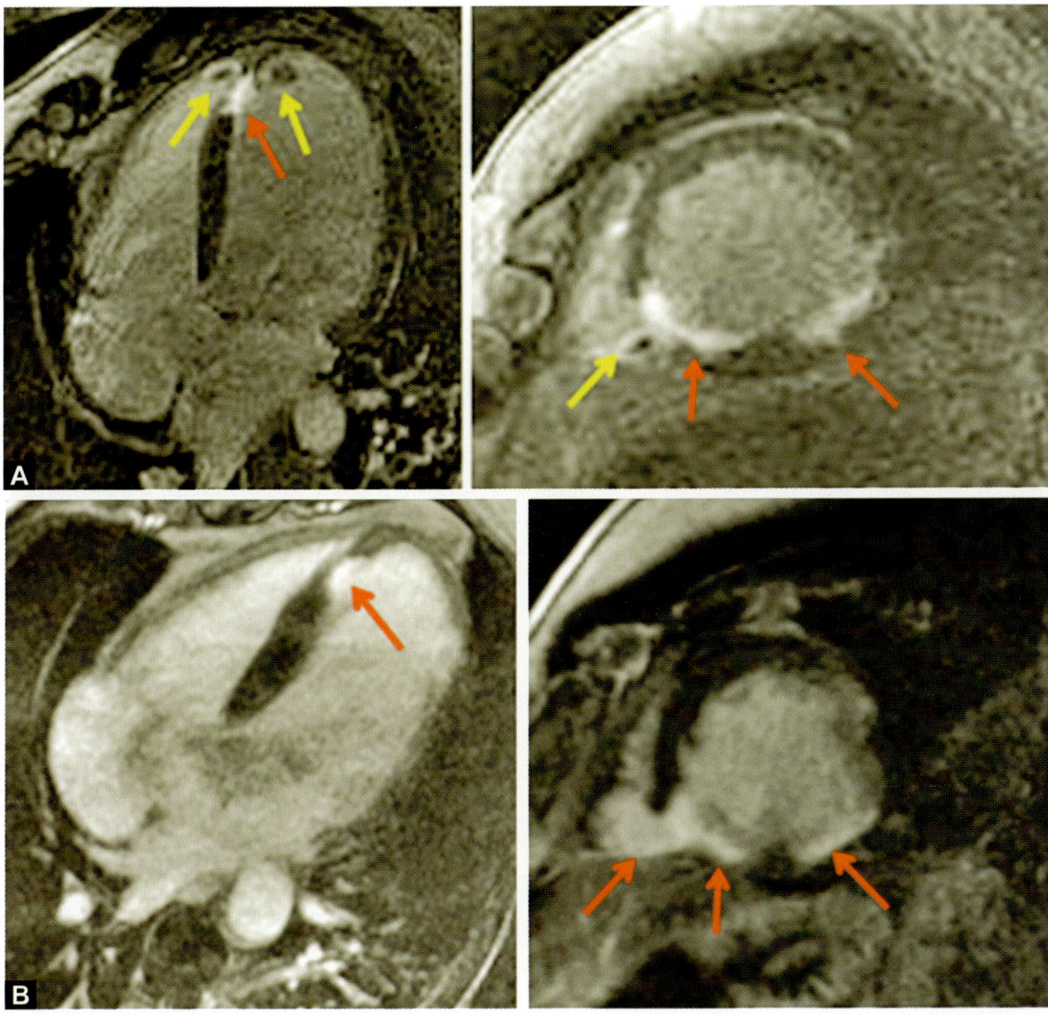

Fig. 5 Dynamics of cardiac magnetic resonance findings in myocarditis. **A,** Magnetic resonance imaging in the acute phase of myocarditis with reduced ejection fraction with left ventricular ejection fraction: 17% in a 39-year-old male patient. Late gadolinium enhancement in the apical, inferoseptal and inferolateral segments (red arrows), as well as thrombi in the right ventricular and the left ventricular (yellow arrows); **B,** Follow-up magnetic resonance image 8 weeks after the initial presentation; left ventricular ejection fraction improved to 38%. Persisting late gadolinium enhancement in the apical, inferoseptal and inferolateral segments (red arrows), indicating left ventricular scar formation. The left ventricular thrombi were not detectable at this stage under anti-coagulation[77]

the clinical relevance of detection and monitoring AMC and DCM by CMR is consolidated.

Autoantibodies

A variety of autoantibodies targeting various myocardial structures has been described for AMC and DCM patients.[4] The detectability of anticardiac autoantibodies has been associated with adverse prognosis in AMC patients.[93] The IgG3 fraction of antibodies might be more important for adverse outcomes of DCM.[94,95] However, disease specificity and "proof of principle" status is controversial for most of these anticardiac antibodies. An interesting model postulated binding of autoantibodies to the Fc receptor of the cardiomyocytes, which thereby induce negative inotropic effects, and eventually contribute to heart failure.[96] So far, no panel of autoantibodies are widely recommended for myocarditis patients, nor are standardized tests widely available for screening approaches.

TREATMENT

Clinical Management and Conventional Heart Failure Treatment; Sudden Cardiac Death Prevention

Patients should be interviewed for the onset and dynamics of their symptoms, and for potentially antecedent viral illness events (mostly respiratory or gastrointestinal tract infections). ST-segment deviations, Q waves, AV block, QRS prolongation and arrhythmias should be documented by ECG. At least one Holter ECG should be considered to detect any arrhythmias, especially AV blocks and/or ventricular tachycardias, since these might be indicative for giant-cell myocarditis.[57] Raised parameters of myocardial damage (creatine kinase, creatine kinase MB, troponins) and indicators of heart failure (natriuretic peptides) are important for the clinical diagnosis of AMC, and may be helpful to differentiate AMC from DCM.[4] However, these parameters have no substantial prognostic impact.[41,97] Monitoring of these patients and telemetry is often applied for this acute stage of overt cardiomyocyte damage; however, we are lacking data confirming a rationale for this measure. The white blood cell count (WBCc; >11Gpt/L) has shown prognostic relevance for DCM patients with LVEDD >70 mm, and might be therefore implemented in the prognostic assessment of the patients. For the laboratory testing, a differential blood analysis should be implemented to cover the rare, but treatable cases with eosinophilic or hypersensitivity myocarditis.[98,99] In the context with myocarditis, echocardiography is mandatory to assess global systolic LV function, regional wall motion abnormalities, edema of the septum, LV thrombus and PE.

For MCPEF, the general prognosis is good.[52] No controlled study is available that favors specific treatment. Off-label use of angiotensin-converting enzyme inhibitor/angiotensin II receptor antagonist (ACEI/ARB) and diuretics to treat heart failure symptoms, and of long-acting nitrates to improve angina pectoris symptoms, may be considered. Beta-blockers and/or ivabradine might be considered for heart rate more than 78/min,[44] especially in cases with sinus tachycardia.

The general guidelines for the treatment of heart failure equally apply to MCREF and DCM, including assist devices and cardiac transplantation as ultima ratio.[100,101] Identified potential cardiotoxic agents (i.e., alcohol, anthracyclines) should be discontinued.[102] In cases with PE (myopericarditis), specific management and treatment should follow the respective recommendations.[103,104]

In AFMC patients, LVEF usually improves dramatically, and LVEDD decreases, and may even normalize under heart failure regimens, with an excellent long-term outcome as compared to lymphocytic myocarditis with mildly or moderately impaired LVEF.[18] Mechanical support inventions such as LVAD, extracorporeal membrane oxygenation (ECMO) or continuous flow pumps (i.e., Impella® pump) may be necessary to bridge this critical status.[105] These invasive supportive solutions may be especially rewarding for the case of AFMC considering the excellent long-term outcome of this specific patient subgroup.[18,106]

Acute myocarditis/dilated cardiomyopathy patients should be followed regularly by clinical assessment and noninvasive examinations, including echocardiography and CMR.[87] Especially in cases with deterioration of LV function parameters, or with failure of improvement despite complete heart failure medication (i.e., within 2 weeks), EMBs should be obtained in these patients and subjected to contemporary diagnostic techniques, preferably in experienced centers.[57] In subjects with high-grade AV block or ventricular tachycardia, giant cell myocarditis must be considered in this particular setting. For the rare cases of giant cell myocarditis detected by EMB, immunosuppressive treatment with corticosteroids and azathioprine or anti-CD3 antibodies is mandatory to prevent from the known deleterious short-term prognosis.[52,56]

Immunomodulatory treatment should be considered especially in such cases not responding to standard CHF care, preferably in experienced centers and/or in the framework of multicenter studies.

Exercise should be avoided during the first weeks after AMC, since SCD is associated with strenuous physical activity.[19,27,107,108] The issue of SCD prevention in the context of AMC primarily affects MCREF; however, SCD can occur in MCPEF patients as well. Although we are lacking precise data on this particular setting, this conclusion may be deduced by the numerous SCD victims during competitive sports, in whom myocarditis was clinically suspected or diagnosed postmortem, and who evidently would not have been able to participate in these athletic events in the presence of heart failure symptoms.[17,109] Absence of strenuous physical activity is therefore highly recommended during the first weeks after AMC regardless of LVEF or NYHA functional class.[4,110,111] Implantation of ICD for primary prevention of SCD is not recommended in AMC/MCREF, as also in every newly diagnosed CHF case of less than 3-month duration, since LVEF can improve substantially during the natural course of the disease under complete CHF medication.[112] Wearable cardioverter defibrillator (WCD) has proven efficacious in primary SCD prevention in new onset DCM, protecting during and bridging the recommended period of 3 months after newly diagnosed DCM.[113,114] The WCD may also possibly prevent from the dilemma of premature ICD implantations in MCREF, especially in AFMC.[112,115] The consideration of WCD is currently recommended by the Heart Rhythm Society (HRS) for the primary SCD prevention for the first 3 months in newly diagnosed nonischemic cardiomyopathies with LVEF less than or equal to 35%.[116] If LVEF does not rise above 35% under continuously optimized standard CHF medication, ICD implantation[117] must be considered after these initial 3 months of WCD bridging. The feasibility and rationale of this algorithm in new onset DCM has been demonstrated in the wearable defibrillator use in heart failure (WIF) registry.[114] A further finding with relevance for SCD prediction may be LGE by CMR, since no SCD events were observed in myocarditis patients without LGE.[41]

The algorithm summarizing these diagnostic and disease management pathways is illustrated in flowchart 1.

Genetic counseling and noninvasive cardiological screening (ECG, echocardiography) is advisable in patients with familial DCM and their first-degree relatives.[118] In a consensus report of the HRS and the European Heart Rhythm Association (EHRA), genetic testing [comprehensive or targeted approach for Lamin A/C (LMNA) and cardiac sodium ion channel (SCN5A) mutations] is recommended for DCM patients with significant cardiac conduction disease (i.e. first-, second-, or third-degree heart block) and/or a family history of premature SCD. Additionally, mutation-specific genetic testing is recommended for family members and relatives after identification of a DCM causative mutation in the index case.[119] Novel studies have aroused some concern on the monogenic pathogenicity of gene mutations

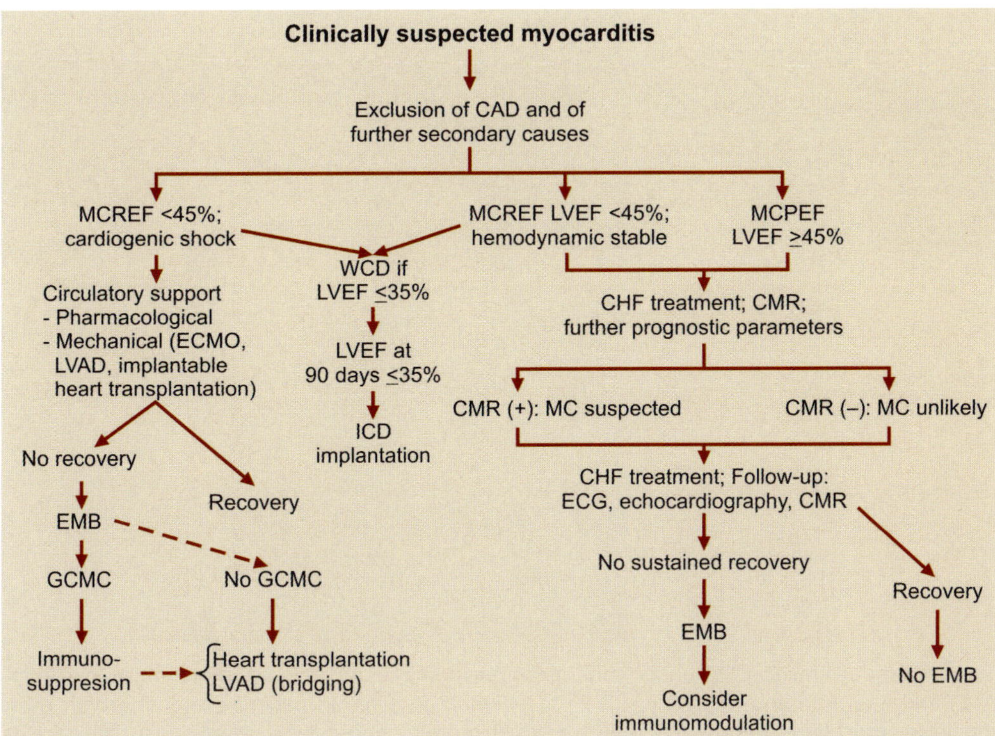

CAD, coronary artery disease; CMR, cardiac magnetic resonance imaging; EMB, endomyocardial biopsy; GCMC, giant cell myocarditis; ICD, implantable cardioverter defibrillator; LVAD, left ventricular assist device; LVEF, left ventricular ejection fraction; MCPEF, clinically suspected myocarditis with preserved ejection fraction; MCREF, clinically suspected myocarditis with reduced ejection fraction; WCD: wearable cardioverter defibrillator; ECMO, extracorporeal membrane oxygenation; CHF, congestive heart failure; MC, myocarditis

Flowchart 1 Management of myocarditis. Proposed algorithm of diagnosis and treatment of patients with clinically suspected myocarditis associated with cardiomyopathies.[120] Treatment of the phenotype, but counseling the genotype is a current concept in this regard.[121]

Immunomodulatory Treatment

The advance of immunomodulatory studies in the past decade has confirmed the vision that the analysis of pathogenic pathways, and the evolution of more refined EMB diagnostics, may ultimately translate to promising therapeutic regimens for myocarditis patients. Except for giant cell myocarditis, the indications for immunomodulation target primarily the chronic status of DCM (differentiated by contemporary EMB diagnostics as DCMi). In general, the natural course of AMC has to be awaited under conventional heart failure regimens. Since the major study endpoints target LVEF, LVEDD, NYHA functional class, need for cardiac transplantation and hospitalization, MCPEF patients are not included in immunomodulatory studies. The DCMi patients without substantial improvement of LVEF and/or CHF, usually after a period of 6 months, may be considered for ongoing clinical trials, registries or for off-label immunomodulation in expert centers. Immunomodulation may be considered also for DCMi patients who experience progressive deterioration of LVEF after MCPEF, or courses of recurrent myocarditis.

Immunosuppression: For histologically diagnosed giant cell myocarditis, immunosuppression is a clear indication, significantly reducing mortality, morbidity, need for cardiac transplantation and the giant cell inflammatory infiltrates (Fig. 6).[56,122,123]

Immunosuppression has proven beneficial effects in patients with immunohistologically confirmed

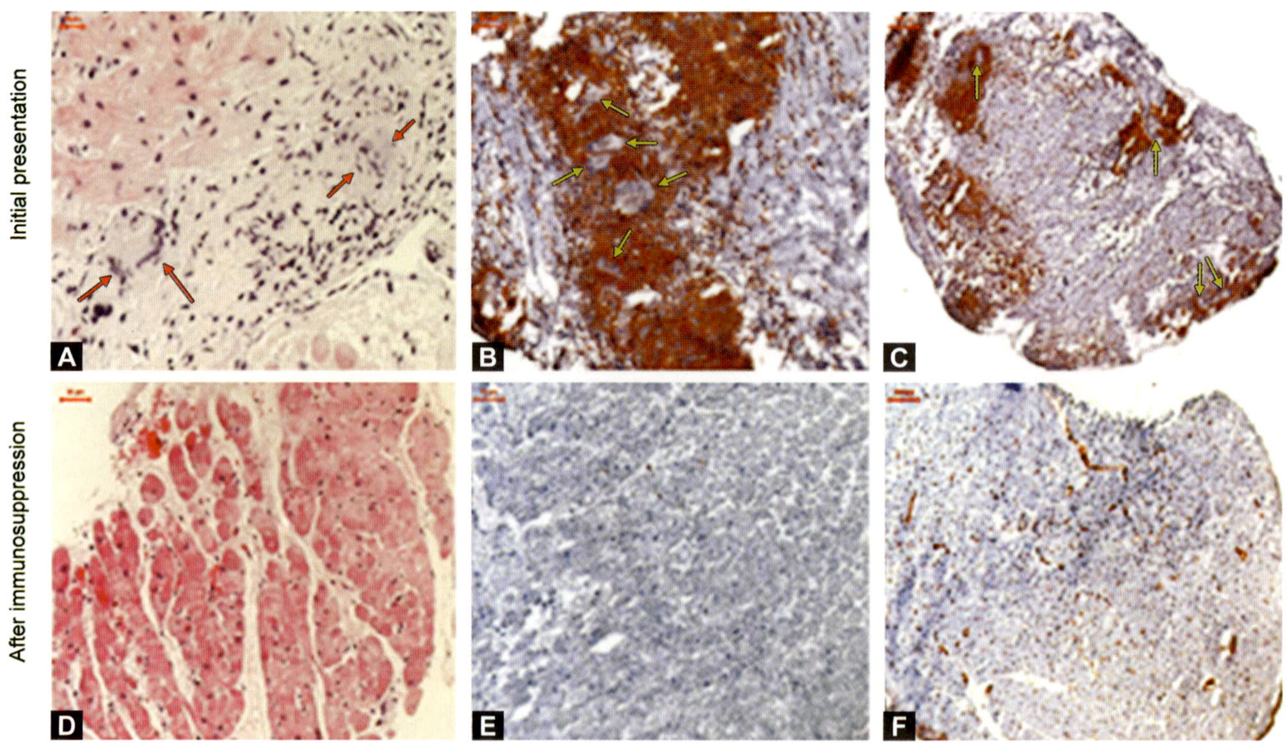

Fig. 6 Resolution of giant cell myocarditis under immunosuppression. Histological and immunohistological findings of EMBs at the initial EMBs (A–C) and after immunosuppression (D–F) in a female 51-year-old patient presenting with myocarditis with reduced ejection fraction, left ventricular ejection fraction 26% and polymorphic nonsustained ventricular tachycardias. **A,** Histology (H & E staining) demonstrated focal lymphocytic infiltration and multinucleated giant cells (arrows; 400x); **B,** Immunohistological staining of focal CD11a/lymphocyte function-associated antigen-1^+ (LFA-1^+) and lymphocytes with giant cells (arrows; 200x); **C,** Focal intracellular adhesion molecule-1 (ICAM-1) abundance pronounced in areas adjacent to giant cells (arrows; 100x); **D,** Histology in the follow-up of endocardial biopsy (EMBs) 6 months after immunosuppression, devoid of any giant cells (200x); **E,** Normal LFA-1^+ infiltration in the follow-up EMBs after immunosuppression (200x); **F,** Baseline ICAM-1 expression in the follow-up of EMBs after immunosuppression (100x)[112]

DCMi, especially in the context of excluded viral genome persistence, in two single center randomized investigations.[60,67]

Beneficial effects of immunosuppression were reported regarding NYHA functional class, LV dimensions and LVEF, and sustained for up to 2 years of follow-up. The immunosuppressive regimens were a 3-month treatment with prednisone (started at 1 mg/kg/day, tapered after off 12 days every 5 days by 5 mg/day until maintenance of 0.2 mg/kg/day for 90 days) and azathioprine (1 mg/kg/day for 100 days),[60] and a 6 months immunosuppressive protocol, respectively.[67] The study by Woijnicz et al. validated also the diagnostic accuracy of CAM abundance for DCMi even in the negligence of lymphocytic infiltration.[14,62] DCMi patients with viral persistence should not be subjected to immunosuppression due to potentially deleterious effects.[80,124] In the Tailored Immunosuppression in Inflammatory Cardiomyopathy (TIMIC) trial, immunosuppressive treatment with prednisone (1 mg/kg/day for 4 weeks, followed by 0.33 mg/kg/day for 5 months), combined with azathioprine (2 mg/kg/day for 6 months) in addition to conventional CHF therapy was associated with a substantial rise of LVEF from 26.5 ± 6.7% to 45.6 ± 9.6%, while the placebo treated group gradually deteriorated regarding LVEF (from 27.7 ± 5.6% to 21.3 ± 5.3%).[67] Immunosuppression is no therapeutic option in myocarditis diagnosed only according to the histological Dallas criteria, in the negligence of viral genome detection.[21,126] This progress highlights the importance of the immunohistological detection of DCMi compared with the histological Dallas criteria.

Intravenous Immunoglobulin Treatment

Intravenous immunoglobulins (IVIG) have multifaceted immunomodulatory (e.g., antiviral, immunoregulatory for overwhelming immune reactions targeting self-antigens) effects.[127-129] In acute DCM, the Intervention in Myocarditis and Acute Cardiomyopathy trial (IMAC; single administration of 2 g/kg IVIG; randomized study design) showed no beneficial effects of IVIG.[130] However, contemporary EMB diagnostics were not available in this study. In contrast, a 26-week course of IVIG treatment was paralleled by a significant improvement of LVEF from 26 ± 2% to 31 ± 3% ($p < 0.01$), and a marked rise of anti-inflammatory mediators [interleukin (IL)-10, IL-1 receptor antagonist] in CHF patients (both ischemic cardiomyopathy and DCM).[131] Dennert et al. reported a significant rise of LVEF (from 34 + 3% to 41 + 3% at 6 months; $p = 0.001$) and an improvement of NYHA functional class (from 2.5 ± 0.1 to 2.1 ± 0.1; $p = 0.004$) in DCM patients with B19V persistence (>250 copies/µg DNA) treated with a high dose of IVIG (2 g/kg).[132] Since no therapy-related complications have been reported for this treatment, an open-label treatment might be considered for AMC/DCM patients.

Antiviral Immunomodulation with Interferon

The antiviral immune response in experimental CBV induced myocarditis is crucially dependent on type I interferons (i.e., IFN-β).[133] A 6-month treatment of 22 DCMi patients with EMB proven enteroviral ($n = 15$) or adenoviral ($n = 7$) persistence, elimination of viral genomes was proven in follow-up EMBs. This course was paralleled by a significant raise of LVEF (from 44.7 ± 15.5% to 53.1 ± 16.8%) and improvement of NYHA functional class.[134] The randomized multicenter Bioferon in Chronic Viral Cardiomyopathy (BICC) trial included also patients with B19V persistence, in whom complete viral elimination could not be confirmed at follow-up EMB. This study has been presented at the American Heart Association (AHA) meeting 2008.[135] However, this trial has not been published thus far. In a further study, IFN-β treatment of 42 DCM patients with PCR proven viral persistence (the majority with B19V persistence) failed to confirm significant beneficial effects on clinical outcome compared with the control group.[136] Interferon-β treatment was safe and well tolerated, and flulike side effects could be efficiently suppressed by NSAID in both studies.[134,136] Zimmermann et al. discussed that the high prevalence of B19V (92%) in the verum treated group might have influenced these negative results. This notion is supported by the known negligible biological relevance of B19V genome persistence in various human tissues, including the myocardium, as detected by PCR alone, neglecting e.g., the pattern of humoral immune response, acute viremia and the B19V viral load.[76,77,79-81,83,132]

Immunoadsorption

The favorable hemodynamic results of immunoadsorption (IA) in DCM patients have been confirmed in several single center investigations, and can be ascribed to multiple mechanisms: removal of autoantibodies;[137] decrease of lymphocytic infiltration and CAM expression;[138] decreased oxidative stress.[139] The effects of IA may be partly due to the restoration of immunoglobulins with 0.5 g/kg polyclonal IgG after IA.[140] 40% of the IA-treated patients show improvement of hemodynamic and clinical parameters.[140] The beneficial effects of IA on LVEF and CHF symptoms are lasting for up to more than 2.5 years after treatment, and contribute to a significant reduction of hospitalization days and morbidity.[141,142] Distinct myocardial gene expression profiles and cardiodepressant autoantibodies may be helpful to differentiate DCM patients who will likely respond favorably to IA.[143] A randomized multicenter IA trial is ongoing for DCM patients (NCT00558584).

CONCLUSION

For myocarditis, heterogeneous clinical presentations and outcomes have been observed. The clinical treatment of myocarditis follows general heart failure guidelines. Recent investigations have identified several conditions that are associated with adverse prognosis, which are important cornerstones for the identification of patients at increased risk. The WCD may be especially important for myocarditis to prevent from SCD, bridging the highly dynamic initial phase of reduced LVEF. CMR imaging has gained substantial importance for the noninvasive diagnosis of myocarditis. Recurrent PEs are responsive to NSAIDs and/or colchicine. Concurrent EMB investigations encompassing histology, immunohistology and virological analyses, are pertinent for the definitive diagnosis of myocarditis. EMB are especially indicated in myocarditis patients with reduced LVEF and/or life-threatening arrhythmias, suggestive of i.e. giant cell myocarditis, which is a proven indication for immunosuppression. Several immunomodulatory studies have shown beneficial effects in selected patient groups, characterized primarily by EMB results. Recent clinical research has vigorously enriched our knowledge on diagnosis, prognosis and immunomodulatory modalities of myocarditis patients, and has partly disenchanted this intriguing conundrum. However, the results of multicenter controlled trials are needed to foster this evidence.

REFERENCES

1. Richardson P, McKenna W, Bristow M, et al. Report of the 1995 World Health Organization/International Society and Federation of Cardiology Task Force on the Definition and Classification of cardiomyopathies. Circulation. 1996;93(5):841-2.
2. D'Ambrosio A, Patti G, Manzoli A, et al. The fate of acute myocarditis between spontaneous improvement and evolution to dilated cardiomyopathy: a review. Heart. 2001;85(5):499-504.
3. Feldman AM, McNamara D. Myocarditis. N Engl J Med. 2000;343(19):1388-98.
4. Noutsias M, Pankuweit S, Maisch B. Myocarditis, cardiac tamponade and pericarditis. In: Tubaro M, Danchin N, Filippatos G, Goldstein P, Vranckx P, Zahger D (Eds). ESC Textbook of Intensive and Acute Cardiac Care. Oxford: Oxford University Press; 2011. pp. 565-77.
5. Mahfoud F, Gartner B, Kindermann M, et al. Virus serology in patients with suspected myocarditis: utility or futility? Eur Heart J. 2011;32(7):897-903.
6. Lurz P, Eitel I, Adam J, et al. Diagnostic performance of CMR imaging compared with EMB in patients with suspected myocarditis. JACC. 2012;5(5):513-24.
7. Noutsias M, Fechner H, de Jonge H, et al. Human coxsackie-adenovirus receptor is colocalized with integrins alpha(v)beta(3) and alpha(v) beta(5) on the cardiomyocyte sarcolemma and upregulated in dilated cardiomyopathy: implications for cardiotropic viral infections. Circulation. 2001;104(3):275-80.
8. Pinkert S, Westermann D, Wang X, et al. Prevention of cardiac dysfunction in acute coxsackievirus B3 cardiomyopathy by inducible expression of a soluble coxsackievirus-adenovirus receptor. Circulation. 2009;120(23):2358-66.
9. Muller-Werdan U, Schumann H, Fuchs R, et al. Tumor necrosis factor alpha (TNF alpha) is cardiodepressant in pathophysiologically relevant concentrations without inducing inducible nitric oxide-(NO)-synthase (iNOS) or triggering serious cytotoxicity. J Mol Cell Cardiol. 1997;29(11):2915-23.
10. Kasner M, Westermann D, Lopez B, et al. Diastolic tissue Doppler indexes correlate with the degree of collagen expression and cross-linking in heart failure and normal ejection fraction. J Am Coll Cardiol. 2011;57(8):977-85.
11. Seko Y, Shinkai Y, Kawasaki A, et al. Expression of perforin in infiltrating cells in murine hearts with acute myocarditis caused by coxsackievirus B3. Circulation. 1991;84(2):788-95.
12. Noutsias M, Pauschinger M, Schultheiss HP, et al. Cytotoxic perforin+ and TIA-1+ infiltrates are associated with cell adhesion molecule expression in dilated cardiomyopathy. Eur J Heart Fail. 2003;5(4):469-79.
13. Seko Y, Yagita H, Okumura K, et al. Expression of vascular cell adhesion molecule-1 in murine hearts with acute myocarditis caused by coxsackievirus B3. J Pathol. 1996;180(4):450-4.
14. Noutsias M, Seeberg B, Schultheiss HP, et al. Expression of cell adhesion molecules in dilated cardiomyopathy: evidence for endothelial activation in inflammatory cardiomyopathy. Circulation. 1999;99(16):2124-31.
15. Kindermann I, Kindermann M, Kandolf R, et al. Predictors of outcome in patients with suspected myocarditis. Circulation. 2008;118(6):639-48.
16. Ilback NG, Fohlman J, Friman G. Exercise in coxsackie B3 myocarditis: effects on heart lymphocyte subpopulations and the inflammatory reaction. Am Heart J. 1989;117(6):1298-302.
17. Basso C, Calabrese F, Corrado D, et al. Postmortem diagnosis in sudden cardiac death victims: macroscopic, microscopic and molecular findings. Cardiovasc Res. 2001;50(2):290-300.
18. McCarthy RE 3rd, Boehmer JP, Hruban RH, et al. Long-term outcome of fulminant myocarditis as compared with acute (nonfulminant) myocarditis. N Engl J Med. 2000;342(10):690-5.
19. Phillips M, Robinowitz M, Higgins JR, et al. Sudden cardiac death in Air Force recruits. A 20-year review. JAMA. 1986;256(19):2696-9.
20. Tomioka N, Kishimoto C, Matsumori A, et al. Effects of prednisolone on acute viral myocarditis in mice. J Am Coll Cardiol. 1986;7(4):868-72.
21. Mason JW, O'Connell JB, Herskowitz A, et al. A clinical trial of immunosuppressive therapy for myocarditis. The Myocarditis Treatment Trial Investigators. N Engl J Med. 1995;333(5):269-75.
22. Kühl U, Pauschinger M, Noutsias M, et al. High prevalence of viral genomes and multiple viral infections in the myocardium of adults with "idiopathic" left ventricular dysfunction. Circulation. 2005;111(7):887-93.
23. Caforio AL, Vinci A, Iliceto S. Anti-heart autoantibodies in familial dilated cardiomyopathy. Autoimmunity. 2008;41(6):462-9.

24. Maisch B, Richter A, Sandmoller A, et al. Inflammatory dilated cardiomyopathy (DCMI). Herz. 2005;30(6):535-44.
25. Gauntt CJ, Arizpe HM, Higdon AL, et al. Molecular mimicry, anti-coxsackievirus B3 neutralizing monoclonal antibodies, and myocarditis. J Immunol. 1995;154(6):2983-95.
26. Esfandiarei M, McManus BM. Molecular biology and pathogenesis of viral myocarditis. Annu Rev Pathol. 2008;3:127-55.
27. Karjalainen J, Heikkila J. Incidence of three presentations of acute myocarditis in young men in military service. A 20-year experience. Eur Heart J. 1999;20(15):1120-5.
28. Andersson B, Caidahl K, Waagstein F. Idiopathic dilated cardiomyopathy among Swedish patients with congestive heart failure. Eur Heart J. 1995;16(1):53-60.
29. Taylor DO, Stehlik J, Edwards LB, et al. Registry of the international society for heart and lung transplantation: twenty-sixth official adult heart transplant report-2009. J Heart Lung Transplant. 2009;28(10):1007-22.
30. Fabre A, Sheppard MN. Sudden adult death syndrome and other non-ischaemic causes of sudden cardiac death. Heart. 2006;92(3):316-20.
31. Doolan A, Langlois N, Semsarian C. Causes of sudden cardiac death in young Australians. Med J Aust. 2004;180(3):110-2.
32. Dec GW Jr, Waldman H, Southern J, et al. Viral myocarditis mimicking acute myocardial infarction. J Am Coll Cardiol. 1992;20(1):85-9.
33. Kühl U, Pauschinger M, Bock T, et al. Parvovirus B19 infection mimicking acute myocardial infarction. Circulation. 2003;108(8):945-50.
34. Lauer B, Niederau C, Kuhl U, et al. Cardiac troponin T in patients with clinically suspected myocarditis. J Am Coll Cardiol. 1997;30(5):1354-9.
35. Pankuweit S, Moll R, Baandrup U, et al. Prevalence of the parvovirus B19 genome in endomyocardial biopsy specimens. Hum Pathol. 2003;34(5):497-503.
36. Di Lenarda A, Pinamonti B, Mestroni L, et al. The natural history of dilated cardiomyopathy: a review of the Heart Muscle Disease Registry of Trieste. Ital Heart J Suppl. 2004;5(4):253-66.
37. Makaryus AN, Revere DJ, Steinberg B. Recurrent reversible dilated cardiomyopathy secondary to viral and streptococcal pneumonia vaccine-associated myocarditis. Cardiol Rev. 2006;14(4):e1-4.
38. Karavidas A, Lazaros G, Noutsias M, et al. Recurrent coxsackie B viral myocarditis leading to progressive impairment of left ventricular function over 8years. Int J Cardiol. 2011;151(2):e65-7.
39. Grogan M, Redfield MM, Bailey KR, et al. Long-term outcome of patients with biopsy-proved myocarditis: comparison with idiopathic dilated cardiomyopathy. J Am Coll Cardiol. 1995;26(1):80-4.
40. Why HJ, Meany BT, Richardson PJ, et al. Clinical and prognostic significance of detection of enteroviral RNA in the myocardium of patients with myocarditis or dilated cardiomyopathy. Circulation. 1994;89(6):2582-9.
41. Grun S, Schumm J, Greulich S, et al. Long-term follow-up of biopsy-proven viral myocarditis: predictors of mortality and incomplete recovery. J Am Coll Cardiol. 2012;59(18):1604-15.
42. Ukena C, Mahfoud F, Kindermann I, et al. Prognostic electrocardiographic parameters in patients with suspected myocarditis. Eur J Heart Fail. 2011;13(4):398-405.
43. Hombach V, Merkle N, Torzewski J, et al. Electrocardiographic and cardiac magnetic resonance imaging parameters as predictors of a worse outcome in patients with idiopathic dilated cardiomyopathy. Eur Heart J. 2009;30(16):2011-8.
44. Mahfoud F, Ukena C, Kandolf R, et al. Blood pressure and heart rate predict outcome in patients acutely admitted with suspected myocarditis without previous heart failure. J Hypertens. 2012;30(6):1217-24.
45. Lehrke S, Lossnitzer D, Schob M, et al. Use of cardiovascular magnetic resonance for risk stratification in chronic heart failure: prognostic value of late gadolinium enhancement in patients with non-ischaemic dilated cardiomyopathy. Heart. 2011;97(9):727-32.
46. Lieberman EB, Hutchins GM, Herskowitz A, et al. Clinicopathologic description of myocarditis. J Am Coll Cardiol. 1991;18(7):1617-26.
47. Holzmann M, Nicko A, Kühl U, et al. Complication rate of right ventricular endomyocardial biopsy via the femoral approach: a retrospective and prospective study analyzing 3048 diagnostic procedures over an 11-year period. Circulation. 2008;118(17):1722-8.
48. Maisch B, Pankuweit S, Karatolios K, et al. Invasive techniques—from diagnosis to treatment. Rheumatology (Oxford). 2006;45 Suppl 4:iv32-8.
49. Yilmaz A, Kindermann I, Kindermann M, et al. Comparative evaluation of left and right ventricular endomyocardial biopsy: differences in complication rate and diagnostic performance. Circulation. 2010;122(9):900-9.
50. Mahrholdt H, Goedecke C, Wagner A, et al. Cardiovascular magnetic resonance assessment of human myocarditis: a comparison to histology and molecular pathology. Circulation. 2004;109(10):1250-8.
51. Aretz HT. Myocarditis: the Dallas criteria. Hum Pathol. 1987;18(6):619-24.
52. Cooper LT Jr. Myocarditis. N Engl J Med. 2009;360(15):1526-38.
53. Strauer BE, Kandolf R, Mall G, et al. Myocarditis—cardiomyopathy. Consensus Report of the German Association for Internal Medicine, presented at the 100th annual meeting, Wiesbaden, 13 April 1994. Acta Cardiol. 1996;51(4):347-71.
54. Shanes JG, Ghali J, Billingham ME, et al. Interobserver variability in the pathologic interpretation of endomyocardial biopsy results. Circulation. 1987;75(2):401-5.
55. Hauck AJ, Kearney DL, Edwards WD. Evaluation of postmortem endo-myocardial biopsy specimens from 38 patients with lymphocytic myocarditis: implications for role of sampling error. Mayo Clin Proc. 1989;64(10):1235-45.
56. Cooper LT Jr, Berry GJ, Shabetai R. Idiopathic giant-cell myocarditis—natural history and treatment. Multicenter Giant Cell Myocarditis Study Group Investigators. N Engl J Med. 1997;336(26):1860-6.
57. Cooper LT, Baughman KL, Feldman AM, et al. The role of endomyocardial biopsy in the management of cardiovascular disease: a scientific statement from the American Heart Association, the American College of Cardiology, and the European Society of Cardiology. Circulation. 2007;116(19):2216-33.
58. Schultheiss HP, Noutsias M, Kühl U, et al. Myocarditis and Viral Cardiomyopathy. In: Camm AJ, Lüscher TF, Serruys PW (Eds). The ESC Textbook of Cardiovascular Medicine. Oxford: Blackwell Publishing Ltd; 2006. pp. 490-501.
59. Noutsias M, Pauschinger M, Schultheiss HP, et al. Advances in the immunohistological diagnosis of inflammatory cardiomyopathy. Eur Heart J Suppl. 2002;4(Supplement I):I54-62.
60. Wojnicz R, Nowalany-Kozielska E, Wojciechowska C, et al. Randomized, placebo-controlled study for immunosuppressive treatment of inflammatory dilated cardiomyopathy: two-year follow-up results. Circulation. 2001; 104(1):39-45.
61. Ino T, Kishiro M, Okubo M, et al. Late persistent expressions of ICAM-1 and VCAM-1 on myocardial tissue in children with lymphocytic myocarditis. Cardiovasc Res. 1997;34(2):323-8.
62. Parrillo JE. Inflammatory cardiomyopathy (myocarditis): which patients should be treated with anti-inflammatory therapy? Circulation. 2001; 104(1):4-6.
63. Kühl U, Noutsias M, Seeberg B, et al. Immunohistological evidence for a chronic intramyocardial inflammatory process in dilated cardiomyopathy. Heart. 1996;75(3):295-300.
64. Maisch B, Bültman B, Factor S, et al. World Heart Federation consensus conferences's definition of inflammatory cardiomyopathy (myocarditis): report from two expert commitees on histology and viral cardiomyopathy. Heartbeat. 1999;4:3-4.
65. Maisch B, Portig I, Ristic A, et al. Definition of inflammatory cardio-myopathy (myocarditis): on the way to consensus. A status report. Herz. 2000;25(3):200-9.

66. Hufnagel G, Pankuweit S, Richter A, et al. The European Study of Epidemiology and Treatment of Cardiac Inflammatory Diseases (ESETCID). First epidemiological results. Herz. 2000;25(3):279-85.
67. Frustaci A, Russo MA, Chimenti C. Randomized study on the efficacy of immunosuppressive therapy in patients with virus-negative inflammatory cardiomyopathy: the TIMIC study. Eur Heart J. 2009;30(16):1995-2002.
68. Baccouche H, Mahrholdt H, Meinhardt G, et al. Diagnostic synergy of non-invasive cardiovascular magnetic resonance and invasive endomyocardial biopsy in troponin-positive patients without coronary artery disease. Eur Heart J. 2009;30(23):2869-79.
69. Pankuweit S, Richter A, Ruppert V, et al. Classification of cardiomyopathies and indication for endomyocardial biopsy revisited. Herz. 2009;34(1):55-62.
70. Noutsias M, Pauschinger M, Ostermann K, et al. Digital image analysis system for the quantification of infiltrates and cell adhesion molecules in inflammatory cardiomyopathy. Med Sci Monit. 2002;8(5):MT59-71.
71. Baboonian C, Treasure T. Meta-analysis of the association of enteroviruses with human heart disease. Heart. 1997;78(6):539-43.
72. Fujioka S, Kitaura Y, Ukimura A, et al. Evaluation of viral infection in the myocardium of patients with idiopathic dilated cardiomyopathy. J Am Coll Cardiol. 2000;36(6):1920-6.
73. Kühl U, Pauschinger M, Seeberg B, et al. Viral persistence in the myocardium is associated with progressive cardiac dysfunction. Circulation. 2005;112(13):1965-70.
74. Kuhl U, Lassner D, von Schlippenbach J, et al. Interferon-Beta improves survival in enterovirus-associated cardiomyopathy. J Am Coll Cardiol. 2012;60(14):1295-6.
75. Kuethe F, Sigusch HH, Hilbig K, et al. Detection of viral genome in the myocardium: lack of prognostic and functional relevance in patients with acute dilated cardiomyopathy. Am Heart J. 2007;153(5):850-8.
76. Streitz M, Noutsias M, Volkmer R, et al. NS1 specific CD8+ T-cells with effector function and TRBV11 dominance in a patient with parvovirus B19 associated inflammatory cardiomyopathy. PLoS One. 2008;3(6):e2361.
77. Bock CT, Klingel K, Kandolf R. Human parvovirus B19-associated myocarditis. N Engl J Med. 2010;362(13):1248-9.
78. Dennert R, Velthuis S, Westermann D, et al. Parvovirus-B19-associated fulminant myocarditis successfully treated with immunosuppressive and antiviral therapy. Antivir Ther. 2010;15(4):681-5.
79. Kuethe F, Lindner J, Matschke K, et al. Prevalence of parvovirus B19 and human bocavirus DNA in the heart of patients with no evidence of dilated cardiomyopathy or myocarditis. Clin Infect Dis. 2009;49(11):1660-6.
80. Schenk T, Enders M, Pollak S, et al. High prevalence of human parvovirus B19 DNA in myocardial autopsy samples from subjects without myocarditis or dilative cardiomyopathy. J Clin Microbiol. 2009;47(1):106-10.
81. Norja P, Hokynar K, Aaltonen LM, et al. Bioportfolio: lifelong persistence of variant and prototypic erythrovirus DNA genomes in human tissue. Proc Natl Acad Sci U S A. 2006;103(19):7450-3.
82. Escher F, Modrow S, Sabi T, et al. Parvovirus B19 profiles in patients presenting with acute myocarditis and chronic dilated cardiomyopathy. Med Sci Monit. 2008;14(12):CR589-97.
83. Lindner J, Noutsias M, Lassner D, et al. Adaptive immune responses against parvovirus B19 in patients with myocardial disease. J Clin Virol. 2009;44(1):27-32.
84. Friedrich MG, Strohm O, Schulz-Menger J, et al. Contrast media-enhanced magnetic resonance imaging visualizes myocardial changes in the course of viral myocarditis. Circulation. 1998;97(18):1802-9.
85. Abdel-Aty H, Boye P, Zagrosek A, et al. Diagnostic performance of cardiovascular magnetic resonance in patients with suspected acute myocarditis: comparison of different approaches. J Am Coll Cardiol. 2005; 45(11):1815-22.
86. Gutberlet M, Spors B, Thoma T, et al. Suspected chronic myocarditis at cardiac MR: diagnostic accuracy and association with immunohistologically detected inflammation and viral persistence. Radiology. 2008;246(2):401-9.
87. Friedrich MG, Sechtem U, Schulz-Menger J, et al. Cardiovascular magnetic resonance in myocarditis: A JACC White Paper. J Am Coll Cardiol. 2009;53(17):1475-87.
88. Noutsias M, Kühl U, Lassner D, et al. Parvovirus B19-associated active myocarditis with biventricular thrombi: results of endomyocardial biopsy investigations and cardiac magnetic resonance imaging. Circulation. 2007;115(13):e378-80.
89. Mahrholdt H, Wagner A, Judd RM, et al. Delayed enhancement cardiovascular magnetic resonance assessment of non-ischaemic cardiomyopathies. Eur Heart J. 2005;26(15):1461-74.
90. Assomull RG, Prasad SK, Lyne J, et al. Cardiovascular magnetic resonance, fibrosis, and prognosis in dilated cardiomyopathy. J Am Coll Cardiol. 2006;48(10):1977-85.
91. Zagrosek A, Abdel-Aty H, Boye P, et al. Cardiac magnetic resonance monitors reversible and irreversible myocardial injury in myocarditis. JACC. 2009;2(2):131-8.
92. Zagrosek A, Wassmuth R, Abdel-Aty H, et al. Relation between myocardial edema and myocardial mass during the acute and convalescent phase of myocarditis: a CMR study. J Cardiovasc Magn Reson. 2008;10(1):19.
93. Caforio AL, Calabrese F, Angelini A, et al. A prospective study of biopsy-proven myocarditis: prognostic relevance of clinical and aetiopathogenetic features at diagnosis. Eur Heart J. 2007;28(11):1326-33.
94. Warraich RS, Noutsias M, Kazak I, et al. Immunoglobulin G3 cardiac myosin autoantibodies correlate with left ventricular dysfunction in patients with dilated cardiomyopathy: immunoglobulin G3 and clinical correlates. Am Heart J. 2002;143(6):1076-84.
95. Staudt A, Bohm M, Knebel F, et al. Potential role of autoantibodies belonging to the immunoglobulin G-3 subclass in cardiac dysfunction among patients with dilated cardiomyopathy. Circulation. 2002;106(19):2448-53.
96. Staudt A, Eichler P, Trimpert C, et al. Fc(gamma) receptors IIa on cardiomyocytes and their potential functional relevance in dilated cardiomyopathy. J Am Coll Cardiol. 2007;49(16):1684-92.
97. Ammann P, Naegeli B, Schuiki E, et al. Long-term outcome of acute myocarditis is independent of cardiac enzyme release. Int J Cardiol. 2003;89(2-3):217-22.
98. Corssmit EP, Trip MD, Durrer JD. Loffler's endomyocarditis in the idiopathic hypereosinophilic syndrome. Cardiology. 1999;91(4):272-6.
99. Spodick DH. Eosinophilic myocarditis. Mayo Clin Proc. 1997;72(10):996.
100. Hunt SA, Baker DW, Chin MH, et al. ACC/AHA Guidelines for the Evaluation and Management of Chronic Heart Failure in the Adult: Executive Summary A Report of the American College of Cardiology/American Heart Association Task Force on Practice Guidelines (Committee to Revise the 1995 Guidelines for the Evaluation and Management of Heart Failure): Developed in Collaboration With the International Society for Heart and Lung Transplantation; Endorsed by the Heart Failure Society of America. Circulation. 2001;104(24):2996-3007.
101. Young JB, Dunlap ME, Pfeffer MA, et al. Mortality and morbidity reduction with Candesartan in patients with chronic heart failure and left ventricular systolic dysfunction: results of the CHARM low-left ventricular ejection fraction trials. Circulation. 2004;110(17):2618-26.
102. Fauchier L, Babuty D, Poret P, et al. Comparison of long-term outcome of alcoholic and idiopathic dilated cardiomyopathy. Eur Heart J. 2000;21(4):306-14.
103. Maisch B, Seferovic PM, Ristic AD, et al. Guidelines on the diagnosis and management of pericardial diseases executive summary; The Task force on the diagnosis and management of pericardial diseases of the European society of cardiology. Eur Heart J. 2004;25(7):587-610.

104. Imazio M, Adler Y. Management of pericardial effusion. Eur Heart J. 2013;34(16):1186-97.
105. Chen YS, Yu HY, Huang SC, et al. Experience and result of extracorporeal membrane oxygenation in treating fulminant myocarditis with shock: what mechanical support should be considered first? J Heart Lung Transplant. 2005;24(1):81-7.
106. Hsu KH, Chi NH, Yu HY, et al. Extracorporeal membranous oxygenation support for acute fulminant myocarditis: analysis of a single center's experience. Eur J Cardiothorac Surg. 2011;40(3):682-8.
107. Drory Y, Turetz Y, Hiss Y, et al. Sudden unexpected death in persons less than 40 years of age. Am J Cardiol. 1991;68(13):1388-92.
108. Wesslen L, Pahlson C, Lindquist O, et al. An increase in sudden unexpected cardiac deaths among young Swedish orienteers during 1979-1992. Eur Heart J. 1996;17(6):902-10.
109. Corrado D, Basso C, Thiene G. Sudden cardiac death in young people with apparently normal heart. Cardiovasc Res. 2001;50(2):399-408.
110. Burke AP, Farb A, Virmani R, et al. Sports-related and non-sports-related sudden cardiac death in young adults. Am Heart J. 1991;121(2 Pt 1): 568-75.
111. Gatmaitan BG, Chason JL, Lerner AM. Augmentation of the virulence of murine coxsackie-virus B-3 myocardiopathy by exercise. J Exp Med. 1970;131(6):1121-36.
112. Al-Khatib SM, Hellkamp A, Curtis J, et al. Non-evidence-based ICD implantations in the United States. JAMA. 2011;305(1):43-9.
113. Chung MK, Szymkiewicz SJ, Shao M, et al. Aggregate national experience with the wearable cardioverter-defibrillator: event rates, compliance, and survival. J Am Coll Cardiol. 2010;56(3):194-203.
114. Kao AC, Krause SW, Handa R, et al. Wearable defibrillator use in heart failure (WIF): results of a prospective registry. BMC Cardiovasc Disord. 2012;12(1):123.
115. Kadish A, Goldberger J. Selecting patients for ICD implantation: are clinicians choosing appropriately? JAMA. 2011;305(1):91-2.
116. Epstein AE, Dimarco JP, Ellenbogen KA, et al. ACC/AHA/HRS 2008 Guidelines for device-based therapy of cardiac rhythm abnormalities. Heart Rhythm. 2008;5(6):e1-62.
117. Bardy GH, Lee KL, Mark DB, et al. Amiodarone or an implantable cardioverter-defibrillator for congestive heart failure. N Engl J Med. 2005;352(3): 225-37.
118. Hershberger RE, Lindenfeld J, Mestroni L, et al. Genetic evaluation of cardiomyopathy—a Heart Failure Society of America practice guideline. J Card Fail. 2009;15(2):83-97.
119. Ackerman MJ, Priori SG, Willems S, et al. HRS/EHRA expert consensus statement on the state of genetic testing for the channelopathies and cardiomyopathies: this document was developed as a partnership between the Heart Rhythm Society (HRS) and the European Heart Rhythm Association (EHRA). Europace. 2011;13(8):1077-109.
120. Andreasen C, Nielsen JB, Refsgaard L, et al. New population-based exome data are questioning the pathogenicity of previously cardiomyopathy-associated genetic variants. Eur J Hum Genet. 2013;21(9):918-28.
121. van der Zwaag PA, van Tintelen JP. Counsel the genotype, treat the phenotype. Eur J Heart Fail. 2011;13(11):1159-60.
122. Cooper LT Jr, Hare JM, Tazelaar HD, et al. Usefulness of immunosuppression for giant cell myocarditis. Am J Cardiol. 2008;102(11):1535-9.
123. Noutsias M, Pauschinger M, Gross U, et al. Giant-cell myocarditis in a patient presenting with dilated cardiomyopathy and ventricular tachycardias treated by immunosuppression: a case report. Int J Cardiol. 2008;128(2):e58-9.
124. Liu PP, Mason JW. Advances in the understanding of myocarditis. Circulation. 2001;104(9):1076-82.
125. Frustaci A, Chimenti C, Calabrese F, et al. Immunosuppressive therapy for active lymphocytic myocarditis: virological and immunologic profile of responders versus nonresponders. Circulation. 2003;107(6):857-63.
126. Maisch B, Camerini F, Schultheiss HP. Immunosuppressive therapy for myocarditis. N Engl J Med. 1995;333(25):1713.
127. Rosen FS. Putative mechanisms of the effect of intravenous gamma-globulin. Clin Immunol Immunopathol. 1993;67(3 Pt 2):S41-3.
128. Takada H, Kishimoto C, Hiraoka Y. Therapy with immunoglobulin suppresses myocarditis in a murine coxsackievirus B3 model. Antiviral and anti-inflammatory effects. Circulation. 1995;92(6):1604-11.
129. Kishimoto C, Takamatsu N, Kawamata H, et al. Immunoglobulin treatment ameliorates murine myocarditis associated with reduction of neurohumoral activity and improvement of extracellular matrix change. J Am Coll Cardiol. 2000;36(6):1979-84.
130. McNamara DM, Holubkov R, Starling RC, et al. Controlled trial of intravenous immune globulin in recent-onset dilated cardiomyopathy. Circulation. 2001;103(18):2254-9.
131. Gullestad L, Aass H, Fjeld JG, et al. Immunomodulating therapy with intravenous immunoglobulin in patients with chronic heart failure. Circulation. 2001;103(2):220-5.
132. Dennert R, Velthuis S, Schalla S, et al. Intravenous immunoglobulin therapy for patients with idiopathic cardiomyopathy and endomyocardial biopsy-proven high PVB19 viral load. Antivir Ther. 2010;15(2): 193-201.
133. Deonarain R, Cerullo D, Fuse K, et al. Protective role for interferon-beta in coxsackievirus B3 infection. Circulation. 2004;110(23):3540-3.
134. Kühl U, Pauschinger M, Schwimmbeck PL, et al. Interferon-beta treatment eliminates cardiotropic viruses and improves left ventricular function in patients with myocardial persistence of viral genomes and left ventricular dysfunction. Circulation. 2003;107(22):2793-8.
135. Coletta AP, Clark AL, Cleland JG. Clinical trials update from the Heart Failure Society of America and the American Heart Association meetings in 2008: SADHART-CHF, COMPARE, MOMENTUM, thyroid hormone analogue study, HF-ACTION, I-PRESERVE, {beta}-interferon study, BACH, and ATHENA. Eur J Heart Fail. 2009;11(2):214-9.
136. Zimmermann O, Rodewald C, Radermacher M, et al. Interferon beta-1b therapy in chronic viral dilated cardiomyopathy-is there a role for specific therapy? J Card Fail. 2010;16(4):348-56.
137. Felix SB, Staudt A, Dorffel WV, et al. Hemodynamic effects of immunoadsorption and subsequent immunoglobulin substitution in dilated cardiomyopathy: three-month results from a randomized study. J Am Coll Cardiol. 2000;35(6):1590-8.
138. Staudt A, Schaper F, Stangl V, et al. Immunohistological changes in dilated cardiomyopathy induced by immunoadsorption therapy and subsequent immunoglobulin substitution. Circulation. 2001;103(22):2681-6.
139. Schimke I, Muller J, Priem F, et al. Decreased oxidative stress in patients with idiopathic dilated cardiomyopathy one year after immunoglobulin adsorption. J Am Coll Cardiol. 2001;38(1):178-83.
140. Felix SB, Staudt A. Non-specific immunoadsorption in patients with dilated cardiomyopathy: mechanisms and clinical effects. Int J Cardiol. 2006;112(1):30-3.
141. Knebel F, Bohm M, Staudt A, et al. Reduction of morbidity by immunoadsorption therapy in patients with dilated cardiomyopathy. Int J Cardiol. 2004;97(3):517-20.
142. Dorffel WV, Wallukat G, Dorffel Y, et al. Immunoadsorption in idiopathic dilated cardiomyopathy, a 3-year follow-up. Int J Cardiol. 2004;97(3): 529-34.
143. Staudt A, Staudt Y, Dorr M, et al. Potential role of humoral immunity in cardiac dysfunction of patients suffering from dilated cardiomyopathy. J Am Coll Cardiol. 2004;44(4):829-36.

Chapter 59

When is Genetic Testing Necessary?

Nupoor Narula, Maurizia Grasso, Alessandra Serio, Takahide Kodama, Eloisa Arbustini

ABSTRACT

Heart failure (HF) is a syndrome caused by many cardiovascular diseases, including cardiomyopathies that have been proven to be monogenic disorders characterized by genetic heterogeneity and phenotype variability in more than 70% of cases. Most cardiomyopathies are inherited as autosomal dominant traits (up to 90% of cases) with a minority assuming autosomal recessive, X-linked, and matrilineal inheritance. Clinically used classifications of cardiomyopathy are phenotype-based, and group cardiomyopathy according to 4 major morphofunctional phenotypes: hypertrophic, restrictive, dilated, and arrhythmogenic, the latter now being recognized as predominantly right, biventricular, or predominantly left. The morphofunctional classification of cardiomyopathy is useful for current clinical management that is based on the phenotype, but does not take into adequate consideration of recent evidence that over 80 known disease genes may cause phenotypically similar but genetically different cardiomyopathies.

Genetic testing is expected to play a major role in the specific diagnosis of cardiomyopathies, thus generating a novel, genetic-based classification of cardiomyopathies. The genetic diagnosis will impact clinical decisions because mutations in different genes may carry different risk, prompting disease-specific medical decisions. A typical example is the high risk of life threatening arrhythmias in patients with mild dilated cardiomyopathy caused by mutations in the *LMNA* gene, not fulfilling the criteria provided by current guidelines for primary prevention of sudden death.

Further, genetic testing may help (i) identify factors that predispose to or worsen HF and (ii) optimize and tailor medical treatments based on the pharmacogenetic make-up of each individual patient. Disease-specific diagnoses, risk stratification, and responsiveness to current treatments are all immediate translational benefits of genetic testing in HF.

INTRODUCTION

Although heart failure (HF) may represent an end-stage syndrome of many cardiovascular diseases,[1-4] the subgroup of primary myocardial diseases, or cardiomyopathies have been proven to be genetic disorders caused by single genetic defects. Both monogenic (or monofactorial) and multifactorial diseases induce similar structural and functional alterations including left ventricular hypertrophy (LVH), matrix remodeling, interstitial fibrosis resulting from activation of the neurohormonal system, and common compensatory mechanisms (Flowchart 1). Genetics is expected to play a major role in the diagnosis of monogenic diseases and identification of genetic factors that predispose or worsen HF. It may also contribute to optimizing and personalizing medical treatments on the basis of pharmacogenetics. In this chapter, we will illustrate when and why genetic testing is necessary in patients with HF caused by idiopathic cardiomyopathies and multifactorial diseases.

CARDIOMYOPATHIES ARE GENETIC DISEASES

Cardiomyopathies are myocardial disorders characterized by structurally and functionally abnormal heart muscle and absence of other diseases sufficient to cause the observed myocardial abnormality.[5] Most cardiomyopathies are genetic diseases inherited as

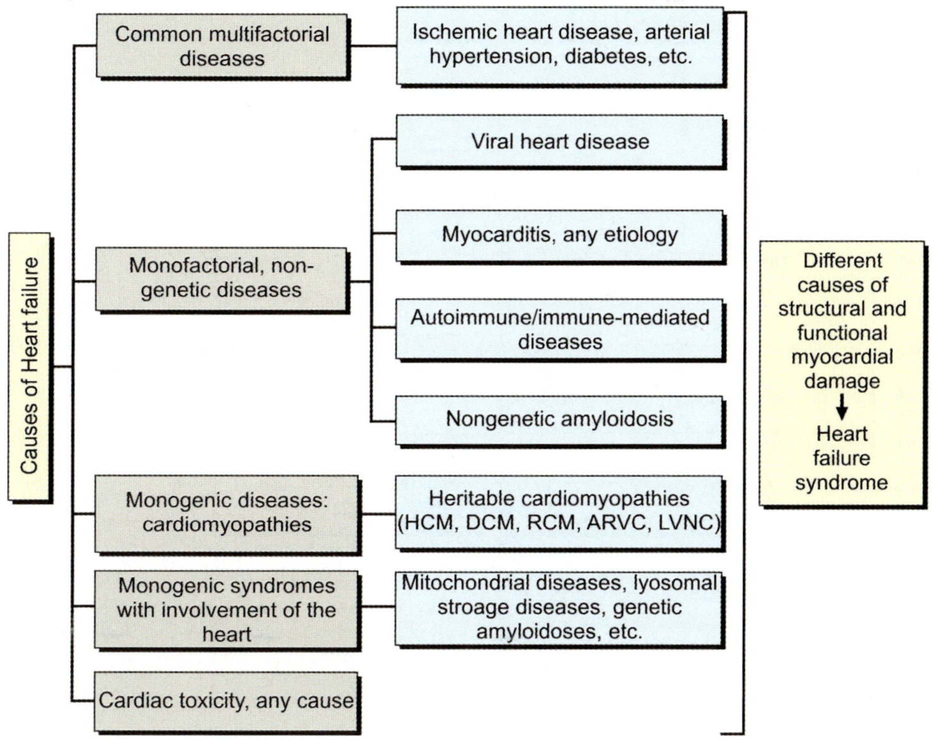

HCM, hypertrophic cardiomyopathy; DCM, dilated cardiomyopathy; RCM, restrictive cardiomyopathy; ARVC, arrhythmogenic right-ventricular cardiomyopathy; LVNC, left ventricular noncompaction

Flowchart 1 Different types of myocardial disorders that may cause heart failure

autosomal dominant (AD) traits in upto 90% of cases with a minority of autosomal recessive, X-linked and matrilineal inheritance.[6] In the last 20 years, the systematic approach to the genetic screening of families has contributed to reassess the proportion of familial cardiomyopathies, to clinically characterize cardiomyopathies and to identity family members that are either symptomatically or asymptomatically affected or predisposed to the development of myocardial dysfunction.[7-13]

The phenotype-based classification of cardiomyopathies continues to offer cardiologists, the feasibility of using a simple and clinically useful diagnostic language. However, categorization by classical hypertrophic cardiomyopathy (HCM), dilated cardiomyopathy (DCM), restrictive cardiomyopathy (RCM), arrhythmogenic right-ventricular cardiomyopathy (ARVC/AVC), or left ventricular noncompaction (LVNC) phenotypes does not uncover the etiologic basis of the disease. Therefore, recently, a working group of the European Society of Cardiology (ESC) recommended to subgrouping each major type of cardiomyopathy into familial and nonfamilial, or genetic and nongenetic forms.[5] The American Heart Association (AHA) further highlighted the importance of genetic characterization and recommended grouping cardiomyopathies into genetic, mixed, and acquired forms, wherein phenotype-based diagnosis was subordinate to the etiologic diagnosis.[14] Both classifications reflect the need of providing cardiologists with a better genetic approach to characterize patients affected by cardiomyopathy as well as their families. There has been an enormous focus on the genetic characterization of heart muscle disorders. The American College of Cardiology (ACC)/AHA classification of HF has included unaffected members of familial cardiomyopathy in stage A of disease.[15] The Heart Failure Society of America (HFSA) published practice guidelines on Genetic Evaluation of Cardiomyopathy[16] and Heart Rhythm Society (HRS)/European Heart Rhythm Association (EHRA) have published a Consensus Statement on the State of Genetic Testing for the channelopathies and cardiomyopathies.[17] A position statement of the Working Group (WG) on myocardial and pericardial diseases of the ESC has recommended a protocol for genetic counseling and testing in cardiomyopathies,[6]

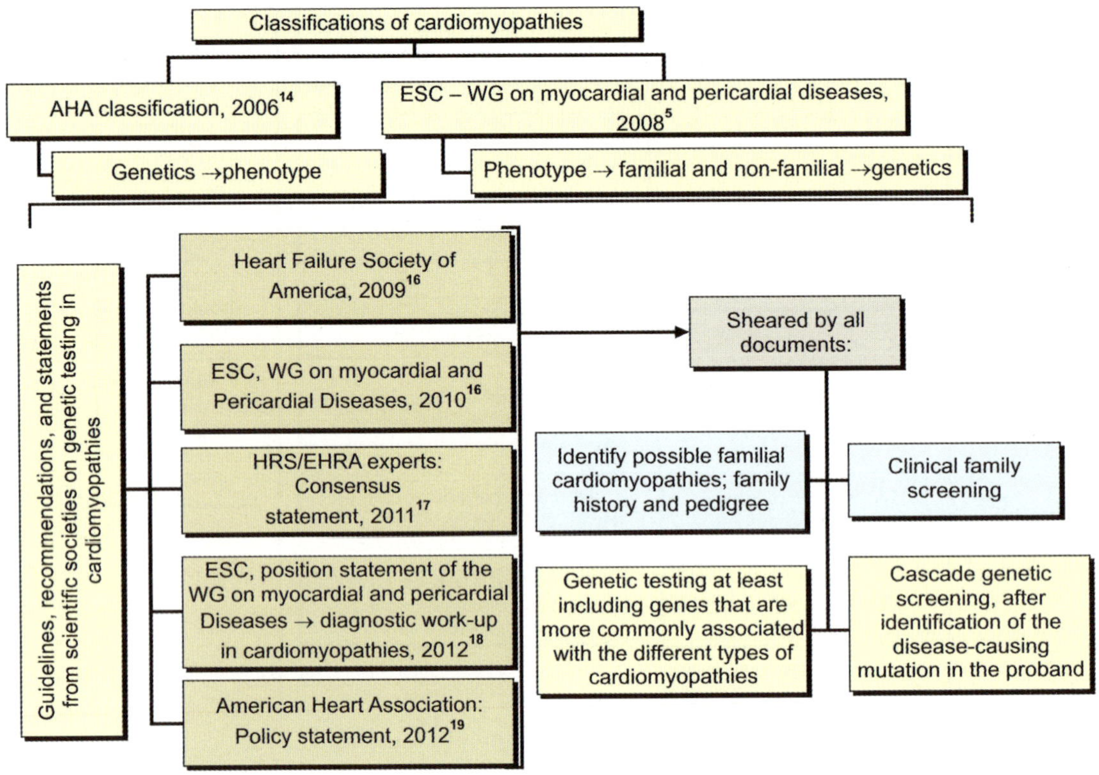

AHA, American Heart Association; ESC, European Society of Cardiology; WG, Working Group; HRS, Heart Rhythm Society; EHRA, European Heart Rhythm Association

Flowchart 2 Both European Society of Cardiology and American Heart Association generated novel classifications of cardiomyopathies. Thereafter, guidelines, recommendations and statements on genetic testing were published; all sharing the evidence that genetic testing is a consolidated step of the diagnostic work-up in cardiomyopathies

followed by a position statement for the diagnostic work-up in cardiomyopathy.[18] Clinical genetics and genetic counseling are expected to play a major role in the overall work-up of cardiomyopathies.[6,18] Flowchart 2 summarizes the list of official guidelines, recommendations, and suggestions from scientific societies. Although each document is different, and provides different indications and suggestions for the major subtypes of cardiomyopathies; they have all emphasized that genetic testing become a part of the diagnostic work-up for cardiomyopathies. The ESC cautiously anticipates a wider applicability of genetic testing when comprehensive parallel sequencing of all disease genes in large clinical series will become available. The ESC statement further underscores the need for correct interpretation of the genetic test results and maintains that interpretation of complex genetic information will require substantial clinical expertise.[6] Further, a policy statement from the AHA suggests the concerted effort of treating physicians and centers of cardiovascular genetics expertise to appropriately initiate, interpret, and implement genetic testing.[19] Overall, the position of all scientific bodies[6,14-19] and of experts on genetic testing in cardiomyopathies[20-23] reflects the clinical need for translation of current scientific knowledge of the genetics of cardiomyopathy into the clinical practice.

GENETIC TEST AND THE DIAGNOSIS OF CARDIOMYOPATHY

Cardiomyopathies are clinically heterogeneous disorders[5,6,18] and enormous variability has been reported in each phenotypic subtype of cardiomyopathies (HCM, DCM, RCM, ARVC, LVNC) pertaining to the age of onset of clinically manifest disease, rate of disease progression, risk of development of HF, and likelihood of sudden death. For instance, in DCM, on one hand while mildly enlarged and mildly dysfunctional left ventricles may be associated with life-threatening ventricular arrhythmias, on the other some patients with substantially dilated and dysfunctional left ventricules (LV) may pose relatively low arrhythmogenic risk.[24,25] Similarly, some HCM patients do not demonstrate syncope or life-threatening arrhythmias even with severe LVH, whereas others with mild or moderate hypertrophy may reveal high arrhythmogenic risk.[26] Although each subtype of cardiomyopathy is defined by its major morphofunctional phenotype, careful evaluation may demonstrate high phenotype variability.[18] For instance, echocardiogram may show variable extent and distribution of hypertrophy, ventricular dilatation and dysfunction, features of restriction and LVNC. Cardiac magnetic resonance (CMR) imaging may show delayed enhancement, or features suggesting infiltrative or intramyocyte storage, or fatty infiltration.[27,28] Electrocardiographic markers, such as atrioventricular block (AVB), pre-excitation syndrome [Wolff-Parkinson-White (WPW)], repolarization abnormalities, or low QRS voltages can be present only in a minority of patients.

Clinical Genetics

Most familial cardiomyopathies are AD diseases, and only a minority are inherited as autosomal recessive, matrilineal, and X-linked recessive diseases (Fig. 1). A recent position statement of the ESC suggests that clinically detectable, low-cost cardiac, and extracardiac markers (red flags) may help generate diagnostic hypothesis about the possible disease causing gene.[18] An integrated framework including pattern of inheritance, major clinical phenotype (HCM or DCM), and biomarkers [increased serum creatine phosphokinase (sCPK) or lactacidemia] may provide a preliminary filter for appropriate genetic testing. Examples include: association of cardiolaminopathies with AVB in upto 80% of cases,[29] association of dystrophinopathies in male patients with increased sCPK (80%) and absence of male-to-male transmission of the disease,[30] relationship of myocardial storage diseases with HCM phenotype

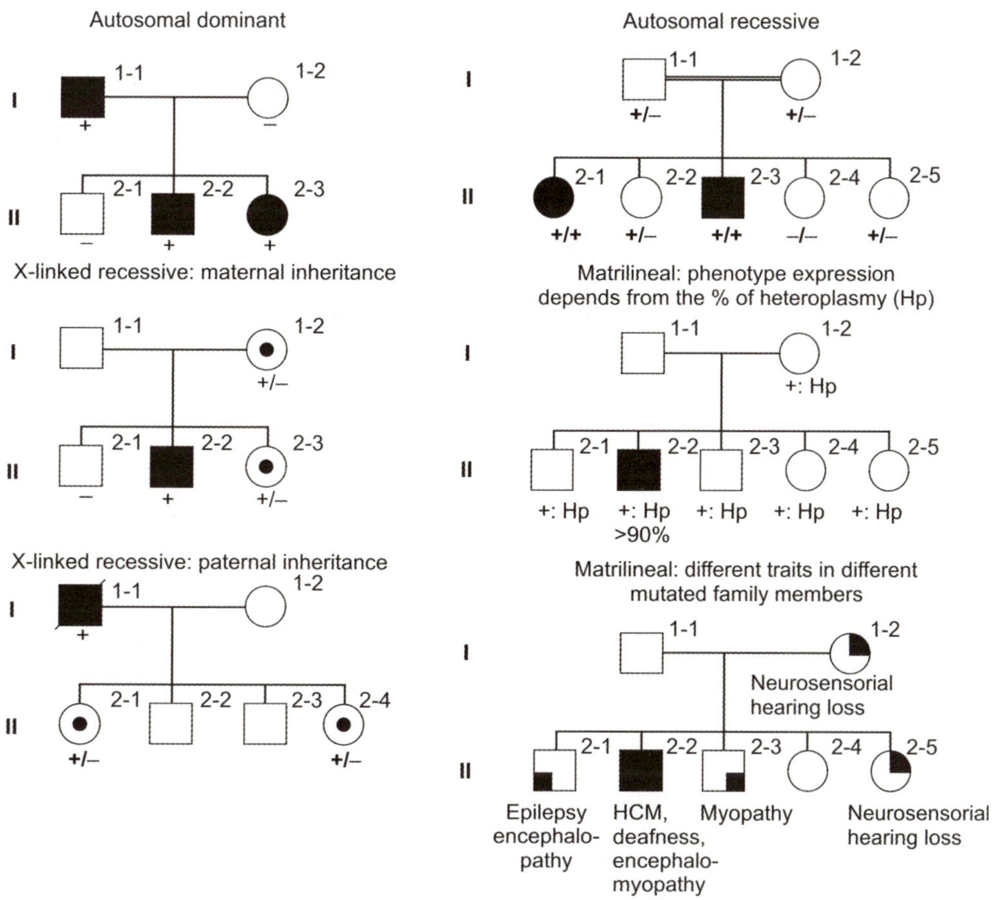

Fig. 1 The pedigrees in autosomal dominant, autosomal recessive, X-linked, and matrilineal inheritance of cardiomyopathies

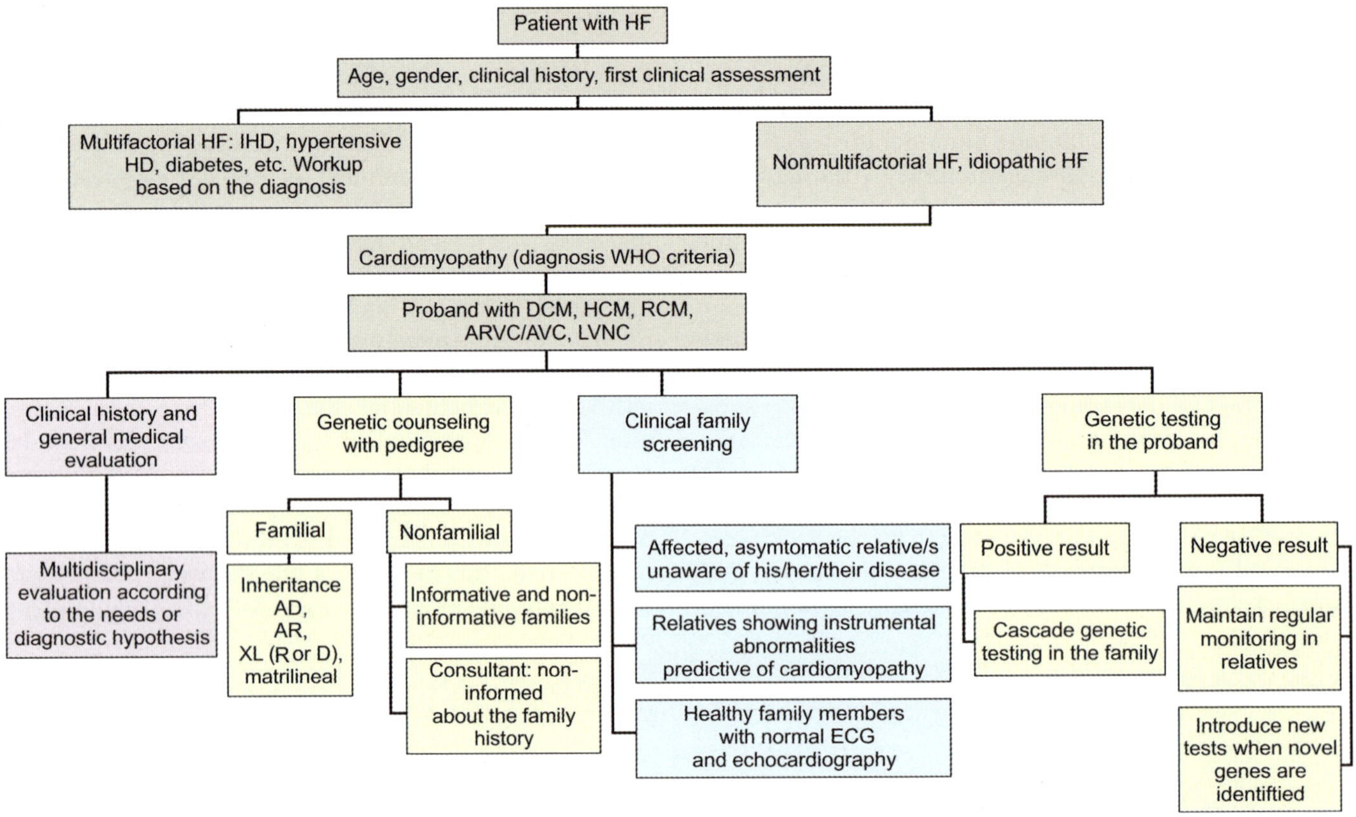

HF, heart failure; IHD, idiopathic heart disease; WHO, World Health Organization; DCM, dilated cardiomyopathy; HCM, hypertrophic cardiomyopathy; RCM, restrictive cardiomyopathy; ARVC, arrhythmogenic right-ventricular cardiomyopathy; LVNC, left ventricular noncompaction; AVC, arrhythmogenic ventricular cardiomyopathy; ECG, electrocardiogram

Flowchart 3 The diagnostic work-up in familial cardiomyopathies, from the diagnosis in the proband to the cascade family screening in the family

and short PR interval,[31] or WPW.[32] Both cardiac and extracardiac traits should be evaluated in each patient with cardiomyopathy.

Family History and Pedigree

A likelihood of heritability of the cardiomyopathy is dependent upon collection of family history to develop a pedigree[6,8,23] (Flowchart 3). The patient often seeks information about the diagnosis, cause, implication for life expectancy, manage options for medical and heart transplantation, and whether offspring will inherit the predisposition to develop the same cardiomyopathy. The counselor should discuss the disease, current knowledge of testable genetic causes, strengths, limitations and possible errors in conducting and interpreting of genetic tests, and the probability of identifying the causative mutation with the consequent necessity of cascade genetic testing in the entire family. After assessing the information in entirety, the consultant must obtain the informed consent for genetic testing. Cascade family screening may uncover family members that are affected, asymptomatic, unaware of their disease, or may show abnormal phenotypic features by various imaging modalities, especially as early markers of disease.[6] Cascade family screening and long-term monitoring of family members may transform a diagnosis of sporadic cardiomyopathy into a diagnosis of familial cardiomyopathy either at the first screening or subsequently in follow-up (Fig. 2).

Genetic Testing

Cardiomyopathies are genetically heterogeneous diseases, with more than 80 disease genes identified. The previous strategy for genetic testing involved the costly and time-consuming Sanger capillary sequencing. The

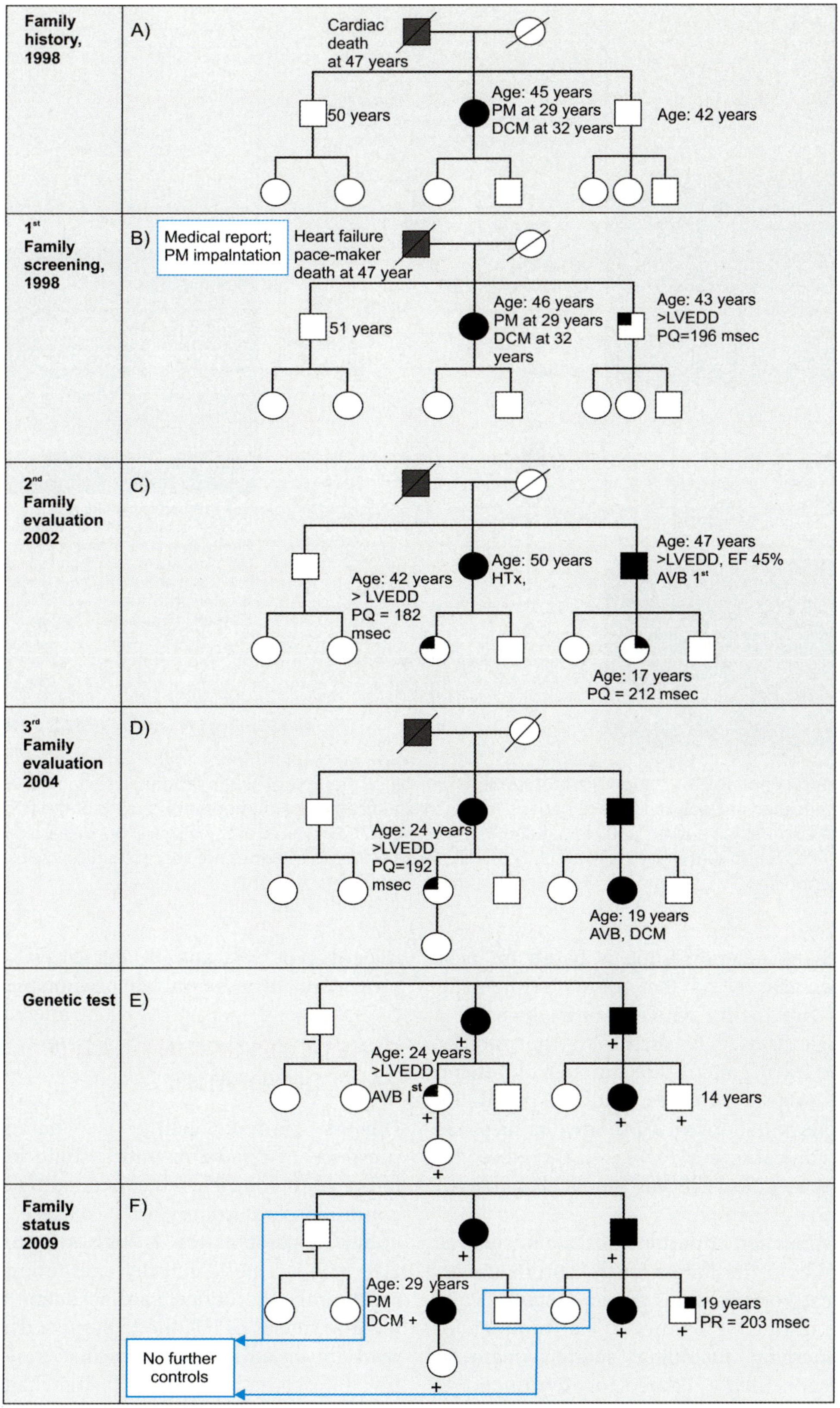

Fig. 2 The diagnostic and monitoring phases and the long-term history of familial dilated cardiolaminopathy

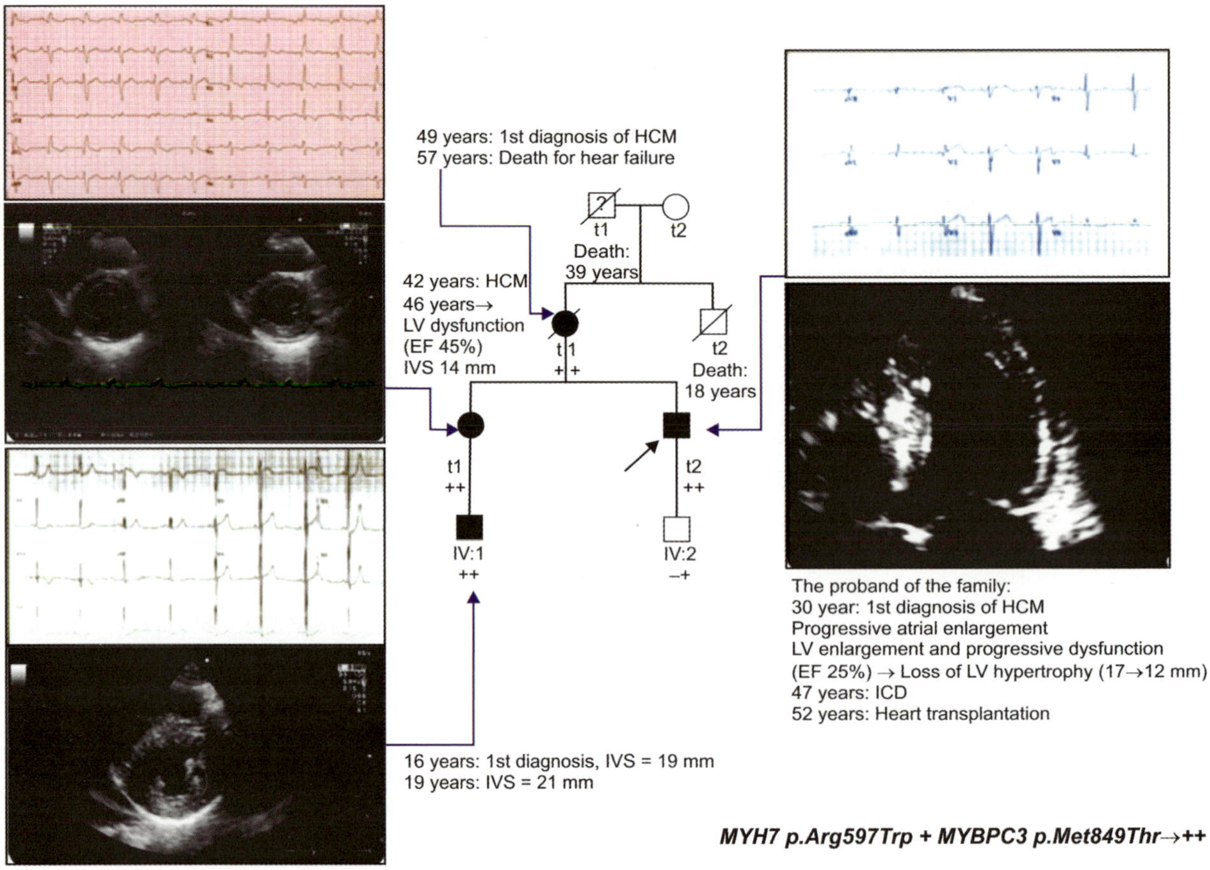

Fig. 3 The identification of double or compound mutations in familial cardiomyopathies is progressively increasing, with the increase of the number of genes that are analyzed in each patient. In this family, all affected members are carriers of the two mutations; the IV:2 only carries the *MYBPC3* mutation and he is still nonaffected. Given the AD inheritance of the disease, the disease causing mutation is in *MYH7*, while the *MYBPC3* is a variant that may eventually modify the phenotype but does not seem to cause, by itself, the hypertrophic cardiomyopathy phenotype

modern approach to genetic testing is based on next generation sequencing (NGS) that allows sequencing of several genes (up to the whole exome) in several patients in a single assay.[33] By increasing the number of tested genes in each patient, the number of genetic variants in each subject increases, and the possibility of double or triple mutations in cardiomyopathies has been reported in clinical series[34,35] (Fig. 3). Therefore, the interpretation of the results is key for genetic diagnosis of the cardiomyopathy.

Current guidelines for important decisions, such as implantable cardiac-defibrillators (ICD) implantation in patients with cardiomyopathies do not systematically include genetic testing.[36-38] However, a number of warnings are emerging; including, sudden death in DCM patients with mildly dilated or dysfunctional left ventricles,[39-41] or in HCM patients with mild LV hypertrophy,[42,43] and underscores the inability to prognosticate based only on phenotypic characterization.

GENETIC TESTING IN DILATED CARDIOMYOPATHY

Dilated cardiomyopathy is characterized by the presence of dilatation and systolic impairment of the left or both ventricles unexplained by abnormal loading conditions or coronary artery disease (CAD).[5] The most common presentation is with symptoms and signs of HF, with a small minority presenting with ventricular arrhythmia or sudden cardiac death. DCM is now the leading causes of HF due to systolic dysfunction and the commonest indication for cardiac transplantation (HTx) in adolescents and adults.[44] The diagnosis of DCM is descriptive and based on morphofunctional imaging.

DCM is defined as familial when two or more related family members are affected and is familial in up to 50% of cases.[5,6] In the majority of patients, the inheritance is AD, in that at least 50% of first-degree relatives of the proband should be affected. In the past, exceptions to this rule were attributed to incomplete or variable penetrance, and in present times, the interpretation should include incomplete genotyping. The latter issue will be effectively addressed by parallel sequencing of all known disease genes or with exome-sequencing of genetically orphan families. Only a minority of DCM is inherited as an autosomal recessive trait, a condition in which parents are healthy and offspring (unique case, sib pairs, trios or more brothers) are affected; parental consanguinity or origin of families from small geographic isolates should be carefully explored. In X-linked recessive inheritance, male patients receive the mutation from a healthy mother or rarely demonstrate a de novo mutation; sons of affected fathers are healthy while daughters are obligate carriers (Flowchart 2). Finally, a small proportion of patients who are carriers of mutations in mitochondrial deoxyribonucleic acid (DNA) develop DCM, which is inherited per matrilineal or maternal inheritance pattern.

Genetic Heterogeneity

More than 40 disease-causing genes have been identified, including nuclear genes encoding proteins of nuclear envelope, sarcolemma, cytoskeleton, sarcomere, desmosome, calcium-handling proteins, and proteins involved in energy generation encoded by nuclear and mitochondrial genes. Age, gender, and inheritance pattern are essential for a preliminary specific diagnostic hypothesis, and the genetic heterogeneity is higher than that of other forms of cardiomyopathies. Difficult issues that often cloud genetic testing include a large number of genes needed to be screened in probands, the correct interpretation of the family history (especially when medical reports of deceased patients are not available), and the lack of comprehensive clinical reports that exclude, for example, an HCM with end-stage evolution through a DCM-like phenotype.[20-22]

Genetic Diagnosis

The genetic work-up in DCM is based on a simple cascade that is similar to the approach suggested earlier. From a practical viewpoint, the genetic heterogeneity constitutes a challenging issue for achieving a gene-specific diagnosis of DCM. It is reasonable to question whether all known disease genes in all probands should be evaluated, or if a pretest hypothesis be developed from the available clinical data? If the test is based on NGS, then all 40 or more genes could theoretically be screened in all patients, but if the test is still based on Sanger sequencing, then a clinically oriented approach becomes necessary.[6,18]

Genetic-based Risk Stratification

The subgroup of dilated cardiac laminopathies deserves special attention because the arrhythmogenic risk does not necessarily correlate with the severity of the DCM. Patients with mildly dilated and dysfunctional left ventricles may develop life-threatening arrhythmias while not fulfilling guideline-based criteria of ICD implantation for primary prevention.[40,41] *LMNA* gene should be screened in all patients with DCM, giving priority to those with AVB, ventricular arrhythmias, and atrial fibrillation, especially when there is a positive family history of sudden death. *Vice versa* the subgroup of dilated cardiodystrophinopathies typically demonstrate extreme LV dilatation and dysfunction (thus fulfilling guideline criteria for ICD implantation) but demonstrate a low arrhythmogenic risk.[30,45] The subgroup of DCM caused by mutations of genes that are typically associated with ARVC/AVC (desmosome genes)[46] may show gene-based high arrhythmogenic risk, independent of the severity of the LV dysfunction, and dilatation or functional class. The three examples above demonstrate that current guidelines do not meet modern risk stratification in DCM and insist that cardiologists should receive genetic information useful for making appropriate decisions for primary prevention of sudden death.

HYPERTROPHIC CARDIOMYOPATHY AND GENETIC TESTING

The Disease

Hypertrophic cardiomyopathy is defined as LVH in the absence of abnormal loading conditions sufficient to explain the observed degree of hypertrophy.[5] The prevalence is high (1:500 affected in adults) and the phenotype is age-dependent with a minority of cases observed in childhood.[47] The disease can be asymptomatic or mildly symptomatic for years or present with symptoms, such as chest pain and dyspnea or with syncope, which can coincide with the clinical onset of the disease.[48] The course of the disease is slow in the long- term; many patients develop progressive symptoms caused by gradual deterioration in LV function or massive hypertrophy,[49] and the end-stage is associated with an annual mortality rate of 10% per year from sudden ventricular arrhythmia, stroke, or diastolic and systolic LV failure.[50] HCM can be broadly grouped into sarcomeric and non-sarcomeric HCM. The former constitutes the majority of HCM, and is caused by mutations in genes coding structural or regulatory proteins of the sarcomere.

Familial Sarcomeric Hypertrophic Cardiomyopathy

Sarcomeric HCM is caused by mutations of genes that code structural or regulatory proteins of the sarcomere.[50,51] The most common pattern of inheritance is AD (Fig. 4).[5,6] Recessive and X-linked inheritance is less common and de novo mutations can also occur.[52] Family screening can

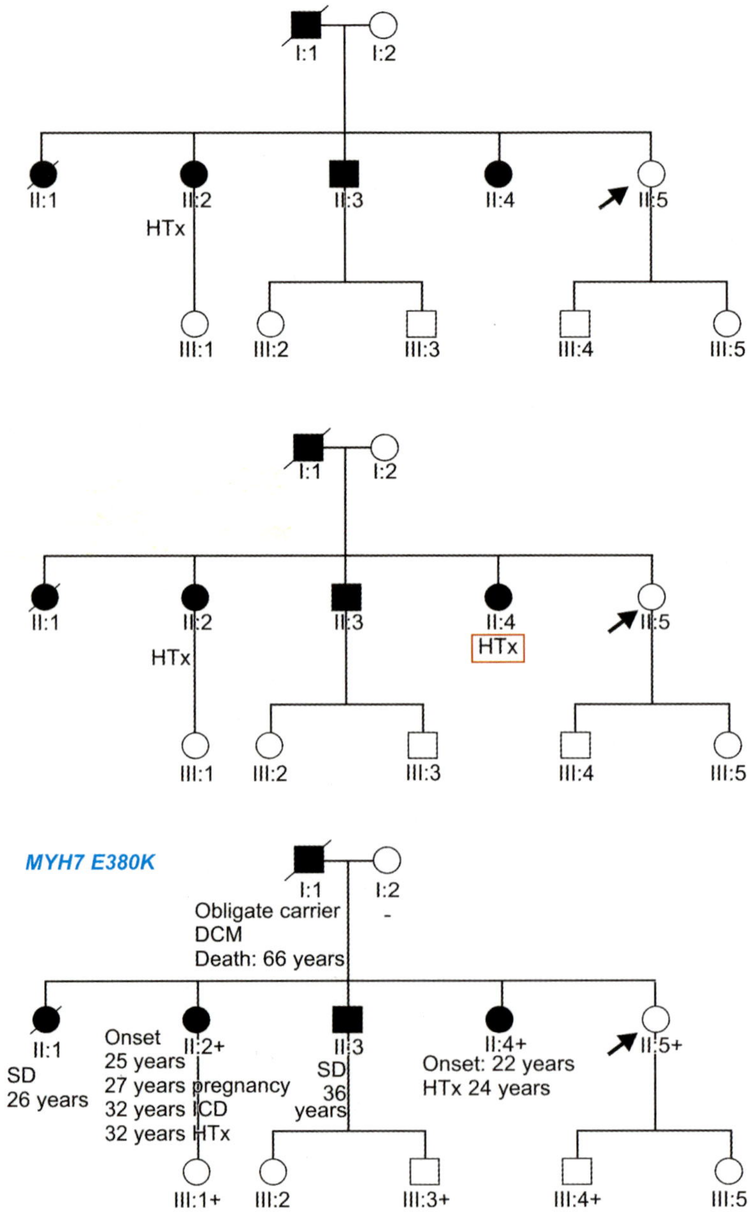

Fig. 4 The typical autosomal dominant inheritance of hypertrophic cardiomyopathy and evolution of the disease as well as clinical history in the family

conveniently help establish the pattern of inheritance and phenotype characteristics in the family. The recurrence of life-threatening events in the family may alert regarding arrhythmogenic risk. The presence of more than one phenotype (HCM, RCM, or HCM with restrictive pattern) in affected members of the same family strongly suggests a sarcomeric HCM.

Genetic Heterogeneity of Sarcomeric Hypertrophic Cardiomyopathy

Sarcomeric HCM is a genetically heterogeneous disease: mutations in *MYH7, MYBPC3, TNNI3,* and *TNNT2* account for upto 70% of cases.[53-55] The extensive screening of all known disease genes may identify an additional number of HCM but the list of disease genes is still incomplete. Nonetheless, a percentage of about 80% of positive genetic testing is a good proportion, especially when all genes are screened in all patients. In fact up to 10% of HCM patients carry double or compound mutations in nuclear genes or in nuclear and mitochondrial genes, a complex genetic condition that is associated with worse prognosis.[56] As recommended by scientific societies, genetic test in patients with HCM should include at least the most common disease genes.

Genetic Testing and Diagnosis

Cardiac and extracardiac markers, which could be potentially useful for guiding genetic testing, are less common in HCM as compared to DCM or even in non-sarcomeric HCM. *MYH7*-related HCM may be associated with fibrillar myopathy and severe LVH;[57] *TNNI3* and *TNNT2*-related HCM commonly show prominent restrictive pattern.[58,59] Genetic testing may include only most common disease genes or screen for all known disease genes, including those responsible for less than 1% of cases. In probands with high probability of genetic disease but negative screening of all known disease genes, exome sequencing can identify novel rare disease genes. Comprehensive genetic testing is the best recommendation. The increasing evidence that more than one mutation can be identified in the same patient or in the same family dictates that even in the presence of a Mendelian inheritance of an established trait, the cascade clinical and genetic family screenings are mandatory to establish the true role of genetic variants identified with genetic tests.[56,60] In relatives, the search for the mutation identified in the probands is easy to perform. However, the interpretation of the significance of the mutation must be based on evidence that the discovered variant is in fact the disease-causing mutation.

Genetics and Risk Stratification

It is important to identify the likelihood of three major untoward outcomes in HCM, including the risk of life-threatening arrhythmias, the evolution through end-stage LV dilatation and dysfunction, and the risk of thromboembolic events.[48,61] Early studies suggested that a genotype to phenotype correlation may exist between the severity of LVH and arrhythmogenic risk;[61] however, these early observations were followed by variable and discordant results that did not confirm reproducible relationships.[26,62,63] For example, troponinopathies carry high risk of sudden death independent of maximal LV wall thickness.[59,64] Therefore, clinical decisions for primary prevention with ICD should be taken in an individual patient based on clinical and genetic data, and family history of sudden death. The evolution to the end-stage disease is more common in patients with complex genetics with two or more mutations.[56,60] On the other hand, thromboembolic risk does not seem to correlate with genetic data but rather with atrial dilatation and arrhythmias.[64]

NON-SARCOMERIC HYPERTROPHIC CARDIOMYOPATHY AND GENETIC TESTING

Up to 10% of patients presenting with idiopathic LVH may mimic sarcomeric HCM, and may include systemic diseases variable extent of extracardiac involvement. Such diseases may result in increased LV wall thickness from an increase in intramyocyte content of organelles or nonmetabolized material, or from extramyocellular interstitial infiltration. The intramyocellular pathology may include mitochondrial diseases (caused either by mutations in mitochondrial DNA or in the nuclear genes coding for mitochondrial proteins) (Flowchart 4),[65] glycogen-storage diseases including other disorders of the glycogen metabolism; lysosomal-storage diseases, such as sphingolipidoses and mucopolysaccharidoses, disorders of glycoproteins and glycosylation metabolism, and abnormalities of amino acid and organic acid metabolism.[66] The most common form of extracellular infiltration is observed in familial amyloidosis.[67] The correct diagnosis of each specific disease is essential for management and prognostication. Several storage diseases can now be treated with enzyme replacement therapy or stem cell transplantation.[68-70] New drugs

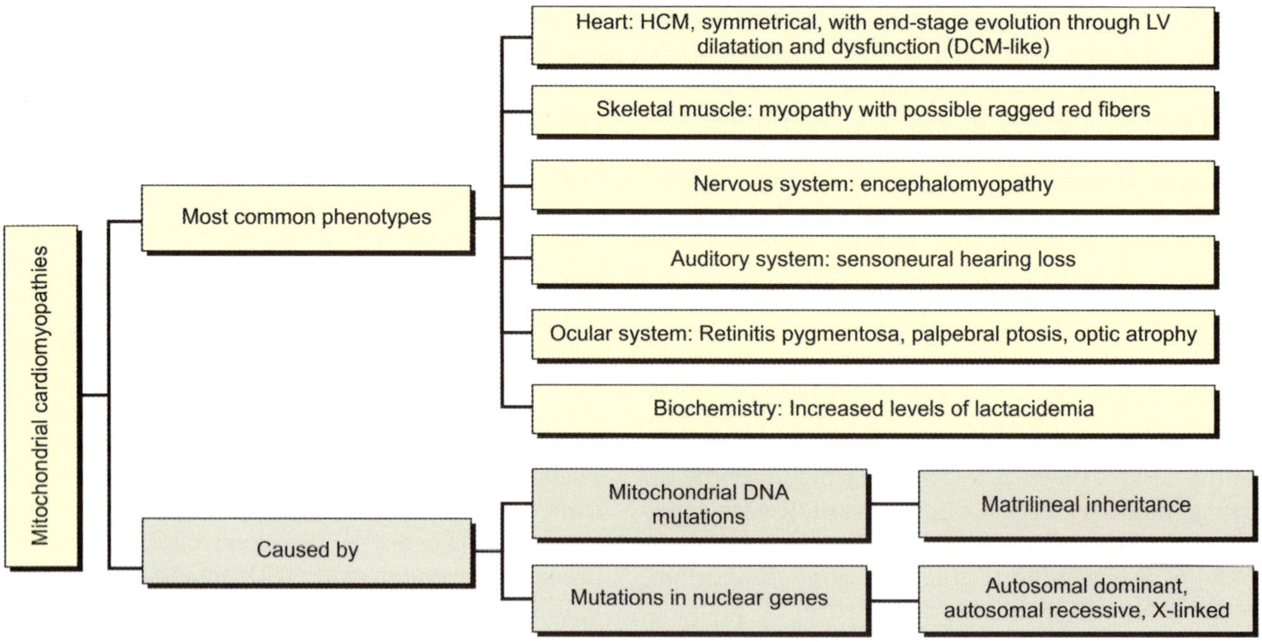

HCM, hypertrophic cardiomyopathy; LV, left ventricular; DCM, dilated cardiomyopathy; DNA, deoxyribonucleic acid

Flowchart 4 The major organ involvement and phenotype traits that may recur in patients with mitochondrial diseases and different patterns of inheritance

are emerging for transthyretin (TTR)-amyloidosis that underscores the importance of correct diagnosis of familial amyloidosis.[71] Patients with mitochondrial disease often show multiorgan or multisystem involvement, including non-thromboembolic stroke-like episodes and epilepsy. The administration of antiepileptic drugs, such as valproate in such patients may cause complications, such as brain pseudoatrophy.[72] On the other hand, stroke-like episodes can be treated (and even probably prevented) with taurine.[73] In non-sarcomeric HCM, a short PR interval or WPW may occur in patients with *PRKAG2*, lysosome-associated membrane protein 2 (*LAMP2*) and alpha-galactosidase (*GLA*) mutations, or in mitochondrial cardiomyopathies;[74-77] in these four conditions, inheritance and traits associated with the HCM phenotypes are characteristically different. *PRKAG2* is AD, *LAMP2* is X-linked with early onset mental retardation in males, *GLA* mutation is X-linked without mental retardation; mitochondrial diseases are either inherited in a matrilineal pattern, or according to Mendelian rules in case of nuclear genes coding mitochondrial proteins. The mitochondrial cardiomyopathies are typically associated with biomarkers (increased lactacidemia) and noncardiac traits [chronic progressive external ophthalmoplegia (CPEO), myopathy and stroke]. In HCM that appears as sporadic (small families or adopted patients or only survivors), the interpretation of cardiac and extracardiac markers is not supported by family data and clinical experience may contribute to the formulation of a specific diagnostic hypothesis.

RESTRICTIVE CARDIOMYOPATHY AND GENETIC TESTING

Pure RCM is a rare condition (1:100,000) clinically characterized by altered relaxation and abnormal LV filling, normal ventricular size, biatrial dilation and absence of significant LV hypertrophy.[5] The major clinical manifestations may consist of diastolic HF, atrial and ventricular arrhythmias, and thromboembolic complications.[78] RCM can be familial or sporadic, the latter often caused by de novo mutations. Sarcomeric RCM are caused by mutations in nuclear genes,[34-79] in particular *TNNI3*,[79] *TNNT2*,[80] and less commonly *MYL3*,[81] and *ACTC1*.[82] Troponinopathies are characterized by high arrhythmogenic risk, which is independent of the LV thickness and rather related to the troponin defects; conduction disease and muscle involvement are uncommon. Phenotype heterogeneity occurs within families with troponinopathies with family members exhibiting typical RCM, others showing HCM with restrictive pathophysiology, and some showing pure RCM.

The association with AVB and myopathy (either clinically overt or subclinical) clinically characterizes a subgroup of RCM caused by mutation of intermediate filament desmin, with intracellular accumulation of desmin aggregates.[83,84] The desmin deposition both in cardiac and skeletal myocytes is a specific marker of disease. Desmin-positive aggregates have been recently reported in intestinal smooth muscle cells[85] that may explain the gastrointestinal involvement in the late phases of the disease. The arrhythmogenic risk in desmin RCM is rather low; in a recent meta-analysis including desmin-related diseases, both myopathies and cardiomyopathies, sudden death was reported only in two of 195 DES-mutation carriers.[86] Complex genetics can be observed in DES families, and a mutation in DES gene has been found in association with variants in two *LQT* genes, *SCN5A* and *KCNH2* in a family with sudden death.[87] The typical evolution is end-stage HF that requires heart transplantation.[83,84,88]

ARRHYTHMOGENIC RIGHT VENTRICULAR CARDIOMYOPATHY/ARRHYTHMOGENIC CARDIOMYOPATHY AND GENETIC TESTING

Although originally termed ARVC because of the typical involvement of the right ventricle, the disease is preferably designated as arrhythmogenic cardiomyopathy (ARC) due to the recent characterization of biventricular and left dominant variants.[89,90] ARC is a heritable myocardial disease with an estimated prevalence that was originally reported as 2:10,000 people and is now close to 1:1,000.[91] ARC is mostly inherited as an AD trait; the penetrance is incomplete, variable, and age-dependent, thus masking the AD inheritance in some families. The rare cardiocutaneous syndromes of Naxos and Carvajal are inherited as autosomal recessive traits.[92,93] Double or compound heterozygosity is common, and contributes to the penetrance complications.[94]

The diagnosis of ARC is based on the presence of characteristic electrocardiogram (ECG) changes, arrhythmias, imaging, and when available, biopsy-verified myocardial fibrofatty replacement.[89] Family screening is contributory; the disease in fact evolves from an early, *concealed* phase (in which the arrhythmogenic risk occurs in structurally and functionally normal hearts) to a fully manifest phase with structural (fibrofatty infiltration of the myocardium, ventricular aneurysms and hypertrabeculation), and functional (wall motion abnormalities) alterations. Family members may also demonstrate an entire clinical spectrum of the disease, with early ECG changes in some relatives to full blown morphofunctional phenotype in others. The major advantage of screening of family members is the identification of family members who may carry a severe arrhythmogenic risk subclinically. In the classic variant with right ventricular predominance, arrhythmias and thromboembolic complications are the major clinical manifestations; HF is uncommonly observed. On the other hand, HF constitutes the major clinical presentation in the biventricular and left-dominant variants. Genetic testing is currently performed, including all disease genes and *LMNA*.[95]

LEFT VENTRICULAR NONCOMPACTION AND GENETIC TESTING

Left ventricular noncompaction is characterized by prominent hypertrabeculations and intertrabecular recesses in the apical and mid-lateral/inferior walls of the LV to confer a spongy morphology to the ventricle.[96] Criteria for the diagnosis of LVNC is entirely based on imaging wherein the ratio of noncompact to compact layer of the myocardium is higher than 2.0.[97] The diagnosis can be incidental or result from clinical evaluation of patients presenting with HF, arrhythmias, or thromboembolic complications. LVNC can be present as an isolated trait or be a part of systemic or neuromuscular disorders. When isolated, the major clinical impact can be related to the potential thromboembolic risk. It can be a marker of disease, which is associated with pattern on inheritance and other abnormalities, may guide the diagnostic hypothesis and, therefore, the genetic testing. LVNC is a typical trait of Barth syndrome and a cardiac variant of tafazzinoapthy.[98,99] Mutations in *CHYPHER-ZASP* (*LDB3*) gene have been reported in patients with LVNC.[100] *LDB3* gene is a causative gene, and is considered a good candidate for explaining LVNC phenotype in patients with HCM or DCM caused by other disease genes.[101] In such cases, the final phenotype is the sum of at least two gene defects but DCM or HCM would occur independent of the *LDB3* mutations.

GENETICS IN HEART FAILURE CAUSED BY MULTIFACTORIAL DISEASES

A majority of the HF cases represent the end-stage manifestation of various multifactorial diseases, such as coronary artery disease, as well as hypertensive, diabetic, and valvular heart diseases.[1] Each multifactorial disease may carry heritable components and the extent of the heritable contribution can be assessed by clinical evaluation of family history and pedigree. Genes associated with increased risk of HF have been identified, but their contribution to the phenotype is highly variable and still a matter of investigation. For multifactorial diseases, such as myocardial infarction (MI), a positive family history of premature MI is a major risk factor independent of risk factors associated with CAD.[102] The relatives of the victim of premature MI often seek genetic counseling for the likelihood of MI, especially in the absence of established risk factors. Simple rules govern current clinical genetics in MI: individuals are expected to be at the highest risk when a closely related family member has experienced premature MI, more than one relative is affected, and when the victim is of the less commonly affected gender (female). Therefore, the son of an affected mother who had premature MI and a sibling of an affected brother carry a very high risk of MI. Family screening in premature MI with more than one affected family member could be the first step in a tailored preventive strategy in clinical practice.[102]

Counseling for the risk of HF should be targeted to the underlying diseases than to the HF syndrome itself. Clinical observations in the families indicate that the relative risk of developing HF for a patient who has one or both parents who suffered HF is less than 2, with slightly higher value for biparental risk.[103] Compared to the contributory role of a single mutation in heritable cardiomyopathies, the heritable component of HF is unlikely to be deterministic.[104] Nonetheless, the role of genetic component of the mechanisms involved in adverse ventricular remodeling seems to be clinically relevant as has been increasingly supported by pharmacogenomics and variable efficacy of drugs used for the clinical management of HF.

Major Molecular Pathways Activated in Heart Failure and Genetic Testing

The syndrome of HF is characterized by upregulation of the neurohumoral axes that contributes to adverse ventricular remodeling,[4,105,106] regardless of the primary cause of HF including multifactorial HF, unique monogenic cardiomyopathies and HF, or monofactorial non-heritable diseases, such as primary amyloidosis. In this molecular context, association studies have investigated variations in one or more genes of the renin-angiotensin-aldosterone (RAAS) and adrenergic systems to decipher the proportion of heritability of HF, risk stratification, and drug responsiveness, especially to angiotensin converting enzyme (ACE) inhibitors and beta (β)-blockers.

Renin-Angiotensin-Aldosterone System

Angiotensin Converting Enzyme Insertion/Deletion Polymorphism

The levels of ACE show familial clustering; about 50% of the variation of ACE plasma levels depend on a common 287 bp insertion (I)/deletion (D) polymorphism in intron 16 of the *ACE* gene. Carriers of homozygous DD have higher ACE levels while carriers of homozygous II have lower ACE levels; heterozygotes (ID) demonstrate intermediate enzyme levels.[107] Several studies have investigated the association of ACE polymorphism with incidence of HF[108] and prognosis,[109,110] drugs responsiveness (D allele carriers seem to have greatest benefit from ACE inhibitors[111]) and correlation with LVH;[112] however, the association between HF and ACE polymorphism has not been established. Scientific documents on HF do not recommend ACE polymorphism testing in HF.

Angiotensin II Type 1 Receptor Gene, *A1166C* Polymorphism

Existing data on the association between *A1166C* single nucleotide polymorphism (SNP) and increased risk of HF are debated with some in favor[113] and others only confirming an association with disease severity and increased mortality.[114] Similar to the ACE polymorphism, there is currently no recommendation to test this SNP in HF.

Angiotensin AGT Polymorphisms and Heart Failure Risk and Mortality

Studies are scarce[115] and do not demonstrate any association of *M235T* and G(-6)A with HF.

Adrenergic System

Adrenergic receptors (ADR) β1 (ARB1) and β2 (ARB2) are expressed in cardiac myocytes with a ratio of about 2:1. The adrenergic stimulation leads to β-ADR coupling to the costimulatory G protein to transduce intracellular signaling by activation of protein kinase A, and adrenergic upregulation during HF leads to downregulation of ARB1 to attenuate the sympathetic toxicity to the myocardium.[116] A recent study tested responses to the β1-receptor agonist dobutamine and the β2-receptor agonist terbutaline using gated blood pool scintigraphy for the efficacy of long-term β-blocker therapy. Changes in heart rate (HR) and cardiac output (CO) with dobutamine were higher in carriers of greater than or equal to 1 β1 Arg389 allele than in homozygous Gly389 allele ($p = 0.02$). Increases in HR, stroke volume (SV), and CO with terbutaline were greater in carriers of the homozygous β2 Glu27 allele than in heterozygous or homozygous carriers of Gln27 allele (HR, $p = 0.048$; CO, $p = 0.034$; SV, $p = 0.045$). The authors proposed that β-receptor gene variants significantly influence inotropic and chronotropic responses to β-agonist exposure in patients on β-blocker therapy.[117] In addition, a study testing a gene-dose interaction with the ADRβ1-389 Arg/Arg versus Gly carriers and β-blocker dose, suggested that patients with the Arg/Arg genotype might require a higher dose of β-blockers to achieve a response similar to that of Gly carriers.[118] Although currently no guidelines have included indications to test SNP in adrenergic receptor genes in HF, testing β1 Arg389Gly could find clinical application to adjust the dose β-blockers in future.

GENOME-WIDE ASSOCIATION STUDIES AND NOVEL CANDIDATE GENES IN CARDIOMYOPATHY AND HEART FAILURE

Genome-Wide Association Studies (GWAS) may not only contribute to the quantitative assessment of the proportion of heritability in multifactorial diseases, but also to identify loci associated with complex traits and novel disease genes.[119-122] GWAS have identified *HSPB7*[123] and a locus located within the *BAG3* sequence (chromosome 10q26) as a risk gene for DCM.[119,120,122] *HSPB7* codes for the cardiovascular heat shock protein that is downregulated in LVH in experimental models.[121]

A meta-analysis from the Cohorts for Heart and Aging Research in Genomic Epidemiology (CHARGE) Consortium identified two loci that were associated with incident HF and exceeded genome-wide significance;[124] one locus was identified at 15q22 chromosome positioned 58.8 kb from Ubiquitin-specific protease 3 (USP3) and 63.9 kb from *CA12* (*Carbonic Anhydrase XII*). USPs play a role in the release of Ubiquitin from degraded proteins: abnormalities in ubiquitin proteasome have been described in HCM and DCM.[125] *CA12* mutations cause the autosomal recessive isolated hyperchlorhidrosis, a condition characterized by visible salt precipitates after sweating, transient hyponatremic dehydration, and slow weight gain in infancy.[126] The second locus was identified in African-ancestry participants at 12q14 located 6.3 kb from the Leucine-Rich Repeats and Immunoglobulin-Like Domains-Containing Protein 3 (*LRIG3*). The *LRIG3* gene is one of the three members of the *LRIG* family of genes; its potential role in HF is still unknown.[124]

Another novel locus at 3p22 in an intron of chemokine-like factor (CKLF) superfamily-MARVEL transmembrane domain containing 7 (*CMTM7*) has been reported to be associated with all-cause mortality among HF patients of European ancestry.[127]

DYNAMIC MOLECULAR TARGETS IN HEART FAILURE

Any physiological or pathological increase in myocardial mass involves differential expression of a large number of genes.[128,129] Epigenetic factors may modulate differential gene expression through modification of chromosomal components without an alteration in the nucleotide sequence of the genome.[130] DNA methylation, chromatin remodeling, and histone modifications modulate the binding of transcription factors to the gene promoters, and may contribute to the regulation of gene expression involved in cardiac hypertrophy, fibrosis, and dilatation. Factors acting at the post-transcriptional levels (microRNA) could potentiate the effects of transcription factors. The above mentioned epigenetic factors may be dynamically and reciprocally interactive,[131] and differential DNA methylation has been reported in HF.[132] Since the final phenotype of HF syndrome is common to all monogenic and multifactorial diseases, it is likely that the modulation of a hub pathway may influence evolution of HF, and either measuring the quantitative expression of genes playing in each known molecular pathway or assay of epigenetic factors and their cross-talk could help identify novel therapeutic targets.[133]

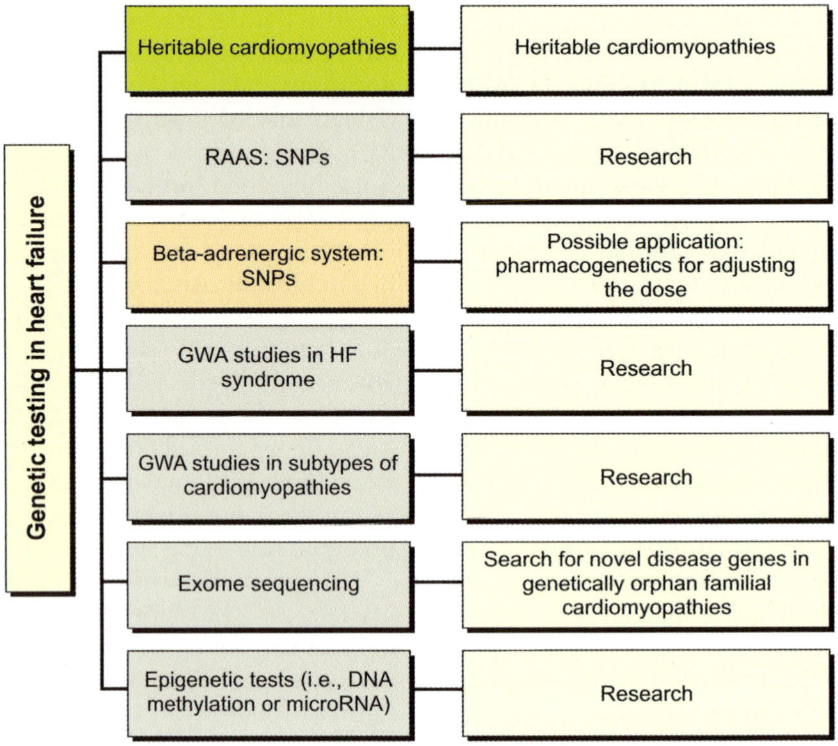

RAAS, renin-angiotensin-aldosterone system; SNPs, single-nucleotide polymorphisms; GWA, Genome-Wide Association Studies; HF, heart failure; DNA, deoxyribonucleic acid

Flowchart 5 The research or diagnostic applications of genetic testing in heart failure

CONCLUSION

Heart failure is a complex syndrome that represents the final evolution of several different diseases, both multifactorial and monogenic-inherited cardiomyopathies. Genetic testing may facilitate clinical work-up of cardiomyopathies with proven benefits to probands and families. The information generated by Sanger-based sequencing although conclusive has not addressed all disease genes in all patients, and has left open the possibility of incomplete genotyping, and a number of genetic variants that either did not segregate in families or have been considered as variants of uncertain significance. NGS will provide more complete genotyping data in patients and families and hopefully help offer correct interpretation of the test results. Genetic testing would become mandatory in heritable cardiomyopathies, but is not indicated in patients with HF caused by multifactorial cardiovascular diseases. The role of genetic polymorphisms for neurohumoral alterations will need further investigation before finding wide applicability (Flowchart 5).

REFERENCES

1. McMurray JJ, Adamopoulos S, Anker SD, et al. ESC guidelines for the diagnosis and treatment of acute and chronic heart failure 2012: The Task Force for the Diagnosis and Treatment of Acute and Chronic Heart Failure 2012 of the European Society of Cardiology. Developed in collaboration with the Heart Failure Association (HFA) of the ESC. Eur Heart J. 2012;14:803-69.
2. Loehr LR, Rosamond WD, Chang PP, et al. Heart failure incidence and survival (from the Atherosclerosis Risk in Communities study). Am J Cardiol. 2008;101(7):1016-22.
3. Cowie MR, Fox KF, Wood DA, et al. Hospitalization of patients with heart failure: a population-based study. Eur Heart J. 2002;23(11):877-85.
4. Braunwald E. Striking improvements in the prognosis of individual cardiac conditions (ACS, severe hypertension, valvular and congenital heart disease) but growing prevalence of Heart Failure. JACC. 2013;1:1-20.
5. Elliott P, Andersson B, Arbustini E, et al. Classification of the cardiomyopathies: a position statement from the European Society of Cardiology Working Group on Myocardial and Pericardial Diseases. Eur Heart J. 2008;29(2):270-6.
6. Charron P, Arad M, Arbustini E, et al. Genetic counselling and testing in cardiomyopathies: a position statement of the European Society of Cardiology Working Group on Myocardial and Pericardial Diseases. Eur Heart J. 2010;3(22):2715-26.
7. Baig MK, Goldman JH, Caforio AL, et al. Familial dilated cardiomyopathy: cardiac abnormalities are common in asymptomatic relatives and may represent early disease. J Am Coll Cardiol. 1998;31(1):195-201.

8. Gavazzi A, Repetto A, Scelsi L, et al. Evidence-based diagnosis of familial non-X-linked dilated cardiomyopathy. Prevalence, inheritance and characteristics. Eur Heart J. 2001;22(1):73-81.
9. Murphy RT, Thaman R, Blanes JG, et al. Natural history and familial characteristics of isolated left ventricular non-compaction. Eur Heart J. 2005;26(2):187-92.
10. Mahon NG, Murphy RT, MacRae CA, et al. Echocardiographic evaluation in asymptomatic relatives of patients with dilated cardiomyopathy reveals preclinical disease. Ann Intern Med. 2005;143(2):108-15.
11. McKenna WJ, Spirito P, Desnos M, et al. Experience from clinical genetics in hypertrophic cardiomyopathy: proposal for new diagnostic criteria in adult members of affected families. Heart. 1997;77(2):130-2.
12. Nava A, Bauce B, Basso C, et al. Clinical profile and long-term follow-up of 37 families with arrhythmogenic right ventricular cardiomyopathy. J Am Coll Cardiol. 2000;36(7):2226-33.
13. Hamid MS, Norman M, Quraishi A, et al. Prospective evaluation of relatives for familial arrhythmogenic right ventricular cardiomyopathy/dysplasia reveals a need to broaden diagnostic criteria. J Am Coll Cardiol. 2002;40(8):1445-50.
14. Maron BJ, Towbin JA, Thiene G, et al. Contemporary definitions and classification of the cardiomyopathies: an American Heart Association Scientific Statement from the Council on Clinical Cardiology, Heart Failure and Transplantation Committee; Quality of Care and Outcomes Research and Functional Genomics and Translational Biology Interdisciplinary Working Groups; and Council on Epidemiology and Prevention. Circulation. 2006;113(14):1807-16.
15. Hunt SA; American College of Cardiology; American Heart Association Task Force on Practice Guidelines. ACC/AHA 2005 guideline update for the diagnosis and management of chronic heart failure in the adult: a report of the American College of Cardiology/American Heart Association Task Force on Practice Guidelines (Writing Committee to Update the 2001 Guidelines for the Evaluation and Management of Heart Failure). J Am Coll Cardiol. 2005;46(6):e1-82.
16. Hershberger RE, Lindenfeld J, Mestroni L, et al. Genetic evaluation of cardiomyopathy—a Heart Failure Society of America practice guideline. J Car Fail. 2009;15(2):83-97.
17. Ackerman MJ, Priori SG, Willems S, et al. HRS/EHRA expert consensus statement on the state of genetic testing for the channelopathies and cardiomyopathies: this document was developed as a partnership between the Heart Rhythm Society (HRS) and the European Heart Rhythm Association (EHRA). Europace. 2011;13(8):1077-109.
18. Rapezzi C, Arbustini E, Caforio AL, et al. Diagnostic work-up in cardiomyopathies: bridging the gap between clinical phenotypes and final diagnosis. A position statement from the ESC Working Group on Myocardial and Pericardial Diseases. Eur Heart J. 2013;34(19):1448-58.
19. Ashley EA, Hershberger RE, Caleshu C, et al. Genetics and cardiovascular disease: a policy statement from the American Heart Association. Circulation. 2012;126(1):142-57.
20. Lopes LR, Elliott PM. New approaches to the clinical diagnosis of inherited heart muscle disease Heart. 2013;99(19):1451-61.
21. Sturm AC. Genetic testing in the contemporary diagnosis of cardiomyopathy. Curr Heart Fail Rep. 2013;10(1):63-72.
22. Morales A, Hershberger RE. Genetic evaluation of dilated cardiomyopathy. Curr Cardiol Rep. 2013;15(7):375.
23. Arbustini E, Cecchi F, Dubourg O, et al. The need for European Registries in inherited cardiomyopathies. Eur Heart J. 2002;23(24):1972-4.
24. Bertrand AT, Chikhaoui K, Yaou RB, et al. Clinical and genetic heterogeneity in laminopathies. Biochem Soc Trans. 2011;39(6):1687-92.
25. Purevjav E, Arimura T, Augustin S, et al. Molecular basis for clinical heterogeneity in inherited cardiomyopathies due to myopalladin mutations. Hum Mol Genet. 2012;21(9):2039-53.
26. Lopes LR, Rahman MS, Elliott PM. A systematic review and meta-analysis of genotype-phenotype associations in patients with hypertrophic cardiomyopathy caused by sarcomeric protein mutations. Heart. 2013;99(24):1800-11.
27. Karamitsos TD, Neubauer S. The prognostic value of late gadolinium enhancement CMR in nonischemic cardiomyopathies. Curr Cardiol Rep. 2013;15(1):326.
28. Quarta G, Sado DM, Moon JC. Cardiomyopathies: focus on cardiovascular magnetic resonance. Br J Radiol. 2011;84(Spec No 3):S296-305.
29. Arbustini E, Pilotto A, Repetto A, et al. Autosomal dominant dilated cardiomyopathy with atrioventricular block: a lamin A/C defect-related disease. J Am Coll Cardiol. 2002;39(6):981-90.
30. Diegoli M, Grasso M, Favalli V, et al. Diagnostic work-up and risk stratification in X-linked dilated cardiomyopathies caused by dystrophin defects. J Am Coll Cardiol. 2011;58(9):925-34.
31. Gambarin FI, Disabella E, Narula J, et al. When should cardiologists suspect Anderson-Fabry disease? Am J Cardiol. 2010;106(10):1492-9.
32. Arad M, Maron BJ, Gorham JM, et al. Glycogen storage diseases presenting as hypertrophic cardiomyopathy. N Engl J Med. 2005;352(4):362-72.
33. Haas J, Katus HA, Meder B. Next-generation sequencing entering the clinical arena. Mol Cell Probes. 2011;25(5-6):206-11.
34. Caleshu C, Sakhuja R, Nussbaum RL, et al. Furthering the link between the sarcomere and primary cardiomyopathies: restrictive cardiomyopathy associated with multiple mutations in genes previously associated with hypertrophic or dilated cardiomyopathy. Am J Med Genet A. 2011;155A(9):2229-35.
35. Arbustini E, Fasani R, Morbini P, et al. Coexistence of mitochondrial DNA and beta myosin heavy chain mutations in hypertrophic cardiomyopathies with late congestive heart failure. Heart. 1998;80(6):548-58.
36. Epstein AE, DiMarco JP, Ellenbogen KA, et al. 2012 ACCF/AHA/HRS focused update incorporated into the ACCF/AHA/HRS 2008 Guidelines for Device-Based Therapy of Cardiac Rhythm Abnormalities: a report of the American College of Cardiology Foundation/American Heart Association Task Force on Practice Guidelines and the Heart Rhythm Society. Developed in collaboration with the American Association for Thoracic Surgery and Society of Thoracic Surgeons. Circulation. 2013;61(3):e6-75.
37. Epstein AE, Di Marco JP, Ellenbogen KA, et al. ACC/AHA/HRS 2008 Guidelines for Device-Based Therapy of Cardiac Rhythm Abnormalities. A report of the American College of Cardiology/American Heart Association Task Force on Practice Guidelines (Writing committee to revise the ACC/AHA/NASPE 2002 guidelines update for implantation of cardiac pacemakers and antiarrhythmic devices): developed in collaboration with the American Association for Thoracic Surgery and Society of Thoracic Surgeons. circulation. 2008;117:e350-408.
38. Russo AM, Steinback RF, Bailey SR, et al. ACCF/HRS/AHA/ASE/HFSA/SCAI/SCCT/SCMR 2013 appropriate use criteria for implantable cardioverter-defibrillator and cardiac resynchronization therapy: a report of the American College of Cardiology Foundation Appropriate Use Criteria Task Force, Heart Rhythm Society, American Heart Association, American Society of Echocardiography, Heart Failure Society of America, Society of Cardiovascular Angiography and Intervention, Society of Cardiovascular Computed Tomography, and Society for Cardiovascular Magnetic Resonance. J Am Coll Cardiol. 2013;61:1323-73.
39. van Berlo JH, de Voogt WG, van der Kooi AJ, et al. Meta-analysis of clinical characteristics of 299 carriers of LMNA gene mutations: do lamin A/C mutations portend a high risk of sudden death? J Mol Med. 2005;83(1):79-83.
40. Pasotti M, Klersy C, Pilotto A, et al. Long-term outcome and risk stratification in dilated cardiolaminopathies. J Am Coll Cardiol. 2008;52(15):1250-60.

41. van Rijsingen IA, Arbustini E, Elliott PM, et al. Risk factors for malignant ventricular arrhythmias in lamin a/c mutation carriers a European cohort study. J Am Coll Cardiol. 2012;59(5):493-500.
42. Christiaans I, Birnie E, Bonsel GJ, et al. Manifest disease, risk factors for sudden cardiac death, and cardiac events in a large nationwide cohort of predictively tested hypertrophic cardiomyopathy mutation carriers: determining the best cardiological screening strategy. Eur Heart J. 2011;32:1161-70.
43. Kaushik S, Subramanian SR, Rafii S, et al. Aborted sudden cardiac death (SCD) in a patient with hypertrophic cardiomyopathy (HCM) with low-risk factors for SCD. BMJ Case Rep. 2013;2013. pii: bcr2012006459.
44. Stehlik J, Edwards LB, Kucheryavaya AY, et al. The Registry of the International Society for Heart and Lung Transplantation: 29th official adult heart transplant report—2012. J Heart Lung Transplant. 2012;31(10):1052-64.
45. Ferlini A, Neri M, Gualandi F. The medical genetics of dystrophinopathies: molecular genetic diagnosis and its impact on clinical practice. Neuromuscul Disord. 2013;23(1):4-14.
46. Garcia-Pavia P, Syrris P, Salas C, et al. Desmosomal protein gene mutations in patients with idiopathic dilated cardiomyopathy undergoing cardiac transplantation: a clinicopathological study. Heart. 2011;97(21):1744-52.
47. Maron BJ, Gardin JM, Flack JM, et al. Prevalence of hypertrophic cardiomyopathy in a general population of young adults: echocardiographic analysis of 4111 subjects in the CARDIA Study. Coronary Artery Risk Development in (Young) Adults. Circulation. 1995;92(4):785-9.
48. Maron MS, Maron BJ. Hypertrophic cardiomyopathy – Authors' reply. Lancet. 2013;381(9876):1457-8.
49. Maron BJ, Olivotto I, Spirito P, et al. Epidemiology of hypertrophic cardiomyopathy-related death: revisited in a large non-referral-based patient population. Circulation. 2000;102(8):858-64.
50. Jacoby D, McKenna WJ. Genetics of inherited cardiomyopathy. Eur Heart J. 2012;33(3):296-304.
51. Frey N, Luedde M, Katus HA. Mechanisms of disease: hypertrophic cardiomyopathy. Nat Rev Cardiol. 2011;9(2):91-100.
52. Olson TM, Karst ML, Whitby FG, et al. Myosin light chain mutation causes autosomal recessive cardiomyopathy with mid-cavitary hypertrophy and restrictive physiology. Circulation. 2002;105(20):2337-40.
53. Morita H, Rehm HL, Menesses A, et al. Shared genetic causes of cardiac hypertrophy in children and adults. N Engl J Med. 2008;358(18):1899-908.
54. Lopes LR, Zekavati A, Syrris P, et al. Genetic complexity in hypertrophic cardiomyopathy revealed by high-throughput sequencing. J Med Genet. 2013;50(4):228-39.
55. Konno T, Chang S, Seidman JG, et al. Genetics of hypertrophic cardiomyopathy. Curr Opin Cardiol. 2010;25(3):205-9.
56. Maron BJ, Maron MS, Semsarian C. Double or compound sarcomere mutations in hypertrophic cardiomyopathy: a potential link to sudden death in the absence of conventional risk factors. Heart Rhythm. 2012;9(1):57-63.
57. Clarke NF, Amburgey K, Teener J, et al. A novel mutation expands the genetic and clinical spectrum of MYH7-related myopathies. Neuromuscul Disord. 2013;23(5):432-6.
58. Chang AN, Parvatiyar MS, Potter JD. Troponin and cardiomyopathy. Biochem Biophys Res Commun. 2008;369(1):74-81.
59. Fiset C, Giles WR. Cardiac troponin T mutations promote life-threatening arrhythmias. J Clin Invest. 2008;118(12):3845-7.
60. Tsoutsman T, Bagnall RD, Semsarian C. Impact of multiple gene mutations in determining the severity of cardiomyopathy and heart failure. Clin Exp Pharmacol Physiol. 2008;35(11):1349-57.
61. Maron BJ, Niimura H, Casey SA, et al. Development of left ventricular hypertrophy in adults with hypertrophic cardiomyopathy caused by cardiac myosin-binding protein C gene mutations. J Am Coll Cardiol. 2001;38(2):315-21.
62. Sorajja P, Elliott PM, McKenna WJ. The molecular genetics of hypertrophic cardiomyopathy: prognostic implications. Europace. 2000;2(1):4-14.
63. Pasquale F, Syrris P, Kaski JP, et al. Long-term outcomes in hypertrophic cardiomyopathy caused by mutations in the cardiac troponin T gene. Circ Cardiovasc Genet. 2012;5(1):10-7.
64 Olivotto I, Maron BJ, Cecchi F. Clinical significance of atrial fibrillation in hypertrophic cardiomyopathy. Curr Cardiol Rep. 2001;3(2):141-6.
65 Chinnery PF, Hudson G. Mitochondrial genetics. Br Med Bull. 2013; 106:135-59.
66 Wicks EC, Elliott PM. Genetics and metabolic cardiomyopathies. Herz. 2012;37(6):598-610.
67 Merlini G, Bellotti V. Molecular mechanisms of amyloidosis. N Engl J Med. 2003;349(6):583-96.
68 Weidemann F, Niemann M, Störk S, et al. Long-term outcome of enzyme-replacement therapy in advanced Fabry disease: evidence for disease progression towards serious complications. J Intern Med. 2013;274(4):331-41.
69 Ohashi T. Enzyme replacement therapy for lysosomal storage diseases. Pediatr Endocrinol Rev. 2012;10(Suppl 1):26-34.
70 de Ru MH, Boelens JJ, Das AM, et al. Enzyme replacement therapy and/or hematopoietic stem cell transplantation at diagnosis in patients with mucopolysaccharidosis type I: results of a European consensus procedure. Orphanet J Rare Dis. 2011;6:55.
71 Penchala SC, Connelly S, Wang Y, et al. AG10 inhibits amyloidogenesis and cellular toxicity of the familial amyloid cardiomyopathy-associated V122I transthyretin. Proc Natl Acad Sci U S A. 2013;110(24):9992-7.
72 Galimberti CA, Diegoli M, Sartori I, et al. Brain pseudoatrophy and mental regression on valproate and a mitochondrial DNA mutation. Neurology. 2006;67(9):1715-7.
73 Rikimaru M, Ohsawa Y, Wolf AM, et al. Taurine ameliorates impaired the mitochondrial function and prevents stroke-like episodes in patients with MELAS. Intern Med. 2012;51(24):3351-7.
74. Gollob MH, Green MS, Tang AS, et al. PRKAG2 cardiac syndrome: familial ventricular preexcitation, conduction system disease, and cardiac hypertrophy. Curr Opin Cardiol. 2002;17(3):229-34.
75. Maron BJ, Roberts WC, Arad M, et al. Clinical outcome and phenotypic expression in LAMP2 cardiomyopathy. JAMA. 2009;301(12):1253-9.
76. Niemann M, Hartmann T, Namdar M, et al. Cross-sectional baseline analysis of electrocardiography in a large cohort of patients with untreated Fabry disease. J Inherit Metab Dis. 2013;36(5):873-9.
77. Sproule DM, Kaufmann P, Engelstad K, et al. Wolff-Parkinson-White syndrome in patients with MELAS. Arch Neurol. 2007;64(11):1625-7.
78. Mogensen J, Arbustini E. Restrictive cardiomyopathy. Curr Opin Cardiol. 2009;24(3):214-20.
79. Parvatiyar MS, Pinto JR, Dweck D, et al. Cardiac troponin mutations and restrictive cardiomyopathy. J Biomed Biotechnol. 2010;2010:350706.
80. Gambarin FI, Tagliani M, Arbustini E. Pure restrictive cardiomyopathy associated with cardiac troponin I gene mutation: mismatch between the lack of hypertrophy and the presence of disarray. Heart. 2008;94(10):1257.
81. Jay A, Chikarmane R, Poulik J, et al. Infantile hypertrophic cardiomyopathy associated with a novel MYL3 mutation. Cardiology. 2013;124(4):248-51.
82. Kaski JP, Syrris P, Burch M, et al. Idiopathic restrictive cardiomyopathy in children is caused by mutations in cardiac sarcomere protein genes. Heart. 2008;94(11):1478-84.
83. Arbustini E, Morbini P, Grasso M, et al. Restrictive cardiomyopathy, atrioventricular block and mild to subclinical myopathy in patients with desmin-immunoreactive material deposits. J Am Coll Cardiol. 1998; 31(3):645-53.

84. Arbustini E, Pasotti M, Pilotto A, et al. Desmin accumulation restrictive cardiomyopathy and atrioventricular block associated with desmin gene defects. Eur J Heart Fail. 2006;8(5):477-83.
85. Ariza A, Coll J, Fernandez-Figueras MT, et al. Desmin myopathy: a multisystem disorder involving skeletal, cardiac, and smooth muscle. Hum Pathol. 1995;26(9):1032-7.
86. van Spaendonck-Zwarts KY, van Hessem L, Jongbloed JD, et al. Desmin-related myopathy. Clin Genet. 2011;80(4):354-66.
87. Sung RK, Ursell PC, Rame JE, et al. QTc prolongation and family history of sudden death in a patient with desmin cardiomyopathy. Pacing Clin Electrophysiol. 2011;34(12):e105-8.
88. Zachara E, Bertini E, Lioy E, et al. Restrictive cardiomyopathy due to desmin accumulation in a family with evidence of autosomal dominant inheritance. G Ital Cardiol. 1997;27(5):436-42.
89. Marcus FI, McKenna WJ, Sherrill D, et al. Diagnosis of arrhythmogenic right ventricular cardiomyopathy/dysplasia: proposed modification of the Task Force Criteria. Eur Heart J. 2010;31(7):806-14.
90. Sen-Chowdhry S, Syrris P, Prasad SK, et al. Left-dominant arrhythmogenic cardiomyopathy: an under-recognized clinical entity. J Am Coll Cardiol. 2008;52(25):2175-87.
91. Azaouagh A, Churzidse S, Konorza T, et al. Arrhythmogenic right ventricular cardiomyopathy/dysplasia: a review and update. Clin Res Cardiol. 2011;100(5):383-94.
92. Protonotarios N, Tsatsopoulou A, Anastasakis A, et al. Genotype-phenotype assessment in autosomal recessive arrhythmogenic right ventricular cardiomyopathy (Naxos disease) caused by a deletion in plakoglobin. J Am Coll Cardiol. 2001;38(5):1477-84.
93. Carvajal-Huerta L. Epidermolytic-palmoplantar keratoderma with woolly hair and dilated cardiomyopathy. J Am Acad Dermatol. 1998;39(3):418-21.
94. Bauce B, Nava A, Beffagna G, et al. Multiple mutations in desmosomal proteins encoding genes in arrhythmogenic right ventricular cardiomyopathy/dysplasia. Heart Rhythm. 2010;7(1):22-9.
95. Quarta G, Syrris P, Ashworth M, et al. Mutations in the Lamin A/C gene mimic arrhythmogenic right ventricular cardiomyopathy. Eur Heart J. 2012;33(9):1128-36.
96. Zaragoza MV, Arbustini E, Narula J. Noncompaction of the left ventricle: primary cardiomyopathy with an elusive genetic etiology. Curr Opin Pediatr. 2007;19(6):619-27.
97. Paterick TE, Umland MM, Jan MF, et al. Left ventricular noncompaction: a 25-year odyssey. J Am Soc Echocardiogr. 2012;25(4):363-75.
98. Rigaud C, Lebre AS, Touraine R, et al. Natural history of Barth syndrome: a national cohort study of 22 patients. Orphanet J Rare Dis. 2013;8:70.
99. Clarke SL, Bowron A, Gonzalez IL, et al. Barth syndrome. Orphanet J Rare Dis. 2013;8:23.
100. Vatta M, Mohapatra B, Jimenez S, et al. Mutations in Cypher/ZASP in patients with dilated cardiomyopathy and left ventricular non-compaction. J Am Coll Cardiol. 2003;42(11):2014-27.
101. Marziliano N, Mannarino S, Nespoli L, et al. Barth syndrome associated with compound hemizygosity and heterozygosity of the TAZ and LDB3 genes. Am J Med Genet A. 2007;143A(9):907-15.
102. Narula N, Rapezzi C, Tavazzi L, et al. My parents died of myocardial infarction: is that my destiny? Med Clin North Am. 2012;96(1):67-86.
103. Lee DS, Pencina MJ, Benjamin EJ, et al. Association of parental heart failure with risk of heart failure in offspring. N Engl J Med. 2006;355(2):138-47.
104. Pasotti M, Repetto A, Tavazzi L, et al. Genetic predisposition to heart failure. Med Clin North Am. 2004;88(5):1173-92.
105. Dube P, Weber KT. Congestive heart failure: pathophysiologic consequences of neurohormonal activation and the potential for recovery: part I. Am J Med Sci. 2011;342(5):348-51.
106. Dube P, Weber KT. Congestive heart failure: pathophysiologic consequences of neurohormonal activation and the potential for recovery: part II. Am J Med Sci. 2011;342(6):503-6.
107. Rigat B, Hubert C, Alhenc-Gelas F, et al. An insertion/deletion polymorphism in the angiotensin I-converting enzyme gene accounting for half the variance of serum enzyme levels. J Clin Invest. 1990;86(4):1343-6.
108. Bai Y, Wang L, Hu S, et al. Association of angiotensin-converting enzyme I/D polymorphism with heart failure: a meta-analysis. Mol Cell Biochem. 2012;361(1-2):297-304.
109. Andersson B, Sylven C. The DD genotype of the angiotensin-converting enzyme gene is associated with increased mortality in idiopathic heart failure. J Am Coll Cardiol. 1996;28(1):162-7.
110. Schut AF, Bleumink GS, Stricker BH, et al. Angiotensin converting enzyme insertion/deletion polymorphism and the risk of heart failure in hypertensive subjects. Eur Heart J. 2004;25(23):2143-8.
111. McNamara DM, Holubkov R, Janosko K, et al. Pharmacogenetic interactions between beta-blocker therapy and the angiotensin-converting enzyme deletion polymorphism in patients with congestive heart failure. Circulation. 2001;103(12):1644-8.
112. Li X, Li Y, Jia N, et al. Angiotensin-converting enzyme gene deletion allele increases the risk of left ventricular hypertrophy: evidence from a meta-analysis. Mol Biol Rep. 2012;39(12):10063-75.
113. Wu CK, Tsai CT, Chang YC, et al. Genetic polymorphisms of the angiotensin II type 1 receptor gene and diastolic heart failure. J Hypertens. 2009;27(3):502-7.
114. Amir O, Amir RE, Paz H, et al. Relation between AT1R gene polymorphism and long-term outcome in patients with heart failure. Cardiology. 2009; 112(2):151-7.
115. Goldbergova M, Spinarova L, Spinar J, et al. Association of two angiotensinogen gene polymorphisms, M235T and G(-6)A, with chronic heart failure. Int J Cardiol. 2003;89(2-3):267-72.
116. Liggett SB. Pharmacogenomics of beta1-adrenergic receptor polymorphisms in heart failure. Heart Fail Clin. 2010;6(1):27-33.
117. McLean RC, Baird SW, Becker LC, et al. Response to catecholamine stimulation of polymorphisms of the beta-1 and beta-2 adrenergic receptors. Am J Cardiol. 2012;110(7):1001-7.
118. Fiuzat M, Neely ML, Starr AZ, et al. Association between adrenergic receptor genotypes and beta-blocker dose in heart failure patients: analysis from the HF-ACTION DNA substudy. Eur J Heart Fail. 2013;15(3):258-66.
119. Villard E, Perret C, Gary F, et al. A genome-wide association study identifies two loci associated with heart failure due to dilated cardiomyopathy. Eur. Heart J. 2011;32(9):1065-76.
120. Norton N, Li D, Rieder MJ, et al. Genome-wide studies of copy number variation and exome sequencing identify rare variants in BAG3 as a cause of dilated cardiomyopathy. Am J Hum Genet. 2011;88(3):273-82.
121. Krief S, Faivre JF, Robert P, et al. Identification and characterization of cvHsp. A novel human small stress protein selectively expressed in cardiovascular and insulin-sensitive tissues. J Biol Chem. 1999;274(51): 36592-600.
122. Arimura T, Ishikawa T, Nunoda S, et al. Dilated cardiomyopathy-associated BAG3 mutations impair Z-disc assembly and enhance sensitivity to apoptosis in cardiomyocytes. Hum Mutat. 2011;32(12):1481-91.
123. Stark K, Esslinger UB, Reinhard W, et al. Genetic association study identifies HSPB7 as a risk gene for idiopathic dilated cardiomyopathy. PLoS Genet. 2010;6(10):e1001167.
124. Smith NL, Felix JF, Morrison AC, et al. Association of genome-wide variation with the risk of incident heart failure in adults of European and African ancestry: a prospective meta-analysis from the Cohorts for Heart and Aging Research in Genomic Epidemiology (CHARGE) consortium. Circ Cardiovasc Genet. 2010;3(3):256-66.

125. Predmore JM, Wang P, Davis F, et al. Ubiquitin proteasome dysfunction in human hypertrophic and dilated cardiomyopathies. Circulation. 2010; 121(8):997-1004.
126. Feldshtein M, Elkrinawi S, Yerushalmi B, et al. Hyperchlorhidrosis caused by homozygous mutation in CA12, encoding carbonic anhydrase XII. Am J Hum Genet. 2010;87(5):713-20.
127. Morrison AC, Felix JF, Cupples LA, et al. Genomic variation associated with mortality among adults of European and African ancestry with heart failure: the cohorts for heart and aging research in genomic epidemiology consortium. Circ Cardiovasc Genet. 2010;3(3):248-55.
128. Stapleton G, Schröder-Bäck P, Townend D. Equity in public health: an epigenetic perspective. Public Health Genomics. 2013;16(4):135-44.
129. Tingare A, Thienpont B, Roderick HL. Epigenetics in the heart: the role of histone modifications in cardiac remodelling. Biochem Soc Trans. 2013;41(3):789-96.
130. Mano H. Epigenetic abnormalities in cardiac hypertrophy and heart failure. Environ Health Prev Med. 2008;13(1):25-9.
131. Udali S, Guarini P, Moruzzi S, et al. Cardiovascular epigenetics: from DNA methylation to microRNAs. Mol Aspects Med. 2013;34(4):883-901.
132. Movassagh M, Vujic A, Foo R. Genome-wide DNA methylation in human heart failure. Epigenomics. 2011;3(1):103-9.
133. Oikonomou E, Siasos G, Tousoulis D, et al. Diagnostic and therapeutic potentials of microRNAs in heart failure. Curr Top Med Chem. 2013; 13(13):1548-58.

Chapter 60

AIDS-induced Cardiac Abnormalities and Heart Failure

Khwaja S Alim, Hermineh Aramin, Minal V Patel, Elizabeth Lee

ABSTRACT

Human immunodeficiency virus (HIV) has become a global epidemic. There are reportedly over 40 million people worldwide living with acquired immunodeficiency syndrome (AIDS), affecting all walks of life. HIV/AIDS affects every part of the body including the myosites, causing dilated cardiomyopathy (CM). The pathophysiology of HIV-induced CM is rather complex. Cytokines including endothelin (ET; particularly ET-1) and tumor necrosis factor α play a major role in the AIDS-induced cardiac dysfunction and chronic heart failure (HF). Certain opportunistic infections can also contribute to CM in this group of people.

The diagnosis and treatment of the AIDS patient with HF is similar to other patients with nonischemic dilated CM. Medical therapy consists of angiotensin converting enzyme inhibitors, beta-blockers, spironolactone, and diuretics for fluid control. In addition, drugs that can cause cardiotoxicity, should be discontinued. Protease inhibitor-sparing regimens may be used, but this decision should be differed to the specialist in HIV medicine.

INTRODUCTION

Human immunodeficiency virus (HIV)/AIDS is an all too familiar topic of discourse in the world of infectious diseases, as health experts and scientists continue to struggle to unveil more of its characteristics and put forth efforts to thwart its progression in the human population. Today, there are reportedly over 40 million people worldwide living with AIDS.[1] While a majority of these belong to Africa, there are numerous others who also contribute to the ever rising number of infected and dying individuals.[2] In the United States of America (USA) and Europe, AIDS has become the primary cause of death amongst young adults. Globally, there are over 1 million children who have acquired this malady and 1,600 infants born with the infection every day.

The first case of dilated cardiomyopathy (CM) in a patient with AIDS was documented in 1986, strongly suggesting the involvement of AIDS in the development of heart muscle disease.[3] In dilated CM, the heart shape is distorted due to ventricular dilation and apical rounding and the weight is increased as a result of fibrosis and myocyte hypertrophy.[4] Dilated CM is the most common cardiovascular complication present in people with late stages of HIV.[5] So far, myocarditis and myocardial infection with HIV-1 are the best studied causes of CM in HIV disease.[6] Because HIV compromises the immune system, the heart may also be affected by other opportunistic pathogens out there, not just by the HIV virus itself. Thus, the pathogenesis of the heart muscle disease in AIDS has still yet to be construed.[7]

Unfortunately, the tide of AIDS shows no signs of receding. Yet there must be hope that we can one day overcome this seemingly indomitable force. The focus of this chapter is to address the pathogenesis, pathophysiology, and prevalence of CM in AIDS, with ultimate goal to diagnose and treat these extremely sick patients.

EPIDEMIOLOGY

At the end of 2011, 34 million HIV affected people were living globally, of which 69% were residents of sub-Saharan Africa and 5 million people from Asia.[8] Amongst this population, cardiovascular diseases (CVDs) have become prevalent, such as myocardial infarction (MI) and CM.[9,10] These numbers do not only represent adults with HIV, but children with HIV/AIDS related heart diseases is increasing as well.[11] HIV infected individuals have higher rates of being by CVD because of any mixture of risk factors, such as fungi, viruses, or protozoa.[3,10]

Most of the pathogens of cardiovascular problems in patients with AIDS are unknown, although cases of CM are prevalent.[4] Cardiac involvement with AIDS was first reported in 1983 along with a CM-related case in 1986.[3,4] Depending on location however, the issues of cardiac problems with AIDS may differ. Pericardial effusion with HIV is the most frequent pericardial disease in Africa.[3] In comparison, 5.1 million individuals are infected with HIV in India, with 28–73% cardiac involvement, such as pericardial effusion, left ventricular (LV) dysfunction, myocarditis, and dilated CM.[12]

A study conducted in Italy showed that about 8% of the population had AIDS CM with 80% of CM individuals having myocarditis.[8] In a study conducted by Milei and colleagues at the University of Buenos Aires, dilated CM affects 10–20% of those with HIV infection and accounts for approximately a third of HIV related deaths.[13]

Though many CVDs occur due to HIV, some diseases can be caused due to the HIV treatment. Some drugs are used to delay heart diseases yet some drugs, such as zidovudine are cardiotoxic.[11] Highly active antiretroviral therapy (HAART) regimens introduction has shown that there is an increase in both peripheral and coronary arterial diseases.[14]

PATHOPHYSIOLOGY OF HIV-INDUCED CARDIAC ABNORMALITIES

With current advances in HIV and AIDS management and increased survival, cardiac muscle disease in association with HIV will become more important and increasingly reported. Four percent of all cases of CM are HIV related. In comparison with idiopathic dilated CM, HIV-related CM results in poor prognosis.[15] Cardiac complications in patients with HIV include direct infection of the heart by HIV-1, systemic circulating toxins, opportunistic pathogens, nutritional disorders, and therapeutic toxins associated with AIDS.[16-18] Additionally, more than one factor plays a role in mortality, and manifestation varies according to treatment regime and stages of the disease (Flowchart 1).

DIAGNOSIS AND TREATMENT OF HEART FAILURE DUE TO HIV/AIDS

Human immunodeficiency virus infected patients can develop several cardiac anomalies including myocarditis, dilated CM, right-sided HF due to pulmonary hypertension (PHT), pericardial effusion and cardiac tamponade (CT), HAART-induced metabolic syndrome, and premature coronary artery disease (CAD).

HIV-induced Cardiomyopathy

Dilated CM, in a patient with HIV is strongly associated with advanced stages of the disease.[19,20] The introduction of HAART, which includes two nucleoside reverse transcriptase inhibitors (NRTIs) and one PI, has significantly reduced the prevalence of HIV CM in developed countries.

The prevalence of this late stage complication continues to remain high in low socioeconomic population due to underdiagnosis of HIV in this group, and also due to noncompliance with the HAART. Of note, there is little evidence that HAART is directly beneficial in HIV-associated CM; however, this therapy prevents development of opportunistic infections which reduces the incidence of HIV-associated heart disease.

Screening

Transthoracic two-dimensional echocardiogram (2D-ECHO) remains the most valuable screening tool for HIV-related CM. It assesses the two independent predictors of all-cause mortality; LV systolic dysfunction and LV hypertrophy.[21] In a recent study using dobutamine stress echocardiography, inotropic contractile reserve (ICR) was found to risk-stratify patients with HIV CM.[22]

Treatment

The treatment of AIDS patient with HF is similar to other patients with nonischemic dilated CM.

Medical therapy: This is consisting of angiotensin-converting enzyme inhibitors (ACEI)/angiotensin receptor blockers (ARB), beta-blockers, and diuretics for fluid control. In addition, drugs that can cause cardiotoxicity should be discontinued. Other opportunistic infections

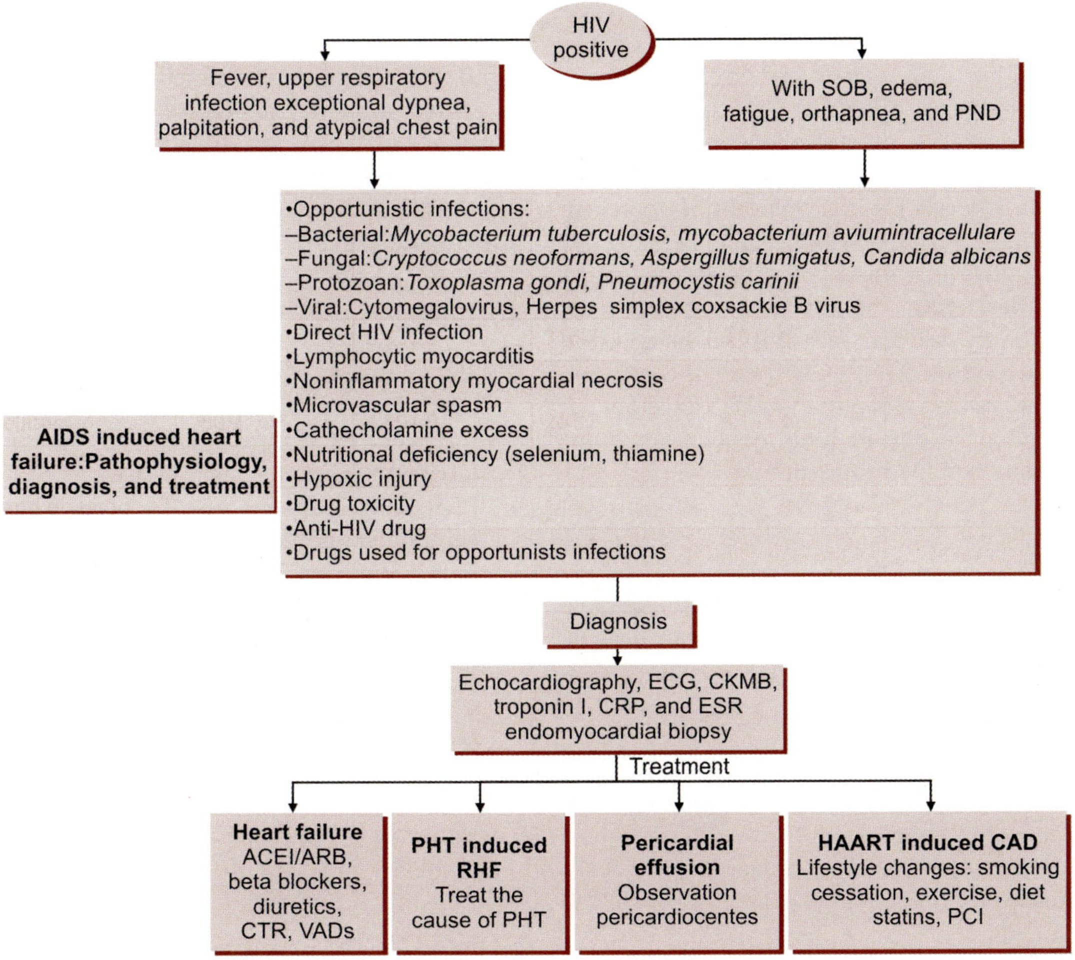

HIV, human immunodeficiency virus; SOB, shortness of breath; PND, paroxysmal nocturnal dyspnea; ECG, electrocardiogram; CK-MB, creatine kinase-MB; CRP, C-reactive protein; ESR, erythrocyte sedimentation rate; ACEI, angiotensin-converting enzyme inhibitor; ARB, angiotensin receptor blockers; CRT, cardiac resynchronization therapy; VAD, ventricular assist device; PHT, pulmonary hypertension; RHF, right heart failure; HAART, highly active antiretroviral therapy; CAD, coronary artery disease; PCI, percutaneous coronary intervention

Flowchart 1 Acquired immunodeficiency syndrome-induced heart failure: Pathophysiology, diagnosis, and treatment

like toxoplasmosis and cytomegalovirus should be treated.

In some studies, monthly infusion of immunoglobulins in HIV-infected children was associated with return to normal LV wall thickness and reduction in peak LV wall stress, suggesting an immunologically mediated etiology of LV dysfunction.[23]

Device-based therapy: Cardiac resynchronization therapy (CRT) should be offered if indicated. In a very carefully selected group of patients with controlled HIV-infection [normal clusters of differentiation (CD)-4 count, undetectable viremia, good compliance and psychosocial support], on a stable regimen of HAART, and with no active opportunistic infections who suffer from end-stage congestive HF refractory to medical management; should be considered as viable candidates for the use of long-term mechanical circulatory support like ventricular assist device (VADs). Indeed, there is considerable apprehension about the placement of a VAD in such patients for fear of infections.

Heart transplant: This option remains rather limited in this group of population.

Right-sided Heart Failure due to Pulmonary Hypertension

Right ventricular hypertrophy usually diagnosed by electrocardiogram (ECG), often accompanies PHT. In most of the cases it presents as a mild asymptomatic condition, but in some cases it can develop into severe cardiac impairment with corpulmonale leading to death.[24] Primary PHT is a rare syndrome characterized by dyspnea, chest pain, and syncope defined by increased pulmonary vascular resistance. It occurs in a disproportionate number of HIV/AIDS patients compared to general population.[25] Secondary PHT develops in HIV-infected patients[26] due to lung infections, venous thromboembolism, and LV dysfunction.

Screening

Two-dimensional ECHO remains the most valuable screening tool. Right heart catheterization can also be performed for further risk stratification.

Treatment

The main focus of therapy is to treat the cause of the PHT. Vasodilator agents like epoprostenol have also been used but it is not clear whether they improve the prognosis, and its administration is generally limited to seriously ill patients.[27,28]

Pericardial Effusion and Cardiac Tamponade

Pericardial effusions may be related to an opportunistic infection or to malignancy but in most of the cases the clear etiology is not found. Survival of AIDS patients with pericardial effusion is significantly shorter than of patients without an effusion.

Screening

Two-dimensional ECHO plays a crucial role in diagnosing the extent of pericardial effusion and ruling out tamponade physiology.

Treatment

Pericardiocentesis is recommended in large poorly tolerated effusions, especially in presence of CT.

HAART-induced Cardiovascular Disease

Lipid abnormalities associated with HAART are related to central adiposity and insulin resistance. The annual incidence of MI among HIV-infected patients on HAART is four to seven times higher when compared to the pre-HAART group. The exposure to the PI therapy is associated with high risk of MI.[29,30]

Treatment

- The patients should be strongly encouraged to make lifestyle changes including smoking cessation, restriction of alcohol intake, and reduction in dietary fat as well as increasing exercise
- PI-sparing regimens may be used, but this decision should be differed to the specialist in HIV medicine
- Lipid lowering medications should be used, if nonpharmacological treatment does not work
- Potential drug interactions should be monitored because most statins are metabolized through the cytochrome P450 3A4 pathway. The inhibition of this pathway by PIs might increase the concentration of statins, with an increase in the risk of skeletal muscle and hepatic toxicity.[31] Pravastatin appears to be the safest agent because it is least influenced by this pathway.

CONCLUSION

Most of the AIDS-related cardiac complications occur in late stages of the disease. Hence, early diagnosis and treatment of this disease with HAART may delay and even prevent these life-threatening conditions.

REFERENCES

1. Zareba KM, Miller TL, Lipshultz SE. Cardiovascular disease and toxicities related to HIV infection and its therapies. Expert Opin Drug Saf. 2005; 4(6):1017-25.
2. Ntsekhe M, Hakim J. Impact of human immunodeficiency virus infection on cardiovascular disease in Africa. Circulation. 2005;112(23):3602-7.
3. Prendergast BD. HIV and cardiovascular medicine. Heart. 2003;89(7):793-800.
4. Lewis W. Cardiomyopathy in AIDS: a pathophysiological perspective. Prog Cardiovasc Dis. 2000;43(2):151-70.
5. Patanè S, Marte F, Sturiale M, et al. Myocarditis and cardiomyopathy HIV associated. Int J Cardiol. 2011;146(3):e56-7.
6. Barbaro G. HIV-associated cardiomyopathy etiopathogenesis and clinical aspects. Herz. 2005;30(6):486-92.
7. Barbaro G, Lipshultz SE. Pathogenesis of HIV-associated cardiomyopathy. Ann N Y Acad Sci. 2001;946:57-81.

8. UNAIDS Report on the Global AIDS Epidemic. (2012). Global Report. Joint United Nations Programme on HIV/AIDS (UNAIDS). [online] Available from: www.unaids.org/en/media/unaids/contentassets/documents/epidemiology/2012/gr2012/20121120_unaids_global_report_2012_with_annexes_en.pdf. [Accessed January, 2014].
9. Boccara F, Lang S, Meuleman C, et al. HIV and coronary heart disease: time for a better understanding. J Am Coll Cardiol. 2013;61(5):511-23.
10. Tseng ZH, Secemsky EA, Dowdy D, et al. Sudden cardiac death in patients with human immunodeficiency virus infection. J Am Coll Cardiol. 2012;59(21):1891-6.
11. Lubega S, Zirembuzi GW, Lwabi P. Heart diseases among children with HIV/AIDS attending the paediatric infectious disease clinic at Mulago Hospital. Afr Health Sci. 2005;5(3):219-26.
12. Singh A, Das S, Dalai RK. Study of Cardiac manifestation in Patients with HIV Infection and their Correlation with CD4 count in Indian population. Int J Clin Med. 2012;178-83.
13. Milei J, Grana D, Fernandez Alonso G, et al. Cardiac involvement in acquired immunodeficiency syndrome--a review to push action. The Committee for the Study of Cardiac Involvement in AIDS. Clin Cardiol. 1998;21(7):465-72.
14. Barbaro G. Cardiovascular manifestations of HIV infection. Circulation. 2002;106(11):1420-5.
15. Barbaro G, Di Lorenzo G, Grisorio B, et al. Incidence of dilated cardiomyopathy and detection of HIV in myocardial cells of HIV-positive patients. Gruppo Italiano per lo Studio Cardiologico dei Pazienti Affetti da AIDS. N Engl J Med. 1998;339(16):1093-9.
16. Kaminski HJ, Katzman M, Wiest PM, et al. Cardiomyopathy associated with the acquired immune deficiency syndrome. J Acquir Immune Defic Syndr. 1988;1(2):105-10.
17. Leidig GA. Clinical, echocardiographic, and electrocardiographic resolution of HIV-related cardiomyopathy. Mil Med. 1991;156(5):260-1.
18. Hecht SR, Berger M, Van Tosh A, et al. Unsuspected cardiac abnormalities in the acquired immune deficiency syndrome. An echocardiographic study. Chest. 1989;96(4):805-8.
19. Currie PF, Jacob AJ, Foreman AR, et al. Heart muscle disease related to HIV infection: prognostic implications. BMJ. 1994;309(6969):1605-7.
20. El Hattaoui M, Charei N, Boumzebra D, et al. [Prevalence of cardiomyopathy in HIV infection: prospective study on 158 HIV patients]. Med Mal Infect. 2008;38(7):387-91.
21. Lipshultz SE, Easley KA, Orav EJ, et al. Cardiac dysfunction and mortality in HIV-infected children: The prospective P2C2 HIV Multicenter Study. Pediatric Pulmonary and Cardiac Complications of Vertically Transmitted HIV Infection (P2C2 HIV) Study Group. Circulation. 2000;102(13):1542-8.
22. Wever-Pinzon O, Bangalore S, Romero J, et al. Inotropic contractile reserve can risk-stratify patients with HIV cardiomyopathy: a dobutamine stress echocardiography study. JACC Cardiovasc Imaging. 2011;4(12):1231-8.
23. Lipshultz SE, Orav EJ, Sanders SP, et al. Immunoglobulins and left ventricular structure and function in pediatric HIV infection. Circulation. 1995;92(8):2220-5.
24. Seoane L, Shellito J, Welsh D, et al. Pulmonary hypertension associated with HIV infection. South Med J. 2001;94(6):635-9.
25. Mesa RA, Edell ES, Dunn WF, et al. Human immunodeficiency virus infection and pulmonary hypertension: two new cases and a review of 86 reported cases. Mayo Clin Proc. 1998;73(1):37-45.
26. Mehmood S, Blais D, Martin S, et al. Heartmate XVE destination therapy for end-stage heart failure in a patient with human immunodeficiency virus. Interact Cardiovasc Thorac Surg. 2009;9(5):909-10.
27. Aguilar RV, Farber HW. Epoprostenol (prostacyclin) therapy in HIV-associated pulmonary hypertension. Am J Respir Crit Care Med. 2000;162(5):1846-50.
28. Felker GM, Thompson RE, Hare JM, et al. Underlying causes and long-term survival in patients with initially unexplained cardiomyopathy. N Engl J Med. 2000;342(15):1077-84.
29. Currier JS. Cardiovascular risk associated with HIV therapy. J Acquir Immune Defic Syndr. 2002;31(Suppl 1):S16-23.
30. Grunfeld C, Kotler DP, Hamadeh R, et al. Hypertriglyceridemia in the acquired immunodeficiency syndrome. Am J Med. 1989;86(1):27-31.
31. Dube MP, Sprecher D, Henry WK, et al. Preliminary guidelines for the evaluation and management of dyslipidemia in adults infected with human immunodeficiency virus and receiving antiretroviral therapy: Recommendations of the Adult AIDS Clinical Trial Group Cardiovascular Disease Focus Group. Clin Infect Dis. 2000;31(5):1216-24.

Chapter 61

Prohormone Levels in Heart Failure

Navaid Iqbal, Rajiv Choudhary, Fatima Iqbal, Erik A Green, Alan S Maisel

ABSTRACT

The use of biomarkers in aiding the care of heart failure (HF) patients has already been established. Their use spans decades of research and clinical applications. However, in long-term management of the disease, in the ability to assess risk and prevent readmission and mortality, there remains much research to be done. In this chapter, several biomarkers valuable in HF are examined: procalcitonin (PCT), a marker of infection; proadrenomedullin (proADM), a potent predictor of mortality; and copeptin, a substitute-marker for arginine vasopressin (AVP). These markers add immense value to a test panel, and enhance the information available to the physician. PCT allows physicians to accurately diagnose an ongoing bacterial infection, and take the appropriate behaviors in response to it. ProADM is an effective predictor of short-term mortality in patients with both acute HF and chronic heart failure (CHF) and elevated levels may require more specific and careful treatment regimen, especially once discharged. Finally, copeptin, acting as a surrogate marker for AVP, allows for a rapid assessment of hyponatremia, the function of the vasopressinergic system and therefore the severity of HF, making it a useful tool in an urgent setting. These three markers all have an important role to play in the future of HF care and their clinical use will continue to expand as we come to know more about them.

INTRODUCTION

Management of chronic conditions such as heart failure (HF) never stops with a hospital discharge. Post-hospitalization events, mortality and readmission continue to plague HF care and be a costly burden on hospitals, providers and patients. Biomarkers are proving to be an excellent method of providing critical information in the long-term management of HF, identifying possible and potentially reversible causes of HF, estimating the disease severity and adding new information for the clinical work-up of these patients. Many studies over the past few decades have shown that biomarkers, especially discharge levels, aid in risk stratification and may add useful prognostic information to help reduce mortality and readmission in chronically ill patients. Although the advent of biomarkers has dramatically improved the overall patient care, the day-to-day management of individual patients with HF continues to be an unaddressed problem. Furthermore, it is still not clear what biomarkers would be most useful in reducing readmissions and what is the best time to measure their levels. Although we rely on the levels measured on the day of hospital discharge, we still need to understand how to use these values and plan treatment strategies in the case of readmission.

Procalcitonin (PCT) has already been discussed as a key marker for infection and its use with dyspneic patients has been delineated. Proadrenomedullin (proADM) and copeptin, as a surrogate for arginine vasopressin (AVP), may both be powerful predictors of mortality in HF patients. Here we shall discuss the use of copeptin, PCT and proADM in post-emergency department (ED) discharge and follow-up care of HF patients.

COPEPTIN

In the recent decade, copeptin has emerged as a novel biomarker to assist physician with decision making and perform relevant therapeutic intervention. AVP, also known as antidiuretic hormone, is one of the key hormones of the hypothalamic-pituitary-adrenal (HPA) axis. Copeptin, a 39-amino-acid peptide, is the C-terminal part of pro-AVP and is released together with AVP in the circulation. During stress, a drop in blood pressure, or a change in osmotic pressure causes copeptin and AVP to be secreted from the posterior pituitary. It is well known that AVP is a major contributor to hyponatremia and is consistently elevated in patients with severe HF, highlighting AVPs potential as a prognostic biomarker. However, AVP has not been widely used in clinical practice due to its rapid clearance and in vitro instability. In contrast to AVP, copeptin is found to be stable in vitro and can be easily measured both in serum and plasma. AVP gets released into the circulation as a result of arteriolar vasoconstriction via the V_1-receptor and mediates an antidiuretic effect in the kidneys via the V_2-receptor.[1] Copeptin works in a similar fashion to AVP, but is considered a more stable marker ex vivo and this feature allows for the precise measurement of copeptin as a surrogate marker for the unstable AVP.

In clinical practice, reliably estimating of the prognosis of HF patients is of immense importance, since prognosis guides the clinicians to intervene accordingly. High levels of copeptin were found to be associated with increased frequencies of typical comorbidities of HF leading to worsening outcomes and increased risk of all-cause death. In the past few years, researchers have found that copeptin may be used to risk-stratify and follow patients with HF decompensation. Multiple studies have reported copeptin to be a significant prognostic biomarker in HF patients. A recent study among elderly patients with symptoms of HF, who were followed for 13 years, provided independent prognostic information that elevated levels of copeptin were associated with increased risk of both all-cause mortality and cardiovascular mortality. Additionally, the combination of elevated concentrations of copeptin and the established biomarker of HF [N-terminal pro-brain natriuretic peptide (NT-proBNP)] added complementary information regarding outcome prediction in these patients.[2] In another study, copeptin and NT-proBNP were compared for prognostic value in patients after an acute myocardial infarction (MI). This study demonstrated that copeptin levels were higher in patients who died or were readmitted with HF than those who survived ($p < 0.0005$). In regression analysis, copeptin ($p < 0.0005$) and NT-proBNP ($p < 0.003$) independently predicted death or HF at 60 days.[3]

Hyponatremia is a common characteristic finding in patients with HF. Neurohumoral activation stimulates AVP release together with copeptin, which parallels the severity of cardiac dysfunction as assessed by left ventricular ejection fraction. Hyponatremia may also be triggered by aggressive diuretic use in the management of HF symptoms. Since copeptin levels are significantly elevated in congestive HF patients who develop hyponatremia, it can be clinically used to identify patients with increased risk of morbidity and mortality. A study by Balling et al.[4] demonstrated that copeptin levels predict both death and hospitalization in outpatients with CHF independently from clinical variables, plasma sodium and loop diuretic doses ($p < 0.019$) but did not predict mortality independently from NT-proBNP. This study also indicates that although NT-proBNP is an excellent marker of mortality, copeptin might be a better marker for hospital admission. However, further studies are required to compare the predictive abilities of NT-proBNP and copeptin.

Heart failure has become one of the growing epidemics around the world, and represents one of the most cost-intensive conditions of industrialized countries. Initiating treatment early in the course of HF provides better outcome and reduces hospitalization. In clinical practice, it is important to reliably estimate the prognosis of an individual patient since it can help in determining urgency and intensity of treatment. Clinically speaking, only natriuretic peptides (NPs) [brain natriuretic peptide (BNP) and NT-proBNP] have been successfully established as simple-to-use diagnostic and prognostic markers. Copeptin's potential as a biomarker resembles how NPs are used to predict HF and other conditions. Higher copeptin levels are linked with poor kidney function, decreased left ventricular ejection fraction and more advanced HF [New York Heart Association (NYHA) class III/IV]. We think that copeptin, a stress hormone involved in water and sodium regulation, can be clinically useful to improve prediction of prognosis in patients with HF.

Measuring copeptin levels in plasma could potentially help in clinical situations where disturbance of vasopressinergic system are suspected. Because of its ability to be measured within an hour, copeptin can be useful when combined with other markers in facilitating level of care decisions, in addition to guiding a physician in answering urgent clinical questions in the acute and critical care settings.

PROCALCITONIN

In patients presenting with dyspnea in the ED, PCT has proven to be a highly effective marker for distinguishing between cardiac and noncardiac patients. Additionally, its ability to detect infectious states in patients, including those with underlying HF, has been established through numerous clinical trials. Using antibiotics unnecessarily creates bacterial resistance with widespread effects, incurring more cost and increasing the risk of adverse events. Research has shown that PCT can be used in diagnosing and managing bacterial infections and aiding physicians in guiding appropriate management whether dyspneic patients are HF or non-HF related. The use of PCT in post-ED care of HF patients is similar to that in the ED. Levels below 0.05 ng/mL indicate a small chance of an infectious state; levels above 0.2 ng/mL point toward a high chance of infection while levels between 0.05 ng/mL and 0.2 ng/mL signifies a possible infection.

If a patient's clinical symptoms show signs of an ongoing infection, a measurement of PCT should be taken before discharge. A level above 0.2 ng/mL requires treatment with antibiotics while a level between 0.05 ng/mL and 0.2 ng/mL should necessitate a follow-up PCT evaluation in 24–48 hours. Several studies have shown treatment guided over several days by PCT to be equal to, or better than, treatment with the standard care guidelines when looking at outcomes such as death, readmission or recurring infection.[5,6] Importantly, PCT-guided therapy can also lower the rates of antibiotic use, helping combat the spread of resistant bacteria, as well as reduce antibiotic exposure and antibiotic-related side-effects in patients. Studies such as the Biomarkers in Acute Heart Failure (BACH) trial[7] demonstrated that HF patients with a low PCT value do better if not treated with a regimen of antibiotics. While overall 90-day mortality did not differ in HF patients treated with, or without antibiotics, those with high PCT levels had greater mortality when not given antibiotics and those with low PCT levels fared worse when given antibiotics. Thus, it is important to treat only when PCT indicates a strong chance of an infectious etiology. PCT is a strong diagnostic tool for identifying ongoing infections and there are indications that it can be an equally strong predictor of the clinical benefit from antibiotic treatment.

PROADRENOMEDULLIN

Adrenomedullin, a 52-amino-acid peptide, plays a significant role in patients with acute HF and CHF.[8] Isolated from human pheochromocytoma cells, ADM levels are increased in proportion to the severity of NYHA functional class serving as a potent vasodilator and natriuretic peptide-mediated intrinsically by cyclic adenosine monophosphate (AMP).[8,9] The ADM messenger ribonucleic acid (mRNA) is upregulated in the cardiomyocytes and fibroblasts in direct response to atrial stretch and increased ventricular wall stretch. Experimental research using canine models demonstrated a positive correlation between plasma ADM levels and pulmonary capillary wedge pressure.[9] The other stimulus for ADM release in HF is linked to the compensatory activation of neurohormones seen in HF exacerbations.[8,9] Moreover, angiotensin II and endothelin-1 have been implicated in triggering ADM release in HF. Extensive research has documented ADM secretions from several other tissues such as the kidneys, adrenal medulla and lungs.[9,10]

Despite the impressive characteristic functions of ADM, it is associated with high plasma clearance rate, short half-life almost equal to 20 minutes and significant *in vitro* instability.[11] The midregional epitope (MR-proADM) consisting of 24–71 amino-acids is found to be more stable in vitro.[11,12] This molecule remains physiologically inactive in the plasma, and has poor affinity to clearance receptors, making it easy to measure. MR-proADM is secreted in equimolar amounts with ADM, and serves as a good surrogate marker for assessing the severity of HF, thus allowing an accurate risk stratification of such patients.[11,12]

von Haehling et al.[11] evaluated MR-proADM levels in 501 patients with mainly NYHA classes II and III CHF. Results revealed that elevated MR-proADM levels were associated with poor survival at 12 months. Receiver-operating characteristic (ROC) curves revealed an area under curve (AUC) of 0.81 at 3 months for MR-proADM compared to 0.79 for NT-proBNP. MR-proADM cutpoint of 0.743 nmol/L achieved 84% sensitivity and 67% specificity in predicting mortality risk at 3 months. Patients with MR-proADM levels 0.870–3.300 nmol/L had the highest number of adverse events.

Potocki et al.[13] conducted a prospective trial of 287 patients with acute dyspnea presenting to the ED with the aim of better understanding the prognostic role of MR-proADM alone and in conjunction with benchmark NPs such as BNP and NT-proBNP. The study concluded that MR-proADM performed better than the NPs in predicting 30-day mortality achieving an ROC-AUC of 0.81 [95% confidence interval (CI) = 0.73–0.90]. Moreover, MR-proADM independently predicted 1-year all-cause mortality demonstrating a poor survival in those with elevated MR-proADM levels ($p < 0.0001$).

The prospective multicenter international BACH trial[14] assessed 1,641 patients with acute dyspnea presenting to the ED. MR-proADM successfully identified those with high 90-day mortality risk in 568 acute HF patients presenting to the ED, achieving an AUC of 0.73 (95% CI = 0.70–0.77) and performing superior to BNP and NT-proBNP. MR-proADM cutpoint of 1.985 nmol/L achieved 74% accuracy, 76% specificity and 53% sensitivity.

Overall, MR-proADM has demonstrated robust evidence in predicting short-term mortality in both acute HF and CHF patients. Thus patients found to have elevated levels of MR-proADM may require a more tailored approach in managing their HF. Moreover, MR-proADM levels can be elevated in other conditions such as sepsis, diabetic nephropathies, malignancies and acute exacerbations of chronic obstructive pulmonary disease (COPD),[15,16] thus its remains imperative to rule out or treat these comorbidities in order to better utilize MR-proADM levels in risk stratification of HF patients.

TABLE 1: Representative overview of biomarker characteristics, mechanism of action and clinical implications in aiding risk stratification of heart failure patients

	Copeptin	*PCT*	*MR-proADM*
Properties	• 39-amino-acid C-terminal fragment of pre-pro-vasopressin	• Peptide precursor of calcitonin	• 24–71 amino acid midregional epitope of ADM
Mechanism	• AVP released from posterior pituitary in response to stress, a drop in blood pressure, or a change in osmotic pressure • Copeptin cleaved from AVP upon release and so serves as a 1:1 surrogate marker • Copeptin degrades in plasma less quickly than AVP	• Precursor of calcitonin, which is synthesized by the parafollicular C cells of the thyroid and normally involved in calcium homeostasis • PCT released by neuroendocrine cells of the lung and intestine in acute inflammatory states, particularly when etiology is bacterial	• Potent vasodilator, hypotensive effects • Secreted in equimolar amounts to ADM • mRNA is upregulated in the cardiomyocytes and fibroblasts in direct response to atrial stretch and increased ventricular wall stretch • Elevated in compensatory response to HF exacerbation • Angiotensin II and endothelin-1 may trigger ADM release
Relevant conditions	Elevated in: • HF • Sepsis • Pneumonia • COPD • Myocardial infarction	• Elevated mainly in bacterial infection and sepsis. Can distinguish from viral and noninfectious inflammation such as autoimmune disease	Elevated in: • HF • Sepsis • Diabetic nephropathies • Malignancies • COPD exacerbations
Laboratory testing	• Stable in vitro, unlike AVP which is cleared rapidly • Can be measured within an hour	• PCT elevated 3–6 hours after bacterial insult	• ADM has a high clearance rate and short half-life. MR-proADM serves as a stable surrogate marker • Poor affinity to clearance receptors makes it easy to measure
Clinical use	• Risk-stratification of HF decompensation • Prognostic after acute HF admission • Predicts death and hospitalization in outpatients with CHF, independent of clinical variables	• Helps distinguish between cardiac and noncardiac dyspneic patients • Aids in determining infectious states, and can guide antibiotic therapy in HF patients: ○ <0.05 ng/mL (low risk) ○ 0.05 ng/mL and 0.2 ng/mL possible risk (follow-up within 48 hours) ○ >0.2 ng/mL (high risk)	• Predicts short-term mortality in both acute HF and CHF patients • When MR-proADM is assessed alongside copeptin, best predictor of mortality after 14 days • May perform superiorly to BNP and NT-proBNP in predicting 30-day mortality

HF, heart failure; AVP, arginine vasopressin; COPD, chronic obstructive pulmonary disease; CHF, chronic heart failure; PCT, procalcitonin; ADM, adrenomedullin; mRNA, messenger ribonucleic acid; MR-proADM, midregional proadrenomedullin; BNP, brain natriuretic peptide; NT-proBNP, amino terminal pro-brain natriuretic peptide

CONCLUSION

The future implications of these new biomarkers in the diagnosis and risk stratification of HF may open new horizons in the field of medicine (Table 1). Entering the foray of multimarker-guided treatment, future application of these biomarkers should be devised from data emerging from recent and ongoing trials. Each of these novel biomarkers are specific to their site of release, and provide specific information regarding ongoing physiological change. Larger randomized controlled clinical trials are required to use these biomarkers in clinical settings in order to reduce hospitalization and improve outcome in HF patients.

REFERENCES

1. Birnbaumer M. Vasopressin receptors. Trends Endocrinol Metab. 2000; 11(10):406-10.
2. Alehagen U, Dahlström U, Rehfeld JF, et al. Association of copeptin and N-terminal proBNP concentrations with risk of cardiovascular death in older patients with symptoms of heart failure. JAMA. 2011;305(20):2088-95.
3. Khan SQ, Dhillon OS, O'Brien RJ, et al. C-terminal provasopresssin (copeptin) as a novel and prognostic marker in acute myocardial infarction: Leicester Acute Myocardial Infarction Peptide (LAMP) study. Circulation. 2007;115(16):2103-10.
4. Balling L, Kistorp C, Schou M, et al. Plasma copeptin levels and prediction of outcome in heart failure outpatients: relation to hyponatremia and loop diuretic doses. J Card Fail. 2012;18(5):351-8.
5. Christ-Crain M, Jaccard-Stolz D, Bingisser R, et al. Effect of procalcitonin-guided treatment on antibiotic use and outcome in lower respiratory tract infections: cluster-randomized, single-blinded intervention trial. Lancet. 2004;363(9409):600-7.
6. Schuetz P, Christ-Crain M, Thomann R, et al. Effect of procalcitonin-based guidelines vs standard guidelines on antibiotic use in lower respiratory tract infections: the ProHOSP randomized controlled trial. JAMA. 2009; 302(10):1059-66.
7. Maisel A, Neath SX, Landsberg J, et al. Use of procalcitonin for the diagnosis if pneumonia in patients presenting with a chief complaint of dyspnea: results from the BACH (Biomarkers in Acute Heart Failure) trial. Eur J Heart Fail. 2012;14(3):278-86.
8. Jougasaki M, Grantham JA, Redfield MM, et al. Regulation of cardiac adrenomedullin in heart failure. Peptides. 2001;22(11):1841-50.
9. Jougasaki M, Stevens TL, Borgeson DD, et al. Adrenomedullin in experimental congestive heart failure: cardiorenal activation. Am J Physiol. 1997;273(4 Pt 2):R1392-9.
10. Daggubati S, Parks JR, Overton RM, et al. Adrenomedullin, endothelin, neuropeptide Y, atrial, brain, and C-natriuretic prohormone peptides compared as early heart failure indicators. Cardiovasc Res. 1997;36(2): 246-55.
11. von Haehling S, Filippatos GS, Papassotiriou J, et al. Mid-regional pro-adrenomedullin as a novel predictor of mortality in patients with chronic heart failure. Euro J Heart Fail. 2010;12(5):484-91.
12. Gumusel B, Chang JK, Hyman A, et al. Adrenotensin: an ADM gene product with the opposite effects of ADM. Life Sci. 1995;57(8):PL87-90.
13. Potocki M, Breidhardt T, Reichlin T, et al. Midregional pro-adrenomedullin in addition to b-type natriuretic peptides in the risk stratification of patients with acute dyspnea: an observational study. Crit Care. 2009; 13(4):R122.
14. Maisel AS, Mueller C, Nowak R, et al. Mid-region pro-hormone markers for diagnosis and prognosis in acute dyspnea: results from the BACH (Biomarkers in Acute Heart Failure) trial. J Am Coll Cardiol. 2010;55(19):2062-76.
15. Lim SC, Morgenthaler NG, Subramaniam T, et al. The relationship between adrenomedullin, metabolic factors, and vascular function in individuals with type 2 diabetes. Diabetes Care. 2007;30(6):1513-9.
16. Cuttitta F, Pio R, Garayoa M, et al. Adrenomedullin functions as an important tumor survival factor in human carcinogenesis. Microsc Res Tech. 2002;57(2):110-9.

Appendix

Heart Failure Admission Checklist

Patient Name: ______________________ Gender: Male/Female

NRIC: ______________________ Age: __________

Admit Date: ______________

Source: Emergency Unit ☐ Clinic ☐ QEH-I ☐ Others: ______________

Underlying Diagnosis: ______________________

Attending Cardiologist: ______________________

Part A (*To be filled by sister or staff nurse in-charge)

Were the following assessments performed?		*Y*	*N*	*Initials*	*Date Performed*	*Comments*
Vital signs (BP, PR, oC, SPO_2, RR, Pain, pulse oximetry)		☐	☐			
Weight taken		☐	☐			
History taken (for co-morbidity)		☐	☐			
Physical examination (for co-morbidity)		☐	☐			
Medical history taken		☐	☐			
Allergy history taken		☐	☐			
Risk stratification:	NYHA Class	☐	☐			
	ACC/AHA Stage	☐	☐			

Part B (*To be filled by attending doctor)

Was the following lab work performed?	*Y*	*N*	*Initials*	*Date Performed*	*Comments*
12-lead ECG	☐	☐			
Echocardiogram/Doppler	☐	☐			
Chest X-ray	☐	☐			
INR. PT/PTT	☐	☐			
BUSE/Creatinine	☐	☐			
FBC w/diff, Platelets	☐	☐			
Cardiac Enzymes (Trop. and/or CK-MB)	☐	☐			
Liver function test	☐	☐			
TFT, iron, TIBC, RUA (if indicated)	☐	☐			

Contd...

Was the following performed/ discussed with the patient?	*Cont' as before*	*D/C*	*Initiated*	*Not Used*	*Initials*	*Date*	*Comments*
I/O totals	☐	☐	☐	☐			
Daily weight	☐	☐	☐	☐			
Low salt diet (<2000 mg/day)	☐	☐	☐	☐			
Fluid restriction: mL/day	☐	☐	☐	☐			
HF patient education pamphlet	☐	☐	☐	☐			

Check the appropriate box for each HF medication	*Cont' as before*	*D/C*	*Initiated*	*Not used*	*Initials*	*Date*	*Comments*
ACE inhibitor	☐	☐	☐	☐			
Angiotensin receptor blocker (if ACEI intolerant or in addition to ACEI)	☐	☐	☐	☐			
B-blocker	☐	☐	☐	☐			
Aldosterone antagonist	☐	☐	☐	☐			
Loop diuretic	☐	☐	☐	☐			
Digoxin	☐	☐	☐	☐			
Supplemental oxygen	☐	☐	☐	☐			
Electrolyte supplement (K, Mg as needed)	☐	☐	☐	☐			
Warfarin (for AF,DCM, MVR, AVR)	☐	☐	☐	☐			
Antiplatelet (CAD, CVD, PVD, DM)	☐	☐	☐	☐			
Statins (CAD, CVD, PVD, DM)	☐	☐	☐	☐			
Diabetes control	☐	☐	☐	☐			
Pain control	☐	☐	☐	☐			
Antiarrhythmics (specific indications)	☐	☐	☐	☐			
Other:	☐	☐	☐	☐			
Other:	☐	☐	☐	☐			
Other:	☐	☐	☐	☐			

Were the following interventions or testing procedures performed planned?	*Performed*	*Planned*	*N/A*	*Initials*	*Date Performed/ Planned*	*Comments*
Echocardiography/Doppler	☐	☐	☐	☐		
Angiography/catherization for possible revascularization	☐	☐	☐	☐		
Biventricular pacing	☐	☐	☐	☐		
Implantable cardioverter/defibrillator	☐	☐	☐	☐		
Other cardiac imaging	☐	☐	☐	☐		

Contd...

Contd...

Were the following secondary prevention measures performed/initiated?	*Performed*	*Planned*	*N/A*	*Initials*	*Date Performed/ Planned*	*Comments*
Fasting lipid profile	☐	☐	☐	☐		
Blood pressure control	☐	☐	☐	☐		
Smoker? If yes, refer to smoking cessation clinic c(QEH-I)	☐	☐	☐	☐		
Diabetic? If yes, HbA1c, glucose, sliding scale insulin	☐	☐	☐	☐		
Atrial fibrillation? If yes, start anticoagulation	☐	☐	☐	☐		
Physiotherapy	☐	☐	☐	☐		
Other:	☐	☐	☐	☐		

Index

Page numbers followed by *f* refer to figure and *t* refer to table.

A

Ablation in
- acute setting 235
- chronic management of VT 236

Abnormal
- mitral inflow Doppler echocardiography pattern 200
- renal 240*t*
  - and liver function 240

Absence of structural heart disease 235
ACE *See* Angiotensin-converting enzyme
ACE inhibitors 393
ACEI *See* Angiotensin-converting enzyme inhibitors
Acetazolamide 119
Acetylsalicylic acid 155
Acquired immunodeficiency syndrome-induced heart failure 543
Actinomyces 507
Activated partial thromboplastin time 241
Active antiretroviral therapy, highly 542
Acute
- agitation/anxiety 410
- aortic regurgitation 59
- atrial fibrillation 27
- cardiac complications 500
- cardiomyopathy trial 517
- care 426
- congestive heart failure, management of 19
- coronary syndrome 44, 151, 154, 294, 299, 426, 494
  - in heart failure 152
    - treatment of 154
  - medications indicated in 156
  - prognostic value in 268
- decompensated heart failure 9, 18, 41, 117, 120, 125, 284
  - national registry 151, 292, 372, 446
- exacerbation of chronic obstructive pulmonary disease 44
- fulminant myocarditis 509
- heart failure 7, 8, 41, 54, 68, 120, 130, 294
  - biomarkers in 110
  - in emergency department, treatment of 15
  - inotropes in different clinical settings of 135*t*
  - management using systolic blood pressure 17
  - prognostic value in 268
  - role of ultrasound in management of 54
  - study 121
  - syndrome 16, 16*t*, 17, 18
  - treatment of 15
  - trial, biomarkers in 548
- ischemic heart disease 199
- kidney injury 47, 48, 141
- maxillary sinusitis 84
- mitral regurgitation 58
- myocardial infarction 4, 87, 178, 226, 285, 291, 430, 508
- myocarditis 506, 508, 509*f*
- pericarditis 200
- pulmonary
  - edema 5, 78
  - embolism 7, 17, 18
- respiratory
  - distress syndrome 178, 179
  - failure 77
- rheumatic fever 389, 390*f*
- ST-elevation myocardial infarction 494
- treatment of sustained ventricular tachycardia 235
- valvular heart disease 57

Acutely decompensated heart failure 80, 127, 181-183
- and hypotension 182
- and worsening renal function 181

Acutely destabilized heart failure 140
Adaptative-pressure-control 77
Adenosine
- diphosphate 156, 341
- monophosphate-activated protein kinase 343
- triphosphat 343

Adenovirus 506, 507
Adequate blood pressure 124
ADH analogues 147
Adherence to guideline-based medications 375
ADHF
- and hypotension 182
- and worsening renal function 182

Administer sliding scale heparin infusion adjustment 171
Adrenergic system 535
Adrenocorticotropic hormone 144
Adrenomedullin 549
Adults with congenital heart disease 98
Advance care planning program 377
Advanced glycation end-products 341
Advanced heart failure 435, 443
AIDS-induced cardiac abnormalities and heart failure 541
Akinesia of mid-ventricle 497*f*
Alcohol
- ablation therapy 492*f*
- consumption, reduction in 394
- septal ablation 491

Aldactone evaluation study, randomized 218
Aldosterone
- antagonists 393
- escape 219

Ambulatory capacity 103
AMC *See* Acute myocarditis
Amiloride 119
Amino N-terminal prohormone 37
Amino-terminal pro-B-type natriuretic peptide 71
Amiodarone 28
Amyloidosis 480
Amyotrophic lateral sclerosis 4
Anderson-Fabry disease 482
Anemia *See* Nutritional deficiencies
Angiotensin
- AGT polymorphisms 534
- converting 354
- converting enzyme 115, 141, 156, 208, 259, 296*f*, 502

deletion polymorphism 534
inhibitors 489, 534, 542
doses of 438
in heart failure 214
insertion polymorphism 534
inhibitors 19, 48, 85, 119, 181, 188, 208, 213, 215, 218, 223, 245, 258, 268, 270, 276, 278, 281, 285, 286, 296, 299, 317, 328, 334, 348, 375, 373, 384, 399, 415, 421, 428-430, 543
receptor blockers 141, 188, 208, 214, 258, 259, 268, 270, 271, 276, 281, 285, 296, 317, 328, 373, 375, 399, 415, 421, 429, 430, 438, 542
therapy 334
treatment algorithm 428
Antiarrhythmic
drugs 147, 228, 229
medications 228
Antibiotics 147
Anticoagulant 156
evaluation of long-term 242
Anticoagulation therapy in heart failure with sinus rhythm 242
Antidepressants 147
Antidiabetic agents 343
Antidiuretic hormone 118
Antihypertensives 147
Antineoplastic agents 147
Antipsychotic drugs 147
Antithrombotic therapy in heart failure patients in sinus rhythm, role of 246
Antiviral immunomodulation with interferon 517
Aortic
pressure 473
regurgitation 59
stenosis, regurgitation 274
valve 455
Apical hypokinesia 497*f*
Apixaban for reduction in stroke 242
Apoptotic myocardial cell death in heart failure 290*f*
Application of natriuretic peptide 109
in diagnostic algorithm for heart failure 111
Arbovirus 507
Arenavirus 507
Arginine vasopressin 144, 546, 549
Arrhythmias 9, 191
Arrhythmic right-ventricular cardiomyopathy/dysplasia 232
Arrhythmogenic
cardiomyopathy 533
right ventricular
cardiomyopathy 95, 477-479, 526, 533
dysplasia 61
Arterial blood gases 6, 13
Artificial hearts 393
ARVC *See* Arrhythmogenic right-ventricular cardiomyopathy
Ascaris 507
Asthma 9, 215
Asymptomatic heart failure 417
Atrial
enlargement 274
fibrillation 21, 225, 227*f*, 229, 281, 313, 354, 358, 359, 373, 439
and heart failure 230
classifications 22
flutter 274
in acute setting 23
in patients with heart failure and preserved, management of 21
natriuretic peptide 32, 34, 41, 109, 110, 219
Atrioventricular dissociation 233*f*
Autoantibodies 513
Autosomal recessive 525*f*
Average volume-assured pressure support 77
AVRC *See* Arrhythmogenic right-ventricular cardiomyopathy

B

Balloon triggering and timing 469
Beats per minute 490
Benzafibrate infarction prevention 245
Beriberi 388
Beta blockers and proper dosing 216*t*
Beta-adrenergic
agonists 131
blocking agent 218, 223
Beta-blocker treatment algorithm 429
Bilateral renal artery stenosis 214
Bilevel positive airway pressure 19, 84
Bioelectrical impedance 66
vector analysis 71
Bioimpedance vector analysis 6, 166, 167
Biopsy 477
Bisoprolol 216
BIV function, assessments of 99
Biva in dyspneic patients, use of 68
Biventricular pacing 264
Bleeding 240, 456
history 240*t*
B-lines 70
Blood
cultures, multiple positive 200
metabolic profile 171
pressure 5, 8, 13, 16, 17, 74, 103, 372, 429, 447, 456
urea
and serum electrolyte 429
nitrogen 13, 17, 18, 82, 103, 174, 410
volume estimation 165
BNP *See* brain natriuretic peptide
Body mass index 44, 372, 448
Bone marrow mononuclear cells 398
Borrelia species 507
Bradycardia 216
Brain natriuretic peptide 16, 70, 71, 103, 104, 109, 189, 298, 298, 303, 316, 417, 488, 490
Breath, shortness of 543
Breathing 23
British National Health Service 365
Brockenbrough sign 487
Broken heart syndrome' 494
Brucella species 507
Brugada criteria 234
B-type natriuretic peptide 32-35, 37, 40, 44, 47, 56, 81, 109, 113, 153, 160, 165, 171, 220, 257, 274, 276, 278, 280, 281, 287, 292, 325
Building blocks of successful ultrafiltration therapy program 168
Bumetanide 119
Burden of heart failure 109
Bystander coronary disease 496

C

CAD *See* Coronary artery disease
Calcified mitral valve 60
Calcium channel blocker 191, 228
Captopril 180, 215
Carbohydrate antigen-125 302
Carbon monoxide 5
Carbonic anhydrase inhibitors 119
Cardiac
abnormalities associated with elevation of B-type natriuretic peptide 274t
arrhythmia 449
catheterization 495
chamber
enlargement 94
size 274
dysfunction 102
function
assessment of 104
heart failure with aldosterone antagonist trial, treatment of 329
implantable electronic devices 261
index 182
intensive care units 73
magnetic resonance 487, 495, 508, 525
diagnosis of myocarditis 512
findings in myocarditis, dynamics of 513*f*
imaging 86-89, 92, 481, 482, 502, 515
in takotsubo cardiomyopathy 499*f*
myosin activators 134
output 167

rehabilitation ward 426
resynchronization 398
therapy 50, 189, 209, 261, 264, 265, 268, 271, 276, 281, 318, 329, 348, 393, 438, 454, 543
recommendation for 265
use of 209
siderosis 482
tamponade 111, 200, 542, 544
case of 57
transplantation 50
troponins 46, 290
in hospitalized patients, recommendations for 293
in management of patients with congestive heart failure 289
in outpatients with heart failure, recommendations for 294
release in patients with heart failure 289
use of 293
Cardiogenic
pulmonary edema 19, 78
sign of 62
shock 8, 130, 181, 182, 444
Cardiomems heart sensor 209
Cardiomyopathies 87, 92, 201, 264, 388, 478
classification of 478
restrictive 478, 480, 532
Cardiopulmonary exercise stress testing 188
Cardiorenal rescue study in acute decompensated heart failure 163
Cardiotoxic drugs, use of 47
Cardiovascular
diseases 101, 312, 387, 542
magnetic resonance 497
risk factors 369
Cardioverter defibrillator 515
therapy 398
Carvedilol 216, 228
CAST *See* cardiac arrhythmia suppression trial
Catecholaminergic polymorphic VT 232
Catheter ablation 229
CCB *See* Calcium channel blocker
Cell adhesion molecules 507
Central
nervous system 143
sleep apnea *See also* Obstructive sleep apnea
Cerebrovascular accident 246
Chest
pain 102
X-ray 16
CHF *See* Chronic heart failure
Chlamydia pneumonia 507
Chlamydophila psittaci 507
Chlorthalidone 119
Chlorthiazide 119
Chordal rupture 57
Chorea minor *See also* Sydenham's chorea
Chronic
constrictive pericarditis 387, 388, 389, 391
dilated cardiomyopathy 506
disease, role of 376
heart failure 19, 33, 38, 185, 273, 285, 286, 298, 322, 402, 549
cause of 151
definition of advanced 438
prognostic value in 267
therapy, outpatient tailored 353
ischemic heart disease 199
kidney disease 191, 219, 333, 388
obstructive pulmonary disease 4, 9, 44, 45, 71, 73, 77, 155, 256, 354, 359, 446, 549
progressive external ophthalmoplegia 532
pulmonary disease 12
renal insufficiency 89
symptomatic heart failure 399, 400
treatment of 400
valvular heart disease 57
ventricular tachycardia, treatment of 236
viral cardiomyopathy 517
CICUS *See* Cardiac intensive care units
Circulation 23
CK-MB *See* Creatine kinase-MB
Classes of inotropes and mechanism of action 131
Claustrophobia 90
Clopidogrel 155
Clostridium tetani 507
CMR *See* Cardiac magnetic resonance imaging
Cohort studies, epidemiological 243*t*
Comet tails 70
Community, prognostic value in 268
Comorbidities, management of other 105
Complaint of dyspnea 4
Complete
blood count 113, 171, 455, 457
metabolic profile 171
Computed tomography 87, 89
Congenital
abnormalities 274
heart disease 87, 98
Congestion
management 208
symptoms of 191
Congestive heart failure 22, 24, 29, 29*t*, 48, 97*f*, 110, 179, 190, 198, 216, 225, 233, 258, 358, 373*f*, 420, 431
evaluation of mechanical assistance for treatment of 444
Randomized evaluation of mechanical assistance for treatment of 451
Constrictive pericarditis 97*f*
Continuous flow left ventricular assist device 458
Continuous positive airway pressure 19, 73, 76, 78, 84
Converting enzyme inhibitors 45
COPD *See* Chronic obstructive pulmonary disease
Coronary
artery
bypass grafting combines with cell transplantation 398
hybrid strategy 398, 399
disease 16, 46, 92, 154, 155, 312, 373, 381, 387, 388, 398, 431, 455, 515, 528
premature 542
ischemia 274
care unit 425
heart disease 312, 314, 447
Corynebacterium diphtheria 507
Coxiella burnetii 507
Coxsackie B virus 506, 507
Coxsackie-adenovirus receptor 507
Coxsackievirus 507
B 512
C-reactive protein 141, 302, 543
Creatine kinase-MB 543
Creatinine 6, 13, 214
Critical pulmonary edema or hypercapnia 22
CRT, cardiac resynchronization therapy 264
CTN *See* Cardiac troponins
Current exacerbation of HF 215
CVD, prevention of 394
Cyanide 5
Cystatin C 301
Cytomegalovirus 507
Cytotoxic T lymphocytes 507

D

DCM *See* Dilated cardiomyopathy
DCMI *See* Dilated cardiomyopathy with inflammation
Decompensated chronic
aortic stenosis 60
valvular heart disease 60
Deep vein thrombosis 243
Delivery of ultrafiltration therapy
choice of location for 169
training of nursing staff in 169
Dengue virus 507
Deoxyribonucleic acid 341, 532, 536
Determining optimal heart failure therapy 317

Device and surgical procedures 393
Device-based therapies 329, 543
Diabetes 314
  management in heart failure 340
  mellitus 22, 24, 152, 155, 191, 225, 354, 359, 371, 373, 382, 431
Diabetic ketoacidosis 4
Diagnosis of chronic heart failure 298
Diagnostic algorithm for dyspneic patients, proposal of 71
Diastolic
  compression of right ventricle 200
  dysfunction 45, 274
    in hypertrophic cardiomyopathy 486
Diet compliance, medication and 191
Digitalis 228
Digoxin 26, 228, 329, 393
Dilated cardiomyopathy 87, 201, 244, 261, 358, 389, 477, 478, 479, 508, 526, 532
  with inflammation 508
Diltiazem 26, 228
Dipeptidyl peptidase-4 inhibitors 344
Direct-current cardioversion 227-229, 235
Disability-adjusted life years 370
Discontinuation of ultrafiltration therapy 175
Disease, patterns of 495
Disposition of emergency department 8
Distal convoluted tubule 118
Distension of inferior vena cava 200
Diuretics 84, 147, 159
  optimization strategies evaluation 158
  pharmacokinetics and dosing of 119*t*
  therapy in hospital 121
  treated heart failure 159
Dizziness 11
DNA *See* Deoxyribonucleic acid
Dobutamine 131, 431
Dofetilide 28
Dopamine 131, 431
Driveline infection 457
Dynamic molecular targets in heart failure 535
Dyspnea 3, 11
  causes of 4*t*
  definition of 3*t*
  in emergency department 34, 42, 49, 50, 268
  resolution 12

E

Echinococcosis 507
Echocardiogram 226
Echocardiographic evaluation 487
Echovirus 507
Edema in lower extremities 410
Effect of mitral regurgitation 246
Effective regurgitant orifice 199
Ejection fraction 188, 219, 249, 313, 324, 328, 359, 376
  preserved 312
Electrical cardioversion 28
Electrocardiogram 16, 113, 193, 226, 233, 294, 363, 495
Electrocardiography 487
EMB *See* Endomyocardial biopsy
Embolus, source of 201
Emergency
  department observation
    chart for patient 83*f*
    unit 80
  department patient with suspected acute heart failure syndrome 16
  heart failure mortality risk grade 10, 10*t*
Enalapril 215
Encephalomyocarditis 507
End-diastole 497*f*
  pressure 473
  volume 473
End-of-life issues 465
Endomyocardial
  biopsy 478, 515
    histology of 510
    immunohistology of 511
    technique 510
  fibrosis 383, 388, 389
Endothelial dysfunction 342
Endotracheal
  intubation 76*f*
  tube 16
End-stage heart failure 443
End-systole 497*f*
Entamoeba histolytica 507
Enteroviruses 506, 507
Epidemiology
  of heart failure in India 387
  study of heart failure in China 396
Epinephrine 131
Eplerenone 119
Eplerenone post-acute myocardial infarction heart failure efficacy and survival study 218
Epstein-Barr virus 506, 507
Erythema marginatum of acute rheumatic fever 390*f*
Erythrocyte sedimentation rate 543
Erythropoiesis-stimulating agents 337
Esmolol 26, 228
ESR *See* Erythrocyte sedimentation rate
Estimated glomerular filtration rate 89, 269
Estimation of
  intracardiac pressures 198
  jugular venous pressure 327*f*
Ethanol septal ablation 491
Euroheart failure survey 348, 359
Evaluating hyponatremia 146
Evidence-based markers of acute heart failure risk 10*t*
Exacerbation 216
Exercise regimen 191
Expiratory positive airway pressure 76
External jugular vein 327*f*
Extracellular
  fluid volume 167
  matrix remodeling 341
Extracorporeal membrane oxygenation 470, 514

F

Familial
  cardiomyopathies 526
  sarcomeric hypertrophic cardiomyopathy 530
Fatigue 410
Female sex category 24
Fibrosis 274
Filling pressures 274
Flavivirus 507
Flecainide 28
Fluid volume 324
  assessment 326
Food and drug administration 46
Forrester's classification 62
Framingham heart study 311
Francisella tularensis 507
Frank-Starling curve 404
Furosemide 119

G

Galectin-3 49, 50, 269, 271, 299
Gastric inhibitory polypeptide 344
GCMC *See* Giant cell myocarditis
Genetic
  and risk stratification 531
  based risk stratification 529
  diagnosis 531
    of cardiomyopathy 524
  diseases 522
  heterogeneity 529
    of sarcomeric hypertrophic cardiomyopathy 531
  in heart failure caused by multifactorial diseases 534
  test of cardiomyopathy 524
  testing 526, 529, 531, 532, 533
    in dilated cardiomyopathy 528
    in heart failure, applications of 536
Geriatric syndrome model of heart failure 323*f*
Giant cell myocarditis 515
Glomerular filtration rate 44, 45, 221, 336
Glycemic control, role of 342

Glyceraldehyde-3-phosphate dehydrogenase 341
Glycoprotein 156
Good death, principles of 463
Guideline-directed medical therapy 265
Guiding heart failure care with natriuretic peptides 273

H

HAART-induced
  cardiovascular disease 544
  metabolic syndrome 542
Haemophilus influenzae 507
Handle
  excessive diuresis 123
  inadequate diuresis 123
HCM *See* Hypertrophic cardiomyopathy
Heart
  attack 504
  block 216
  disease
    preclinical structural 236, 370
    right 201
  failure 4, 27, 40, 48, 54, 80, 87, 89, 101, 104, 143, 182, 183, 198, 203, 204, 210, 213, 215, 219, 223, 238, 249, 261, 275, 284, 286, 292, 311, 322, 324, 325, 336, 337, 340, 347, 351, 353, 377, 388, 396, 402, 415, 426, 427, 429, 430, 439, 447, 451, 461, 522, 526, 536, 546, 549
    advanced 377
    and acute coronary syndrome 151
    and atrial fibrillation 239
    causes of 388
    classification of 81
    clinic 429
    daycare 409, 432
    disease management 410
      in nursing homes 408
      in nursing homes 408, 411
    disposition 8
    education 206
    epidemiology 426
    etiology 245, 312
    in China 396
      registery study of 396
    in diabetes, pathophysiology of 341
    in Europe 347
    in hospital 107
    in India 380, 387
    in primary care 348
    in southeast Asia 369
    long-term antithrombotic study 246
    management of 333
      congestive 80
      symptomatic 375, 376
    managing adults with 417
    morbidity, reduction of 220
    multinational study in 268
    outpatients with 348, 445
    pathophysiology of 375
    patient
      daily review chart 430*t*
      discharge planning 432
      with symptomatic 420
    prevention strategies 318
    progressive 508
    readmission 205*f*
    relevant structural 256
    risk
      and mortality 534
      stratification for inpatients with 446
    rule out acute 37
    signs
      of advanced 439*t*
      typical of 256
    stage
      B 370
      C 371
    surgical management of 398
    survival score 446, 447
    symptomatic 371
    symptoms of 256
      advanced 439*t*
    therapies for 276*t*
    to HIV/AIDS
      diagnosis of 542
      treatment of 542
    treatment of 324
    ultrafiltration therapy orders 170
    with normal ejection fraction 257, 353
    with preserved ejection fraction 255, 256, 256*f*, 259, 277, 374
      management of patient with 255
      treatment of 259
    with preserved systolic function 56, 295
    with reduced ejection fraction 223, 255, 437
  rate 16, 399, 429, 490
  rhythm abnormalities 274
  transplant 366, 393
  transplantation 443
    in China 399
    role of 377
Heartmate vented electric left ventricular assist system 377
Heartware ventricular assist device 377
Helminthic diseases 507
Hematocrit monitoring, technical aspects of 174
Hematologic function 449
Hemodynamics 56, 57, 448
  and pulmonary congestion 62
  congestion 62
  instability/shock 197
Hemorrhagic shock 6
Heparin-induced thrombocytopenia 171, 173, 455
Hepatic function 449
Hepatitis
  B virus 507
  C virus 507
  virus 507
Hepatojugular reflux 121
Heterophile-blocking tubes 290
HF *See* Heart failure
HFPEF, management of 329
High blood
  glucose 370, 371
  pressure 370, 371
High cholesterol 370, 371
High dependency unit 426
High flow nasal cannula 77
High sensitivity
  cardiac troponin 300
  troponins 46
High-dose chemotherapy 296
HIV *See* Human immunodeficiency virus
HIV-induced
  cardiac abnormalities, pathophysiology of 542
  cardiomyopathy 542
HNCM *See* Hypertrophic nonobstructive cardiomyopathy
HOCM *See* Hypertrophic obstructive cardiomyopathy
Home-based palliative disease management 377
Human
  herpes-virus type 6 506
  herpes-virus type 7 506
  immunodeficiency virus 541, 543
Hydralazine 180
Hydrochlorthiazide 119
Hydrogram 66
Hydrograph 66
Hyperglycemia, without 145
Hyperkalemia 214, 219
Hyperkinesia of apical and basal regions 497*f*
Hyperlipidemia 152
Hypertension 9, 22, 24, 44, 103, 152, 155, 182, 191, 225, 240, 240*t*, 311, 313, 326, 353, 358, 359, 373, 382, 389
Hypertensive
  acute heart failure syndrome pathway 17
  and normotensive acute heart failure, therapies for 19
  heart disease 371
Hypertrophic
  cardiomyopathy 87, 92, 201, 232, 262, 477, 478, 479, 485, 489, 490, 526, 529, 532

treatment of 490, 491
nonobstructive cardiomyopathy 491
obstructive cardiomyopathy 447, 485, 491, 492*f*
Hypertrophy 274
Hyperuricemia 125
Hypokalemia 6
Hyponatremia 143, 145
in heart failure 143
treatment of 146
in HF, presence of 146
in stage d heart failure 148
treatment of 145
Hypotensive acute heart failure syndrome pathway 18
Hypothalamic-pituitary-adrenal axis 547

I

ICD *See* Implantable cardioverter defibrillator
Iceberg phenomenon 190
Idiopathic
heart disease 526
pulmonary arterial hypertension 250
IHD *See* Idiopathic heart disease
Immunoadsorption 517
Immunohistological aspects of dilated cardiomyopathy with inflammation 511*f*
Immunomodulatory treatment 516
Immunosuppression 516
Impaired excitation contraction coupling 341
Impella 472, 473*f*
Implantable
cardiac-defibrillator 50, 528
cardioverter defibrillator 9, 189, 236, 250, 261, 262, 329, 376, 408, 438, 454, 459, 489, 510, 515, 532
Inappropriate antidiuretic hormone, syndrome of 146
Infectious agents 507*t*
Infective endocarditis 391*f*
Inferior vena cava 57, 198
Infiltrative
cardiomyopathies 480
diseases 274
Initiation of angiotensin-converting enzyme inhibitors 213
Inotropes 130
dependency, weaning of 136
in AHF 134
weaning of 136
Inotropic
agents, treatment with 136
contractile reserve 542
Inspiratory positive airway pressure 76
Intensive care unit 16-18, 141, 179, 299
Internal
cardiac defibrillators 318
jugular vein 325
International
normalized ratio 221, 240, 455
registry for heart and lung transplantation 399, 447
Interpretation of natriuretic peptide values in ambulatory heart failure 274
Intra-aortic balloon 469
counterpulsation 468, 502, 503
pump 181, 182, 469*f*
support for myocardial infarction with cardiogenic shock 504
Intravenous
immunoglobulin treatment 517
nitroglycerin 127
non-potassium sparing loop diuretics 19
pyelogram 84
Invasive
blood pressure monitoring 136
diagnostics 488
Iodinated contrast for computed tomography 90
Iron
deficiency anemia 334
overload cardiomyopathy 97
Ischemic
cardiomyopathy 244, 262, 478
evaluation 234
heart disease 199, 274, 353, 354, 358, 359, 371
surgical treatment for 93
Isosorbide dinitrate 180

J

Jugular venous 71
distension 15, 16, 81, 121, 122
pressure elevation 419
pressure 16, 192, 324, 325

K

Kaplan-Meier
analysis 294*f*
curves 296, 440*f*
Kidney injury molecule 301

L

Labile international normalized ratios 240
Late gadolinium enhancement 94, 499
LBBB, left bundle branch block 264
Left
anterior descending 496
coronary artery 490
atrial, pressure 486
bundle branch block 261, 265, 318
sided HF 81
ventricular 94, 152, 315, 458, 502, 526, 532
aneurysm 246
assist device 183, 250, 451, 452*f*, 454, 458, 510, 515
candidacy evaluation 183
in China 399
infection 457
versus transplantation 443
diastolic function 56
dysfunction
studies of 244, 315
trial, studies of 341
ejection 359
fraction, reduced 218
fractions 63, 92, 236, 242, 255, 257, 262-265, 268, 285, 294, 296, 313, 343, 374, 393, 399, 445, 454, 478, 485, 515
end diastolic
diameter 509
pressure 127, 257, 290, 486
volume index 257
end-systolic volume 478
filing pressures 62
hypertrophy 18, 226, 313, 315, 480, 486, 522
mass 370
masses and thrombus, evaluation of 97
noncompaction 479, 480, 533
outflow tract 56, 490
obstruction 486, 492*f*, 496, 502, 503
suction event 459
support 444
systolic
dysfunction 214, 225, 278, 348, 353, 354
function 55
thrombus 246
Legionella pneumophila 507
Leishmaniasis 507
Leptospira 507
Levosimendan 133
Lightheadedness 410
Lipid-lowering therapy 156
Lisinopril 215
Liver function 240*t*
Long QT syndrome 232
Low left ventricular ejection fraction 244
Low-density lipoprotein 156
Low-dose dobutamine stress magnetic resonance 93
Lower natriuretic peptide concentrations 281
Lupus erythematosus 152
Lutz frankenstein 364

LVAD *See* Left ventricular assist device
LVEDP *See* Left ventricular end-diastolic pressure
LVEF *See* Left ventricular ejection fraction
LVNC *See* Left ventricular
LVOTO *See* Left ventricular outflow tract obstruction

M

Magnetic resonance angiography 399
Major histocompatibility complex 511
Malaria 507
Malignant arrhythmias 507
Management and conventional heart failure treatment 514
Matrilineal inheritance of cardiomyopathies 525*f*
Matrix metalloproteinase-9 140
Mean
  arterial blood pressure 509
  corpuscular hemoglobin 336
  corpuscular volume 336
  pulmonary
    artery pressure 182
    capillary wedge pressure 257
  rehospitalization equivalents 162*f*
Mechanical
  circulatory support 250, 443, 447
    duration of 452
  ventilation in acute heart failure 73
Medication 268
  exacerbate hyponatremia 147
  optimization of 208
  reconciliation 208
Messenger ribonucleic acid 303, 548, 549
Metallic implants 88
Metalloproteinase-9 140
Metastatic renal cell carcinoma 90*f*
Meteor 145
Metformin 343
Metolazone 119
Metoprolol 26, 228
  CR/XL 216
Mid-region
  proadrenomedullin 103, 300, 549
  proatrial natriuretic peptide 32, 34, 109, 110
  prohormone atrial natriuretic peptide 35
    versus B-type natriuretic peptide 35*t*
Milrinone 133, 431
Mineralocorticoid
  antagonists 438
  receptor 223
    antagonist 218, 270, 271, 274, 276, 278, 281
      in patients with heart failure 218
Ministry of Health 425*t*
Minnesota living with heart failure questionnaire 376
Mitral
  regurgitation 219, 359, 486
  stenosis, regurgitation 274
  valve 58, 455
Moderate-to-severe respiratory distress 76*f*
Molecular
  genetics 488
  pathways activated in heart failure and genetic testing, major 534
Monitor during diuresis 123
Monitoring
  devices 194
  of trends and determinants in cardiovascular disease 316
MRNA *See* Messenger ribonucleic acid
Mr-Proadm *See* Midregional proadrenomedullin
MR-ProANP *See* Mid-region proatrial natriuretic peptide
MRSA, methicillin-resistant staphylococcus aureus 457
Multicenter
  automatic defibrillator implantation trial ii 262
  INSYNC ICD randomized clinical evaluation 264
Multidisciplinary
  chronic disease management program 376
  teams 206
Multisystem organ failure 444
Myocardial
  infarction 8, 29, 87, 140, 179, 198, 223, 244, 249, 263, 264, 284, 341, 353, 426, 431, 478
  ischemia 9, 426
  processes 274
Myocarditis 388, 506
  management of 515
  proof of 510*f*
  with preserved ejection fraction 508
Myopericarditis 514

N

National
  Cardiovascular Database 426
  Health and Nutrition Examination Survey 109
  Heart, Lung and Blood Institute 257, 311, 451
Natriuretic peptides 9, 10, 32, 40, 44, 69, 71, 109, 113, 152, 165, 274
  for emergency department 43
  for guiding heart failure management 276
  function 42
  in acute coronary syndrome 47
  in Emergency Department 32, 35
  in general inpatient setting 114
  in inpatient setting 109
  in intensive care unit, use of 114, 115
  pathophysiology 41
  role for 12
Nebivolol 216
Negative predictive value 43, 109
Neisseri 507
Nephrotic syndrome 143
Nesiritide 128
  use of 19
  versus dobutamine in heart failure 293
Neutrophil gelatinase-associated lipocalin 41, 47, 48, 102, 103, 139, 140, 141, 301
  augments 140*f*
New biomarkers in emergency department 40
New cardiovascular disease biomarkers in hospital medicine 139
Newer inotropes 133
Next generation sequencing 528
Nicotinamide adenine dinucleotide phosphate 341
Nighttime
  shortness of breath 410
  urination, increase in *See also* Nighttime shortness of breath
Nitric oxide 182
  inhaled 182
Nitroglycerin 17, 127, 128
Nitroprusside 128
NIV with acute pulmonary edema 78
Nomenclature of indication of mechanical circulatory support 453
Non-cardiogenic dyspnea 61
Noncommunicable diseases, prevalence of 426
Noncompaction cardiomyopathy 98
Noncompliance to medications 426
Noninvasive
  ventilation 16, 19, 73, 78, 128
    in acute heart failure 77
    modalities of 75
    role of 73
Nonischemic cardiomyopathies 94, 262, 479
  treatment evaluation, defibrillators in 262
Nonpharmacological measures 394
Non-sarcomeric hypertrophic cardiomyopathy 531
Non-ST-elevation
  acute coronary syndrome 47, 285
  myocardial infarction 154, 285

Non-steroidal anti-inflammatory drugs 47, 48, 103, 215, 222, 439
Nonsteroidal anti-inflammatory drugs *See also* Calcium channel blocker
Non-ST-segment elevation myocardial infarction 46, 47
Nonsustained ventricular tachycardia 262
Nonsustained VT 232
Noradrenaline 431
Norepinephrine 131
Normal sinus rhythm 454
Normotensive acute heart failure syndrome pathway 18
Novel
  anticoagulant agents 240
  oral anticoagulants 240
NSAIDs *See* Nonsteroidal anti-inflammatory drugs
NSTEMI *See* Non-ST-segment elevation myocardial infarction
N-terminal 13
  pro-brain natriuretic peptide 490
  pro-B-type natriuretic peptide 34, 47, 110, 113, 269, 271, 299
  prohormone
    B-type natriuretic peptide 35
    of brain natriuretic peptide 274*t*, 275, 276, 280
NT-ProBNP *See* N-terminal pro-B-type natriuretic peptide
Nuclear imaging 481
Nurse
  management of asymptomatic heart failure 420
  training and role 416
Nutrition 456
Nutritional deficiencies 388
  markers of 456*t*

O

Obesity 45, 152, 314, 370
Obstructive
  pulmonary disease 60
  sleep apnea 190
Optimal
  cutpoints for N-terminal pro-B type natriuretic peptide 43*t*
  pharmacological therapy 262
Optivolemic B-type natriuretic peptide 45
Oral anticoagulants 229, 240, 244
Orthopnea 11, 102
Osler's nodes 391, 391*f*
Overweight 370
Oxidative stress 341
Oxygen 24
  saturation 103
  supplementation 82
  therapy 78, 82

P

Painkillers 147
Palliation and end-of-life care 423, 461
  during illness trajectory 462
  in heart failure 461
Palliative care 329, 461, 465
  in heart failure trajectory f 465
Paragonimus westermani 507
Parasternal long axis 57
Paroxysmal nocturnal dyspnea 81, 323, 543
Partial thromboplastin time 171, 455
PASP *See* Pulmonary artery systolic pressures
Patent foramen ovale 455
Pathogenesis of virus-induced acute cardiomyopathy 508*f*
Patient self care 206
Patient-centered heart failure care 466*f*
Peak expiratory flow rate 12
Pedigrees in autosomal dominant 525*f*
Percutaneous
  coronary intervention 141, 155, 425
  extracorporeal membrane oxygenator 470, 470*f*
  mechanical circulatory support in cardiogenic shock 468
  transluminal septal myocardial ablation 491
Pericardial
  constriction 201
  diseases 200, 274
  effusion 57, 200, 544
    pleural and 58*f*
Peripheral
  arterial disease 29
  artery disease 225
  vascular resistance 501, 503
Pharmacologic cardioversion 28
Phosphodiesterase III inhibitors 133
Physical inactivity 370
Pleural effusion 6
Pneumonia 6, 48
Pneumothorax 6
Polyarteritis nodosum 152
Polymerase chain reaction 506
Polymorphic VT 233
Poor perfusion, symptoms of 191
Positive
  end expiratory pressure 76, 78, 115
  predictive value 43
Post HOC analyses of clinical trials 244
Postdischarge management 105
Post-myocardial infarction 218
Potassium-sparing diuretics 119
Potential
  candidates for ultrafiltration 164
  noncardiac of NPS in ICU 114
Prasugrel 155
Pressure assisted-controlled ventilation 76
Pressure support 76, 78
  ventilation f 76
Pretransplant evalution 182
Primary care physician 354
Proadrenomedullin 548
Procainamide 28
Procalcitonin 48, 300, 546, 548, 549
Prohormone levels in heart failure 546
Propafenone 28
Proportional assist ventilation 76
Prothrombin time 455
  and international normalized ratio 171
Proximal convoluted tubule 118
PTSMA *See* Percutaneous transluminal septal myocardial ablation
Pulmonary
  arterial hypertension 98, 250
    pathophysiology of 250
  artery catheter 178, 179, 181, 182, 183
    in heart failure 179
      patients, uses of 182*t*
    monitoring 136
    trials of 179*t*
  artery
    systolic pressures 57
    wedge pressure 33*f*
  capillary wedge pressure 56, 180, 189
  congestion 61, 62
  disease 45
  embolism 179
  function 448
  hypertension 121, 178, 250, 542
  interstitial edema 62
  vasodilator challenge 182
Pulmonic stenosis 274
Pulsatile index 458
Pump
  endocarditis 457
  pocket infection 457
  thrombus 459

Q

Quality of life 179

R

RAAS *See* Renin-angiotensin-aldosterone system
Ramipril 215
Randomized controlled trial 179
Rapid
  Emergency Department Heart Failure Outpatient 42
  ventricular response 13
Rate
  control efficacy in permanent atrial fibrillation 227
  versus rhythm control 24

Reactive oxygen species 341
Recent European Society of Cardiology Guidelines 333
Recurrent congestion 125
Red blood cell 336
REDHOT *See* Rapid Emergency Department Heart Failure Outpatient
Reduced
- ejection fraction 218, 312, 508
- left ventricular ejection fraction 218, 508

Refractory heart failure symptoms 441
Regional wall motion abnormalities 198
Relative dyspnea score 4
REMATCH trial 162
Renal
- biomarkers 301
- dysfunction 45
  - use of 47
- function 10, 268, 447
  - assessment 103
- impairment 313

Renin-angiotensin
- aldosterone 534
  - system 42, 110, 118, 143, 158, 218, 534, 536
- system 314, 315
  - blockade 328

Resolution of giant cell myocarditis under immunosuppression 516*f*
Restrictive cardiomyopathy 477, 526
Reverse transcriptase inhibitors 542
Revolution acute respiratory failure 76*f*
RHD, prevention of 394
Rheumatic heart disease 382, 388, 389, 426
Rheumatoid arthritis *See also* Polyarteritis nodosum
Rhythm
- control
  - agents 28*t*
  - treatment 27
- diagnostics 488

Riet dierckx 363
Right ventricular 94, 458
- presence of 61
- stroke work index 183
- support 444
- systolic pressure 57

Right-sided
- heart failure to pulmonary hypertension 544
- versus left-sided heart failure 81

S

Sarcoidosis 481
Saturated oxygen 13, 24
Scar 274
Schistosoma species 507
Seattle heart failure model 446, 447
Secondary
- comorbidities 102
- medical issues, treatment of 103

Senile systemic amyloidosis 480
Serum
- amyloid P component scintigraphy 481
- neutrophil gelatinase-associated lipocalin levels, management based on 141*t*
- sodium 149

Severe
- asymptomatic hypotension 214
- cases with cardiogenic shock 502
- chronic heart failure 218
- systolic dysfunction 400

Sex differences in
- clinical presentation 315
- heart failure 311

Short QT syndrome 232
Simpson's rule 55
Singapore heart failure outcomes and phenotypes 374
Single-nucleotide polymorphisms 536
Sinus rhythm
- maintaining 228
- restoring 228

Slow continuous ultrafiltration 167
Smoking cessation 394
SMT, standard medical therapy 264
SNPS *See* Single-nucleotide polymorphisms
Soap 431
Social welfare contribution 363
Socioeconomic factors 204
Sodium 13, 175
- nitroprusside 128

Soluble
- guanylyl cyclase 375
- transferrin receptor 337

Sotalol 28
Spironolactone 119, 219
Stage heart failure 369
Stamatia prapa 365
Standard operational procedures 427
Staphylococcus aureus bacteremia 201
Steady-state free precession 88
ST-elevation myocardial infarction 154, 284, 285
Stenotic lesions 274
Stepped pharmacologic therapy 163
Stroke 22, 24, 240, 240*t*
- prevention 29

Strongyloides stercoralis 507
ST-segment elevation myocardial infarction 16, 291
Suboptimal TTE images 201
Subxiphoid of pericardial effusion 7*f*
Sudden cardiac death 95, 232, 261, 398, 486, 490, 507
- in heart failure 262
  - trial 244, 245
- prevention 514

Sudden death in heart failure trial 262
Sulfa-based diuretics 181
Sulfonylureas 343
Supraventricular tachycardias 233, 234, 486
Sydenham's chorea 390
Sympathico-adrenergic system 315
Symptomatic
- hypertrophic
  - nonobstructive cardiomyopathy patients 489
  - obstructive cardiomyopathy patients 491
- hypervolemic hyponatremia 148
- hypotension 214

Systemic vascular resistance 180, 182
Systolic
- anterior
  - motion 201
  - movement 486
- blood pressure 13, 17, 18, 82, 84, 128, 130, 183, 214, 354, 429
- dysfunction 274
- function, preserved 312
- heart failure 92
- pulmonary artery pressure 198
- versus diastolic dysfunction 82

T

Taenia solium 507
Takayasu arteritis 383
Takotsubo cardiomyopathy 494, 497*f*, 504
- complicated by cardiogenic shock 503
- management priorities in 502

Tandemheart 471
Tandemheart® system and pump 471*f*
TASH *See* Transcoronary ablation of septal hypertrophy
Teach-back method concepts 194
TEE, transesophageal echocardiography 457
Telemonitoring 209
Telemonitoring to improve heart failure outcomes 209
Therapeutic
- algorithms 488
- range 240
- window for noninvasive ventilation 76*f*

Therapy-related factors 204
Thiazide diuretics 119
Thiazolidinediones 343
Thibaud damy 363
Thick ascending limb 118
Thoracis ultrasound 71
Thromboembolic events 242
Thrombolysis in myocardial infarction 155

score for unstable angina 155*t*
Ticagrelor 155
Tissue Doppler imaging 56
Tolvaptan 119
Torsades de pointes 28, 317, 495, 500
Torsemide 119
Toxic conditions with acute myocarditis 507*t*
Toxoplasma gondii 507
Traditional biomarkers 298
Trajectories of decline 462*f*
Trandolapril 215
Transcoronary ablation of septal hypertrophy 491
Transesophageal echocardiogram 98, 197, 201, 227, 229
Transient ischemic attack 29
Transition
care nursing roles 422
from intravenous to oral drug regimens 125
to end-of-life care 412
Transthoracic echocardiogram 54, 193, 54, 200
Triamterene 119
Trichinella spiralis 507
Trichinosis 507
Tricuspid
annular plane systolic excursion 61
regurgitation 55, 198, 274
velocity of 198
valve 455
Troponin peptide 9
Troubleshooting left ventricular assist device patients 183
Trypanosoma cruzi 507
Tuberculosis prevention 394

U

Ultrafiltration 159
clinical specialist, role of 168
in fluid-overloaded heart failure patients 160, 162
therapy in heart failure in china 398
United Network for Organ Sharing 1a Status, maintenance of 183
Universal health literacy principles 194
US carvedilol heart failure program 215
Utility in emergency department 42

V

VAD, ventricular assist device 457
Valsartan heart failure trial 268
Valvular
abnormalities 274
disease 455
disorders 45
dysfunction 57
function 197
heart disease 199, 201, 388
Vascular
abnormalities. 239
disease 22, 24, 225, 342
Vasodilator-heart failure trial 244, 245
Vasodilators 19, 85
in acute heart failure 127
induced
decrease in blood pressure, management of 129
hypotension 129
recommended dose of 128*t*
Vasopressin
and heart failure 144
antagonists 119
levels of 144
receptor antagonists 120
role of 144
Venoarterial extracorporeal membrane oxygenation 504
Venous access 172
Ventilator associated pneumonia 74
Ventricle, right 61, 163
Ventricular
arrhythmias 459
assist device 393, 443, 448, 543
role of 377
enlargement 274
fibrillation 263
function, right 448, 454, 456
rate control 227
systolic function 197
tachycardia 232, 233*f*, 234, 235, 263, 447, 490
done right 232
types of 236
Ventriculography of
classic apical pattern of takotsubo cardiomyopathy 496*f*
midventricular variant of takotsubo cardiomyopathy 497*f*
Verapamil 26, 228
Veterans health administration 402
Virological analyses of endomyocardial biopsy 512
Vital signs 4
Vitamin K antagonists 240

W

Warfarin
and antiplatelet therapy in chronic heart failure 247
in nonvalvular atrial fibrillation 242
versus aspirin in reduced cardiac ejection fraction 247
Well's criteria 7*t*
Wet versus dry natriuretic peptide levels 113*t*
Wide complex tachycardias 233, 234
Wolff-Parkinson-White syndrome 226
Worsening renal function 9, 181, 182
WPW syndrome *See* Wolff-Parkinson-White syndrome

Z

Zidovudine 336